POTENTIAL INTERACTIONS BETWEEN PHYSICAL AGENTS AND THERAPEUTIC DRUGS

Listed here are some potential interactions between physical agents used in rehabilitation and various pharmacological agents. It is impossible to list all the possible relationships between the vast array of therapeutic drugs and the interventions used in physical therapy and occupational therapy. However, some of the more common interactions are identified here.

Modality	Desired Therapeutic Effect	Drugs With Complementary/ Synergistic Effects	Drugs With Antagonistic Effects	Other Drug-Modality Interactions
Cryotherapy				
Cold/ice packs Ice massage Cold bath Vapocoolant sprays	Decreased pain, edema, and inflammation	Anti-inflammatory steroids (glucocorticoids); nonsteroidal anti-inflammatory analgesics (aspirin and similar NSAIDs)	Peripheral vasodilators may exacerbate acute local edema.	Some forms of cryotherapy may produce local vasoconstriction that temporarily impedes diffusion of drugs to the site of inflammation.
	Muscle relaxation and decreased spasticity	Skeletal muscle relaxants	Nonselective cholinergic agonists may stimulate the neuromuscular junction.	—
Superficial and Deep Heat				
Local application Hot packs Paraffin Infrared Fluidotherapy Diathermy Ultrasound	Decreased muscle/ joint pain and stiffness	NSAIDs; opioid analgesics; local anesthetics	—	—
	Decreased muscle spasms	Skeletal muscle relaxants	Nonselective cholinergic agonists may stimulate the neuromuscular junction.	—
	Increased blood flow to improve tissue healing	Peripheral vasodilators	Systemic vasoconstrictors (e.g., alpha-1 agonists) may decrease perfusion of peripheral tissues.	—
Systemic Heat				
Large whirlpool Hubbard tank	Decreased muscle/joint stiffness in large areas of the body	Opioid and nonopioid analgesics; skeletal muscle relaxants	—	Severe hypotension may occur if systemic hot whirlpool is administered to patients taking peripheral vasodilators and some antihypertensive drugs (e.g., alpha-1 antagonists, nitrates, direct-acting vasodilators, calcium channel blockers).
Ultraviolet Radiation	Increased wound healing	Various systemic and topical antibiotics	—	Antibacterial drugs generally increase cutaneous sensitivity to ultraviolet light (i.e., photosensitivity).
	Management of skin disorders (acne, rashes)	Systemic and topical antibiotics and anti-inflammatory steroids (glucocorticoids)	Many drugs may cause hypersensitivity reactions that result in skin rashes, itching.	Photosensitivity with antibacterial drugs
Transcutaneous Electrical Nerve Stimulation (TENS)	Decreased pain	Opioid and nonopioid analgesics; certain antiseizure drugs (e.g., gabapentin, pregabalin)	Opioid antagonists (naloxone, naltrexone)	—
Functional Neuromuscular Electrical Stimulation	Increased skeletal muscle strength and endurance	Low-dose androgens in certain populations (e.g., androgen-deficient men)	Skeletal muscle relaxants	—
	Decreased spasticity and muscle spasms	Skeletal muscle relaxants	Nonselective cholinergic agonists may stimulate the neuromuscular junction.	—

Pharmacology in Rehabilitation

FIFTH EDITION

Contemporary Perspectives in Rehabilitation

Contemporary Perspectives in Rehabilitation

Steven L. Wolf, PT, PhD, FAPTA, Editor-in-Chief

Pharmacology in Rehabilitation, Fifth Edition
Charles D. Ciccone, PT, PhD, FAPTA

Vestibular Rehabilitation, Fourth Edition
Susan J. Herdman, PT, PhD, FAPTA, and Richard Clendaniel, PT, PhD

Modalities for Therapeutic Intervention, Fifth Edition
Susan L. Michlovitz, PT, PhD, CHT, James W. Bellew, PT, EdD, and Thomas P. Nolan, Jr., PT, MS, OCS

Fundamentals of Musculoskeletal Imaging, Fourth Edition
Lynn N. McKinnis, PT, OCS

Wound Healing: Alternatives in Management, Fourth Edition
Joseph M. McCulloch, PT, PhD, CWS, FACCWS, FAPTA, and
Luther C. Kloth, PT, MS, CWS, FACCWS, FAPTA

For more information on each title in the Contemporary Perspectives in Rehabilitation series, go to www.fadavis.com.

Charles D. Ciccone, PT, PhD, FAPTA
Professor
Department of Physical Therapy
School of Health Sciences and Human Performance
Ithaca College
Ithaca, New York

Pharmacology in Rehabilitation

FIFTH EDITION

JAYPEE The Health Sciences Publisher

F.A. Davis Company • Philadelphia

FIRST INDIAN EDITION 2016

Pharmacology in Rehabilitation, 5th edn

As new scientific information becomes available through basic and clinical research, recommended treatments and drug therapies undergo changes. The author(s) and publisher have done everything possible to make this book accurate, up to date, and in accord with accepted standards at the time of publication. The author(s), editors, and publisher are not responsible for errors or omissions or for consequences from application of the book, and make no warranty, expressed or implied, in regard to the contents of the book. Any practice described in this book should be applied by the reader in accordance with professional standards of care used in regard to the unique circumstances that may apply in each situation. The reader is advised always to check product information (package inserts) for changes and new information regarding dose and contraindications before administering any drug. Caution is especially urged when using new or infrequently ordered drugs.

Printed in India

Published by
Jaypee Brothers Medical Publishers (P) Ltd

Corporate Office
4838/24, Ansari Road, Daryaganj, **New Delhi** 110002, India, Phone: +91-11-43574357

Registered Office
B-3, EMCA House, 23/23B, Ansari Road, Daryaganj, **New Delhi** 110002, India
Phones: +91-11-23272143, +91-91-23272703, +91-11-23282021, +91-11-23245672
Rel: +91-11-32558559, Fax: +91-11-23276490, +91-11-23245683
e-mail: jaypee@jaypebrothers.com, Website: www.jaypeebrothers.com

Branches
- **Ahmedabad** e-mail: ahmedabad@jaypeebrother.com
- **Bengaluru** e-mail: bangalore@jaypeebrothers.com
- **Chennai** e-mail: chennai@jaypeebrothers.com
- **Lucknow** e-mail: lucknow@jaypeebrothers.com
- **Hyderabad** e-mail: hyderabad@jaypeebrother.com
- **Kochi** e-mail: kochi@jaypeebrothers.com
- **Kolkata** e-mail: kolkata@jaypeebrothers.com
- **Mumbai** e-mail: mumabi@jaypeebrothers.com
- **Nagpur** e-mail: nagpur@jaypeebrothers.com

ISBN 978-93-86322-08-1

Dedicated to Penny, Kate, Alex, and Rosemary.
I continue to be inspired by your faith and support throughout the years.

Foreword to the Fourth Edition

There are very peculiar ways in which one can mark time. We often do so by observing the rate at which our siblings, children, or grandchildren grow, especially when we are not in daily contact, or by how we inevitably underestimate the length of time transpired since we last encountered an old friend. In this context, it seems remarkable that over 13 years have transpired since I first discussed with Chuck Ciccone the prospects for a text on pharmacology for our *Contemporary Perspectives in Rehabilitation.* The realization that the first edition of *Pharmacology in Rehabilitation* appeared more than a decade ago is even more astounding. The basis for the genesis of such a book was founded on the belief that rehabilitation specialists received little formal training about drug interactions and how any single pharmacological agent could impact either treatment plans or outcomes. Chuck took it upon himself to generate a text that would address this educational and clinical shortcoming. The result is very clear. *Pharmacology in Rehabilitation* is the "gold standard" among all texts addressing this content for nonphysician rehabilitation specialists.

So why is it important to create a fourth edition within one decade? Why is a more superficial compendium of information about drugs and their actions inadequate? The answer to these questions is directly related to the rapidly emerging responsibilities incumbent upon rehabilitation specialists. During the past 5 years, the advent of clinical doctoral programs in physical and occupational therapy has heralded a rapid transformation in these educational arenas. Several attributes now take on a meaning that previously might have been underappreciated. First, the label of "doctor" implies an ***expectation*** on the part of the consumer that the practitioner is the penultimate expert on providing an analysis and treatment plan for improving upon the pathology of any system's movement, whether muscle, joint, pulmonary, etc. Second, given the status associated with the professional label, there is an associated ***obligation*** on the part of the practitioner to address all aspects of the patients' signs and symptoms. This obligation requires that the clinician differentiate patient responses to treatment from patient responses to pharmacy. As one physical therapist so astutely told me, her recognition that a patient was not responding to pain medication taken well above the specified dosage, in the absence of any evidence for malingering behavior, resulted in the subsequent detection and successful removal of a renal tumor. Third, as practitioners, the DPT or DOT now assumes a greater ***responsibility*** for keeping a contemporary knowledge base about the interface between treatment plan and concurrent synergies or exacerbations that might result from single or multiple medications taken by the patient.

This collection of attributes can be best appreciated if the student is first informed and the clinician is educated about the most recent medications, their pharmokinetics, and the interactions they have with patients with specific diagnoses. Since the drug industry is arguably one of the most dynamic corporate structures in the world, changes in pharmacy occur at an alarmingly fast rate, one that will increase even more dramatically as transplants and the sequelae resulting from genetic engineering (as two examples) take on greater roles in medicine. Such rapid changes, then, call for contemporary and comprehensive updates in available information. Such updates must be presented in a manner that is compelling, yet easy to understand.

Inclusive in this perception is the absolute requirement that the student or clinician be able to relate to the text meaningfully. Toward this important goal, the 4th edition of *Pharmacology in Rehabilitation* is designed to address rehabilitation relevance in every clinical chapter as well as to present important case histories to reinforce this relevance. New materials on agents used in or even as complementary and alternative medicines have been added. Moreover, we have made efforts to add to the appeal of the book through the addition of colorization, use of double columns, and encasing the text within a newly designed hard cover. These changes are in contradistinction to one standard that remains immutable—Dr. Ciccone's remarkable gift for taking complex material and making it easy to understand.

For those clinicians who have in their possession early editions of this book, I invite you to compare your copy to the 4th edition as validation for the assertions made in this Foreword. We have not compromised the comprehensive nature of this volume in favor of a "simpler" approach to understanding pharmacology. We believe that the topic, by its very nature and from the implications inherent in its knowledge base, requires a comprehensive, yet user-friendly, delivery. This belief system remains unhindered in this latest edition; yet the problem-solving and evidence-based nature of the content is preserved and enhanced.

The thought of having a reference text for rehabilitation specialists was considered by us to be a unique concept 13 years ago. Today, many doctoral programs include pharmacology as a separate course or as an important component in teaching the rationale for treatment approaches and their assessment. There is much gratification to be gained from recognizing this transformation and in knowing that the content of this book contributes to the evolving maturation of our educational programs and our clinical services.

Steven L. Wolf, PT, PhD, FAPTA
Series Editor

Preface

As in the past, I was excited, albeit somewhat apprehensive, to start working on a new edition of this book. I always joke that I should have written a text on gross anatomy—human structures have not changed much in the few years since the last edition. Pharmacology, however, continues to change and expand as new drugs are developed and we explore how patients respond to various drug regimens. Pharmacology has likewise taken advantage of scientific developments in other areas to enhance patient outcomes. For example, the Human Genome Project, nanotechnology, and creation of monoclonal antibodies were still in their infancy when I began working on the first edition of this text. These and other scientific breakthroughs are now an important part of drug development, and they continue to contribute to innovative and clinically relevant advances in pharmacotherapy.

Given all the advancements in pharmacology, I tried to maintain the basic ideas presented in previous editions—that is, I describe drug therapy from the perspective of how specific drugs work and how they can provide beneficial effects as well as adverse effects in patients undergoing physical rehabilitation. As in previous editions, I relied heavily on the peer-reviewed literature to provide current information, while trying to distill the wealth of information to the issues that are most relevant to our patients.

This edition starts with several chapters that address basic pharmacological principles, followed by chapters that deal with drugs used to treat specific disorders or achieve certain clinical outcomes. The text, figures, and tables were all updated, and new figures were added to several chapters to illustrate drug actions and effects. Case studies appear at the end of chapters that deal with specific clinical disorders. I revised all the case studies and changed the format so that several questions are posed within the case. Answers to these questions appear in an appendix at the end of the book. This change will hopefully engage readers and encourage application of information gleaned from the respective chapters.

Finally, I always appreciate the opportunity to write a new edition of this book. Pharmacology has certainly become an integral part of contemporary health care, and we must have a working knowledge of how drugs affect our patients. I hope that I have provided students and clinicians with a useful resource on this topic and that this text will ultimately help guide your practice when treating patients in a rehabilitation setting.

Charles D. Ciccone

Acknowledgments

I am grateful to all of the people who provided input and support as this book evolved through five editions. I must once again thank Barbara MacDermott Costa, Linda D. Crane, John F. Decker, Susan S. Glenney, Gary Gorniak, Mark Greve, Helen Wruble Hakim, Sandra B. Levine, Donald L. Merrill, Grace Minerbo, Peter Panus, Jeffrey Rothman, and Steven R. Tippett. Their expert advice when reviewing previous editions of this book has proven invaluable in laying the foundation for the current edition.

As always, the staff at F. A. Davis Company has been incredibly supportive in the development of this edition. I would like to especially thank Melissa Duffield, senior acquisitions editor, for her advice and encouragement while I was working on this project. Thanks also to production manager, Bob Butler; director of art and design, Carolyn O'Brien; and everyone else at F.A. Davis who helped bring this book to completion. I am likewise extremely grateful to Dean DeChambeau, who was the developmental editor on this project. Dean's suggestions, ideas, and careful attention to detail will undoubtedly make this a stronger and more clinically relevant text.

Finally, Steve Wolf has served as editor of the CPR series since its inception, and I remain indebted to him for his wisdom and support over the years. Likewise, all the students and clinicians I have worked with have unknowingly contributed to this book by asking good questions and reminding me how drug therapy is related to clinical practice. Their dedication to clinical practice is outstanding, and I hope I can repay their efforts with a book that is interesting, useful, and relevant.

Reviewers

Dina Brooks, PhD, MSc, BSc (PT)
Physical Therapy
University of Toronto
Toronto, Ontario, Canada

Douglas Haladay, DPT, MHS, OCS, CSCS
Physical Therapy Department
University of Scranton
Scranton, Pennsylvania

Kristen Klyczek, PT, PhD
Physical Therapy
Daemen College
Amherst, New York

Michael Moran, PT, DPT, ScD
Physical Therapy Department
Misericordia University
Dallas, Pennsylvania

Brief Contents

SECTION 1

General Principles of Pharmacology, 1

1 Basic Principles of Pharmacology, 3

2 Pharmacokinetics I: Drug Administration, Absorption, and Distribution, 15

3 Pharmacokinetics II: Drug Elimination, 31

4 Drug Receptors, 43

SECTION 2

Pharmacology of the Central Nervous System, 57

5 General Principles of Central Nervous System Pharmacology, 59

6 Sedative-Hypnotic and Antianxiety Drugs, 69

7 Drugs to Treat Affective Disorders: Depression and Bipolar Syndrome, 83

8 Antipsychotic Drugs, 101

9 Antiepileptic Drugs, 115

10 Pharmacological Management of Parkinson Disease, 131

11 General Anesthetics, 149

12 Local Anesthetics, 165

SECTION 3

Drugs Affecting Skeletal Muscle, 177

13 Skeletal Muscle Relaxants, 179

SECTION 4

Drugs Used to Treat Pain and Inflammation, 199

14 Opioid Analgesics, 201

15 Nonsteroidal Anti-Inflammatory Drugs, 219

16 Pharmacological Management of Rheumatoid Arthritis and Osteoarthritis, 237

17 Patient-Controlled Analgesia, 261

SECTION 5

Autonomic and Cardiovascular Pharmacology, 277

18 Introduction to Autonomic Pharmacology, 279

19 Cholinergic Drugs, 289

20 Adrenergic Drugs, 301

21 Antihypertensive Drugs, 315

22 Treatment of Angina Pectoris, 335

23 Treatment of Cardiac Arrhythmias, 349

24 Treatment of Congestive Heart Failure, 359

25 Treatment of Coagulation Disorders and Hyperlipidemia, 375

SECTION 6

Respiratory and Gastrointestinal Pharmacology, 397

26 Respiratory Drugs, 399

27 Gastrointestinal Drugs, 421

SECTION 7

Endocrine Pharmacology, 433

28 Introduction to Endocrine Pharmacology, 435

29 Adrenocorticosteroids, 447

30 Male and Female Hormones, 465

31 Thyroid and Parathyroid Drugs: Agents Affecting Bone Mineralization, 491

32 Pancreatic Hormones and the Treatment of Diabetes Mellitus, 507

SECTION 8

Chemotherapy of Infectious and Neoplastic Diseases, 529

33 Treatment of Infections I: Antibacterial Drugs, 531

34 Treatment of Infections II: Antiviral Drugs, 557

35 Treatment of Infections III: Antifungal and Antiparasitic Drugs, 581

36 Cancer Chemotherapy, 599

37 Immunomodulating Agents, 625

38 Complementary and Alternative Medications, 641

Appendix A Drugs Administered by Iontophoresis and Phonophoresis, 657

Appendix B Drugs of Abuse, 659

Appendix C Answers to Case Study Questions, 661

Glossary, 673

Index, 681

Contents

SECTION 1

General Principles of Pharmacology, 1

CHAPTER 1. Basic Principles of Pharmacology, **3**

Relevance of Pharmacology in Rehabilitation, 3
Drug Nomenclature, 4
Substitution of Generic Drugs for Brand-Name Products, 5
What Constitutes a Drug: Development and Approval of Therapeutic Agents, 6
Drug Approval Process, 6
Orphan Drugs, 7
Off-Label Prescribing, 8
Prescription Versus Over-the-Counter Medication, 8
Controlled Substances, 9
Basic Concepts in Drug Therapy, 9
Dose-Response Curves and Maximal Efficacy, 9
Potency, 10
Elements of Drug Safety, 11
Quantal Dose-Response Curves and the Median Effective Dose, 11
Median Toxic Dose, 11
Therapeutic Index, 12
Summary, 12
References, 12

CHAPTER 2. Pharmacokinetics I: Drug Administration, Absorption, and Distribution, **15**

Routes of Administration, 15
Enteral, 15
Parenteral, 17
Transdermal, 18
Bioavailability and Drug Absorption Across the Cell Membrane, 19
Membrane Structure and Function, 19
Movement Across Membrane Barriers, 20
Distribution of Drugs Within the Body, 23
Factors Affecting Distribution, 23
Volume of Distribution, 24
Drug Storage, 24
Storage Sites, 24
Adverse Consequences of Drug Storage, 25
Newer Techniques for Drug Delivery, 25
Controlled-Release Preparations, 25
Implanted Drug Delivery Systems, 25
Targeting Drug Delivery to Specific Cells and Tissues, 26
Summary, 26
References, 27

CHAPTER 3. Pharmacokinetics II: Drug Elimination, **31**

Biotransformation, 31
Cellular Mechanisms of Drug Biotransformation, 31
Organs Responsible for Drug Biotransformation, 33
Enzyme Induction, 33
Drug Excretion, 33
Drug Elimination Rates, 34
Clearance, 34
Half-Life, 35
Dosing Schedules and Plasma Concentration, 35
Variations in Drug Response and Metabolism, 36
Genetics, 36
Disease, 37
Drug Interactions, 37
Age, 38
Diet, 38

Sex, 38
Other Factors, 39
Summary, 39
References, 39

CHAPTER 4. Drug Receptors, **43**

Receptors Located on the Cell's Surface, 43
Surface Receptors Linked Directly to Ion Channels, 43
Surface Receptors Linked Directly to Enzymes, 44
Surface Receptors Linked to Regulatory (G) Proteins and the Role of the Second Messenger, 44
Intracellular Receptors, 46
Drug-Receptor Interactions, 46
Functional Aspects of Drug-Receptor Interactions, 47
Drug Selectivity and Receptor Subtypes, 47
Dose-Response, 48
Classification of Drugs: Agonist Versus Antagonist, 49
Competitive Versus Noncompetitive Antagonists, 49
Partial Agonists, 50
Mixed Agonist-Antagonists and Inverse Agonists, 50
Receptor Regulation, 51
Receptor Desensitization and Down-Regulation, 51
Receptor Supersensitivity, 52
Nonreceptor Drug Mechanisms, 52
Summary, 52
References, 53

SECTION 2

Pharmacology of the Central Nervous System, 57

CHAPTER 5. General Principles of Central Nervous System Pharmacology, **59**

CNS Organization, 59
Cerebrum, 59
Basal Ganglia, 59
Diencephalon, 60
Mesencephalon and Brainstem, 60
Cerebellum, 60
Limbic System, 61
Spinal Cord, 61
The Blood-Brain Barrier, 61
CNS Neurotransmitters, 62
Acetylcholine, 63
Monoamines, 63
Amino Acids, 63
Peptides, 63
Other Transmitters, 64
The General Mechanisms of CNS Drugs, 64
Summary, 66
References, 66

CHAPTER 6. Sedative-Hypnotic and Antianxiety Drugs, **69**

Sedative-Hypnotic Drugs, 69
Benzodiazepines, 69
Nonbenzodiazepines, 72
Pharmacokinetics, 73
Problems and Adverse Effects of Sedative-Hypnotics, 73
Antianxiety Drugs, 75
Benzodiazepines, 75
Buspirone, 76
Use of Antidepressants in Anxiety, 76
Other Antianxiety Drugs, 77
Problems and Adverse Effects of Anxiolytics, 78
Special Concerns for Rehabilitation Patients, 78
Case Study, 79
Sedative-Hypnotic Drugs, 79
Summary, 80
References, 80

CHAPTER 7. Drugs to Treat Affective Disorders: Depression and Bipolar Syndrome, **83**

Depression, 83
Pathophysiology of Depression, 84
Antidepressant Drugs, 86
Pharmacokinetics of Antidepressants, 90
Problems and Adverse Effects, 90
Antidepressants and Chronic Pain, 92
Bipolar Disorder, 93
Lithium, 94
Other Drugs for Bipolar Disorder, 95
Special Concerns for Rehabilitation Patients, 95
Case Study, 97
Antidepressant Drugs, 97
Summary, 97
References, 97

CHAPTER 8. Antipsychotic Drugs, **101**

Schizophrenia, 101
Pathogenesis of Schizophrenia, 102
Neurotransmitter Changes in Schizophrenia, 102
Antipsychotics Mechanism of Action, 103
Antipsychotic Drugs, 105
Traditional Antipsychotics, 105
Atypical Antipsychotics, 105
Pharmacokinetics, 106
Other Uses of Antipsychotics, 106
Problems and Adverse Effects, 107
Extrapyramidal Symptoms, 107

Nonmotor Effects, 109
Other Side Effects, 110
Special Concerns for Rehabilitation Patients, 110
Case Study, 111
Antipsychotic Drugs, 111
Summary, 111
References,111

CHAPTER 9. Antiepileptic Drugs, **115**

Classification of Epileptic Seizures, 116
Rationale for Drug Treatment, 117
Antiseizure Drugs, 118
First-Generation Antiseizure Drugs, 118
Second-Generation Agents, 121
Selection of a Specific Antiepileptic Agent, 124
Pharmacokinetics, 125
Special Precautions During Pregnancy, 125
Treatment of Status Epilepticus, 126
Withdrawal of Antiseizure Medications, 126
Special Concerns for Rehabilitation Patients, 127
Case Study, 127
Antiepileptic Drugs, 127
Summary, 128
References, 128

CHAPTER 10. Pharmacological Management of Parkinson Disease, **131**

Pathophysiology of Parkinson Disease, 132
Etiology of Parkinson Disease: Genetic and Environmental Factors, 133
Genetic Factors, 133
Environmental Factors, 134
Therapeutic Agents in Parkinsonism, 134
Levodopa, 135
Pharmacokinetics of Levodopa, 135
Use of Peripheral Decarboxylase Inhibitors, 136
Problems and Adverse Effects of Levodopa Therapy, 137
Drug Holidays From Levodopa, 139
Other Drugs to Treat Parkinson Disease, 140
Dopamine Agonists, 140
Anticholinergic Drugs, 141
Amantadine, 141
Monoamine Oxidase B Inhibitors, 141
Catechol-O-Methyltransferase Inhibitors, 142
Clinical Course of Parkinson Disease: When to Use Specific Drugs, 142
Neurosurgical Interventions in Parkinson Disease, 143
Special Concerns For Rehabilitation Patients, 144
Case Study, 144
Anti-Parkinson Drugs, 144
Summary, 145
References, 145

CHAPTER 11. General Anesthetics, **149**

Requirements for General Anesthesia, 149
Induction Stages of General Anesthesia, 150
General Anesthetic Agents: Classification and Use According to Route of Administration, 150
Inhalation Anesthetics, 150
Intravenous Anesthetics, 153
Pharmacokinetics, 154
Mechanisms of Action, 154
Adjuvants in General Anesthesia, 156
Preoperative Medications, 156
Neuromuscular Blockers, 157
Nondepolarizing Blockers, 159
Depolarizing Blocker, 159
Special Concerns for Rehabilitation Patients, 160
Case Study, 160
General Anesthetics, 160
Summary, 161
References, 161

CHAPTER 12. Local Anesthetics, **165**

Types of Local Anesthetics, 165
Pharmacokinetics, 167
Clinical Use of Local Anesthetics, 167
Topical Administration, 167
Transdermal Administration, 167
Infiltration Anesthesia, 168
Peripheral Nerve Block, 168
Central Neural Blockade, 168
Sympathetic Blockade, 169
Intravenous Regional Anesthesia (Bier Block), 170
Mechanism of Action, 170
Differential Nerve Block, 171
Systemic Effects of Local Anesthetics, 172
Special Concerns for Rehabilitation Patients, 173
Case Study, 174
Local Anesthetics, 174
Summary, 174
References, 174

SECTION 3

Drugs Affecting Skeletal Muscle, 177

CHAPTER 13. Skeletal Muscle Relaxants, **179**

Increased Muscle Tone: Spasticity Versus Muscle Spasms, 179
Antispasm Drugs, 180
Diazepam, 180
Centrally Acting Antispasm Drugs, 181

Antispasticity Drugs, 183
Baclofen, 183
Intrathecal Baclofen, 184
Dantrolene Sodium, 185
Diazepam, 186
Gabapentin, 186
Tizanidine, 187
Use of Botulinum Toxin as a Muscle Relaxant, 187
Mechanism of Action, 188
Clinical Use of Botulinum Toxin, 189
Limitations and Adverse Effects, 190
Pharmacokinetics, 191
Special Concerns for Rehabilitation Patients, 191
Case Study, 193
Muscle Relaxants, 193
Summary, 193
References, 194

SECTION 4

Drugs Used to Treat Pain and Inflammation, 199

CHAPTER 14. Opioid Analgesics, 201

Sources of Opioid Analgesics, 201
Endogenous Opioid Peptides and Opioid Receptors, 202
Endogenous Opioids, 202
Opioid Receptors, 202
Classification of Specific Agents, 203
Strong Agonists, 203
Mild-to-Moderate Agonists, 205
Mixed Agonist–Antagonists, 206
Antagonists, 206
Pharmacokinetics, 206
Mechanism of Action, 207
Sites of Opioid Effects, 207
Effects of Opioids on Synaptic Activity, 209
Clinical Applications, 210
Treatment of Pain, 210
Use of Opioids in Patient-Controlled Analgesia, 211
Other Opioid Uses, 211
Problems and Adverse Effects, 211
Concepts of Addiction, Tolerance, and Physical Dependence, 211
Tolerance, 212
Physical Dependence, 212
Tolerance and Dependence During Therapeutic Opioid Use, 213
Opioid-Induced Hyperalgesia, 213
Pharmacological Treatment of Opioid Addiction, 214
Special Concerns for Rehabilitation Patients, 214
Case Study, 215
Opioid Analgesics, 215
Summary, 216
References, 216

CHAPTER 15. Nonsteroidal Anti-Inflammatory Drugs, 219

Aspirin and Other NSAIDs: General Aspects, 219
Prostaglandins, Thromboxanes, and Leukotrienes, 220
Eicosanoid Biosynthesis, 220
Role of Eicosanoids in Health and Disease, 220
Mechanism of NSAID Action: Inhibition of Prostaglandin and Thromboxane Synthesis, 222
Aspirin: The Prototypical NSAID, 223
Clinical Applications of Aspirinlike Drugs, 224
Treatment of Pain and Inflammation, 224
Treatment of Fever, 224
Treatment of Vascular Disorders, 224
Prevention of Cancer, 224
Problems and Adverse Effects of Aspirinlike Drugs, 224
Gastrointestinal Problems, 224
Cardiovascular Problems, 225
Other Side Effects, 226
Comparison of Aspirin With Other NSAIDs, 227
COX-2 Selective Drugs, 229
COX-2 Drugs and the Risk of Heart Attack and Stroke, 230
Acetaminophen, 230
Pharmacokinetics of NSAIDS and Acetaminophen, 232
Special Concerns for Rehabilitation Patients, 232
Case Study, 233
Nonsteroidal Anti-Inflammatory Drugs, 233
Summary, 233
References, 233

CHAPTER 16. Pharmacological Management of Rheumatoid Arthritis and Osteoarthritis, 237

Rheumatoid Arthritis, 237
Immune Basis for Rheumatoid Arthritis, 239
Overview of Drug Therapy in Rheumatoid Arthritis, 239
NSAIDs, 240
Glucocorticoids, 241
Disease-Modifying Antirheumatic Drugs, 242
Traditional (Nonbiological) DMARDs, 243
Biological DMARDs, 247
Other DMARDs, 249
DMARD Combinations Used in Rheumatoid Arthritis, 249
Dietary Implications for Rheumatoid Arthritis, 250
Osteoarthritis, 250
Acetaminophen and NSAIDs, 251
Viscosupplementation, 251
Glucosamine and Chondroitin Sulfate, 252
Special Concerns for Rehabilitation Patients, 253

Case Study, 253
Rheumatoid Arthritis, 253
Summary, 254
References, 254

CHAPTER 17. Patient-Controlled Analgesia, **261**

Pharmacokinetic Basis for PCA, 261
PCA Dosing Strategies and Parameters, 262
Types of Analgesics Used for PCA, 263
PCA Pumps, 264
Administration Routes During PCA, 265
IV PCA, 265
Epidural PCA, 266
Regional PCA, 267
Transdermal PCA, 267
Other Potential Administration Routes for PCA, 268
Comparison of PCA to Other Methods of Analgesic Administration, 268
Comparison of PCA to Continuous Nerve Blocks, 269
Problems and Adverse Effects of PCA, 270
Pharmacological Adverse Effects, 270
Problems With PCA Delivery, 270
Special Concerns for Rehabilitation Patients, 271
Case Study, 272
Patient-Controlled Analgesia, 272
Summary, 272
References, 272

SECTION 5

Autonomic and Cardiovascular Pharmacology, 277

CHAPTER 18. Introduction to Autonomic Pharmacology, **279**

Anatomy of the Autonomic Nervous System: Sympathetic and Parasympathetic Divisions, 279
Preganglionic and Postganglionic Neurons, 280
Sympathetic Organization, 280
Parasympathetic Organization, 280
Functional Aspects of the Sympathetic and Parasympathetic Divisions, 280
Function of the Adrenal Medulla, 282
Autonomic Integration and Control, 282
Autonomic Neurotransmitters, 283
Acetylcholine and Norepinephrine, 283
Other Autonomic Neurotransmitters, 283
Autonomic Receptors, 284
Cholinergic Receptors, 284
Adrenergic Receptors, 286
Pharmacological Significance of Autonomic Receptors, 287
Summary, 288
References, 288

CHAPTER 19. Cholinergic Drugs, **289**

Cholinergic Receptors, 289
Cholinergic Stimulants, 290
Direct-Acting Cholinergic Stimulants, 290
Indirect-Acting Cholinergic Stimulants, 291
Clinical Applications of Cholinergic Stimulants, 292
Problems and Adverse Effects of Cholinergic Stimulants, 293
Anticholinergic Drugs, 293
Source and Mechanism of Action of Antimuscarinic Anticholinergic Drugs, 294
Clinical Applications of Antimuscarinic Drugs, 294
Problems and Adverse Effects of Anticholinergic Drugs, 297
Summary, 297
References, 298

CHAPTER 20. Adrenergic Drugs, **301**

Adrenergic Receptor Subclassifications, 302
Adrenergic Agonists, 303
Alpha-1-Selective Agonists, 303
Alpha-2-Selective Agonists, 304
Beta-1-Selective Agonists, 305
Beta-2-Selective Agonists, 305
Drugs With Mixed Alpha- and Beta-Agonist Activity, 306
Adrenergic Antagonists, 307
Alpha Antagonists, 307
Beta Antagonists, 309
Other Drugs That Inhibit Adrenergic Neurons, 312
Summary, 313
References, 313

CHAPTER 21. Antihypertensive Drugs, **315**

Normal Control of Blood Pressure, 316
Pathogenesis of Hypertension, 316
Essential Versus Secondary Hypertension, 316
Possible Mechanisms in Essential Hypertension, 317
Drug Therapy, 318
Diuretics, 318
Sympatholytic Drugs, 320
Vasodilators, 323
Renin-Angiotensin System Inhibitors, 324
Calcium Channel Blockers, 326
Drug Selection for Specific Patients With Hypertension, 327
Nonpharmacological Treatment of Hypertension, 328
Special Concerns for Rehabilitation Patients, 329
Case Study, 329
Hypertension, 329

Summary, 330
References, 330

CHAPTER 22. Treatment of Angina Pectoris, **335**

Drugs Used to Treat Angina Pectoris, 335
Organic Nitrates, 335
Beta-Adrenergic Blockers, 338
Calcium Channel Blockers, 339
Other Drugs Affecting Myocardial Oxygen Balance in Angina Pectoris, 340
Use of Anticoagulants in Angina Pectoris, 341
Treatment of Specific Types of Angina Pectoris, 341
Stable Angina, 341
Variant Angina (Prinzmetal Ischemia), 343
Unstable Angina, 343
Nonpharmacologic Management of Angina Pectoris, 344
Special Concerns for Rehabilitation Patients, 344
Case Study, 345
Antianginal Drugs, 345
Summary, 346
References, 346

CHAPTER 23. Treatment of Cardiac Arrhythmias, **349**

Cardiac Electrophysiology, 349
Cardiac Action Potentials, 349
Normal Cardiac Rhythm, 350
Normal Conduction of the Cardiac Action Potential, 351
Mechanisms of Cardiac Arrhythmias, 351
Types of Arrhythmias, 352
Classification of Antiarrhythmic Drugs, 352
Class I: Sodium Channel Blockers, 352
Class II: Beta Blockers, 354
Class III: Drugs That Prolong Repolarization, 354
Class IV: Calcium Channel Blockers, 355
Other Drugs Used to Treat Arrhythmias, 355
Nonpharmacological Treatment of Arrhythmias, 355
Special Concerns for Rehabilitation Patients, 356
Case Study, 356
Antiarrhythmic Drugs, 356
Summary, 357
References, 357

CHAPTER 24. Treatment of Congestive Heart Failure, **359**

Pathophysiology of Congestive Heart Failure, 360
The Vicious Cycle of Heart Failure, 360
Congestion in Left and Right Heart Failure, 361
Pharmacotherapy, 362
Drugs That Increase Myocardial Contraction Force (Positive Inotropic Agents), 362
Digitalis, 362
Phosphodiesterase Inhibitors, 365
Dopamine and Dobutamine, 366
Agents That Decrease Cardiac Workload, 367
Drugs Affecting the Renin-Angiotensin System, 367
Adverse Effects of Drugs Affecting the Renin-Angiotensin System, 368
Beta Blockers, 368
Diuretics, 369
Vasodilators, 370
Special Concerns for Rehabilitation Patients, 371
Case Study, 371
Congestive Heart Failure, 371
Summary, 372
References, 372

CHAPTER 25. Treatment of Coagulation Disorders and Hyperlipidemia, **375**

Normal Mechanism of Blood Coagulation, 376
Clot Formation, 376
Clot Breakdown, 377
Drugs Used to Treat Overactive Clotting, 377
Anticoagulants, 377
Antiplatelet Drugs, 381
Fibrinolytics, 383
Treatment of Clotting Deficiencies, 385
Hemophilia, 385
Deficiencies of Vitamin K–Dependent Clotting Factors, 386
Antifibrinolytics, 386
Agents Used to Treat Hyperlipidemia, 387
HMG-CoA Reductase Inhibitors (Statins), 387
Fibric Acids, 388
Other Lipid-Lowering Agents, 389
Adverse Effects of Antihyperlipidemic Agents, 389
Special Concerns for Rehabilitation Patients, 390
Case Study, 391
Clotting Disorders, 391
Summary, 391
References, 392

SECTION 6

Respiratory and Gastrointestinal Pharmacology, 397

CHAPTER 26. Respiratory Drugs, **399**

Drugs Used to Treat Respiratory Tract Irritation and Control Respiratory Secretions, 399
Antitussives, 399
Decongestants, 400
Antihistamines, 401
Mucolytics and Expectorants, 402
Drugs Used to Maintain Airway Patency in Obstructive Pulmonary Disease, 403
Beta-Adrenergic Agonists, 403
Xanthine Derivatives, 406

Anticholinergic Drugs, 407
Glucocorticoids, 408
Cromones, 409
Leukotriene Inhibitors, 409
Treatment of Bronchial Asthma, 410
Pathophysiology of Bronchial Asthma, 410
Long-Term Management of Asthma, 410
Treatment of Reversible Bronchospasm in COPD, 412
Treatment of Respiratory Problems in Cystic Fibrosis, 412
Special Concerns for Rehabilitation Patients, 413
Case Study, 414
Respiratory Drugs, 414
Summary, 415
References, 415

CHAPTER 27. Gastrointestinal Drugs, **421**

Drugs Used to Control Gastric Acidity and Secretion, 421
Antacids, 422
H_2 Receptor Blockers, 423
Proton Pump Inhibitors, 423
Treatment of Helicobacter Pylori Infection in Gastric Ulcer Disease, 425
Other Agents Used to Control and Treat Gastric Ulcers, 425
Antidiarrheal Agents, 426
Opioid Derivatives, 426
Bismuth Salicylate, 427
Miscellaneous Agents Used to Treat Diarrhea, 427
Laxatives and Cathartics, 428
Specific Agents and Mechanism of Action, 428
Adverse Effects, 429
Miscellaneous Gastrointestinal Drugs, 429
Digestants, 429
Emetics, 429
Antiemetics, 429
Cholelitholytic Agents, 430
Special Concerns for Rehabilitation Patients, 430
Case Study, 430
Gastrointestinal Drugs, 430
Summary, 431
References, 431

SECTION 7

Endocrine Pharmacology, 433

CHAPTER 28. Introduction to Endocrine Pharmacology, **435**

Primary Endocrine Glands and Their Hormones, 435
Hypothalamus and Pituitary Gland, 436
Thyroid Gland, 437
Parathyroid Gland, 438
Pancreas, 438
Adrenal Gland, 438
Gonads, 439
Endocrine Physiology and Pharmacology, 439
Hormone Chemistry, 439
Synthesis and Release of Hormones, 440
Feedback Control Mechanisms in Endocrine Function, 440
Hormone Transport, 441
Hormone Effects on the Target Cell, 441
Clinical Use of Endocrine Drugs, 443
Replacement Therapy, 443
Diagnosis of Endocrine Disorders, 443
Treatment of Excessive Endocrine Function, 443
Exploitation of Beneficial Hormone Effects, 444
Use of Hormones to Alter Normal Endocrine Function, 444
Use of Hormones in Nonendocrine Disease, 444
Summary, 444
References, 444

CHAPTER 29. Adrenocorticosteroids, **447**

Steroid Synthesis, 447
Glucocorticoids, 449
Role of Glucocorticoids in Normal Function, 449
Mechanism of Action of Glucocorticoids, 450
Physiological Effects of Glucocorticoids, 450
Clinical Uses of Glucocorticoids, 453
Glucocorticoid Use in Endocrine Disorders, 454
Glucocorticoid Use in Nonendocrine Conditions, 454
Adverse Effects of Glucocorticoids, 455
Adrenocortical Suppression, 456
Drug-Induced Cushing Syndrome, 456
Breakdown of Supporting Tissues, 456
Other Adverse Effects, 457
Drugs That Inhibit Adrenocortical Hormone Biosynthesis, 457
Mineralocorticoids, 457
Regulation of Mineralocorticoid Secretion, 458
Mechanism of Action and Physiological Effects of Mineralocorticoids, 458
Therapeutic Use of Mineralocorticoid Drugs, 459
Adverse Effects of Mineralocorticoid Agonists, 459
Mineralocorticoid Antagonists, 460
Special Concerns for Rehabilitation Patients, 460
Case Study, 461
Adrenocorticosteroids, 461
Summary, 462
References, 462

CHAPTER 30. Male and Female Hormones, **465**

Androgens, 465
Source and Regulation of Androgen Synthesis, 465
Physiological Effects of Androgens, 467
Clinical Use of Androgens, 467
Replacement Therapy, 467
Catabolic States, 467
Delayed Puberty, 468

Breast Cancer, 468
Anemia, 468
Hereditary Angioedema, 468
Specific Agents, 468
Adverse Effects of Clinical Androgen Use, 469
Antiandrogens, 469
Androgen Abuse, 470
Effects of Androgens on Athletic Performance, 471
Adverse Effects of Androgen Abuse, 472
Estrogen and Progesterone, 472
Effects of Estrogen and Progesterone on Sexual Maturation, 473
Regulation and Effects of Hormonal Synthesis During the Menstrual Cycle, 473
Female Hormones in Pregnancy and Parturition, 475
Pharmacological Use of Estrogen and Progesterone, 475
Conditions Treated With Estrogen and Progesterone, 475
Use of Hormone Replacement Therapy Following Menopause, 476
Specific Agents, 477
Adverse Effects of Estrogen and Progesterone, 477
Other Drugs That Affect Estrogen and Progesterone Activity, 478
Selective Estrogen Receptor Modulators, 478
Antiestrogens, 479
Antiprogestins, 479
Hormonal Contraceptives, 480
Types of Contraceptive Preparations, 480
Mechanism of Contraceptive Action, 482
Adverse Effects of Hormonal Contraceptives, 482
Case Study, 483
Male and Female Hormones, 483
Special Concerns for Rehabilitation Patients, 484
Summary, 484
References, 485

CHAPTER 31. Thyroid and Parathyroid Drugs: Agents Affecting Bone Mineralization, **491**

Hormones of the Thyroid Gland, 491
Synthesis of Thyroid Hormones, 491
Regulation of Thyroid Hormone Release, 493
Physiological Effects of Thyroid Hormones, 493
Mechanism of Action of Thyroid Hormones, 493
Treatment of Thyroid Disorders, 494
Hyperthyroidism, 494
Hypothyroidism, 496
Parathyroid Hormone, 497
Regulation of Bone Mineral Homeostasis, 498
Parathyroid Hormone and Bone Formation, 498
Vitamin D, 498
Calcitonin, 498
Other Hormones, 499
Pharmacological Control of Bone Mineral Homeostasis, 499
Calcium Supplements, 501
Vitamin D, 501
Bisphosphonates, 501
Calcitonin, 502
Estrogen Therapy, 503
Other Agents That Promote Bone Mineral Content, 503
Special Concerns for Rehabilitation Patients, 504
Case Study, 504
Agents Affecting Bone Mineral Metabolism, 504
Summary, 505
References, 505

CHAPTER 32. Pancreatic Hormones and the Treatment of Diabetes Mellitus, **507**

Structure and Function of the Endocrine Pancreas, 507
Insulin, 508
Effects of Insulin on Carbohydrate Metabolism, 508
Effects of Insulin on Protein and Lipid Metabolism, 508
Cellular Mechanism of Insulin Action, 508
Glucagon, 509
Control of Insulin and Glucagon Release, 510
Diabetes Mellitus, 510
Type 1 Diabetes, 511
Type 2 Diabetes, 511
Effects and Complications of Diabetes Mellitus, 512
Use of Insulin in Diabetes Mellitus, 513
Therapeutic Effects and Rationale for Use, 513
Insulin Preparations, 513
Administration of Insulin, 515
Intensive Insulin Therapy, 516
Adverse Effects of Insulin Therapy, 516
Primary Agents in Type 2 Diabetes, 517
Drugs That Stimulate Insulin Secretion and Supply, 517
Insulin Sensitizers, 519
Other Antidiabetics, 520
Prevention of Type 1 Diabetes Mellitus: The Potential Role of Immune-Based Therapies, 520
Nonpharmacological Intervention in Diabetes Mellitus, 521
Dietary Management and Weight Reduction, 521
Exercise, 521
Tissue Transplants and Gene Therapy, 521
Special Concerns for Rehabilitation Patients, 522
Case Study, 523
Diabetes Mellitus, 523
Summary, 523
References, 523

SECTION 8

Chemotherapy of Infectious and Neoplastic Diseases, 529

CHAPTER 33. Treatment of Infections I: Antibacterial Drugs, **531**

Bacteria: Basic Concepts, 532
Bacterial Structure and Function, 532
Pathogenic Effects of Bacteria, 532
Bacterial Nomenclature and Classification, 532
Spectrum and Activity of Antibacterial Drugs, 533
Spectrum of Antibacterial Activity, 533
Bactericidal Versus Bacteriostatic Activity, 533
Basic Mechanisms of Antibacterial Drugs, 533
Inhibition of Bacterial Cell Wall Synthesis and Function, 534
Inhibition of Bacterial Protein Synthesis, 534
Inhibition of Bacterial DNA/RNA Synthesis and Function, 535
Specific Antibacterial Agents, 535
Antibacterial Drugs That Inhibit Bacterial Cell Wall Synthesis and Function, 535
Penicillins, 536
Cephalosporins, 537
Carbapenems, 538
Other Agents That Inhibit Bacterial Cell Wall Synthesis, 538
Use of Beta-Lactamase Inhibitors, 539
Drugs That Inhibit Bacterial Protein Synthesis, 539
Aminoglycosides, 539
Erythromycin and Other Macrolides, 540
Other Agents That Inhibit Bacterial Protein Synthesis, 541
Drugs That Inhibit Bacterial DNA/RNA Synthesis and Function, 543
Aminosalicylic Acid, 543
Clofazimine, 543
Dapsone, 543
Fluoroquinolones, 543
Metronidazole, 544
Mupirocin, 544
Rifamycins, 544
Sulfonamides, 545
Trimethoprim, 545
Other Antibacterial Drugs, 545
Capreomycin, 545
Daptomycin, 546
Isoniazid, 546
Methenamine, 546
Nitrofurantoin, 546
Pyrazinamide, 546
Clinical Use of Antibacterial Drugs: Relationship to Specific Bacterial Infections, 546
Resistance to Antibacterial Drugs, 549
Special Concerns for Rehabilitation Patients, 551
Case Study, 551
Antibacterial Drugs, 551
Summary, 552
References, 552

CHAPTER 34. Treatment of Infections II: Antiviral Drugs, **557**

Viral Structure and Function, 557
Classification of Viruses, 557
Characteristics of Viruses, 558
Viral Replication, 559
Specific Antiviral Drugs, 560
Acyclovir and Valacyclovir, 561
Amantadine and Rimantadine, 561
Cidofovir, 562
Docosanol, 563
Dolutegravir, Elvitegravir, and Raltegravir, 563
Enfuvirtide and Maraviroc, 563
Famciclovir and Penciclovir, 564
Foscarnet, 564
Ganciclovir and Valganciclovir, 564
Imiquimod, 565
Trifluridine, 565
Oseltamivir and Zanamivir, 565
Protease Inhibitors, 565
Reverse Transcriptase Inhibitors, 566
Ribavirin, 567
Viral Resistance, 568
Interferons, 568
Synthesis and Cellular Effects of Interferons, 568
Pharmacological Applications of Interferons, 569
Adverse Effects of Interferons, 570
Control of Viral Infection With Vaccines, 570
HIV and the Treatment of AIDS, 571
Inhibition of HIV Proliferation in Infected Individuals, 571
Anti-HIV Drug Combinations: Use of Highly Active Antiretroviral Therapy, 573
HIV Vaccines, 574
Management of Opportunistic Infections, 574
Special Concerns for Rehabilitation Patients, 576
Case Study, 576
Antiviral Drugs, 576
Summary, 577
References, 577

CHAPTER 35. Treatment of Infections III: Antifungal and Antiparasitic Drugs, **581**

Antifungal Agents, 581
Systemic Antifungal Agents, 584
Topical Antifungal Agents, 586
Antiprotozoal Agents, 587
Antimalarial Agents, 588
Drugs Used to Treat Protozoal Infections in the Intestines and Other Tissues, 591
Other Antiprotozoal Drugs, 593
Anthelmintics, 593
Albendazole, 593
Diethylcarbamazine, 594
Ivermectin, 594
Mebendazole, 594
Praziquantel, 594
Pyrantel Pamoate, 595
Thiabendazole, 595
Other Anthelmintics, 595
Special Concerns for Rehabilitation Patients, 595
Case Study, 596
Antifungal Drugs, 596
Summary, 596
References, 596

CHAPTER 36. Cancer Chemotherapy, **599**

General Principles, 600
Cytotoxic Strategy, 600
Cell-Cycle–Specific Versus Cell-Cycle–Nonspecific Drugs, 600
Concepts of Growth Fraction and Cell Kill, 600
Prevalence and Management of Adverse Effects, 601
Specific Anticancer Drugs, 602
Alkylating Agents, 602
Antimetabolites, 603
Anticancer Antibiotics, 605
Antimicrotubule Agents, 605
Topoisomerase Inhibitors, 608
Anticancer Hormones, 608
Targeted and Biological Therapies, 610
Platinum Coordination Complexes, 613
Aspirin and Other NSAIDs, 613
Miscellaneous Agents, 614
Combination Chemotherapy, 616
Use of Anticancer Drugs With Other Treatments, 617
Success of Anticancer Drugs, 617
Resistance to Anticancer Drugs, 618
Future Perspectives, 618
Special Concerns for Rehabilitation Patients, 619
Case Study, 620
Cancer Chemotherapy, 620
Summary, 621
References, 621

CHAPTER 37. Immunomodulating Agents, **625**

Overview of the Immune Response, 626
Pharmacological Suppression of the Immune Response, 627
Specific Immunosuppressive Agents, 627
Azathioprine, 627
Cyclophosphamide, 629
Cyclosporine, 629
Glucocorticoids, 629
Methotrexate, 630
Mycophenolate Mofetil, 630
Sulfasalazine, 631
Sirolimus and Other mTOR Inhibitors, 631
Tacrolimus, 631
Other Methods of Immunosuppression, 632
Immunostimulants, 634
Bacille Calmette-Guérin, 634
Immune Globulin, 634
Other Immunomodulators, 635
Special Concerns for Rehabilitation Patients, 635
Case Study, 636
Immunomodulating Agents, 636
Summary, 637
References, 637

CHAPTER 38. Complementary and Alternative Medications, **641**

Problems Associated With CAMs, 641
Misconceptions About CAM Safety, 641
Failure to Report CAM Use, 642
Lack of Standards for Quality and Purity of CAMs, 642
Delayed Use of Conventional Medications, 642
Potential Adverse Effects of CAMs, 643
Specific CAMs, 643
Bee Venom, 643
Echinacea, 644
Garlic, 644
Ginger, 645
Ginkgo Biloba, 645
Ginseng, 645
Glucosamine and Chondroitin, 645
Kava, 646

Melatonin, 646
Saw Palmetto, 646
St. John's Wort, 647
Valerian, 647
Vitamins and Minerals, 647
Vitamins, 647
Minerals, 649
Special Concerns for Rehabilitation Patients, 650
Case Study, 651
Complementary and Alternative Medications, 651
Summary, 652
References, 652

APPENDIX A: Drugs Administered by Iontophoresis and Phonophoresis, **657**

APPENDIX B: Drugs of Abuse, **659**

APPENDIX C: Answers to Case Study Questions, **661**

Glossary, **673**

Index, **681**

SECTION

1

General Principles of Pharmacology

CHAPTER 1

Basic Principles of Pharmacology

Pharmacology is the study of drugs. In its broadest definition, a drug can be described as "any substance that, when taken into a living organism, may modify one or more of its functions."[1] In this sense, a drug includes any substance that alters physiological function in the organism, regardless of whether the effect is beneficial or harmful. In terms of clinical pharmacology, it has traditionally been the beneficial or therapeutic effects that have been of special interest.

For centuries, people have used naturally occurring chemicals to relieve pain or treat disease. Almost everyone, for example, has been administered some form of natural product or home remedy that was handed down from generation to generation when trying to resolve a minor illness or painful condition. However, these natural cures and home remedies are understandably limited in how well they can treat more serious conditions. Within the past 100 years, medical practitioners have therefore expanded their use of natural, semisynthetic, and synthetic chemical agents to the point where many diseases can be prevented or cured, and the general health and well-being of many individuals has dramatically improved through therapeutic drug use. Current medical practitioners who prescribe and administer drugs (i.e., physicians and nurses) are expected to know the drugs and the basic mechanisms of their actions. It is now recognized that members of other health-related professions must have a fundamental knowledge of pharmacology as well.

RELEVANCE OF PHARMACOLOGY IN REHABILITATION

As a physical therapist, occupational therapist, or other rehabilitation specialist, you can expect that your patient will be using therapeutic medications. When you know how the various drugs may affect a patient and the mechanisms behind those effects, you can apply that knowledge to get an optimal response from the patient's therapy treatment. For instance, you can improve a patient's therapy session dramatically by scheduling the therapy when certain drugs reach their peak effect, such as drugs that decrease pain (analgesics) or improve the patient's motor skills (anti-Parkinson drugs). Conversely, some therapy sessions that require the patient's active participation can be rendered useless if scheduled when medications such as sedatives reach their peak effect. Also, when you understand a drug's pharmacological aspects, you can avoid or control any adverse responses from occurring due to direct interaction between the therapy treatment and certain medications. For example, a patient who is taking a peripheral vasodilator may experience a profound decrease in blood pressure in a hot whirlpool. By understanding the implications of such an interaction, you can be especially alert for any detrimental effects on the patient, or you may institute a different therapy treatment for them.

Pharmacology is a broad topic, so it is often subdivided into several areas of interest to help describe the discipline (Fig. 1-1). **Pharmacotherapeutics**

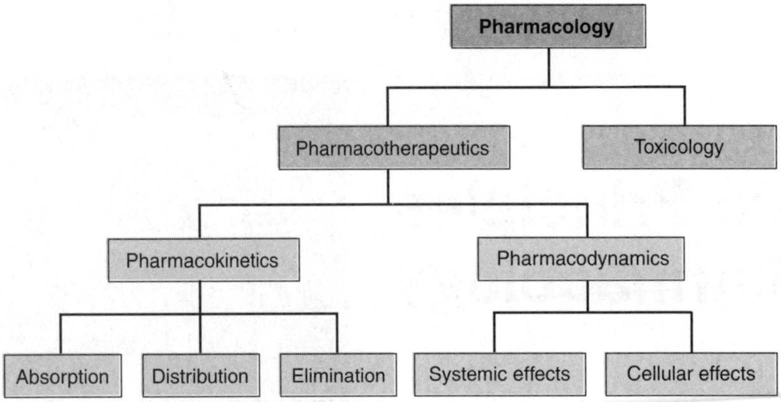

Figure ■ 1-1
Areas of study within pharmacology.

is the area of pharmacology that refers to the use of specific drugs to prevent, treat, or diagnose a disease. This text's primary concern is of the effects of drugs on humans, with animal pharmacology mentioned only in reference to drug testing and research in animals.

If we are to use therapeutic drugs safely, it is crucial to know how the body interacts with the drug and what effect it has on an individual. Consequently, pharmacotherapeutics is divided into two functional areas: pharmacokinetics and pharmacodynamics (see Fig. 1-1). **Pharmacokinetics** is the study of how the body absorbs, distributes, and eliminates the drug. **Pharmacodynamics** is the analysis of what the drug does to the body, including the mechanism by which the drug exerts its effect. Chapters 2 and 3 outline the basic principles of pharmacokinetics, and the pharmacodynamics and pharmacokinetics of specific drugs will be discussed in their respective chapters.

Toxicology is the study of the harmful effects of chemicals. Although it can be viewed as a subdivision of pharmacology, toxicology has evolved into a separate area of study. Toxicology is therefore considered a distinct discipline because of the scope of all the therapeutic agents' adverse effects, environmental toxins, and poisons. However, because virtually every medication can produce adverse effects, a discussion of toxicology must be included in pharmacotherapeutics. This text limits the discussions of drug toxicity to the unwanted effects that occur when therapeutic drugs reach excessively high (toxic) levels. The toxic side effects of individual drugs are covered in the chapters describing the therapeutic effects of that drug.

Pharmacy deals with the preparation and dispensing of medications. Although pharmacy is also frequently considered a subdivision of pharmacology, this area has evolved into a distinct professional discipline. The terms *pharmacy* and *pharmacology* refer to different areas of study and should not be used interchangeably.

Pharmacogenetics is a relatively new area of pharmacology.[2] It deals with the genetic basis for drug responses, especially variations in drug response from person to person. We know that individual differences in specific genes can alter pharmacokinetic and pharmacodynamic variables. These differences provide one reason why various people might react differently to the same drug. Examining the genetic code for a given patient could help predict which drugs might be most effective for that patient and which drugs should be avoided because of potentially harmful side effects. This process could help eliminate some of the trial and error that occurs when trying to find the best drug for that patient. Pharmacogenetics promises to play an increasing role in determining how drugs can be used safely and effectively.

Pharmacology is therefore an important aspect of health care that has direct relevance to patients in a rehabilitation setting. This chapter provides an overview of how drugs are named, classified, developed, and approved, and it will introduce concepts that help us compare the safety and effects of various drugs. Subsequent chapters will draw on this information when considering the effects of specific drugs on our patients.

DRUG NOMENCLATURE

One of the most potentially confusing aspects of pharmacology is the variety of names given to different drugs or even to the same compound. Students of pharmacology, as well as clinicians, are often faced with myriad terms representing the same drug.[3,4] Many problems in drug terminology arise from the fact that each drug can be identified according to its *chemical*, *generic*, or *trade* name (Table 1-1).[4] **Chemical names** refer to the specific compound's structure and are usually fairly long and cumbersome. The **generic name** (also known as the *official* or **nonproprietary name**) tends to be somewhat shorter and is often derived from the chemical name. A **trade name** (also known as the *brand name*) is assigned to the compound by the pharmaceutical company and may or may not bear any reference to the chemical and generic terminology. An additional problem with trade names is that several manufacturers may be marketing the same compound under different names, adding to the confusion. Different drug companies may market the same drug if there is no existing patent for that compound or if the patent has expired.[5] For practical purposes, the generic name is often the easiest and most effective way to refer to a drug, and we will use this terminology frequently in this text.

Drug nomenclature is also a source of confusion and potential errors when different drugs have names that look or sound alike.[6] Practitioners could accidentally select and prescribe the wrong drug if its name sounds or looks like a different drug. This fact seems especially true for drugs with similar brand names.[7] Consider, for example, the confusion that could occur when trying to differentiate between the following three brand-name products: Celebrex, Cerebyx, and Celexa.[8] These three brand names correspond to an analgesic (see Chapter 15), an antiseizure drug (see Chapter 9), and an antidepressant (see Chapter 7), respectively. Despite their similar brand names, these three products represent three distinct pharmacological classes that are used in very different clinical situations. Hence, practitioners need to be especially careful when documenting the use of specific medications and make sure that the correct drug name is used to identify each product. In addition, patients are often concerned that a generic drug may represent a different and less effective product than its trade (brand) name counterpart. We address the issue of substituting generic products in the next section.

SUBSTITUTION OF GENERIC DRUGS FOR BRAND-NAME PRODUCTS

A common question among practitioners and patients is whether the generic form of a drug can be substituted for the brand-name product. The **generic drug** is typically less expensive than its brand-name counterparts, and substitution of a generic drug can help reduce health-care costs.[9] The generic form of the drug should be as safe and effective as the original brand-name product, provided that the generic form satisfies certain criteria.[10,11] Specifically, the generic form should undergo testing to establish that it has the same type and amount of the active ingredient(s), the same administration route, the same pharmacokinetic profile (e.g., drug absorption plasma levels, metabolism), and the same therapeutic effects as the brand-name drug.[12] If such testing is done, the two drugs are said to be "bioequivalent."[12]

Unless bioequivalence is established, however, it can only be assumed that substituting a generic drug will produce therapeutic effects that are similar to the brand-name drug. Likewise, establishing bioequivalence of a generic form does not guarantee that a given patient will not experience different effects from the generic form compared with the brand-name product. Some patients might simply respond differently to the generic form of a drug because of differences in their ability to absorb and metabolize certain generic

Table 1-1
EXAMPLES OF DRUG NOMENCLATURE

Chemical	Generic (Nonproprietary)	Trade/Brand-Name (Proprietary)
N-acetyl-*p*-aminophenol	Acetaminophen	Tylenol, Panadol, many others
3,4-Dihydroxyphenyl-L-alanine	Levodopa	Larodopa
5,5-Phenylethylbarbituric acid	Phenobarbital	Luminal, Eskabarb
7-Chloro-1,3-dihydro-1-methyl-5-phenyl-2*H*-1, 4-benzodiazepin-2-one	Diazepam	Valium

products, even if these products were shown to be similar to their brand-name counterpart during bioequivalence testing. This seems especially true for drugs that tend to produce a wider range of therapeutic and adverse effects when tested in a specific patient or within a group of patients (i.e., drugs with more intrasubject and intersubject variability).[13] If generic forms of such drugs are used clinically, the overall health-care costs may actually increase because of decreased therapeutic effects and a higher incidence of adverse effects.[14,15]

Hence, there are many issues that practitioners consider before a generic drug is substituted. Nonetheless, rehabilitation specialists should be able to explain the rationale for why a generic form of the drug might be prescribed but should also refer their patient to the physician or pharmacist if the patient has additional concerns about the effects of the generic drug.

WHAT CONSTITUTES A DRUG: DEVELOPMENT AND APPROVAL OF THERAPEUTIC AGENTS

In the United States, the Food and Drug Administration (FDA) is responsible for monitoring the use of existing drugs and for developing and approving new ones.[5,16] The analogous body in Canada is the Health Products and Food Branch of the Department of National Health and Welfare. The two primary concerns of these agencies are (1) whether the drug is effective in treating a certain condition and (2) whether the drug is reasonably safe for human use.

Drug Approval Process

The development of a new drug involves extensive preclinical (animal) and clinical (human) studies.[5,17] The basic procedure for testing a new drug is outlined here and summarized in Table 1-2. Details about the drug approval process can also be found on the FDA website (www.fda.gov/Drugs/DevelopmentApprovalProcess/).

Animal (Preclinical) Studies

Drugs are typically tested in animals initially, often using several different species. The animal trials provide preliminary information on the pharmacokinetic and pharmacodynamic properties of the compound and information on dosage and toxicity.

Human (Clinical) Studies

If the results from animal trials are favorable, the drug sponsor files an investigational new drug (IND) application with the FDA. If the drug is approved as an IND, the sponsor may begin testing it in humans.

Table 1-2
DRUG DEVELOPMENT AND APPROVAL

Testing Phase	Purpose	Subjects	Usual Time Period
Preclinical testing	Initial laboratory tests to determine drug effects and safety	Laboratory animals	1–2 yrs
Investigational New Drug (IND) Application			
Human (clinical) testing:			
Phase I	Determine effects, safe dosage, pharmacokinetics	Small number (less than 100) of healthy volunteers	Less than 1 yr
Phase II	Assess drug's effectiveness in treating a specific disease/disorder	Limited number of patients (200–300) with target disorder	2 yrs
Phase III	Assess safety and effectiveness in a larger patient population	Large number of patients (1,000–3,000) targeted	3 yrs
New Drug Application (NDA) Approval			
Phase IV (postmarketing surveillance)	Monitor any problems that occur after NDA approval	General patient population	Indefinite

Human, or "clinical," testing is divided into three primary phases:

Phase I. The drug is usually tested in a relatively small number of healthy volunteers. The purpose of this phase is to obtain some initial information about the pharmacological actions and the drug's possible toxic effects in humans. In general, between 10 and 100 subjects are studied in phase I, but the actual number of subjects will vary according to the drug,

Phase II. The drug is tested in a relatively small sample (50 to 500 people) with a specific disease or pathological condition. The primary goal of phase II is to evaluate the dosage range and effectiveness of the drug and to assess the side effects and other risks.

Phase III. The clinical evaluation is expanded to include more patients (several hundred to several thousand) and more evaluators. The larger patient population provides additional information regarding the drug's safety and effectiveness.

At the end of phase III, the drug sponsor applies for a new drug application (NDA). The FDA extensively reviews the results from clinical testing, and if found favorable, the NDA is approved. At this point, the drug can be marketed and prescribed for use in the general population.

Postmarketing Surveillance

Although it is not always required, a fourth phase, known as *postmarketing surveillance*, is often instituted after the NDA is approved. Postmarketing surveillance refers to all of the methods used to continue monitoring drug safety and effectiveness after approval for public use.[18,19] These methods often consist of reports from health-care providers that describe specific rare adverse effects that were not discovered during clinical testing.[18] For example, a drug might cause a specific adverse effect in only 1 in 10,000 patients taking the drug.[20] It is very likely that such an adverse effect could be missed during phases I through III of the clinical trials because the drug is typically tested only in a few thousand subjects (e.g., 1,000 to 3,000 people). In addition to monitoring adverse effects, postmarketing surveillance can use more formal research methods to obtain information about how a specific drug is used in clinical practice and how that drug compares to similar drugs on the market.[19] Hence, many experts believe that postmarketing surveillance is critical in ensuring that the safety and efficacy of the drug continues to be monitored when it is used by the general patient population.[18,20]

The development of a new drug in the United States is an extremely expensive and time-consuming process.[20] The time for the entire testing process from the beginning of animal trials to the end of phase III human testing may be as long as 7 to 9 years. However, the FDA has made provisions to shorten the development and review process for drugs designed to treat serious and life-threatening conditions, especially if the drug shows substantial benefits over existing treatments or if no drugs are currently available for these conditions.[21,22] This expedited review consists of several FDA programs such as fast-track review, priority review, and accelerated approval. Drug companies can request that these programs be considered for drugs that show promise in treating conditions such as cancer or AIDS.

The exact amount of time that is saved by expedited review and approval depends on which provisions are granted for each drug and how well the drug meets the terms of the acceleration process. Likewise, these expedited drugs may be made available for patient use even before formal clinical testing is completed.[23] However, the FDA will often require that the drug sponsor continue drug testing even after the drug is approved to ensure that it actually provides the therapeutic benefits that were initially promised.[24,25] The approval process can also be expedited if a drug has already received approval for treating one condition but is now being considered for use in other "supplemental" conditions.[5]

The process of drug testing and approval does seem to be fairly rigorous in its ability to screen out ineffective or potentially harmful drugs. Out of thousands of newly synthesized compounds that begin preclinical (animal) trials, only one will ever be released as a prescription drug for use in humans.[5]

Orphan Drugs

The FDA also makes provisions for the development, approval, and production of drugs that treat rare diseases.[26,27] These **orphan drugs** may be indicated for only the relatively small population with the disease—that is, fewer than 200,000 people in the United States. Research into the development of these drugs may be difficult, and the cost of developing these drugs may be prohibitive given the relatively small amount of people who will eventually use the drug.[26] Hence, the FDA takes into account the complexity of testing orphan drugs, and additional funding from various sources may be available for the development of these drugs.[26] Since 1983, the FDA has facilitated the approval and marketing of over 300 orphan drugs used to treat more than 80 rare diseases.[20,27]

Off-Label Prescribing

Off-label prescribing is the use of a drug to treat conditions other than those that the drug was originally approved to treat.[28,29] When the FDA approves a drug, the approval is only for treating the conditions that were indicated in the New Drug Application, the one or two conditions that were tested during phase II and III clinical trials. However, clinical observation and additional studies of the drug's effects occasionally determine that the drug may also be helpful in treating other conditions. For example, antiseizure drugs such as gabapentin (Neurontin) and antidepressants such as fluoxetine (Prozac) are often prescribed off-label for treating chronic pain. Practitioners have the ability to prescribe the drug for other conditions based on their judgment and evidence from additional research. Off-label prescribing is permitted because the FDA cannot dictate how physicians and other qualified clinicians prescribe medications if the clinician has justification that the drug could benefit a given patient.[5]

It is estimated that off-label prescribing constitutes a substantial portion of all drug prescriptions in the United States. But problems arise when insurance companies fail to recognize the use of a drug beyond the approved indications and might therefore refuse to reimburse the cost of the drug. Practitioners may also be subjected to more rigorous legal prosecution if a patient experiences serious adverse effects during off-label drug use. There has likewise been considerable debate about whether a drug company can market the drug for off-label applications or if drugs can only be advertised to treat conditions approved by the FDA.[30,31] Despite these problems, off-label prescribing commonly occurs in clinical practice, and reasonable use of drugs beyond their original indications can allow more extensive therapeutic applications to a wider group of patients.

Prescription Versus Over-the-Counter Medication

In the United States, pharmacotherapeutic agents are divided into drugs requiring a prescription for use and drugs available as nonprescription, or **over-the-counter (OTC) drugs.**[28] Nonprescription drugs can be purchased directly by the consumer, whereas prescription medications must be ordered or dispensed only by an authorized practitioner (i.e., physician, dentist, or other appropriate health-care provider). Prescription and nonprescription drug classification falls under the jurisdiction of the FDA.[32] In general, OTC medications are used to treat relatively minor problems and to make the consumer more comfortable until the condition is resolved. These medications have been judged to be safe for use by the consumer without direct medical supervision, and the chances of toxic effects are usually small when the medications are taken in the recommended amounts.[33] Of course, the patient may ingest more than the recommended amount, and in the case of an overdose, the danger always exists for potentially harmful effects, even if the drug is nonprescription in nature.[34,35]

The choice of OTC products in the health-care market has expanded dramatically in recent years.[36,37] Many drugs that were formerly available only by prescription are now available in a nonprescription form. Some common examples include ibuprofen (Advil, Motrin; see Chapter 15), loratadine (Claritin; see Chapter 26), and cimetidine (Tagamet; see Chapter 27). Transition of a prescription drug to an OTC product usually occurs when the drug's marketing company applies to the FDA and receives approval to develop and market it in a nonprescription form. FDA approval is based on the drug having an adequate safety profile, and the FDA may require other stipulations such as lowering the drug dosage in the OTC product.

The fact that more and more prescription drugs are now available in a nonprescription form offers some obvious benefits. The increased availability of OTC products can make it easier for consumers to gain access to these medications.[38] In addition, OTC products are typically less expensive than prescription drugs, and the purported savings might help contain overall medication costs. The actual cost to the patient, however, might be greater for an OTC product because the patient must pay directly out of pocket;[39] that is, health-care programs with prescription drug plans may cover the majority of a prescription drug's cost, whereas the patient often must pay directly for the entire cost of an OTC product. Hence the overall benefits of OTC products on health-care costs remains complex.[39]

Despite the potential benefits of OTC products, there are some obvious concerns about their increased use and emphasis on self-care that permeates today's health-care market. Consumers must realize that these products are important therapeutic medications and must be used appropriately.[38,40] There is also the chance that inappropriate OTC use can cause serious interactions with a patient's prescription medications, or they may lack adequate therapeutic effects and thus delay the use of more effective medications.[41,42] The impact of such OTC compounds is discussed in this text in the appropriate chapters.

It is clear that consumers need to be educated about the use of such medications and reminded that OTC products can produce substantial benefits and adverse effects.[43] All health-care providers, including physical therapists and occupational therapists, are in a position to help educate and counsel their patients about the benefits and drawbacks of such medications. While therapists should not directly prescribe or administer OTC products, therapists can provide information about the proper use and potential benefits of these medications.

Controlled Substances

In 1970, federal legislation was enacted to help control the abuse of legal and illegal drugs. The Comprehensive Drug Abuse Prevention and Control Act (or Controlled Substances Act) placed drugs into specific categories, or "schedules," according to their potential for abuse.[7] The schedules for controlled drugs can be found on the FDA website (www.fda.gov/regulatoryinformation/legislation/ucm148726.htm) and are briefly described here:

Schedule I. These drugs are regarded as having the highest potential for abuse and are not typically used as an acceptable medical treatment in the United States. Legal use of agents in this category is typically restricted to research studies by properly approved and registered researchers. Examples of schedule I drugs include heroin, lysergic acid diethylamide (LSD), psilocybin, mescaline, peyote, and several other hallucinogens.

Schedule II. Drugs in this category are approved for specific therapeutic purposes but still have a high potential for abuse and possible addiction. Examples include opioids, such as morphine and fentanyl, and drugs containing amphetamine derivatives.

Schedule III. Although these drugs have a lower abuse potential than those in schedules I and II, there is still the possibility of developing mild to moderate physical dependence, strong psychological dependence, or both. Drugs in schedule III include certain opioids (e.g., codeine) that are combined in a limited dosage with other nonopioid drugs. Other drugs in this category include anabolic steroids, certain barbiturates, and amphetamines that are not included in schedule II.

Schedule IV. These drugs supposedly have a lower potential for abuse than schedule III drugs, with only a limited possibility of physical dependence, psychological dependence, or both. Examples include certain antianxiety drugs (meprobamate), certain barbiturates (barbital, phenobarbital), and a variety of other depressants and stimulants.

Schedule V. These drugs have the lowest relative abuse potential. Drugs in this category consist primarily of low doses of opioids that are used in cough medications and antidiarrheal preparations.

Several other criteria relate to the different controlled substance schedules, such as restrictions on prescription renewal and penalties for illegal possession of drugs in different schedules. For a deeper discussion of **controlled substances**, the references at the end of this chapter include additional sources.[7]

BASIC CONCEPTS IN DRUG THERAPY

All drugs exert their beneficial effects by reaching some specific target cell or tissue. The drug in some way changes the function of the cell either to help restore normal physiological function or to prevent a disease process from occurring. In general, the dose of a drug must be large enough to allow an adequate concentration to reach the target site and produce a beneficial response. However, the administered dosage must not be so excessive that it produces toxicological effects. Some key aspects of the relationship between dose and response are discussed here.

Dose-Response Curves and Maximal Efficacy

A dose-response curve illustrates several important characteristics of a drug (Fig. 1-2). In particular, a **dose-response curve** provides information about the dosage range over which the drug is effective, as well as the peak response that can be expected from the drug. Typically, very low doses do not produce

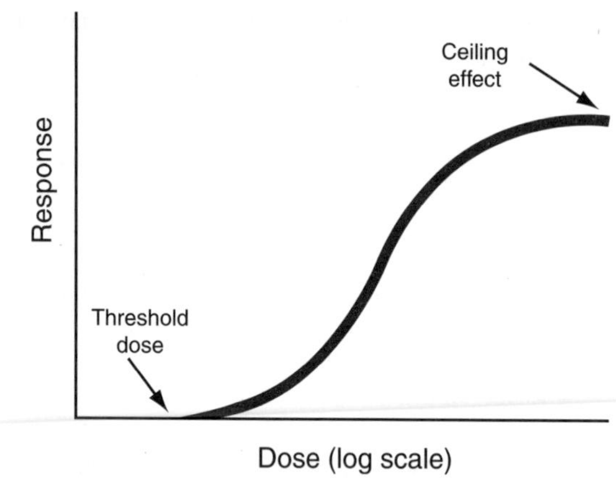

Figure ■ 1-2
Dose-response curve.

any observable effect. At some threshold dose, the response begins to occur and continues to increase in magnitude before reaching a plateau. The plateau indicates that there will be no further increment in the response, even if the dosage continues to be increased. The point at which there is no further increase in the response is known as the *ceiling effect*, or *maximal effect*, of the drug.[44]

In addition, the characteristic shape of the dose-response curve and the presence of the plateau associated with maximal efficacy can be used to indicate specific information about the binding of the drug to cellular receptors. The relevance of dose-response curves to drug-receptor interactions is discussed further in Chapter 4.

Potency

One criterion used frequently when comparing drugs is the concept of potency. **Potency** is related to the dose that produces a given response in a specific amplitude.[45] When two drugs are compared, the more potent drug requires a lower dose to produce the same effect as a higher dose of the second drug. For instance, in Figure 1-3, a dose of 10 mg of drug A would lower blood pressure by 25 percent, whereas 80 mg of drug B would be required to produce the same response. Consequently, drug A would be described as being more potent. It should be noted that potency is not synonymous with maximal efficacy. Drug B is clearly able to exert a greater maximal effect than drug A. Consequently, the term *potency* is often taken to be much more significant than it really is.[45] The potency of a drug is often misinterpreted by the layperson as an indication of the drug's overall therapeutic benefits, whereas potency really just means that less of the compound is required to produce a given response. In fact, neither potency nor maximal efficacy fully indicates a drug's therapeutic potential. Other factors, such as the therapeutic index (described

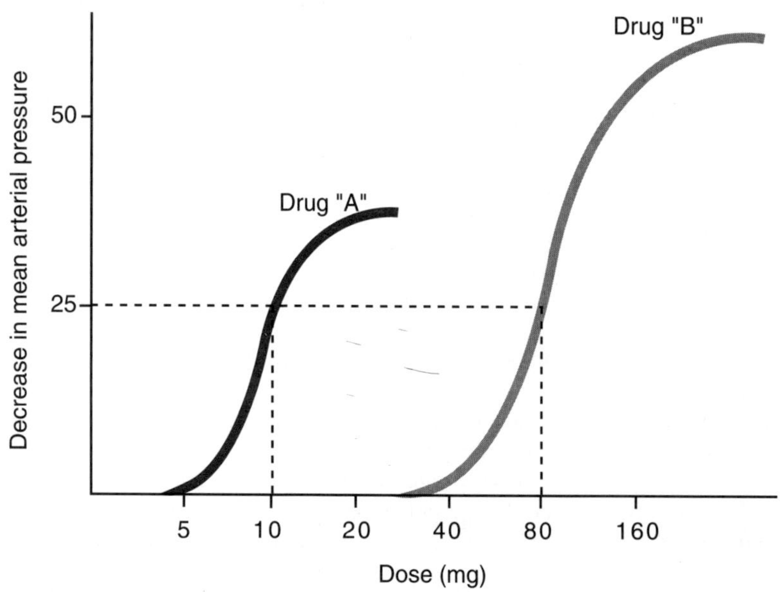

Figure ■ 1-3
Relative potency and maximal efficacy of two drugs. Drug A is more potent, and drug B has a greater maximal efficacy.

further on) and drug selectivity (see Chapter 4), are also important in comparing and ultimately choosing the best medication for a given problem.

ELEMENTS OF DRUG SAFETY

Drugs are often compared in terms of whether one drug is safer and less toxic than its counterparts. What follows is a brief description of the primary ways that the relative safety of a drug can be determined.

Quantal Dose-Response Curves and the Median Effective Dose

The dose-response curves shown in Figures 1-2 and 1-3 represent the graded response to a drug as it would occur in a single individual or in a homogeneous population. In reality, individual differences in the clinical population cause variations in drug responses that need to be considered when trying to assess whether a drug is safe as well as effective. Consequently, the relationship between the dose of the drug and the occurrence of a certain response is measured in a large group of people (or animals if the drug is being tested preclinically). When plotted, this relationship yields a cumulative, or quantal, dose-response curve (Fig. 1-4).[45] This curve differs from the dose-response curve discussed previously, as it is not the magnitude of the response that increases with a higher dosage but the percentage of the population that exhibits a specific response as the dosage is increased. The response is not graded; it is either present or it is absent in each member of the population. For example, a headache medication is administered in an increasing dosage to 1,000 people. At a certain dose, some of the individuals will respond to the drug and report the absence of their headache. As the dosage is increased, more and more individuals will experience pain relief because of the medication, until finally 100 percent of the population report that their headaches are gone. Again, it is the percentage of the population that responds in a specific way (e.g., reporting loss of their headaches) that is measured relative to the dose of the drug. An important reference point in this type of cumulative dose-response curve is the **median effective dose (ED_{50})**.[46] This is the dose at which 50 percent of the population responds to the drug in a specified manner.

Median Toxic Dose

In the aforementioned example, relief from pain was the desired response, which is often termed the *beneficial effect*. However, as dosages of the drug continue to be increased, adverse or toxic effects may become

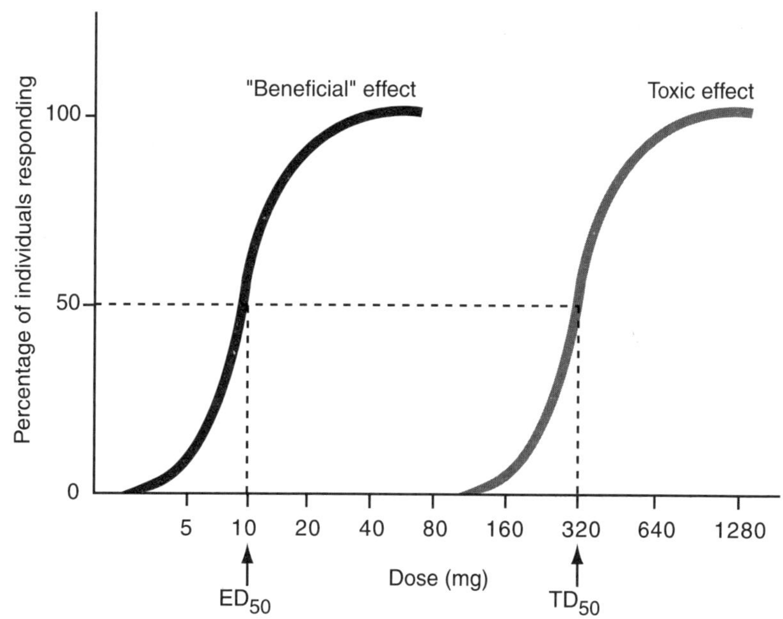

Figure ■ 1-4
Cumulative dose-response curve. The median effective dose (ED_{50}) is 10 mg, and the median toxic dose (TD_{50}) is 320 mg. The therapeutic index for this drug is 32.

apparent. To continue the earlier example, higher doses of the same medication may be associated with the appearance of a specific toxic effect, such as acute gastric hemorrhage. As the dosage is increased, more and more individuals will then begin to exhibit that particular adverse effect. The dose at which 50 percent of the group exhibits the adverse effect is termed the **median toxic dose (TD_{50})**. In animal studies, the toxic effect studied is often the death of the animal. In these cases, high doses of the drug are used to determine the **median lethal dose (LD_{50})**—the dose that causes death in 50 percent of the animals studied.[45] Of course, the LD_{50} is not a relevant term in clinical use of the drug in humans, but it does serve to provide some indication of the drug's safety in preclinical animal trials. The median effective and toxic doses are used to determine the therapeutic index (TI).[46]

Therapeutic Index

The **therapeutic index** is used as an indicator of the drug's safety.[45] The greater the value of the TI, the safer the drug is considered to be. In essence, a large TI indicates that it takes a much larger dose to evoke a toxic response than it does to cause a beneficial effect.

The TI is calculated as the ratio of the TD_{50} to the ED_{50}:

$$TI = TD_{50} \div ED_{50}$$

In animal studies in which the median lethal dose is known, the TI is often calculated using the LD_{50} in place of the TD_{50}.

It should be noted that the TI is a relative term. Acetaminophen, a nonprescription analgesic, has a TI of approximately 27 (i.e., the ratio of the median toxic dose to the median effective dose equals 27). Prescription agents tend to have lower TIs. For instance, the narcotic analgesic meperidine (Demerol) has a TI of 8, and the sedative-hypnotic diazepam (Valium) has a TI equal to 3. Other prescription agents such as cancer chemotherapeutics (methotrexate, vincristine, etc.) may have very low TIs, some close to 1. However, a low TI is often acceptable in these agents, considering the critical nature of cancer and similar serious conditions. The consequences of not using the drug outweigh the risks of some of the toxic effects.

To help keep the risk of toxicity to a minimum with low-TI drugs, it is generally advisable to periodically monitor blood levels. Monitoring helps prevent concentrations from quickly reaching toxic levels. This precaution is usually not necessary with high-TI drugs, because there is a greater margin of error (i.e., blood levels can rise quite a lot above the therapeutic concentration before becoming dangerous).

SUMMARY

In its broadest sense, pharmacology is the study of the effects of chemicals on living organisms. As addressed in this chapter, clinical pharmacology deals primarily with the beneficial effects of specific drugs on humans and the manner in which these drugs exert their therapeutic effects. Because all drugs have the potential to produce unwanted or toxic responses, we must also be aware that the drug's adverse effects will influence our patients and their responses to physical rehabilitation. This chapter also addressed the strategies used to name drugs and described the distinction between generic and trade (brand) names for a given drug. Furthermore, clinicians should know that drugs used therapeutically are subjected to extensive testing prior to approval for use in humans and that they are classified as either prescription or over-the-counter, depending on their dosage, effectiveness, and safety profile. Finally, this chapter described certain characteristic relationships between the dose of a drug and the response or effect it produces. Such relationships can provide useful information about drug efficacy and potency and about the relative safety of different compounds.

REFERENCES

1. *Taber's Cyclopedic Medical Dictionary*. 22nd ed. Philadelphia, PA: FA Davis; 2013.
2. Relling MV, Giacomini KM. Pharmacogenetics. In: Brunton LL, et al., eds. *The Pharmacological Basis of Therapeutics*. 12th ed. New York: McGraw Hill; 2011.
3. Steinman MA, Chren MM, Landefeld CS. What's in a name? Use of brand versus generic drug names in United States outpatient practice. *J Gen Intern Med*. 2007;22:645-648.
4. Wick JY. Why is it called that? Tongue-twisting taxonomy. *Consult Pharm*. 2011;26:544-552.
5. Rivera SM, Gilman AG. Drug invention and the pharmaceutical industry. In: Brunton LL, et al., eds. *The Pharmacological Basis of Therapeutics*. 12th ed. New York: McGraw Hill; 2011.
6. Emmerton LM, Rizk MF. Look-alike and sound-alike medicines: risks and "solutions." *Int J Clin Pharm*. 2012;34:4-8.
7. Buxton ILO. Principles of prescription order writing and patient compliance. In: Brunton LL, et al., eds. *The Pharmacological Basis of Therapeutics*. 12th ed. New York: McGraw Hill; 2011.

8. Hoffman JM, Proulx SM. Medication errors caused by confusion of drug names. *Drug Saf.* 2003;26:445-452.
9. Shrank WH, Choudhry NK, Liberman JN, Brennan TA. The use of generic drugs in prevention of chronic disease is far more cost-effective than thought, and may save money. *Health Aff.* 2011;30:1351-1357.
10. Davit BM, Nwakama PE, Buehler GJ, et al. Comparing generic and innovator drugs: a review of 12 years of bioequivalence data from the United States Food and Drug Administration. *Ann Pharmacother.* 2009;43:1583-1597.
11. Howland RH. Evaluating the bioavailability and bioequivalence of generic medications. *J Psychosoc Nurs Ment Health Serv.* 2010;48:13-16.
12. Howland RH. What makes a generic medication generic? *J Psychosoc Nurs Ment Health Serv.* 2009;47:17-20.
13. Tothfalusi L, Endrenyi L, Arieta AG. Evaluation of bioequivalence for highly variable drugs with scaled average bioequivalence. *Clin Pharmacokinet.* 2009;48:725-743.
14. Duh MS, Cahill KE, Paradis PE, Cremieux PY, Greenberg PE. The economic implications of generic substitution of antiepileptic drugs: a review of recent evidence. *Expert Opin Pharmacother.* 2009;10:2317-2328.
15. Wu EQ, Yu AP, Lauzon V, et al. Economic impact of therapeutic substitution of a brand selective serotonin reuptake inhibitor with an alternative generic selective serotonin reuptake inhibitor in patients with major depressive disorder. *Ann Pharmacother.* 2011;45:441-451.
16. Borchers AT, Hagie F, Keen CL, Gershwin ME. The history and contemporary challenges of the US Food and Drug Administration. *Clin Ther.* 2007;29:1-16.
17. Howland RH. How are drugs approved? Part 3. The stages of drug development. *J Psychosoc Nurs Ment Health Serv.* 2008;46:17-20.
18. Vlahović-Palčevski V, Mentzer D. Postmarketing surveillance. *Handb Exp Pharmacol.* 2011;205:339-351.
19. Woodcock J, Behrman RE, Dal Pan GJ. Role of postmarketing surveillance in contemporary medicine. *Annu Rev Med.* 2011; 62:1-10.
20. Katzung BG. Development and regulation of drugs. In: Katzung BG, ed. *Basic and Clinical Pharmacology.* 12th ed. New York: Lange Medical Books/McGraw Hill; 2012.
21. Cole P. Accelerating drug development and approval. *Drug News Perspect.* 2010;23:37-47.
22. Graul AI. Promoting, improving and accelerating the drug development and approval processes. *Drug News Perspect.* 2008; 21:36-43.
23. Richey EA, Lyons EA, Nebeker JR, et al. Accelerated approval of cancer drugs: improved access to therapeutic breakthroughs or early release of unsafe and ineffective drugs? *J Clin Oncol.* 2009;27:4398-4405.
24. Johnson JR, Ning YM, Farrell A, Justice R, Keegan P, Pazdur R. Accelerated approval of oncology products: the food and drug administration experience. *J Natl Cancer Inst.* 2011;103:636-644.
25. Meyer RJ. Regulatory considerations for determining post-marketing study commitments. *Clin Pharmacol Ther.* 2007;82: 228-230.
26. Pariser AR, Xu K, Milto J, Coté TR. Regulatory considerations for developing drugs for rare diseases: orphan designations and early phase clinical trials. *Discov Med.* 2011;11:367-375.
27. Thorat C, Xu K, Freeman SN, et al. What the Orphan Drug Act has done lately for children with rare diseases: a 10-year analysis. *Pediatrics.* 2012;129:516-521.
28. Lofholm PW, Katzung BG. Rational prescribing and prescription writing. In: Katzung BG, ed. *Basic and Clinical Pharmacology.* 12th ed. New York: Lange Medical Books/McGraw Hill; 2012.
29. Spector RA, Marquez E. "Off-label" prescribing, the Physician's Desk Reference and the court. *J La State Med Soc.* 2011; 163:276-280.
30. Gilhooley M. Commercial speech and off-label drug uses: what role for wide acceptance, general recognition and research incentives? *Am J Law Med.* 2011;37:258-277.
31. Greenwood K. The ban on "off-label" pharmaceutical promotion: constitutionally permissible prophylaxis against false or misleading commercial speech? *Am J Law Med.* 2011;37: 278-298.
32. Corelli RL. Therapeutic and toxic potential of over-the-counter agents. In: Katzung BG, ed. *Basic and Clinical Pharmacology.* 12th ed. New York: Lange Medical Books/McGraw Hill; 2012.
33. Rainsford KD. Ibuprofen: pharmacology, efficacy and safety. *Inflammopharmacology.* 2009;17:275-342.
34. Conca AJ, Worthen DR. Nonprescription drug abuse. *J Pharm Pract.* 2012;25:13-21.
35. Lavonas EJ, Fries JF, Furst DE, et al. Comparative risks of non-prescription analgesics: a structured topic review and research priorities. *Expert Opin Drug Saf.* 2012;11:33-44.
36. Bednar B. OTC medication-induced nephrotoxicity in the elderly and CKD patient. *Nephrol News Issues.* 2009;23:36, 38-40, 43-44.
37. Hemwall EL. Increasing access to nonprescription medicines: a global public health challenge and opportunity. *Clin Pharmacol Ther.* 2010;87:267-269.
38. Ruiz ME. Risks of self-medication practices. *Curr Drug Saf.* 2010;5:315-323.
39. Brass EP. Changing the status of drugs from prescription to over-the-counter availability. *N Engl J Med.* 2001;345: 810-816.
40. Colebatch AN, Marks JL, Edwards CJ. Safety of non-steroidal anti-inflammatory drugs, including aspirin and paracetamol (acetaminophen) in people receiving methotrexate for inflammatory arthritis (rheumatoid arthritis, ankylosing spondylitis, psoriatic arthritis, other spondyloarthritis). *Cochrane Database Syst Rev.* 2011;CD008872.
41. Hersh EV, Pinto A, Moore PA. Adverse drug interactions involving common prescription and over-the-counter analgesic agents. *Clin Ther.* 2007; 29(suppl):2477-2497.
42. Vassilev ZP, Kabadi S, Villa R. Safety and efficacy of over-the-counter cough and cold medicines for use in children. *Expert Opin Drug Saf.* 2010;9:233-242.
43. Brass EP, Lofstedt R, Renn O. Improving the decision-making process for nonprescription drugs: a framework for benefit-risk assessment. *Clin Pharmacol Ther.* 2011;90:791-803.
44. Holford NHG. Pharmacokinetics and pharmacodynamics: rational dosing and the time course of drug action. Katzung BG, ed. *Basic and Clinical Pharmacology.* 12th ed. New York: Lange Medical Books/McGraw Hill; 2012.
45. Blumenthal DK, Garrison JC. Pharmacodynamics: molecular mechanisms of drug action. In: Brunton LL, et al., eds. *The Pharmacological Basis of Therapeutics.* 12th ed. New York: McGraw Hill; 2011.
46. von Zastrow M. Drug receptors and pharmacodynamics. Katzung BG, ed. *Basic and Clinical Pharmacology.* 12th ed. New York: Lange Medical Books/McGraw Hill; 2012.

CHAPTER 2

Pharmacokinetics I: Drug Administration, Absorption, and Distribution

Pharmacokinetics is the study of how the body absorbs, distributes, and eventually eliminates pharmacological compounds. In other words, what does the body do with the drug? This area includes the manner in which the drug is administered.

An introduction to pharmacokinetic principles will help you understand why specific drugs are administered in certain ways. Why, for example, can some drugs be administered orally while others need to be administered by injection, inhalation, or other non-oral routes? Likewise, drugs must reach a specific organ or "target" tissue to exert therapeutic effects, and various pharmacokinetic variables must be taken into account to maximize the drug's ability to reach these tissues. Finally, it is critical to know how the body metabolizes and eliminates a drug so that you can be aware of problems that might arise if drug metabolism is altered by illness, disease, or other factors. This chapter will begin by considering various routes of administration. Other pharmacokinetic issues, such as drug absorption, distribution, and storage, will then be addressed. Drug metabolism will be covered in the next chapter.

ROUTES OF ADMINISTRATION

In general, drugs can be administered via two primary routes: the alimentary canal (**enteral administration**) or the nonalimentary routes (parenteral administration). Each route has several variations, and each offers distinct advantages and disadvantages. The key features of various routes are discussed here (see Table 2-1). For a more detailed description of the specific methodology involved in drug administration, the references at the end of this chapter include several excellent resources on this topic.[1-3]

Enteral

Oral

The most common method of enteral medication administration is through the oral route, which offers several distinct advantages. Oral administration is the easiest method for taking medications, especially when self-administration is necessary or desired. The oral route is also relatively safe because drugs enter the system in a fairly controlled manner. This avoids a large, sudden increase in plasma drug levels, which can occur when the drug is administered by other methods such as IV injection. Most medications that are administered orally are absorbed from the small intestine, thus utilizing the large surface area of the intestinal microvilli to enhance their entry into the body.

Several disadvantages may preclude drugs from being given orally. Drugs that are administered by mouth must have a relatively high degree of lipid solubility in order to pass through the gastrointestinal (GI) mucosa and into the bloodstream. Large, nonlipid-soluble compounds are absorbed very poorly from the alimentary canal and will eventually be lost through the feces. Absorption of some nonlipid-soluble substances

Table 2-1
ROUTES OF DRUG ADMINISTRATION

Route	Advantages	Disadvantages	Examples
Enteral			
Oral	Easy, safe, convenient	Limited or erratic absorption of some drugs; chance of first-pass inactivation in liver	Analgesics; sedative-hypnotics; many others
	Rapid onset; not subject to first-pass inactivation	Drug must be easily absorbed from oral mucosa	Nitroglycerin
Rectal	Alternative to oral route; local effect on rectal tissues	Poor or incomplete absorption; chance of rectal irritation	Laxatives; suppository forms of other drugs
Parenteral			
Inhalation	Rapid onset; direct application for respiratory disorders; large surface area for systemic absorption	Chance of tissue irritation; patient compliance sometimes a problem	General anesthetics; antiasthmatic agents
Injection	Provides more direct administration to target tissues; rapid onset	Chance of infection if sterility is not maintained	Insulin; antibiotics; anticancer drugs; narcotic analgesics
Topical	Local effects on surface of skin	Only effective in treating outer layers of skin	Antibiotic ointments; creams used to treat minor skin irritation and injury
Transdermal	Introduces drug into body without breaking the skin; can provide steady, prolonged delivery via medicated patch	Drug must be able to pass through dermal layers intact	Nitroglycerin; motion sickness medications; drugs used with phonophoresis and iontophoresis

(peptides, small proteins) can be enhanced to some extent by encapsulating these agents in lipid vesicles (liposomes) or biodegradable polymers. This encapsulating technique enables the oral administration of drugs that were formerly administered only through injection or some other parenteral route.[4,5]

Other drawbacks to the oral route include the fact that certain medications may irritate the stomach and cause discomfort, vomiting, or even damage to the gastric mucosa. The acidic environment and digestive proteases in the stomach may also degrade and destroy various compounds prior to absorption from the GI tract.[4]

Drugs that are given orally are subject to a phenomenon known as the **first-pass effect**.[1,6] After absorption from the alimentary canal, the drug is transported directly into the liver via the portal vein, where a significant amount of the drug may be metabolized and destroyed prior to reaching its site of action. The dosage of the orally administered drug must be sufficient enough to allow an adequate amount of the compound to survive hepatic degradation and to eventually reach the target tissue.[1] Some drugs—such as nitroglycerin—undergo such extensive inactivation from the first-pass effect that it is usually preferable to administer them through non-oral routes.[7]

A final limitation of the oral route is that the amount and rate at which the drug eventually reaches the bloodstream is somewhat less predictable compared with more direct routes, such as injection. Factors that affect intestinal absorption (e.g., intestinal infection, presence of food, rate of gastric emptying, and amount of visceral blood flow) can alter the usual manner in which the body absorbs a drug from the GI tract.[1,8,9]

Sublingual and Buccal

Sublingual drugs are administered by placing the drug under the tongue. **Buccal** administration is when the drug is placed between the cheek and gums. The drugs are absorbed transmucosally (through the oral mucosa) into the venous system that is draining the mouth region. These veins eventually carry blood to the superior vena cava, which in turn carries blood to the heart. Consequently, a drug administered sublingually or buccally can reach the systemic circulation without being subjected to first-pass inactivation in the liver.[10,11] This provides an obvious advantage for drugs such as nitroglycerin that would be destroyed in the liver when absorbed from the stomach or intestines.

Sublingual and buccal routes can also provide faster effects than swallowing the drug and may be preferred for treating conditions such as acute angina and other types of acute or "breakthrough" pain.[12,13] These routes also offer a means of enteral administration to people who have difficulty swallowing or to patients who cannot be given drugs rectally.[14] However, the amount of drug that can be administered through sublingual and buccal routes is somewhat limited, and the drug must be able to pass easily through the oral mucosa in order to reach the venous drainage of the mouth.[11]

Rectal

A final method of enteral administration is via the rectum using rectal suppositories. This method is less favorable because many drugs are absorbed poorly or incompletely, and irritation of the rectal mucosa may occur.[1] Rectal administration does offer the advantage of allowing drugs to be given to a patient who is unconscious or when vomiting prevents drugs from being taken orally. However, the rectal route is used most often for treating local conditions such as hemorrhoids.

Parenteral

All methods of drug administration that do not use the GI tract are termed **parenteral**. Parenteral administration generally delivers the drug to the target site more directly, and the quantity of the drug that actually reaches the target site is often more predictable.[1] Also, drugs given parenterally are not usually subject to first-pass inactivation in the liver. Other advantages and disadvantages of various parenteral routes are discussed later in this section.

Inhalation

Drugs that exist in a gaseous or volatile state or that can be suspended as tiny droplets in an aerosol form may be given via inhalation. Pulmonary administration is advantageous because of the large (alveolar) surface area for diffusion of the drug into the pulmonary circulation, and it is generally associated with rapid entry of the drug into the bloodstream.[1,15] Anesthesia providers use the pulmonary route extensively when administering volatile general anesthetics (e.g., halothane). It is also advantageous when applying medications directly to the bronchial and alveolar tissues for the treatment of specific pulmonary pathologies.[1] The pulmonary route has also been explored as a way to administer larger nonlipid-soluble agents such as peptides, small proteins (including insulin), and DNA.[16-18]

One limitation of inhalation is that the drug could irritate the alveoli or other areas of the respiratory tract. Also, some patients have trouble administering drugs by this route, and drug particles tend to be trapped by cilia and mucus in the respiratory tract. Both of these factors can limit the ability to predict exactly how much of the drug eventually reaches the lungs. Efforts continue to advance the use of inhaled drugs by improving the physicochemical properties of these drugs and the devices used to deliver them (i.e., inhalers).[19-21] Chapter 26 on respiratory medications covers the technological advancements in inhaled drugs in more detail.

Injection

Various types of injection can be used to introduce the drug either systemically or locally. If sterility is not maintained, all types of injection can cause infection, and certain types of injection are more difficult, if not impossible, for the patient to self-administer. Specific types of injection include IV, intra-arterial, subcutaneous, intramuscular, and intrathecal.

IV. The bolus injection of a medication into a peripheral vein allows an accurate, known quantity of the drug to be introduced into the bloodstream over a short period of time, frequently resulting in peak levels of the drug appearing almost instantaneously in the peripheral circulation and thus reaching the target site rapidly. This characteristic is advantageous in emergency situations when it is necessary for the medication to exert an immediate effect. Of course, adverse reactions may also occur because of the sudden appearance of large titers of the drug in the plasma. Any unexpected side effects or miscalculations in the amount of the administered drug are often difficult to handle after the full dose has been injected. In certain situations such as hospitals, an indwelling IV cannula (IV "line") can be used to allow the prolonged, steady infusion of a drug into the venous system. This method prevents large fluctuations in the plasma concentration of the drug and allows the dosage to be maintained at a specific level for as long as desired.

Intra-arterial. Injecting a drug directly into an artery is a difficult and dangerous procedure. This method permits a large dose of the medication to reach a given site, such as a specific organ, and may be used to focus the administration of drugs into certain tissues. Intra-arterial injections are used occasionally in chemotherapy to administer the anticancer drug directly to the tumor site with minimal exposure of the drug to healthy tissues. This route may also be used to focus the administration of other substances such as radiopaque dyes for various diagnostic procedures.

Subcutaneous (SC). Injecting medications directly beneath the skin is used when a local response is desired, such as in certain situations requiring local anesthesia. Also, an SC injection can permit a slower, more prolonged release of the medication into the systemic circulation. A primary example is insulin injection in a patient with diabetes mellitus. SC administration provides a relatively easy route of parenteral injection that patients can perform by themselves, providing they are properly trained.

The SC route can also be used when a drug needs to be slowly dispersed from the injection site and absorbed into the bloodstream for several weeks or months.[1] A common example of this is the use of hormonal contraceptive products (e.g., medroxyprogesterone; see Chapter 30).[22] Other methods of controlled or prolonged-release drug preparations are addressed in more detail later in this chapter.

On the other hand, SC injection can deliver only a small amount of drug. Furthermore, the injected drug must not irritate or inflame the SC tissues.

Intramuscular (IM). The large quantity of skeletal muscle in the body allows this route to be easily accessible for parenteral administration. IM injections are useful for treating a problem located directly in the injected muscle. For example, botulinum toxin and other substances can be injected directly into hyperexcitable muscles to control certain types of muscle spasms or spasticity (see Chapter 13).[23,24] Alternatively, IM injection can provide a relatively steady, prolonged release of the drug into the systemic circulation to control conditions such as psychosis[25] or to administer certain vaccines.[26]

IM injection provides a relatively rapid effect (i.e., within a few minutes) while avoiding the sudden, large increase in plasma levels seen with IV injection. The major problem with IM administration is that many drugs injected directly into a muscle cause significant amounts of local pain and prolonged soreness, which tends to limit the use of this route for repeated injections.

Intrathecal. Intrathecal injections deliver the medication within a sheath, such as the spinal subarachnoid space (i.e., the space between the arachnoid membrane and the pia mater that helps form the meninges surrounding the spinal cord). Injecting into the spinal subarachnoid space allows practitioners to apply such drugs as narcotic analgesics, local anesthetics, and antispasticity drugs directly to an area adjacent to the spinal cord, thereby allowing these drugs to gain better access to the cord.[27-29] Also, intrathecal injections allow certain drugs—for example, antibiotics and anticancer drugs—to bypass the blood-brain barrier and reach the central nervous system (CNS) (see Chapter 5).[1] Other intrathecal injections include administration of the drug within a tendon sheath or bursa, which may be used to treat a local condition such as inflammation within those structures.

Topical

Drugs given topically are applied to the surface of the skin or mucous membranes. Topical medications primarily help treat problems that exist on the skin itself, because most medications applied directly to the skin are absorbed fairly poorly through the epidermis and into the systemic circulation. Common examples of topical drugs include antibiotics to treat cutaneous infections, anti-inflammatory steroids to reduce skin inflammation, and various topical products to promote wound healing.[30-33] To treat various ophthalmological and otic problems, medications are often applied topically via eyedrops and eardrops, respectively.[34,35]

Topical application to mucous membranes is also often used to treat problems on the membrane itself.[36,37] However, significant amounts of the drug can be readily absorbed through the mucous membrane and into the bloodstream. Topical application of drugs to mucous membranes can therefore provide a fairly easy and convenient way to administer drugs systemically. Certain medications, for example, can be administered to the nasal mucosa via nasal spray[38,39] or to other mucous membranes to facilitate systemic absorption and treat disorders throughout the body.[1] Nonetheless, the potential for adverse systemic effects must also be considered if large amounts of topically administered drugs are absorbed inadvertently into the body.[37]

Transdermal

Unlike topical administration, transdermal application consists of applying drugs directly to the surface of the skin with the intent that they *will* be absorbed through the dermal layers and into either the subcutaneous tissues or the peripheral circulation. A transdermally administered drug must possess two basic properties: (1) It must be able to penetrate the skin, and (2) It must not be degraded to any major extent by drug-metabolizing enzymes located in the dermis.[40] Absorption may be enhanced by mixing the drug in an oily base or in some other chemical enhancer, thus increasing solubility and permeability through the dermis.[41,42]

Transdermal administration provides a slow, controlled release of the drug into the body that is effective in maintaining plasma levels of the drug at a relatively constant level for prolonged periods of time.[43] Drugs administered transdermally are often delivered through medicated "patches" adhered to the skin, much like a small adhesive bandage. This method allows the prolonged administration of drugs such as nitroglycerin and some motion-sickness medications such as scopolamine. Transdermal patches can also deliver other medications such as hormonal agents (estrogen, testosterone), local anesthetics (lidocaine), opioid analgesics (fentanyl),[44,45] and nicotine patches.[46] Researchers continue to explore the use of the transdermal route, and the use of transdermal patches has gained acceptance as a safe and effective method of administering many medications.

Iontophoresis and phonophoresis also use the transdermal route to administer drugs. In iontophoresis, an electric current "drives" the ionized form of the medication through the skin.[47,48] Phonophoresis (also known as *sonophoresis*) uses ultrasound waves to enhance transmission of the medication through the dermis.[48,49] Physical therapists often use phonophoresis and iontophoresis to treat pain and inflammation by transmitting specific medications to subcutaneous tissue such as a muscle, tendon, or bursa. The physical therapist follows a physician's prescription for an analgesic or anti-inflammatory and uses iontophoresis or phonophoresis techniques to enhance the movement of that medication through the skin. Specific medications that can be administered via iontophoresis or phonophoresis are listed in Appendix A. The references at the end of this chapter include several additional sources that provide a more detailed description of how these transdermal routes are employed.[47,50,51]

BIOAVAILABILITY AND DRUG ABSORPTION ACROSS THE CELL MEMBRANE

Although several routes exist for the administration of drugs, merely introducing the drug into the body does not ensure that the compound will reach all tissues uniformly or that the drug will even reach the appropriate target site. For instance, oral administration of a drug that affects the myocardium will not have any pharmacological effect unless the drug is absorbed from the GI tract into the bloodstream. The extent to which the drug reaches the systemic circulation is referred to as **bioavailability**, which is a parameter expressed as the percentage of the drug administered that reaches the bloodstream.[1] For instance, if 100 mg of a drug is given orally and 50 mg eventually make it into the systemic circulation, the drug is said to be 50 percent bioavailable. If 100 mg of the same compound were injected IV, the drug would be 100 percent bioavailable by that route.

Consequently, bioavailability depends on the route of administration and the drug's ability to cross membrane barriers. Once in the systemic circulation, further distribution into peripheral tissues may also be important in allowing the drug to reach the target site. Many drugs must eventually leave the systemic capillaries and enter other cells. Thus, drugs have to move across cell membranes and tissue barriers if they are to be distributed within the body. This section discusses the ability of these membranes to affect absorption and distribution of drugs.

Membrane Structure and Function

Biological membranes throughout the body act as barriers that permit some substances to pass freely, while others pass through with difficulty or not at all. This differential separation serves an obvious protective effect and limits the distribution of the substance within the body. In effect, the body is separated into various "compartments" by these membranes. In the case of pharmacotherapeutics, a drug often needs to cross one or more of these membrane barriers to reach the target site.

The ability of the membrane to act as a selective barrier is related to the membrane's normal structure and physiological function. The **cell membrane** is composed primarily of lipids and proteins. Membrane lipids are actually phospholipids, which are composed of a polar, hydrophilic "head" (containing a phosphate group) and a lipid, hydrophobic "tail" (Fig. 2-1). The phospholipids appear to be arranged in a bilayer, with the hydrophobic tails of the molecule oriented toward the membrane's center and the hydrophilic heads facing away from the center of the membrane. Interspersed throughout the lipid bilayer are membrane proteins, which can exist primarily in the outer or inner portion of the membrane or can span the entire width of the cell membrane (see Fig. 2-1).

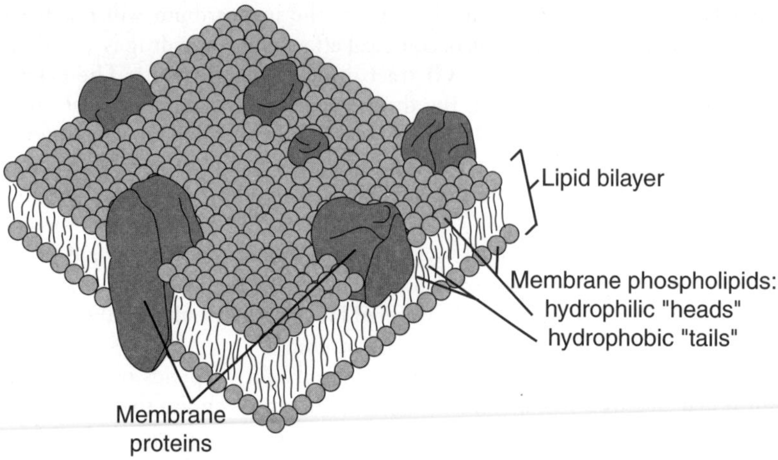

Figure ■ 2-1
Schematic diagram of the cell membrane.

Recent evidence also suggests that the distribution of phospholipids and proteins within the cell membrane is not random, and certain areas of the cell membrane are organized into special regions or "domains."[52,53] In particular, certain domains appear to consist primarily of lipids such as cholesterol and sphingolipids.[54,55] These lipid domains are often described as lipid "rafts" that move freely about the cell membrane and these lipid rafts appear to be important in controlling various cell functions, including cell signaling, endocytosis, and ion channel function.[53,54] Future research will help further define the role of the lipid rafts and other specific domains within the cell membrane and how these domains affect drug absorption and distribution.

The lipid bilayer that composes the basic structure of the cell membrane acts as a water barrier. The lipid portion of the membrane is essentially impermeable to water and other nonlipid-soluble substances (electrolytes, glucose). Lipid-soluble compounds (including most drugs) are able to pass directly through the membrane by dissolving in the lipid bilayer. Nonlipid-soluble substances, including water, can pass through from one side of the membrane to the other because of the presence of membrane pores.[56] Small holes or channels exist in the membrane, thereby allowing certain substances to pass from one side of the membrane to the other. These channels are typically formed by some of the membrane proteins that span the width of the membrane.[57] The ability of a substance to pass through a specific pore depends primarily on the size, shape, and electrical charge of the molecule. Also, in excitable membranes (nerve, muscle), some of these pores are dynamic in nature and can "open" and "close" to regulate the flow of ions, such as sodium, potassium, and chloride, in and out of the cell.[58-60] These dynamic ion channels are especially important in pharmacology because many drugs can affect their ability to open and close. By regulating the movement of ions across the cell membrane, the drugs can alter cell excitability.[60-62]

Movement Across Membrane Barriers

Drugs and other substances that pass through biological membranes usually do so via passive diffusion, active transport, facilitated diffusion, or a cytosis process such as endocytosis (Fig. 2-2). Each of these mechanisms is discussed here.

Passive Diffusion

Drugs and other substances will pass through a membrane by way of diffusion if two essential criteria are met. First, there must be some type of difference or "gradient" on one side of the membrane compared with the other. A concentration gradient, for example, occurs when the concentration of the substance differs on one side of the membrane compared to that on the other side. When this gradient occurs, the diffusing substance can move "downhill" from the area of high concentration to that of low concentration. In addition to a concentration difference, diffusion can also occur because of a pressure gradient or, in the case of charged particles, an electrical potential gradient. The rate of diffusion is dependent on several factors, including the magnitude of the gradient, the size of the diffusing substance, the distance over which diffusion occurs,

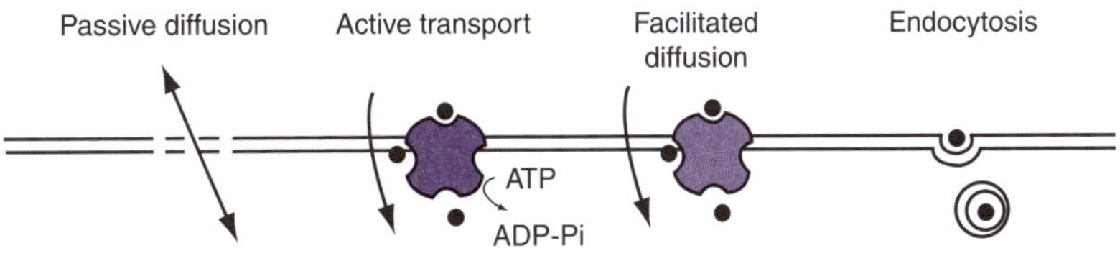

Figure ■ 2-2
A summary of drug movement across biological membranes. Energy is expended during active transport by hydrolyzing adenosine triphosphate (ATP) into adenosine diphosphate (ADP) and inorganic phosphate (Pi). The three other mechanisms do not require any net energy expenditure.

and the temperature at which diffusion occurs.[63] The term *passive diffusion* is often used to emphasize the fact that this movement occurs without expending any energy. The driving forces in passive diffusion are the electrical, chemical, and pressure differences on the two sides of the membrane.

The second essential factor for passive diffusion to occur is that the membrane must be permeable to the diffusing substance. As mentioned earlier, nonlipid-soluble compounds must diffuse through the membrane via specific pores. Some nonlipid-soluble drugs such as lithium are small enough to diffuse through these pores. Many drugs, however, are able to diffuse directly through the lipid bilayer because they are fairly lipid soluble. Passive lipid diffusion is nonselective, and a drug with a high degree of lipid solubility can gain access to many tissues. As indicated earlier, certain nonlipid-soluble substances—including some proteins—can be encapsulated in lipid vesicles, thereby enhancing their lipid solubility and increasing their ability to cross lipid membranes by passive diffusion

Effect of Ionization on Lipid Diffusion. Passive lipid diffusion of certain drugs is also dependent on whether the drug is ionized. Drugs will diffuse more readily through the lipid layer if they are in their neutral, nonionized form while ionization decreases their lipid solubility. Most drugs are weak acids or weak bases,[63] meaning they have the potential to become positively charged or negatively charged, depending on the pH of certain body fluids. In the plasma and in most other fluids, most drugs remain in their neutral, nonionized form because of the relatively neutral pH of these fluids. But in specific fluids, a drug may exist in an ionized state, and its absorption will be affected. For instance, when a weak acid drug is in an acidic environment (e.g., gastric secretions of the stomach), it tends to be in its neutral, nonionized form. The same drug will become positively charged if the pH of the solution increases and becomes more basic (e.g., the digestive fluids in the duodenum). For instance, aspirin is a weak acid and nonionized while it is in the stomach. The aspirin is absorbed fairly easily from the stomach because of its lipid solubility (Fig. 2-3). This same drug, on the other hand, will be poorly absorbed if it reaches the basic pH of the duodenum and becomes ionized. Conversely, a weak base drug is ionized in the acidic environment of the stomach and poorly absorbed, but when it reaches the duodenum, the same drug becomes nonionized and lipid soluble, allowing it to be absorbed from the proximal small intestine.

Diffusion Trapping. Changes in lipid solubility caused by ionization can also be important when the body attempts to excrete a drug in the urine. Here the

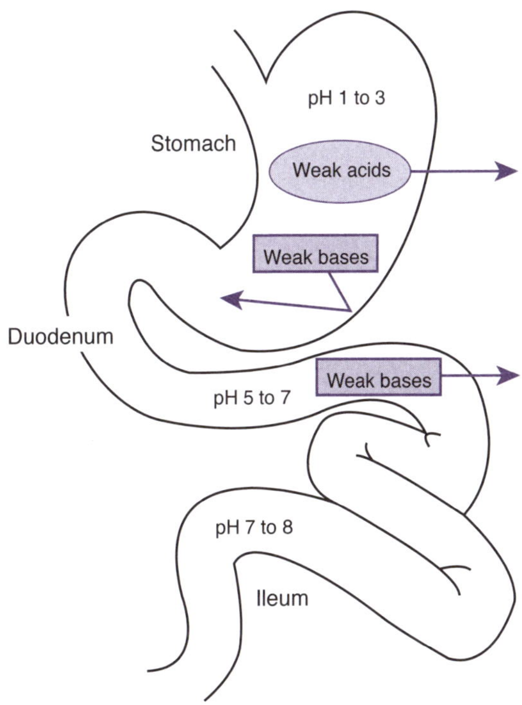

Figure ■ 2-3
Effect of pH and ionization on absorption of drugs from the GI tract. Weak acids and bases are absorbed from the stomach and duodenum, respectively, when they are in their neutral, nonionized form.

situation becomes slightly more complex because the urine can sometimes be acidic and at other times basic. In either situation, it is often desirable for the drug to remain ionized while in the urine so that the body will excrete the drug. If the drug becomes nonionized while in the nephron, it may be reabsorbed back into the body because of its increased lipid solubility. However, an ionized form of the drug is "trapped" in the nephron and eventually excreted in the urine.[63] Essentially, if the urine is basic, weak acids are trapped in the nephron and excreted more readily, but if the urine is acidic, weak bases are excreted better. The importance of the kidneys in excreting drugs from the body is discussed in Chapter 3.

Diffusion Between Cell Junctions. So far, the discussion has focused on the diffusion of drugs and other substances through individual cell membranes. Often, groups of cells join to form a barrier that separates one body compartment from another. In some locations, cells form "tight junctions" with each other and do not allow any appreciable space to exist between adjacent cells. In these cases, the primary way that a drug may diffuse across the barrier is by diffusing first into and then out of the other side of the cells comprising the barrier. Such locations include the epithelial lining of the GI tract and the capillary endothelium of the brain (one of the structures of the blood-brain barrier). In other tissues such as peripheral capillaries, there are relatively large gaps between adjacent cells. Here, large substances with molecular weights as high as 30,000 can cross the barrier by diffusing between adjacent cells.

Osmosis. This refers to when the diffusing substance is water. In this situation, water moves from an area where it is highly concentrated to an area of low concentration. Of course, permeability is still a factor when osmosis occurs across a membrane or tissue barrier. During osmosis, certain drugs may simply travel with the diffusing water, thus crossing the membrane by the process of "bulk flow." This is usually limited to osmosis through the gaps between adjacent cells because membrane pores are often too small to allow the passage of the drug molecule along with the diffusing water.

Active Transport

Active or carrier-mediated transport involves using membrane proteins to transport substances across the cell membrane (see Fig. 2-2). Membrane proteins that span the entire membrane may serve as some sort of carrier that shuttles substances from one side of the membrane to the other.[1] Characteristics of active transport include the following:

- *Carrier specificity.* The protein carrier exhibits some degree of specificity for certain substances, usually discriminating among different compounds according to their shape and electrical charge. This specificity is not absolute, and some compounds that resemble one another will be transported by the same group of carriers.
- *Expenditure of energy.* The term *active transport* implies that some energy must be used to fuel the carrier system. This energy is usually in the form of adenosine triphosphate (ATP) hydrolysis.
- *Ability to transport substances against a concentration gradient.* Carrier-mediated active transport carries substances "uphill"—that is, from areas of low concentration to areas of high concentration.

The role of active transport in moving drugs across cell membranes has some important implications. Essentially, the drug will be affected by one of the body's active transport systems if the drug resembles some endogenous substance that the transport system routinely carries. For example, drugs that resemble amino acids and small peptides can be absorbed from the GI tract via active transport proteins that normally absorb these substances into the body. Active transport systems in the kidneys, liver, brain, intestines, and placenta are likewise responsible for the movement of organic ions, peptides, and other substances across cell membranes, and these transport systems play an important role in the disposition of certain drugs within these tissues.[1,64,65] In some cases, transporters can increase a drug's effects by enhancing uptake into a specific tissue, whereas other transporters may remove drugs from the tissue, thereby reducing the drug's effects.[1]

Some drugs also may exert their effect by either facilitating or inhibiting endogenous transport systems that affect cellular homeostasis. For example, some of the drugs used to treat excess gastric acid secretion (e.g., **proton pump** inhibitors; see Chapter 27) inhibit the active transport of hydrogen ions into the stomach, thus reducing the formation of hydrochloric acid within the stomach.[66] Hence, medications can interact with the body's active transport systems in several ways, and researchers continue to develop new methods to enhance a drug's effects by using or modifying active transport pathways.

Facilitated Diffusion

Facilitated diffusion bears some features of both active transport and passive diffusion. An assisting protein carrier is present, but no net energy is expended in transporting the substance across the cell membrane during facilitated diffusion.[1] As a result, in most cases of facilitated diffusion, there is an inability to transport substances uphill against a concentration gradient. The entry of glucose into skeletal muscle cells via facilitated diffusion is probably the best example of this type of transport in the body.[67] As in active transport, the movement of drugs across membranes through facilitated diffusion is fairly infrequent, but certain medications may affect the rate at which endogenous facilitated diffusion occurs.

Endocytosis and Exocytosis

Certain cells can transport substances across their membranes through processes such as endocytosis. Here the drug is engulfed by the cell via an invagination of the cell membrane. Although limited in scope, this method does allow certain large, nonlipid-soluble drugs to enter the cell. Exocytosis is the opposite phenomenon, where substances synthesized within the cell can be encapsulated in vesicles, merged with the inner surface of the cell membrane, and extruded through the membrane and out of the cell. Drugs are not usually transported out of cells by exocytosis, and exocytosis is typically used to release endogenously produced products (proteins, neurotransmitters) from the cell.

DISTRIBUTION OF DRUGS WITHIN THE BODY

It is often necessary to know how and where a drug is distributed within the body. Why, for example, are some drugs distributed evenly throughout all the body tissues, while other drugs are concentrated in a specific compartment such as the plasma or in a specific tissue or organ? The next section addresses the primary factors that affect drug distribution, and the subsequent section describes volume of distribution, which is a calculation often used to assess where a drug is distributed within the body.

Factors Affecting Distribution

Following administration, the extent to which a drug is uniformly distributed throughout the body or sequestered in a specific body compartment depends on several factors:

Tissue permeability. A drug's ability to pass through membranes radically affects the extent to which it moves around within the body. A highly lipid-soluble drug can potentially reach all of the different body compartments and enter virtually every cell it reaches.[68] A large nonlipid-soluble compound will remain primarily in the compartment or tissue to which it is administered. Also, certain tissues such as the brain capillary endothelium have special characteristics that limit the passage of drugs. This blood-brain barrier limits the movement of drugs out of the bloodstream and into the CNS tissue.

Blood flow. If a drug is circulating in the bloodstream, it will gain greater access to highly perfused tissues. More of the drug will reach organs that receive a great deal of blood flow—such as the brain, kidneys, and exercising skeletal muscle—than will other, less active tissues such as adipose stores.[1] Similarly, diseases that reduce blood flow to specific tissues and organs will result in less drug being delivered to those tissues.[8]

Binding to plasma proteins. Certain drugs will form reversible bonds to circulating proteins in the bloodstream such as albumin.[1] This fact is significant because only the unbound or "free" drug can reach the target tissue and exert a pharmacological effect. Basically, the fraction of the drug that remains bound to the circulating proteins is sequestered within the vascular system and is not available for therapeutic purposes in other tissues and organs.

Binding to subcellular components. Similar to plasma protein binding, drugs that are bound within specific cells cannot be distributed throughout other fluid compartments. Several drugs, for instance, bind to subcellular organelles such as the lysosome, thus trapping the drug within the cell. Examples of this type of subcellular binding include certain antidepressants, antipsychotics, and other drugs with a relatively high pH that are attracted by the acidic environment found inside the lysosome.[69]

Volume of Distribution

The distribution of a given drug within the body is often described by calculating its **volume of distribution (V_d)**.[70] V_d is the ratio of the amount of drug administered to the concentration of drug in the plasma:

$$V_d = \text{amount of drug administered} \div \text{concentration of drug in plasma.}$$

V_d is used to estimate a drug's distribution by comparing the calculated V_d with the total amount of body water in a healthy person. A healthy 70-kg man has a total body fluid content of approximately 42 L (5.5 L blood, 12 L extracellular fluid, 24.5 L intracellular fluid). If the calculated V_d of a drug is approximately equal to the total amount of body water, then the drug is distributed uniformly throughout all of the body's fluids. If the drug's V_d is far less than 42 L, then the drug is retained in the bloodstream due to factors such as plasma protein binding. A V_d much greater than 42 L indicates that the drug is being concentrated in the tissues. It should be noted that V_d is not a real value—that is, it does not indicate the actual amount of fluid in the body but is merely an arbitrary figure that reflects the apparent distribution of a drug using total body water as a reference point. Table 2-2 gives some examples of calculating the V_d for three different types of drugs.

DRUG STORAGE

Most drugs are meant to enter a specific tissue or organ, exert their therapeutic effects, and then be removed by various metabolic processes (see the next chapter). Sometimes, however, drugs are stored temporarily in various tissues, which can have adverse effects on those tissues. Potential sites for drug storage and the possible adverse effects on these tissues are addressed in the next two sections.

Storage Sites

Following administration and absorption, many drugs are stored to some extent at certain locations in the body;[1] that is, prior to drug elimination, the drug may be sequestered in its active form in a relatively inert tissue that may be different from the target site. Some storage sites include the following:

Adipose. The primary site for drug storage in the body is adipose tissue. Because many drugs are lipid soluble, fat deposits throughout the body can serve as a considerable reservoir for these compounds. In some individuals, the amount of fat in the body can reach as high as 40 to 50 percent of body weight, thus creating an extensive storage compartment. Once drugs have been stored in adipose tissue, they tend to remain there for long periods of time because of the low metabolic rate and poor blood perfusion of these tissues. Examples of drugs that tend to be stored in fat include highly lipid-soluble anesthetics such as the barbiturates (thiopental) and inhalation anesthetics (halothane).

Bone. Bone acts as a storage site for several toxic agents, especially heavy metals like lead. Also, drugs such as the tetracyclines, which bind to and form molecular complexes with the crystal components in the skeletal matrix, are stored within bone.

Muscle. Binding of drugs to components within the muscle may lead to the long-term storage of these compounds. It is possible for various agents,

Table 2-2
EXAMPLES OF VOLUME OF DISTRIBUTION

Drug	Amount Administered	Plasma Concentration	Volume of Distribution	Indication	Examples
A	420 mg	0.01 mg/mL	420 mg ÷ 0.01 mg/mL = 42,000 mL = 42 L	Uniform distribution	Erythromycin; lithium
B	420 mg	0.05 mg/mL	420 mg ÷ 0.05 mg/mL = 8,400 mL = 8.4 L	Retained in plasma	Aspirin; valproic acid
C	420 mg	0.001 mg/mL	420 mg ÷ 0.001 mg/mL = 420,000 mL = 420 L	Sequestered in tissues	Morphine; quinidine

actively transported into the muscle cell, to form reversible bonds to intracellular structures such as proteins, nucleoproteins, or phospholipids. An example is the antimalarial drug quinacrine.

Organs. Drugs are often stored within certain organs such as the liver and kidneys. As in muscle cells, the drug enters the organ cells passively or by active transport and then forms bonds to subcellular components; examples include antimicrobial aminoglycoside agents (e.g., gentamicin and streptomycin), which accumulate in renal proximal tubular cells.

Adverse Consequences of Drug Storage

High concentrations of drugs, drug metabolites, and toxic compounds stored within tissues can cause local damage to these tissues. This is particularly true for toxic compounds that are incorporated and stored in the matrix of bone or that are highly concentrated within specific organs. Lead poisoning, for example, causes several well-known and potentially devastating effects when this metal accumulates in the CNS, bone, GI tract, and several other tissues.

Exposing various organs to high concentrations of therapeutic drugs can also result in a myriad of problems. For instance, acetaminophen is normally metabolized in the liver to form several highly reactive by-products or metabolites (see Chapter 15). When normal doses of acetaminophen are metabolized in a reasonably healthy liver, these metabolites are rapidly inactivated in the liver and subsequently excreted by the kidneys. However, very high doses of acetaminophen form excessive amounts of a toxic metabolite that can react with hepatic proteins and cause severe liver damage.[71] Hence, organs such as the liver and the kidneys are often subjected to local damage when these organs must deal with high concentrations of therapeutic and toxic agents.

Another problem with drug storage occurs when a reservoir "soaks up" the drug and prevents it from reaching the target site. For instance, a highly lipid-soluble drug such as a general anesthetic must be administered at a sufficient dose to ensure that there will be enough drug available to reach the CNS, despite the tendency for much of the drug to be sequestered in the body's fat stores.

Storage sites may also be responsible for the redistribution of drugs. The drug can leak out of the reservoir after plasma levels of the drug have begun to diminish. In this way, the storage site reintroduces the drug to the target site long after the original dose should have been eliminated. This redistribution may explain why certain individuals experience prolonged effects of the drug or extended adverse side effects.

NEWER TECHNIQUES FOR DRUG DELIVERY

Basic and clinical pharmacologists are always looking for better ways to administer medications and provide optimal therapeutic effects. Innovative techniques such as controlled-release preparations, implanted drugs, and targeted drug delivery can enhance drug delivery to specific tissues and possibly result in better drug effects with fewer side effects.

Controlled-Release Preparations

Controlled-release preparations, also known as *timed-release*, *sustained-release*, *extended-release*, or *prolonged-action preparations*, are generally designed to permit a slower and more prolonged absorption of the drug from the GI tract and other routes of administration.[72,73] This technique offers several advantages, such as decreasing the number of doses needed each day, preventing large fluctuations in the amount of drug appearing in the plasma, and sustaining plasma levels throughout the night.[73,74] This type of preparation is used with many types of drugs, including cardiovascular medications (beta blockers, calcium channel blockers),[75,76] narcotic analgesics such as morphine and hydromorphone,[77,78] and anti-parkinsonism medications that contain L-dopa.[79,80]

Implanted Drug Delivery Systems

The surgically implanted drug "reservoir" is a small container placed under the skin in the abdomen. The container releases a small, measured dose of a drug on a preprogrammed schedule.[1] Alternatively, the reservoir can be controlled electronically from outside of the body through the use of small, remote-controlled devices, thus allowing the patient to regulate release of the drug as needed. In some cases, the drug reservoir may be connected by a small cannula to a specific body compartment—such as the subarachnoid space or epidural space—so that the drug can be delivered directly into that space. This type of system can be very helpful in applying drugs such as analgesics, anesthetics, and muscle relaxants into the area around the spinal cord.[28,29,81]

Another type of implantable system incorporates the drug into a biodegradable or nonbiodegradable substance such as a polymer matrix or gel.[82-84] The drug-polymer complex is then implanted in the body and the drug is slowly released into surrounding tissues (nonbiodegradable), or it is released as the matrix gradually dissolves (biodegradable). This type of system was used in the past with only limited success to deliver contraceptive hormones such as progesterone (Norplant; see Chapter 30). Nonetheless, these implants have been used on an experimental basis to deliver other medications, such as local anesthetics, insulin, and vaccines.[83]

Improvements in the technology of this drug delivery will hopefully permit increased clinical applications of these systems in the near future. The use of implantable drug delivery systems with specific types of medications will be discussed in more detail when these medications are addressed in subsequent chapters.

Targeting Drug Delivery to Specific Cells and Tissues

Several innovative strategies can target specific drugs to specific tissues, thereby focusing the drug's effects and reducing its side effects. For instance, researchers can synthesize specific types of antibodies (monoclonal antibodies) and attach them to drugs such as the cytotoxic agents often used in cancer chemotherapy.[85,86] The antibodies are attracted to antigens located on the surface of the tumor cells and thereby carry the anticancer drugs directly to these cells. This strategy offers the distinct advantage of focusing the drug more directly on the cancerous cells rather than on healthy tissues.

Drug manufacturers can also use various techniques to modify a drug so that it is activated only after it reaches a specific organ or tissue. A compound might, for instance, be administered in an inactive form or "prodrug," with the intent of converting it to the active form of the drug by specific enzymes or other biochemical properties within the target tissue.[87,88] An example is the use of a prodrug to treat colon problems; it is administered orally but does not become activated until it reaches the colon.[89,90]

Finally, new advances in nanotechnology may prove useful for drug delivery.[91] Nanotechnology involves the use of very small particles (i.e., particles between 1 and 1,000 nanometers) with physical properties that facilitate drug absorption or distribution within the body.[92] Some examples of nanoparticles include biological substances such as viruslike components and lipid vesicles (liposomes)[93-95] or nonbiological particles such as polymers and small metal structures.[96] These nanoparticles may be able to enhance drug movement across specific membranes. Nanoparticles could, for example, allow drugs that do not ordinarily cross the blood-brain barrier to reach the brain and thus treat CNS disorders.[95] Likewise, researchers are investigating nanotechnology as a way to facilitate absorption of insulin and other proteins from the GI tract.[97,98]

In addition, nanoparticles could help direct the drug to a specific type of cell. For instance, nanotechnology could help target cancer chemotherapy drugs to only the cancerous cells, thereby reducing the drug's toxic effects on healthy cells.[99,100] It may also be possible to activate the nanoparticle after it reaches certain tissues[92,93]or even target the drug to specific subcellular organelles such as the mitochondria.[101,102] Clearly, there are many potential benefits for using nanotechnology to enhance drug delivery, and these benefits will continue to be realized as researchers further explore this technology.

SUMMARY

In order for any drug to be effective, it must be able to reach specific target tissues. The goal of drug administration is to deliver the drug in the least complicated manner while still allowing sufficient concentrations of the active form of the drug to arrive at the desired site. Each route of administration has certain advantages and disadvantages that will determine how much and how fast the drug is delivered to specific tissues. The distribution of the drug within the body must also be taken into account. Simply introducing the drug into certain body fluids such as the bloodstream does not ensure its entry into the desired tissues. Factors such as tissue permeability and protein binding may influence how the drug is dispersed within the various fluid compartments in the body. Some drugs also have a tendency to be stored in certain tissues for prolonged periods of time. This storage may produce serious toxic effects if high concentrations of the compound damage the cells in which it is stored. Finally, controlled-release preparations and implantable delivery systems can provide a more sustained and predictable administration of certain drugs, and various technological advancements may help deliver the drug specifically to the tissues where the drug exerts its primary therapeutic effects.

REFERENCES

1. Buxton ILO, Benet LZ. Pharmacokinetics: the dynamics of drug absorption, distribution, metabolism, and elimination. In: Brunton LL, et al., eds. *The Pharmacological Basis of Therapeutics*. 12th ed. New York: McGraw Hill; 2011.
2. Kee J, Hayes E, McCuistion L. *Pharmacology: A Nursing Process Approach*. 7th ed. New York: Elsevier Saunders; 2012.
3. Woo TM, Wynne AL. *Pharmacotherapeutics for Nurse Practitioner Prescribers*. 3rd ed. Philadelphia, PA: FA Davis; 2012.
4. Singh R, Singh S, Lillard JW Jr. Past, present, and future technologies for oral delivery of therapeutic proteins. *J Pharm Sci*. 2008;97:2497-2523.
5. Slomkowski S, Gosecki M. Progress in nanoparticulate systems for peptide, proteins and nucleic acid drug delivery. *Curr Pharm Biotechnol*. 2011;12:1823-1839.
6. Mathias NR, Hussain MA. Non-invasive systemic drug delivery: developability considerations for alternate routes of administration. *J Pharm Sci*. 2010;99:1-20.
7. Katzung BG. Vasodilators and the treatment of angina pectoris. In: Katzung BG, ed. *Basic and Clinical Pharmacology*. 12th ed. New York: Lange Medical Books/McGraw Hill; 2012.
8. Smith BS, Yogaratnam D, Levasseur-Franklin KE, et al. Introduction to drug pharmacokinetics in the critically ill patient. *Chest*. 2012;141:1327-1336.
9. Yasuji T, Kondo H, Sako K. The effect of food on the oral bioavailability of drugs: a review of current developments and pharmaceutical technologies for pharmacokinetic control. *Ther Deliv*. 2012;3:81-90.
10. Goswami T, Jasti B, Li X. Sublingual drug delivery. *Crit Rev Ther Drug Carrier Syst*. 2008;25:449-484.
11. Sohi H, Ahuja A, Ahmad FJ, Khar RK. Critical evaluation of permeation enhancers for oral mucosal drug delivery. *Drug Dev Ind Pharm*. 2010;36:254-282.
12. Mercadante S. Pharmacotherapy for breakthrough cancer pain. *Drugs*. 2012;72:181-190.
13. Paech MJ, Bloor M, Schug SA. New formulations of fentanyl for acute pain management. *Drugs Today*. 2012;48:119-132.
14. Stubbs J, Haw C, Dickens G. Dose form modification—a common but potentially hazardous practice. A literature review and study of medication administration to older psychiatric inpatients. *Int Psychogeriatr*. 2008;20:616-627.
15. Noymer P, Biondi S, Myers D, Cassella J. Pulmonary delivery of therapeutic compounds for treating CNS disorders. *Ther Deliv*. 2011;2:1125-1140.
16. Hohenegger M. Novel and current treatment concepts using pulmonary drug delivery. *Curr Pharm Des*. 2010;16:2484-2492.
17. Patton JS, Brain JD, Davies LA, et al. The particle has landed—characterizing the fate of inhaled pharmaceuticals. *J Aerosol Med Pulm Drug Deliv*. 2010;23(suppl 2):S71-S87.
18. Zarogoulidis P, Papanas N, Kouliatsis G, et al. Inhaled insulin: too soon to be forgotten? *J Aerosol Med Pulm Drug Deliv*. 2011;24:213-223.
19. Donovan MJ, Gibbons A, Herpin MJ, et al. Novel dry powder inhaler particle-dispersion systems. *Ther Deliv*. 2011;2:1295-1311.
20. Islam N, Cleary MJ. Developing an efficient and reliable dry powder inhaler for pulmonary drug delivery—a review for multidisciplinary researchers. *Med Eng Phys*. 2012;34:409-427.
21. Kaur G, Narang RK, Rath G, Goyal AK. Advances in pulmonary delivery of nanoparticles. *Artif Cells Blood Substit Immobil Biotechnol*. 2012;40:75-96.
22. Benagiano G, Gabelnick H, Farris M. Contraceptive devices: subcutaneous delivery systems. *Expert Rev Med Devices*. 2008;5:623-637.
23. Lim EC, Quek AM, Seet RC. Accurate targeting of botulinum toxin injections: how to and why. *Parkinsonism Relat Disord*. 2011;17(suppl 1):S34-39.
24. Olvey EL, Armstrong EP, Grizzle AJ. Contemporary pharmacologic treatments for spasticity of the upper limb after stroke: a systematic review. *Clin Ther*. 2010;32:2282-2303.
25. Sanford M, Scott LJ. Intramuscular aripiprazole: a review of its use in the management of agitation in schizophrenia and bipolar I disorder. *CNS Drugs*. 2008;22:335-352.
26. Petousis-Harris H. Vaccine injection technique and reactogenicity—evidence for practice. *Vaccine*. 2008;26:6299-6304.
27. Hayek SM, Deer TR, Pope JE, et al. Intrathecal therapy for cancer and non-cancer pain. *Pain Physician*. 2011;14:219-248.
28. Francisco GE, Saulino MF, Yablon SA, Turner M. Intrathecal baclofen therapy: an update. *PM R*. 2009;1:852-858.
29. Moore JM. Continuous spinal anesthesia. *Am J Ther*. 2009;16:289-294.
30. Castela E, Archier E, Devaux S, et al. Topical corticosteroids in plaque psoriasis: a systematic review of efficacy and treatment modalities. *J Eur Acad Dermatol Venereol*. 2012;26(suppl 3):36-46.
31. Drucker CR. Update on topical antibiotics in dermatology. *Dermatol Ther*. 2012;25:6-11.
32. Hsu AR, Hsu JW. Topical review: skin infections in the foot and ankle patient. *Foot Ankle Int*. 2012;33:612-619.
33. Papanas N, Eleftheriadou I, Tentolouris N, Maltezos E. Advances in the topical treatment of diabetic foot ulcers. *Curr Diabetes Rev*. 2012;8:209-218.
34. Rawas-Qalaji M, Williams CA. Advances in ocular drug delivery. *Curr Eye Res*. 2012;37:345-356.
35. Wall GM, Stroman DW, Roland PS, Dohar J. Ciprofloxacin 0.3%/dexamethasone 0.1% sterile otic suspension for the topical treatment of ear infections: a review of the literature. *Pediatr Infect Dis J*. 2009;28:141-144.
36. Sankar V, Hearnden V, Hull K, et al. Local drug delivery for oral mucosal diseases: challenges and opportunities. *Oral Dis*. 2011;17(suppl 1):73-84.
37. Sastre J, Mosges R. Local and systemic safety of intranasal corticosteroids. *J Investig Allergol Clin Immunol*. 2012;22:1-12.
38. Veldhorst-Janssen NM, Fiddelers AA, van der Kuy PH, et al. A review of the clinical pharmacokinetics of opioids, benzodiazepines, and antimigraine drugs delivered intranasally. *Clin Ther*. 2009;31:2954-2987.
39. Wong JP, Christopher ME, Viswanathan S, et al. Aerosol and nasal delivery of vaccines and antiviral drugs against seasonal and pandemic influenza. *Expert Rev Respir Med*. 2010;4:171-177.

40. Paudel KS, Milewski M, Swadley CL, et al. Challenges and opportunities in dermal/transdermal delivery. *Ther Deliv.* 2010;1:109-131.
41. Aungst BJ. Absorption enhancers: applications and advances. *AAPS J.* 2012;14:10-18.
42. Subedi RK, Oh SY, Chun MK, Choi HK. Recent advances in transdermal drug delivery. *Arch Pharm Res.* 2010;33:339-351.
43. Wohlrab J, Kreft B, Tamke B. Skin tolerability of transdermal patches. *Expert Opin Drug Deliv.* 2011;8:939-948.
44. Cachia E, Ahmedzai SH. Transdermal opioids for cancer pain. *Curr Opin Support Palliat Care.* 2011;5:15-19.
45. Studd J. Treatment of premenstrual disorders by suppression of ovulation by transdermal estrogens. *Menopause Int.* 2012;18: 65-67.
46. Shiffman S, Sweeney CT, Ferguson SG, et al. Relationship between adherence to daily nicotine patch use and treatment efficacy: secondary analysis of a 10-week randomized, double-blind, placebo-controlled clinical trial simulating over-the-counter use in adult smokers. *Clin Ther.* 2008;30:1852-1858.
47. Ciccone CD. Electrical stimulation for delivery of medications: iontophoresis. In: Robinson AJ, Snyder-Mackler L, eds. *Clinical Electrophysiology: Electrotherapy and Electrophysiologic Testing.* 3rd ed. Baltimore, MD: Lippincott, Williams & Wilkins; 2007.
48. Herwadkar A, Banga AK. An update on the application of physical technologies to enhance intradermal and transdermal drug delivery. *Ther Deliv.* 2012;3:339-355.
49. Polat BE, Hart D, Langer R, Blankschtein D. Ultrasound-mediated transdermal drug delivery: mechanisms, scope, and emerging trends. *J Control Release.* 2011;152:330-348.
50. Dhote V, Bhatnagar P, Mishra PK, et al. Iontophoresis: a potential emergence of a transdermal drug delivery system. *Sci Pharm.* 2012;80:1-28.
51. Rao R, Nanda S. Sonophoresis: recent advancements and future trends. *J Pharm Pharmacol.* 2009;61:689-705.
52. Cornely R, Rentero C, Enrich C, et al. Annexin A6 is an organizer of membrane microdomains to regulate receptor localization and signalling. *IUBMB Life.* 2011;63:1009-1017.
53. Kusumi A, Fujiwara TK, Morone N, et al. Membrane mechanisms for signal transduction: the coupling of the meso-scale raft domains to membrane-skeleton-induced compartments and dynamic protein complexes. *Semin Cell Dev Biol.* 2012;23: 126-144.
54. Lingwood D, Simons K. Lipid rafts as a membrane-organizing principle. *Science.* 2010;327:46-50.
55. Simons K, Sampaio JL. Membrane organization and lipid rafts. *Cold Spring Harb Perspect Biol.* 2011;3:a004697.
56. Törnroth-Horsefield S, Hedfalk K, Fischer G, et al. Structural insights into eukaryotic aquaporin regulation. *FEBS Lett.* 2010;584:2580-2588.
57. Fuertes G, Giménez D, Esteban-Martin S, et al. Role of membrane lipids for the activity of pore forming peptides and proteins. *Adv Exp Med Biol.* 2010;677:31-55.
58. French RJ, Zamponi GW. Voltage-gated sodium and calcium channels in nerve, muscle, and heart. *IEEE Trans Nanobioscience.* 2005;4:58-69.
59. Goldfarb M. Voltage-gated sodium channel-associated proteins and alternative mechanisms of inactivation and block. *Cell Mol Life Sci.* 2012;69:1067-1076.
60. Judge SI, Smith PJ, Stewart PE, Bever CT Jr. Potassium channel blockers and openers as CNS neurologic therapeutic agents. *Recent Pat CNS Drug Discov.* 2007;2:200-228.
61. Arcangeli A, Pillozzi S, Becchetti A. Targeting ion channels in leukemias: a new challenge for treatment. *Curr Med Chem.* 2012;19:683-696.
62. Pexton T, Moeller-Bertram T, Schilling JM, Wallace MS. Targeting voltage-gated calcium channels for the treatment of neuropathic pain: a review of drug development. *Expert Opin Investig Drugs.* 2011;20:1277-1284.
63. Katzung BG. Introduction. In: Katzung BG, ed. *Basic and Clinical Pharmacology.* 12th ed. New York: Lange Medical Books/ McGraw Hill; 2012.
64. Lepist EI, Ray AS. Renal drug-drug interactions: what we have learned and where we are going. *Expert Opin Drug Metab Toxicol.* 2012;8:433-448.
65. Müller F, Fromm MF. Transporter-mediated drug-drug interactions. *Pharmacogenomics.* 2011;12:1017-1037.
66. Boparai V, Rajagopalan J, Triadafilopoulos G. Guide to the use of proton pump inhibitors in adult patients. *Drugs.* 2008;68: 925-947.
67. Thorens B, Mueckler M. Glucose transporters in the 21st century. *Am J Physiol Endocrinol Metab.* 2010;298:E141-145.
68. Burton PS, Goodwin JT. Solubility and permeability measurement and applications in drug discovery. *Comb Chem High Throughput Screen.* 2010;13:101-111.
69. Daniel WA. Mechanisms of cellular distribution of psychotropic drugs. Significance for drug action and interactions. *Prog Neuropsychopharmacol Biol Psychiatry.* 2003;27:65-73.
70. Holford NHG. Pharmacokinetics and pharmacodynamics: rational dosing and the time course of drug action. In: Katzung BG, ed. *Basic and Clinical Pharmacology.* 12th ed. New York: Lange Medical Books/McGraw Hill; 2012.
71. Jaeschke H, McGill MR, Ramachandran A. Oxidant stress, mitochondria, and cell death mechanisms in drug-induced liver injury: lessons learned from acetaminophen hepatotoxicity. *Drug Metab Rev.* 2012;44:88-106.
72. Prinderre P, Sauzet C, Fuxen C. Advances in gastro retentive drug-delivery systems. *Expert Opin Drug Deliv.* 2011;8: 1189-1203.
73. Tran PH, Tran TT, Park JB, Lee BJ. Controlled release systems containing solid dispersions: strategies and mechanisms. *Pharm Res.* 2011;28:2353-2378.
74. Balmayor ER, Azevedo HS, Reis RL. Controlled delivery systems: from pharmaceuticals to cells and genes. *Pharm Res.* 2011;28:1241-1258.
75. Fonarow GC. Role of carvedilol controlled-release in cardiovascular disease. *Expert Rev Cardiovasc Ther.* 2009;7:483-498.
76. Snider ME, Nuzum DS, Veverka A. Long-acting nifedipine in the management of the hypertensive patient. *Vasc Health Risk Manag.* 2008;4:1249-1257.
77. Guay DR. Oral hydromorphone extended-release. *Consult Pharm.* 2010;25:816-828.
78. Jegu J, Gallini A, Soler P, et al. Slow-release oral morphine for opioid maintenance treatment: a systematic review. *Br J Clin Pharmacol.* 2011;71:832-843.
79. Contin M, Martinelli P. Pharmacokinetics of levodopa. *J Neurol.* 2010;257(suppl 2):S253-261.
80. Fabbrini G, Di Stasio F, Bloise M, Berardelli A. Soluble and controlled-release preparations of levodopa: do we really need them? *J Neurol.* 2010;257(suppl 2):S292-297.
81. Upadhyay SP, Mallick PN. Intrathecal drug delivery system (IDDS) for cancer pain management: a review and updates. *Am J Hosp Palliat Care.* 2012;29:388-398.

82. Cabral J, Moratti SC. Hydrogels for biomedical applications. *Future Med Chem.* 2011;3:1877-1888.
83. McInnes SJ, Voelcker NH. Silicon-polymer hybrid materials for drug delivery. *Future Med Chem.* 2009;1:1051-1074.
84. Pritchard EM, Kaplan DL. Silk fibroin biomaterials for controlled release drug delivery. *Expert Opin Drug Deliv.* 2011; 8(6):797-811.
85. Dienstmann R, Markman B, Tabernero J. Application of monoclonal antibodies as cancer therapy in solid tumors. *Curr Clin Pharmacol.* 2012;7:137-145.
86. Prabhu S, Boswell CA, Leipold D, et al. Antibody delivery of drugs and radionuclides: factors influencing clinical pharmacology. *Ther Deliv.* 2011;2:769-791.
87. Huttunen KM, Raunio H, Rautio J. Prodrugs—from serendipity to rational design. *Pharmacol Rev.* 2011;63:750-771.
88. Lin C, Sunkara G, Cannon JB, Ranade V. Recent advances in prodrugs as drug delivery systems. *Am J Ther.* 2012;19:33-43.
89. Jain SK, Jain A. Target-specific drug release to the colon. *Expert Opin Drug Deliv.* 2008;5:483-498.
90. Patel M, Amin A. Recent trends in microbially and/or enzymatically driven colon-specific drug delivery systems. *Crit Rev Ther Drug Carrier Syst.* 2011;28:489-552.
91. Doane TL, Burda C. The unique role of nanoparticles in nanomedicine: imaging, drug delivery and therapy. *Chem Soc Rev.* 2012;41:2885-2911.
92. Liu Y, Tan J, Thomas A, et al. The shape of things to come: importance of design in nanotechnology for drug delivery. *Ther Deliv.* 2012;3:181-194.
93. Elizondo E, Moreno E, Cabrera I, et al. Liposomes and other vesicular systems: structural characteristics, methods of preparation, and use in nanomedicine. *Prog Mol Biol Transl Sci.* 2011;104:1-52.
94. Ma Y, Nolte RJ, Cornelissen JJ. Virus-based nanocarriers for drug delivery. *Adv Drug Deliv Rev.* 2012;64:811-825.
95. Micheli MR, Bova R, Magini A, et al. Lipid-based nanocarriers for CNS-targeted drug delivery. *Recent Pat CNS Drug Discov.* 2012;7:71-86.
96. He Q, Wu Z, Huang C. Hollow magnetic nanoparticles: synthesis and applications in biomedicine. *J Nanosci Nanotechnol.* 2012;12:2943-2954.
97. Herrero EP, Alonso MJ, Csaba N. Polymer-based oral peptide nanomedicines. *Ther Deliv.* 2012;3:657-668.
98. Reis CP, Damgé C. Nanotechnology as a promising strategy for alternative routes of insulin delivery. *Methods Enzymol.* 2012;508:271-294.
99. Dreaden EC, Austin LA, Mackey MA, El-Sayed MA. Size matters: gold nanoparticles in targeted cancer drug delivery. *Ther Deliv.* 2012;3:457-478.
100. Kolhe S, Parikh K. Application of nanotechnology in cancer: a review. *Int J Bioinform Res Appl.* 2012;8:112-125.
101. Durazo SA, Kompella UB. Functionalized nanosystems for targeted mitochondrial delivery. *Mitochondrion.* 2012;12: 190-201.
102. Paulo CS, Pires das Neves R, Ferreira LS. Nanoparticles for intracellular-targeted drug delivery. *Nanotechnology.* 2011;22: 494002.

CHAPTER 3

Pharmacokinetics II: Drug Elimination

All drugs eventually must be eliminated from the body to terminate their effect and to prevent excessive accumulation of the drug. The body can usually eliminate the drug by biotransformation—chemically altering the original compound so that it is no longer active—by excreting the active form of the drug, or by a combination of biotransformation and excretion.

Eliminating a drug and terminating its effects after it is no longer needed are often essential. For instance, the effects of general and local anesthetics must eventually wear off, allowing the patient to resume normal functioning. Although termination of drug activity can occur when the active form of the drug is excreted from the body via organs such as the kidneys, excretory mechanisms are often too slow to effectively terminate any activity within a reasonable time period. If excretion were the only way to terminate drug activity, some compounds would continue to exert their effects for several days or even weeks. Drug biotransformation into an inactive form usually occurs within a matter of minutes or hours, thus reducing the chance for toxic effects caused by drug accumulation or prolonged drug activity. Excretion can then remove any metabolic by-products that remain after biotransformation, further reducing the risk that these by-products might accumulate and cause toxicity.

Biotransformation and excretion are therefore essential in eliminating specific drugs from the body. This is important, considering the large number of patients who have altered liver function, kidney function, or other physiological changes that affect drug elimination. This chapter will introduce you to the ways that drugs are normally eliminated and how drug metabolism and excretion can be influenced by disease, age, genetics, and other factors. This information will set the stage for subsequent chapters that address how specific drugs are eliminated after being administered to treat various conditions.

BIOTRANSFORMATION

Biotransformation, or drug metabolism, refers to chemical changes that take place in the drug following administration. Biotransformation typically results in an altered version of the original compound, known as a **metabolite**, which is usually inactive or has a greatly reduced level of pharmacological activity. Occasionally, the metabolite has a higher level of activity than the original compound. In these cases, the drug may be given in an inactive, or "prodrug," form that will activate via biotransformation following administration. However, after it has exerted its pharmacological effect, drug termination is the primary function of biotransformation.[1]

Cellular Mechanisms of Drug Biotransformation

The chemical changes that occur during drug metabolism are usually caused by oxidation, reduction, hydrolysis, or conjugation of the original compound.[1] Examples of each type of reaction are listed in Table 3-1.

Table 3-1
EXAMPLES OF DRUG BIOTRANSFORMATION REACTIONS

I. Oxidation	Examples
A. Side chain (aliphatic) hydroxylation	
$RCH_2CH_3 \xrightarrow{[O]} RCH(OH)CH_3$	Ibuprofen
B. N-oxidation	
$(R)_2NH \xrightarrow{[O]} (R)_2NOH$	Acetaminophen
C. Deamination	
$RCH_2NH_2 \xrightarrow{[O]} RCHO + NH_3$	Diazepam
II. Reduction	
A. Nitro reductions	
$RNO_2 \rightarrow RNH_2$	Dantrolene
B. Carbonyl reductions	
$RC(=O)R' \rightarrow RCH(OH)R'$	Methadone
III. Hydrolysis	
A. Esters	
$RC(=O)OR' \rightarrow RCOOH + R'OH$	Aspirin
B. Amides	
$RC(=O)NR' \rightarrow RCOOH + R'NH2$	Lidocaine
IV. Conjugation	
A. Acetylation	
$RNH_2 + AcetylCoA \rightarrow RNHC(=O)CH_3 + CoA\text{-}SH$	Clonazepam
B. Glycine conjugation	
$RCOOH \rightarrow RC(=O)SCoA + NH_2CH_2COOH \rightarrow RC(=O)NHCH_2COOH + CoA\text{-}SH$	Benzoic acid

Parent drug compounds are represented by the letter 'R'. Examples are types of drugs that undergo biotransformation via the respective type of chemical reaction.

Enzymes that are located within specific tissues are responsible for catalyzing changes in the drug's structure and subsequently altering the drug's pharmacological properties. The type of reaction and the enzymes catalyzing the reaction include the following:

Oxidation. Oxidation occurs when either oxygen is added or hydrogen is removed from the original compound. Oxidation reactions comprise the predominant method of drug biotransformation in the body, and the primary enzymes that catalyze these reactions are known collectively as the cytochrome P450 monooxygenases.[2-4] These enzymes are located primarily on the smooth endoplasmic reticulum of specific cells and are sometimes referred to as the **drug microsomal metabolizing system** (DMMS). Figure 3-1 shows the general scheme of drug oxidation as catalyzed by the DMMS.

Reduction. Reduction reactions remove oxygen or add hydrogen to the original compound. Enzymes that are located in the cell cytoplasm are usually responsible for drug reduction.

Hydrolysis. The original compound is broken into separate parts. The enzymes responsible for this are located at several sites within the cell (i.e., the endoplasmic reticulum and cytoplasm) and extracellularly (e.g., circulating in the plasma).

Conjugation. In conjugation reactions, the intact drug or the metabolite of one of the reactions described earlier is coupled to an endogenous substance such as acetyl coenzyme A (acetyl CoA), glucuronic acid, or an amino acid. Enzymes catalyzing drug conjugations are found in the cytoplasm and on the endoplasmic reticulum.

The chemical reactions involved in drug biotransformation are classified as either phase I or phase II reactions.[1,5] Phase I reactions consist of those using oxidation, reduction, or hydrolysis. Phase II reactions involve conjugation of the parent drug or the

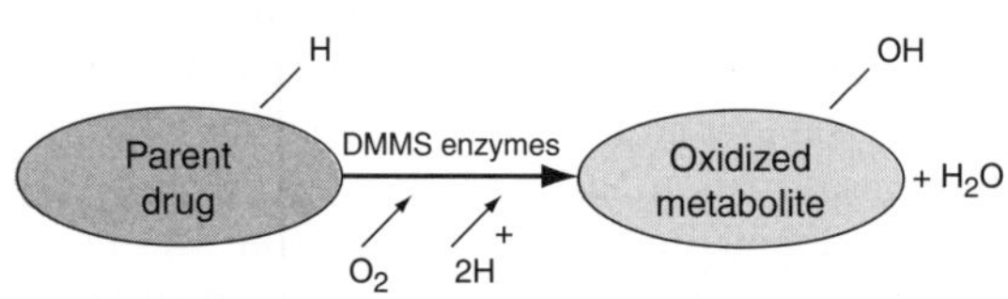

Figure ■ 3-1
Drug oxidation catalyzed by drug microsomal metabolizing system (DMMS) enzymes.

metabolite of a drug that was already metabolized using a phase I reaction.

Regardless of the type of chemical reaction used, biotransformation also helps in metabolite excretion from the body by creating a more polar compound.[1,6] After one or more of the reactions just described occurs, the remaining drug metabolite usually tends to be ionized in the body's fluids. The ionized metabolite is more water soluble and thus transported more easily in the bloodstream to the kidneys. Upon reaching the kidneys, the polar metabolite can be excreted through the urine.

Organs Responsible for Drug Biotransformation

The primary location for drug metabolism is the liver.[1,7] Enzymes responsible for drug metabolism, such as the cytochrome P450 enzymes, are abundant on the hepatic smooth endoplasmic reticulum. Liver cells also contain cytoplasmic enzymes responsible for drug reduction and hydrolysis. Other organs that contain metabolizing enzymes and exhibit considerable drug transformation abilities include the lungs, kidneys, gastrointestinal (GI) epithelium, and skin. Drug metabolism can be radically altered in conditions where these tissues are damaged. For instance, inactivation of certain drugs may be significantly delayed in the patient with hepatitis, cirrhosis, or other liver disorders.[8,9] As expected, dosages in these patients must be adjusted accordingly to prevent drug accumulation and toxicity.

Enzyme Induction

A frequent problem in drug metabolism is enzyme induction.[10,11] Prolonged use of certain drugs "induces" the body to adjust and enzymatically destroy the drug more rapidly than expected, usually because either more metabolizing enzymes are being manufactured or fewer are being degraded. The induction decreases the drugs' therapeutic effect. This may be one reason why tolerance to some drugs occurs when they are used for extended periods. **Tolerance** is the need for increased drug dosages to produce the same effect. Long-term ingestion or inhalation of other exogenous compounds such as alcohol, cigarette smoke, herbal products, or environmental toxins may also cause enzyme induction.[12-14] Medicinal drugs may be more rapidly metabolized even when they are first administered because of the preexisting enzyme induction.

DRUG EXCRETION

The kidneys are the primary sites for drug excretion.[15,16] The functional unit of the kidney is the nephron (Fig. 3-2), and each kidney is composed of approximately 1 million nephrons. Usually, the metabolized or conjugated version of the original drug reaches the nephron and is then filtered at the glomerulus. Following filtration, the compound traverses the proximal convoluted tubule, loop of Henle, and distal convoluted tubule before reaching the collecting ducts in the renal medulla. If a compound is not reabsorbed while moving through the nephron, it will ultimately leave the body in the urine.

As discussed earlier, biotransformation plays a significant role in creating a polar, water-soluble metabolite that can reach the kidneys through the bloodstream. Only relatively polar drugs or their metabolites will be excreted in significant amounts by the kidneys because the ionized metabolite is relatively impermeable to the epithelium lining. The metabolite tends to remain "trapped" in the nephron and not be reabsorbed into the body (see Fig. 3-2).[1] In contrast, the nonpolar compounds filtered by the kidneys are relatively lipophilic and can easily be reabsorbed back into the body passively by diffusing through the wall of the nephron.

Some drugs may be secreted into the nephron by active transport mechanisms located in the proximal convoluted tubule. These drugs can be transported by one of several distinct types of transport proteins that secrete organic cations (e.g., uric acid), organic anions (e.g., choline, histamine), prostaglandins, conjugated drug metabolites, and a variety of other compounds.[15,17,18] For example, penicillin G is actively secreted via the transport system for organic acids, and morphine is secreted by the organic base transport system. In these cases, elimination of the drug is enhanced by the combined effects of tubular secretion and filtration in delivering the drug to the urine.

Other routes for drug excretion include the lungs and GI tract. The lungs play a significant role in excreting volatile drugs—that is, drugs that are usually

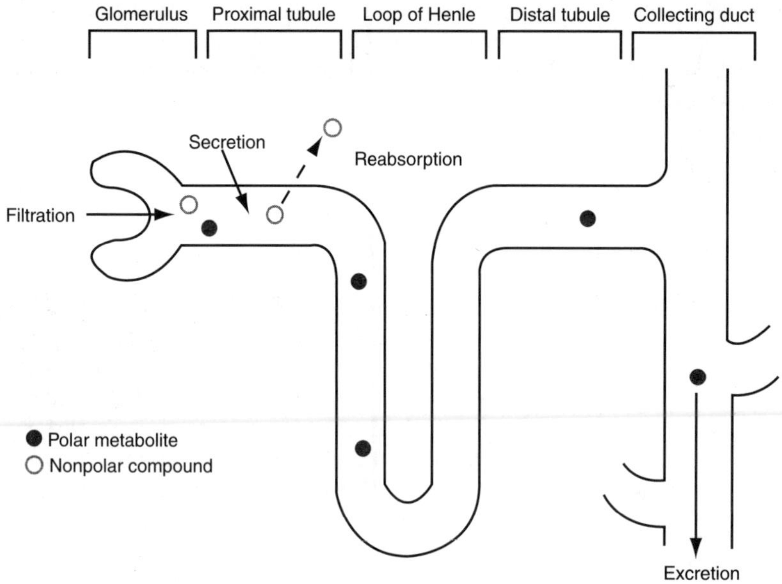

Figure ■ 3-2
Drug excretion at the nephron. Compounds reach the nephron by either filtration, secretion, or both. Polar metabolites remain trapped in the nephron and are eventually excreted. Nonpolar compounds are able to diffuse back into the body (reabsorption).

administered by inhalation, such as gaseous anesthetics. Consequently, the lungs serve as the route of both drug administration and excretion. The GI tract usually plays only a minor role in drug excretion. Certain drugs can be excreted by the liver into the bile and subsequently reach the duodenum via the bile duct. If the drug remains in the GI tract, it will eventually be excreted in the feces. However, most of the secreted bile is reabsorbed, and drugs contained in it are often reabsorbed simultaneously.

Other minor routes for drug excretion include the sweat, saliva, and breast milk of lactating mothers. Although drugs excreted via lactation are considered a relatively minor route with regard to loss from the mother, the possibility that the infant may imbibe substantial concentrations of the drug does exist. Careful consideration for the welfare of the nursing infant must always be a factor when administering medications to the lactating mother.[19,20]

DRUG ELIMINATION RATES

The rate at which a drug is eliminated is significant in determining the amount and frequency of its dosage. If a drug is administered much faster than it is eliminated, the drug will accumulate excessively in the body and reach toxic levels. Conversely, if elimination greatly exceeds the rate of delivery, the concentration in the body may never reach therapeutic levels. Several parameters are used to indicate the rate at which a drug is usually eliminated so that dosages may be adjusted accordingly. Two of the primary measurements are *clearance* and *half-life*.[5,21]

Clearance

Clearance of a drug (CL) can be described either in terms of all organs' and tissues' ability to eliminate the drug (systemic clearance) or in terms of a single organ or tissue's ability to eliminate the drug.[21,22] To calculate clearance from a specific organ, two primary factors must be considered. First, the blood flow to the organ (Q) determines how much drug will be delivered to the organ for elimination. Second, the fraction of drug removed from the plasma as it passes through the organ must be known. This fraction, termed the *extraction ratio*, is equal to the difference in the concentration of drug entering (Ci) and exiting (Co) the organ, divided by the entering concentration (Ci). Clearance by an individual organ is summarized by the following equation:

$$CL = Q \times [(Ci - Co) \div Ci].$$

The calculation of clearance is illustrated by the following example. Aspirin is metabolized primarily in the liver. Normal hepatic blood flow (Q) equals 1,500 mL/min. If the blood entering the liver contains 200 μg/mL of aspirin (Ci) and the blood leaving the liver contains 134 μg/mL (Co), hepatic clearance of aspirin is calculated as follows:

$$CL_{hepatic} = Q \times [(Ci - Co) \div Ci]$$

$$= 1{,}500 \text{ mL/min} \times [(200 \ \mu\text{g/mL} - 134 \ \mu\text{g/mL}) \div 200 \ \mu\text{g/mL}]$$

$$= 495 \text{ mL/min.}$$

This example illustrates that clearance is actually the amount of plasma from which the drug can be totally removed per unit time. As calculated here, the liver would be able to completely remove aspirin from 495 mL of blood each minute. Tetracycline, a common antibacterial drug, has a clearance equal to 130 mL/min, indicating that this drug would be completely removed from approximately 130 mL of plasma each minute.

Clearance is dependent on the organ or tissue's ability to extract the drug from the plasma as well as the perfusion of the organ. Some tissues may have an excellent ability to remove the drug from the bloodstream, but clearance is limited because only a small amount of blood reaches the organ. Conversely, highly perfused organs may be ineffective in removing the drug, thus prolonging its activity.

In terms of drug elimination from the entire body, systemic clearance is calculated as the sum of all individual clearances from all organs and tissues (i.e., systemic CL = hepatic CL + renal CL + lung CL, etc.). Note that the elimination of the drug includes the combined processes of drug loss from the body (excretion) and inactivation of the drug through biotransformation.[21]

Half-Life

In addition to clearance, the half-life of the drug is important in describing the compound's duration of activity. **Half-life** is defined as the amount of time required for 50 percent of the drug remaining in the body to be eliminated.[21,23] Most drugs are eliminated in a manner such that a fixed portion of the drug is eliminated in a given time period. For example, acetaminophen has a half-life of 2 hours, which indicates that in each 2-hour period, 50 percent of the acetaminophen still in the body will be eliminated (Fig. 3-3).

Half-life is a function of both clearance and volume of distribution (V_d);[21] that is, the time it takes

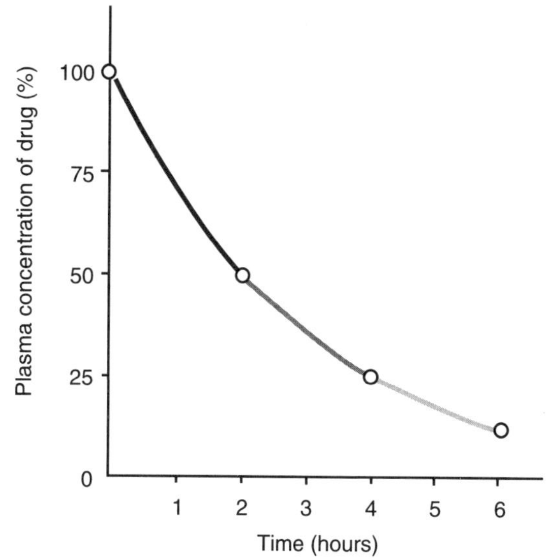

Figure ■ 3-3
Elimination of a drug with a half-life of 2 hours. Fifty percent of the drug remaining in the bloodstream is eliminated in each 2-hour period.

to eliminate 50 percent of the drug depends on the ability of the organ(s) to remove the drug from the plasma and on the distribution or presence of the drug in the plasma (see Chapter 2 for a description of V_d). A drug that undergoes extensive inactivation in the liver may have a long half-life if it is sequestered intracellularly in skeletal muscle. Also, disease states that affect either clearance or V_d will affect the drug's half-life, so prescribers must alter the dosages.

DOSING SCHEDULES AND PLASMA CONCENTRATION

With most medications, it is desirable to bring plasma concentrations of the drug up to a certain level and maintain it there. If the drug is administered by continuous IV administration, this can be done fairly easily by matching the rate of administration with the rate of drug elimination (clearance) once the desired plasma concentration is achieved (Fig. 3-4). In situations where the drug is given at specific intervals, the dosage must be adjusted to provide an average plasma concentration over the dosing period. Figure 3-4

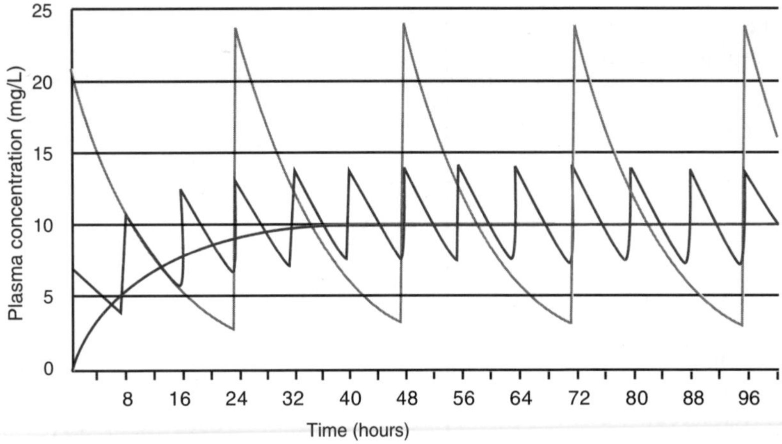

Figure 3-4
Relationship between dosing interval and plasma concentrations of the antiasthmatic drug theophylline. A constant IV infusion (shown by the smoothly rising line) yields a desired plasma level of 10 mg/L. The same *average* plasma concentration is achieved when a dose of 224 mg is taken every 8 hours, or a dose of 672 mg every 24 hours. However, note the fluctuations in plasma concentration seen when doses are taken at specific hourly intervals.

illustrates that if the dosing interval is relatively long (e.g., 12 hours), the dose must be considerably large to provide the same relative plasma concentration that would exist in a shorter dosing interval (e.g., 8 hours). Note also that larger doses given farther apart result in greater plasma fluctuations—that is, greater maximum and minimum plasma levels over the dosing period. Giving smaller doses more frequently provides an equivalent average concentration without the extreme peaks and valleys associated with longer intervals.

VARIATIONS IN DRUG RESPONSE AND METABOLISM

The fact that different people react differently to the same relative drug dosage is an important and often critical aspect of pharmacology. Two patients who are given the same drug may exhibit different magnitudes of a beneficial response as well as different adverse effects. Several of the primary factors that are responsible for variations in the response to drugs include genetics, disease, drug interactions, age, diet, and sex.

Genetics

Genetic variability can result in altered drug pharmacokinetics in certain individuals. In extreme cases, genetic variations may result in abnormal or absent drug-metabolizing enzymes.[4,24] This deficiency can be harmful or even fatal if the drug is not metabolized and begins exerting toxic effects due to accumulation or prolonged pharmacological activity. For example, some individuals lack the appropriate plasma cholinesterase to break down circulating acetylcholine and acetylcholine-like compounds.[25] Succinylcholine is a neuromuscular blocking agent that an anesthesia provider usually administers with general anesthesia to ensure muscular relaxation during surgery. Normally, the succinylcholine is quickly degraded by plasma cholinesterase; however, individuals lacking the appropriate form of cholinesterase may suffer respiratory paralysis because the succinylcholine exerts its effect much longer than the expected period of time.

In addition to the extreme case described above, we know that many people have subtle but important differences in the genes controlling the synthesis of many drug-related proteins. These differences—known as *genetic polymorphisms*—will result in the production of proteins that are somewhat different in structure and function.[4,24] From this, various aspects of drug disposition and response will be affected.[26,27] For example, differences in proteins that transport drugs across membranes will result in altered absorption, distribution, and excretion of drugs using these transport systems. Differences in the genetic control of drug-metabolizing proteins (enzymes) will likewise result in altered metabolism and biotransformation of specific drugs. Finally, differences in the proteins that function as drug receptors on specific cells and target tissues (see Chapter 4) might cause variability in the tissues' responses.

The study of potential influences of genetic variability on drug responses and metabolism has actually evolved into a branch of genetics known as *pharmacogenetics* or *pharmacogenomics*.[28,29] Research in pharmacogenetics will continue to expand as more details emerge about human genetic makeup (i.e., from the Human Genome Project). Prescribers can tailor drug therapy more specifically for patients by realizing how specific genetic differences might influence drug responses.[26,27,30] That is, doses can be adjusted to account for genetic differences in drug disposition, and certain drugs can be avoided altogether in people who lack the appropriate enzymes for these drugs. Drug regimens that take into account genetic variability will ultimately result in better drug effects with fewer side effects.

Disease

Structural or functional damage to an organ or tissue responsible for drug metabolism or excretion presents an obvious problem in pharmacology. Diseases initiating change in tissue function or blood flow to specific organs like the liver and kidneys can dramatically affect the elimination of various drugs.[31,32] Certain diseases may also impair the absorption and distribution of the drug, further complicating the problem of individualized response. The significance of disease in affecting the patient's response is crucial because response to a medication may be affected by the very same pathology that the drug is being used to treat. For instance, renal excretion of antibiotics, such as the aminoglycosides, is altered radically in many types of bacterial infection, but these drugs are typically administered to treat the same infections altering their own excretion.[31] Consequently, prescribers must take great care to adjust the dosage accordingly when administering medications in conditions where drug disposition might be altered by various diseases.[32,33]

Drug Interactions

When two or more drugs are present in the body at the same time, the chance exists that they may interact and alter each other's effects and metabolism.[34,35] The majority of drug–drug interactions are insignificant and do not result in any clinically meaningful adverse effects.[36,37] Likewise, certain drug combinations and interactions can be beneficial because two or more compounds might act synergistically to produce a cumulative effect that is greater than each drug would produce alone. For example, several drugs are often administered simultaneously so that they augment each other when treating conditions such as hypertension, cancer, and HIV. However, certain combinations can lead to serious adverse effects and interactions. For instance, two or more drugs can have additive effects that cause an adverse response, even if each drug is given in a nontoxic dose. For example, taking two central nervous system (CNS) depressants simultaneously (e.g., barbiturates and alcohol) may cause such severe CNS inhibition that the additive effects are lethal.

In contrast to an additive effect, drugs with opposite actions may essentially cancel each other out, thus negating or reducing the beneficial effects of one or both medications. A drug that causes bronchodilation (i.e., for the treatment of asthma) will be negated by an agent that constricts the bronchioles.

Some of the most serious drug interaction problems occur when one drug delays the biotransformation of the other. If a second compound inhibits the enzymes that normally metabolize a drug, the original drug will exert its effect for prolonged periods, possibly leading to toxic effects.[38] For instance, the antifungal drug miconazole (Monistat, others) inhibits the hepatic metabolism of oral anticoagulants such as warfarin (Coumadin). Taking these two drugs together tends to cause elevated plasma levels of the anticoagulant, which may slow blood clotting and lead to a possible hemorrhage. Another type of interaction occurs when two or more drugs alter each other's absorption and distribution; this can occur when they compete for the same active transport carrier or bind to the same plasma proteins. An example is the interaction between aspirin and methotrexate, a drug used to treat cancer and rheumatoid arthritis. Aspirin can displace methotrexate from its binding site on plasma proteins, thus allowing relatively high amounts of unbound or "free" methotrexate to exist in the bloodstream. The increased levels of free methotrexate may lead to toxic effects.

Considering the large number of drugs on the market, it is well beyond the scope of this text to discuss all of the clinically relevant drug interactions. The prescribing physician and pharmacist must carefully evaluate the potential for drug interactions. Likewise, physical therapists, occupational therapists, and other individuals dealing with patients taking medications must be alert for any abnormal symptoms or untoward effects because they may indicate a possible drug interaction.

Age

In general, older patients are more sensitive to drugs.[39,40] Drugs are usually not metabolized as quickly in the elderly, primarily because of decreases in liver and kidney function that typically accompany the aging process.[41,42] Therefore, decreased drug elimination often results in higher plasma levels in older adults than those occurring in younger adults given equivalent doses.[43,44] Older adults also suffer more illnesses and consequently receive more drugs than younger adults; this fact further increases their vulnerability to altered drug responses.[41,44] Various other age-related changes in physiology (e.g., increased body fat, decreased cardiovascular function, etc.) can affect pharmacokinetics and pharmacodynamics in older adults.[39,42] However, there is large variability among older patients regarding the extent to which drug metabolism changes with advanced age. These changes may be minimal in some older adults, while others exhibit a substantial decline in drug metabolism due to multiple organ disease, inactivity, genetic influences, other drugs they are taking, and many other factors.[43] Hence, drug disposition is certainly subject to change in older adults, but the extent to which these changes affect metabolism and other pharmacokinetic variables may vary greatly among older individuals.

Children are also subject to problems and variability in drug metabolism.[45] Because liver and kidney function is immature, newborns may be deficient in specific drug-metabolizing enzymes, thus prolonging the effects of drugs.[45,46] Infants also differ from adults in several other key factors affecting drug disposition, including differences in membrane function, plasma proteins, regional blood flow, and body composition (i.e., percentage of body fat and total body water).[47] Consequently, drug absorption, distribution, and elimination will be altered in infants, which is especially problematic in infants who are born prematurely. Moreover, drug metabolism and other pharmacokinetic variables change rapidly in the first few months of life as the liver, kidneys, and other organ systems begin to grow and mature.[48,49] Thus, drug dosages must be adjusted frequently to keep pace with these changes throughout infancy and early childhood.[50] Safe and effective dosing in neonates and infants is one of the more difficult and complex aspects of clinical pharmacology.

Diet

Diet is shown to affect the absorption, metabolism, and response to many drugs.[51,52] Animal and human studies indicate that the total caloric input and the percentage of calories obtained from different sources (carbohydrates, proteins, and fats) influence drug pharmacokinetics.[51,53] Specific dietary constituents such as cruciferous vegetables and charcoal-broiled beef can also alter drug metabolism.[12,54]

Fortunately, most food–drug interactions are not serious and will not alter the clinical effects of the drug. However, there are a few well-known food–drug combinations that people should avoid because of their potentially serious interaction. For example, grapefruit juice inhibits the enzymes that metabolize certain drugs as they are absorbed from the gastrointestinal (GI) tract. As a result, taking these drugs orally with grapefruit juice will result in *increased* drug bioavailability because more of the drug's active form will reach the bloodstream.[55,56] This increased bioavailability will result in plasma levels that are higher than expected, thereby increasing the risk of side effects and adverse reactions.

Another important food–drug interaction involves foods such as fermented cheese and wine.[57,58] These foods may contain high amounts of tyramine, which stimulates the release of catecholamines (norepinephrine, epinephrine) within the body. Hence, these foods should not be ingested with drugs that inhibit the monoamine oxidase (MAO) enzyme. MAO-inhibiting drugs work by suppressing the destruction of catecholamines, thus allowing higher levels of norepinephrine and epinephrine to occur. (MAO inhibitors are frequently used in the treatment of depression; see Chapter 7). Consequently, when MAO inhibitors are taken with tyramine-containing foods, excessive levels of catecholamines may develop, leading to a dangerous increase in blood pressure (hypertensive crisis).

Many other potential food–drug interactions occur,[51,59] but it is beyond the scope of this text to discuss all of them. Clinicians should be aware of these well-known interactions and be on the alert for others as new drugs arrive on the market.

Sex

Men and women may have distinct differences in the way that certain drugs are absorbed, distributed, and metabolized.[60,61] This idea makes sense when one considers that sex-related differences in body composition, GI function, enzyme activity, and various other systems can potentially affect pharmacokinetic variables.[60,62] The cyclic hormonal variations occurring during the menstrual cycle may also influence drug disposition in women, whereas men do not typically undergo such routine hormonal fluctuations.[63]

Pharmacokinetics can clearly differ between men and women, and future research is needed to determine how sex-related differences affect the therapeutic outcomes of specific drugs.[61,62,64]

Other Factors

Several additional factors may alter the patient's predicted response to a drug. As discussed earlier, environmental and occupational hazards may produce certain toxins that change drug absorption and metabolism.[12,13] Factors such as cigarette smoking and alcohol consumption have been shown to influence the metabolism of specific compounds.[65,66] Drug distribution and metabolism may be altered in the obese patient[67] or in response to chronic and acute exercise.[68] Individuals with spinal cord injuries exhibit changes in drug absorption, distribution, and clearance depending on the level of spinal cord injury and related changes in GI activity, body composition, and kidney function.[69,70] Likewise, patients with extensive burn injuries may have changes in plasma protein levels, total body water, renal blood flow, and gastrointestinal absorption that dramatically affect the distribution and bioavailability of certain drugs; these changes will depend on several factors, including the type of burn, the extent of the area burned, and the stage of recovery after the burn injury.[71]

There are therefore many factors that influence the way each individual responds to a medication, and these factors must be taken into account whenever possible. Clinicians should also realize that these factors are not mutually exclusive. For example, premature infants with genetic polymorphisms might present an extremely complex pharmacological dilemma because of their very young age and genetic variability.[72] In older adults, the combined effects of old age and disease can likewise increase the complexity of pharmacokinetic variability. Hence, special care must be taken in observing a patient's response to medication in any situation where the predicted responses to drug therapy might be altered by one or more of the factors described.

SUMMARY

Drug elimination occurs because of the combined effects of drug metabolism and excretion. Elimination is essential in terminating drug activity within a reasonable and predictable time frame. Various tissues and organs (especially the liver and kidneys) are involved in drug elimination, and injury or disease of these tissues can markedly alter the response to certain drugs. In cases of disease or injury, dosages must frequently be adjusted to prevent adverse side effects from altered elimination rates. Many other environmental, behavioral, and genetic factors may also alter drug metabolism and disposition, and possible variability in the patient's response should always be a matter of concern when treating a patient.

REFERENCES

1. Correia MA. Drug biotransformation. In: Katzung BG, ed. *Basic and Clinical Pharmacology.* 12th ed. New York: Lange Medical Books/McGraw Hill; 2012.
2. Chen Q, Zhang T, Wang JF, Wei DQ. Advances in human cytochrome p450 and personalized medicine. *Curr Drug Metab.* 2011;12:436-444.
3. Davydov DR, Halpert JR. Allosteric P450 mechanisms: multiple binding sites, multiple conformers or both? *Expert Opin Drug Metab Toxicol.* 2008;4:1523-1535.
4. Lee IS, Kim D. Polymorphic metabolism by functional alterations of human cytochrome P450 enzymes. *Arch Pharm Res.* 2011;34:1799-1816.
5. Buxton ILO, Benet LZ. Pharmacokinetics: the dynamics of drug absorption, distribution, metabolism, and elimination. In: Brunton LL, et al, eds. *The Pharmacological Basis of Therapeutics.* 12th ed. New York: McGraw Hill; 2011.
6. Smith DA, Obach RS. Metabolites: have we MIST out the importance of structure and physicochemistry? *Bioanalysis.* 2010;2:1223-1233.
7. Sahi J, Grepper S, Smith C. Hepatocytes as a tool in drug metabolism, transport and safety evaluations in drug discovery. *Curr Drug Discov Technol.* 2010;7:188-198.
8. Buechler C, Weiss TS. Does hepatic steatosis affect drug metabolizing enzymes in the liver? *Curr Drug Metab.* 2011;12: 24-34.
9. Sease JM. Portal hypertension and cirrhosis. In: DiPiro JT, et al, eds. *Pharmacotherapy: A Pathophysiologic Approach.* 8th ed. New York: McGraw-Hill; 2011.
10. Mohutsky MA, Romeike A, Meador V, et al. Hepatic drug-metabolizing enzyme induction and implications for preclinical and clinical risk assessment. *Toxicol Pathol.* 2010;38:799-809.
11. Zhu BT. On the general mechanism of selective induction of cytochrome P450 enzymes by chemicals: some theoretical considerations. *Expert Opin Drug Metab Toxicol.* 2010;6:483-494.

12. Elsherbiny ME, Brocks DR. The ability of polycyclic aromatic hydrocarbons to alter physiological factors underlying drug disposition. *Drug Metab Rev.* 2011;43:457-475.
13. Krämer SD, Testa B. The biochemistry of drug metabolism—an introduction: part 7. Intra-individual factors affecting drug metabolism. *Chem Biodivers.* 2009;6:1477-1660.
14. Rahimi R, Abdollahi M. An update on the ability of St. John's wort to affect the metabolism of other drugs. *Expert Opin Drug Metab Toxicol.* 2012;8:691-708.
15. Masereeuw R, Russel FG. Therapeutic implications of renal anionic drug transporters. *Pharmacol Ther.* 2010;126:200-216.
16. Verbeeck RK, Musuamba FT. Pharmacokinetics and dosage adjustment in patients with renal dysfunction. *Eur J Clin Pharmacol.* 2009;65:757-773.
17. Burckhardt G. Drug transport by Organic Anion Transporters (OATs). *Pharmacol Ther.* 2012;136:106-130.
18. El-Sheikh AA, Masereeuw R, Russel FG. Mechanisms of renal anionic drug transport. *Eur J Pharmacol.* 2008;585:245-255.
19. Fortinguerra F, Clavenna A, Bonati M. Psychotropic drug use during breastfeeding: a review of the evidence. *Pediatrics.* 2009;124:e547-556.
20. Mitrano JA, Spooner LM, Belliveau P. Excretion of antimicrobials used to treat methicillin-resistant Staphylococcus aureus infections during lactation: safety in breastfeeding infants. *Pharmacotherapy.* 2009;29:1103-1109.
21. Holford NHG. Pharmacokinetics and pharmacodynamics: rational dosing and the time course of drug action. Katzung BG, ed. *Basic and Clinical Pharmacology.* 12th ed. New York: Lange Medical Books/McGraw Hill; 2012.
22. Benet LZ. Clearance (née Rowland) concepts: a downdate and an update. *J Pharmacokinet Pharmacodyn.* 2010;37:529-539.
23. Patel K, Kirkpatrick CM. Pharmacokinetic concepts revisited—basic and applied. *Curr Pharm Biotechnol.* 2011;12:1983-1990.
24. Yoo HD, Lee YB. Interplay of pharmacogenetic variations in ABCB1 transporters and cytochrome P450 enzymes. *Arch Pharm Res.* 2011;34:1817-1828.
25. Soliday FK, Conley YP, Henker R. Pseudocholinesterase deficiency: a comprehensive review of genetic, acquired, and drug influences. *AANA J.* 2010;78:313-320.
26. Kirchheiner J, Seeringer A. Clinical implications of pharmacogenetics of cytochrome P450 drug metabolizing enzymes. *Biochim Biophys Acta.* 2007;1770:489-494.
27. Schwaiblmair M, Behr W, Foerg W, Berghaus T. Cytochrome P450 polymorphisms and drug-induced interstitial lung disease. *Expert Opin Drug Metab Toxicol.* 2011;7:1547-1560.
28. Blakey JD, Hall IP. Current progress in pharmacogenetics. *Br J Clin Pharmacol.* 2011;71:824-831.
29. Cordero P, Ashley EA. Whole-genome sequencing in personalized therapeutics. *Clin Pharmacol Ther.* 2012;91:1001-1009.
30. Ingelman-Sundberg M, Sim SC. Pharmacogenetic biomarkers as tools for improved drug therapy; emphasis on the cytochrome P450 system. *Biochem Biophys Res Commun.* 2010;396:90-94.
31. Roberts DM. The relevance of drug clearance to antibiotic dosing in critically ill patients. *Curr Pharm Biotechnol.* 2011;12: 2002-2014.
32. Ulldemolins M, Roberts JA, Lipman J, Rello J. Antibiotic dosing in multiple organ dysfunction syndrome. *Chest.* 2011;139: 1210-1220.
33. Eyler RF, Mueller BA; Medscape. Antibiotic dosing in critically ill patients with acute kidney injury. *Nat Rev Nephrol.* 2011;7:226-235.
34. Baneyx G, Fukushima Y, Parrott N. Use of physiologically based pharmacokinetic modeling for assessment of drug-drug interactions. *Future Med Chem.* 2012;4:681-693.
35. Hines LE, Murphy JE. Potentially harmful drug-drug interactions in the elderly: a review. *Am J Geriatr Pharmacother.* 2011;9:364-377.
36. Boulenc X, Barberan O. Metabolic-based drug-drug interactions prediction, recent approaches for risk assessment along drug development. *Drug Metabol Drug Interact.* 2011;26:147-168.
37. Spina E, Trifirò G, Caraci F. Clinically significant drug interactions with newer antidepressants. *CNS Drugs.* 2012;26:39-67.
38. Thi L, Shaw D, Bird J. Warfarin potentiation: a review of the "FAB-4" significant drug interactions. *Consult Pharm.* 2009;24:227-230.
39. Ciccone CD. Geriatric pharmacology. In: Guccione AA, Wong R, Avers D, eds. *Geriatric Physical Therapy.* 3rd ed. St Louis, MO: CV Mosby; 2012.
40. Trifirò G, Spina E. Age-related changes in pharmacodynamics: focus on drugs acting on central nervous and cardiovascular systems. *Curr Drug Metab.* 2011;12:611-620.
41. Corsonello A, Pedone C, Incalzi RA. Age-related pharmacokinetic and pharmacodynamic changes and related risk of adverse drug reactions. *Curr Med Chem.* 2010;17:571-584.
42. Klotz U. Pharmacokinetics and drug metabolism in the elderly. *Drug Metab Rev.* 2009;41:67-76.
43. McLachlan AJ, Pont LG. Drug metabolism in older people—a key consideration in achieving optimal outcomes with medicines. *J Gerontol A Biol Sci Med Sci.* 2012;67:175-180.
44. Shi S, Klotz U. Age-related changes in pharmacokinetics. *Curr Drug Metab.* 2011;12:601-610.
45. Yokoi T. Essentials for starting a pediatric clinical study (1): Pharmacokinetics in children. *J Toxicol Sci.* 2009;34(suppl 2): SP307-312.
46. de Wildt SN. Profound changes in drug metabolism enzymes and possible effects on drug therapy in neonates and children. *Expert Opin Drug Metab Toxicol.* 2011;7:935-948.
47. Allegaert K, Verbesselt R, Naulaers G, et al. Developmental pharmacology: neonates are not just small adults. *Acta Clin Belg.* 2008;63:16-24.
48. Anderson BJ. My child is unique; the pharmacokinetics are universal. *Paediatr Anaesth.* 2012;22:530-538.
49. Smits A, Kulo A, de Hoon JN, Allegaert K. Pharmacokinetics of drugs in neonates: pattern recognition beyond compound specific observations. *Curr Pharm Des.* 2012;18:3119-3146
50. Young TE. Therapeutic drug monitoring—the appropriate use of drug level measurement in the care of the neonate. *Clin Perinatol.* 2012;39:25-31.
51. Boullata JI, Hudson LM. Drug-nutrient interactions: a broad view with implications for practice. *J Acad Nutr Diet.* 2012;112:506-517.
52. Ruggiero A, Cefalo MG, Coccia P, et al. The role of diet on the clinical pharmacology of oral antineoplastic agents. *Eur J Clin Pharmacol.* 2012;68:115-122.
53. Mason P. Important drug-nutrient interactions. *Proc Nutr Soc.* 2010;69:551-557.
54. Scott O, Galicia-Connolly E, Adams D, Surette S, Vohra S, Yager JY. The safety of cruciferous plants in humans: a systematic review. *J Biomed Biotechnol.* 2012; 2012:503241.
55. Hanley MJ, Cancalon P, Widmer WW, Greenblatt DJ. The effect of grapefruit juice on drug disposition. *Expert Opin Drug Metab Toxicol.* 2011;7:267-286.

56. Seden K, Dickinson L, Khoo S, Back D. Grapefruit-drug interactions. *Drugs*. 2010;70:2373-2407.
57. Bonnin-Jusserand MM, Grandvalet CC, Rieu AA, et al. Tyrosine-containing peptides are precursors of tyramine produced by lactobacillus plantarum strain IR BL0076 isolated from wine. *BMC Microbiol.* 2012;12:199.
58. Finberg JP, Gillman K. Selective inhibitors of monoamine oxidase type B and the "cheese effect." *Int Rev Neurobiol.* 2011;100:169-190.
59. Yasuji T, Kondo H, Sako K. The effect of food on the oral bioavailability of drugs: a review of current developments and pharmaceutical technologies for pharmacokinetic control. *Ther Deliv.* 2012;3:81-90.
60. Soldin OP, Mattison DR. Sex differences in pharmacokinetics and pharmacodynamics. *Clin Pharmacokinet.* 2009;48:143-157.
61. Soldin OP, Chung SH, Mattison DR. Sex differences in drug disposition. *J Biomed Biotechnol.* 2011;2011:187103.
62. Franconi F, Carru C, Malorni W, et al. The effect of sex/gender on cardiovascular pharmacology. *Curr Pharm Des.* 2011;17:1095-1107.
63. Mitchell SC, Smith RL, Waring RH. The menstrual cycle and drug metabolism. *Curr Drug Metab.* 2009;10:499-507.
64. Franconi F, Brunelleschi S, Steardo L, Cuomo V. Gender differences in drug responses. *Pharmacol Res.* 2007;55:81-95.
65. Lennernäs H. Ethanol-drug absorption interaction: potential for a significant effect on the plasma pharmacokinetics of ethanol vulnerable formulations. *Mol Pharm.* 2009;6:1429-1440.
66. Yue J, Khokhar J, Miksys S, Tyndale RF. Differential induction of ethanol-metabolizing CYP2E1 and nicotine-metabolizing CYP2B1/2 in rat liver by chronic nicotine treatment and voluntary ethanol intake. *Eur J Pharmacol.* 2009;609:88-95.
67. Brill MJ, Diepstraten J, van Rongen A, et al. Impact of obesity on drug metabolism and elimination in adults and children. *Clin Pharmacokinet.* 2012;51:277-304.
68. Lenz TL. The effects of high physical activity on pharmacokinetic drug interactions. *Expert Opin Drug Metab Toxicol.* 2011;7:257-266.
69. Lee JP, Dang AT. Evaluation of methods to estimate glomerular filtration rate versus actual drug clearance in patients with chronic spinal cord injury. *Spinal Cord.* 2011;49:1158-1163.
70. Mestre H, Alkon T, Salazar S, Ibarra A. Spinal cord injury sequelae alter drug pharmacokinetics: an overview. *Spinal Cord.* 2011;49:955-960.
71. Blanchet B, Jullien V, Vinsonneau C, Tod M. Influence of burns on pharmacokinetics and pharmacodynamics of drugs used in the care of burn patients. *Clin Pharmacokinet.* 2008;47:635-654.
72. Allegaert K, Rochette A, Veyckemans F. Developmental pharmacology of tramadol during infancy: ontogeny, pharmacogenetics and elimination clearance. *Paediatr Anaesth.* 2011;21:266-273.

CHAPTER 4

Drug Receptors

A receptor is a component on or within a cell that a substance can bind to.[1] Most drugs exert their effect by binding to and activating one of these receptors.[1] The receptors can be any cellular macromolecule, but many receptors have been identified as proteins or protein complexes that are located on or within the cell.[1,2] When a drug binds to a receptor, it initiates a chain of biochemical events that brings about some change in the physiological function of the cell.

This chapter will help you understand how drugs interact with specific receptors, and how these interactions cause changes in cell function. Drug–receptor interactions at the cellular level ultimately cause the physiological changes that we observe in our patients in response to drug therapy. Likewise, abnormal drug responses can sometimes be explained by changes in the way that drugs interact with their receptors. Hence, this chapter will help you understand how drugs addressed in subsequent chapters act on specific cells, and why these drugs cause various responses in patients.

RECEPTORS LOCATED ON THE CELL'S SURFACE

Receptors that recognize endogenous and exogenous compounds often have a binding site for these compounds that is located on the outer surface of the cell membrane.[1] By placing the binding site of the receptor on its outer surface, the cell is able to differentiate and respond to specific substances that approach the cell, without actually allowing these substances to enter. The receptor can then transmit a message through the cell membrane to cause some change in the activity within the cell. Hence, many surface receptors are "transmembrane" proteins that span the width of the cell membrane and can relay information from the binding site of the outer surface to some intracellular mechanism that causes a change within the cell.

Surface receptors are primarily responsive to specific amino acid, peptide, or amine compounds. These receptors typically affect cell function in one of three ways:

- By acting as an ion channel and directly altering membrane permeability
- By acting enzymatically to directly influence function within the cell
- By being linked to regulatory proteins that control other chemical and enzymatic processes within the cell

Each of these is addressed here.

Surface Receptors Linked Directly to Ion Channels

Membrane receptors may be involved directly in the cellular response to the drug by acting as an ion pore, which changes the membrane permeability.[3] Perhaps the most well-known example is the acetylcholine receptor located on the postsynaptic membrane of the neuromuscular junction[2,4] (Fig. 4-1). When bound by acetylcholine molecules, the receptor activates and opens a pore through the cell membrane, thereby increasing the permeability of the muscle cell to sodium.[5,6] This action results in depolarization and excitation of the cell because of sodium influx. Another important example of a receptor-ion channel system is the **gamma-aminobutyric acid (GABA)**-benzodiazepine-chloride ion channel complex found on neuronal membranes in the central nervous system.[7,8] In this situation, the membrane's permeability to chloride is increased by the binding of both the neurotransmitter GABA and benzodiazepine drugs such as diazepam (Valium) and chlordiazepoxide (Librium). The function of this chloride ion channel complex is discussed in more detail in Chapter 6. Pharmacologists have identified surface receptors for other ions (e.g., potassium, calcium) and amino acids (glutamate) that are likewise linked directly to ion channels that control permeability of the cell membrane.[9,10]

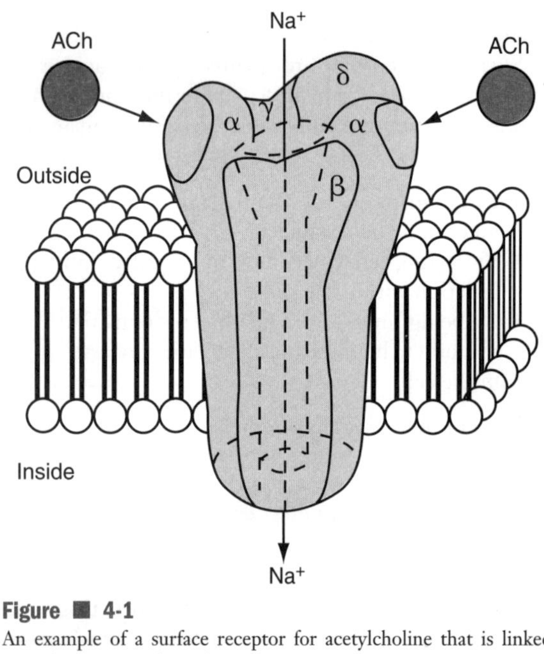

Figure ■ 4-1
An example of a surface receptor for acetylcholine that is linked directly to an ion channel.

Surface Receptors Linked Directly to Enzymes

Some proteins that span the entire width of the cell membrane may have an extracellular receptor site (binding domain) and an intracellular enzymatic component (catalytic domain)[1] (Fig. 4-2). Drugs and endogenous chemicals that bind to the receptor site can change the enzyme activity of the intracellular catalytic component, thus altering the biochemical function within the cell.[11] A common example of a receptor-enzyme system is the receptor tyrosine kinase protein. In this system, binding of an appropriate substance to the outer (receptor) component initiates the phosphorylation of certain tyrosine amino acids on the inner (catalytic) component of the protein, which in turn increases the enzyme (kinase) activity of the intracellular component.[11,12] The activated enzymatic component of the protein then catalyzes the activation of other substrates within the cell.

It appears that insulin and certain growth factors may exert their effects by acting through this type of receptor tyrosine kinase system.[13] Insulin, for example, binds to the extracellular component of a protein located on skeletal muscle cells, thereby initiating activation of this protein's enzymatic activity on the inner surface of the cell membrane. This change in enzyme function causes further changes in cell activity, which ultimately results in increased glucose uptake in the muscle cell. The function of insulin receptors and their role in the cause and treatment of diabetes mellitus are discussed in more detail in Chapter 32.

Surface Receptors Linked to Regulatory (G) Proteins and the Role of the Second Messenger

Rather than directly affecting membrane permeability or directly influencing enzyme activity, other membrane receptors affect cell function by linking to an intermediate regulatory protein that is located on the inner surface of the cell's membrane.[14] These regulatory proteins are activated by binding guanine nucleotides; hence they are often termed **G proteins.**[1] When an appropriate substance binds to the surface receptor, the receptor undergoes a specific conformational (shape) change that causes the receptor to attach to a nearby G protein.[15,16] This attachment activates the G protein, which in turn alters the activity of an intracellular effector (such as an enzyme or ion channel), ultimately leading to a change in cell function.[11]

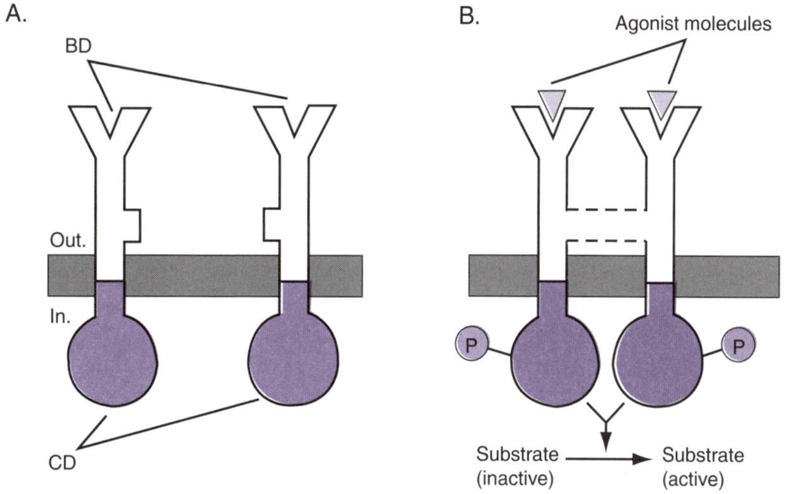

Figure ■ 4-2 An example of a surface receptor that is linked directly to intracellular enzyme activity. **A.** The receptor exists in an inactive state as two subunits: each subunit has a binding domain (BD) on the outer surface and a catalytic domain (CD) on the inner surface. **B.** Binding of agonist molecules to the BDs causes the subunits to join together and induces phosphorylation (P) of tyrosine receptors on the CD. Tyrosine phosphorylation initiates enzymatic activity of the catalytic units, which then causes substrate activation within the cell.

Receptors that are linked to G proteins, also called *G protein–coupled receptors* (GPCRs), represent one of the largest groups of surface receptors.[17] Therefore, these GPCRs represent the primary way that signals from the surface receptor are transduced into the appropriate response within various cells. There likewise appears to be several classes and types of regulatory G proteins.[17] For example, a stimulatory G protein (G_s) increases the response of certain cells to substances such as epinephrine, histamine, serotonin, and several hormones, whereas several types of inhibitory (G_i) proteins may mediate a decrease in cell activity in response to other chemicals such as acetylcholine and opioid analgesics.[1]

Drugs that bind to GPCRs exert specific effects depending on the type of G protein. A drug that stimulates a receptor that is linked to a G_s protein will activate the G_s protein, which in turn activates the effector system that opens an ion channel or activates a specific enzyme. Conversely, a drug that binds to a receptor that is linked to a G_i protein inhibits channel opening or intracellular enzyme activity.

Hence, regulatory G proteins help account for how drugs can bind to one type of receptor and stimulate cell function, whereas drugs that bind to a different receptor on the same cell can inhibit cell activity. In addition to G_s and G_i proteins, other types of G proteins are found on certain cells, and these proteins mediate specific responses associated with vision, olfaction, and other specific responses.

G proteins also seem to be important in mediating the other cell responses to stimulation or inhibition. For instance, cell function may continue to be affected through the action of G proteins even after the drug has left the binding site on the cell's surface;[1] that is, the drug may bind to the cell for only a short period, but long enough to initiate the interaction of the G protein with the intracellular effector system. Sustained influence of the G protein on the effector system helps explain why the cell may continue to exhibit a response even after the drug has dissociated from it, or even after the drug has been eliminated from the body completely.

As indicated earlier, many G protein–coupled receptors are linked directly to an intracellular enzyme. Drugs and other substances that exert their effects through receptor–G protein–enzyme systems often form (or inhibit the formation of) an intracellular compound known as a **second messenger**. In effect, the drug acts as the first messenger, which triggers a biochemical change in the cell, but the drug itself does not enter. The second messenger, which is the substance produced inside the cell, actually mediates the change in function.

The primary example of this second messenger strategy is the **adenylate cyclase–cyclic adenosine monophosphate (cAMP)** system present in many cells (Fig. 4-3).[18,19] Adenylate cyclase, an enzyme located on the inner surface of the cell membrane, is responsible for hydrolyzing adenosine triphosphate (ATP) into cAMP. Cyclic AMP acts as the second messenger in this system by activating other enzymes (i.e., protein kinases) throughout the cell. Drugs that bind to a surface receptor linked to a G_s protein will

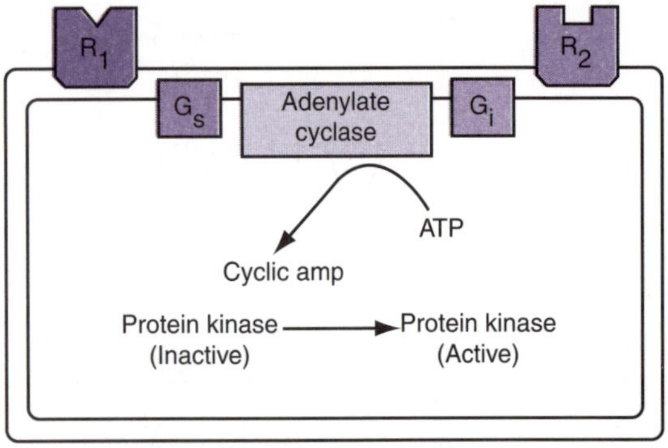

Figure ■ 4-3

A surface receptor–second messenger system. In this example, the second messenger is cAMP, which is synthesized from ATP by the adenylate cyclase enzyme. The enzyme is linked to surface receptors (R_1 and R_2) by regulatory G proteins. G_S stimulates the enzyme and G_i inhibits enzyme activity. Thus, a drug binding to R_1 will increase production of cAMP, while a different drug binding to R_2 will inhibit cAMP production.

increase adenylate cyclase activity, resulting in increased production of cAMP within the cell. Other drugs bound to a different receptor linked to a G_i protein will inhibit adenylate cyclase activity, resulting in decreased production of cAMP.

The adenylate cyclase–cAMP system is associated with specific membrane receptors such as the beta-adrenergic receptors.[20] Other surface receptors may also be linked to this particular effector–second messenger system, or they may be linked to other intracellular processes that use different second messengers, including:

- Cyclic guanine monophosphate (cGMP)
- Cyclic adenosine diphosphoribose (cADPR)
- Diacylglycerol, phosphoinositides
- Nicotinic acid adenine dinucleotide phosphate (NAADP)
- Calcium ions[21-27]

Finally, alterations in the synthesis, function, and regulation of G proteins have been identified in certain pathological conditions, including alcoholism, diabetes mellitus, heart failure, and certain tumors.[28-33] This illustrates the fact that G proteins seem to play an integral role in mediating the cell's response to various substances in both normal and disease states. The importance of these regulatory proteins will almost certainly continue to emerge as additional information about their structure and function becomes available.

INTRACELLULAR RECEPTORS

Receptors have been identified within the cell's cytoplasm and the nucleus.[34-36] These intracellular receptors are specific for certain endogenous hormones, and hormone-like drugs exert some of their effects by acting on these receptors. For instance, steroid and steroid-like compounds cause some of their effects by initially interacting with a receptor that is located in the cytoplasm.[36-38] Specifically, these hormones form a complex with the receptor in the cytoplasm, and the hormone-receptor complex then moves to the cell's nucleus, where it affects the function of specific genes. Thyroid hormones (thyroxin, triiodothyronine) likewise exert some of their effects by binding directly to a receptor located on the chromatin in the cell's nucleus.[34,35] In either case, cell function is altered because the hormone-receptor complex affects specific genes in the DNA and causes changes in gene expression and messenger RNA transcription. Altered transcription of specific genes results in altered cellular protein synthesis, which ultimately results in altered cell function.[38] Hence, certain endogenous hormones and hormone-like drugs exert some of their effects by acting on receptors located within the cell.

It has become clear that certain endogenous hormones and hormone-like drugs might also exert some of their effects by binding to a second set of receptors located on the cell surface.[34,39,40] That is, surface receptors have been identified for steroid and thyroid hormones, and stimulation of these surface receptors might complement or exaggerate the effects of the intracellular receptors.[34,41] The role of intracellular receptors, and their analogous surface receptors, is discussed further in this text in the chapters that deal with specific drugs that bind to these cellular components.

DRUG–RECEPTOR INTERACTIONS

The drug's ability to bind to any receptor depends on the drug's size and shape relative to the configuration of the receptor's binding site. The electrostatic attraction between the drug and the receptor may also be important in determining the extent to which the drug binds to the receptor. This drug–receptor interaction is somewhat analogous to a key fitting into a lock. The drug acts as a "key" that will only fit into certain receptors. Once inserted into a suitable receptor, the drug activates it, much like a key turning and "activating" the appropriate lock. To carry this analogy one step further, unlocking a door to a room would increase the "permeability" of the room in a manner similar to the direct effect of certain activated membrane receptors (e.g., the acetylcholine receptor on the neuromuscular junction). Other types of key–lock interactions would be "linked" to some other event, such as using a key to start an automobile engine. This is analogous to linking a surface receptor to some intracellular enzymatic process that would affect the internal "machinery" of the cell.

Although the key–lock analogy serves as a crude example of drug–receptor interactions, the attraction between a drug and any receptor is much more complex.[42] Binding a drug to a receptor is not an all-or-none phenomenon but is graded depending on the drug in question. Some drugs will bind readily to the receptor, some moderately, some very little, or some not at all. The term **affinity** is used to describe the amount of attraction between a drug and a receptor.[43] Affinity is actually related to the drug amount that is required to bind to the unoccupied receptors.[1] A drug with a high affinity binds readily to the open receptors, even if the concentration of the drug is relatively low. Drugs with moderate or low affinity require a higher concentration in the body before the receptors become occupied.

In addition to the relative degree of affinity of different drugs for a receptor, the status of the receptor can also vary under specific conditions. Receptors may exist in variable affinity states (super-high, high, low), depending on the influence of local regulators such as guanine nucleotides, ammonium ions, and divalent cations.[44-46] These local regulators are also known as **allosteric modulators**, which can bind to specific sites on the receptor that are distinct from the primary (drug) binding site and thereby increase or decrease the affinity for the drug.[44,47] Membrane receptors may also be influenced by the local environment of the lipid bilayer. The amount of flexibility or "fluidity" of the cell membrane is critical in providing a suitable environment in which membrane constituents such as receptors can optimally function. Physical and chemical factors (including other drugs) may change the membrane's fluidity and organization, thereby disrupting the normal orientation of the receptor and subsequently altering its affinity state and ability to interact with a drug.[48-50]

The exact way in which a drug activates a receptor has been the subject of considerable debate. Binding a drug to the receptor is hypothesized to cause the receptor to undergo some sort of temporary change in its shape or conformation. The change in structure of the activated receptor then mediates a change in cell function, either directly or by linking to some effector system. Studies have suggested that certain receptor proteins, such as the acetylcholine receptor, undergo a specific change in structure after binding with specific chemicals.[2,51] This certainly seems plausible because most receptors have been identified as protein molecules, and proteins are known to be able to reversibly change their shape and conformation as part of normal physiological function.[42] However, this should not rule out other possible ways in which an activated receptor may mediate changes in cell function. Future research will continue to clarify the role of conformational changes and other possible mechanisms of receptor activation.

FUNCTIONAL ASPECTS OF DRUG–RECEPTOR INTERACTIONS

The interaction between the drug and the receptor dictates several important aspects of pharmacology. Concepts such as drug selectivity, the relationship between dose and response, and the ability of a drug to block the effects of other chemicals can often be explained by how a drug interacts with its receptor. These concepts are addressed briefly here.

Drug Selectivity and Receptor Subtypes

A drug is said to be *selective* if it affects only one type of cell or tissue and produces a specific physiological response. For instance, a drug that is cardioselective will affect heart function without affecting other tissues such as the gastrointestinal tract or respiratory system. The selectivity of a particular drug is a function of its ability to interact with specific receptors on the target tissue and not with other receptors on the target tissue or on other tissues (Fig. 4-4). In reality, *drug selectivity* is a relative term because no drug produces only one effect. But drugs can be compared to one another with the more selective drug being able to affect one type of tissue or organ with only a minimum of other responses.

Drug selectivity is related closely to the fact that many receptor populations can be divided into

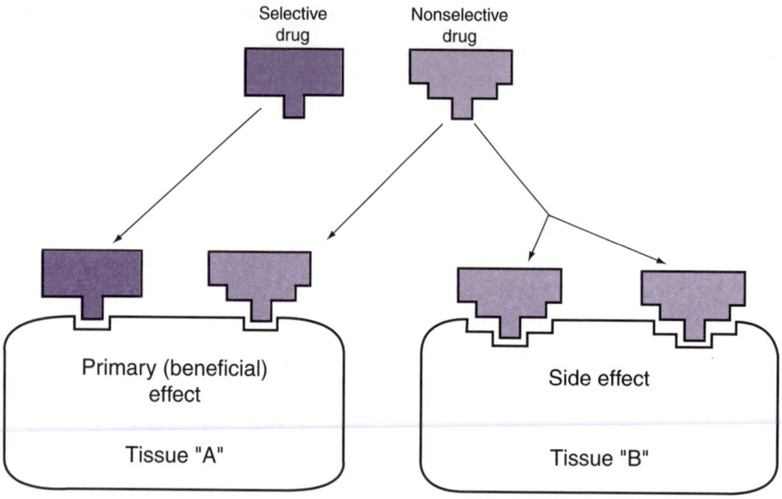

Figure ■ 4-4
Drug selectivity. The diagram represents an ideal situation where the selective drug produces only beneficial effects and the nonselective drug exerts both beneficial and nonbeneficial effects. *Drug selectivity* is a relative term, because all drugs produce some side effects; however, a selective drug produces fewer side effects than a nonselective agent.

various subtypes according to specific structural and functional differences between subgroups of the receptor. A primary example is the cholinergic (acetylcholine) receptor found on various tissues throughout the body. These receptors can be classified into two primary subtypes: muscarinic and nicotinic. Acetylcholine will bind to either subtype, but drugs such as nicotine will bind preferentially to the nicotinic subtype, and muscarine (a toxin found in certain mushrooms) will bind preferentially to the muscarinic subtype.

Other types of receptors can be divided and subdivided in a similar manner. For example, the adrenergic receptor (i.e., the receptor for epinephrine or "adrenaline") is divided into two primary subtypes (alpha and beta), with each subtype having two primary divisions (alpha-1 and alpha-2; beta-1 and beta-2). Epinephrine will stimulate all adrenergic receptor subtypes, but certain drugs will affect only one of the primary divisions (e.g., a beta-selective drug) or even one subtype within each division (e.g., a beta-1 selective drug). The functional significance of adrenergic and cholinergic receptors is discussed in more detail in Chapter 18. Receptor subtypes also exist for other substances (opioids, dopamine, GABA, hormones, etc.); the significance of these will be addressed in their respective chapters in this text.

The fact that we can classify many receptors into subtypes means we can develop drugs that will affect only one receptor subtype and therefore produce fairly selective effects with fewer side effects.[52-56] For example, a beta-1 selective drug will primarily affect the heart because the heart has a preponderance of the beta-1 subtype of adrenergic receptor, and other tissues (e.g., lungs, arterioles) contain other subtypes of adrenergic receptors. Research is ongoing to learn more about the structure and function of receptor populations and their subtypes.

Dose-Response

The shape of the typical dose-response curve (discussed in Chapter 1) is related to the number of receptors that are bound by the drug, because within certain limits of the drug concentration, the response is essentially proportional to the number of receptors occupied by the drug (see Fig. 1-2).[57,58] At low dosages, for example, only a few receptors are bound by the drug, so the effect is relatively small. As the dosage (and drug concentration) increases, more receptors become occupied and the response increases. Finally, at a certain dosage, all available receptors will be occupied, and the response will be maximal. Increasing the dosage beyond the point at which the maximal effect is reached will not produce any further increase in response because all the receptors are bound by the drug. However, the relationship between drug receptors and drug response is not a simple linear relationship for many drugs. For instance, a drug that occupies half the available receptors may produce a response that is greater than 50 percent of the maximal response.[59] Clearly, other factors influence the absolute magnitude of the response, including factors that affect the relative affinity for the drug and how well the occupied receptor can transmit the signal to the cell's effector mechanisms. Nonetheless, it is essentially true that increasing or decreasing the amount of drug available to the appropriate receptors will cause a concomitant increase or decrease in the response to that drug.[57,60]

Classification of Drugs: Agonist Versus Antagonist

So far, we have used drug–receptor interactions to describe the process by which a drug occupies a receptor and in some way activates it. The activated receptor then brings about a change in cell function. A drug that can bind to a receptor and initiate a change in the cell's function is referred to as an **agonist**. An agonist is identified as having affinity and efficacy.[59,61] As discussed earlier, *affinity* refers to the attraction, or desire, of the drug to bind to a given receptor. The second characteristic, *efficacy*, indicates that the drug will activate the receptor and change the function of the cell. Whereas an agonist has both affinity and efficacy, an **antagonist** has only affinity. This means the drug will bind to the receptor, but it will not cause any direct change in the function of the receptor or cell (Fig. 4-5). Antagonists are significant because, by occupying the receptor, they prevent the agonistic compound from having any effect on the cell. Antagonists are often referred to as *blockers* because of their ability to block the effect of another chemical. The primary pharmacological significance of these antagonists has been their use in blocking the effects of certain endogenous compounds. A classic example is the use of beta blockers, which occupy specific receptors on the myocardium, thus preventing circulating catecholamines from increasing heart rate and contractility. Other examples of antagonistic drugs are discussed in their appropriate chapters.

Competitive Versus Noncompetitive Antagonists

Pharmacological antagonists are generally divided into two categories depending on whether they are competing with the agonist for the receptor.[59,62,63] Competitive antagonists are so classified because they vie for the same receptor as the agonist. In other words, both the agonist and antagonist have an equal opportunity to occupy the receptor. Whichever drug concentration is greater tends to have the predominant effect. If the number of competitive antagonist molecules far exceeds the number of agonist molecules, the antagonists will occupy most of the receptors and the overall effect will be inhibition of the particular response. Conversely, a high concentration of an agonist relative to an antagonist will produce a pharmacological effect, because the agonist will occupy most of the receptors. In fact, raising the concentration of the agonist with a competitive antagonist present can actually overcome

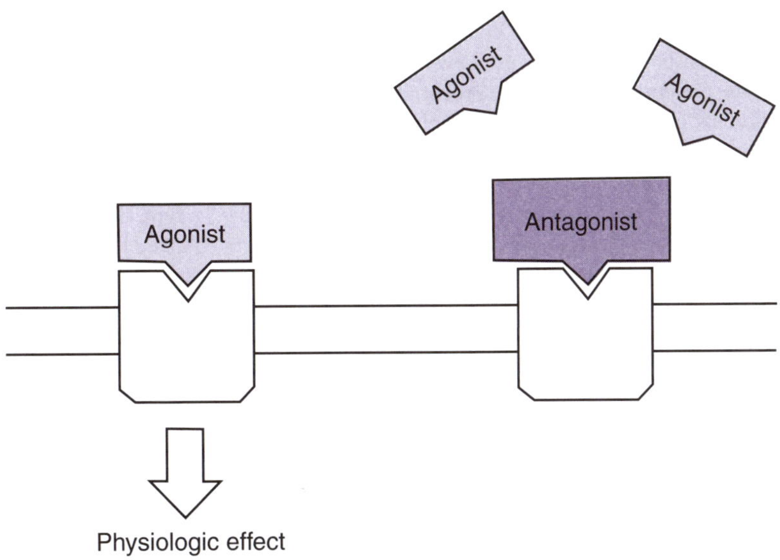

Figure ■ 4-5
Agonist versus antagonist drug classifications. The antagonist (blocker) prevents the agonist from binding to the receptor and exerting a physiological effect.

the original inhibition, because the competitive antagonists form rather weak bonds with the receptor and can be displaced from it by a sufficient concentration of agonist molecules.[1] This is an important advantage of competitive antagonists because, if necessary, the inhibition caused by the antagonist can be overcome simply by administering high concentrations of the agonist.

In contrast to competitive antagonists, *noncompetitive antagonists* form strong, essentially permanent, bonds to the receptor. Noncompetitive antagonists, also called *irreversible antagonists*, either have an extremely high affinity for the receptor or form irreversible covalent bonds to it.[1] Once bound to the receptor, the noncompetitive antagonist cannot be displaced by the agonist, regardless of how much agonist is present. Thus the term *noncompetitive* refers to the inability of the agonist to compete with the antagonist for the receptor site. The obvious disadvantage to this type of receptor blocker is that the inhibition cannot be overcome in cases of an overdose of the antagonist. Also, noncompetitive antagonists often remain bound for the receptor's life span, and their effect is terminated only after the receptor has been replaced as part of the normal protein turnover within the cell. Consequently, the inhibition produced by a noncompetitive blocker tends to remain in effect for long periods (i.e., several days).

Partial Agonists

Drugs are classified as *partial agonists* when they do not evoke a maximal response compared to a strong agonist. This classification is used even though the partial agonist occupies all available receptors.[1] In fact, partial agonists can be thought of as having an efficacy that lies somewhere between that of a full agonist and a full noncompetitive antagonist. The lack of a maximal response is not caused by decreased drug–receptor affinity. On the contrary, partial agonists often have a high affinity for the receptor. The decreased efficacy may occur because the partial agonist does not completely activate the receptor after it binds, and that binding results in a lower level of any postreceptor events (e.g., less activation of G proteins, smaller changes in enzyme function).

The realization that certain drugs act as partial agonists has led to the idea that a range of efficacy can exist, depending on how specific drugs interact with their respective receptors.[1] At one end of this range are the drugs that bind strongly and produce a high degree of efficacy (strong agonists), while the other end of the spectrum contains drugs that bind strongly and produce no effect (strong antagonists). Agents that fall between these two extremes (partial agonists) can have varying degrees of agonistic activity. Likewise, a new concept has emerged regarding "biased" agonists. These agents may activate receptors in such a way as to activate only certain signaling pathways, as opposed to the full or unbiased agonist that activates all signaling pathways related to that receptor.[64,65] Partial agonists and biased agonists can also have certain clinical advantages. For instance, certain beta blockers with biased agonism may produce preferential cardiac effects, and antipsychotic drugs that function as partial agonists may reduce psychotic episodes without excessive side effects.[61,64]

Mixed Agonist–Antagonists and Inverse Agonists

Some agents will stimulate certain receptor subtypes while simultaneously blocking the effects of endogenous substances on other receptor subtypes (the concept of receptor subtypes was addressed earlier in this section). These agents are known as *mixed agonist–antagonists*, and they are especially useful in certain clinical situations.[66,67,68] In some women, for example, it is often beneficial to stimulate estrogen receptors on bone to prevent osteoporosis, while simultaneously blocking the effects of estrogen on breast tissues to prevent cancer. Certain drugs known as **selective estrogen receptor modulators** (SERMs; see Chapters 30, 31, and 36) can differentiate between the subtypes of estrogen receptors on these two tissues and act as an agonist on bone and an antagonist on breast tissues.[68] These agents are a good example of drugs with mixed agonist–antagonist activity, and other drugs with this type of mixed activity will be discussed in their respective chapters throughout this text.

Finally, pharmacologists have proposed that some drugs could function as inverse agonists.[52,69] As this classification implies, these drugs would bind to the same receptor as the agonist but have the *opposite* effect of the agonist on cellular function. This effect is different from a traditional, or neutral, antagonist that binds to the tissue and simply prevents an increase in the agonist's effect. By creating the opposite effect, inverse agonists could bring about a decrease in activity in situations where the receptor is too active or overstimulated.[52,70] Pharmacologists are currently developing various inverse agonists for specific clinical situations, and studies are ongoing to determine how inverse agonists might be useful as therapeutic agents.

RECEPTOR REGULATION

Receptor responses are not static but are regulated by endogenous and exogenous factors. In general, a prolonged increase in the stimulation of various receptors will lead to a *decrease* in receptor function, and decreased stimulation will lead to an *increase* in receptor numbers or sensitivity (Fig. 4-6). The mechanisms and significance of these receptor changes are described here.

Receptor Desensitization and Down-Regulation

As presented in Figure 4-6, overstimulation of postsynaptic receptors by endogenous substances (neurotransmitters, hormones) or by exogenous agonists (drugs) may lead to a functional decrease in the appropriate receptor population.[59] In effect, the cell becomes less responsive to the prolonged stimulation by decreasing the number of active receptors. The term **desensitization** is typically used to describe a fairly brief and transient decrease in responsiveness.[59,71] Desensitization is believed to occur because of the addition of phosphate residues (phosphorylation) or some other chemical modification to the receptor protein.[71,72] Adding a phosphate molecule seems to cause some membrane receptors to uncouple from their intermediate regulatory proteins and consequently from the rest of the cell's biochemical machinery.[72] Phosphorylation may also cause the receptor to be withdrawn from the cell membrane by endocytosis and sequestered temporarily within the cell; this process is known commonly as *receptor internalization*.[71,73] Receptor desensitization and internalization contribute to the decrease in response that may be seen even though the agonist remains present in high concentration in the body. However, the decrease in responsiveness caused by desensitization and internalization is usually fairly brief, and a return to normal response may occur within a few minutes after the agonist is removed.

Receptor **down-regulation** describes a slower, more prolonged process in which the number of available receptors is diminished.[59] Although the exact mechanisms responsible for down-regulation are not fully understood, it appears that prolonged exposure of the agonist causes increased receptor removal, decreased receptor synthesis, or a combination of increased removal and decreased synthesis.[1,74] The cell undergoes a decrease in responsiveness that remains in effect long after the agonist is removed (i.e., several days). Normal sensitivity to the agonist will be reestablished

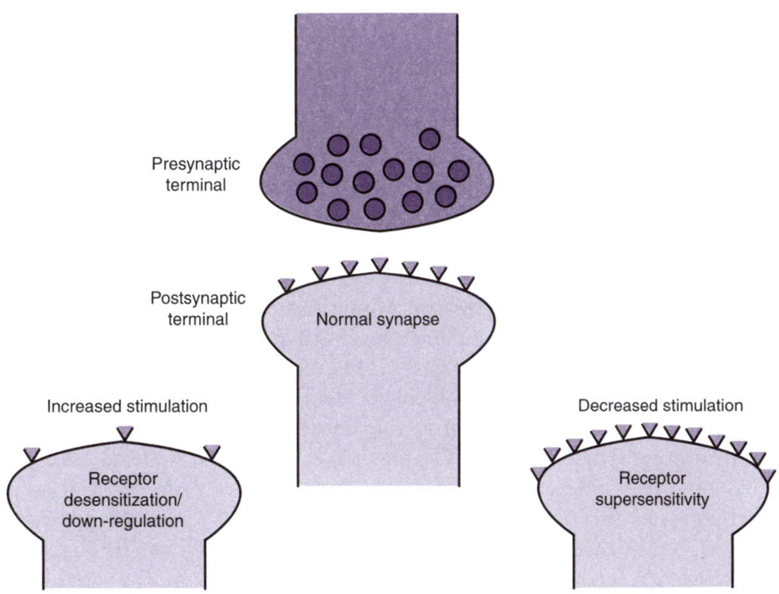

Figure ■ 4-6
Receptor regulation. Functionally active receptor sites are represented by a "▼." Increased stimulation results in a decrease in receptor numbers (desensitization/ down-regulation), while decreased stimulation causes increased receptor numbers (supersensitivity).

only when the cell has the chance to replace and restore the receptors that were eliminated during down-regulation.

Receptor desensitization and down-regulation appear to be examples of a negative feedback system used by the cell to prevent overstimulation by an agonist. The cell appears to selectively decrease its responsiveness to a particular stimulus to protect itself from excessive perturbation. Receptor down-regulation is important pharmacologically because it may be one of the primary reasons that a decrease in drug responsiveness occurs when patients use certain drugs for prolonged periods.[75,76] Drug tolerance, which is defined as the need to progressively increase the dose to achieve therapeutic effects, may be due in part to changes in receptor sensitivity and function. Drug tolerance, however, is a very complex process that may involve other changes in cell function besides just a change in receptor activity. On the other hand, receptor desensitization and down-regulation have been linked to several pathological situations, including acute CNS injury, cardiac disease, or viral infections. Drugs that prevent these decreases in receptor function could prove useful in these conditions.[77-80] Conversely, some drugs, such as antidepressants, may exert their beneficial effects by intentionally causing receptor down-regulation and desensitization in certain neural pathways that cause clinical depression. These drugs are discussed in detail in Chapter 7.

Receptor Supersensitivity

A prolonged decrease in the stimulation of the postsynaptic receptors can result in a functional increase in receptor sensitivity. The best example of this is the denervation supersensitivity seen when a peripheral nerve is severed.[81] The lack of presynaptic neurotransmitter release results in a compensatory increase in postsynaptic receptor numbers on the muscle cell. Similarly, the loss of the endogenous neurotransmitter dopamine in neurodegenerative conditions such as Parkinson disease can result in supersensitivity of receptors for that neurotransmitter.[82] This increased receptor sensitivity becomes problematic because administration of dopamine-like drugs can cause excessive or untoward responses (see Chapter 10).[83]

A somewhat different type of denervation supersensitivity can also occur when a patient uses receptor antagonist drugs for prolonged periods. Here the postsynaptic receptors are blocked by the antagonistic drug and are unavailable for stimulation by the appropriate agonist. The postsynaptic neuron interprets this as the synapse being denervated and responds by manufacturing more receptors, resulting in a compensatory *increase* in function at the synapse that was supposed to be blocked by the antagonist. Again, drug therapy could be affected in this situation because the dose of the blocker will need to be altered to cope with the new, larger population of receptors.

NONRECEPTOR DRUG MECHANISMS

Certain drugs appear to exert their effects through mechanisms that do not involve binding to a specific cellular component.[59] For example, some cancer chemotherapeutic agents act as "antimetabolites" by becoming incorporated into the manufacture of specific cellular components. The drug acts as an improper ingredient in the biosynthesis of the component, so that the cell does not manufacture harmful or unwanted materials. In addition, many common antacids work by directly neutralizing stomach acid—that is, these drugs act via a chemical reaction rather than through a specific receptor molecule. Other drugs may affect cell function without first binding to a receptor by directly altering enzyme function or by acting as "chelating agents," which bind to harmful compounds such as heavy metals and prevent them from exerting toxic effects. Additional nonreceptor-mediated mechanisms of specific compounds are discussed when those drugs are examined in their respective chapters.

SUMMARY

Many drugs and endogenous chemicals exert their effects by first binding to and activating a cellular receptor. Cellular receptors are proteins located on the cell surface or at specific locations within the cell. The primary role of the receptor is to recognize specific chemicals from the vast number of compounds that are introduced to the cell and to initiate a change in cell function by interacting with a specific agent. Activated receptors mediate a change in function by altering cell permeability or modifying the biochemical function within the cell, or both. The exact mechanism by which a receptor affects cell function depends on the type and location of the receptor.

Drug–receptor interactions are significant pharmacologically because they account for some of the basic pharmacodynamic principles such as drug selectivity and the relationship between drug dose and response. Also, the development of chemical agents that block specific receptors (antagonists) has been useful in moderating the effects of endogenous compounds on specific physiological processes. Finally, changes in receptor number and sensitivity are important in the altered response seen in certain drugs with prolonged use. Information about the relationship between drugs and cellular receptors has been, and will continue to be, critical to our understanding of how drugs work and in helping researchers develop new compounds.

REFERENCES

1. von Zastrow M. Drug receptors and pharmacodynamics. In: Katzung BG, ed. *Basic and Clinical Pharmacology.* 12th ed. New York: Lange Medical Books/McGraw Hill; 2012.
2. Sine SM. End-plate acetylcholine receptor: structure, mechanism, pharmacology, and disease. *Physiol Rev.* 2012;92:1189-1234.
3. Araud T, Wonnacott S, Bertrand D. Associated proteins: the universal toolbox controlling ligand gated ion channel function. *Biochem Pharmacol.* 2010;80:160-169.
4. Leach K, Simms J, Sexton PM, Christopoulos A. Structure-function studies of muscarinic acetylcholine receptors. *Handb Exp Pharmacol.* 2012;208:29-48.
5. Fagerlund MJ, Eriksson LI. Current concepts in neuromuscular transmission. *Br J Anaesth.* 2009;103:108-114.
6. Martyn JA, Fagerlund MJ, Eriksson LI. Basic principles of neuromuscular transmission. *Anaesthesia.* 2009;64(suppl 1):1-9.
7. Sankar R. GABA(A) receptor physiology and its relationship to the mechanism of action of the 1,5-benzodiazepine clobazam. *CNS Drugs.* 2012;26:229-244.
8. Trincavelli ML, Da Pozzo E, Daniele S, Martini C. The GABAA-BZR complex as target for the development of anxiolytic drugs. *Curr Top Med Chem.* 2012;12:254-269.
9. Chakravarti B, Chattopadhyay N, Brown EM. Signaling through the extracellular calcium-sensing receptor (CaSR). *Adv Exp Med Biol.* 2012;740:103-142.
10. Fagni L. Diversity of metabotropic glutamate receptor-interacting proteins and pathophysiological functions. *Adv Exp Med Biol.* 2012;970:63-79.
11. Choura M, Rebaï A. Receptor tyrosine kinases: from biology to pathology. *J Recept Signal Transduct Res.* 2011;31:387-394.
12. Takeuchi K, Ito F. Receptor tyrosine kinases and targeted cancer therapeutics. *Biol Pharm Bull.* 2011;34:1774-1780.
13. Siddle K. Signalling by insulin and IGF receptors: supporting acts and new players. *J Mol Endocrinol.* 2011;47:R1-10.
14. Chun L, Zhang WH, Liu JF. Structure and ligand recognition of class C GPCRs. *Acta Pharmacol Sin.* 2012;33:312-323.
15. Deupi X, Standfuss J. Structural insights into agonist-induced activation of G-protein-coupled receptors. *Curr Opin Struct Biol.* 2011;21:541-551.
16. Trzaskowski B, Latek D, Yuan S, Ghoshdastider U, Debinski A, Filipek S. Action of molecular switches in GPCRs—theoretical and experimental studies. *Curr Med Chem.* 2012;19:1090-1109.
17. Millar RP, Newton CL. The year in G protein-coupled receptor research. *Mol Endocrinol.* 2010;24:261-274.
18. Antoni FA. New paradigms in cAMP signalling. *Mol Cell Endocrinol.* 2012;353:3-9.
19. Bai G, Knapp GS, McDonough KA. Cyclic AMP signalling in mycobacteria: redirecting the conversation with a common currency. *Cell Microbiol.* 2011;13:349-358.
20. Pierre S, Eschenhagen T, Geisslinger G, Scholich K. Capturing adenylyl cyclases as potential drug targets. *Nat Rev Drug Discov.* 2009;8:321-335.
21. Balla T, Szentpetery Z, Kim YJ. Phosphoinositide signaling: new tools and insights. *Physiology.* 2009;24:231-244.
22. Giusto NM, Pasquaré SJ, Salvador GA, et al. Lipid second messengers and related enzymes in vertebrate rod outer segments. *J Lipid Res.* 2010;51:685-700.
23. Guse AH. Linking NAADP to ion channel activity: a unifying hypothesis. *Sci Signal.* 2012;5:pe18.
24. Konieczny V, Keebler MV, Taylor CW. Spatial organization of intracellular Ca2+ signals. *Semin Cell Dev Biol.* 2012;23:172-180.
25. Kots AY, Bian K, Murad F. Nitric oxide and cyclic GMP signaling pathway as a focus for drug development. *Curr Med Chem.* 2011;18:3299-3305.
26. Rah SY, Mushtaq M, Nam TS, Kim SH, Kim UH. Generation of cyclic ADP-ribose and nicotinic acid adenine dinucleotide phosphate by CD38 for Ca2+ signaling in interleukin-8-treated lymphokine-activated killer cells. *J Biol Chem.* 2010;285:21877-21887.
27. Smolenski A. Novel roles of cAMP/cGMP-dependent signaling in platelets. *J Thromb Haemost.* 2012;10:167-176.
28. Kowluru A. Small G proteins in islet beta-cell function. *Endocr Rev.* 2010;31:52-78.
29. Lappano R, Maggiolini M. GPCRs and cancer. *Acta Pharmacol Sin.* 2012;33:351-362.
30. Lymperopoulos A, Rengo G, Koch WJ. GRK2 inhibition in heart failure: something old, something new. *Curr Pharm Des.* 2012;18:186-191.
31. Reinkober J, Tscheschner H, Pleger ST, et al. Targeting GRK2 by gene therapy for heart failure: benefits above β-blockade. *Gene Ther.* 2012;19:686-693.
32. Ruby CL, Adams CA, Knight EJ, et al. An essential role for adenosine signaling in alcohol abuse. *Curr Drug Abuse Rev.* 2010;3:163-174.
33. Talukdar S, Olefsky JM, Osborn O. Targeting GPR120 and other fatty acid-sensing GPCRs ameliorates insulin resistance and inflammatory diseases. *Trends Pharmacol Sci.* 2011;32:543-550.
34. Cheng SY, Leonard JL, Davis PJ. Molecular aspects of thyroid hormone actions. *Endocr Rev.* 2010;31:139-170.
35. McEwan IJ. Nuclear receptors: one big family. *Methods Mol Biol.* 2009;505:3-18.
36. Vandevyver S, Dejager L, Libert C. On the trail of the glucocorticoid receptor: into the nucleus and back. *Traffic.* 2012;13:364-374.
37. Heitzer MD, Wolf IM, Sanchez ER, et al. Glucocorticoid receptor physiology. *Rev Endocr Metab Disord.* 2007;8:321-330.
38. Revollo JR, Cidlowski JA. Mechanisms generating diversity in glucocorticoid receptor signaling. *Ann NY Acad Sci.* 2009;1179:167-178.

39. Krug AW, Pojoga LH, Williams GH, Adler GK. Cell membrane-associated mineralocorticoid receptors? New evidence. *Hypertension*. 2011;57:1019-1025.
40. Levin ER. Minireview: Extranuclear steroid receptors: roles in modulation of cell functions. *Mol Endocrinol.* 2011;25:377-384.
41. Groeneweg FL, Karst H, de Kloet ER, Joëls M. Mineralocorticoid and glucocorticoid receptors at the neuronal membrane, regulators of nongenomic corticosteroid signalling. *Mol Cell Endocrinol.* 2012;350:299-309.
42. Spyrakis F, BidonChanal A, Barril X, Luque FJ. Protein flexibility and ligand recognition: challenges for molecular modeling. *Curr Top Med Chem.* 2011;11:192-210.
43. Frecer V. Theoretical prediction of drug-receptor interactions. *Drug Metabol Drug Interact.* 2011;26:91-104.
44. Kumar R, McEwan IJ. Allosteric modulators of steroid hormone receptors: structural dynamics and gene regulation. *Endocr Rev.* 2012;33:271-299.
45. Li M, Li C, Allen A, Stanley CA, Smith TJ. The structure and allosteric regulation of mammalian glutamate dehydrogenase. *Arch Biochem Biophys*. 2012;519:69-80.
46. Yevenes GE, Zeilhofer HU. Allosteric modulation of glycine receptors. *Br J Pharmacol.* 2011;164:224-236.
47. Digby GJ, Shirey JK, Conn PJ. Allosteric activators of muscarinic receptors as novel approaches for treatment of CNS disorders. *Mol Biosyst.* 2010;6:1345-1354.
48. Brzeszczynska J, Pieniazek A, Gwozdzinski L, et al. Structural alterations of erythrocyte membrane components induced by exhaustive exercise. *Appl Physiol Nutr Metab.* 2008;33: 1223-1231.
49. Maccarrone M, Bernardi G, Agrò AF, Centonze D. Cannabinoid receptor signaling in neurodegenerative diseases: a potential role for membrane fluidity disturbance. *Br J Pharmacol.* 2011; 163:1379-1390.
50. Tavolari S, Munarini A, Storci G, et al. The decrease of cell membrane fluidity by the non-steroidal anti-inflammatory drug Licofelone inhibits epidermal growth factor receptor signalling and triggers apoptosis in HCA-7 colon cancer cells. *Cancer Lett.* 2012;321(2):187-194.
51. Jadey S, Auerbach A. An integrated catch-and-hold mechanism activates nicotinic acetylcholine receptors. *J Gen Physiol.* 2012;140:17-28.
52. Atack JR. GABAA receptor subtype-selective modulators. II. α5-selective inverse agonists for cognition enhancement. *Curr Top Med Chem.* 2011;11:1203-1214.
53. Baker JG, Hill SJ, Summers RJ. Evolution of β-blockers: from anti-anginal drugs to ligand-directed signalling. *Trends Pharmacol Sci.* 2011;32:227-234.
54. Bubser M, Byun N, Wood MR, Jones CK. Muscarinic receptor pharmacology and circuitry for the modulation of cognition. *Handb Exp Pharmacol.* 2012;208:121-166.
55. Conn PJ, Jones CK, Lindsley CW. Subtype-selective allosteric modulators of muscarinic receptors for the treatment of CNS disorders. *Trends Pharmacol Sci*. 2009;30:148-155.
56. Shanle EK, Xu W. Selectively targeting estrogen receptors for cancer treatment. *Adv Drug Deliv Rev.* 2010;62:1265-1276.
57. Church MK, Gillard M, Sargentini-Maier ML, Poggesi I, Campbell A, Benedetti MS. From pharmacokinetics to therapeutics. *Drug Metab Rev.* 2009;41:455-474.
58. Nord M, Farde L. Antipsychotic occupancy of dopamine receptors in schizophrenia. *CNS Neurosci Ther.* 2011;17:97-103.
59. Blumenthal DK, Garrison JC. Pharmacodynamics: molecular mechanisms of drug action. In: Brunton LL, et al, eds. *The Pharmacological Basis of Therapeutics.* 12th ed. New York: McGraw Hill; 2011.
60. Sparshatt A, Taylor D, Patel MX, Kapur S. Relationship between daily dose, plasma concentrations, dopamine receptor occupancy, and clinical response to quetiapine: a review. *J Clin Psychiatry.* 2011;72:1108-1123.
61. Strange PG. Agonist binding, agonist affinity and agonist efficacy at G protein-coupled receptors. *Br J Pharmacol.* 2008;153:1353-1363.
62. Helm S, Trescot AM, Colson J, Sehgal N, Silverman S. Opioid antagonists, partial agonists, and agonists/antagonists: the role of office-based detoxification. *Pain Physician.* 2008;11:225-235.
63. Meltzer HY, Horiguchi M, Massey BW. The role of serotonin in the NMDA receptor antagonist models of psychosis and cognitive impairment. *Psychopharmacology*. 2011;213:289-305.
64. Andresen BT. A pharmacological primer of biased agonism. *Endocr Metab Immune Disord Drug Targets.* 2011;11:92-98.
65. Reiter E, Ahn S, Shukla AK, Lefkowitz RJ. Molecular mechanism of β-arrestin-biased agonism at seven-transmembrane receptors. *Annu Rev Pharmacol Toxicol.* 2012;52:179-197.
66. Kojetin DJ, Burris TP, Jensen EV, Khan SA. Implications of the binding of tamoxifen to the coactivator recognition site of the estrogen receptor. *Endocr Relat Cancer.* 2008;15:851-870.
67. Sterniczuk R, Stepkowski A, Jones M, Antle MC. Enhancement of photic shifts with the 5-HT1A mixed agonist/antagonist NAN-190: intra-suprachiasmatic nucleus pathway. *Neuroscience*. 2008;153:571-580.
68. McDonnell DP, Wardell SE. The molecular mechanisms underlying the pharmacological actions of ER modulators: implications for new drug discovery in breast cancer. *Curr Opin Pharmacol.* 2010;10:620-628.
69. Fong TM, Heymsfield SB. Cannabinoid-1 receptor inverse agonists: current understanding of mechanism of action and unanswered questions. *Int J Obes.* 2009;33:947-955.
70. Ito C. Histamine H3-receptor inverse agonists as novel antipsychotics. *Cent Nerv Syst Agents Med Chem.* 2009;9:132-136.
71. Vasudevan NT, Mohan ML, Goswami SK, Naga Prasad SV. Regulation of β-adrenergic receptor function: an emphasis on receptor resensitization. *Cell Cycle*. 2011;10:3684-3691.
72. Evron T, Daigle TL, Caron MG. GRK2: multiple roles beyond G protein-coupled receptor desensitization. *Trends Pharmacol Sci.* 2012;33:154-164.
73. Koch T, Höllt V. Role of receptor internalization in opioid tolerance and dependence. *Pharmacol Ther.* 2008;117:199-206.
74. Menon KM, Menon B. Structure, function and regulation of gonadotropin receptors—a perspective. *Mol Cell Endocrinol.* 2012;356(1-2):88-97.
75. Chu J, Zheng H, Zhang Y, et al. Agonist-dependent mu-opioid receptor signaling can lead to heterologous desensitization. *Cell Signal.* 2010;22:684-696.
76. Dang VC, Christie MJ. Mechanisms of rapid opioid receptor desensitization, resensitization and tolerance in brain neurons. *Br J Pharmacol.* 2012;165:1704-1716.
77. Huang ZM, Gold JI, Koch WJ. G protein-coupled receptor kinases in normal and failing myocardium. *Front Biosci.* 2011;16:3047-3060.
78. Kamal FA, Smrcka AV, Blaxall BC. Taking the heart failure battle inside the cell: small molecule targeting of Gβγ subunits. *J Mol Cell Cardiol.* 2011;51:462-467.

79. Sherrill JD, Miller WE. Desensitization of herpesvirus-encoded G protein-coupled receptors. *Life Sci.* 2008;82:125-134.
80. Suo WZ, Li L. Dysfunction of G protein-coupled receptor kinases in Alzheimer's disease. *Scientific World Journal.* 2010; 10:1667-1678.
81. Katzung BG. Introduction to autonomic pharmacology. In: Katzung BG, ed. *Basic and Clinical Pharmacology.* 12th ed. New York: Lange Medical Books/McGraw Hill; 2012.
82. Prieto GA, Perez-Burgos A, Fiordelisio T, et al. Dopamine D(2)-class receptor supersensitivity as reflected in Ca2+ current modulation in neostriatal neurons. *Neuroscience.* 2009;164: 345-350.
83. Iravani MM, McCreary AC, Jenner P. Striatal plasticity in Parkinson's disease and L-dopa induced dyskinesia. *Parkinsonism Relat Disord.* 2012;18(suppl 1):S123-125.

SECTION

2

Pharmacology of the Central Nervous System

CHAPTER 5

General Principles of Central Nervous System Pharmacology

The central nervous system (CNS) is responsible for controlling bodily functions, and it is the center for behavioral and intellectual abilities. Neurons within the CNS are organized into highly complex patterns that mediate information through synaptic interactions. Clinicians prescribe CNS drugs to modify the activity of these neurons in order to treat specific disorders or to alter the general level of arousal of the CNS. This chapter presents a simplified introduction to the organization of the CNS and the general drug strategies medical practitioners use to alter activity within the brain and spinal cord. This chapter is not intended to be an extensive review of neuroanatomy and neurophysiology; the references at the end of this chapter include several excellent resources on this topic.[1-3] However, this chapter will review certain neuroanatomical and neurophysiological concepts that will help you understand how drugs can affect CNS function. These concepts will likewise be important when we examine the actions of specific CNS drugs in the next several chapters in this book.

CNS ORGANIZATION

The CNS can be grossly divided into the brain and spinal cord (Fig. 5-1). The brain is subdivided according to anatomic or functional criteria. The following is a brief overview of the general organization of the brain and spinal cord, with some indication of where particular CNS drugs tend to exert their effects.

Cerebrum

The largest and most rostral aspect of the brain is the cerebrum (see Fig. 5-1). The cerebrum consists of bilateral hemispheres, with each hemisphere divided anatomically into several lobes (frontal, temporal, parietal, and occipital). The outer cerebrum, or cerebral cortex, is the highest order of conscious function and integration in the CNS. Specific cortical areas are responsible for sensory and motor functions as well as intellectual and cognitive abilities. Other cortical areas are involved in short-term memory and speech. The cortex also operates in a somewhat supervisory capacity regarding lower brain functioning and may influence the control of other activities, such as the autonomic nervous system.

Most CNS therapeutic medications tend to affect cortical function indirectly by first altering the function of lower brain and spinal cord structures. An exception is the group of drugs used to treat epilepsy, which are often targeted directly for hyperexcitable neurons in the cerebral cortex. In addition, drugs that attempt to enhance cognitive function in conditions such as Alzheimer disease (cholinergic stimulants; see Chapter 19) might also exert their primary effects in the cerebrum.

Basal Ganglia

A group of specific areas located deep within the cerebral hemispheres is collectively termed the *basal*

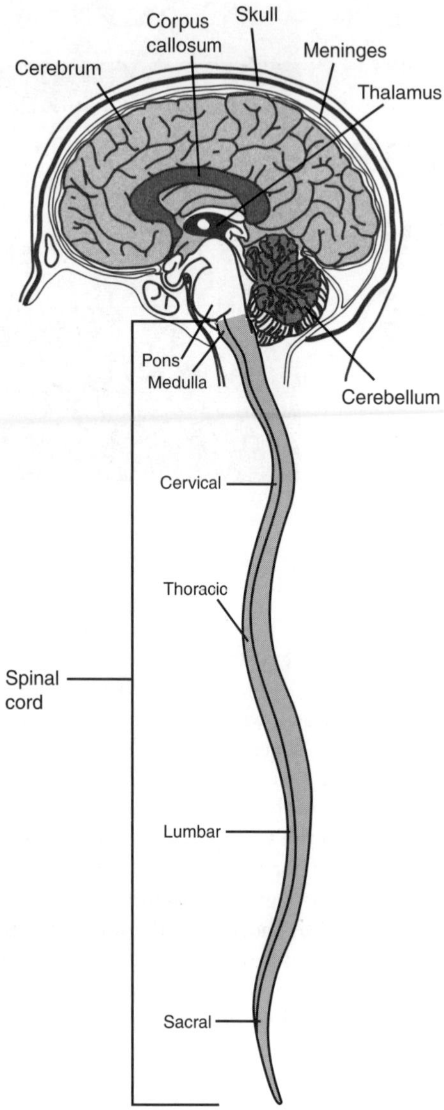

Figure ■ 5-1
General organization of the CNS.

ganglia. Its components include the caudate nucleus, putamen, globus pallidus, lentiform nucleus, and substantia nigra. The basal ganglia are primarily involved in the control of motor activities; deficits in this area are significant in movement disorders such as Parkinson disease and Huntington chorea. Certain medications that treat these movement disorders exert their effects by interacting with basal ganglia structures.

Diencephalon

The area of the brain enclosing the third ventricle is the diencephalon, which consists of several important structures, including the thalamus and hypothalamus. The thalamus contains distinct nuclei that are crucial in the integration of certain types of sensations and their relay to other areas of the brain (such as the somatosensory cortex). The hypothalamus is involved in the control of diverse body functions, including temperature control, appetite, water balance, and certain emotional reactions. The hypothalamus is also significant in its control over the function of hormonal release from the pituitary gland. Several CNS drugs affecting sensation and control of the body functions listed manifest their effects by interacting with the thalamus and hypothalamus.

Mesencephalon and Brainstem

The *mesencephalon*, or *midbrain*, serves as a bridge between the higher areas of the brain (cerebrum and diencephalon) and the *brainstem*. The brainstem consists of the pons and the medulla oblongata. In addition to serving as a pathway between the higher brain and spinal cord, the midbrain and brainstem are the locations of centers responsible for controlling respiration and cardiovascular function (vasomotor center).

The reticular formation is also located in the midbrain and brainstem. The reticular formation is comprised of a collection of neurons that extend from the reticular substance of the upper spinal cord through the midbrain and the thalamus. The reticular formation monitors and controls consciousness and is important in regulating the amount of arousal or alertness in the cerebral cortex. Consequently, CNS drugs that affect the individual's arousal state tend to exert their effects on the reticular formation. Sedative-hypnotics and general anesthetics tend to decrease activity in the reticular formation, whereas certain CNS stimulants (e.g., caffeine, amphetamines) may increase arousal through a stimulatory effect on reticular formation neurons.

Cerebellum

The cerebellum lies posterior to the brainstem and is separated from it by the fourth ventricle. Anatomically it is divided into two hemispheres, each consisting of three lobes (anterior, posterior, and flocculonodular). The cerebellum helps plan and coordinate motor activity and is responsible for comparing the actual movement with the intended motor pattern. The cerebellum interprets various sensory input and helps modulate motor output so that the actual movement closely resembles the intended motor program. The cerebellum also controls the vestibular mechanisms responsible for maintaining balance and posture. Therapeutic medications are not usually targeted directly for the cerebellum, but incoordination and other movement disorders may result if a drug exerts a toxic side effect on the cerebellum.

Limbic System

So far, all of the structures described have been grouped primarily by their anatomic relationships with the brain. The limbic system is comprised of several structures that are dispersed throughout the brain but are often considered as a functional unit or system within the CNS. Major components of the limbic system include cortical structures (e.g., the amygdala, hippocampus, and cingulate gyrus), the hypothalamus, certain thalamic nuclei, mamillary bodies, septum pellucidum, and several other structures and tracts. These structures are involved in the control of emotional and behavioral activity. Certain aspects of motivation, aggression, sexual activity, and instinctive responses may be influenced by activity within the limbic system. CNS drugs affecting these aspects of behavior, including some antianxiety and antipsychotic medications, are believed to exert their beneficial effects primarily by altering activity in the limbic structures.

Spinal Cord

At the caudal end of the brainstem, the CNS continues distally as the spinal cord. The spinal cord is cylindrically shaped and consists of centrally located gray matter that is surrounded by white matter. The gray matter serves as an area for synaptic connections between various neurons. The white matter consists of the myelinated axons of neurons, which are grouped into tracts ascending or descending between the brain and specific levels of the cord.

Certain CNS drugs exert some or all of their effects by modifying synaptic transmission in specific areas of gray matter, while other CNS drugs, such as narcotic analgesics, may exert an effect on synaptic transmission in the gray matter of the cord as well as on synapses in other areas of the brain. Some drugs may be specifically directed toward the white matter of the cord. Drugs such as local anesthetics can block action potential propagation in the white matter so that ascending or descending information is interrupted (e.g., a spinal block).

THE BLOOD-BRAIN BARRIER

The **blood-brain barrier** refers to the unique structure and function of CNS capillaries, which act as a selective filter and protects the CNS by limiting the substances that enter the brain and spinal cord.[4,5] Certain substances are not able to pass from the bloodstream into the CNS, even though these substances are able to pass without difficulty from the systemic circulation into other peripheral tissues. This is because CNS capillaries have a unique structure and function that prevents many substances from entering the brain and spinal cord—hence the term *blood-brain barrier*. This barrier effect is caused primarily by the tight junctions that occur between capillary endothelial cells. In fact, CNS capillaries lack the gaps and fenestrations that are seen in peripheral capillaries. Also, non-neuronal cells in the CNS (e.g., astrocytes) and the capillary basement membrane seem to contribute to the relative impermeability of this barrier.

The blood-brain barrier obviously plays an important role in clinical pharmacotherapeutics. To exert their effects, drugs targeted for the CNS must be able to pass from the bloodstream into the brain and spinal cord. In general, nonpolar, lipid-soluble drugs are able to cross the blood-brain barrier by passive diffusion.[6] Polar and lipophobic compounds are usually unable to enter the brain, but exceptions occur because of the presence of carrier-mediated transport systems in the blood-brain barrier.[7] Some substances (such as glucose) are transported via facilitated diffusion, while other compounds (including some drugs) may be able to enter the brain by active transport or by endocytosis. There has been considerable effort to develop or re-engineer specific drugs to take advantage of these endogenous transport systems, thus providing a way for these drugs to enter the brain.[8-10] Other chemical modifications of the drug, including the use of nanotechnology (see Chapter 2), can increase lipophilicity, which would allow the drug to enter the brain by passive lipid diffusion.[8] As a result of this research, many drugs that previously could not cross the blood-brain barrier can now reach the CNS, and future technological advancements will explore other ways to enhance the transport of specific drugs into the CNS.[11,12]

Several active transport systems also exist on the blood-brain barrier that are responsible for *removing* drugs and toxins from the brain.[13,14] That is, certain drugs can enter the brain easily via diffusion or another process, but these drugs are then rapidly and efficiently transported out of the brain and back into the systemic circulation.[14] This effect creates an obvious problem because these drugs will not reach therapeutic levels within the CNS and will not be beneficial. Again, there has been considerable research exploring ways to inhibit drug efflux so that meaningful amounts of the drug remain in the CNS.[15,16]

The blood-brain barrier has many structural and functional characteristics that influence CNS drugs. Researchers continue to examine how these characteristics can be modified to ensure adequate drug delivery to the brain and spinal cord.

CNS NEUROTRANSMITTERS

Neurons often release a specific chemical to transmit a signal to another neuron in the CNS. These chemicals are known as *neurotransmitters*. Likewise, the majority of neural connections in the human brain and spinal cord are characterized as chemical synapses, meaning that a chemical neurotransmitter propagates the nervous impulse across the gap that exists between two neurons. Several distinct chemicals have been identified as neurotransmitters within the brain and spinal cord (Table 5-1). Groups of neurons within the CNS tend to use one of these neurotransmitters to produce either excitation or inhibition of the other neurons. Although each neurotransmitter can be generally described as either excitatory or inhibitory within the CNS, some transmitters may have different effects, depending on the nature of the postsynaptic receptor involved. As discussed in Chapter 4, the interaction of the transmitter and the receptor dictates the effect on the postsynaptic neuron.

The fact that several distinct neurotransmitters exist and that neurons using specific transmitters are organized functionally within the CNS has important pharmacological implications. Certain drugs may alter the transmission in pathways using a specific neurotransmitter while having little or no effect on other transmitter pathways. This allows the drug to exert a rather specific effect on the CNS, so many disorders may be rectified without radically altering other CNS functions. Other drugs may have a much more general effect and may alter transmission in many CNS regions. The major categories of CNS neurotransmitters are acetylcholine, monoamines, amino acids, and peptides. This section discusses their general functions, locations, and effects.

Table 5-1
CENTRAL NEUROTRANSMITTERS

Transmitter	Primary CNS Location	General Effect
Acetylcholine	Cerebral cortex (many areas); basal ganglia; limbic and thalamic regions; spinal interneurons	Excitation
Norepinephrine	Neurons originating in brainstem and hypothalamus that project throughout other areas of brain	Inhibition
Dopamine	Basal ganglia; limbic system	Inhibition
Serotonin	Neurons originating in brainstem that project upward (to hypothalamus) and downward (to spinal cord)	Inhibition
GABA (gamma-aminobutyric acid)	Interneurons throughout the spinal cord, cerebellum, basal ganglia, cerebral cortex	Inhibition
Glycine	Interneurons in spinal cord and brainstem	Inhibition
Glutamate, aspartate	Interneurons throughout brain and spinal cord	Excitation
Substance P	Pathways in spinal cord and brain that mediate painful stimuli	Excitation
Enkephalins	Pain suppression pathways in spinal cord and brain	Excitation

Acetylcholine

Acetylcholine is in many areas of the brain and in the periphery (e.g., skeletal neuromuscular junction and some autonomic synapses). Acetylcholine is abundant in the cerebral cortex and seems to play a critical role in cognition and memory.[17,18] Neurons originating in the large pyramidal cells of the motor cortex and many neurons originating in the basal ganglia also secrete acetylcholine from their terminal axons. In general, acetylcholine synapses in the CNS are excitatory in nature.

Monoamines

Monoamines are a group of structurally similar CNS neurotransmitters that include the catecholamines (dopamine, norepinephrine) and 5-hydroxytryptamine (serotonin).[19] Dopamine exerts different effects at various locations within the brain.[20,21] Within the basal ganglia, dopamine is secreted by neurons that originate in the substantia nigra and project to the corpus striatum. As such, it is important in regulating motor control, and the loss of these dopaminergic neurons results in symptoms commonly associated with Parkinson disease (see Chapter 10). Dopamine also influences mood and emotions, primarily via its presence in the hypothalamus and other structures within the limbic system. Although its effects within the brain are very complex, dopamine generally inhibits the neurons onto which it is released.

Norepinephrine is secreted by neurons that originate in the locus caeruleus of the pons and projects throughout the reticular formation. Norepinephrine is generally regarded as an inhibitory transmitter within the CNS, but the overall effect following activity of norepinephrine synapses is often general excitation of the brain, probably because norepinephrine directly inhibits other neurons that produce inhibition. This phenomenon of *disinhibition* causes excitation by removing the influence of inhibitory neurons.

Serotonin (5-hydroxytryptamine) is released by cells originating in the midline of the pons and brainstem and is projected to many different areas, including the dorsal horns of the spinal cord and the hypothalamus. Serotonin is considered to be a strong inhibitor in most areas of the CNS and is believed to be important in mediating the inhibition of painful stimuli. It is also involved in controlling many aspects of mood and behavior, and problems with serotonergic activity have been implicated in several psychiatric disorders, including depression and anxiety.[22,23] The roles of serotonin and the other monoamines in psychiatric disorders are discussed in Chapters 6 through 8.

Amino Acids

Several amino acids, such as glycine and gamma-aminobutyric acid (GABA), are important inhibitory transmitters in the brain and spinal cord. Certain interneurons located throughout the spinal cord seem to use glycine for the inhibitory transmitter, and this amino acid also causes inhibition in certain areas of the brain.[24,25] Likewise, GABA is found throughout the CNS and is believed to be the primary neurotransmitter used to cause inhibition at presynaptic and postsynaptic neurons in the brain and spinal cord.[26-28] Other amino acids such as aspartate and glutamate have been found in high concentrations throughout the brain and spinal cord; these substances cause excitation of CNS neurons.[29,30] These excitatory amino acids have received a great deal of attention because they may also produce neurotoxic effects when released in large amounts during CNS injury and certain neurological disorders (e.g., epilepsy, neuropathic pain, amyotrophic lateral sclerosis, etc.).[29,31,32]

Peptides

Many peptides are CNS neurotransmitters.[33,34] One peptide that is important from a pharmacological standpoint is substance P, which is an excitatory transmitter that is involved in spinal cord pathways transmitting pain impulses.[34] Increased activity at substance P synapses in the cord serves to mediate the transmission of painful sensations, and certain drugs such as the opioid analgesics may decrease activity at these synapses. Other peptides that have important pharmacological implications include three families of compounds: the endorphins, enkephalins, and dynorphins.[35] These peptides, also known as the *endogenous opioids*, are excitatory transmitters in certain brain synapses that inhibit painful sensations and thus decrease the central perception of pain when they are produced within the body. The interaction of these compounds with exogenous opioid drugs is discussed in Chapter 14.

Finally, peptides such as galanin, leptin, neuropeptide Y, vasoactive intestinal polypeptide (VIP), and pituitary adenylate cyclase–activating polypeptide (PACAP) have been identified in various areas of the

CNS. These and other peptides may affect various CNS functions, either by acting directly as neurotransmitters or by acting as cotransmitters moderating the effects of other neurotransmitters.[36-38]

Other Transmitters

In addition to the well-known substances, other chemicals are continually being identified as potential CNS neurotransmitters. Purines such as adenosine and adenosine triphosphate (ATP) are now recognized as transmitters or modulators of neural transmission in specific areas of the brain and in the autonomic nervous system.[39,40] Many other chemicals that are traditionally associated with functions outside the CNS are being identified as possible CNS transmitters or neuromodulators, including histamine, nitric oxide, and certain hormones (vasopressin, oxytocin).[41-43] As the function of these chemicals and other new transmitters becomes clearer, the pharmacological significance of drugs that affect these synapses will undoubtedly be considered.

THE GENERAL MECHANISMS OF CNS DRUGS

The majority of CNS drugs work by modifying synaptic transmission in some way. Figure 5-2 shows a typical chemical synapse that is found in the CNS. Most drugs that attempt to rectify CNS-related disorders do so by either increasing or decreasing transmission at specific synapses. For instance, psychotic behavior has been associated with overactivity in central synapses that use dopamine as a neurotransmitter (see Chapter 8). Drug therapy in this situation consists of agents that decrease activity at central dopamine synapses. Conversely, Parkinson disease results from a decrease in activity at specific dopamine synapses (see Chapter 10). Antiparkinsonian drugs attempt to increase dopaminergic transmission at these synapses and bring synaptic activity back to normal levels.

A drug that modifies synaptic transmission must somehow alter the quantity of the neurotransmitter that is released from the presynaptic terminal or affect the stimulation of postsynaptic receptors, or both. When considering a typical synapse, such as the one shown in Figure 5-2, there are several distinct sites at which a drug may alter activity in the synapse. There are also specific ways a drug may modify synaptic transmission:

Presynaptic action potential. The arrival of an action potential at the presynaptic terminal initiates neurotransmitter release. Certain drugs, such as local anesthetics, block propagation along neural axons so that the action potential fails to reach the presynaptic terminal, which effectively eliminates activity at that particular synapse. Also, the amount of depolarization or the height of the action potential arriving at the

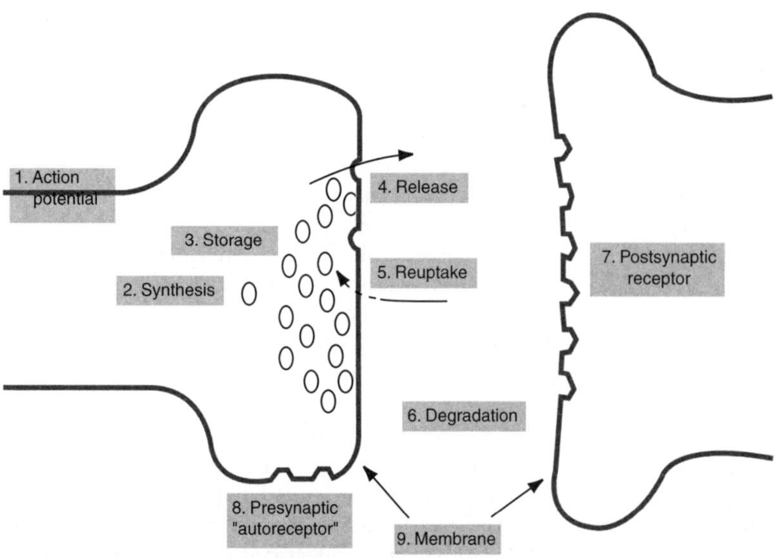

Figure ■ 5-2
Sites at which drugs can alter transmission at a CNS synapse.

presynaptic terminal is directly related to the amount of transmitter released. Any drug or endogenous chemical that limits the amount of depolarization occurring in the presynaptic terminal will inhibit the synapse because less neurotransmitter is released. In certain situations, this is referred to as *presynaptic inhibition*, because the site of this effect is at the presynaptic terminal. The endogenous neurotransmitter GABA is believed to exert some of its inhibitory effects via this mechanism.

Synthesis of neurotransmitter. Drugs that block the synthesis of a neurotransmitter will eventually deplete the presynaptic terminal and impair transmission. For example, metyrosine (Demser) inhibits an enzyme that is essential for catecholamine biosynthesis in the presynaptic terminal. Treatment with metyrosine results in decreased synthesis of transmitters such as dopamine and norepinephrine.

Storage of neurotransmitter. A certain amount of chemical transmitter is stored in presynaptic vesicles. Drugs that impair this storage will decrease the synapse's ability to continue transmitting information for extended periods. An example of this is the antihypertensive drug reserpine (Novoreserpine, Reserfia), which impairs the ability of adrenergic terminals to sequester and store norepinephrine in presynaptic vesicles.

Release. Certain drugs will increase synaptic activity by directly increasing the release of the neurotransmitter from the presynaptic terminal. Amphetamines appear to exert their effects on the CNS primarily by increasing the presynaptic release of catecholamine neurotransmitters (e.g., norepinephrine). Conversely, other compounds may inhibit the synapse by directly decreasing the amount of transmitter released during each action potential. An example is botulinum toxin (Botox), which can be used as a skeletal muscle relaxant because of its ability to impair the release of acetylcholine from the skeletal neuromuscular junction (see Chapter 13).

Reuptake. After the neurotransmitter is released, some chemical synapses terminate activity primarily by transmitter reuptake. Reuptake involves the movement of the transmitter molecule back into the presynaptic terminal. A drug that impairs the reuptake of transmitter allows more of it to remain in the synaptic cleft and continue to exert an effect. Consequently, blocking reuptake actually increases activity at the synapse. For instance, tricyclic antidepressants (see Chapter 7) impair the reuptake mechanism that pumps amine neurotransmitters back into the presynaptic terminal, which allows the transmitter to continue to exert its effect and prolong activity at the synapse.

Degradation. Some synapses rely primarily on the enzymatic breakdown of the released transmitter to terminate synaptic activity. Inhibition of the enzyme responsible for terminating the transmitter allows more of the active transmitter to remain in the synaptic cleft, thereby increasing activity at the synapse. An example is using a drug that inhibits the **cholinesterase** enzyme as a method of treating myasthenia gravis. In myasthenia gravis, there is a functional decrease in activity at the skeletal neuromuscular junction. Anticholinesterase drugs such as neostigmine (Prostigmin) and pyridostigmine (Mestinon) inhibit acetylcholine breakdown, allowing more of the released neurotransmitter to continue to exert an effect at the neuromuscular synapse.

Postsynaptic receptor. As discussed in Chapter 4, chemical antagonists can block the postsynaptic receptor, thus decreasing synaptic transmission. The best-known example of this is the use of beta blockers. These agents are antagonists that are specific for the beta-adrenergic receptors on the myocardium, and they are frequently used to treat hypertension, cardiac arrhythmias, and angina pectoris. Other drugs may improve synaptic transmission by affecting the receptor directly, so there is a tendency for increased neurotransmitter binding or improved receptor–effector coupling, or both. For instance, benzodiazepines (e.g., diazepam [Valium], chlordiazepoxide [Librium, others]) appear to enhance the postsynaptic effects of the inhibitory neurotransmitter GABA.

Presynaptic autoreceptors. In addition to postsynaptic receptors, there are also receptors on the presynaptic terminal of some types of chemical synapses. These presynaptic receptors seem to serve as a method of negative feedback in controlling neurotransmitter release.[44,45] During high levels of synaptic activity, the accumulation of neurotransmitter in the synaptic cleft may allow binding to the presynaptic receptors and limit further release of chemical transmitter. Certain drugs may also be able to attenuate synaptic activity through presynaptic autoreceptors.

For instance, clonidine (Catapres) may exert some of its antihypertensive effects by binding to presynaptic receptors on sympathetic postganglionic neurons and impairing the release of norepinephrine onto the peripheral vasculature. However, the use of drugs that alter synaptic activity by binding to these autoreceptors is still somewhat new, and the full potential for this area of pharmacology remains to be determined.

Membrane effects. Drugs may alter synaptic transmission by affecting membrane organization and fluidity. Membrane fluidity is the amount of flexibility or mobility of the lipid bilayer. Drugs that alter the fluidity of the presynaptic membrane could affect the way that presynaptic vesicles fuse with and release their neurotransmitter. Drug-induced changes in the postsynaptic membrane would affect the receptor environment and thereby alter receptor function. Membrane modification will result in either increased or decreased synaptic transmission, depending on the drug in question and the type and magnitude of membrane change. Alcohol (ethanol) and general anesthetics were originally thought to exert their effects by producing reversible changes in the fluidity and organization of the cell membranes of central neurons. Although this idea has been challenged somewhat, these drugs may still exert some of their effects via neuronal membranes.

A CNS drug does not have to adhere specifically to only one of these methods of synaptic modification. Some drugs may affect the synapse in two or more ways. For example, the antihypertensive agent guanethidine (Ismelin) impairs both presynaptic storage and release of norepinephrine. Other drugs such as barbiturates may affect both the presynaptic terminal and the postsynaptic receptor in CNS synapses.

SUMMARY

Therapeutic CNS drugs tend to exert their effects on particular CNS structures, and drugs need to cross the blood-brain barrier to reach the CNS. Neurotransmitters produce either excitation or inhibition of the other neurons. Drugs affecting the brain and spinal cord usually exert their effects by somehow modifying synaptic transmission. In some instances, drugs may be targeted for specific synapses in an attempt to rectify some problem with transmission at that particular synapse. Other drugs may increase or decrease the excitability of CNS neurons in an attempt to have a more general effect on the overall level of consciousness of the individual. This information will help you understand the actions of specific CNS drugs when these drugs are discussed in succeeding chapters.

REFERENCES

1. Brodal P. *The Central Nervous System*. 4th ed. New York: Oxford University Press; 2010.
2. Kandel ER, Schwartz JH, Jessell TM, Siegelbaum S, Hudspeth AJ. *Principles of Neural Science*. 5th ed. New York: McGraw-Hill; 2012.
3. Waxman SG. *Clinical Neuroanatomy*. 26th ed. New York: McGraw-Hill; 2009.
4. Nico B, Ribatti D. Morphofunctional aspects of the blood-brain barrier. *Curr Drug Metab*. 2012;13:50-60.
5. Potschka H. Targeting the brain—surmounting or bypassing the blood-brain barrier. *Handb Exp Pharmacol*. 2010;197:411-431.
6. Soni V, Jain A, Khare P, et al. Potential approaches for drug delivery to the brain: past, present, and future. *Crit Rev Ther Drug Carrier Syst*. 2010;27:187-236.
7. Ueno M, Nakagawa T, Wu B, et al. Transporters in the brain endothelial barrier. *Curr Med Chem*. 2010;17:1125-1138.
8. Gagliardi M, Bardi G, Bifone A. Polymeric nanocarriers for controlled and enhanced delivery of therapeutic agents to the CNS. *Ther Deliv*. 2012;3:875-887.
9. Pardridge WM, Boado RJ. Reengineering biopharmaceuticals for targeted delivery across the blood-brain barrier. *Methods Enzymol*. 2012;503:269-292.
10. Pavan B, Dalpiaz A, Ciliberti N, et al. Progress in drug delivery to the central nervous system by the prodrug approach. *Molecules*. 2008;13:1035-1065.
11. Patel MM, Goyal BR, Bhadada SV, et al. Getting into the brain: approaches to enhance brain drug delivery. *CNS Drugs*. 2009;23:35-58.
12. Stenehjem DD, Hartz AM, Bauer B, Anderson GW. Novel and emerging strategies in drug delivery for overcoming the blood-brain barrier. *Future Med Chem*. 2009;1:1623-1641.
13. Mahringer A, Ott M, Reimold I, et al. The ABC of the blood-brain barrier—regulation of drug efflux pumps. *Curr Pharm Des*. 2011;17:2762-2770.
14. Shen S, Zhang W. ABC transporters and drug efflux at the blood-brain barrier. *Rev Neurosci*. 2010;21:29-53.
15. Miller DS, Bauer B, Hartz AM. Modulation of P-glycoprotein at the blood-brain barrier: opportunities to improve central nervous system pharmacotherapy. *Pharmacol Rev*. 2008;60:196-209.
16. Potschka H. Targeting regulation of ABC efflux transporters in brain diseases: a novel therapeutic approach. *Pharmacol Ther*. 2010;125:118-127.
17. Bentley P, Driver J, Dolan RJ. Cholinergic modulation of cognition: insights from human pharmacological functional neuroimaging. *Prog Neurobiol*. 2011;94:360-388.
18. Robinson L, Platt B, Riedel G. Involvement of the cholinergic system in conditioning and perceptual memory. *Behav Brain Res*. 2011;221:443-465.

19. Walther DJ, Stahlberg S, Vowinckel J. Novel roles for biogenic monoamines: from monoamines in transglutaminase-mediated post-translational protein modification to monoaminylation deregulation diseases. *FEBS J.* 2011;278:4740-4755.
20. Liss B, Roeper J. Individual dopamine midbrain neurons: functional diversity and flexibility in health and disease. *Brain Res Rev.* 2008;58:314-321.
21. Nitsche MA, Monte-Silva K, Kuo MF, Paulus W. Dopaminergic impact on cortical excitability in humans. *Rev Neurosci.* 2010;21:289-298.
22. Hale MW, Shekhar A, Lowry CA. Stress-related serotonergic systems: implications for symptomatology of anxiety and affective disorders. *Cell Mol Neurobiol.* 2012;32:695-708.
23. Hung AS, Tsui TY, Lam JC, et al. Serotonin and its receptors in the human CNS with new findings—a mini review. *Curr Med Chem.* 2011;18:5281-5288.
24. Keck T, White JA. Glycinergic inhibition in the hippocampus. *Rev Neurosci.* 2009;20:13-22.
25. Xu TL, Gong N. Glycine and glycine receptor signaling in hippocampal neurons: diversity, function and regulation. *Prog Neurobiol.* 2010;91:349-361.
26. Gajcy K, Lochy_ski S, Librowski T. A role of GABA analogues in the treatment of neurological diseases. *Curr Med Chem.* 2010; 17:2338-2347.
27. Ramamoorthi K, Lin Y. The contribution of GABAergic dysfunction to neurodevelopmental disorders. *Trends Mol Med.* 2011; 17:452-462.
28. Roth FC, Draguhn A. GABA metabolism and transport: effects on synaptic efficacy. *Neural Plast.* 2012;2012:805830.
29. Javitt DC, Schoepp D, Kalivas PW, et al. Translating glutamate: from pathophysiology to treatment. *Sci Transl Med.* 2011;3:102mr2..
30. Dobrek L, Thor P. Glutamate NMDA receptors in pathophysiology and pharmacotherapy of selected nervous system diseases. *Postepy Hig Med Dosw (Online).* 2011;65:338-346.
31. Ghasemi M, Schachter SC. The NMDA receptor complex as a therapeutic target in epilepsy: a review. *Epilepsy Behav.* 2011; 22:617-640.
32. Zhou HY, Chen SR, Pan HL. Targeting N-methyl-D-aspartate receptors for treatment of neuropathic pain. *Expert Rev Clin Pharmacol.* 2011;4:379-388.
33. Greco R, Tassorelli C, Sandrini G, et al. Role of calcitonin gene-related peptide and substance P in different models of pain. *Cephalalgia.* 2008;28:114-126.
34. Seybold VS. The role of peptides in central sensitization. *Handb Exp Pharmacol.* 2009;194:451-491.
35. Bodnar RJ. Endogenous opiates and behavior: 2010. *Peptides.* 2011;32:2522-2552.
36. Opland DM, Leinninger GM, Myers MG Jr. Modulation of the mesolimbic dopamine system by leptin. *Brain Res.* 2010;1350:65-70.
37. Mechenthaler I. Galanin and the neuroendocrine axes. *Cell Mol Life Sci.* 2008;65:1826-1835.
38. Tan YV, Waschek JA. Targeting VIP and PACAP receptor signalling: new therapeutic strategies in multiple sclerosis. *ASN Neuro.* 2011;3:e00065.
39. Burnstock G. Purinergic signalling: Its unpopular beginning, its acceptance and its exciting future. *Bioessays.* 2012;34: 218-225.
40. Burnstock G, Krügel U, Abbracchio MP, Illes P. Purinergic signalling: from normal behaviour to pathological brain function. *Prog Neurobiol.* 2011;95:229-274.
41. Laranjinha J, Santos RM, Lourenço CF, et al. Nitric oxide signaling in the brain: translation of dynamics into respiration control and neurovascular coupling. *Ann NY Acad Sci.* 2012; 1259:10-18.
42. Tiligada E, Kyriakidis K, Chazot PL, Passani MB. Histamine pharmacology and new CNS drug targets. *CNS Neurosci Ther.* 2011;17:620-628.
43. Viviani D, Stoop R. Opposite effects of oxytocin and vasopressin on the emotional expression of the fear response. *Prog Brain Res.* 2008;170:207-218.
44. Feuerstein TJ. Presynaptic receptors for dopamine, histamine, and serotonin. *Handb Exp Pharmacol.* 2008;184:289-338.
45. Langer SZ. Presynaptic autoreceptors regulating transmitter release. *Neurochem Int.* 2008;52:26-30.

CHAPTER 6

Sedative-Hypnotic and Antianxiety Drugs

Sedative-hypnotic and antianxiety drugs are among the most commonly used drugs worldwide. These agents exert a calming effect and help relax the patient.[1] At higher doses, the same drug can produce drowsiness and initiate a relatively normal state of sleep (hypnosis). At still higher doses, some sedative-hypnotics (especially barbiturates) will eventually bring on a state of general anesthesia. Because of their general central nervous system (CNS)–depressant effects, some sedative-hypnotic drugs are also used for other functions, such as treating epilepsy or producing muscle relaxation.

While producing sedation, many drugs will also decrease the level of anxiety in a patient. Of course, these anxiolytic properties often cause a decrease in the level of alertness in the individual. However, certain agents are available that can reduce anxiety without an overt sedative effect. Hence, these agents are classified as antianxiety drugs because they produce less sedation than their sedative-hypnotic counterparts. However, this distinction is relative because most antianxiety drugs produce some level of sedation, especially at higher doses.

It is estimated that insomnia affects between 10 to 15 percent of the general population, and pharmacological management can be helpful in promoting normal sleep.[2] Moreover, people who are ill or who have recently been relocated to a new environment (hospital, nursing home) will often have difficulty sleeping and might need some form of sedative-hypnotic agent.[3,4] A person who sustains an injury or illness will certainly have some apprehension concerning his or her welfare.[2,5] If necessary, this apprehension can be controlled to some extent by using antianxiety drugs during the course of rehabilitation.

As a rehabilitation specialist, you will encounter many physical therapy and occupational therapy patients who are taking sedative-hypnotic and antianxiety agents. It is important that you understand the basic pharmacology of these agents and their adverse effects.

SEDATIVE-HYPNOTIC DRUGS

Sedative-hypnotics fall into two general categories: benzodiazepines and nonbenzodiazepines (Table 6-1). These agents are used to promote sleep, especially in relatively acute or short-term situations where sleep has been disturbed by illness, injury, or other factors. We will address the benzodiazepines first, followed by a description of the nonbenzodiazepine hypnotics.

Benzodiazepines

Benzodiazepines are a family of compounds that share the same basic chemical structure and pharmacological effects. Although the more famous members of this family are associated with treating anxiety (e.g., diazepam [Valium]; see later in this chapter), several benzodiazepines are indicated specifically to promote sleep (see Table 6-1). These agents have hypnotic effects similar to those of nonbenzodiazepines—such

Table 6-1
COMMON SEDATIVE-HYPNOTIC DRUGS

Generic Name	Trade Name	Sedative Oral Adult Dose (mg)	Hypnotic* Oral Adult Dose (mg)
Barbiturates			
Amobarbital	Amytal	30–50 bid or tid	65–200
Pentobarbital	Nembutal	20 tid or qid	100
Phenobarbital	Luminal, Solfoton, Ancalixir	15–40 bid or tid	100–320
Secobarbital	Novosecobarb, Seconal	30–50 tid or qid	100
*Benzodiazepines***			
Estazolam	ProSom	______	1–2
Flurazepam	Dalmane	______	15–30
Quazepam	Doral	______	7.5–15
Temazepam	Restoril	______	7.5–30
Triazolam	Halcion	______	0.125–0.25
Others			
Chloral hydrate	Noctec	250 tid	500–1,000
Eszopiclone	Lunesta	______	2–3
Ramelteon	Rozerem	______	8
Zaleplon	Sonata	______	5–20
Zolpidem	Ambien	______	10

**Hypnotic doses are typically administered as a single dose at bedtime.*

***Benzodiazepines listed here are indicated specifically as hypnotic agents and are not approved for other uses (antianxiety, anticonvulsant, etc.). Virtually all benzodiazepines have sedative-hypnotic effects, and other benzodiazepines may be administered to produce sedation or sleep, depending on the dosage and the patient.*

as the barbiturates—but benzodiazepines are generally regarded as safer because there is less of a chance for lethal overdose.[6,7] But benzodiazepines are not without their drawbacks, and they can cause residual effects the day after they are administered; prolonged use can also cause tolerance and physical dependence (see "Problems and Adverse Effects of Sedative-Hypnotics," later in this chapter).[8,9]

Mechanism of Benzodiazepine Effects

The benzodiazepines work by increasing the inhibitory effects at CNS synapses that use the neurotransmitter gamma-aminobutyric acid (GABA).[1,10] GABA is the primary neurotransmitter that causes inhibition at presynaptic and postsynaptic neurons throughout the brain and spinal cord.[11-13] In other words, benzodiazepines enhance relaxation and sleep by boosting the effect of the brain's endogenous inhibitory neurotransmitter (GABA).

Benzodiazepines bind to a specific receptor located at certain inhibitory synapses in the reticular formation of the CNS. The receptor primarily affected by benzodiazepines contains three principal components: (1) binding site(s) for GABA, (2) a binding site for benzodiazepines, and (3) an ion channel that is specific for chloride ions (Fig. 6-1).[10,14] It is the presence of this GABA-benzodiazepine–chloride ion channel receptor that accounts for the specific mechanism of action.

GABA typically exerts its inhibitory effects by binding to its receptor site or sites (GABA may bind in more than one location) and by initiating an increase in chloride conductance through the channel. Increased chloride conductance facilitates chloride entry into the neuron and results in hyperpolarization, or a decreased ability to raise the neuron to its firing threshold. By binding to their own respective site on the receptor, benzodiazepines potentiate the effects of GABA and increase the inhibition at these synapses. These drugs exert other beneficial effects by enhancing GABA

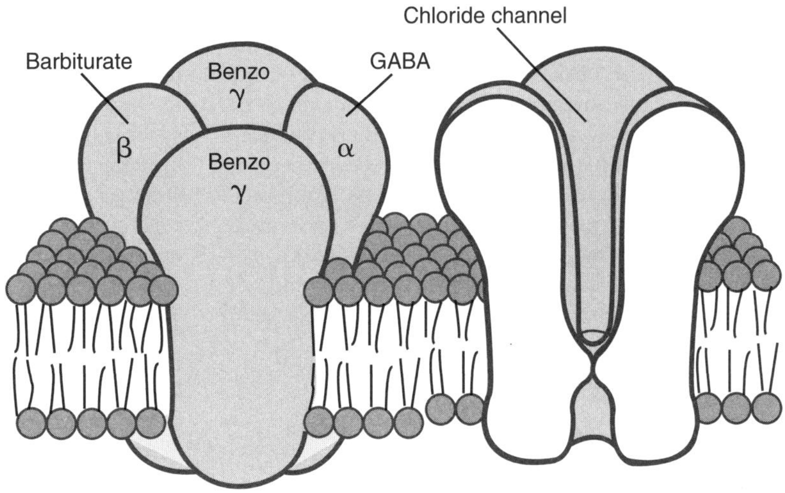

Figure ■ 6-1
Simplified structure of the $GABA_A$ receptor located on CNS neurons. Binding of GABA to specific sites on the receptor opens a centrally located chloride ion channel, thus increasing chloride entry and inhibition of the neuron. Benzodiazepines (BZD) bind to other parts (subunits) of the receptor, thus enhancing the inhibitory effects of GABA. Other sedative-hypnotic and antianxiety drugs (barbiturates, eszopiclone, zaleplon, zolpidem) bind to other sites on or within the receptor and increase GABA inhibition.

inhibition in other areas of the CNS to treat anxiety, decrease seizures (Chapter 9), use in general anesthesia (Chapter 11), and use for skeletal muscle relaxation (Chapter 13). Clearly, benzodiazepines are very versatile and important therapeutic agents.

Research has also indicated that there are at least three types of GABA receptors, and these receptors are classified as $GABA_A$, $GABA_B$, and $GABA_C$ according to their structural and functional characteristics.[15] $GABA_A$ and $GABA_C$ receptors, for example, cause inhibition by increasing chloride entry as described above, whereas $GABA_B$ receptors may cause inhibition by affecting potassium channels and decreasing calcium entrance into CNS neurons.[15,16] It appears that benzodiazepines act primarily on the $GABA_A$ class, and the therapeutic effects of these drugs (i.e., sedation, hypnosis, decreased anxiety) are mediated through the $GABA_A$ receptor, which is found in the brain (see Fig. 6-1).[1,11] Hence, clinically used benzodiazepines are basically $GABA_A$ receptor agonists.

Furthermore, the $GABA_A$ receptor is composed of several subunits (alpha, beta, gamma), with each subunit having several subdivisions (alpha-1, beta-2, beta-3, gamma-2, etc.). It appears that individual subunits on this receptor mediate specific effects.[10,17] Sedation, for example, seems to be mediated by the alpha-1, beta-2, and gamma-2 subunits, whereas other beneficial effects such as decreased anxiety might be mediated by the alpha-2, beta-3, and gamma-2 subunits. Benzodiazepines seem to affect most or all of these subunits, hence their ability to produce sedative and antianxiety effects.[10,15] However, these drugs might also cause certain side effects (e.g., tolerance, dependence) by affecting other subunits on the $GABA_A$ receptor. But a drug that is selective for only the alpha-1 subunit might exert sedative effects without producing as many side effects.[1,18] These types of drugs are addressed later in this chapter.

Because of these new advances, scientists continue to study the molecular physiology of the $GABA_A$ receptor and clarify how benzodiazepines affect these receptors. Likewise, differences between the principal GABA receptor classes (A, B, C) have encouraged the development of drugs that are more selective to GABA receptors located in certain areas of the CNS. For example, the muscle relaxant baclofen (Lioresal) may be somewhat more selective for $GABA_B$ receptors in the spinal cord than for other $GABA_A$ or $GABA_C$ receptors that are found in the brain (see Chapter 13). Future drug development will continue to exploit the differences between the GABA receptor classes and subtypes within these classes so that drugs are more selective and can produce more specific beneficial effects with fewer side effects.

Finally, the discovery of a CNS receptor that is specific for benzodiazepines has led to some interesting speculation as to the possible existence of some type of endogenous sedative-like agent—that is, the presence of a certain type of receptor usually indicates that the body produces an appropriate agonist for that receptor. For instance, the discovery of opiate receptors initiated the search for endogenous opiate-like substances, which culminated in the discovery of the enkephalins. It has been surmised that certain endogenous neurosteroids such as allopregnanolone (a metabolic by-product of progesterone) can bind to the $GABA_A$ receptors in the CNS and produce sedative-hypnotic effects.[19] It remains to be determined exactly why allopregnanolone is produced in humans and whether its effect on $GABA_A$ receptors is physiologically important. Nonetheless, continued research in this area may someday reveal why steroids and other endogenous substances affect $GABA_A$ receptors, and the focus of pharmacological treatment can then be directed toward stimulating the release of endogenous sedative-hypnotic agents.

Nonbenzodiazepines

Barbiturates

The barbiturates are a group of CNS depressants that share a common chemical origin: barbituric acid. The potent sedative-hypnotic properties of these drugs have been recognized for some time, and their status as the premier medication used to promote sleep went unchallenged for many years. However, barbiturates are associated with a relatively small therapeutic index; approximately 10 times the therapeutic dose can often be fatal. These drugs are also very addictive, and their prolonged use often leads to drug abuse. Consequently, the lack of safety of the barbiturates and their strong potential for addiction and abuse necessitated the development of alternative nonbarbiturate drugs such as the benzodiazepines. Still, some barbiturates are occasionally used for their hypnotic properties; these drugs are listed in Table 6-1.

Despite their extensive use in the past, the exact mechanism of the barbiturates remains somewhat unclear. When used in sedative-hypnotic doses, barbiturates may function in a similar fashion to the benzodiazepines in that they also potentiate the inhibitory effects of GABA.[20] This idea suggests that barbiturates may affect the GABA-benzodiazepine–chloride ion channel receptor described above.[1] Indeed, considerable evidence exists that barbiturates bind directly to the $GABA_A$ receptor at a site that is different from the binding site for GABA or benzodiazepines (see Fig. 6-1).[1] However, barbiturates may also exert effects that are not mediated through an effect on the GABA-benzodiazepine–chloride ion channel receptor. At higher doses, for instance, barbiturates may directly increase the release of inhibitory transmitters such as glycine and reduce the effects of excitatory transmitters such as glutamate.[7] Regardless of their exact mechanism, barbiturates are effective sedative-hypnotics because of their specificity for neurons in the midbrain portion of the reticular formation as well as some limbic system structures. At higher doses, barbiturates also depress neuronal excitability in other areas of the brain and spinal cord. We discuss their role in producing general anesthesia by this more extensive CNS depression in Chapter 11.

Nonbenzodiazepine Sedative-Hypnotics

Pharmacologists have developed several drugs, including zolpidem (Ambien), zaleplon (Sonata), and eszopiclone (Lunesta) as sedative-hypnotics (see Table 6-1).[18,21] These drugs are chemically different from the benzodiazepines but still seem to affect the $GABA_A$ receptors in the brain—that is, they bind to the $GABA_A$ receptor, which then causes GABA to bind more effectively, thus increasing chloride conductance and the level of inhibition in the neuron. Increased inhibition in certain areas of the brain results in less arousal and the promotion of sleep.

These $GABA_A$ drugs appear to be as effective as the benzodiazepines in promoting sleep. The drugs also seem to have a lower risk of producing certain side effects and causing problems when discontinued (see "Problems and Adverse Effects," below).[18,22] This difference might be explained by the fact that nonbenzodiazepine drugs bind preferentially to the alpha-1 subunit of the $GABA_A$ receptor.[1,22] As discussed earlier, stimulation of this particular subunit seems to mediate sedation without producing other side effects. These drugs likewise tend to have a shorter duration of action than traditional benzodiazepines, thus decreasing the chance of residual or "hangover" effects the next day.[18,21] Hence, drugs like zolpidem, zaleplon, and eszopiclone can be used instead of benzodiazepines to treat sleep disorders, and efforts continue to develop other nonbenzodiazepine drugs that selectively affect the $GABA_A$ receptor.

Ramelteon (Rozerem) is another drug that can be used as an alternative to traditional sedative-hypnotic benzodiazepines.[23] Rather than having GABA-like effects, ramelteon is similar in structure and function to melatonin. Melatonin, an endogenous neurohormone produced in the pineal gland, binds to melatonin receptors in the hypothalamus. Melatonin seems to be important in controlling sleep cycles and plays a key role in bringing about the onset of sleep.[24,25] Hence, by acting like melatonin, ramelteon has been especially helpful in facilitating sleep onset and in maintaining normal sleep patterns in certain individuals. This drug may also have a lower risk of side effects, including a reduced incidence of next day "hangover" symptoms and less tolerance and physical dependence during long-term use.[23,26] Ramelteon therefore offers another valuable strategy for treating certain sleep disorders in people with chronic insomnia.

Other Nonbenzodiazepines

Practitioners can prescribe several other nonbenzodiazepine compounds for their sedative-hypnotic properties. These compounds are chemically dissimilar from one another but share the ability to promote relaxation and sleep via depressing the CNS. Cyclic ethers and alcohols (including ethanol) can be included in this category, but their use specifically as sedative-hypnotics is fairly limited at present. The recreational use of ethanol in alcoholic beverages is an important topic in terms of abuse and long-term effects. However, since this area is much too extensive to be addressed here, only their sedative-hypnotic effect is considered.

Alcohol (ethanol) and substances with alcohol-like properties (e.g., chloral hydrate, see Table 6-1), work through mechanisms that are poorly understood. In the past, it was thought that alcohols exerted their CNS-depressant effects directly on neuronal membrane composition and fluidity. These and other highly lipid-soluble substances could simply dissolve in the lipid bilayer and inhibit neuronal excitability by temporarily disrupting membrane structures in the presynaptic and postsynaptic regions of CNS neurons.[27] However, recent evidence suggests that alcohols may act on protein receptors much in the same way as the benzodiazepines and barbiturates—that is, alcohols may exert some of their effects by activating $GABA_A$ receptors and increasing GABA-mediated inhibition in the CNS.[28,29] But alcohols produce many other effects on several other types of receptors and neurotransmitters throughout the CNS, and it is difficult to determine the exact molecular mechanism by which alcohols produce sedative-hypnotic effects. In any event, alcohols and similar agents decrease neuronal transmission; this causes fairly widespread CNS depression, which accounts for the subsequent sedative effects of such compounds.

Lastly, practitioners can prescribe many other sedation-causing drugs to facilitate sleep in specific situations. For example, certain antihistamines (see Chapter 26) can cause profound sedation, and these drugs are often used in over-the-counter products that are promoted as "sleep aids."[30] Antidepressants (Chapter 7), antipsychotics (Chapter 8), anticonvulsants (Chapter 9), and opioid analgesics (Chapter 14) with sedative properties may be used in limited situations to promote sleep.[31,32] A patient who is in acute pain, for instance, might receive the dual benefit of analgesia and sedation if given an opioid drug. Sedation, however, is usually a side effect of these other medications, and these drugs are not typically advocated for treating classic insomnia or chronic sleep problems.

Pharmacokinetics

Benzodiazepine and nonbenzodiazepine sedative-hypnotics are usually highly lipid soluble (Table 6-2). They are typically administered orally and are absorbed easily and completely from the gastrointestinal (GI) tract. Distribution is fairly uniform throughout the body, and these drugs reach the CNS readily because of their high degree of lipid solubility. Sedative-hypnotics are metabolized primarily by the oxidative enzymes of the drug-metabolizing system in liver cells. Termination of their activity is accomplished either by hepatic enzymes or by storage of these drugs in non-CNS tissues—that is, sequestering the drugs in adipose and other peripheral tissues negates their CNS-depressant effects. However, when the drugs slowly leak out of their peripheral storage sites, they can be redistributed to the brain and can cause low levels of sedation. This occurrence may help explain the "hangover" frequently reported the day after taking sedative-hypnotic drugs. Finally, excretion of these drugs occurs through the kidney after their metabolism in the liver. As with most drug biotransformations, metabolism of sedative-hypnotics is essential in creating a polar metabolite that is readily excreted by the kidney.

Problems and Adverse Effects of Sedative-Hypnotics

Residual Effects

The primary problem associated with sedative-hypnotic use is the residual effects that can occur the day after administration. Individuals who take a sedative-hypnotic to sleep at night sometimes complain of

Table 6-2
PHARMACOKINETIC PROPERTIES OF COMMON SEDATIVE-HYPNOTICS

Drug	Time to Peak Plasma Concentration (hr)*	Relative Half-Life	Comments
Estazolam (ProSom)	2	Intermediate	Well absorbed after oral administration
Eszopiclone (Lunesta)	1	Short	Rapidly absorbed after oral administration
Flurazepam (Dalmane)	0.5–1	Long	Long elimination half-life because of active metabolites
Quazepam (Doral)	2	Long	Daytime drowsiness more likely than with other benzodiazepines
Ramelteon (Rozerem)	0.5–1.5	Short	Rapid oral absorption, but low bioavailability due to extensive first-pass metabolism
Temazepam (Restoril)	1–2	Short–intermediate	Slow oral absorption
Triazolam (Halcion)	Within 2	Short	Rapid inactivation; residual (daytime) effects may be disturbing
Zaleplon (Sonata)	Unknown	Short	Rapidly absorbed after oral administration
Zolpidem (Ambien)	0.5–2	Short	Rapid oral absorption; may cause complex nocturnal behaviors (sleepwalking, sleep driving)

**Adult oral hypnotic dose.*

drowsiness and decreased motor performance the next day.[33-35] This hangover may be caused by the drug being redistributed to the CNS from peripheral storage sites or may occur simply because the drug has not been fully metabolized. Residual effects can result in serious or catastrophic problems when the patient must react quickly the next morning while driving a car, avoiding a fall, or performing other activities that require rapid motor responses.[35-37]

Anterograde amnesia is another problem sometimes associated with sedative-hypnotic use.[38] The patient may have trouble recalling details of events that occurred for a certain period of time before the drug was taken. Although usually a minor problem, this can become serious if the drug-induced amnesia exacerbates an already existing memory problem, as might occur in some elderly patients.

The residual problems can be resolved somewhat by taking a smaller dose or by using a drug with a shorter half-life (see Table 6-2).[34] Also, nonbenzodiazepine agents such as zolpidem, zaleplon, eszopiclone, and ramelteon appear to have milder effects, perhaps because of their relatively short half-life and limited duration of action.[18,21,33] These newer drugs have therefore been advocated in people who are prone to residual effects (e.g., older adults) and people who need to use these drugs for an extended period of time. Nonetheless, residual effects may continue to be a problem even with these milder nonbenzodiazepine drugs, and patients should still be careful about driving and performing other activities that require quick responses until the effects of these drugs have worn off.

Tolerance and Physical Dependence

Another potential problem with long-term sedative-hypnotic drug use is that prolonged administration may cause tolerance and physical dependence. *Drug tolerance* is the need to take more of a drug to exert the same effect. *Dependence* is the onset of withdrawal symptoms if drug administration is ceased. Although these problems were originally thought to be limited to barbiturates, benzodiazepines and other sedative-hypnotics are now recognized as also causing tolerance and dependence when taken continually for several weeks.[8,9,39]

The manner and severity of withdrawal symptoms varies according to the type of drug and the extent of physical dependence.[18,40] Withdrawal after short-term benzodiazepine use may be associated with problems such as sleep disturbances (i.e., rebound insomnia).[39,41] As discussed earlier, withdrawal effects seem to be milder with the nonbenzodiazepine agents (e.g., zolpidem, zaleplon, eszopiclone, ramelteon).[18,33] However, these agents are not devoid of these problems and care should be taken with prolonged use, especially in people with psychiatric disorders or a history of substance abuse.[21]

Consequently, the long-term use of these drugs should be avoided, and other nonpharmacological methods of reducing stress and promoting relaxation (e.g., mental imagery, biofeedback, cognitive behavioral therapies) should be instituted before tolerance and physical dependence can occur.[42-44] If the sedative-hypnotic drug has been used for an extended period, tapering off the dosage rather than abruptly stopping it has been recommended as a safer way to terminate administration.[41]

Complex Behaviors

Some people taking certain sedative-hypnotics have exhibited complex motor behaviors, including sleepwalking and driving a car while asleep (sleep driving).[45] Other behaviors such as eating large amounts of food while asleep have also been reported.[45,46] In most cases, the patient has no memory of these events and cannot recall anything that occurred when the drug was in effect. These complex behaviors seem to be most prevalent with some of the nonbenzodiazepine drugs, especially zolpidem (Ambien). Although the reasons for these behaviors are not fully understood, they may be more likely to occur if the patient has taken an excessive dose of the drug or has combined the drug with alcohol or other CNS depressants.[47]

Regardless of the cause, these behaviors are understandably of great concern because patients could injure themselves and others while engaging in activities such as sleepwalking and sleep driving. Hence, patients taking these drugs should be monitored as closely as possible to ensure that they do not engage in such behaviors, and evidence of any strange activities should be brought to the attention of the physician immediately.

Other Side Effects

Other side effects such as GI discomfort (nausea and vomiting), dry mouth, sore throat, and muscular incoordination have been reported, but these occur fairly infrequently and vary according to the exact drug used. Cardiovascular and respiratory depression may also occur, but these problems are dose-related and are usually not significant, except in cases of overdose.

ANTIANXIETY DRUGS

Anxiety can be described as a fear or apprehension over a situation or event that an individual feels is threatening. These events can range from a change in employment or family life to somewhat irrational phobias concerning everyday occurrences. Anxiety disorders can also be classified in several clinical categories, including generalized anxiety disorder, social anxiety disorder, panic disorder, obsessive-compulsive disorder, and posttraumatic stress syndrome.[48] Antianxiety drugs can help decrease the tension and nervousness associated with many of these syndromes until the situation is resolved or until the individual is counseled effectively in other methods of dealing with his or her anxiety.

Many drugs—including sedative-hypnotics—have the ability to decrease anxiety levels, but this is usually at the expense of an increase in sedation. Frequently, alleviating anxiety without producing excessive sedation is desirable so that the individual can function at home, on the job, and so on. Consequently, certain drugs are available that have significant anxiolytic properties at doses that produce minimal sedation. We discuss benzodiazepine drugs and other nonbenzodiazepine strategies for dealing with anxiety below.

Benzodiazepines

As discussed previously, because of their relative safety, the benzodiazepines are often the primary drugs used to treat many forms of anxiety.[49,50] In terms of anxiolytic properties, diazepam (Valium) is the prototypical antianxiety benzodiazepine (Fig. 6-2). The extensive use of this drug in treating nervousness and apprehension has made the trade name of this compound virtually synonymous with a decrease in tension and anxiety. When prescribed in anxiolytic dosages, diazepam and certain other benzodiazepines will decrease anxiety without

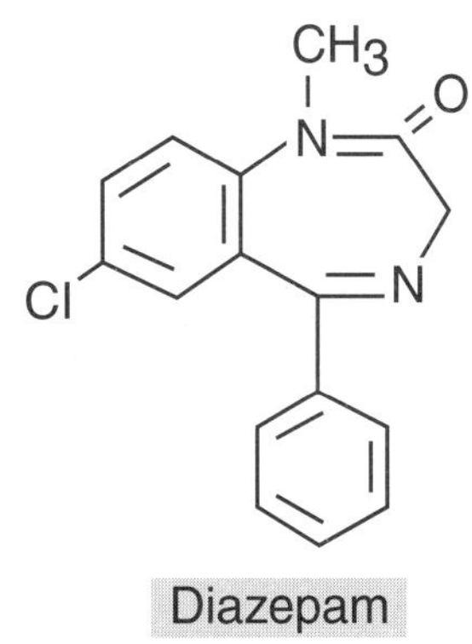

Figure ■ 6-2
Diazepam (Valium).

major sedative effects (Table 6-3). Some sedation, however, may occur even at anxiolytic dosages.

The antianxiety properties of benzodiazepines involve a mechanism similar or identical to their sedative-hypnotic effects (i.e., potentiating GABAergic transmission).[10] Benzodiazepines also seem to increase inhibition in the spinal cord, which produces some degree of skeletal muscle relaxation, which may contribute to their antianxiety effects by making the individual feel more relaxed. Chapter 13 provides further discussion on the use of these drugs as skeletal muscle relaxants.

Buspirone

Buspirone (BuSpar) is an antianxiety agent (approved in 1986) used to treat general anxiety disorder.[51] This agent belongs in a drug class known as the *azapirones*.[52] Buspirone does not act on the GABA receptor but exerts its antianxiety effects by increasing the effects of 5-hydroxytryptamine (serotonin) in certain areas of the brain.[51] Buspirone is basically a serotonin agonist that stimulates specific serotonin receptors, especially the 5-HT1A serotonin receptor subtype.[51] This increase in serotonergic influence is beneficial in treating general anxiety disorder and possibly panic disorder, obsessive-compulsive disorder, post-traumatic stress disorder, and various other disorders that may benefit from increased CNS serotonin activity.[52]

More importantly, buspirone has a much better side-effect profile than traditional antianxiety drugs. It produces less sedation and psychomotor impairment than benzodiazepine agents.[1,52] There is a much smaller risk of developing tolerance and dependence to buspirone, and the potential for abuse is much lower than with other anxiolytics.[1] However, buspirone has only moderate efficacy, and this drug may not take effect as quickly in patients with severe anxiety.[1] Nonetheless, buspirone offers a safer alternative to traditional antianxiety drugs such as benzodiazepines, especially if patients need to receive treatment for an extended period of time. Buspirone may also be helpful in treating depression, in reducing the side effects of Parkinson treatment, and in helping decrease behavioral problems related to attention deficit disorder, dementia, and traumatic brain injury.[51] Buspirone therefore remains a possible alternative to other antianxiety drugs and may also gain acceptance in treating other neurological disorders that are influenced by serotonin levels in the brain.

Use of Antidepressants in Anxiety

Many patients with anxiety also have symptoms of depression.[53,54] It therefore seems reasonable to include antidepressant drugs as part of the pharmacological regimen in these patients. Hence, patients with a combination of anxiety and depression often take a traditional antianxiety agent such as a benzodiazepine along with an antidepressant, especially if anxiety is resistant to treatment with only one agent.[55] The pharmacology of the antidepressants is addressed in Chapter 7.

Antidepressant drugs, however, can have direct antianxiety effects. In particular, antidepressants such as paroxetine (Paxil), venlafaxine (Effexor), and similar agents (Table 6-4) are often considered the first-line treatment for long-term management of generalized

Table 6-3
BENZODIAZEPINE ANTIANXIETY DRUGS

Generic Name	Trade Name	Antianxiety Dose (mg)*	Relative Half-Life
Alprazolam	Xanax, others	0.25–0.5 bid or tid	Short–intermediate
Chlordiazepoxide	Librium, others	5–25 tid or qid	Long
Clonazepam	Klonopin	0.50 tid	Intermediate
Clorazepate	Tranxene, others	7.5–15 bid to qid	Long
Diazepam	Valium, others	2–10 bid to qid	Long
Lorazepam	Ativan, others	1–3 bid or tid	Short–intermediate
Oxazepam	Serax, others	10–30 tid or qid	Short–intermediate

**Dose refers to initial adult oral dose used to treat generalized anxiety disorder. Dosage is adjusted depending on the patient's response. Doses are likewise often lower in elderly or debilitated patients.*

Table 6-4
ANTIDEPRESSANTS USED TO TREAT ANXIETY DISORDERS

Generic Name	Trade Name	Approved Use(s)*	Unlabeled Use(s)**
Duloxetine	Cymbalta	Generalized anxiety disorder	———
Escitalopram	Lexapro	Generalized anxiety disorder	Panic disorder, obsessive-compulsive disorder, post-traumatic stress disorder, social anxiety disorder
Paroxetine	Paxil, others	Generalized anxiety disorder, obsessive-compulsive disorder, social anxiety disorder, post-traumatic stress disorder	———
Sertraline	Zoloft	Panic disorder, obsessive-compulsive disorder, post-traumatic stress disorder, social anxiety disorder	Generalized anxiety disorder
Venlafaxine	Effexor XR	Generalized anxiety disorder, social anxiety disorder, panic disorder	———

**Approved by the Food and Drug Administration (FDA) to treat depression and the specific anxiety disorders indicated here.*
***Unlabeled use(s) (known also as off-label prescribing; see Chapter 1) are additional indications that are not FDA approved but may benefit from the drug.*

anxiety disorders and for other anxiety problems such as panic disorder and social anxiety disorder.[55-57] These antidepressants affect either serotonin or serotonin-norepinephrine balance in the brain, and their mechanism of action is addressed in more detail in Chapter 7. Although it is not clear exactly how these effects on serotonin and norepinephrine can help resolve anxiety disorders, there is ample evidence that these drugs are effective in many patients.[58]

Hence, certain antidepressants listed in Table 6-4 are now advocated as the primary way to treat certain anxiety disorders. Although benzodiazepines may take effect more quickly and are still often used to treat acute symptoms of anxiety, antidepressants tend to have fewer side effects and a lower risk of physical dependence and addiction.[55,56] The antidepressants described here have therefore emerged as a more effective and tolerable way to treat chronic anxiety problems. Future clinical research will continue to clarify how antidepressants can be used alone or in combination with other antianxiety drugs when managing the symptoms of specific anxiety disorders.

Other Antianxiety Drugs

The ideal antianxiety agent is nonaddictive, safe (i.e., relatively free from harmful side effects and potential for lethal overdose), and not associated with any sedative properties. Drugs such as meprobamate (Miltown) and barbiturates are not currently used to any great extent because they do not meet any of these criteria and are no more effective in reducing anxiety than benzodiazepines. Buspirone and certain antidepressants currently offer an effective and somewhat safer method of treating anxiety.

Another option includes the beta-adrenergic antagonists (beta blockers, see Chapter 20), because these drugs can decrease situational anxiety without producing sedation.[59] In particular, some musicians and other performing artists who experience intense stage fright use beta blockers such as propranolol (Inderal) to decrease the cardiac palpitations, muscle tremors, hyperventilation, and other manifestations of anxiety that tend to occur before an important performance.[60] These drugs may blunt the symptoms of performance anxiety without actually diminishing the anticipation and excitement that is requisite for a strong performance. Beta blockers probably exert their antianxiety effects through their ability to decrease activity in the sympathetic nervous system—that is, through their sympatholytic effects. These drugs may exert peripheral sympatholytic effects (e.g., blockade of myocardial beta-1 receptors) and decrease central sympathetic tone. In any event, beta blockers may offer a suitable alternative to decrease the effects of nervousness without a concomitant decrease in levels of alertness or motivation.[60] Beta blockers such as propranolol have also been used to treat anxiety related to post-traumatic stress disorder, and these drugs may provide a useful alternative to more traditional antianxiety drugs in people with various trauma-related anxiety.[61,62]

Finally, several other drugs, including antipsychotics such as quetiapine (see Chapter 8), anticonvulsants such as gabapentin and pregabalin (see Chapter 9), and antihistamines such as hydroxyzine (see Chapter 26) can be used as alternative agents to treat specific patients with anxiety. These drugs work in different ways to reduce excitation levels in the brain and may be helpful in patients who have not responded to more traditional antianxiety drugs.

Problems and Adverse Effects of Anxiolytics

Most of the problems that occur with benzodiazepine anxiolytic drugs are similar to those mentioned regarding the use of these agents as sedative-hypnotics. Sedation is still the most common side effect of anxiolytic benzodiazepines, even though this effect is not as pronounced as with their sedative-hypnotic counterparts.[55] Still, even short-term use of these drugs can produce psychomotor impairment, especially during activities that require people to remain especially alert, such as driving a car.[39] Addiction and abuse are problems with chronic benzodiazepine use, and withdrawal from these drugs can be a serious problem.[9,39] Also, anxiety can return to or exceed pretreatment levels when benzodiazepines are suddenly discontinued, a problem known as *rebound anxiety*.[38] The fact that chronic benzodiazepine use can cause these problems reinforces the idea that these drugs are not curative and should be used only for limited periods of time as an adjunct to nonpharmacological treatment such as psychological counseling.[63,64]

Problems and side effects associated with buspirone include dizziness, headache, nausea, and restlessness. Antidepressants such as paroxetine and venlafaxine also produce several side effects (described in Chapter 7), depending on the specific agent. Nonetheless, these nonbenzodiazepine anxiolytics tend to produce less sedation, and their potential for addiction is lower compared to benzodiazepines. Consequently, nonbenzodiazepine drugs might be an attractive alternative, especially in patients who are prone to sedation (e.g., older adults), patients with a history of substance abuse, or people who need chronic anxiolytic treatment.

Special Concerns for Rehabilitation Patients

Although sedative-hypnotic and antianxiety drugs are not used to directly influence the rehabilitation of musculoskeletal or other somatic disorders, the prevalence of their use in patient populations is high. Any time a patient is injured or hospitalized for treatment of a disorder, a substantial amount of apprehension and concern exists. The foreign environment of the institution and a change in the individual's daily routine can understandably result in sleep disturbances.[3,4] Likewise, older adults often have trouble sleeping, and the use of sedative-hypnotic agents is common, especially in patients living in nursing homes or other facilities.[65,66] Individuals who are involved in rehabilitation programs, both as inpatients and outpatients, may also have a fairly high level of anxiety because of concern about their health and ability to resume normal functioning.[2,5] Acute and chronic illnesses can create uncertainty about a patient's future family and job obligations as well as doubts about his or her self-image. The tension and anxiety produced may necessitate pharmacological management.

The administration of sedative-hypnotic and antianxiety drugs has several direct implications for the rehabilitation session. Obviously the patient will be much calmer and more relaxed after taking an antianxiety drug, thus offering the potential benefit of gaining the patient's full cooperation during physical therapy or occupational therapy interventions. Anxiolytic benzodiazepines, for example, typically reach peak blood levels 2 to 4 hours after oral administration, so scheduling the rehabilitation session during that time may improve the patient's participation in treatment. Of course, this rationale will backfire if the drug produces significant hypnotic effects. Therapy sessions that require the patient to actively participate in activities such as gait training or therapeutic exercise will be essentially useless and even hazardous if the patient is extremely drowsy. Consequently, scheduling patients

Special Concerns for Rehabilitation Patients (Continued)

for certain types of rehabilitation within several hours after administration of sedative-hypnotics or sedative-like anxiolytics is counterproductive and should be avoided.

Benzodiazepines and other drugs used to treat sleep disorders and anxiety are often associated with falls and subsequent trauma, including hip fractures, especially in older adults.[67,68] The risk of falls is greater in people who have a history of doing so or who have other problems that would predispose them to falling (e.g., vestibular disorders, impaired vision, etc.). Therapists can identify such people and intervene to help prevent this through balance training, environmental modifications (e.g., removing cluttered furniture, throw rugs, etc.), and similar activities.

Finally, therapists can help plan and implement nonpharmacological interventions to help decrease anxiety and improve sleep. Interventions such as regular exercise, massage, relaxation techniques, yoga, and other complementary therapies may be very helpful in reducing stress levels, decreasing anxiety, and promoting normal sleep.[69-72] Therapists can also review the patient's sleep habits and suggest improvements in sleep "hygiene," such as decreasing caffeine intake and establishing a consistent prebedtime routine.[73,74] By helping patients explore nonpharmacological methods for resolving insomnia and decreasing anxiety, clinicians can help reduce the need for drugs and improve the patient's quality of life by decreasing drug-related side effects.

CASE STUDY

SEDATIVE-HYPNOTIC DRUGS

Brief History. R.S. is a 34-year-old construction worker who sustained a fracture-dislocation of the vertebral column in an automobile accident. He was admitted to an acute care facility, where a diagnosis of complete paraplegia was made at the T-12 spinal level. Surgery was performed to stabilize the vertebral column. During the next 3 weeks, his medical condition improved. At the end of 1 month, he was transferred to a rehabilitation facility to begin an intensive program of physical therapy and occupational therapy. Rehabilitation included strengthening and range-of-motion (ROM) exercises, as well as training in wheelchair mobility, transfers, and activities of daily living (ADLs). However, upon arriving at the new institution, R.S. complained of difficulty sleeping. Flurazepam (Dalmane) was prescribed at a dosage of 30 mg administered orally each night at bedtime.

Problem/Influence of Medication. During his daily rehabilitation regimen, the therapists noted that R.S.'s performance and level of attentiveness were markedly poor during the morning sessions. He was excessively lethargic and drowsy, and his speech was slurred. These symptoms were present to a much greater extent than the normal slow start that occurs in some patients on wakening in the morning. The therapists also found that when ADL or mobility training was taught during the morning sessions, there was poor carryover from day to day regarding these activities.

1. *What is the most likely reason for R.S.'s poor performance in the morning rehabilitation sessions?*
2. *What would be the likely solution?*

See Appendix C, "Answers to Case Study Questions."

SUMMARY

Sedative-hypnotic and antianxiety drugs play a prominent role in today's society. The normal pressures of daily life often result in tension and stress, which affects an individual's ability to relax or cope with problems. These issues are compounded when there is some type of illness or injury present. As would be expected, many patients seen in a rehabilitation setting are taking these drugs. Benzodiazepines have long been the premier agents used to treat sleep disorders and anxiety; they all share a common mechanism of action, and they potentiate the inhibitory effects of GABA in the CNS. Benzodiazepines such as flurazepam and triazolam are commonly used to promote sleep because of their sedative-hypnotic effects. Although benzodiazepines are generally safer than their forerunners, they are not without their problems. Nonbenzodiazepine sedative-hypnotics such as zolpidem, zaleplon, eszopiclone, and ramelteon may also be effective in treating sleep disorders, and these agents may be somewhat safer than their benzodiazepine counterparts. Benzodiazepines such as diazepam (Valium) are also used frequently to reduce anxiety, but the introduction of newer drugs such as buspirone and specific antidepressants (paroxetine, venlafaxine) have provided an effective and somewhat safer alternative for treating anxiety. Because of the potential for physical and psychological dependence, sedative-hypnotic and antianxiety drugs should not be used indefinitely. These drugs should be prescribed judiciously as an adjunct to helping patients deal with the source of their problems.

REFERENCES

1. Trevor AJ, Way WL. Sedative-hypnotic drugs. In: Katzung BG, ed. *Basic and Clinical Pharmacology.* 12th ed. New York: Lange Medical Books/McGraw Hill; 2012.
2. Kraus SS, Rabin LA. Sleep America: managing the crisis of adult chronic insomnia and associated conditions. *J Affect Disord.* 2012; 138:192-212.
3. Gay PC. Sleep and sleep-disordered breathing in the hospitalized patient. *Respir Care.* 2010;55:1240-1254.
4. Young JS, Bourgeois JA, Hilty DM, Hardin KA. Sleep in hospitalized medical patients, part 1: factors affecting sleep. *J Hosp Med.* 2008;3:473-482.
5. Walker JR, Graff LA, Dutz JP, Bernstein CN. Psychiatric disorders in patients with immune-mediated inflammatory diseases: prevalence, association with disease activity, and overall patient well-being. *J Rheumatol Suppl.* 2011;88:31-35.
6. Licata SC, Rowlett JK. Abuse and dependence liability of benzodiazepine-type drugs: GABA(A) receptor modulation and beyond. *Pharmacol Biochem Behav.* 2008;90:74-89.
7. Mihac SJ, Harris RA. Hypnotics and sedatives. In: Brunton LL, et al, eds. *The Pharmacological Basis of Therapeutics.* 12th ed. New York: McGraw Hill; 2011.
8. Authier N, Balayssac D, Sautereau M, et al. Benzodiazepine dependence: focus on withdrawal syndrome. *Ann Pharm Fr.* 2009; 67:408-413.
9. Tan KR, Rudolph U, Lüscher C. Hooked on benzodiazepines: GABAA receptor subtypes and addiction. *Trends Neurosci.* 2011;34:188-197.
10. Trincavelli ML, Da Pozzo E, Daniele S, Martini C. The GABAA-BZR complex as target for the development of anxiolytic drugs. *Curr Top Med Chem.* 2012;12:254-269.
11. Carter CR, Kozuska JL, Dunn SM. Insights into the structure and pharmacology of GABA(A) receptors. *Future Med Chem.* 2010;2:859-875.
12. Gajcy K, Lochy_ski S, Librowski T. A role of GABA analogues in the treatment of neurological diseases. *Curr Med Chem.* 2010;17:2338-2347.
13. Roth FC, Draguhn A. GABA metabolism and transport: effects on synaptic efficacy. *Neural Plast.* 2012;2012:805-830.
14. Sigel E, Lüscher BP. A closer look at the high affinity benzodiazepine binding site on GABAA receptors. *Curr Top Med Chem.* 2011;11:241-246.
15. Molinoff PB. Neurotransmission and the central nervous system. In: Brunton LL, et al, eds. *The Pharmacological Basis of Therapeutics.* 12th ed. New York: McGraw Hill; 2011.
16. Lujan R, Ciruela F. GABAB receptors-associated proteins: potential drug targets in neurological disorders? *Curr Drug Targets.* 2012;13:129-144.
17. Sieghart W, Ramerstorfer J, Sarto-Jackson I, et al. A novel GABA(A) receptor pharmacology: drugs interacting with the α(+) β(-) interface. *Br J Pharmacol.* 2012;166:476-485.
18. Richey SM, Krystal AD. Pharmacological advances in the treatment of insomnia. *Curr Pharm Des.* 2011;17:1471-1475.
19. Melcangi RC, Panzica G, Garcia-Segura LM. Neuroactive steroids: focus on human brain. *Neuroscience.* 2011;191:1-5.
20. D'Hulst C, Atack JR, Kooy RF. The complexity of the GABAA receptor shapes unique pharmacological profiles. *Drug Discov Today.* 2009;14:866-875.
21. Zammit G. Comparative tolerability of newer agents for insomnia. *Drug Saf.* 2009;32:735-748.
22. Nutt DJ, Stahl SM. Searching for perfect sleep: the continuing evolution of GABAA receptor modulators as hypnotics. *J Psychopharmacol.* 2010;24:1601-1612.
23. Liu J, Wang LN. Ramelteon in the treatment of chronic insomnia: systematic review and meta-analysis. *Int J Clin Pract.* 2012;66:867-873.
24. Rios ER, Venâncio ET, Rocha NF, et al. Melatonin: pharmacological aspects and clinical trends. *Int J Neurosci.* 2010;120: 583-590.
25. Srinivasan V, Zakaria R, Othaman Z, et al. Melatonergic drugs for therapeutic use in insomnia and sleep disturbances of mood disorders. *CNS Neurol Disord Drug Targets.* 2012;11:180-189.
26. Cardinali DP, Srinivasan V, Brzezinski A, Brown GM. Melatonin and its analogs in insomnia and depression. *J Pineal Res.* 2012;52:365-375.
27. Melgaard B. The neurotoxicity of ethanol. *Acta Neurol Scand.* 1983;67:131-142.

28. Kumar S, Porcu P, Werner DF, et al. The role of GABA(A) receptors in the acute and chronic effects of ethanol: a decade of progress. *Psychopharmacology*. 2009;205:529-564.
29. Schuckit MA. Ethanol and methanol. In: Brunton LL, et al, eds. *The Pharmacological Basis of Therapeutics*. 12th ed. New York: McGraw Hill; 2011.
30. Morin AK, Jarvis CI, Lynch AM. Therapeutic options for sleep-maintenance and sleep-onset insomnia. *Pharmacotherapy*. 2007;27:89-110.
31. McCall C, McCall WV. What is the role of sedating antidepressants, antipsychotics, and anticonvulsants in the management of insomnia? *Curr Psychiatry Rep*. 2012;14:494-502.
32. Ramakrishnan K, Scheid DC. Treatment options for insomnia. *Am Fam Physician*. 2007;76:517-526.
33. Bogan RK. Treatment options for insomnia—pharmacodynamics of zolpidem extended-release to benefit next-day performance. *Postgrad Med*. 2008;120:161-171.
34. Vermeeren A. Residual effects of hypnotics: epidemiology and clinical implications. *CNS Drugs*. 2004;18:297-328.
35. Vermeeren A, Coenen AM. Effects of the use of hypnotics on cognition. *Prog Brain Res*. 2011;190:89-103.
36. Mets MA, de Vries JM, de Senerpont Domis LM, et al. Next-day effects of ramelteon (8 mg), zopiclone (7.5 mg), and placebo on highway driving performance, memory functioning, psychomotor performance, and mood in healthy adult subjects. *Sleep*. 2011;34:1327-1334.
37. Verster JC, Spence DW, Shahid A, et al. Zopiclone as positive control in studies examining the residual effects of hypnotic drugs on driving ability. *Curr Drug Saf*. 2011;6:209-218.
38. Uzun S, Kozumplik O, Jakovljević M, Sedić B. Side effects of treatment with benzodiazepines. *Psychiatr Danub*. 2010;22:90-93.
39. Lader M. Benzodiazepines revisited—will we ever learn? *Addiction*. 2011;106:2086-2109.
40. Zisapel N. Drugs for insomnia. *Expert Opin Emerg Drugs*. 2012;17:299-317.
41. Lader M, Tylee A, Donoghue J. Withdrawing benzodiazepines in primary care. *CNS Drugs*. 2009;23:19-34.
42. Pigeon WR. Treatment of adult insomnia with cognitive-behavioral therapy. *J Clin Psychol*. 2010;66:1148-1160.
43. Sánchez-Ortuño MM, Edinger JD. Cognitive-behavioral therapy for the management of insomnia comorbid with mental disorders. *Curr Psychiatry Rep*. 2012;14:519-528.
44. Young JS, Bourgeois JA, Hilty DM, Hardin KA. Sleep in hospitalized medical patients, part 2: behavioral and pharmacological management of sleep disturbances. *J Hosp Med*. 2009;4:50-59.
45. Hoque R, Chesson AL Jr. Zolpidem-induced sleepwalking, sleep related eating disorder, and sleep-driving: fluorine-18-flourodeoxyglucose positron emission tomography analysis, and a literature review of other unexpected clinical effects of zolpidem. *J Clin Sleep Med*. 2009;5:471-476.
46. Najjar M. Zolpidem and amnestic sleep related eating disorder. *J Clin Sleep Med*. 2007;3:637-638.
47. Pressman MR. Sleep driving: sleepwalking variant or misuse of z-drugs? *Sleep Med Rev*. 2011;15:285-292.
48. McTeague LM, Lang PJ. The anxiety spectrum and the reflex physiology of defense: from circumscribed fear to broad distress. *Depress Anxiety*. 2012;29:264-281.
49. López-Muñoz F, Alamo C, García-García P. The discovery of chlordiazepoxide and the clinical introduction of benzodiazepines: half a century of anxiolytic drugs. *J Anxiety Disord*. 2011;25:554-562.
50. Ravindran LN, Stein MB. The pharmacologic treatment of anxiety disorders: a review of progress. *J Clin Psychiatry*. 2010; 71:839-854.
51. Loane C, Politis M. Buspirone: what is it all about? *Brain Res*. 2012;1461:111-118.
52. Chessick CA, Allen MH, Thase M, et al. Azapirones for generalized anxiety disorder. *Cochrane Database Syst Rev*. 2006; 3:CD006115.
53. Beattie E, Pachana NA, Franklin SJ. Double jeopardy: Comorbid anxiety and depression in late life. *Res Gerontol Nurs*. 2010;3:209-220.
54. Goldberg D, Fawcett J. The importance of anxiety in both major depression and bipolar disorder. *Depress Anxiety*. 2012;29: 471-478.
55. Melton ST, Kirkwood CK. Anxiety disorders I: generalized anxiety, panic, and social anxiety disorders. In: DiPiro JT, et al, eds. *Pharmacotherapy: A Pathophysiologic Approach*. 8th ed. New York: McGraw-Hill; 2011.
56. Baldwin DS, Ajel KI, Garner M. Pharmacological treatment of generalized anxiety disorder. *Curr Top Behav Neurosci*. 2010; 2:453-467.
57. Reinhold JA, Mandos LA, Rickels K, Lohoff FW. Pharmacological treatment of generalized anxiety disorder. *Expert Opin Pharmacother*. 2011;12:2457-2467.
58. Baldwin DS, Waldman S, Allgulander C. Evidence-based pharmacological treatment of generalized anxiety disorder. *Int J Neuropsychopharmacol*. 2011;14:697-710.
59. Beversdorf DQ, White DM, Chever DC, et al. Central beta-adrenergic modulation of cognitive flexibility. *Neuroreport*. 2002;13:2505-2507.
60. Brugués AO. Music performance anxiety-part 2. A review of treatment options. *Med Probl Perform Art*. 2011;26: 164-171.
61. Bell J. Propranolol, post-traumatic stress disorder and narrative identity. *J Med Ethics*. 2008;34:e23.
62. Donovan E. Propranolol use in the prevention and treatment of posttraumatic stress disorder in military veterans: forgetting therapy revisited. *Perspect Biol Med*. 2010;53:61-74.
63. Archer J, Bower P, Gilbody S, et al. Collaborative care for depression and anxiety problems. *Cochrane Database Syst Rev*. 2012;10:CD006525.
64. Bower P, Knowles S, Coventry PA, Rowland N. Counselling for mental health and psychosocial problems in primary care. *Cochrane Database Syst Rev*. 2011;9:CD001025.
65. Crowley K. Sleep and sleep disorders in older adults. *Neuropsychol Rev*. 2011;21:41-53.
66. Vance DE, Heaton K, Eaves Y, Fazeli PL. Sleep and cognition on everyday functioning in older adults: implications for nursing practice and research. *J Neurosci Nurs*. 2011;43: 261-271.
67. Huang AR, Mallet L, Rochefort CM, et al. Medication-related falls in the elderly: causative factors and preventive strategies. *Drugs Aging*. 2012;29:359-376.
68. Khong TP, de Vries F, Goldenberg JS, et al. Potential impact of benzodiazepine use on the rate of hip fractures in five large European countries and the United States. *Calcif Tissue Int*. 2012;91:24-31.
69. Herring MP, Jacob ML, Suveg C, et al. Feasibility of exercise training for the short-term treatment of generalized anxiety disorder: a randomized controlled trial. *Psychother Psychosom*. 2012; 81:21-28.

70. Kozasa EH, Hachul H, Monson C, et al. Mind-body interventions for the treatment of insomnia: a review. *Rev Bras Psiquiatr.* 2010;32:437-443.
71. Sarris J, Byrne GJ. A systematic review of insomnia and complementary medicine. *Sleep Med Rev.* 2011;15:99-106.
72. Yang PY, Ho KH, Chen HC, Chien MY. Exercise training improves sleep quality in middle-aged and older adults with sleep problems: a systematic review. *J Physiother.* 2012;58:157-163.
73. Kaku A, Nishinoue N, Takano T, et al. Randomized controlled trial on the effects of a combined sleep hygiene education and behavioral approach program on sleep quality in workers with insomnia. *Ind Health.* 2012;50:52-59.
74. Sin CW, Ho JS, Chung JW. Systematic review on the effectiveness of caffeine abstinence on the quality of sleep. *J Clin Nurs.* 2009;18:13-21.

CHAPTER 7

Drugs to Treat Affective Disorders: Depression and Bipolar Syndrome

Affective disorders comprise the group of mental conditions that includes depression, bipolar syndrome (manic-depression), and several others that are characterized by a marked disturbance in a patient's mood.[1] Patients with an affective disorder typically present with an inappropriate disposition, feeling unreasonably sad and discouraged (major depressive disorder), or fluctuating between periods of depression and excessive excitation and elation (bipolar disorder).

Because these forms of mental illness are relatively common, many rehabilitation specialists will work with patients who are receiving drug therapy for an affective disorder. Also, serious injury or illness may precipitate an episode of depression in the patient undergoing physical rehabilitation. Consequently, this chapter will discuss the pharmacological management of affective disorders and how antidepressant and antimanic drugs may influence the patient involved in physical therapy and occupational therapy.

DEPRESSION

Depression is a form of mental illness characterized by intense feelings of sadness and despair. It is considered to be the most prevalent mental illness in the United States, with approximately 15 to 20 percent of adults experiencing major depression at some point in their lives.[2,3] Likewise, the incidence of depression varies in different age groups, and women tend to be approximately twice as likely to experience depression during their lifetime compared to men.[3] While a certain amount of disappointment and sadness is part of everyday life, a diagnosis of clinical depression indicates that these feelings are increased in both intensity and duration to an incapacitating extent.

Depressive disorders are characterized by a general dysphoric mood (sadness, irritability, feeling "down in the dumps") and by a general lack of interest in previously pleasurable activities. Other symptoms include anorexia, sleep disorders (either too much or too little), fatigue, lack of self-esteem, somatic complaints, and irrational guilt. Recurrent thoughts of death and suicide may also help lead to a diagnosis of depression. To initiate effective treatment, a proper diagnosis must be made; depression must not be confused with other mental disorders that also may influence mood and behavior (e.g., schizophrenia). The American Psychiatric Association has outlined specific criteria for diagnosis in order to standardize the terminology and aid in recognizing depression.[4] Depressive disorders can also be subclassified according to the type, duration, and intensity of the patient's symptoms.[5-7] For the purpose of this chapter, we use the term *depression* to indicate major depressive disorder, but you should be aware that the exact type of depression may vary somewhat from person to person.

The causes of depression seem to be complex and unclear. Although a recent stressful incident, misfortune, or illness can certainly exacerbate an episode of depression, some patients may become depressed for no apparent reason. The role of genetic factors in depression has been explored but remains uncertain.

Over the past few decades, it has been suggested that a central nervous system (CNS) neurochemical imbalance may be the underlying feature in depression and in other forms of mental illness. The importance of these findings as related to pharmacological treatment will be discussed later. However, factors responsible for initiating these changes in CNS function are unclear. Depression is undoubtedly caused by the complex interaction of genetic, environmental, and biochemical factors.[8-11]

Treatment of depression is essential in minimizing the disruptive influence that this disease has on patients' quality of life and on their relationships with their family and job. Effective treatment of depression can also help improve outcomes in people with back pain, stroke, and other conditions seen commonly in physical therapist and occupational therapist practice.[12-14] Depending on the severity and type of depression, treatment can include various procedures ranging from psychotherapy to electroconvulsive treatment. However, antidepressant drugs are the primary method for alleviating and preventing the occurrence of major depression.

Pathophysiology of Depression

It appears that depression is related to a disturbance in CNS neurotransmission involving certain chemicals know as *amine neurotransmitters*. These transmitters include 5-hydroxytryptamine (serotonin), norepinephrine, and dopamine. Amine neurotransmitters are found in many areas of the brain and are important in controlling many aspects of mood and behavior.

However, the exact problem in CNS amine neurotransmission remains a subject of much debate. An early theory focused on the idea that depression may be caused by an *increased* sensitivity of the presynaptic or postsynaptic receptors for these transmitters (Fig. 7-1). That is, the neurochemistry of the brain has been changed in some way to make the amine receptors *more* sensitive to their respective amine neurotransmitters (norepinephrine, serotonin, and to a lesser extent, dopamine).[15] This receptor sensitivity theory was based primarily on the finding that antidepressant drugs prolong the activity of amine neurotransmission in the brain, thereby causing a compensatory decrease in the sensitivity of the amine receptors.[3,15]

Antidepressant drugs increase amine transmission by a variety of methods, thereby bringing about overstimulation of the postsynaptic receptor. (The exact method by which these drugs increase amine stimulation is discussed later in this chapter.) Overstimulation of the postsynaptic receptor then leads to a compensatory down-regulation and decreased sensitivity of the receptor. As discussed in Chapter 4, this down-regulation is a normal response to overstimulation by either endogenous or exogenous agonists. As receptor sensitivity decreases, the clinical symptoms of depression might be resolved.

On the other hand, other research suggested that the primary problem in depression is an increased

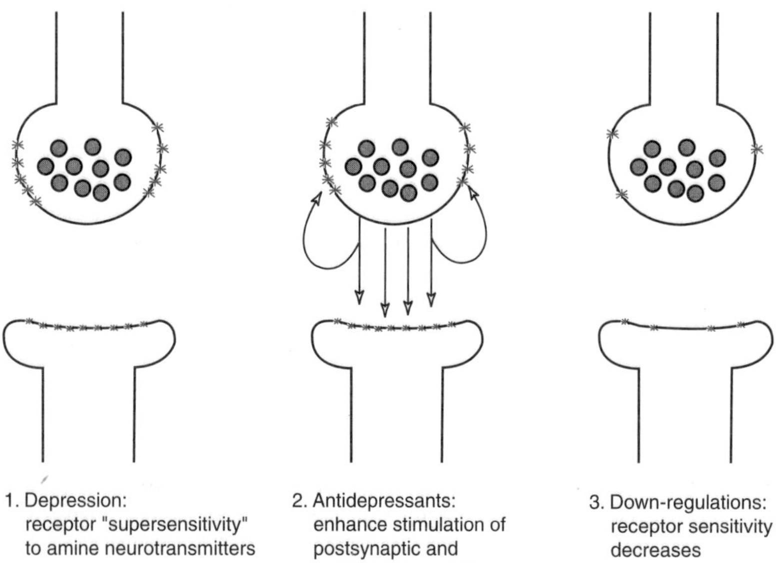

Figure 7-1
Receptor sensitivity theory of depression. Functionally active receptor sites are indicated by an asterisk (*). Depression is believed to be initiated by increased postsynaptic or presynaptic receptor sensitivity. Drugs that enhance stimulation of these receptors ultimately lead to receptor down-regulation, which normalizes synaptic activity and may bring about positive changes in the function and growth of postsynaptic neurons, thus resolving the depression.

sensitivity to receptors that are located on the *presynaptic* terminals of amine synapses.[15,16] These presynaptic "autoreceptors" normally regulate and limit the release of amine transmitters, such as norepinephrine or serotonin, from the presynaptic terminal. Increasing their sensitivity could result in a relative lack of adequate neurotransmitter release at these synapses. By causing overstimulation of these presynaptic receptors, antidepressant drugs could eventually normalize their sensitivity and help reestablish proper control and regulation of these amine synapses.[15]

More recently, it has been hypothesized that depression may be caused by decreased formation of new neurons (neurogenesis) and impaired formation of synaptic connections in areas of the brain such as the hippocampus[17,18] (Fig. 7-2). That is, factors such as stress, trauma, environmental influences, and genetic predisposition may inhibit neurogenesis in the hippocampus, thus leading to symptoms of depression. Likewise, glucocorticoids such as cortisol may impair neurogenesis and synaptic function in the hippocampus, thus leading to depression. Indeed, high levels of cortisol are often found in the bloodstream of certain people with depression.[19] This makes sense because cortisol is often released from the adrenal cortex in response to stress, and prolonged or severe stress can be a precipitating factor in certain forms of depression (see Chapter 28 for a description of cortisol production).[19,20] Hence, the "neurogenesis" hypothesis of depression is based on the idea that emotional, environmental, and hormonal factors can act together to bring about impaired neuronal growth and function in the hippocampus of susceptible individuals.

Antidepressant drug treatment may also be consistent with the neurogenesis basis for depression. By altering amine neurotransmitter activity, antidepressant drugs may help restore chemical signals that enhance neurogenesis and the formation of synaptic connections in the brain.[17,21] In particular, a protein known as **brain-derived neurotrophic factor (BDNF)** seems to be important in sustaining neuronal growth and activity in the brain.[22,23] BDNF may be decreased in people with depression, and antidepressant drugs may ultimately increase production of BDNF to help restore neuronal growth and synaptic

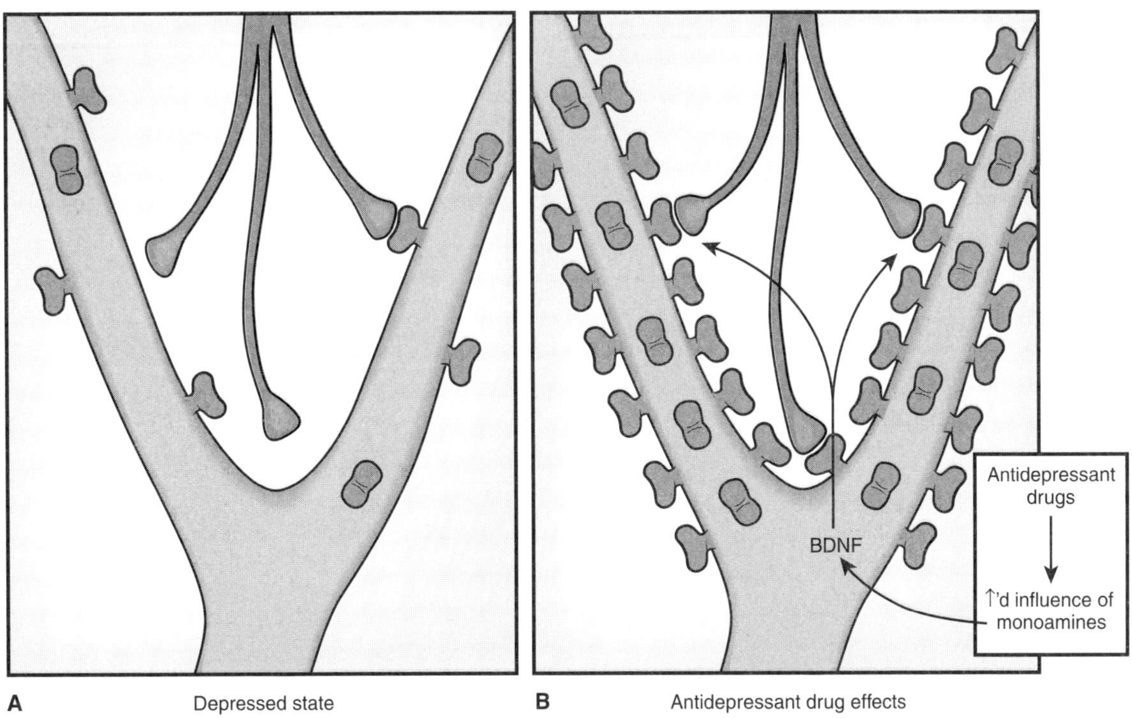

Figure 7-2
Neurogenesis hypothesis of depression. **A.** Depressed state results from decreased synaptic connections in the hippocampus. **B.** Antidepressants increase monoamine transmitter influence, which in turn increases synthesis of brain-derived neurotrophic factor (BDNF). BDNF increases hippocampal neuronal growth and synaptic connections.

connections in the hippocampus.[18,24] Researchers continue to evaluate the exact role of BDNF and the ability of antidepressant drugs to restore this important factor. Future research should help clarify the neurochemical changes that underlie depression.

It must be emphasized that it is difficult to prove the neurochemical changes responsible for depression, and the way that antidepressant drugs help resolve depression remains theoretical at present. Still, certain aspects of drug therapy tend to support the amine hypothesis and the putative changes in receptor sensitivity induced by drug therapy. For instance, there is usually a time lag of approximately 2 to 4 weeks before antidepressant drugs begin to work.[18] This latency period would be necessary for a compensatory change in receptor sensitivity or neurogenesis to take place after drug therapy is initiated.[3]

In essence, complex neurochemical changes seem to occur in certain areas of the brain in people with depression, and these changes may vary depending on each person and the specific type of depression. Likewise, changes in other brain chemicals—such as gamma-aminobutyric acid (GABA), glutamate, neuropeptides (substance P, vasopressin, others), and intracellular second messengers (cyclic adenosine monophosphate, cyclic guanosine monophosphate)—may also play a role in the pathophysiology of depression.[25-28] Future research will continue to clarify the exact cellular and subcellular events that occur during depression and how these events can be resolved pharmacologically. Drugs currently used to treat depression are discussed next.

Antidepressant Drugs

The drugs that are currently used to treat depression are grouped into several categories, according to chemical or functional criteria (Table 7-1):

- Selective serotonin reuptake inhibitors
- Serotonin-norepinephrine reuptake inhibitors
- Tricyclics
- Monoamine oxidase (MAO) inhibitors
- Other compounds

These drugs all attempt to increase aminergic transmission, but by different mechanisms (Fig. 7-3). The pharmacological effects of the primary antidepressant drug categories are discussed below.

Table 7-1
COMMON ANTIDEPRESSANT DRUGS

Prescribing Generic Name	Trade Name	Initial Adult Dose* (mg/day)	Limits* (mg/day)
Serotonin Selective Reuptake Inhibitors			
Citalopram	Celexa	20	60
Escitalopram	Lexapro	10	20
Fluoxetine	Prozac	20	80
Fluvoxamine	Luvox	50	300
Paroxetine	Paxil	20	50
Sertraline	Zoloft	50	200
Serotonin-Norepinephrine Reuptake Inhibitors			
Desvenlafaxine	Pristiq	50	50
Duloxetine	Cymbalta	40–60	60
Venlafaxine	Effexor	75	375
Tricyclics			
Amitriptyline	Elavil, Endep, others	75	300
Amoxapine	Asendin	100–150	600
Clomipramine	Anafranil	75	300
Desipramine	Norpramin	100–200	300

Table 7-1
COMMON ANTIDEPRESSANT DRUGS—cont'd

Prescribing Generic Name	Trade Name	Initial Adult Dose* (mg/day)	Limits* (mg/day)
Doxepin	Sinequan	75	300
Imipramine	Norfranil, Tofranil, others	75–200	300
Nortriptyline	Aventyl, Pamelor	75–100	150
Protriptyline	Vivactil	15–40	60
Trimipramine	Surmontil	75	300
Monoamine Oxidase (MAO) Inhibitors			
Isocarboxazid	Marplan	20	60
Phenelzine	Nardil	45	90
Tranylcypromine	Parnate	30	60
Others			
Bupropion	Wellbutrin	150	450
Mirtazapine	Remeron	15	45
Nefazodone	Serzone	200	600
Trazodone	Desyrel	150	600

**Dosages typically refer to immediate-release preparations versus extended-release products. Some total daily doses are divided into two to four smaller doses. Upper limits may reflect dosages administered to patients with severe depression who are being treated as inpatients.*

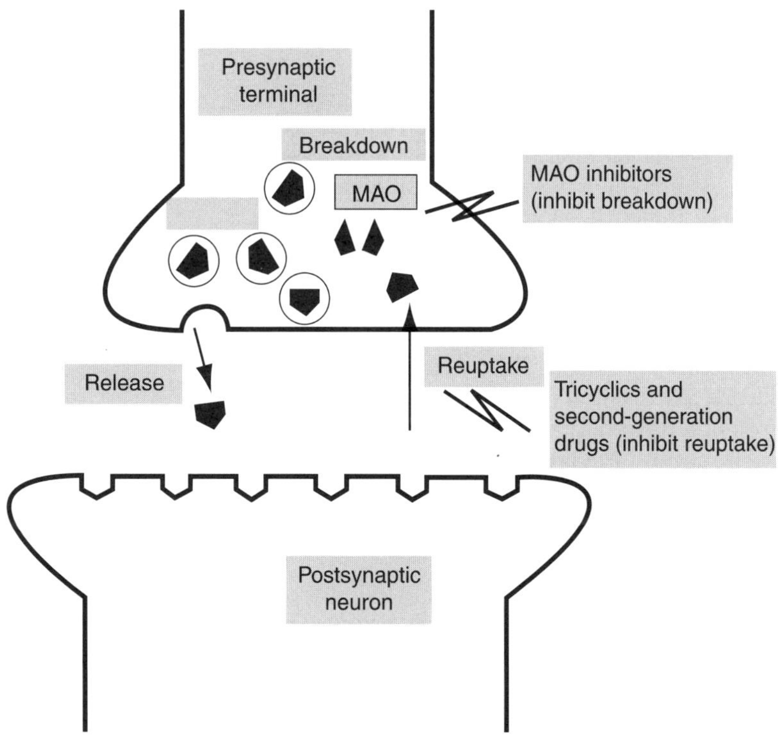

Figure ■ 7-3
Effects of antidepressant drugs on amine synapses. All three types of drugs increase the presence of amine transmitters (norepinephrine, dopamine, serotonin) in the synaptic cleft. Increased transmitter stimulation leads to receptor down-regulation/desensitization (receptor sensitivity theory), facilitates synaptic connections in the hippocampus (neurogenesis hypothesis), or causes other effects that may help restore function in postsynaptic neuronal pathways.

Selective Serotonin Reuptake Inhibitors

As indicated earlier, serotonin (5-hydroxytryptamine) seems to be one of the key amine neurotransmitters that helps regulate mood and depression. Drugs have therefore been developed that are relatively selective for synapses that use serotonin, rather than synapses involving the other two primary amine neurotransmitters (i.e., norepinephrine, dopamine).[29] These drugs, known collectively as *selective serotonin reuptake inhibitors* (SSRIs), have become a mainstay in treating depression. This group likewise includes some of the most well-known antidepressants such as fluoxetine (Prozac), paroxetine (Paxil), and sertraline (Zoloft) (Table 7-2).

As their name suggests, SSRIs work by blocking the reuptake of serotonin into the presynaptic terminal at key locations within the brain.[29,30] At these synapses, 50 to 80 percent of the released transmitter is removed from the synaptic cleft by "reuptake," which occurs when the neurotransmitter is actively transported back into the presynaptic terminal. By inhibiting the enzyme responsible for this active transport (reuptake), SSRIs allow the released serotonin to remain in the synaptic cleft and continue to exert its effects for a longer period of time. The prolonged effects of serotonin will hopefully lead to the beneficial changes in receptor sensitivity or neuronal growth and function as described earlier (see the "Pathophysiology of Depression" section above).

Hence, SSRIs are distinguished from other antidepressants by their relatively selective effect on serotonin. As a result, certain patients may experience greater antidepressant effects with SSRIs compared to nonselective drugs, presumably because a serotonin imbalance is the primary problem in those patients. Likewise, some SSRIs may produce fewer and less bothersome side effects than their nonselective counterparts in some patients, thus improving compliance and adherence to drug treatment.[31] Side effects, however, are highly variable depending on the patient and specific drug used[32] (see "Problems and Adverse Effects" later in this chapter). Hence, SSRIs remain very popular as a first choice when treating depression, but selection of the best drug for a given patient will depend on many factors, including how effective the drug is in reducing depression relative to the side effects that occur in that patient.

Serotonin-Norepinephrine Reuptake Inhibitors

Some of the newest antidepressants can decrease serotonin and norepinephrine reuptake without an appreciable effect of dopamine synapses.[33,34] These drugs, known as the *serotonin-norepinephrine reuptake inhibitors* (SNRIs), include duloxetine (Cymbalta), venlafaxine (Effexor), and desvenlafaxine (Pristiq) (see Tables 7-1 and 7-2). Milnacipran (Savella) is an SNRI that is used as an antidepressant in other countries but is approved only for treating fibromyalgia in the United States.[35] In general, SNRIs appear to be similar to other common antidepressants in terms of safety and antidepressant effects. Nonetheless, certain patients seem to experience optimal effects from the SNRIs compared to more established agents such as the SSRIs or tricyclic drugs.[33,34] Again, treatment of depression is highly variable from patient to patient, and it seems reasonable that SNRIs will be the drugs of choice in a specific subgroup of people with major depression.[36] SNRIs have also received considerable attention for their beneficial effects in treating other conditions, especially chronic pain associated with osteoarthritis, peripheral neuropathies, and fibromyalgia (see "Antidepressants and Chronic Pain" later in this chapter). Future studies will continue to determine how SNRIs can best be used to treat specific types of depression and other conditions such as chronic pain.

Tricyclics

Drugs in this category share a common three-ring chemical structure, hence the name *tricyclic*. These drugs work by blocking the reuptake of amine neurotransmitters into the presynaptic terminal.[30] However, they are not very selective in their effects and tend to affect synapses using all three of the primary amines: serotonin, norepinephrine, and dopamine.

In the past, tricyclic drugs such as amitriptyline and nortriptyline were the most commonly used antidepressants and were the standard against which other antidepressants were measured.[30] The use of tricyclic drugs as the initial treatment of depression has diminished somewhat in favor of some of the newer, more selective drugs such as the SSRIs and SNRIs. Due to their relatively nonselective effects, tricyclics tend to have more interactions with other drugs and may also be more harmful during overdose.[37,38] Nonetheless, tricyclic agents remain an important component in the management of depressive disorders but are usually reserved for patients who have failed to respond to other antidepressants, such as the SSRIs.[39]

Monoamine Oxidase Inhibitors

Monoamine oxidase (MAO) is an enzyme located at amine synapses that helps remove released transmitters through enzymatic destruction. Drugs that inhibit this enzyme allow more of the transmitter to remain in the synaptic cleft and continue to exert an effect.[40,41] As

Table 7-2
RELATIVE EFFECTS OF COMMON ANTIDEPRESSANTS*

Drug	Mechanism (Amine Selectivity)	Advantages	Disadvantages
Selective Serotonin Reuptake Inhibitors			
Citalopram (Celexa)	Strong, selective inhibition of serotonin reuptake	Low incidence of sedation and anticholinergic effects; does not cause orthostatic hypotension or cardiac arrhythmias	May cause sexual dysfunction (decreased libido, impotence)
Escitalopram (Lexapro)	Strong, selective inhibition of serotonin reuptake	Similar to citalopram	Similar to citalopram
Fluoxetine (Prozac)	Moderate, selective inhibition of serotonin reuptake	No sedative, anticholinergic, or cardiovascular side effects; helpful in obsessive-compulsive disorder	May cause anxiety, nausea, insomnia; long half-life can lead to accumulation
Fluvoxamine (Luvox)	Strong, selective inhibition of serotonin reuptake	Similar to fluoxetine	Similar to fluoxetine
Paroxetine (Paxil)	Strong, selective inhibition of serotonin reuptake	Similar to citalopram	Similar to citalopram
Sertraline (Zoloft)	Strong, selective inhibition of serotonin reuptake	Similar to fluoxetine	Similar to fluoxetine
Serotonin-Norepinephrine Reuptake Inhibitors			
Desvenlafaxine (Pristiq)	Strong inhibition of norepinephrine and serotonin reuptake	Low risk of orthostatic hypotension, sedation, and anticholinergic side effects	May cause GI problems (nausea, constipation) and male sexual dysfunction (decreased libido, impotence)
Duloxetine (Cymbalta)	Strong inhibition of norepinephrine and serotonin reuptake	Low risk of sedation, seizures, cardiovascular effects, and GI problems	Slightly higher risk of agitation or increased mania
Venlafaxine (Effexor)	Strong inhibition of norepinephrine and serotonin reuptake	Similar to desvenlafaxine	Similar to desvenlafaxine
Others			
Bupropion (Wellbutrin, Zyban)	Primarily inhibits dopamine reuptake; little effect on norepinephrine or serotonin	Low sedative, anticholinergic, and cardiovascular side effects; also used as an intervention to quit cigarette smoking	May cause overstimulation (insomnia, tremor) and induce psychotic symptoms
Mirtazapine (Remeron)	Exact mechanism unclear; may increase norepinephrine and serotonin activity by blocking inhibitory presynaptic autoreceptors	Low incidence of sedative, anticholinergic, and cardiovascular side effects	May cause agitation, anxiety, other mood changes
Nefazodone (Serzone)	Slight inhibition of serotonin and norepinephrine reuptake; may also block CNS serotonin receptors	Sedating: useful in agitation	May cause orthostatic hypotension because of antagonistic effect on vascular alpha-1 receptors
Trazodone (Desyrel)	Slight inhibition of serotonin reuptake	Sedating: useful in agitation; lower relative risk of overdose	May cause orthostatic hypotension (similar to nefazodone); serious problems related to priapism may also occur in men

**Drugs listed here are newer or "second-generation" antidepressants; these agents are generally more selective for specific amine neurotransmitters compared to older, more traditional drugs such as the tricyclics and MAO inhibitors.*

with the tricyclics, MAO inhibitors directly increase activity at amine synapses, which can bring about beneficial changes in receptor sensitivity and neuronal function at these synapses. However, MAO inhibitors are not usually the drugs of choice in depression; they are associated with a relatively higher incidence of side effects, and they can be dangerous if taken with foods that contain tyramine (reasons for dietary restrictions during MAO inhibitor use are addressed in the "Problems and Adverse Effects" section later in this chapter).

Nonetheless, MAO inhibitors may be helpful if patients do not respond to other agents (SSRIs, SNRIs, tricyclics).[42] Likewise, pharmacologists have developed MAO inhibitors that can be administered transdermally, which may provide a safer and more effective alternative to traditional oral MAO inhibitors.[40,43] Clinical studies will continue to determine if these newer transdermal MAO inhibitors might offer advantages over other drugs when treating depression.

Another issue affecting the use of MAO inhibitors is that the MAO enzyme exists in two primary forms or subtypes: MAO type A and MAO type B.[40,44] These two subtypes are differentiated according to their ability to degrade specific amines and to the ability of various drugs that inhibit one or both subtypes of the MAO enzyme. Preliminary evidence suggests that selective inhibition of MAO type A may be desirable in treating depression,[44] whereas inhibition of MAO type B may be more important in prolonging the effects of dopamine in Parkinson disease (see Chapter 10). Regardless, the MAO inhibitors currently used as antidepressants are relatively nonselective, meaning that they inhibit MAO A and MAO B fairly equally. Development of new MAO inhibitors may produce agents that are more selective for the MAO A subtype and may therefore produce better antidepressant effects with fewer adverse reactions.[44]

Other Antidepressants

Several other compounds that are not members of the groups listed above can also be used to treat depression. Trazodone (Desyrel) and nefazodone (Serzone) block serotonin receptors while simultaneously inhibiting serotonin reuptake.[45] These actions have a complex effect on serotonin balance, and these drugs may therefore help decrease depression in certain patients by normalizing serotonin influence in the brain. Trazodone also has several non-approved (off-label) uses and is commonly prescribed to treat insomnia and various other conditions such as anxiety, chronic pain, sexual dysfunction, and eating disorders.[46,47]

Another atypical antidepressant is bupropion (Wellbutrin). This drug is unique because it is the only antidepressant that does not seem to have a significant effect on serotonin but acts primarily as a dopamine and norepinephrine reuptake inhibitor.[48] Again, this effect may be helpful in a subgroup of people with depression who are influenced primarily by dopamine and norepinephrine imbalances. Bupropion is also marketed under the trade name Zyban as an adjunct to helping people quit cigarette smoking and overcome nicotine addiction.[49]

These other antidepressants typically play a secondary role in treating depression—that is, they are not usually the drug of choice but may be helpful if other treatments have not been successful. Efforts are ongoing to develop other atypical antidepressants and determine how these newer agents might be most effective in treating specific types of depression.

In the past, sympathomimetic stimulants such as the amphetamine drugs were also used on a limited basis to treat depression. However, these drugs produce powerful CNS excitation and have a high risk for addiction and overdose. Hence, use of amphetamine-like drugs to treat depression has essentially been replaced by the safer alternatives described above.

Pharmacokinetics of Antidepressants

Antidepressants are usually administered orally. Dosages vary depending on each drug and on each individual. Initial dosages generally start out low and are increased slowly within the therapeutic range until beneficial effects are observed. Distribution within the body also varies with each type of antidepressant, but all eventually reach the brain to exert their effects. Metabolism takes place primarily in the liver, and metabolites of several drugs continue to show significant antidepressant activity. This fact may be responsible for prolonging the drug's effects, even after it has undergone hepatic biotransformation. Elimination takes place by biotransformation and renal excretion.

Problems and Adverse Effects

Table 7-3 provides a summary of the antidepressants' common side effects and the relative incidence of these side effects in specific antidepressants. As indicated in this table, different groups of antidepressants are associated with specific problems and clusters of adverse symptoms. The primary side effects of each group are summarized next.

Table 7-3
SIDE EFFECTS OF ANTIDEPRESSANT DRUGS*

Drug	Sedation	Anticholinergic Effects	Orthostatic Hypotension	Cardiac Arrhythmias	Seizures
Selective Serotonin Reuptake Inhibitors					
Citalopram	+	0	0	0	++
Escitalopram	0	0	0	0	0
Fluoxetine	0	0	0	0	++
Fluvoxamine	0	0	0	0	++
Paroxetine	+	+	0	0	++
Sertraline	0	0	0	0	++
Serotonin-Norepinephrine Reuptake Inhibitors					
Desvenlafaxine	+	+	0	+	++
Duloxetine	0	+	+	0	0
Venlafaxine	+	+	0	+	++
Tricyclic Drugs					
Amitriptyline	++++	++++	+++	+++	+++
Amoxapine	++	+++	++	++	+++
Clomipramine	++++	++++	++	+++	++++
Desipramine	++	++	++	++	++
Doxepin	++++	+++	++	++	+++
Imipramine	+++	+++	++++	+++	+++
Nortriptyline	++	++	+	++	++
Protriptyline	+	++	++	+++	++
Trimipramine	++++	++++	+++	+++	+++
Monoamine Oxidase (MAO) Inhibitors					
Phenelzine	++	+	++	+	+
Tranylcypromine	+	+	++	+	+
Others					
Bupropion	0	+	0	+	++++
Mirtazapine	++	+	++	+	+
Nefazodone	+++	0	+++	+	++
Trazodone	++++	0	+++	+	++

**Zero denotes no side effect, + a very low incidence, ++ a low incidence, +++ a moderate incidence, and ++++ a high incidence.*

Source: Adapted from Teter, et al. Major depressive disorders. In: DiPiro JT, et al, eds. Pharmacotherapy: A Pathophysiologic Approach. 8th ed. New York: McGraw-Hill; 2011:1179, with permission.

Serotonin and Serotonin-Norepinephrine Reuptake Inhibitors

Gastrointestinal (GI) symptoms such as nausea, vomiting, and diarrhea or constipation are the most common side effects associated with SSRIs and SNRIs.[3,50] However, these drugs tend to cause less sedation compared to the tricyclic antidepressants and drugs like trazodone and nefazodone (see Table 7-3). Likewise, SSRIs and SNRIs tend to have a fairly low incidence of cardiovascular problems (e.g., **arrhythmias**, orthostatic hypotension) and anticholinergic effects (e.g., dry mouth, constipation, urinary retention, confusion). Hence, the SSRIs and SNRIs are often well tolerated compared to older, more traditional agents like the tricyclics and MAO inhibitors.

But SSRIs and SNRIs may cause a serious and potentially fatal adverse effect known as *serotonin syndrome*.[51,52] This syndrome can occur with all antidepressant drugs but often happens when SSRIs or SNRIs are used in high doses or when two or more antidepressants are administered concurrently.[51] Because they inhibit serotonin reuptake, antidepressants cause serotonin to accumulate in brain tissues. If serotonin reaches excessive levels, serotonin syndrome occurs and is characterized by an array of symptoms such as sweating, agitation, restlessness, shivering, increased heart rate (tachycardia), and neuromuscular hyperexcitability (i.e., tremor, clonus, hyperreflexia, fasciculations, rigidity).[53] These symptoms typically disappear if the drug is discontinued, but they should be identified early or this syndrome could progress to seizures, coma, and death.[51,53]

Tricyclics

A major problem with the tricyclic antidepressants is sedation (see Table 7-3). Although a certain degree of sedation may be desirable in some patients who are agitated and depressed, feelings of lethargy and sluggishness may impair patient adherence to drug therapy and result in a failure to take their medication. A second major problem is that these drugs tend to have significant anticholinergic properties—that is, they act as if they are blocking certain central and peripheral acetylcholine receptors (see Table 7-3). Impairment of central acetylcholine transmission may cause confusion and delirium. The peripheral anticholinergic properties produce a variety of symptoms, including dry mouth, constipation, urinary retention, confusion, and tachycardia. Other cardiovascular problems include arrhythmias and orthostatic hypotension, with the latter being particularly common in elderly patients. These drugs also increase seizure activity, and they must be used cautiously in patients who are at risk for developing seizures.[54] Finally, tricyclics have the highest potential for lethal overdose from an antidepressant, primarily because high doses can cause fatal cardiac arrhythmias.[55] This leads to a serious problem when one considers the risk of suicide among depressed patients. These drugs must be used cautiously in patients who have suicidal thoughts or a history of suicidal behaviors.

MAO Inhibitors

In contrast to the tricyclics, MAO inhibitors tend to produce CNS excitation, which can result in restlessness, irritability, agitation, and sleep loss. These drugs also produce some central and peripheral anticholinergic effects (e.g., tremor, confusion, dry mouth, and urinary retention), but these tend to occur to a lesser extent than with the tricyclics (see Table 7-3). Because of the systemic MAO inhibition, excess activity at peripheral sympathetic adrenergic terminals may cause a profound increase in blood pressure, leading to a hypertensive crisis. This situation is exacerbated if other drugs that increase sympathetic nervous activity are being taken concurrently. Also, there is a distinct interaction between the MAO inhibitors used as antidepressants (i.e., the MAO type A inhibitors) and certain foods such as fermented cheese and wines.[56,57] These fermented foods contain tyramine, which stimulates the release of endogenous epinephrine and norepinephrine (the "cheese effect").[56] The additive effect of increased catecholamine release (because of the ingested tyramine) and decreased catecholamine breakdown (because of MAO inhibition) can lead to excessive catecholamine levels, thereby causing a hypertensive crisis that leads to heart attack or stroke.[57]

Antidepressants and Chronic Pain

Many chronic pain syndromes (e.g., neuropathic pain, fibromyalgia, chronic low back pain, etc.) can be treated more effectively if antidepressants are included in the treatment regimen, as clinical depression is present in many patients with chronic pain.[58-63] A decrease in depression symptoms will certainly increase the chance that the patient will simply feel better and be more responsive to other interventions. However, there is considerable evidence that antidepressants will help patients with chronic pain even if no symptoms of depression are present—that is, improvements in pain have been noted even when there has been no observed effect on the patient's mood.

Antidepressants that can be used to treat chronic pain are listed in Table 7-4. Traditional tricyclic medications such as amitriptyline and nortriptyline have long been considered a valuable option in the pharmacotherapy for chronic pain.[59,63] Newer drugs such as the SSRIs (e.g., paroxetine) and SNRIs (e.g., duloxetine, venlafaxine) might also be considered for some patients with fibromyalgia, neuropathies, and other forms of chronic pain.[59,60]

Table 7-4
ANTIDEPRESSANTS USED TO TREAT CHRONIC PAIN

Drug	Possible Indication(s)*
Amitriptyline (Elavil, Endep, others)	Fibromyalgia, neuropathic pain, headache, low back pain
Amoxapine (Asendin)	Neuropathic pain, other chronic pain syndromes
Clomipramine (Anafranil)	Neuropathic pain, other chronic pain syndromes
Doxepin (Sinequan)	Chronic pain syndromes
Duloxetine (Cymbalta)	Diabetic neuropathic pain, fibromyalgia, osteoarthritis, back pain
Fluoxetine (Prozac)	Diabetic neuropathic pain, fibromyalgia, Raynaud's phenomenon
Imipramine (Norfranil, Tofranil, others)	Chronic pain syndromes, vascular headache prophylaxis, cluster headache
Nortriptyline (Aventyl, Pamelor)	Chronic neurogenic pain
Trazodone (Desyrel)	Diabetic neuropathic pain, other chronic pain syndromes

**Except for duloxetine; antidepressants are not FDA approved to treat chronic pain but may be prescribed off-label for various chronic pain syndromes (see Chapter 1 for a description of off-label prescribing). Drugs listed here have been reported by the manufacturer to be useful in treating the conditions listed above; other antidepressants may also be used as adjuncts for chronic pain in specific clinical situations.*

Antidepressants probably affect chronic pain by their actions on CNS monoamine neurotransmitters. As indicated earlier, these drugs have the ability to modulate the effects of serotonin, norepinephrine, and dopamine, and their effects on chronic pain may be related to the influence on monoamine transmission in critical pain pathways in the brain.[64,65] In particular, serotonin seems especially important in regulating certain pathways that may be important in inhibiting pain. Studies in animal models suggest that decreased activity in descending (efferent) serotonergic pathways that inhibit pain may lead to chronic pain syndromes.[65] By restoring serotonin influence in these pathways, antidepressants could help resolve the neurophysiological changes that initiate and sustain chronic pain. Hence, the exact way that antidepressants affect pain pathways remains under investigation, and future studies may help clarify how antidepressants affect chronic pain.

Antidepressants may therefore be successful as an adjunct or as a primary medication in the treatment of patients with chronic pain, including those who have been resistant to more traditional pain treatments.[66] But the response to these drugs varies considerably from patient to patient, and there is still extensive debate about exactly how effective these drugs are in treating different types of chronic pain.[58,59] Future research should help clarify how specific antidepressants can be used most effectively as part of a comprehensive regimen for treating various types of chronic pain.

BIPOLAR DISORDER

The form of depression discussed previously is often referred to as *major depressive disorder* or *unipolar depression*, in contrast to *bipolar* or *manic-depressive disorder*. As the term *manic-depressive* implies, bipolar syndrome is associated with mood swings from one extreme (mania) to the other (depression).[67] Manic episodes are characterized by euphoria, hyperactivity, and talkativeness, and depressive episodes are similar to those described previously. Bipolar disorder can also be subclassified as bipolar I disorder in people who exhibit alternating episodes of mania and major depression, and bipolar II disorder if depressive episodes are interspersed with less severe manic symptoms (hypomania).[4,68]

As in unipolar depression, the exact causes of bipolar disorder are unknown. One theory is that genetic and environmental factors conspire to alter neurotransmitter balance in the brain.[69] However, exactly which neurotransmitters are most influential in causing bipolar syndrome remains to be determined. It seems likely that bipolar disorder may be caused by an imbalance between inhibitory neurotransmitters (serotonin, GABA) and excitatory neurotransmitters (norepinephrine, dopamine, glutamate, aspartate).[67,70] Other neurotransmitters (acetylcholine), hormones (thyroid hormones, cortisol), membrane ions (sodium, potassium, calcium), and dysfunction of neuronal second messenger systems have also been implicated as playing a role in the pathophysiology of bipolar syndrome.[67]

Clearly, the causes of bipolar disorder are complex and not fully understood. It is well beyond the scope of this chapter to address all the theories that try to explain the genetic and nongenetic factors that underlie this disorder. Nonetheless, treatment of bipolar disorder often focuses on preventing the start of these pendulum-like mood swings by preventing the manic episodes. Hence, drugs used in the long-term management of bipolar disorder are often mood stabilizers or "antimanic drugs." The classic strategy used to stabilize mood and prevent or treat bipolar syndrome consists of administering lithium salts (i.e., lithium carbonate, lithium citrate).[71,72]

Lithium

Lithium has been the primary drug used to treat bipolar disorder for over 60 years. Lithium (Li^+) is actually a monovalent cation included in the alkali metal group of the periodic table. Because of its small size (molecular weight 7) and single positive charge, lithium may influence neural excitability by competing with other cations, including sodium, potassium, and calcium.[73] Lithium, however, can affect many other aspects of neuronal function, including effects on enzymes such as protein kinase C, glycogen synthetase kinase-3 beta, and inositol monophosphatase; regulation of second messenger systems involving cAMP and phosphoinositol; direct effects on the release of neurotransmitters such as serotonin, norepinephrine, and dopamine; and the ability to normalize sensitivity of receptors for these and other neurotransmitters.[74,75] Many of these effects are interconnected—that is, changes in one aspect of neuronal activity can produce a domino-like effect on other neurophysiological properties.[75] Still, it is not clear which, if any, of these neurochemical changes can account for how this drug is able to stabilize mood and prevent the manic episodes associated with bipolar disorder.[74]

It has been proposed that lithium can help prevent neuronal degeneration and sustain neuronal function in certain areas of the brain.[76] That is, one or more of the actions described above may enable lithium to have neuroprotective effects, thus preventing neuronal damage that may be responsible for mood swings in bipolar disorder.[75,77] Lithium may likewise increase production of factors that enhance neuronal growth and survival, such as brain-derived neurotrophic factor (BDNF; discussed earlier in this chapter).[78]

The idea that lithium has neuroprotective effects has helped unify theories about the cause and treatment of bipolar disorder.[76] Medical researchers have identified many neuronal changes in this disorder, and it seems likely that these changes all conspire to cause damage to certain neurons in the brain. By counteracting this neuronal damage, lithium can prevent manic episodes and stabilize mood during long-term treatment. Nevertheless, exactly how lithium exerts neuroprotective effects remains to be determined, and studies will continue to investigate how this drug might affect neuronal survival in bipolar disorder and other neurodegenerative diseases.[78]

Pharmacokinetics

Lithium is administered orally and is readily absorbed from the GI tract; it is then completely distributed throughout all the tissues in the body. During an acute manic episode, it may be necessary to administer a relatively high dose in order to achieve blood serum concentrations between 1 and 1.5 mEq/L. Maintenance doses are somewhat lower, and serum concentrations that range from 0.6 to 1.2 mEq/L are often adequate to control bipolar symptoms.[67]

Problems and Adverse Effects of Lithium

A major problem with lithium use is the danger of accumulation within the body.[73] Lithium is not metabolized, and drug elimination takes place almost exclusively through excretion in the urine. Consequently, lithium tends to accumulate in the body, and toxic levels can frequently be reached during administration.

Symptoms of lithium toxicity are summarized in Table 7-5. These symptoms are related to the amount of lithium in the bloodstream. Mild toxic symptoms may be present when serum levels approach the high end of the therapeutic range (1.5 mEq/l).[79] However, toxic side effects reach moderate to severe levels when serum concentrations exceed 1.5 mEq/L and typically require medical intervention when serum levels exceed 2 mEq/L.[67,73] As indicated in Table 7-5, progressive accumulation of lithium can lead to serious neurological complications, including seizures, coma, and even death.

Consequently, clinicians should be aware of any changes in behavior in patients taking lithium that may

Table 7-5
SYMPTOMS OF LITHIUM TOXICITY

Physiological System	Symptoms	
	*Mild Toxicity**	*Moderate-Severe Toxicity***
CNS	Fine hand tremor, fatigue, weakness, dizziness, blurred vision, slurred speech	Ataxia, fasciculations, nystagmus, confusion, stupor, seizures, coma
GI	Nausea, loss of appetite, dry mouth, abdominal pain	Vomiting, diarrhea
Cardiovascular	ECG changes (T wave flattening, appearance of U waves)	Syncope, bradycardia, A-V block, other atrial and ventricular arrhythmias
Renal	Polyuria, polydipsia (due to decreased ability to concentrate urine)	Renal insufficiency; possible permanent kidney damage and decreased glomerular filtration

**Symptoms seen in mild toxicity typically increase progressively and become more prominent as toxicity approaches moderate to severe levels.*

***Some moderate to severe symptoms may also occur at lower plasma levels in elderly or debilitated patients, or in patients with specific comorbidities.*

indicate the drug is reaching toxic levels. If symptoms of toxicity occur, alert the physician as soon as possible so that lithium levels in the body fluids can be measured. The patient's medical practitioner can usually resolve toxicity by adjusting the dosage or prescribing a sustained-release form of lithium.[80] Also, the medical practitioner can continue to periodically monitor the patient's serum titers of lithium to ensure that blood levels remain within the therapeutic range, especially in older adults or other patients who are at risk for lithium toxicity.[67,81]

Other Drugs for Bipolar Disorder

Although lithium remains the cornerstone of treatment for bipolar disorder, it is now recognized that other agents may be helpful, especially during manic episodes. In particular, antiseizure medications such as carbamazepine, valproic acid, gabapentin, and lamotrigine may help stabilize mood and limit manic symptoms.[82,83] Antipsychotic medications, especially the newer "atypical" antipsychotics such as aripiprazole, clozapine, and risperidone, may also be helpful as antimanic drugs.[84,85] Antipsychotic and antiseizure drugs (see Chapters 8 and 9, respectively) are believed to help because they act directly on CNS neurons to help prevent the neuronal excitation that seems to precipitate manic symptoms.[85,86] Hence, these drugs can be used initially, along with lithium, to decrease manic mood swings or to simply stabilize mood at baseline levels and to prevent mood swings that characterize bipolar disorder. These additional drugs may be discontinued when the mood is stabilized, or they may be administered alone or with lithium treatment as maintenance therapy, especially in patients who have not responded well to treatment with only lithium.[87,88]

Special Concerns for Rehabilitation Patients

Patients receiving physical therapy and occupational therapy for any number of acute or chronic illnesses may be taking antidepressants to improve their mood and general well-being. Some amount of depression will be present with a catastrophic injury or illness, and medical practitioners frequently prescribe these drugs to patients with a spinal cord injury, stroke, severe burn, multiple sclerosis, amputation, and so on. Of course, therapists working in a psychiatric facility will deal with many patients taking antidepressant drugs, and severe depression may be the primary reason the patient is institutionalized in the first place.

Therapists must realize that depression is a serious and complex psychological disorder and that it is very difficult to treat effectively. Even with

Continued on following page

Special Concerns for Rehabilitation Patients (Continued)

optimal pharmacological and psychological intervention, it is estimated that up to one-third of patients with depression may not respond adequately.[3] The effects of drug treatment also vary greatly from individual to individual. It is therefore imperative that the physician and other health-care professionals work closely with the patient and the patient's family to find the drug that produces optimal results with a minimum of side effects. Again, this task is complicated by many issues, including the complex interplay of factors causing depression in each patient and the unpredictable response to each type of antidepressant.

However, antidepressant and antimanic agents can be extremely beneficial in helping to improve a patient's outlook for the rehabilitation process. The patient may become more optimistic regarding the future and may assume a more active role and interest in the rehabilitation process. This attitude can be invaluable in increasing patient cooperation and improving compliance with rehabilitation goals. However, certain side effects can be troublesome during rehabilitation treatments. Sedation, lethargy, and muscle weakness can occur with the tricyclics and lithium, which can present a problem if the patient's active cooperation is required. Other unpleasant side effects, such as nausea and vomiting, can also be disturbing during treatments. A more common and potentially more serious problem is the orthostatic hypotension that occurs predominantly with the tricyclics. This hypotension can cause syncope and subsequent injury if patients fall during gait training. Conversely, MAO inhibitors can increase blood pressure, and care should be taken to avoid a hypertensive crisis, especially during therapy sessions that tend to increase blood pressure (e.g., certain forms of exercise). Hence, patients should also be monitored regularly to detect an increase or decrease in blood pressure, depending on the drug and the patient.

Rehabilitation specialists should also be aware that there may be a substantial delay between when antidepressant drug therapy is initiated and when the patient actually notices an improvement in mood. Although some improvement in mood may occur within 2 weeks after beginning antidepressant drug treatment, these agents must often be administered for 1 month or more before an appreciable improvement in symptoms occurs.[3,89] Patients may need to be reminded of this fact, especially if they become discouraged because these drugs do not seem to be helping to resolve their depression.

Drug therapy may actually precipitate an increase in depression during the initial treatment period, including increased thoughts of suicide.[90] Increased risk of suicidal behaviors is especially important when antidepressants are given to children, teenagers, and young adults through their early 20s.[91] Likewise, suicide risk increases substantially in patients with bipolar disorder who are in the depressive phase.[92,93] Rehabilitation specialists should therefore keep alert for any signs that a patient is becoming more depressed and possibly suicidal, especially during the first few weeks after antidepressant drug therapy is initiated. Increased awareness seems particularly important in high-risk patients such as younger individuals and patients with a history of suicidal tendencies.

Finally, clinicians can help guide patients toward nonpharmacological interventions that might help prevent and treat depression. In particular, regular exercise has been shown to be very effective in helping reduce depression in many individuals.[94-96] Therapists can design and implement such exercise programs or refer patients to other exercise specialists with expertise in this area. Clinicians can also suggest and encourage patients to participate in other programs such as counseling, support groups, and cognitive-behavioral therapies. These interventions may help reduce the need for antidepressant drugs and ultimately be used as an effective nonpharmacological way to treat depression and improve quality of life in various patient populations.

CASE STUDY

ANTIDEPRESSANT DRUGS

Brief History. J.G., a 71-year-old retired pharmacist, was admitted to the hospital with a chief complaint of an inability to move his right arm and leg. He was also unable to speak at the time of admission. The clinical impression was right hemiplegia caused by left-middle cerebral artery thrombosis. The patient also had a history of hypertension and had been taking cardiac beta blockers for several years. J.G.'s medical condition stabilized, and the third day after admission he was seen for the first time by a physical therapist. Speech therapy and occupational therapy were also soon initiated. The patient's condition improved rapidly, and motor function began to return in the right side. Balance and gross motor skills increased until he could transfer from his wheelchair to his bed with minimal assistance, and gait training activities were initiated. J.G. was able to comprehend verbal commands, but his speech remained markedly slurred and difficult to understand. During his hospitalization, J.G. showed signs of severe depression. Symptoms increased until cooperation with the rehabilitation and nursing staff was compromised. Imipramine (Tofranil) was prescribed at a dosage of 150 mg/day.

Problem/Influence of Medication. Imipramine is a tricyclic antidepressant, and these drugs are known to produce orthostatic hypotension during the initial stages of drug therapy. Because the patient is expressively aphasic, he will have trouble telling the therapist that he feels dizzy or faint. Also, the cardiac beta blockers will blunt any compensatory increase in cardiac output if blood pressure drops during postural changes.

1. ***How can the therapist reduce the risk of orthostatic hypotension during rehabilitation sessions?***
2. ***Will clinicians notice an immediate improvement in J.G.'s mood after starting this antidepressant drug?***

See Appendix C, "Answers to Case Study Questions."

SUMMARY

Affective disorders such as depression and bipolar disorder are found frequently in the general population and in rehabilitation patients. Drugs commonly prescribed in the treatment of unipolar depression include newer agents such as the selective serotonin reuptake inhibitors and serotonin-norepinephrine reuptake inhibitors, as well as more traditional drugs like the tricyclics and MAO inhibitors. Lithium is the drug of choice for treating bipolar disorder. All of these drugs seem to exert their principal effects by modifying synaptic transmission and neuronal growth/function in CNS pathways that use amine neurotransmitters. The exact manner in which these drugs affect neuronal activity has shed some light on the possible neurochemical changes that underlie these forms of mental illness. Effective treatment of depression and bipolar disorder can improve the patient's attitude and participation during rehabilitation. However, therapists should be aware that drug responses often vary greatly from patient to patient and that certain drug side effects may alter the patient's physical and mental behavior.

REFERENCES

1. Duberstein PR, Heisel MJ. Personality traits and the reporting of affective disorder symptoms in depressed patients. *J Affect Disord.* 2007;103:165-171.
2. Hirschfeld RM. The epidemiology of depression and the evolution of treatment. *J Clin Psychiatry.* 2012;73(suppl 1):5-9.

3. Teter CJ, Kando JC, Wells BG. Major depressive disorder. In: DiPiro JT, et al, eds. *Pharmacotherapy: A Pathophysiologic Approach*. 8th ed. New York: McGraw-Hill; 2011.
4. American Psychiatric Association. *Diagnostic and Statistical Manual of Mental Disorders*. 4th edition, Text Revision. Arlington, VA: American Psychiatric Association; 2000.
5. Ayuso-Gutiérrez JL. Depressive subtypes and efficacy of antidepressive pharmacotherapy. *World J Biol Psychiatry*. 2005;6 (suppl 2):31-37.
6. Mitchell AJ. Clinical utility of screening for clinical depression and bipolar disorder. *Curr Opin Psychiatry*. 2012;25:24-31.
7. Pae CU, Tharwani H, Marks DM, et al. Atypical depression: a comprehensive review. *CNS Drugs*. 2009;23:1023-1037.
8. Kristensen P, Weisæth L, Heir T. Bereavement and mental health after sudden and violent losses: a review. *Psychiatry*. 2012;75: 76-97.
9. Palazidou E. The neurobiology of depression. *Br Med Bull*. 2012;101:127-145.
10. Saveanu RV, Nemeroff CB. Etiology of depression: genetic and environmental factors. *Psychiatr Clin North Am*. 2012;35:51-71.
11. Sullivan PF, Daly MJ, O'Donovan M. Genetic architectures of psychiatric disorders: the emerging picture and its implications. *Nat Rev Genet*. 2012;13:537-551.
12. Hill JC, Fritz JM. Psychosocial influences on low back pain, disability, and response to treatment. *Phys Ther*. 2011;91:712-721.
13. Mead GE, Hsieh CF, Lee R, et al. Selective serotonin reuptake inhibitors (SSRIs) for stroke recovery. *Cochrane Database Syst Rev*. 2012;11:CD009286.
14. Taylor D, Meader N, Bird V, et al. Pharmacological interventions for people with depression and chronic physical health problems: systematic review and meta-analyses of safety and efficacy. *Br J Psychiatry*. 2011;198:179-188.
15. Elhwuegi AS. Central monoamines and their role in major depression. *Prog Neuropsychopharmacol Biol Psychiatry*. 2004; 28:435-451.
16. Nutt DJ. The neuropharmacology of serotonin and noradrenaline in depression. *Int Clin Psychopharmacol*. 2002;17(suppl 1):S1-12.
17. Bambico FR, Belzung C. Novel insights into depression and antidepressants: a synergy between synaptogenesis and neurogenesis? *Curr Top Behav Neurosci*. 2013;15:243-291.
18. Masi G, Brovedani P. The hippocampus, neurotrophic factors and depression: possible implications for the pharmacotherapy of depression. *CNS Drugs*. 2011;25:913-931.
19. Piwowarska J, Chimiak A, Matsumoto H, et al. Serum cortisol concentration in patients with major depression after treatment with fluoxetine. *Psychiatry Res*. 2012;198:407-411.
20. Dienes KA, Hazel NA, Hammen CL. Cortisol secretion in depressed, and at-risk adults. Psychoneuroendocrinology. 2013; 38:927-940.
21. Tang SW, Helmeste D, Leonard B. Is neurogenesis relevant in depression and in the mechanism of antidepressant drug action? A critical review. *World J Biol Psychiatry*. 2012;13:402-412.
22. Numakawa T, Suzuki S, Kumamaru E, et al. BDNF function and intracellular signaling in neurons. *Histol Histopathol*. 2010; 25:237-258.
23. Yu H, Chen ZY. The role of BDNF in depression on the basis of its location in the neural circuitry. *Acta Pharmacol Sin*. 2011;32:3-11.
24. Autry AE, Monteggia LM. Brain-derived neurotrophic factor and neuropsychiatric disorders. *Pharmacol Rev*. 2012;64: 238-258.
25. Esposito K, Reierson GW, Luo HR, et al. Phosphodiesterase genes and antidepressant treatment response: a review. *Ann Med*. 2009;41:177-185.
26. Madaan V, Wilson DR. Neuropeptides: relevance in treatment of depression and anxiety disorders. *Drug News Perspect*. 2009;22:319-324.
27. Mathews DC, Henter ID, Zarate CA. Targeting the glutamatergic system to treat major depressive disorder: rationale and progress to date. *Drugs*. 2012;72:1313-1333.
28. Möhler H. The GABA system in anxiety and depression and its therapeutic potential. *Neuropharmacology*. 2012;62:42-53.
29. Sghendo L, Mifsud J. Understanding the molecular pharmacology of the serotonergic system: using fluoxetine as a model. *J Pharm Pharmacol*. 2012;64:317-325.
30. López-Muñoz F, Alamo C. Monoaminergic neurotransmission: the history of the discovery of antidepressants from 1950s until today. *Curr Pharm Des*. 2009;15:1563-1586.
31. Cipriani A, La Ferla T, Furukawa TA, et al. Sertraline versus other antidepressive agents for depression. *Cochrane Database Syst Rev*. 2010;1:CD006117.
32. Kok RM, Heeren TJ, Nolen WA. Continuing treatment of depression in the elderly: a systematic review and meta-analysis of double-blinded randomized controlled trials with antidepressants. *Am J Geriatr Psychiatry*. 2011;19:249-255.
33. Carter NJ, McCormack PL. Duloxetine: a review of its use in the treatment of generalized anxiety disorder. *CNS Drugs*. 2009;23:523-541.
34. Perry R, Cassagnol M. Desvenlafaxine: a new serotonin-norepinephrine reuptake inhibitor for the treatment of adults with major depressive disorder. *Clin Ther*. 2009;31(pt 1):1374-1404.
35. Derry S, Gill D, Phillips T, Moore RA. Milnacipran for neuropathic pain and fibromyalgia in adults. *Cochrane Database Syst Rev*. 2012;3:CD008244.
36. Reddy S, Kane C, Pitrosky B, Musgnung J, et al. Clinical utility of desvenlafaxine 50 mg/d for treating MDD: a review of two randomized placebo-controlled trials for the practicing physician. *Curr Med Res Opin*. 2010;26:139-150.
37. Flanagan RJ. Fatal toxicity of drugs used in psychiatry. *Hum Psychopharmacol*. 2008;23(suppl 1):43-51.
38. Spina E, Trifirò G, Caraci F. Clinically significant drug interactions with newer antidepressants. *CNS Drugs*. 2012;26:39-67.
39. Connolly KR, Thase ME. If at first you don't succeed: a review of the evidence for antidepressant augmentation, combination and switching strategies. *Drugs*. 2011;71:43-64.
40. VanDenBerg CM. The transdermal delivery system of monoamine oxidase inhibitors. *J Clin Psychiatry*. 2012;73(suppl 1): 25-30.
41. Wimbiscus M, Kostenko O, Malone D. MAO inhibitors: risks, benefits, and lore. *Cleve Clin J Med*. 2010;77:859-882.
42. Culpepper L. The use of monoamine oxidase inhibitors in primary care. *J Clin Psychiatry*. 2012;73(suppl 1):37-41.
43. Cohen LJ, Sclar DA. Issues in adherence to treatment with monoamine oxidase inhibitors and the rate of treatment failure. *J Clin Psychiatry*. 2012;73(suppl 1):31-36.
44. O'Donnell JM, Shelton RC. Drug therapy of depression and anxiety disorders. In: Brunton LL, et al, eds. *The Pharmacological Basis of Therapeutics*. 12th ed. New York: McGraw Hill; 2011.
45. Stahl SM. Mechanism of action of trazodone: a multifunctional drug. *CNS Spectr*. 2009;14:536-546.
46. Bossini L, Casolaro I, Koukouna D, et al. Off-label uses of trazodone: a review. *Expert Opin Pharmacother*. 2012;13:1707-1717.

47. Mittur A. Trazodone: properties and utility in multiple disorders. *Expert Rev Clin Pharmacol.* 2011;4:181-196.
48. Moreira R. The efficacy and tolerability of bupropion in the treatment of major depressive disorder. *Clin Drug Investig.* 2011;31(suppl 1):5-17.
49. Mills EJ, Wu P, Lockhart I, et al. Comparisons of high-dose and combination nicotine replacement therapy, varenicline, and bupropion for smoking cessation: a systematic review and multiple treatment meta-analysis. *Ann Med.* 2012;44:588-597.
50. Mottram P, Wilson K, Strobl J. Antidepressants for depressed elderly. *Cochrane Database Syst Rev.* 2006;1:CD003491.
51. Ables AZ, Nagubilli R. Prevention, recognition, and management of serotonin syndrome. *Am Fam Physician.* 2010;81:1139-1142.
52. Sun-Edelstein C, Tepper SJ, Shapiro RE. Drug-induced serotonin syndrome: a review. *Expert Opin Drug Saf.* 2008;7:587-596.
53. Dvir Y, Smallwood P. Serotonin syndrome: a complex but easily avoidable condition. *Gen Hosp Psychiatry.* 2008;30:284-287.
54. Montgomery SA. Antidepressants and seizures: emphasis on newer agents and clinical implications. *Int J Clin Pract.* 2005;59:1435-1440.
55. Taylor D. Antidepressant drugs and cardiovascular pathology: a clinical overview of effectiveness and safety. *Acta Psychiatr Scand.* 2008;118:434-442.
56. Finberg JP, Gillman K. Selective inhibitors of monoamine oxidase type B and the "cheese effect." *Int Rev Neurobiol.* 2011;100:169-190.
57. Flockhart DA. Dietary restrictions and drug interactions with monoamine oxidase inhibitors: an update. *J Clin Psychiatry.* 2012;73(suppl 1):17-24.
58. Chou R, Huffman LH; American Pain Society; American College of Physicians. Medications for acute and chronic low back pain: a review of the evidence for an American Pain Society/American College of Physicians clinical practice guideline. *Ann Intern Med.* 2007;147:505-514.
59. Dworkin RH, O'Connor AB, Audette J, et al. Recommendations for the pharmacological management of neuropathic pain: an overview and literature update. *Mayo Clin Proc.* 2010;85 (3 suppl):S3-14.
60. Mease PJ, Dundon K, Sarzi-Puttini P. Pharmacotherapy of fibromyalgia. *Best Pract Res Clin Rheumatol.* 2011;25:285-297.
61. Thaler KJ, Morgan LC, Van Noord M, et al. Comparative effectiveness of second-generation antidepressants for accompanying anxiety, insomnia, and pain in depressed patients: a systematic review. *Depress Anxiety.* 2012;29:495-505.
62. Barkin RL, Barkin SJ, Irving GA, Gordon A. Management of chronic noncancer pain in depressed patients. *Postgrad Med.* 2011;123:143-154.
63. Häuser W, Wolfe F, Tölle T, et al. The role of antidepressants in the management of fibromyalgia syndrome: a systematic review and meta-analysis. *CNS Drugs.* 2012;26:297-307.
64. Bardin L. The complex role of serotonin and 5-HT receptors in chronic pain. *Behav Pharmacol.* 2011;22:390-404.
65. Liu FY, Qu XX, Ding X, et al. Decrease in the descending inhibitory 5-HT system in rats with spinal nerve ligation. *Brain Res.* 2010;1330:45-60.
66. Bair MJ, Sanderson TR. Coanalgesics for chronic pain therapy: a narrative review. *Postgrad Med.* 2011;123:140-150.
67. Drayton SJ. Bipolar disorder. In: DiPiro JT, et al, eds. *Pharmacotherapy: A Pathophysiologic Approach.* 8th ed. New York: McGraw-Hill; 2011.
68. Rapoport SI, Basselin M, Kim HW, Rao JS. Bipolar disorder and mechanisms of action of mood stabilizers. *Brain Res Rev.* 2009;61:185-209.
69. Offord J. Genetic approaches to a better understanding of bipolar disorder. *Pharmacol Ther.* 2012;133:133-141.
70. Nikolaus S, Hautzel H, Heinzel A, Müller HW. Key players in major and bipolar depression—a retrospective analysis of in vivo imaging studies. *Behav Brain Res.* 2012;232:358-390.
71. Licht RW. Lithium: still a major option in the management of bipolar disorder. *CNS Neurosci Ther.* 2012;18:219-226.
72. Malhi GS, Tanious M, Das P, Berk M. The science and practice of lithium therapy. *Aust N Z J Psychiatry.* 2012;46:192-211.
73. Meyer JM. Pharmacotherapy of psychosis and mania. In: Brunton LL, et al, eds. *The Pharmacological Basis of Therapeutics.* 12th ed. New York: McGraw Hill; 2011.
74. Marmol F. Lithium: bipolar disorder and neurodegenerative diseases Possible cellular mechanisms of the therapeutic effects of lithium. *Prog Neuropsychopharmacol Biol Psychiatry.* 2008;32:1761-1771.
75. Pasquali L, Busceti CL, Fulceri F, et al. Intracellular pathways underlying the effects of lithium. *Behav Pharmacol.* 2010;21:473-492.
76. Machado-Vieira R, Manji HK, Zarate CA Jr. The role of lithium in the treatment of bipolar disorder: convergent evidence for neurotrophic effects as a unifying hypothesis. *Bipolar Disord.* 2009;11(suppl 2):92-109.
77. Quiroz JA, Machado-Vieira R, Zarate CA Jr, Manji HK. Novel insights into lithium's mechanism of action: neurotrophic and neuroprotective effects. *Neuropsychobiology.* 2010;62:50-60.
78. Chiu CT, Chuang DM. Molecular actions and therapeutic potential of lithium in preclinical and clinical studies of CNS disorders. *Pharmacol Ther.* 2010;128:281-304.
79. Thompson JW, Johnson AC. Acute lithium intoxication: properly directing an index of suspicion. *South Med J.* 2011;104:371-372.
80. Grandjean EM, Aubry JM. Lithium: updated human knowledge using an evidence-based approach. Part II: Clinical pharmacology and therapeutic monitoring. *CNS Drugs.* 2009;23:331-349.
81. D'Souza R, Rajji TK, Mulsant BH, Pollock BG. Use of lithium in the treatment of bipolar disorder in late-life. *Curr Psychiatry Rep.* 2011;13:488-492.
82. Bialer M. Why are antiepileptic drugs used for nonepileptic conditions? *Epilepsia.* 2012;53(suppl 7):26-33.
83. Grunze HC. Anticonvulsants in bipolar disorder. *J Ment Health.* 2010;19:127-141.
84. de Bartolomeis A, Perugi G. Combination of aripiprazole with mood stabilizers for the treatment of bipolar disorder: from acute mania to long-term maintenance. *Expert Opin Pharmacother.* 2012;13:2027-2036.
85. Dhillon S. Aripiprazole: a review of its use in the management of mania in adults with bipolar I disorder. *Drugs.* 2012;72:133-162.
86. Johannessen Landmark C. Antiepileptic drugs in non-epilepsy disorders: relations between mechanisms of action and clinical efficacy. *CNS Drugs.* 2008;22:27-47.
87. Gitlin M, Frye MA. Maintenance therapies in bipolar disorders. *Bipolar Disord.* 2012;14(suppl 2):51-65.
88. Poon SH, Sim K, Sum MY, et al. Evidence-based options for treatment-resistant adult bipolar disorder patients. *Bipolar Disord.* 2012;14:573-584.
89. Nakajima S, Suzuki T, Watanabe K, et al. Accelerating response to antidepressant treatment in depression: a review and clinical suggestions. *Prog Neuropsychopharmacol Biol Psychiatry.* 2010;34:259-264.

90. Kupfer DJ, Frank E, Phillips ML. Major depressive disorder: new clinical, neurobiological, and treatment perspectives. *Lancet.* 2012;379:1045-1055.
91. Reeves RR, Ladner ME. Antidepressant-induced suicidality: an update. *CNS Neurosci Ther.* 2010;16:227-234.
92. Novick DM, Swartz HA, Frank E. Suicide attempts in bipolar I and bipolar II disorder: a review and meta-analysis of the evidence. *Bipolar Disord.* 2010;12:1-9.
93. Rihmer Z, Gonda X. The effect of pharmacotherapy on suicide rates in bipolar patients. *CNS Neurosci Ther.* 2012;18:238-242.
94. Bridle C, Spanjers K, Patel S, et al. Effect of exercise on depression severity in older people: systematic review and meta-analysis of randomised controlled trials. *Br J Psychiatry.* 2012;201:180-185.
95. Herring MP, Puetz TW, O'Connor PJ, Dishman RK. Effect of exercise training on depressive symptoms among patients with a chronic illness: a systematic review and meta-analysis of randomized controlled trials. *Arch Intern Med.* 2012;172:101-111.
96. Rimer J, Dwan K, Lawlor DA, et al. Exercise for depression. *Cochrane Database Syst Rev.* 2012;7:CD004366.

CHAPTER 8

Antipsychotic Drugs

Psychosis is the term used to describe the more severe forms of mental illness. Psychoses are actually a group of mental disorders characterized by marked thought disturbance and an impaired perception of reality. The most common form of psychosis by far is schizophrenia; it is estimated that 1 percent of the world population has this disorder.[1] Other psychotic disorders include schizoaffective disorder, delusional disorder, brief psychotic disorder, and shared psychotic disorder. In the past, strong, sedative-like drugs were the primary method of treating patients with psychosis. The goal was to pacify these patients so they were no longer combative and abusive to themselves and others. These drugs were commonly referred to as *major tranquilizers* and had the obvious disadvantage of sedating a patient so that his or her cognitive and motor skills were compromised.

As researchers learned more about the neurochemical changes involved in psychosis, pharmacologists developed drugs to specifically treat disorders rather than simply sedate the patient. These antipsychotic drugs, or **neuroleptics** as they were sometimes called in the past, represented a major breakthrough in the treatment of schizophrenia and other psychotic disorders. Today, antipsychotic drugs often have positive effects on the quality of life in people with psychosis and have enabled many of them to live in the community rather than be institutionalized for long periods of time.[2,3] This observation does not imply that these drugs cure schizophrenia. Schizophrenia and other psychoses are believed to be incurable, and psychotic episodes can recur throughout a patient's lifetime. But these drugs can normalize the patient's behavior and thinking during an acute psychotic episode, and maintenance dosages are believed to help prevent the recurrence of psychosis. Consequently, the ability of people with psychosis to take care of themselves and cooperate with others is greatly improved.

Physical therapists and occupational therapists frequently encounter patients taking antipsychotics. Therapists employed in a psychiatric facility will routinely treat patients taking these medications. Therapists who practice in nonpsychiatric settings may still encounter these patients for various reasons. For instance, a patient on an antipsychotic medication who sustains a fractured hip may be seen at an orthopedic facility. Consequently, knowledge of antipsychotic pharmacology will be useful to all rehabilitation specialists.

Because of the prevalence of schizophrenia, this chapter concentrates on the treatment of this psychotic disorder. Also, the pathogenesis and subsequent treatment of other forms of psychosis are similar to those of schizophrenia, so we use this specific condition as an example of the broader range of psychotic conditions.

SCHIZOPHRENIA

The *Diagnostic and Statistical Manual of Mental Disorders* lists several distinct criteria necessary for a diagnosis of schizophrenia,[4] including delusions, hallucinations, disorganized speech, and grossly disorganized or catatonic behavior. Also, a decreased level of function in work, social relations, and self-care may be present. Other factors include the duration of these and additional symptoms (at least 6 months) and a differential diagnosis from other forms of mental illness (such as affective disorders and organic brain syndrome).

Pathogenesis of Schizophrenia

The exact cause of schizophrenia has been the subject of extensive research. It appears that genetic factors (i.e., chromosomal changes that cause deviations in brain structure and function) may set the stage for developing psychosis. These genetic factors might be due to variations in DNA sequences that result in altered expression of neurotransmitter receptors and other specific cellular proteins.[5,6] Likewise, other factors that modify gene expression without a change in gene sequence (**epigenetic factors**) have been implicated as an underlying cause of psychosis.[7,8] Epigenetic factors include chemical modifications, such as adding a methyl group (methylation) to the DNA or to the proteins (histones) that help package DNA within the chromosomes.[9] Individuals with these genetic and epigenetic factors are then at risk for developing psychosis when exposed to specific environmental triggers, such as prenatal or childhood brain injury, other forms of childhood or adult trauma, social stresses, and so forth.[10-12] The exact genetic changes and specific environmental triggers may vary considerably from person to person.[13] Hence, psychosis seems to be caused by a complex interplay between genetic and environmental factors, and the exact way that these factors interact in specific people with psychosis continues to be elucidated.[14,15]

Neurotransmitter Changes in Schizophrenia

Schizophrenia appears to be caused by an overactivity of dopamine pathways in certain parts of the brain, such as the limbic system.[16,17] This idea is based primarily on the fact that most antipsychotics block dopamine receptors to some extent, thereby reducing dopaminergic hyperactivity in mesolimbic pathways and other limbic structures (see the next section of this chapter). The increased dopamine influence underlying psychosis could be caused by excessive dopamine synthesis and release by the presynaptic neuron, decreased dopamine breakdown at the synapse, increased postsynaptic dopamine receptor sensitivity, or a combination of these and other factors.

Consequently, increased dopamine transmission in areas such as the limbic system seems to be the primary neurochemical change associated with schizophrenia and other psychotic syndromes. However, given the complexity of central neurotransmitter interaction, changes in dopamine activity in the limbic system will almost certainly be associated with changes in other neurotransmitters in other parts of the brain. Indeed, there is substantial evidence that increased serotonin activity may also play a key role in the pathophysiology of psychosis.[3] This idea is based on the finding that some of the newer antipsychotics affect serotonin receptors as well as dopamine receptors.[18] It seems likely that serotonin may help moderate the effects of dopamine in specific parts of the brain and that overactivity in one or both of these systems may cause psychosis.

Finally, other neurotransmitters such as glutamate and gamma-aminobutyric acid (GABA) may be involved in the pathogenesis of psychosis.[3,19,20] Glutamate is an amino acid that typically produces excitation in the brain, and GABA is an inhibitory neurotransmitter that often moderates the effects of glutamate. Preliminary evidence suggests that a defect in GABA's ability to control glutamate could lead to overexcitation, thus resulting in symptoms of psychosis.[21] Likewise, researchers identified decreased sensitivity to acetylcholine as a possible factor in psychosis, and an imbalance in acetylcholine may also contribute to the complex neurochemical changes in schizophrenia and related disorders.[22,23]

In essence, it appears that increased dopamine activity in certain limbic pathways is a key factor in schizophrenia and other forms of psychosis. However, increased dopamine activity is not the only neurochemical change underlying psychosis, and excessive dopamine influence may bring about subsequent changes in serotonin, amino acids, and other neurotransmitters. Conversely, the increased dopamine activity may be a result of altered serotonin activity, amino acid imbalances, or changes in other neurochemicals.[17,24] Regardless of the initiating factors, resolving all these neurochemical changes might ultimately provide optimal treatment for people with schizophrenia and other forms of psychosis. For now, however, the mechanism of action for antipsychotic drugs is focused primarily on normalizing dopamine and serotonin activity in specific parts of the brain.

ANTIPSYCHOTICS MECHANISM OF ACTION

Drugs originally developed to treat psychosis all acted as strong antagonists (blockers) of specific dopamine receptors in mesolimbic pathways in the brain—that is, these traditional or first-generation antipsychotics (Table 8-1) have a high affinity for the dopamine type 2 (D2) receptor located within the limbic system.[1,25] Dopamine receptors exist in several subtypes throughout the body, and these subtypes are identified as D1, D2, D3, and so on.[3] The clinical effects and side effects of specific antipsychotic medications are therefore related to their ability to affect certain dopamine receptor populations. Again, the receptor that appears to be most important in mediating antipsychotic effects is the D2 receptor subtype, and most antipsychotic medications therefore have some ability to block the D2 receptor[3] (Fig. 8-1).

In the 1990s, a second major group of antipsychotics appeared on the market. These agents are known collectively as *second-generation antipsychotics*, or *atypical*

Table 8-1
COMMON ANTIPSYCHOTIC DRUGS AND THEIR SIDE EFFECTS*

Drug	Sedation	Extrapyramidal Effects	Anticholinergic Effects
Traditional Antipsychotics			
Chlorpromazine	++++	+++	+++
Fluphenazine	+	++++	+
Haloperidol	+	++++	+
Loxapine	+++	+++	++
Molindone	+	+++	++
Perphenazine	++	+++	++
Prochlorperazine	++	++++	+
Thioridazine	++++	+++	++++
Thiothixene	+	++++	+
Trifluoperazine	++	+++	++
Triflupromazine	+++	+++	++++
Atypical Antipsychotics			
Aripiprazole	++	+	+
Clozapine	++++	+	++++
Iloperidone	+	+	++
Olanzapine	++	++	++
Paliperidone	+	++	+
Quetiapine	++	+	+
Risperidone	+	++	+
Ziprasidone	++	++	+

**Incidence of side effects are classified as follows: + a very low incidence, ++ a low incidence, +++ a moderate incidence, and ++++ a high incidence.*

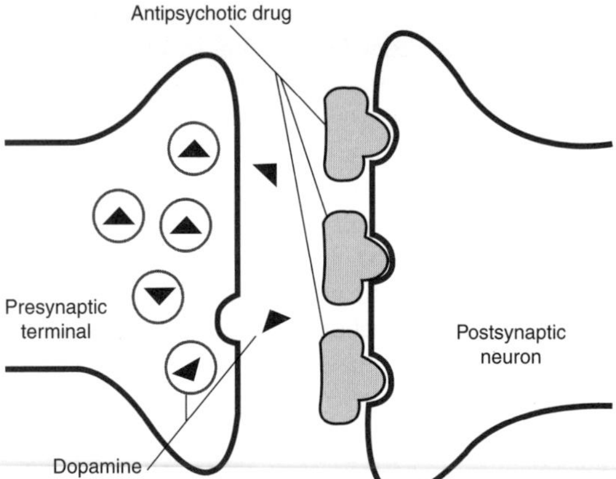

Figure ■ 8-1
Basic effect of antipsychotic drugs on dopamine synapses. All antipsychotics act as antagonists at postsynaptic dopamine type 2 (D2) receptors and block the effects of overactive dopamine transmission in specific CNS pathways. Some antipsychotics may also block other pre- and postsynaptic dopamine receptor subtypes, and newer/atypical agents may also block serotonin receptors in these pathways.

antipsychotics, because of different effects and side effects compared to the traditional drugs (Table 8-2). Specifically, these atypical agents are only weak antagonists at D2 receptors but are usually strong blockers of specific 5-hydroxytryptamine (serotonin) receptors (i.e., the 5-HT_2 receptor).[18,26] Some of the newer agents may also affect other serotonin receptor subtypes, but it is their ability to block the 5-HT_2 receptor that differentiates these drugs from traditional or first-generation antipsychotics.[18] As discussed later in this chapter, these newer drugs may produce antipsychotic effects with a lower risk of certain side effects compared with the traditional agents.

Many of the antipsychotics that are currently in clinical use have the ability to block dopamine receptors or to block serotonin and dopamine receptors in specific pathways within the brain. Again, changes in the activity of other neurotransmitters such as glutamate, GABA, and acetylcholine may also be important in psychosis, and the use of drugs to control these other neurotransmitters is currently under investigation.

Table 8-2
TRADITIONAL AND ATYPICAL ANTIPSYCHOTIC DRUGS AND THEIR DOSAGE

Generic Name	Common Trade Name(s)	Usual Target Dosage Range (mg/d)*	Maximum Recommended Dosage (mg/d)**
Traditional Antipsychotics			
Chlorpromazine	Thorazine	100–200	1,000
Fluphenazine	Permitil, Prolixin	2–20	40
Haloperidol	Haldol	2–20	100
Loxapine	Loxitane	60–100	225
Molindone	Moban	15–100	225
Perphenazine	Trilafon	8–64	64
Prochlorperazine	Compazine	15–150	150
Thioridazine	Mellaril	100–800	800
Thiothixene	Navane	4–40	60
Trifluoperazine	Stelazine	5–40	40
Atypical Antipsychotics			
Aripiprazole	Abilify	10–30	30
Clozapine	Clozaril	300–450	900
Iloperidone	Fanapt	12–24	24
Lurasidone	Latuda	40-80	80

Table 8-2
TRADITIONAL AND ATYPICAL ANTIPSYCHOTIC DRUGS AND THEIR DOSAGE—cont'd

Generic Name	Common Trade Name(s)	Usual Target Dosage Range (mg/d)*	Maximum Recommended Dosage (mg/d)**
Olanzapine	Zyprexa	10–20	20
Paliperidone	Invega	3–12	12
Quetiapine	Seroquel	200–600	800
Risperidone	Risperdal	4–8	16
Ziprasidone	Geodon	40–160	160

Dosage range represents typical adult oral maintenance dose. Initial doses may be lower and then increased gradually to achieve therapeutic effects. Lower maintenance dosages may also be indicated for older or debilitated patients.

***Maximum recommended dosage represents the typical upper limit that can be administered each day. Slightly higher daily doses may be administered for short periods of time to control severe psychotic symptoms, usually in hospitalized patients.*

The neurochemical changes underlying psychosis are complex, and psychotic symptoms probably occur because of imbalances in several neurotransmitter pathways. We address the specific drugs currently used to help resolve these imbalances and treat psychosis next.

ANTIPSYCHOTIC DRUGS

Antipsychotic medications comprise a somewhat diverse group in terms of their chemical background and potency—that is, the dosage range typically needed to achieve antipsychotic effects (see Table 8-1). As indicated earlier, these agents all block D2 dopamine receptors to some extent, despite their chemical diversity. In addition to their chemical differences, antipsychotics can be classified as either traditional agents or newer "atypical" antipsychotics according to their effects on different neurotransmitter pathways and their side effect profiles (see Table 8-2). Differences between these two classes are described here.

Traditional Antipsychotics

Traditional antipsychotics are associated with more side effects than their newer counterparts, including an increased incidence of movement disorders and motor side effects (see "Problems and Adverse Effects" later in this chapter). This increased risk may be due to the traditional agents' tendencies to bind to several types of central nervous system (CNS) dopamine receptors, including those that influence motor function in the basal ganglia. This seems especially true for high-potency traditional agents such as haloperidol (Haldol) and fluphenazine (Prolixin). These agents have a strong affinity for CNS dopamine receptors and can exert beneficial effects when used in low dosages (see Table 8-2). Other traditional agents such as chlorpromazine (Thorazine) and thioridazine (Mellaril) have lower potency and must be used in high dosages to exert an antipsychotic effect. These low-potency agents tend to cause fewer motor side effects but are associated with an increased incidence of other problems, such as sedative and anticholinergic side effects (e.g., dry mouth, constipation, urinary retention). These side effects and their possible long-term implications are discussed further in this chapter.

Traditional agents are also somewhat less predictable, and there tends to be more patient-to-patient variability in the beneficial (antipsychotic) effects of these medications.[16] Newer, atypical drugs may be somewhat safer and more predictable, and these agents are described next.

Atypical Antipsychotics

Pharmacologists have developed several newer antipsychotic medications that are different or "atypical," compared with their predecessors. These agents include clozapine (Clozaril), risperidone (Risperdal), and several others listed in Tables 8-1 and 8-2. Although there is some debate about what exactly defines these drugs as "atypical," the most distinguishing feature is that they have a much better side-effect profile, including a decreased risk of producing movement disorders and motor side effects.[18]

As indicated earlier, atypical agents seem to affect dopamine and serotonin receptor subtypes differently than the older, more conventional drugs. In particular, the atypical agents do not block dopamine D2 receptors as strongly as traditional antipsychotics, but instead strongly block the 5-HT_2 serotonin receptors in specific limbic system pathways. Dopamine is, of course, important in controlling motor function in other areas of the brain such as the basal ganglia. Antipsychotics that strongly affect dopamine receptors in the limbic system may inadvertently affect dopamine receptors in the basal ganglia, thereby producing motor side effects.[27,28] Because atypical agents do not affect dopamine receptors as strongly, they have a lower tendency to affect dopamine activity in the basal ganglia and therefore have a lower risk of producing motor side effects. There is also evidence that these drugs might have beneficial effects on other neurotransmitters, including glutamate, GABA, and acetylcholine.[29,30] These additional effects might add to their antipsychotic benefits by improving cognition and reducing the incidence of other problems such as social withdrawal.[27,31]

The newer atypical agents seem to be at least as effective as the traditional drugs, but the atypical drugs may be associated with a lower incidence of relapse compared to traditional agents.[32] The risk of relapse may be lower because the atypical drugs are better tolerated—that is, patients will continue taking the atypical drugs on a regular basis if they are not subjected to side effects such as movement disorders.[32,33] Nonetheless, there is still considerable debate about which drugs should be the first-choice or "front-line" treatment of psychosis. Presently, there does not seem to be a clearly superior choice in terms of efficacy; atypical and traditional antipsychotic drugs are both fairly similar in their ability to reduce psychotic symptoms.[34] Drug selection is therefore based primarily on potential side effects; hence, the atypical drugs are often used as a first choice because of a somewhat more favorable side-effect profile.[3,16] If the first choice is not effective, or if side effects are problematic, the physician may consider switching the patient to a more traditional drug.[16]

PHARMACOKINETICS

Antipsychotics are usually administered orally. During the acute stage of a psychotic episode, the daily dosage is often divided into three or four equal amounts. Maintenance doses are usually lower and can often be administered once each day. Under certain conditions, antipsychotics can be given intramuscularly (IM). During acute episodes, IM injections tend to reach the bloodstream faster than an orally administered drug and may be used if the patient is especially agitated.

Conversely, certain forms of IM antipsychotics that enter the bloodstream slowly have been developed. This method of "depot administration" may prove helpful if the patient has poor self-adherence to drug therapy and neglects to take his or her medication regularly.[35,36] For example, depot preparations of conventional antipsychotics such as fluphenazine decanoate and haloperidol decanoate can be injected every 3 to 4 weeks, respectively, and serve as a method of slow, continual release during the maintenance phase of psychosis.[37] More recently, an injectable form of risperidone, an atypical antipsychotic, has been developed. This preparation is typically administered IM every 2 weeks and appears to provide beneficial long-term effects with fewer motor side effects.[36,38]

Metabolism of antipsychotics is through two mechanisms: conjugation with glucuronic acid and oxidation by hepatic microsomal enzymes. Both mechanisms of metabolism and subsequent inactivation take place in the liver. Prolonged use of antipsychotics may create some degree of enzyme induction, which may be responsible for increasing the rate of metabolism of these drugs.

OTHER USES OF ANTIPSYCHOTICS

Occasionally, antipsychotics are prescribed for conditions other than classic psychosis. As discussed in Chapter 7, an antipsychotic can be used alone or combined with lithium during an acute manic phase of bipolar disorder.[39] In particular, aripiprazole (Abilify) has received considerable attention in treating bipolar disorder.[40,41] This drug is somewhat different than other atypical antipsychotics because it partially activates certain dopamine and serotonin receptors (i.e., the D2, D3, and $5HT_{1a}$ subtypes), while blocking the

$5\text{-}HT_{2a}$ serotonin receptor.[40] Hence, these complex effects differentiate aripiprazole from other antipsychotics and may help explain why this drug is successful in treating bipolar disorder and similar mood disorders.

Some traditional antipsychotics like prochlorperazine (Compazine) are also effective in decreasing nausea and vomiting and can be used as antiemetics in various situations such as cancer chemotherapy or when dopamine agonists and precursors are administered to treat Parkinson disease. The antiemetic effect of antipsychotics is probably caused by their ability to block dopamine receptors located on the brainstem that cause vomiting when stimulated by dopamine.

Medical practitioners often prescribe antipsychotics for Alzheimer disease and other cases of dementia to help control aggression and agitation.[42,43] However, these agents should be used carefully in patients with Alzheimer disease and should not be used merely as "chemical restraints" to sedate them. Likewise, older adults are at greater risk for developing movement disorders when taking antipsychotics, and these drugs may also increase mortality in the elderly due to stroke and other cardiovascular events.[44,45] Ideally, patients with Alzheimer disease and other forms of dementia should use antipsychotics for only short periods of time to control the acute or severe aggressive behaviors.[43] Clinicians can guide patients toward nonpharmacological interventions that help calm the patient and reduce aggression whenever possible to avoid the risks of long-term antipsychotic use. For example, surrounding the patient with familiar items can decrease feelings of disorientation and alienation. Likewise, engaging the patient in structured activities throughout the day can help decrease agitation, thereby reducing the need for antipsychotic drugs.

PROBLEMS AND ADVERSE EFFECTS

Extrapyramidal Symptoms

One of the more serious problems occurring from the use of antipsychotics is the production of abnormal movement patterns.[46,47] Many of the aberrant movements are similar to those seen in patients with lesions of the extrapyramidal system and are often referred to as *extrapyramidal side effects*. Motor problems occur because dopamine is an important neurotransmitter in motor pathways, especially in the integration of motor function that takes place in the basal ganglia, and antipsychotic drugs block CNS dopamine receptors. The unintentional antagonism of dopamine receptors in areas of motor integration (as opposed to the beneficial blockade of behaviorally related receptors) results in a neurotransmitter imbalance that creates several distinct types of movement problems. Thus, most traditional antipsychotics are associated with an increased risk of motor side effects because these drugs are relatively nonselective in their ability to block CNS dopamine receptors.

The newer (atypical) agents such as clozapine and risperidone, on the other hand, are not associated with as high an incidence of extrapyramidal side effects.[48] Several hypotheses exist to explain the lower incidence, including the idea that the atypical antipsychotics block serotonin receptors more than the D2 receptors associated with motor side effects.[49] Alternatively, it has been proposed that atypical agents block dopamine receptors long enough to cause a therapeutic effect, but not long enough to cause receptor supersensitivity and other changes that result in motor side effects.[50] However, the exact reasons for their lower incidence of extrapyramidal side effects is not known. Although the risk of extrapyramidal side effects is generally lower with the atypical drugs, some patients may still develop motor problems when taking these drugs.[46,51]

The extrapyramidal side effects continue to be one of the major drawbacks of antipsychotic medications. The primary types of extrapyramidal side effects, the manifestations of each type, and the relative time of their onset are shown in Figure 8-2. Some factors involved in patient susceptibility and possible treatment of these side effects are discussed here.

Tardive Dyskinesia

Tardive dyskinesia is the most feared side effect of antipsychotic drugs because it may be irreversible.[3,52] Tardive dyskinesia is characterized by several involuntary and fragmented movements.[52] In particular, rhythmic movements of the mouth, tongue, and jaw occur, and the patient often produces involuntary sucking and smacking noises. Because this condition typically involves the tongue and orofacial musculature, serious swallowing disorders (dysphagia) may also occur.[53] Other symptoms include choreoathetoid movements of the extremities and dystonias of the neck and trunk. As indicated in Table 8-2, a greater risk of extrapyramidal effects (including tardive dyskinesia) is associated with certain traditional high-potency

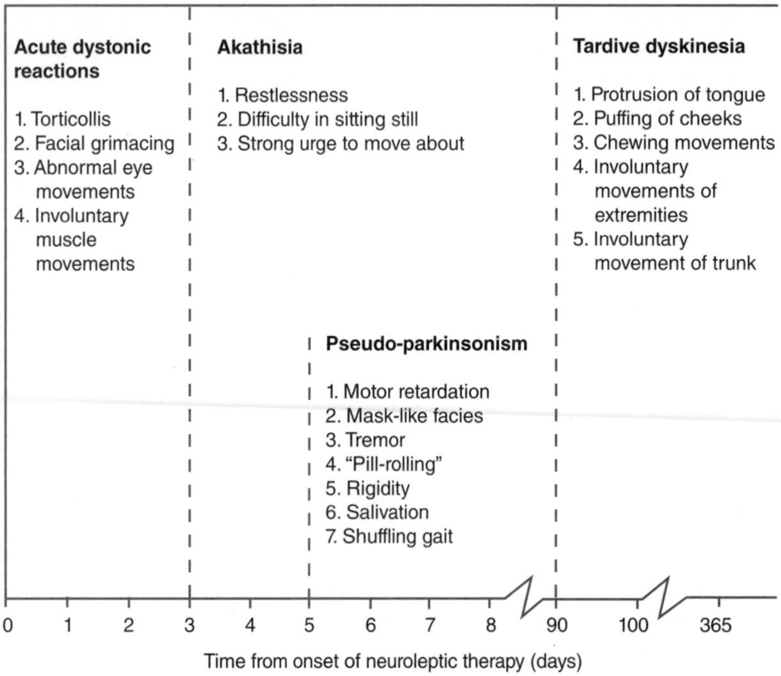

Figure ■ 8-2
Extrapyramidal side effects and their relative onset after beginning antipsychotic drug therapy.

antipsychotics. In fact, tardive dyskinesia is relatively common in patients taking traditional antipsychotics, with an estimated prevalence of 20 to 25 percent in people undergoing long-term treatment with these drugs.[16]

Other risk factors include advanced patient age, genetic predisposition, affective mood disorders, diabetes mellitus, history of alcohol abuse, and continual use of the drug for 6 months or longer.[51,54,55] The risk of tardive dyskinesia is generally lower with the newer atypical agents, and the exact incidence varies considerably depending on the specific drug, the dosage used, and other factors such as the patient's age and previous exposure to antipsychotics.[51,56]

Tardive dyskinesia induced by antipsychotic drugs may be caused by "disuse supersensitivity" of the dopamine receptor.[57,58] Although the presynaptic neurons are still intact, drug blockade of the postsynaptic receptor induces the postsynaptic neuron to respond by "up-regulating" the number or sensitivity of the receptors. This increase in receptor sensitivity causes a functional increase in dopaminergic influence, leading to a neurotransmitter imbalance between dopamine and other central neurotransmitters such as acetylcholine and GABA. In addition, changes in the structure of striatonigral neurons and other brain structures accompany the functional changes in neurotransmitter sensitivity.[59] These functional and structural changes result in the symptoms of tardive dyskinesia.

Physicians can deal with the motor symptoms of tardive dyskinesia by lowering the drug dosage or by substituting an antipsychotic that produces fewer extrapyramidal side effects (see Table 8-2). In some patients, the symptoms will disappear if the drug is stopped or if the dosage is decreased, but this can take several weeks to several years to occur, and may never disappear in some individuals. This is especially disturbing because the antipsychotic drug has created a permanent motor problem that can affect swallowing and has generated abnormal orofacial movements that are embarrassing to the patient and can further affect the patient's psychosocial well-being.[52,53] To prevent the occurrence of tardive dyskinesia, the physician should prescribe the lowest effective dose of the antipsychotic, especially during the maintenance phase of drug therapy.[51] Patients taking these drugs for 3 months or more should undergo periodic reevaluation for any symptoms of tardive dyskinesia.[16] Early intervention is generally believed to be the most effective way of preventing the permanent changes associated with antipsychotic-induced tardive dyskinesia.[51]

Physicians can administer other drugs to alleviate the symptoms of drug-induced tardive dyskinesia.[60-63]

Agents such as anticholinergic drugs (e.g., atropine-like drugs), GABA-enhancing drugs (e.g., benzodiazepines), vitamin E, and calcium channel blockers can be used to attempt to rectify the transmitter imbalance or the cellular changes created by the increased dopamine sensitivity. Drugs like reserpine and tetrabenazine can also be used in some patients because of the drug's ability to deplete presynaptic stores of dopamine, thus limiting the influence of this neurotransmitter. However, these additional agents have been only marginally successful in reducing the **dyskinesia** symptoms, and their use adds complexity to the drug management of patients with psychoses. Thus, the best course of action continues to be judicious administration of antipsychotic drugs, using the lowest effective dose, and early recognition and intervention if extrapyramidal symptoms appear.[16,51]

Pseudoparkinsonism

The motor symptoms seen in Parkinson disease (see Chapter 10) are caused by a deficiency in dopamine transmission in the basal ganglia. Because antipsychotic drugs block dopamine receptors, some patients may experience symptoms similar to those seen in Parkinson disease, including resting tremor, bradykinesia, and rigidity. Elderly patients are more susceptible to these drug-induced parkinsonian-like symptoms, probably because dopamine content (and therefore dopaminergic influence) tends to be lower in older individuals.[64] The outcome of antipsychotic-induced parkinsonism is usually favorable, and these symptoms normally disappear when the dosage is adjusted or the drug is withdrawn. Anticholinergic drugs used as adjuncts in treating Parkinson disease (e.g., benztropine mesylate, diphenhydramine) may also be administered to deal with parkinsonian-like side effects.[16] However, primary antiparkinsonian drugs such as levodopa and dopamine agonists are not typically used to treat these side effects because they tend to exacerbate the psychotic symptoms.

Akathisia

Patients taking antipsychotics may experience sensations of motor restlessness and may complain of an inability to sit or lie still. This condition is known as **akathisia**.[16,65] Patients may also appear agitated, may pace the floor, and may have problems with insomnia. Akathisia can usually be dealt with by altering the dosage or type of medication. If this is unsuccessful, beta-2 adrenergic receptor blockers (propranolol) may help decrease the restlessness associated with akathisia by a mechanism involving central adrenergic receptors.[16,66] Medical practitioners may also use anticholinergic drugs to treat akathisia, but it is not clear if these drugs actually reduce symptoms associated with akathisia.[16]

Dyskinesia and Dystonias

Patients may exhibit a broad range of movements in the arms, legs, neck, and face, including torticollis, oculogyric crisis, and opisthotonos.[16] These movements are involuntary and uncoordinated and may begin fairly soon after initiating antipsychotic therapy (even after a single dose).[16] If the movements persist during therapy, other drugs such as antiparkinsonian adjuncts or benzodiazepines (e.g., diazepam) can be used to try to combat the aberrant motor symptoms.

Neuroleptic Malignant Syndrome

Patients taking relatively high doses of the more potent antipsychotics may experience a serious disorder known as neuroleptic malignant syndrome (NMS).[67,68] Symptoms of NMS include catatonia, stupor, rigidity, tremors, and fever.[16,69] These symptoms are severe and can lead to death if left untreated.[67] Clinicians should seek emergency medical attention if the patient exhibits these symptoms during rehabilitation sessions, especially if the symptoms occur suddenly or increase rapidly. Treatment typically consists of stopping the antipsychotic drug and providing supportive care. The exact causes of NMS are unclear, but the risk of developing this syndrome is increased in patients who are agitated, who have impaired mental function, or when traditional antipsychotics are administered at high doses or via intramuscular injection.[16]

Nonmotor Effects

Metabolic Effects

The newer, atypical antipsychotics can produce metabolic side effects that result in substantial weight gain, increased plasma lipids, and diabetes mellitus in some patients.[70,71] The risk of metabolic side effects varies according to each drug, with the highest risk associated with clozapine and olanzapine; moderate risk with iloperidone, paliperidone, quetiapine, and risperidone; and lowest risk with aripiprazole, lurasidone, and ziprasidone.[71] The reasons for these metabolic effects are not clear and probably occur because of a complex interaction between genetic factors and the ability of these drugs to affect serotonin, dopamine, and other CNS receptors.[72] Thus, these newer drugs pose less risk of motor symptoms but can cause side effects that ultimately produce serious cardiovascular and endocrine problems.[73] Medical practitioners should screen their patients for cardiovascular or metabolic disorders before starting an atypical antipsychotic, and these drugs should probably be avoided in people with preexisting metabolic or cardiovascular diseases.

Sedation

Antipsychotics have varying degrees of sedative properties. Contrary to previous beliefs, sedative properties do not enhance the antipsychotic efficacy of these drugs. Consequently, sedative side effects offer no benefit and can be detrimental in withdrawn patients.

Anticholinergic Effects

Some antipsychotics also decrease acetylcholine function in various physiological systems throughout the body. These anticholinergic effects are manifested by a variety of symptoms such as blurred vision, dry mouth, constipation, and urinary retention. Fortunately, these problems are usually self-limiting as many patients become tolerant to the anticholinergic side effects while remaining responsive to the antipsychotic properties.

Other Side Effects

Orthostatic hypotension is a frequent problem during the initial stages of antipsychotic therapy. This problem usually disappears after a few days. Certain antipsychotic drugs such as chlorpromazine are associated with photosensitivity, and care should be taken when exposing these patients to ultraviolet irradiation. Finally, abrupt withdrawal of antipsychotic drugs after prolonged use often results in nausea and vomiting, so it is advisable for medical practitioners to decrease dosage gradually rather than to suddenly stop administration.

Special Concerns for Rehabilitation Patients

Antipsychotic drugs have been a great benefit to patients seen in various rehabilitation facilities. Regardless of the reason these individuals are referred to physical therapy and occupational therapy, the drug therapy will hopefully enhance the patient's cooperation during rehabilitation. Because these drugs tend to normalize patient behavior, the withdrawn patient often becomes more active and amiable, while the agitated patient becomes calmer and more engaged. Also, remission of some confusion and impaired thinking will enable the patient to follow instructions more easily. Patients with paranoid symptoms may have fewer delusions of persecution and will feel less threatened by the entire therapy environment.

The benefits of antipsychotic drugs must be weighed against their side effect risks. The less serious side effects such as sedation and some of the anticholinergic effects (e.g., blurred vision, dry mouth, constipation) can be bothersome during the treatment session. Orthostatic hypotension should be guarded against, especially during the first few days after drug therapy is initiated. However, the major problems have to do with the antipsychotic drug's extrapyramidal motor effects. Therapists treating patients on antipsychotic medications should remain alert for early signs of motor involvement. Chances are good that the therapist may be the first person to notice a change in posture, balance, or involuntary movements. Even subtle problems in motor function should be brought to the attention of the medical staff immediately. This early intervention may diminish the risk of long-term or even permanent motor dysfunction.

CASE STUDY

ANTIPSYCHOTIC DRUGS

Brief History. R.F., a 63-year-old woman, has been receiving treatment for schizophrenia intermittently for many years. She was last hospitalized for an acute episode 7 months ago and has since been on a maintenance dosage of haloperidol (Haldol), 25 mg/d. She is also being seen as an outpatient for treatment of rheumatoid arthritis in both hands. Her current treatment consists of gentle heat and active range-of-motion exercises, three times each week. She is being considered for possible metacarpophalangeal joint replacement.

Problem/Influence of Medication. During the course of physical therapy, the therapist noticed the onset and slow, progressive increase in writhing gestures of both upper extremities. Extraneous movements of her mouth and face were also observed, including chewing-like jaw movements and tongue protrusion.

1. ***Why might antipsychotic drugs cause these abnormal movements?***
2. ***What specific movement disorder might be indicated by these symptoms?***
3. ***Why is it critical to resolve this situation as soon as possible?***

See Appendix C, "Answers to Case Study Questions."

SUMMARY

Antipsychotic drugs represent one of the major advances in the management of mental illness. Drugs are currently available that diminish the symptoms of psychosis and improve a patient's ability to cooperate with others and to administer self-care. Despite their chemical diversity, antipsychotics all seem to exert beneficial effects by blocking central dopamine receptors. Therefore, psychoses such as schizophrenia may be caused by an overactivity of CNS dopaminergic pathways. Other neurotransmitters such as serotonin may also play a role in psychosis, and some of the newer antipsychotics also moderate serotonin activity in the brain.

Because of their potential to block dopaminergic receptors, antipsychotics are associated with several adverse side effects. The most serious of these are abnormal movement patterns that resemble tardive dyskinesia, Parkinson disease, and other lesions associated with the extrapyramidal system. In some cases, these aberrant motor activities may become irreversible and persist even after drug therapy is terminated. Rehabilitation specialists may play a critical role in recognizing the early onset of these motor abnormalities. When identified early, potentially serious motor problems can be dealt with by altering the dosage or type of antipsychotic agent.

REFERENCES

1 Meyer JM. Pharmacotherapy of psychosis and mania. In: Brunton LL, et al., eds. *The Pharmacological Basis of Therapeutics.* 12th ed. New York: McGraw Hill; 2011.
2. de Araújo AN, de Sena EP, de Oliveira IR, Juruena MF. Antipsychotic agents: efficacy and safety in schizophrenia. *Drug Healthc Patient Saf.* 2012;4:173-180.
3. Meltzer H. Antipsychotic agents and lithium. In: Katzung BG, ed. *Basic and Clinical Pharmacology.* 12th ed. New York: Lange Medical Books/McGraw Hill; 2012.
4. American Psychiatric Association. *Diagnostic and Statistical Manual of Mental Disorders.* 4th ed. Text Revision. Arlington, VA: American Psychiatric Association; 2000.
5. Lee KW, Woon PS, Teo YY, Sim K. Genome wide association studies (GWAS) and copy number variation (CNV) studies of the major psychoses: what have we learnt? *Neurosci Biobehav Rev.* 2012;36:556-571.
6. Itokawa M, Arinami T, Toru M. Advanced research on dopamine signaling to develop drugs for the treatment of mental disorders: Ser311Cys polymorphisms of the dopamine D2-receptor gene and schizophrenia. *J Pharmacol Sci.* 2010;114:1-5.

7. Labrie V, Pai S, Petronis A. Epigenetics of major psychosis: progress, problems and perspectives. *Trends Genet.* 2012;28: 427-435.
8. Peter CJ, Akbarian S. Balancing histone methylation activities in psychiatric disorders. *Trends Mol Med.* 2011;17:372-379.
9. Pidsley R, Mill J. Epigenetic studies of psychosis: current findings, methodological approaches, and implications for postmortem research. *Biol Psychiatry.* 2011;69:146-156.
10. Brown AS. The environment and susceptibility to schizophrenia. *Prog Neurobiol.* 2011;93:23-58.
11. Clarke MC, Kelleher I, Clancy M, Cannon M. Predicting risk and the emergence of schizophrenia. *Psychiatr Clin North Am.* 2012;35:585-612.
12. Schäfer I, Fisher HL. Childhood trauma and posttraumatic stress disorder in patients with psychosis: clinical challenges and emerging treatments. *Curr Opin Psychiatry.* 2011;24:514-518.
13. Wermter AK, Laucht M, Schimmelmann BG, et al. From nature versus nurture, via nature and nurture, to gene x environment interaction in mental disorders. *Eur Child Adolesc Psychiatry.* 2010;19:199-210.
14. Baune BT, Thome J. Translational research approach to biological and modifiable risk factors of psychosis and affective disorders. *World J Biol Psychiatry.* 2011;12(suppl 1):28-34.
15. Holtzman CW, Shapiro DI, Trotman HD, Walker EF. Stress and the prodromal phase of psychosis. *Curr Pharm Des.* 2012; 18:527-533.
16. Crismon ML, Argo TR, Buckley PF. Schizophrenia. In: DiPiro JT, et al., eds. *Pharmacotherapy: A Pathophysiologic Approach.* 8th ed. New York: McGraw-Hill; 2011.
17. Lodge DJ, Grace AA. Hippocampal dysregulation of dopamine system function and the pathophysiology of schizophrenia. *Trends Pharmacol Sci.* 2011;32:507-513.
18. Meltzer HY, Massey BW. The role of serotonin receptors in the action of atypical antipsychotic drugs. *Curr Opin Pharmacol.* 2011;11:59-67.
19. Coyle JT, Basu A, Benneyworth M, et al. Glutamatergic synaptic dysregulation in schizophrenia: therapeutic implications. *Handb Exp Pharmacol.* 2012;213:267-295.
20. Vinson PN, Conn PJ. Metabotropic glutamate receptors as therapeutic targets for schizophrenia. *Neuropharmacology.* 2012; 62:1461-1472.
21. Field JR, Walker AG, Conn PJ. Targeting glutamate synapses in schizophrenia. *Trends Mol Med.* 2011;17:689-698.
22. Bolbecker AR, Shekhar A. Muscarinic agonists and antagonists in schizophrenia: recent therapeutic advances and future directions. *Handb Exp Pharmacol.* 2012;208:167-190.
23. Dean B. Selective activation of muscarinic acetylcholine receptors for the treatment of schizophrenia. *Curr Pharm Biotechnol.* 2012;13:1563-1571.
24. Grace AA. Dopamine system dysregulation by the hippocampus: implications for the pathophysiology and treatment of schizophrenia. *Neuropharmacology.* 2012;62:1342-1348.
25. Mailman RB, Murthy V. Third generation antipsychotic drugs: partial agonism or receptor functional selectivity? *Curr Pharm Des.* 2010;16:488-501.
26. Miyake N, Miyamoto S, Jarskog LF. New serotonin/dopamine antagonists for the treatment of schizophrenia: are we making real progress? *Clin Schizophr Relat Psychoses.* 2012;6:122-133.
27. Newman-Tancredi A. The importance of 5-HT1A receptor agonism in antipsychotic drug action: rationale and perspectives. *Curr Opin Investig Drugs.* 2010;11:802-812.
28. Thomasson-Perret N, Pénélaud PF, Théron D, et al. Markers of D(2) and D(3) receptor activity in vivo: PET scan and prolactin. *Therapie.* 2008;63:237-242.
29. López-Gil X, Artigas F, Adell A. Unraveling monoamine receptors involved in the action of typical and atypical antipsychotics on glutamatergic and serotonergic transmission in prefrontal cortex. *Curr Pharm Des.* 2010;16:502-515.
30. Sanger DJ. The search for novel antipsychotics: pharmacological and molecular targets. *Expert Opin Ther Targets.* 2004;8: 631-641.
31. Newman-Tancredi A, Kleven MS. Comparative pharmacology of antipsychotics possessing combined dopamine D2 and serotonin 5-HT1A receptor properties. *Psychopharmacology.* 2011; 216:451-473.
32. Nasrallah HA, Lasser R. Improving patient outcomes in schizophrenia: achieving remission. *J Psychopharmacol.* 2006;20(suppl): 57-61.
33. Thomas P, Alptekin K, Gheorghe M, et al. Management of patients presenting with acute psychotic episodes of schizophrenia. *CNS Drugs.* 2009;23:193-212.
34. Crossley NA, Constante M, McGuire P, Power P. Efficacy of atypical v. typical antipsychotics in the treatment of early psychosis: meta-analysis. *Br J Psychiatry.* 2010;196:434-439.
35. Baweja R, Sedky K, Lippmann S. Long-acting antipsychotic medications. *Curr Drug Targets.* 2012;13:555-560.
36. Cañas F, Möller HJ. Long-acting atypical injectable antipsychotics in the treatment of schizophrenia: safety and tolerability review. *Expert Opin Drug Saf.* 2010;9:683-697.
37. Citrome L, Jaffe A, Levine J. Treatment of schizophrenia with depot preparations of fluphenazine, haloperidol, and risperidone among inpatients at state-operated psychiatric facilities. *Schizophr Res.* 2010;119:153-159.
38. Rosa F, Schreiner A, Thomas P, Sherif T. Switching patients with stable schizophrenia or schizoaffective disorder from olanzapine to risperidone long-acting injectable. *Clin Drug Investig.* 2012;32:267-279.
39. Price AL, Marzani-Nissen GR. Bipolar disorders: a review. *Am Fam Physician.* 2012;85:483-493.
40. Dhillon S. Aripiprazole: a review of its use in the management of mania in adults with bipolar I disorder. *Drugs.* 2012;72: 133-162.
41. Goodwin GM, Abbar M, Schlaepfer TE, et al. Aripiprazole in patients with bipolar mania and beyond: an update of practical guidance. *Curr Med Res Opin.* 2011;27:2285-2299.
42. Ballard C, Corbett A. Management of neuropsychiatric symptoms in people with dementia. *CNS Drugs.* 2010;24:729-739.
43. Ballard C, Waite J. The effectiveness of atypical antipsychotics for the treatment of aggression and psychosis in Alzheimer's disease. *Cochrane Database Syst Rev.* 2006;1:CD003476.
44. Ballard C, Creese B, Corbett A, Aarsland D. Atypical antipsychotics for the treatment of behavioral and psychological symptoms in dementia, with a particular focus on longer term outcomes and mortality. *Expert Opin Drug Saf.* 2011;10:35-43.
45. Herrmann N, Gauthier S. Diagnosis and treatment of dementia: 6. Management of severe Alzheimer disease. *CMAJ.* 2008;179:1279-1287.
46. Cha DS, McIntyre RS. Treatment-emergent adverse events associated with atypical antipsychotics. *Expert Opin Pharmacother.* 2012;13:1587-1598.
47. Tandon R. Antipsychotics in the treatment of schizophrenia: an overview. *J Clin Psychiatry.* 2011;72(suppl 1):4-8.

48. Haddad PM, Das A, Keyhani S, Chaudhry IB. Antipsychotic drugs and extrapyramidal side effects in first episode psychosis: a systematic review of head-head comparisons. *J Psychopharmacol.* 2012;26(suppl):15-26.
49. Nord M, Farde L. Antipsychotic occupancy of dopamine receptors in schizophrenia. *CNS Neurosci Ther.* 2011;17:97-103.
50. Vauquelin G, Bostoen S, Vanderheyden P, Seeman P. Clozapine, atypical antipsychotics, and the benefits of fast-off D2 dopamine receptor antagonism. *Naunyn Schmiedebergs Arch Pharmacol.* 2012;385:337-372.
51. Tarsy D, Lungu C, Baldessarini RJ. Epidemiology of tardive dyskinesia before and during the era of modern antipsychotic drugs. *Handb Clin Neurol.* 2011;100:601-616.
52. van Harten PN, Tenback DE. Tardive dyskinesia: clinical presentation and treatment. *Int Rev Neurobiol.* 2011;98:187-210.
53. Baheshree RD, Jonas SS. Dysphagia in a psychotic patient: diagnostic challenges and a systematic management approach. *Indian J Psychiatry.* 2012;54:280-282.
54. Lerner V, Miodownik C. Motor symptoms of schizophrenia: is tardive dyskinesia a symptom or side effect? A modern treatment. *Curr Psychiatry Rep.* 2011;13:295-304.
55. Tenback DE, van Harten PN. Epidemiology and risk factors for (tardive) dyskinesia. *Int Rev Neurobiol.* 2011;98:211-230.
56. Rummel-Kluge C, Komossa K, Schwarz S, et al. Second-generation antipsychotic drugs and extrapyramidal side effects: a systematic review and meta-analysis of head-to-head comparisons. *Schizophr Bull.* 2012;38:167-177.
57. Kostrzewa RM, Huang NY, Kostrzewa JP, et al. Modeling tardive dyskinesia: predictive 5-HT2C receptor antagonist treatment. *Neurotox Res.* 2007;11:41-50.
58. Seeman P. All roads to schizophrenia lead to dopamine supersensitivity and elevated dopamine D2 (high) receptors. *CNS Neurosci Ther.* 2011;17:118-132.
59. Margolese HC, Chouinard G, Kolivakis TT, et al. Tardive dyskinesia in the era of typical and atypical antipsychotics. Part 1: pathophysiology and mechanisms of induction. *Can J Psychiatry.* 2005;50:541-547.
60. Alabed S, Latifeh Y, Mohammad HA, Rifai A. Gamma-aminobutyric acid agonists for neuroleptic-induced tardive dyskinesia. *Cochrane Database Syst Rev.* 2011;4:CD000203.
61. Desmarais JE, Beauclair L, Margolese HC. Anticholinergics in the era of atypical antipsychotics: short-term or long-term treatment? *J Psychopharmacol.* 2012;26:1167-1174.
62. Essali A, Deirawan H, Soares-Weiser K, Adams CE. Calcium channel blockers for neuroleptic-induced tardive dyskinesia. *Cochrane Database Syst Rev.* 2011;11:CD000206.
63. Soares-Weiser K, Maayan N, McGrath J. Vitamin E for neuroleptic-induced tardive dyskinesia. *Cochrane Database Syst Rev.* 2011;2:CD000209.
64. Thanvi B, Treadwell S. Drug induced parkinsonism: a common cause of parkinsonism in older people. *Postgrad Med J.* 2009;85:322-326.
65. Kane JM, Barnes TR, Correll CU, et al. Evaluation of akathisia in patients with schizophrenia, schizoaffective disorder, or bipolar I disorder: a post hoc analysis of pooled data from short- and long-term aripiprazole trials. *J Psychopharmacol.* 2010;24:1019-1029.
66. Koliscak LP, Makela EH. Selective serotonin reuptake inhibitor-induced akathisia. *J Am Pharm Assoc.* 2009;49:e28-36.
67. Gillman PK. Neuroleptic malignant syndrome: mechanisms, interactions, and causality. *Mov Disord.* 2010;25:1780-1790.
68. Trollor JN, Chen X, Sachdev PS. Neuroleptic malignant syndrome associated with atypical antipsychotic drugs. *CNS Drugs.* 2009;23:477-492.
69. Margetić B, Aukst-Margetić B. Neuroleptic malignant syndrome and its controversies. *Pharmacoepidemiol Drug Saf.* 2010; 19:429-435.
70. Das C, Mendez G, Jagasia S, Labbate LA. Second-generation antipsychotic use in schizophrenia and associated weight gain: a critical review and meta-analysis of behavioral and pharmacologic treatments. *Ann Clin Psychiatry.* 2012;24:225-239.
71. Hasnain M, W Victor RV, Hollett B. Weight gain and glucose dysregulation with second-generation antipsychotics and antidepressants: a review for primary care physicians. *Postgrad Med.* 2012;124:154-167.
72. Roerig JL, Steffen KJ, Mitchell JE. Atypical antipsychotic-induced weight gain: insights into mechanisms of action. *CNS Drugs.* 2011;25:1035-1059.
73. Leung JY, Barr AM, Procyshyn RM, et al. Cardiovascular side-effects of antipsychotic drugs: the role of the autonomic nervous system. *Pharmacol Ther.* 2012;135:113-122.

CHAPTER 9

Antiepileptic Drugs

Epilepsy is a chronic neurological disorder characterized by recurrent seizures.[1,2] Seizures are episodes of sudden, transient disturbances in cerebral excitation that occur when a sufficient number of cerebral neurons begin to fire rapidly and in synchronized bursts.[3] Depending on the type of seizure, neuronal activity may remain localized in a specific area of the brain, or it may spread to other areas of the brain. In some seizures, neurons in the motor cortex are activated, leading to skeletal muscle contraction via descending neuronal pathways. These involuntary, paroxysmal skeletal muscle contractions seen during certain seizures are referred to as *convulsions*. However, convulsions are not associated with all types of epilepsy, and other types of seizures are characterized by a wide variety of sensory or behavioral symptoms.

Epilepsy is associated with the presence of a group or focus of cerebral neurons that are hyperexcitable, or "irritable." The spontaneous discharge of these irritable neurons initiates the epileptic seizure. The reason for the altered excitability of these focal neurons, and thus the cause of epilepsy, varies depending on the patient.[4,5] In some patients, a specific incident such as a stroke, tumor, encephalopathy, head trauma, or other CNS injury probably damaged certain neurons, resulting in their altered threshold.[6-9] In other patients, the reason for seizures may be less distinct or unknown, perhaps relating to a congenital abnormality, birth trauma, or genetic factor.[10-12] A systemic metabolic disorder such as infection, hypoglycemia, hypoxia, or uremia may precipitate seizure activity.[13-15] Once the cause of the seizures is identified in this last group of individuals, the epilepsy can often be treated by resolving the metabolic disorder.

The exact prevalence of epilepsy is difficult to determine and varies considerably from country to country and when different criteria and survey techniques are used to assess people with epilepsy. Nonetheless, it is estimated that about 3 percent of the U.S. population that lives to 80 years of age is diagnosed with epilepsy, making this one of the most common neurological disorders.[1]

Because epilepsy is rather prevalent, you will frequently encounter patients with this disorder. Likewise, you will see many patients with specific conditions such as traumatic brain injury, stroke, and cerebral palsy that increase the likelihood that they will have seizures. You must adjust their treatments accordingly to try to prevent the seizures. Moreover, a patient may have a seizure during a rehabilitation session, and you should understand how to deal with it. Seizures are a common and important comorbidity that affects your ability to work with patients who have epilepsy or other seizure disorders.

Although some innovative approaches using surgery, neural stimulation, and dietary control have been reported,[16-19] drug therapy remains the primary method for treating epilepsy. In general, antiepileptic medications are successful in eliminating seizures in 50 percent of the patient population and can reduce seizure activity substantially in an additional 25 percent of patients with epilepsy.[3] On the other hand, at least 25 percent of patients with epilepsy do not receive adequate seizure control using the drugs that are currently available.[20] Hence, many experts feel that there is a critical need for safer, more effective antiseizure drugs. Nonetheless, epileptic medications have been a mainstay in treating seizures in many people. Some of these drugs have also been used to treat bipolar disorder (see Chapter 7), and certain antiseizure agents such as gabapentin and pregabalin are useful in treating peripheral neuropathies, fibromyalgia, and other chronic pain syndromes.[21] This chapter will focus primarily on the use of these medications to resolve seizure disorders.

Several types of drugs are currently available, and certain compounds work best in specific types of epilepsy. Consequently, the type of epilepsy must be determined by observing the patient and using diagnostic tests such as electroencephalography (EEG).[22] The classification system most commonly used in characterizing epilepsy is discussed here.

CLASSIFICATION OF EPILEPTIC SEIZURES

In an attempt to standardize the terminology used in describing various forms of epilepsy, the International League Against Epilepsy[23] proposed the classification scheme outlined in Table 9-1. Seizures are divided into two major categories: generalized seizures and focal seizures. The latter category was formerly called *partial*

Table 9-1
CLASSIFICATION OF SEIZURES

Seizure Class and Subclasses	Typical Symptoms
Generalized Seizures	
Tonic-clonic	Major convulsions of entire body; sustained contraction of all muscles (tonic phase) followed by powerful rhythmic contractions (clonic phase); loss of consciousness
Absence (petit mal) seizures Typical Atypical Absence with special features Myoclonic absence Eyelid myoclonia	Sudden, brief loss of consciousness; motor signs may be absent or may range from rapid eye-blinking to symmetrical jerking movements of entire body
Myoclonic seizure Myoclonic Myoclonic atonic Myoclonic tonic	Sudden, brief, “shocklike” contractions of muscles in the face and trunk or in one or more extremities; contractions may be single or multiple; consciousness may be impaired
Clonic seizures	Rhythmic, synchronized contractions throughout the body; loss of consciousness
Tonic seizures	Generalized sustained muscle contractions throughout body; loss of consciousness
Atonic seizures	Sudden loss of muscle tone in the head and neck, one limb, or throughout the entire body; consciousness may be maintained or lost briefly
Focal Seizures*	
Simple partial seizures	Consciousness remains intact, but there are observable motor or autonomic responses, including convulsions confined to one limb or specific sensory hallucinations
Complex partial seizures	Consciousness or awareness is impaired and may include a wide variety of other manifestations and bizarre behaviors
Secondary generalized seizures	Symptoms progressively increase to a bilateral, convulsive seizure, including tonic, clonic, or tonic-clonic components
Unknown	

**Organized by their former subclassifications. The current system does not subclassify focal seizure but uses descriptors that correspond to the older classifications.*
Source: Modified from Report of the ILAE Commission on Classification and Terminology, 2005-2009, p 678, with permission.

seizures, and this term is still used commonly when referring to antiepileptic drug indications. A third category of "unknown" seizures is sometimes included to encompass additional seizure types not fitting into the two major groups. Originally devised in the 1980s, this classification system has been revised periodically, and it will undoubtedly continue to be revised as more is learned about the cause and symptoms of specific seizures.[24]

In focal (partial) seizures, only part of the brain (i.e., one cerebral hemisphere) is involved, whereas in generalized seizures the whole brain is involved (Fig. 9-1).

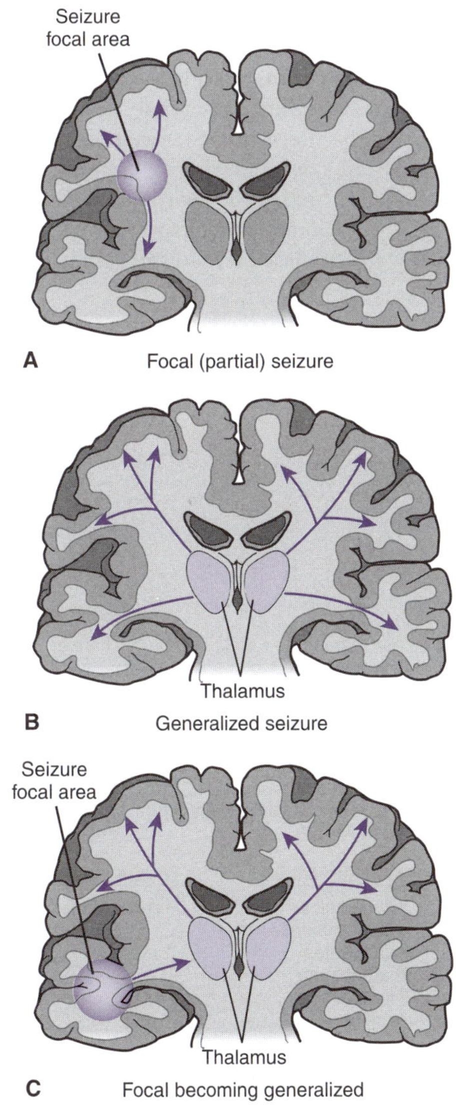

Figure ■ 9-1
Initiation and spread of seizure activity in the brain.

Focal seizures that spread throughout the entire brain are referred to as *focal becoming generalized* or *secondarily generalized seizures*.

Seizures are also classified and subclassified depending on the specific symptoms that occur during the epileptic seizure (see Table 9-1). As a rule, the outward manifestations of the seizure depend on the area of the brain involved. Focal seizures that remain localized within the motor cortex for the right hand may cause involuntary, spasmlike movements of only the right hand. Other focal seizures produce motor and sensory symptoms and can also affect consciousness and memory. According to earlier terminology, focal seizures were subclassified as *simple partial seizures* if patients remained fully conscious during the seizure, and they were called *complex partial seizures* if consciousness was altered during the seizure. Again, this earlier terminology is still commonly used, and the terms *simple* and *complex partial seizures* will be used elsewhere in this chapter when describing the indications for specific antiepileptic drugs.

Generalized seizures are subclassified depending on the type and degree of motor involvement and other factors such as EEG recordings. The most well-known and dramatic seizure of the generalized group is the tonic-clonic, or "grand mal," seizure. Absence, or "petit mal," seizures also fall into the generalized seizure category. Drug therapy for generalized and focal seizures is discussed later in "Antiseizure Drugs."

RATIONALE FOR DRUG TREATMENT

Even in the absence of drug therapy, individual seizures are usually self-limiting. Brain neurons are often unable to sustain a high level of synaptic activity for more than a few minutes, and the seizure ends spontaneously. However, the uncontrolled recurrence of seizures is believed to cause further damage to the already injured neurons and can be potentially harmful to healthy cells.[25] In particular, excessive neuronal excitation can initiate a cascade of biochemical changes involving the production of harmful proteins and oxidative stress in the affected neurons.[26-28] These biochemical changes damage the mitochondria and other cellular components, which ultimately leads to programmed cell death (apoptosis) in these neurons.[25] Certain seizures can therefore cause structural and functional changes in neuronal pathways, resulting in impaired cerebral activity and increased susceptibility to additional seizures.[27,29]

Certain types of seizures will also be harmful if the patient loses consciousness or goes into convulsions and gets injured during a fall. Certain types of convulsions are potentially fatal if cardiac irregularities result and the individual goes into cardiac arrest. Even relatively minor seizures may be embarrassing to a person, and social interaction may be compromised if the individual is afraid of having a seizure in public. Consequently, a strong effort is made to find effective medications to control or eliminate the incidence of seizures.

ANTISEIZURE DRUGS

Antiseizure drugs all share a common goal: suppress the excitability of neurons that initiate the seizure. To achieve this goal, specific drugs typically use one of the strategies illustrated in Figure 9-2—that is, increase the activity of CNS inhibitory neurons, decrease the activity of CNS excitatory neurons, or stabilize the opening and closing of neuronal sodium or calcium channels. Drugs commonly used to treat seizures are presented here.

First-Generation Antiseizure Drugs

Table 9-2 lists drugs commonly used to treat epilepsy according to their chemical classes and mechanisms of action. These drugs represent some of the original antiseizure medications and are sometimes referred to as *first-generation drugs* to differentiate them from the newer second-generation drugs that are discussed later in this chapter. As indicated in Table 9-2, the first-generation drugs generally try to inhibit firing of certain cerebral neurons, usually by increasing the inhibitory effects of gamma-aminobutyric acid (GABA), by decreasing the effects of excitatory amino acids (glutamate, aspartate), or by altering the movement of ions (sodium, calcium) across the neuronal membrane[21,30,31] (see Fig. 9-2). Some antiepileptic drugs probably work by several of these mechanisms simultaneously.[31]

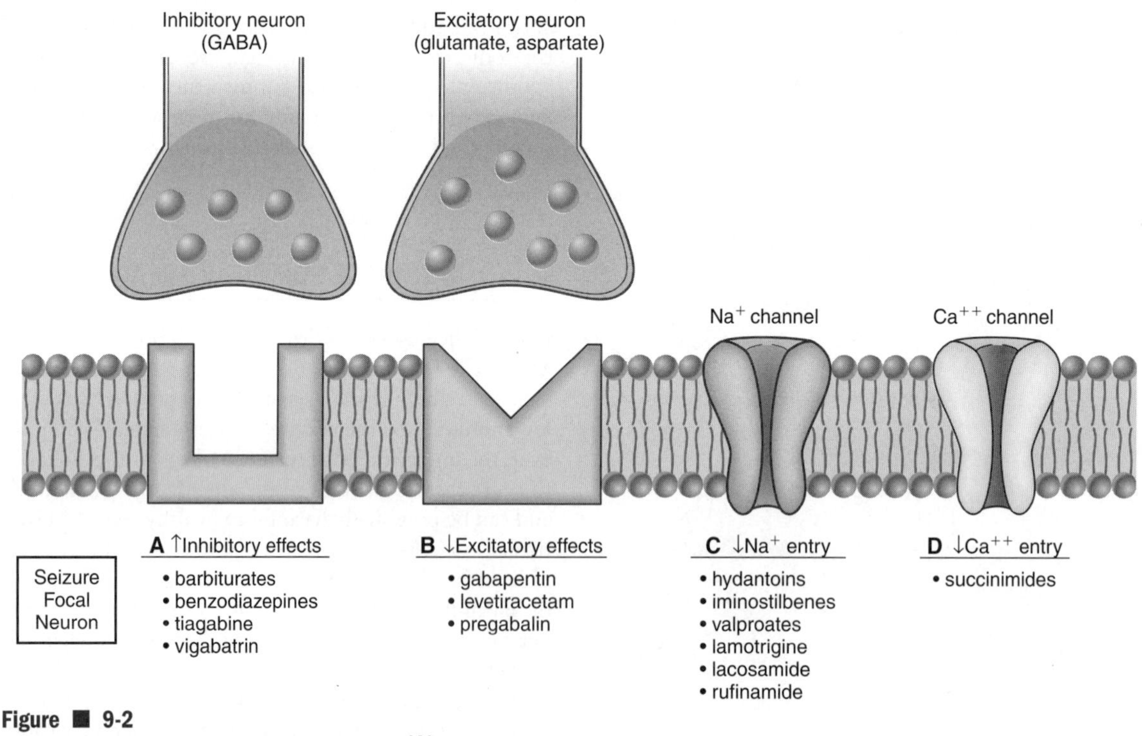

Figure ■ 9-2

Antiseizure drug mechanisms. Specific drugs can **(A)** increase the inhibitory effects at synapses that use gamma-aminobutyric acid (GABA); **(B)** decrease the excitatory effects of synapses that use glutamate or aspartate; **(C)** decrease sodium (Na^+) entry into sodium channels that are opening/closing too rapidly; or **(D)** decrease calcium (Ca^{++}) entry into calcium channels that are opening/closing too rapidly. The primary effect of each drug is listed here; some drugs may decrease seizures by multiple mechanisms.

Table 9-2
CHEMICAL CLASSIFICATION AND ACTIONS OF ANTIEPILEPTIC AGENTS

Chemical Class	Possible Mechanism of Action
Barbiturates	
Pentobarbital (Nembutal)* Phenobarbital (Solfoton, others) Primidone (Mysoline)	Potentiate inhibitory effects of GABA;** may also decrease the release of excitatory glutamate
Benzodiazepines	
Clonazepam (Klonopin) Clorazepate (Tranxene) Diazepam (Valium)* Lorazepam (Ativan)*	Potentiate inhibitory effects of GABA
Hydantoins	
Fosphenytoin (Cerebyx)* Phenytoin (Dilantin)	Primary effect is to stabilize membrane by blocking sodium channels in rapid-firing neurons; higher concentrations may also influence potassium and calcium channels and may increase concentrations of inhibitory neurotransmitters such as GABA
Iminostilbenes	
Carbamazepine (Tegretol) Oxcarbazepine (Trileptal)	Similar to hydantoins. May also inhibit the presynaptic uptake and release of norepinephrine
Succinimides	
Ethosuximide (Zarontin)	Affects calcium channels; appears to inhibit spontaneous firing in thalamic neurons by limiting calcium entry
Valproates	
Valproic acid (Depakene, others) Valproate sodium (Depacon) Divalproex (Depakote, others)	Unclear; may inhibit sodium channels (similar to phenytoin, ethosuximide); may also hyperpolarize neurons through an effect on potassium channels; higher concentrations increase CNS GABA concentrations

**Usually administered parentally (IV injection) to stop severe seizures, especially during status epilepticus.*
***GABA = gamma-aminobutyric acid.*

In some cases, however, the exact way that antiepileptic drugs exert their beneficial effects is obscure or unknown.[32] Details of each chemical class of drugs are covered here. Because these drugs tend to have many adverse side effects, only the frequently occurring or more serious problems are listed for each category.

Barbiturates

In the past, barbiturates were commonly used to treat seizure disorders, but their use is often limited because of their strong tendency to produce sedation and other adverse effects.[33] As discussed in Chapter 6, these drugs also have a small therapeutic index, and overdose can lead to fatalities. Hence, barbiturate use in epilepsy has declined somewhat in favor of newer agents. However, barbiturates remain very effective in controlling seizures, including those that have not responded to other drugs. Because of their relatively low cost, these drugs are commonly used to treat seizure disorders in underdeveloped countries.[33]

At the present time, phenobarbital (various trade names) is the primary barbiturate used in the treatment of epilepsy. This drug is effective in virtually all types of adult seizures but seems to be especially effective in generalized tonic-clonic and simple and complex partial (focal) seizures. Pentobarbital (Nembutal, others) is a powerful barbiturate that is sometimes administered via IV to stop severe, uncontrolled seizures that fail to respond to other drugs (see "Treatment of Status Epilepticus" later in this chapter). Primidone (Mysoline) is another barbiturate-like drug that is recommended in several types of epilepsy but is particularly useful in generalized tonic-clonic seizures, complex partial seizures, and focal seizures that have not responded to other drugs.

Mechanism of Action. Barbiturates are known to increase the inhibitory effects of GABA (see Chapter 6), and this effect is probably the primary way that these drugs decrease seizure activity. Barbiturates may also produce some of their antiseizure effects by inhibiting calcium entry into excitatory presynaptic nerve terminals, thereby decreasing the release of excitatory neurotransmitters such as glutamate.[34]

Adverse Side Effects. Sedation (primary problem), nystagmus, ataxia, folate deficiency, vitamin K deficiency, and skin problems are typical side effects. A paradoxical increase in seizures and an increase in hyperactivity may occur in some children.

Benzodiazepines

Several members of the benzodiazepine group are effective in treating epilepsy, but most are limited because of problems with sedation and tolerance. Some agents such as diazepam (Valium) and lorazepam (Ativan) are typically used in the acute treatment of status epilepticus, a condition addressed later in this chapter, but only a few benzodiazepines are used in the long-term treatment of epilepsy. Clonazepam (Klonopin, others) is recommended in specific forms of absence seizures and may also be useful in minor generalized seizures, such as akinetic spells and myoclonic seizures. Clorazepate (Tranxene, others) is occasionally used as an adjunct in simple partial seizures.

Mechanism of Action. These drugs are known to potentiate the inhibitory effects of GABA in the brain (see Chapter 6), and their antiepileptic properties are probably exerted through this mechanism.

Adverse Side Effects. Sedation, ataxia, and behavioral changes can be observed.

Hydantoins

Phenytoin (Dilantin, Phenytek) is the primary hydantoin used clinically. It is often the first drug considered in treating many types of epilepsy, and it is especially effective in treating partial seizures and generalized tonic-clonic seizures. Although not FDA approved, this drug is sometimes prescribed off-label to treat neuropathic pain, including trigeminal neuralgia. Fosphenytoin (Cerebyx) may be administered parenterally by intramuscular or IV injection for short periods of time (5 days or less) to help control severe seizures, or in the acute treatment of status epilepticus, a condition addressed later in this chapter. Other hydantoins such as ethotoin (Peganone) and mephenytoin (Mesantoin) are no longer widely used because of their relatively high toxicity.

Mechanism of Action. Phenytoin stabilizes neural membranes and decreases neuronal excitability by decreasing sodium entry into rapidly firing neurons. This drug basically inhibits the ability of sodium channels to reset from an inactive to active state after the neuron has fired an action potential. By inhibiting the reactivation of sodium channels, phenytoin prolongs the time between action potentials (absolute refractory period) so that neurons must slow their firing rate to a normal level. At higher doses, phenytoin may also decrease neuronal excitability by increasing the effects of GABA and by influencing the movement of potassium and calcium across the nerve membrane. These nonsodium effects generally occur at higher drug concentrations than those used therapeutically to control seizures. Less is known about the molecular mechanisms of the other drugs in this category, but they probably work by a similar effect on the sodium channels.

Adverse Side Effects. Gastric irritation, confusion, sedation, dizziness, headache, cerebellar signs (nystagmus, ataxia, dysarthria), gingival hyperplasia, increased body and facial hair (hirsutism), and skin disorders are typical adverse effects.

Iminostilbenes

The primary drugs in this category are carbamazepine (Tegretol, others) and oxcarbazepine (Trileptal). Carbamazepine has been shown to be effective in treating all types of epilepsy except absence seizures, and it is often considered the primary agent for treating partial seizures and tonic-clonic seizures. Carbamazepine is regarded as equivalent to phenytoin in efficacy and side effects and may be substituted for that drug, depending on patient response. Alternatively, oxcarbazepine can be used alone (monotherapy) or with other antiepileptics to treat partial seizures in adults, as monotherapy to treat partial seizures in children between the ages 4 and 16, and as an adjunct to other antiepileptics in children age 2 and older. Like phenytoin, oxcarbazepine in sometimes used off-label to manage trigeminal neuralgia.

Mechanism of Action. These drugs are believed to exert their primary antiepileptic effects in a manner similar to phenytoin—that is, they stabilize the neuronal membrane by slowing the recovery of sodium channels firing too rapidly. Carbamazepine may also inhibit the presynaptic uptake and release of norepinephrine, and this effect may contribute to its antiseizure activity.

Adverse Side Effects. Dizziness, drowsiness, ataxia, blurred vision, anemia, water retention (because of abnormal antidiuretic hormone [ADH] release), cardiac arrhythmias, and congestive heart failure can occur with use of these drugs.

Succinimides

The primary drug in this category is ethosuximide (Zarontin), which is used commonly to treat absence (petit mal) seizures. Other succinimides such as methsuximide (Celontin) and phensuximide (Milontin) are no longer used clinically.

Mechanism of Action. Ethosuximide seems to exert antiseizure effects by decreasing calcium influx in certain thalamic neurons. Like sodium, calcium entry into neurons can depolarize the neuron and cause it to fire an action potential. Repetitive and excessive calcium entry into thalamic neurons may be responsible for initiating absence seizures, and ethosuximide can help prevent seizure onset by blunting calcium influx.

Adverse Side Effects. Gastrointestinal (GI) distress (nausea, vomiting), headache, dizziness, fatigue, lethargy, movement disorders (dyskinesia, bradykinesia), and skin rashes and itching are common side effects.

Valproates

Valproates such as valproic acid (Depakene, others), valproate sodium (Depacon), and divalproex sodium (Depakote, others) are often used in several seizure disorders. These drugs can be used alone or with other agents to treat simple and complex absence seizures, complex partial seizures, or as an adjunct in patients with multiple seizure types. These drugs are also used to treat bipolar disorder (manic-depression), especially during the acute manic phase (see Chapter 7), and may be prescribed off-label to treat migraine headaches.

Mechanism of Action. Valproates exert some or most of their effects in a manner similar to phenytoin and ethosuximide—that is, they limit sodium entry into rapidly firing neurons. High concentrations of valproates are also associated with increased levels of GABA in the brain, and this increase in GABAergic inhibition may be responsible for some of their antiepileptic effects. However, lower concentrations are still effective in limiting seizures and do not increase CNS GABA, raising questions about whether the effects on GABA are clinically important. These drugs may also increase potassium conductance and efflux from certain neurons, thereby hyperpolarizing the neuron and decreasing its excitability. Hence, the exact way that valproates affect seizures remains to be determined, and these drugs may actually work through a combination of several different molecular mechanisms.

Adverse Side Effects. GI distress, temporary hair loss, weight gain or loss, and impaired platelet function are documented adverse reactions.

Second-Generation Agents

The medications described earlier have been on the market for many years and have been used routinely for decreasing seizure activity. Beginning with the introduction of felbamate in 1993, several new, or "second-generation," drugs have been approved by the FDA and are currently in use (Table 9-3). In most cases, these newer drugs are not more effective than their predecessors.[35] However, they generally have favorable pharmacokinetic characteristics (e.g., absorption, distribution, metabolism, etc.) and have relatively mild side effects that allow their use along with the more traditional antiseizure medications.[36-38]

The development of the newer antiseizure medications has advanced the strategy of using these drugs as adjuncts or "add-on" therapy.[39,40] In the past, an effort was made to use only one drug (primary agent), with an additional drug (secondary agent) being added only if the epilepsy was especially resistant to management with the primary medication.[40] The use of a single drug (monotherapy) offered several advantages, including fewer side effects, lower cost, no interactions with other antiseizure drugs, better patient adherence to the drug regimen, and better seizure control because the patient was able to tolerate a higher dose of a single agent.[41] Likewise, management of adverse side effects in single-drug therapy was easier because there was no question about which anti-seizure drug was producing the adverse effect. However, the newer drugs have relatively predictable pharmacokinetic and side-effect profiles; they can often be added to traditional medications without excessive complications and risk to the patient.[38,40] The combinations often allow adequate seizure control in patients who did not respond to a single traditional antiseizure agent. As more is learned about these newer drugs, some are being used alone as the initial treatment or in certain types of seizures that are resistant to other drugs.[42,43] Second-generation antiseizure medications currently available are described here.

Felbamate (Felbatol)

Felbamate is indicated for treatment of partial seizures in adults and children as well as multiple seizure types associated with Lennox-Gastaut syndrome in children. Felbamate appears to bind to specific receptors in the brain (the *N*-methyl-D-aspartate receptor) and blocks the effects of excitatory amino acids such as glutamate. Reduced influence of these excitatory amino acids results in decreased seizure activity. As

Table 9-3
SECOND-GENERATION ANTIEPILEPTICS

Generic Name	Trade Name	Primary Indication(s)
Felbamate	Felbatol	Used alone or as an adjunct in partial seizures in adults; treatment adjunct in partial and generalized seizures associated with Lennox-Gastaut syndrome in children
Gabapentin	Neurontin	Treatment adjunct in partial seizures in adults and children over age 3
Lacosamide	Vimpat	Treatment adjunct in partial-onset seizures in adults
Lamotrigine	Lamictal	Use alone or as a treatment adjunct in partial seizures in adults over age 16; treatment adjunct in generalized seizures associated with Lennox-Gastaut syndrome in adults and children over age 2
Levetiracetam	Keppra	Treatment adjunct in partial onset seizures in adults, generalized tonic-clonic seizures in patients 6 years of age and older, and myoclonic seizures in adults.
Pregabalin	Lyrica	Treatment adjunct in partial onset seizures in adults
Rufinamide	Banzel	Seizures associated with Lennox-Gastaut syndrome in adults and children ages 4 and older
Tiagabine	Gabitril	Treatment adjunct in partial seizures in adults and children over age 12
Topiramate	Topamax	Use alone or as a treatment adjunct in partial-onset seizures in adults or as an adjunct in adults and children with partial seizures, generalized tonic-clonic seizures, and seizures associated with Lennox-Gastaut syndrome
Vigabatrin	Sabril	Treatment adjunct in complex partial seizures in adults
Zonisamide	Zonegran	Treatment adjunct in partial seizures in adults

indicated, this drug first appeared on the market in 1993 and represented the first "new-generation" antiseizure agent. It was soon recognized, however, that felbamate could cause severe toxic effects such as aplastic anemia and liver failure.[44] Felbamate is therefore not widely prescribed and is typically used only in patients with severe epilepsy who fail to respond to other antiseizure drugs. Other common side effects include insomnia, headache, dizziness, and GI problems (anorexia, nausea, and vomiting).

Gabapentin (Neurontin)

Gabapentin is typically used with other antiseizure drugs to treat partial seizures in adults and children who have not responded to other treatments. As the name implies, gabapentin was designed to act as a GABA agonist. However, this drug probably works by inhibiting specific calcium channels in presynaptic terminals. This effect limits calcium entry into the presynaptic terminal, thus decreasing the release of glutamate and other excitatory neurotransmitters from those neurons.[45,46] Decreased influence of excitatory neurotransmitters can help reduce excessive neuronal activity in seizure disorders. Gabapentin may also help reduce excitation in pathways responsible for specific types of chronic pain, and this drug has been used extensively to treat neuropathic pain and other chronic pain syndromes.[21] The primary side effects of this drug are sedation, fatigue, dizziness, and ataxia.

Lacosamide (Vimpat)

This drug was approved in 2008 as an adjunct in treating partial-onset seizures in adults. Like several other antiepileptic drugs, lacosamide inhibits neuronal sodium channel activity. However, this drug enhances the slow inactivation of sodium channels, compared to other drugs like carbamazepine, phenytoin, and lamotrigine that affect rapid inactivation of the sodium channel.[47] Hence, lacosamide may prolong sodium channel inactivation and limit sodium entry in a different manner than other antiepileptics. This action may help supplement the effects of other drugs in decreasing the repetitive firing that initiates certain types of partial-onset seizures. Lacosamide is usually well tolerated, with dizziness, headache, nausea, and double vision being the most frequent side effects.

Lamotrigine (Lamictal)

Lamotrigine is used primarily as an adjunct to other medications in adults with partial seizures, although it has also been used alone to treat partial seizures, generalized tonic-clonic seizures, and seizures due to Lennox-Gastaut syndrome in adults and children. This drug exerts some of its effects by stabilizing sodium channels in a manner similar to carbamazepine and phenytoin.[48] In particular, lamotrigine may decrease seizure activity by stabilizing sodium channels on excitatory neurons that release glutamate.[49] The primary side effects include dizziness, headache, ataxia, vision problems, and skin rash.

Levetiracetam (Keppra)

Levetiracetam is typically used in conjunction with traditional antiseizure drugs to treat partial-onset seizures in adults, generalized tonic-clonic seizures in patients 6 years of age and older, and myoclonic seizures in adults. Although the exact mechanism of this drug is not known, it does not appear to decrease seizure activity via one of the common antiseizure mechanisms (i.e., stabilize sodium channels, increase GABA inhibition, etc.). Levetiracetam may instead work by a complex mechanism that involves inhibition of presynaptic proteins, intraneuronal calcium release, presynaptic calcium influx, and other chemicals that cause repetitive, synchronous neuronal firing.[50] Levetiracetam is usually well tolerated, although some patients may experience sedation, dizziness, and generalized weakness.

Pregabalin (Lyrica)

This drug was originally approved as an adjunct for treating partial-onset seizures in adults. It later received considerable attention for treating chronic pain and is now approved for the treatment of fibromyalgia, diabetic peripheral neuropathy, and postherpetic neuralgia.[21] Pregabalin works in a manner similar to gabapentin—that is, it inhibits calcium channels in presynaptic terminals of specific neurons, thus limiting calcium entry into those neurons and decreasing the release of excitatory neurotransmitters such as glutamate.[51] This drug therefore helps decrease seizure activity by decreasing excitatory neurotransmitter influence on neurons that start the seizure. Pregabalin probably acts in a similar manner in chronic pain—that is, it decreases activity in hyperactive neurons involved in specific pain pathways. Primary side effects include dizziness, drowsiness, and peripheral edema. These side effects are usually mild and often disappear within a week or two of continuous treatment.

Rufinamide (Banzel)

Rufinamide is another drug approved as an adjunct in treating seizures associated with Lennox-Gastaut syndrome in adults and children ages 4 and older. This drug seems to work in a manner similar to lacosamide in that it enhances the slow inactivation of sodium channels, thereby prolonging sodium channel inactivation and limiting sodium entry into rapidly firing neurons.[52] Dizziness, drowsiness, headache, nausea, and fatigue are the most common side effects of this drug.

Tiagabine (Gabitril)

Tiagabine is used primarily as an adjunct to other drugs in adults and children over age 12 with partial seizures that are poorly controlled by traditional drug therapy. This drug inhibits the reuptake of GABA after it is released from presynaptic terminals, thereby inhibiting seizure activity by enabling GABA to remain active in the synaptic cleft for longer periods.[53] The primary side effects of this drug are dizziness, weakness, and a slight tendency for psychiatric disturbances (e.g., anxiety, depression).

Topiramate (Topamax)

Topiramate is used alone or as an adjunct to other medications in adults and children with partial seizures, generalized tonic-clonic seizures, and seizures associated with Lennox-Gastaut syndrome. This drug is also FDA approved to prevent migraine headaches. Topiramate appears to limit seizure activity through several complementary mechanisms, including inhibition of sodium channel opening, stimulation of GABA receptors, and decreased responsiveness of receptors for excitatory amino acids such as glutamate.[3,32] Primary side effects include sedation, dizziness, fatigue, and ataxia.

Vigabatrin (Sabril)

This drug is used to supplement the effects of other antiepileptic drugs in adults with complex partial seizures who have not responded adequately to alternative treatments. Vigabatrin may also be used to treat infantile spasms—that is, specific seizures that cause spontaneous, uncontrolled muscular contractions of the trunk and extremities in infants and children under 2 years of age. However, vigabatrin has been associated with possible damage to the retina, which can cause visual field defects and permanent loss of peripheral vision.[54] This drug must therefore be used very cautiously, and only in cases where its antiseizure effects justify its risk.[55] Vigabatrin inhibits the enzyme that breaks down GABA, thus prolonging the effects of this inhibitory neurotransmitter.[56] Its antiseizure effects are therefore related to increased GABA inhibition of neurons that initiate or sustain seizure activity. In addition to potentially harmful effects on vision, this drug is associated with suicidal thoughts, and it can cause several other side effects such as confusion, drowsiness, fatigue, incoordination, weight gain, and joint pain.

Zonisamide (Zonegran)

Zonisamide is used primarily to treat partial seizures in adults. This drug stabilizes sodium channels in a manner similar to carbamazepine and phenytoin—that is, it limits sodium entry into rapidly firing neurons that initiate seizure activity.[57] Zonisamide may also exert some of its antiseizure effects by inhibiting calcium entry into rapidly firing neurons, increasing GABA release, and inhibiting the release of glutamate.[57] Zonisamide is fairly well tolerated, although side effects may include sedation, ataxia, loss of appetite, and fatigue.

SELECTION OF A SPECIFIC ANTIEPILEPTIC AGENT

Although a fairly large number of drugs can be used to treat epileptic seizures (see Tables 9-2 and 9-3), it is apparent that certain drugs are often considered first when treating specific types of seizures. These agents comprise a fairly small group. Table 9-4 lists some of the more common types of seizures and the primary and alternative agents used to treat each seizure type. It is important to note that while Table 9-4 indicates general guidelines for drug selection, selection of the best agent must be done on a patient-by-patient basis. Some patients will understandably exhibit a better response to agents that are not typically used as the first or second choice for a specific type of seizure. Hence, some trial and error may occur before the best drug is found, and drug selection may need to be altered periodically throughout the patient's lifetime to achieve optimal results.[2]

The preferred drugs and their relevant dosing parameters are listed in Table 9-5. Again, alternative antiseizure drugs can be used if commonly used drugs are ineffective or poorly tolerated. As indicated earlier, one of the newer agents can also be added to traditional drugs if patients do not respond to single-drug therapy.

Table 9-4
DRUGS OF CHOICE FOR SPECIFIC SEIZURE DISORDERS

Seizure Type	First-Line Drug	Alternate Drugs*
Focal Seizures		
Partial (focal) seizures (newly diagnosed)	Carbamazepine Gabapentin Lamotrigine Oxcarbazepine Phenobarbital Phenytoin Topiramate Valproic acid	Levetiracetam
Refractory partial seizures	Lamotrigine Oxcarbazepine Topiramate	Gabapentin Lamotrigine Levetiracetam Oxcarbazepine Tiagabine Topiramate Zonisamide
Generalized Seizures		
Absence seizures (newly diagnosed)	Ethosuximide Lamotrigine Valproic acid	Ethosuximide Lamotrigine Valproic acid
Tonic-clonic seizures	Lamotrigine Topiramate Valproic acid	Carbamazepine Lamotrigine Oxcarbazepine Phenobarbital Phenytoin Topiramate Valproic acid
Juvenile myoclonic epilepsy	Valproic acid	Clonazepam Lamotrigine Levetiracetam Topiramate Valproic acid Zonisamide

**Alternate drugs can be substituted if the first-line drug is not effective, or alternate drugs can be added as adjuncts to the first-line drug. Selection of a first-line or alternative drug will vary, depending on the patient's symptoms, age, comorbidities, and so forth.*

Source: adapted from Rogers SJ, Cavazos JE. Epilepsy. In: DiPiro JT, et al, eds. Pharmacotherapy: A Pathophysiologic Approach. 8th ed. New York: McGraw-Hill; 2011:985.

Table 9-5
DOSAGES OF COMMON ANTIEPILEPTIC DRUGS*

Drug	Initial Dose (mg)	Increment** (mg)	Maintenance (mg/d)
Carbamazepine	200 bid	200 q wk	600–1,800
Clonazepam	0.5 tid	0.05–1 q 3d	Up to 20
Ethosuximide	250 bid	250 q 4–7d	20–40 mg/kg/d
Felbamate	1,200 qd	600 q 2 wk	Up to 3,600
Gabapentin	300 qd	300 q 3–7 d	1,200–3,600
Lacosamide	50 qd	100 q wk	300–600
Lamotrigine	6.25–12.5 qd to qod	12.5–25 q 2 wk	100–400
Levetiracetam	500 qd	500 q wk	2,000–4,000
Oxcarbazepine	300 qd	300 q wk	900–2,400
Phenobarbital	30–60 qd	30 q 1–2 wk	60–120
Phenytoin	200 qd	100 q wk	200–300
Pregabalin	50 qd	50 q 3–7 d	150–600
Primidone	100–125 qd for the first 3 d	100–125 bid for 3 d; 100–125 tid for the next 3d	250 tid or qid
Tiagabine	4 qd	4–8 q wk	Up to 56 qd
Topiramate	25 qd	25 q 1–2 wk	200–400
Valproic acid	250 qd	250 q 3–7 d	750–3,000
Vigabatrin	500 qd	500 q wk	Up to 1.5 bid
Zonisamide	100 qd	100 q 2 wk	200–400

Abbreviations: qd = every day; qod = every other day; bid = twice a day; tid = three times a day; qid = 4 times a day.

**Dosages reflect monotherapy in adults. Dosages may vary if combining the drug with other antiseizure agents or other drugs that affect liver enzyme function. Doses for children are typically lower and adjusted according to the child's age and body weight.*

***Increments reflect the rate that dosage can typically be increased when trying to find the appropriate therapeutic dose.*

Source: Dobrin S. Seizures and epilepsy in adolescents and adults. In: Bope ET, Kellerman RD, eds. Conn's Current Therapy 2013. *New York: Elsevier/Saunders; 2013:650; Ciccone CD.* Davis's Drug Guide for Rehabilitation Professionals. *Philadelphia: FA Davis; 2013.*

PHARMACOKINETICS

When given for the long-term control of epilepsy, these drugs are normally administered orally. Daily oral doses are usually divided into three or four equal quantities, and the amount of each dose varies widely depending on the specific drug and the severity of the seizures. Distribution within the body is fairly extensive, with all antiepileptic drugs eventually reaching the brain to exert their beneficial effects. Drug biotransformation usually occurs via liver microsomal oxidases, and this is the primary method of drug termination.

SPECIAL PRECAUTIONS DURING PREGNANCY

Most women with epilepsy continue to take their antiseizure medications when they become pregnant and eventually give birth to normal, healthy babies.[58] Nonetheless, the incidence of birth defects is increased in children of mothers with epilepsy compared with children of mothers who are not epileptic.[59-61] For example, it is estimated that the risk of a major congenital malformation is approximately doubled in children born to mothers who took a single antiseizure drug during pregnancy, and the risk of malformation may be three times higher if multiple antiepileptics are taken throughout pregnancy.[61,62] Such congenital malformations include cleft palate, cardiac defects, microencephaly, and neural tube defects. Other problems such as stillbirth, developmental delays, mental retardation, and infant seizures also occur more frequently in children born to women who took antiseizure drugs during pregnancy. These problems are probably related to the in utero exposure to antiepileptic drugs rather than a sequela of the mother's epilepsy.[63] Because there is at least some concern that fetal malformations may be a drug side effect, some mothers may choose to discontinue drug therapy during their pregnancies.[64] This action obviously places the mother at risk for uncontrolled seizures, which may be even more harmful to the mother and unborn child.

Hence, women taking antiepileptic drugs should discuss the potential risks with their family members and physician, and consider whether they will continue taking their medication.[65,66] If an expectant mother continues to take her medication, using one drug (monotherapy) at the lowest effective dose will help reduce the risk of harmful effects on the fetus.[65,67] Certain drugs such as the valproates also appear to be associated with a higher risk of congenital defects and should probably be avoided whenever possible.[67,68] In addition, mothers should receive optimal prenatal care (i.e., folic acid supplementation, proper amounts of exercise, rest, etc.) to help ensure the baby's health.[64,69] After delivery, the baby should be monitored initially for drug-related effects such as withdrawal symptoms and should be subsequently evaluated for neurodevelopmental delays that might become apparent later in childhood.[63]

TREATMENT OF STATUS EPILEPTICUS

Status epilepticus is a series of seizures occurring without any appreciable period of recovery between individual seizures.[70,71] Essentially the patient experiences a continuous seizure of 30 minutes or more, or a series of seizures where the patient does not regain consciousness between each seizure.[71] This may be brought on by a number of factors such as sudden withdrawal from antiepileptic drugs, cerebral infarct, systemic or intracranial infection, or withdrawal from addictive drugs, including alcohol.[72,73] If untreated, status epilepticus will result in permanent damage or death, especially if the seizures are severe and resistant to treatment.[74] Consequently, this event is regarded as a medical emergency that should be resolved as rapidly as possible.

Treatment begins with standard emergency procedures such as maintaining an airway, administering oxygen, monitoring blood pressure, assessing for injury, testing blood gases and toxicology, and starting an IV line for drug administration.[70,71] The first drugs administered are usually benzodiazepines: lorazepam (Ativan) or diazepam (Valium) given intravenously. This approach is followed by IV administration of phenytoin or fosphenytoin. The phenytoin or fosphenytoin is given concurrently with or immediately after the benzodiazepine so that seizures are controlled when the relatively short-acting benzodiazepine is metabolized. If seizures continue despite these drugs, phenobarbital or valproic acid may be given intravenously. If all other attempts fail, general anesthesia (e.g., midazolam, pentobarbital, or propofol; see Chapter 11) is administered intravenously and then slowly tapered off over 12 hours. When status epilepticus is eventually controlled, an attempt is made to begin or reinstitute chronic antiepileptic therapy.

WITHDRAWAL OF ANTISEIZURE MEDICATIONS

Many people with seizure disorders will need to adhere to a regimen of antiseizure medications throughout their lifetime. However, there appears to be a certain percentage of patients who can discontinue their medications once their seizures are under control.[75] Although the exact success rate after discontinuation is difficult to determine, it is estimated that approximately 60 to 70 percent of people can remain seizure-free after their medication is withdrawn.[2] Factors associated with successful medication withdrawal include being free of seizures for at least 2 years while on medication, having good control of seizures within 1 year after seizures begin, having a normal neurological examination prior to withdrawal, and having had the initial onset of seizures during childhood.[3] Some patients, of course, are not good candidates for withdrawal, and the risk and consequences of seizure recurrence must be considered in each patient before withdrawing antiseizure drugs.[76]

Withdrawal of medication must be done under close medical supervision. Medications are usually tapered off over an extended period of time (3 to 6 months) rather than being suddenly discontinued.[77] Nonetheless, it appears that a large proportion of people with epilepsy may be able to maintain seizure-free status once their seizures are controlled by the appropriate medications.

Special Concerns for Rehabilitation Patients

Rehabilitation specialists must always be cognizant of their patients who have a history of seizures and who are taking antiepileptic drugs. Patients being treated for conditions unrelated to epilepsy (e.g., the outpatient with low back pain) should be identified as potentially at risk for a seizure during the therapy session. This knowledge will better prepare the therapist to recognize and deal with such an episode. Therefore, it is important that therapists have a thorough medical history of all patients.

Therapists also may help determine the efficacy of antiepileptic drug therapy. The primary goal in any patient taking antiepileptic drugs is maintaining the drug dosage within a therapeutic window. Dosage must be high enough to adequately control seizure activity but not so high as to invoke serious side effects. By constantly observing and monitoring patient progress, rehabilitation specialists can help determine if this goal is being met. By noting changes in either seizure frequency or side effects, physical therapists, occupational therapists, and other rehabilitation personnel may help the medical staff arrive at an effective dosing regimen. This information can be invaluable in helping achieve optimal patient care with a minimum of adverse side effects.

Some of the more frequent side effects may affect physical therapy and other rehabilitation procedures. Headache, dizziness, sedation, and gastric disturbances (nausea, vomiting) may be bothersome during the therapy session. Often, therapists can address these reactions by scheduling therapy at a time of day when these problems are relatively mild. The optimal treatment time will vary from patient to patient, depending on the particular drug, dosing schedule, and age of the patient. Cerebellar side effects such as ataxia also occur frequently and may impair the patient's ability to participate in various functional activities. If ataxia persists despite efforts to alter drug dosage or substitute another agent, coordination exercises may help resolve this problem. Skin conditions (e.g., dermatitis, rashes, etc.) are another frequent problem in long-term antiepileptic therapy. The therapist should discontinue any therapeutic modalities that might exacerbate these conditions.

Finally, in some patients, seizures tend to be triggered by environmental stimuli such as lights and sound. In such patients, conducting the therapy session in a busy, noisy clinic may precipitate a seizure, especially if the epilepsy is poorly controlled by drug therapy. Also, certain patients may have a history of increased seizure activity at certain times of the day, which may be related to when the antiepileptic drug is administered. Consequently, these patients may benefit if the therapy session is held in a relatively quiet setting at a time when the chance of a seizure is minimal.

CASE STUDY

ANTIEPILEPTIC DRUGS

Brief History. F.B. is a 43-year-old man who works in the shipping department of a large company. He was diagnosed in childhood as having generalized tonic-clonic epilepsy, and his seizures have been managed successfully with various drugs over the years. Most recently, he has been taking carbamazepine (Tegretol), 800 mg/d (i.e., one 200-mg tablet, qid). One month ago, he began complaining of dizziness and blurred vision, so the dosage was reduced to 600 mg/d (one 200 mg tablet tid).

Continued on following page

CASE STUDY (Continued)

He usually takes his antiseizure medication after meals. F.B. also takes an antihypertensive (lisinopril, 10 mg/day) and a cholesterol-lowering drug (simvastatin, 20 mg/day). Two weeks ago, he injured his back while lifting a large box at work. He was evaluated in physical therapy as having an acute lumbosacral strain. He attends physical therapy daily as an outpatient. Treatment includes heat, ultrasound, and manual therapy, and he is also receiving instruction in proper body mechanics and lifting technique. F.B. continues to work at his normal job, but he avoids heavy lifting. He attends therapy on his way home from work, at about 5:00 p.m.

Problem/Influence of Medication. F.B. arrived at physical therapy the first afternoon stating that he had had a particularly long day. He was positioned prone on a treatment table, and hot packs were placed over his low back. As the heat was applied, he began to drift off to sleep. Five minutes into the treatment, he had a seizure. Because of a thorough initial evaluation, the therapist was aware of his epileptic condition and protected him from injury during the seizure. The patient regained consciousness and rested quietly until he felt able to go home. No long-term effects were noted from the seizure.

1. ***What factors may have precipitated F.B.'s seizure?***
2. ***What precautions can be taken to prevent additional seizures and guard against injuries if a seizure occurs during a rehabilitation session?***

See Appendix C, "Answers to Case Study Questions."

SUMMARY

Epilepsy is a chronic condition characterized by recurrent seizures. Causes of this disorder range from a distinct traumatic episode to obscure or unknown origins. Seizures are categorized according to the clinical and electrophysiological manifestations that occur during the seizure. Fortunately, most individuals with epilepsy (up to 75 percent) can be treated successfully with antiepileptic drugs. Although these drugs do not cure this disorder, reduction or elimination of seizures will prevent further CNS damage.

The primary antiseizure drugs are classified as either traditional (first-generation) or newer (second-generation) drugs. These drugs vary in terms of their effects, indications, safety, and pharmacokinetic variables. Certain antiseizure drugs are also important in managing the prolonged, uncontrolled seizures that pose serious harm in a condition called status epilepticus. Although many patients on antiepileptic drugs must take these drugs indefinitely, these drugs can sometimes be withdrawn in carefully selected patients who meet specific clinical criteria.

As in any area of pharmacotherapeutics, antiepileptic drugs are associated with adverse side effects. Some of these may become a problem in rehabilitation patients, so therapists should be ready to alter the time and type of treatment as needed to accommodate these side effects. Likewise, these drugs can increase the risk of birth defects, and expectant mothers should discuss these risks with their medical practitioners. Physical therapists and other rehabilitation personnel should also be alert for any behavioral or functional changes in the patient that might indicate a problem in drug therapy. Insufficient drug therapy (as evidenced by increased seizures) or possible drug toxicity (as evidenced by increased side effects) should be brought to the physician's attention so that these problems can be rectified.

REFERENCES

1. Kandel ER, Scwartz JH, Jessell TM, et al. Seizures and epilepsy. In: *Principles of Neural Science*. 5th ed. New York: McGraw-Hill; 2013.
2. Rogers SJ, Cavazos JE. Epilepsy. In: DiPiro JT, et al, eds. *Pharmacotherapy: A Pathophysiologic Approach*. 8th ed. New York: McGraw-Hill; 2011.

3. McNamara JO. Pharmacotherapy of the epilepsies. In: Brunton LL, et al, eds. *The Pharmacological Basis of Therapeutics*. 12th ed. New York: McGraw Hill; 2011.
4. Beleza P. Acute symptomatic seizures: a clinically oriented review. *Neurologist*. 2012;18:109-119.
5. Bhalla D, Godet B, Druet-Cabanac M, Preux PM. Etiologies of epilepsy: a comprehensive review. *Expert Rev Neurother*. 2011;11:861-876.
6. Christensen J. Traumatic brain injury: risks of epilepsy and implications for medicolegal assessment. *Epilepsia*. 2012;53 (suppl 4):43-47.
7. Covanis A. Epileptic encephalopathies (including severe epilepsy syndromes). *Epilepsia*. 2012;53(suppl 4):114-126.
8. Gilad R. Management of seizures following a stroke: what are the options? *Drugs Aging*. 2012;29:533-538.
9. You G, Sha Z, Jiang T. The pathogenesis of tumor-related epilepsy and its implications for clinical treatment. *Seizure*. 2012;21:153-159.
10. Guerrini R, Pellacani S. Benign childhood focal epilepsies. *Epilepsia*. 2012;53(suppl 4):9-18.
11. Michelucci R, Pasini E, Riguzzi P, et al. Genetics of epilepsy and relevance to current practice. *Curr Neurol Neurosci Rep*. 2012;12:445-455.
12. Pandolfo M. Genetics of epilepsy. *Semin Neurol*. 2011;31: 506-518.
13. Lai MC, Yang SN. Perinatal hypoxic-ischemic encephalopathy. *J Biomed Biotechnol*. 2011;2011:609813.
14. Michael BD, Solomon T. Seizures and encephalitis: clinical features, management, and potential pathophysiologic mechanisms. *Epilepsia*. 2012;53(suppl 4):63-71.
15. Verrotti A, Scaparrotta A, Olivieri C, Chiarelli F. Seizures and type 1 diabetes mellitus: current state of knowledge. *Eur J Endocrinol*. 2012;167:749-758.
16. Fridley J, Thomas JG, Navarro JC, Yoshor D. Brain stimulation for the treatment of epilepsy. *Neurosurg Focus*. 2012;32:E13.
17. Kunieda T, Kikuchi T, Miyamoto S. Epilepsy surgery: surgical aspects. *Curr Opin Anaesthesiol*. 2012;25:533-539.
18. Levy RG, Cooper PN, Giri P. Ketogenic diet and other dietary treatments for epilepsy. *Cochrane Database Syst Rev*. 2012;3: CD001903.
19. Wiebe S, Jetté N. Epilepsy surgery utilization: who, when, where, and why? *Curr Opin Neurol*. 2012;25:187-193.
20. Dalkara S, Karakurt A. Recent progress in anticonvulsant drug research: strategies for anticonvulsant drug development and applications of antiepileptic drugs for non-epileptic central nervous system disorders. *Curr Top Med Chem*. 2012;12:1033-1071.
21. Bialer M. Why are antiepileptic drugs used for nonepileptic conditions? *Epilepsia*. 2012;53(suppl 7):26-33.
22. Kennett R. Modern electroencephalography. *J Neurol*. 2012;259: 783-789.
23. Berg AT, Berkovic SF, Brodie MJ, et al. Revised terminology and concepts for organization of seizures and epilepsies: report of the ILAE Commission on Classification and Terminology, 2005-2009. *Epilepsia*. 2010;51:676-685.
24. Panayiotopoulos CP. The new ILAE report on terminology and concepts for organization of epileptic seizures: a clinician's critical view and contribution. *Epilepsia*. 2011;52:2155-2160.
25. Chen SD, Chang AY, Chuang YC. The potential role of mitochondrial dysfunction in seizure-associated cell death in the hippocampus and epileptogenesis. *J Bioenerg Biomembr*. 2010; 42:461-465.
26. Aguiar CC, Almeida AB, Araújo PV, et al. Oxidative stress and epilepsy: literature review. *Oxid Med Cell Longev*. 2012; 2012:795259.
27. Chuang YC. Mitochondrial dysfunction and oxidative stress in seizure-induced neuronal cell death. *Acta Neurol Taiwan*. 2010; 19:3-15.
28. Engel T, Plesnila N, Prehn JH, Henshall DC. In vivo contributions of BH3-only proteins to neuronal death following seizures, ischemia, and traumatic brain injury. *J Cereb Blood Flow Metab*. 2011;31:1196-1210.
29. Huff JS, Fountain NB. Pathophysiology and definitions of seizures and status epilepticus. *Emerg Med Clin North Am*. 2011;29:1-13.
30. Gitto R, De Luca L, De Grazia S, Chimirri A. Glutamatergic neurotransmission as molecular target of new anticonvulsants. *Curr Top Med Chem*. 2012;12:971-993.
31. White HS, Smith MD, Wilcox KS. Mechanisms of action of antiepileptic drugs. *Int Rev Neurobiol*. 2007;81:85-110.
32. Landmark CJ. Targets for antiepileptic drugs in the synapse. *Med Sci Monit*. 2007;13:RA1-7.
33. Zhang LL, Zeng LN, Li YP. Side effects of phenobarbital in epilepsy: a systematic review. *Epileptic Disord*. 2011;13:349-365.
34. Holtkamp M, Meierkord H. Anticonvulsant, antiepileptogenic, and antiictogenic pharmacostrategies. *Cell Mol Life Sci*. 2007;64:2023-2041.
35. Löscher W, Schmidt D. Modern antiepileptic drug development has failed to deliver: ways out of the current dilemma. *Epilepsia*. 2011;52:657-678.
36. Bialer M, White HS. Key factors in the discovery and development of new antiepileptic drugs. *Nat Rev Drug Discov*. 2010;9:68-82.
37. Cramer JA. Tolerability of antiepileptic drugs: can we determine differences? *Epilepsy Behav*. 2012;23:187-192.
38. Privitera M. Current challenges in the management of epilepsy. *Am J Manag Care*. 2011;17(suppl 7):S195-203.
39. Pulman J, Marson AG, Hutton JL. Tiagabine add-on for drug-resistant partial epilepsy. *Cochrane Database Syst Rev*. 2012;5: CD001908.
40. Stephen LJ, Brodie MJ. Antiepileptic drug monotherapy versus polytherapy: pursuing seizure freedom and tolerability in adults. *Curr Opin Neurol*. 2012;25:164-172.
41. Faught E. Monotherapy in adults and elderly persons. Neurology. 2007;69(suppl 3):S3-9.
42. Glauser T, Ben-Menachem E, Bourgeois B, et al. Updated ILAE evidence review of antiepileptic drug efficacy and effectiveness as initial monotherapy for epileptic seizures and syndromes. *Epilepsia*. 2013;54:551-563.
43. Wilby J, Kainth A, Hawkins N, et al. Clinical effectiveness, tolerability and cost-effectiveness of newer drugs for epilepsy in adults: a systematic review and economic evaluation. *Health Technol Assess*. 2005;9:1-157.
44. Borowicz KK, Piskorska B, Kimber-Trojnar Z, et al. Is there any future for felbamate treatment? *Pol J Pharmacol*. 2004;56:289-294.
45. Bockbrader HN, Wesche D, Miller R, et al. A comparison of the pharmacokinetics and pharmacodynamics of pregabalin and gabapentin. *Clin Pharmacokinet*. 2010;49:661-669.
46. Striano P, Striano S. Gabapentin: a Ca2+ channel alpha 2-delta ligand far beyond epilepsy therapy. *Drugs Today*. 2008;44: 353-368.
47. Biton V. Lacosamide for the treatment of partial-onset seizures. *Expert Rev Neurother*. 2012;12:645-655.

48. Mantegazza M, Curia G, Biagini G, et al. Voltage-gated sodium channels as therapeutic targets in epilepsy and other neurological disorders. *Lancet Neurol.* 2010;9:413-424.
49. Seo HJ, Chiesa A, Lee SJ, et al. Safety and tolerability of lamotrigine: results from 12 placebo-controlled clinical trials and clinical implications. *Clin Neuropharmacol.* 2011;34:39-47.
50. Lyseng-Williamson KA. Spotlight on levetiracetam in epilepsy. *CNS Drugs.* 2011;25:901-905.
51. Taylor CP, Angelotti T, Fauman E. Pharmacology and mechanism of action of pregabalin: the calcium channel alpha2-delta (alpha2-delta) subunit as a target for antiepileptic drug discovery. *Epilepsy Res.* 2007;73:137-150.
52. Wisniewski CS. Rufinamide: a new antiepileptic medication for the treatment of seizures associated with Lennox-Gastaut syndrome. *Ann Pharmacother.* 2010;44:658-667.
53. Schousboe A, Madsen KK, White HS. GABA transport inhibitors and seizure protection: the past and future. *Future Med Chem.* 2011;3:183-187.
54. Heim MK, Gidal BE. Vigabatrin-associated retinal damage: potential biochemical mechanisms. *Acta Neurol Scand.* 2012; 126:219-228.
55. Pellock JM. Balancing clinical benefits of vigabatrin with its associated risk of vision loss. *Acta Neurol Scand Suppl.* 2011;192:83-91.
56. Ben-Menachem E. Mechanism of action of vigabatrin: correcting misperceptions. *Acta Neurol Scand Suppl.* 2011;192:5-15.
57. Holder JL Jr, Wilfong AA. Zonisamide in the treatment of epilepsy. *Expert Opin Pharmacother.* 2011;12:2573-2581.
58. Burakgazi E, Pollard J, Harden C. The effect of pregnancy on seizure control and antiepileptic drugs in women with epilepsy. *Rev Neurol Dis.* 2011;8:16-22.
59. Borthen I, Gilhus NE. Pregnancy complications in patients with epilepsy. *Curr Opin Obstet Gynecol.* 2012;24:78-83.
60. Tomson T, Battino D. Teratogenic effects of antiepileptic drugs. *Lancet Neurol.* 2012;11:803-813.
61. Wlodarczyk BJ, Palacios AM, George TM, Finnell RH. Antiepileptic drugs and pregnancy outcomes. *Am J Med Genet A.* 2012;158A:2071-2090.
62. Hill DS, Wlodarczyk BJ, Palacios AM, Finnell RH. Teratogenic effects of antiepileptic drugs. *Expert Rev Neurother.* 2010;10: 943-959.
63. Banach R, Boskovic R, Einarson T, Koren G. Long-term developmental outcome of children of women with epilepsy, unexposed or exposed prenatally to antiepileptic drugs: a meta-analysis of cohort studies. *Drug Saf.* 2010;33:73-79.
64. Yerby MS. Teratogenicity and antiepileptic drugs: potential mechanisms. *Int Rev Neurobiol.* 2008;83:181-204.
65. Crawford PM. Managing epilepsy in women of childbearing age. *Drug Saf.* 2009;32:293-307.
66. Shallcross R, Winterbottom J, Bromley R. Prenatal exposure to anti-epileptic drugs: the need for preconception counselling. *Pract Midwife.* 2011;14:20-21.
67. Harden CL, Meador KJ, Pennell PB, et al. Management issues for women with epilepsy—focus on pregnancy (an evidence-based review): II. Teratogenesis and perinatal outcomes: Report of the Quality Standards Subcommittee and Therapeutics and Technology Subcommittee of the American Academy of Neurology and the American Epilepsy Society. *Epilepsia.* 2009;50:1237-1246.
68. Jentink J, Loane MA, Dolk H, et al. Valproic acid monotherapy in pregnancy and major congenital malformations. *N Engl J Med.* 2010 ;362:2185-2193.
69. Harden CL, Pennell PB, Koppel BS, et al. Management issues for women with epilepsy—focus on pregnancy (an evidence-based review): III. Vitamin K, folic acid, blood levels, and breast-feeding: Report of the Quality Standards Subcommittee and Therapeutics and Technology Assessment Subcommittee of the American Academy of Neurology and the American Epilepsy Society. *Epilepsia.* 2009;50:1247-1255.
70. Mastrangelo M, Celato A. Diagnostic work-up and therapeutic options in management of pediatric status epilepticus. *World J Pediatr.* 2012;8:109-115.
71. Phelps SJ, Hoving CA, Wheless JW. Status epilepticus. In: DiPiro JT, et al, eds. *Pharmacotherapy: A Pathophysiologic Approach.* 8th ed. New York: McGraw-Hill; 2011.
72. Nair PP, Kalita J, Misra UK. Status epilepticus: why, what, and how. *J Postgrad Med.* 2011;57:242-252.
73. Trinka E, Höfler J, Zerbs A. Causes of status epilepticus. *Epilepsia.* 2012;53(suppl 4):127-138.
74. Shorvon S, Ferlisi M. The outcome of therapies in refractory and super-refractory convulsive status epilepticus and recommendations for therapy. *Brain.* 2012;135(pt 8):2314-2328.
75. Beghi E. AED discontinuation may not be dangerous in seizure-free patients. *J Neural Transm.* 2011;118:187-191.
76. Schmidt D. AED discontinuation may be dangerous for seizure-free patients. *J Neural Transm.* 2011;118:183-186.
77. Lossius MI, Hessen E, Mowinckel P, et al. Consequences of antiepileptic drug withdrawal: a randomized, double-blind study (Akershus Study). *Epilepsia.* 2008;49:455-463.

CHAPTER 10

Pharmacological Management of Parkinson Disease

Parkinson disease is a movement disorder characterized by resting tremor, bradykinesia, rigidity, and postural instability.[1,2] In Parkinson disease, there is a slow, progressive degeneration of certain dopamine-secreting neurons in the basal ganglia.[1,3] Several theories have been proposed to explain this spontaneous neuronal degeneration, including the possibility that the disease may be caused by a combination of genetic and environmental factors (see "Etiology of Parkinson Disease: Genetic and Environmental Factors").[4-6] However, the precise initiating factor in Parkinson disease is still unknown.

The clinical syndrome of parkinsonism (i.e., rigidity, bradykinesia) may be caused by other factors such as trauma, infectious agents, antipsychotic drugs, cerebrovascular disease, and various forms of cortical degeneration, including Alzheimer disease.[7-10] However, the most frequent cause of parkinsonism is the spontaneous slow, selective neuronal degeneration characteristic of Parkinson disease itself.[1] Also, the drug management of parkinsonism caused by these other factors closely resembles the management of Parkinson disease.[1] Consequently, this chapter will address the idiopathic onset and pharmacological treatment of Parkinson disease.

Parkinson disease usually begins in the fifth or sixth decade, and symptoms progressively worsen over a period of 10 to 20 years. It is estimated that more than 1 percent of the U.S. population older than 65 years is afflicted with Parkinson disease, making it one of the most prevalent neurological disorders affecting elderly individuals.[1] In addition to the symptoms of bradykinesia and rigidity, a patient with advanced Parkinson disease maintains a flexed posture and speaks in a low, soft voice (microphonia). If left untreated, the motor problems associated with this illness eventually lead to total incapacitation. Parkinson disease is also associated with a wide variety of nonmotor symptoms such as depression, cognitive impairment, memory loss, sleep disorders, impulsiveness, fatigue, and chronic pain.

Fortunately, the pharmacological management of Parkinson disease has evolved to where the symptoms associated with this disorder can be greatly diminished in many patients. The use of levodopa (L-dopa) alone or in combination with other drugs can improve motor function and general mobility well into the advanced stages of this disease. Drugs used in treating Parkinson disease do not cure this condition, and motor function often tends to slowly deteriorate regardless of when drug therapy is initiated.[11,12] However, by alleviating the motor symptoms (i.e., bradykinesia and rigidity), drug therapy can allow patients with Parkinson disease to continue to lead relatively active lifestyles, thus improving their overall physiological and psychological well-being.

Likewise, effective drug treatment can dramatically increase the patient's ability to participate in physical rehabilitation. Antiparkinson drugs help improve motor function so that the patient can be actively involved in cardiovascular conditioning, balance training, fine motor tasks, and various other rehabilitation interventions. What follows is a brief discussion of the neurochemical changes and possible causative factors in Parkinson disease. This review will help you better understand the rationale for using various antiparkinson drugs. The positive and negative aspects of specific drugs are then addressed, with the final part of this chapter lending some insight into future pharmacological and nonpharmacological treatments for Parkinson disease.

PATHOPHYSIOLOGY OF PARKINSON DISEASE

During the past 50 years, researchers established the specific neuronal changes and related neurotransmitter imbalances in the basal ganglia that are responsible for the symptoms of Parkinson disease.[13,14] The basal ganglia are groups of nuclei located in the brain that are involved in the coordination and regulation of motor function. One such nucleus, the substantia nigra, contains the cell bodies of neurons that project to other areas such as the putamen and caudate nucleus (known collectively as the *corpus striatum*). The neurotransmitter used in this nigrostriatal pathway is **dopamine**. The primary neurochemical change in Parkinson disease is the degeneration of dopamine-producing cells in the substantia nigra, resulting in the eventual loss of dopaminergic input into the corpus striatum.[3,13,15]

Consequently, the decrease in striatal dopamine seems to be the initiating factor in the symptom onset associated with Parkinson disease. The loss of dopamine influence is believed to then cause changes in neuronal activity within the basal ganglia, which causes changes in neuronal pathways that project from the basal ganglia to the thalamus and cortex. These neuronal pathway changes are complex, and we present only a brief synopsis (Fig. 10-1). The references at the end of this chapter provide several sources for more detailed descriptions of the neurochemical basis for Parkinson disease.[1,14,16]

Dopaminergic neurons that originate in the basal ganglia's substantia nigra pars compacta project to the corpus striatum (see Fig.10-1). Dopamine released from these neurons binds to the dopamine type 1 (D1) receptor in the corpus striatum. These D1 receptors are excitatory, and they activate a direct pathway that inhibits other basal ganglia structures such as the globus pallidus interna and the substantia nigra pars reticulata. Outflow from these other structures would inhibit the ventroanterior and ventrolateral nuclei in the thalamus, which would result in less excitation of the cerebral cortex. However, the D1-mediated activation of this direct pathway reduces the ability of the globus pallidus interna and the substantia nigra pars reticulata to inhibit thalamic nuclei, thus allowing the thalamus to excite the cortex.

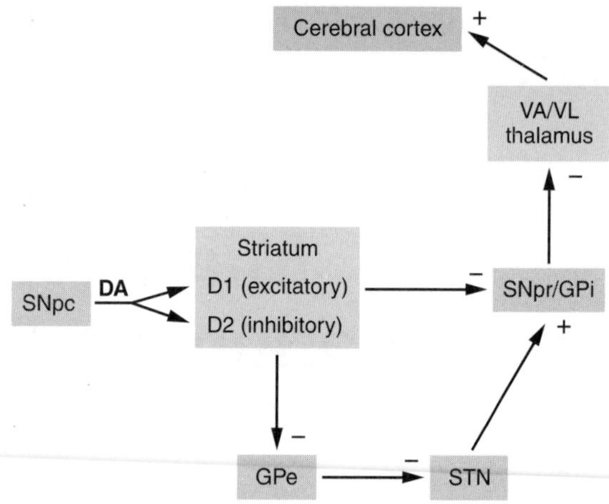

Figure ■ 10-1
Simplified diagram of the neural connections between the basal ganglia, thalamus, and cerebral cortex. Excitatory pathways are indicated by "+"; inhibitory pathways are indicated by "-". Normally, dopamine (DA) input to the striatum affects two subtypes of dopamine receptors (D1, D2) that control two different pathways. The D1 receptors are excitatory and turn on the direct pathway that inhibits outflow from the SNpr/GPi, resulting in less inhibition of thalamic nuclei and more excitation of the cerebral cortex. The D2 receptors are inhibitory and turn off the indirect pathway that would otherwise excite the SNpr/GPi and allow these structures to inhibit the thalamus and reduce cortical excitation. In Parkinson disease, decreased dopaminergic input to the striatum reduces the ability of both pathways to inhibit the SNpr/GPi, thus allowing the SNpr/GPi to inhibit the thalamus and reduce thalamic stimulation of the cortex. (SNpc: substantia nigra pars compacta; GPe: globus pallidus externa; STN: subthalamic nucleus; SNpr: substantia nigra pars reticulate; GPi: globus pallidus interna; VA: ventroanterior nucleus of the thalamus; VL: ventrolateral nucleus of the thalamus).

Dopamine also binds to striatal D2 receptors, which are inhibitory—that is, when dopamine binds to D2 receptors, activity is reduced in a second or "indirect" pathway that affects outflow from the basal ganglia (see Fig. 10-1). Increased activity in this indirect pathway increases inhibitory outflow from the globus pallidus interna and the substantia nigra pars reticulata, which inhibits the thalamus and reduces cortical excitation. However, when dopamine binds to the D2 receptors, activity in the indirect pathway is inhibited, thus reducing this pathway's ability to inhibit the thalamus and cortex.

Because dopamine acts on two complementary pathways to moderate outflow from the basal ganglia, the thalamus can exert its normal excitatory influence on the cerebral cortex. But in Parkinson disease, decreased dopamine influence on striatal D1 and D2 receptors results in decreased activity in the direct and indirect pathways, respectively. Decreased activity in the direct pathway removes the inhibitory effect on the globus pallidus interna and the substantia nigra pars reticulata, thus allowing these structures to inhibit thalamic nuclei and reduce the thalamus's ability to excite the cortex. Likewise, dopamine can no longer activate the D2 receptors that normally inhibit the indirect pathway, thereby allowing this pathway to excite the globus pallidus interna and the substantia nigra pars reticulata. Again, increased outflow from these structures inhibits the thalamus, reducing its ability to excite the cortex (see Fig. 10-1).

The loss of dopamine influence in the corpus striatum results in a complex series of changes in other neuronal pathways that ultimately affect higher (cortical) brain function. The fact that several other neuronal pathways are involved in Parkinson disease suggests that neurotransmitters other than dopamine may also be affected by this disease. This idea is certainly true for neurotransmitters such as acetylcholine, because interneurons within the corpus striatum release acetylcholine that helps moderate the activity of the neuronal pathways described above. An imbalance between striatal dopamine and acetylcholine may therefore be responsible for some of the symptoms in Parkinson disease.[17,18] The effects of amino acid neurotransmitters such as GABA (inhibition) and glutamate (excitation) are also important at the synaptic connections within basal ganglia pathways, at synapses between neurons projecting from the basal ganglia to the thalamus, and at the connections between thalamic neurons and the cortex. Alterations in the release of, or receptor responses to, these amino acids have been implicated in the neurochemical changes seen in Parkinson disease.[19,20] Finally, neurotransmitters such as serotonin and norepinephrine may also be affected, and altered activity of these neurotransmitters may be responsible for some symptoms of Parkinson disease and perhaps the dyskinesias and other side effects associated with certain anti-Parkinson drugs.[21,22]

Essentially, we now understand that Parkinson disease occurs when the loss of dopamine in the basal ganglia results in a domino effect that disrupts other neuronal pathways involving several other neurotransmitters. Drugs that help normalize dopamine activity in the basal ganglia will hopefully resolve the initial problem, thus allowing other neurochemical disruptions to return to normal levels. Likewise, some anti-Parkinson drugs may also directly affect acetylcholine or other neurotransmitters, thus helping to maintain the balance between dopamine and other neurotransmitters in motor pathways. Drugs that affect dopamine activity and the activity of other neurotransmitters are discussed later in this chapter.

ETIOLOGY OF PARKINSON DISEASE: GENETIC AND ENVIRONMENTAL FACTORS

As stated previously, the exact factors that initiate the loss of striatal dopamine are unknown in most patients with Parkinson disease. However, recent evidence suggests that genetic factors may interact with environmental factors to make certain individuals susceptible to the destruction of dopaminergic neurons in the substantia nigra.[4-6]

Genetic Factors

Researchers have identified mutations of several genes that might play a causative role in Parkinson disease.[23,24] Some of these genes are responsible for controlling the production of alpha-synuclein (a small presynaptic protein) and other neuronal proteins.[25] Defects in the genes regulating the production of these proteins appear to lead to the overproduction and abnormal accumulation of proteins in neuronal tissues, especially in people with certain forms of Parkinson disease such as early onset parkinsonism and other familial forms.[25,26] As proteins accumulate, they can damage specific cellular components such as the mitochondria and cell membrane.[27-29] Indeed, Parkinson disease and several other neurodegenerative disorders are associated with the formation of Lewy bodies, which are clumps of proteins found in the neuronal tissues.[25,30]

Abnormal protein accumulation therefore seems to play a role in the degenerative changes seen in Parkinson disease. The actual neuronal death, however, may be caused by the formation of harmful by-products of oxygen metabolism, known commonly as *reactive oxygen species* (ROS) or *oxygen free radicals*.[31] A free radical is a chemical species that has an unpaired electron in its outer shell.[32] In order to become more stable, the free radical steals an electron from some other cellular component such as a protein, DNA molecule, or membrane phospholipid. In this process, the free radical damages the cellular component, subsequently damaging the cell. Free radicals, for example, might initiate or accelerate the abnormal accumulation and aggregation of alpha-synuclein and other proteins within the neuron.[33] Conversely, production of free radicals may be the result of abnormal protein accumulation—that is, alpha-synuclein may initiate damage to the cell, causing increased production of free radicals, which then cause the actual cell death. Regardless of which factor occurs first, cells subjected to free radical–induced damage are said to undergo oxidative stress because loss of electrons (oxidation) of proteins and other cellular components leads to harmful effects on the cell.[34]

Hence, oxygen free radicals might ultimately be responsible for causing the degeneration and death of substantia nigra neurons. Production of these free radicals appears to be increased in people with Parkinson disease, either in response to protein accumulation or because of a primary defect in the synthesis of free radicals by the mitochondria or by other enzymatic reactions within the cell.[35-37] Regardless of the initiating factor, excess production of free radicals in the basal ganglia could lead to a vicious cycle whereby the free radicals accelerate protein accumulation and damage the mitochondria, which in turn causes more free radical production, and so on.[31] It therefore appears that neurons in the substantia nigra might ultimately be destroyed because genetic factors lead to neuronal protein accumulation and free radical–induced oxidative stress that causes the degeneration and death of these neurons.

Environmental Factors

The idea that environmental factors may play a role in Parkinson disease was discovered in an interesting way. In 1982, several young adults in their 20s and 30s developed permanent, severe parkinsonism.[38] Because the sudden onset of Parkinson disease before age 40 is extremely rare, these individuals aroused a great deal of interest. Upon close investigation, all of these individuals were found to have experimented with synthetic opioid-like drugs. These so-called designer drugs were manufactured by drug dealers in an attempt to create an illicit supply of narcotics for heroin addicts. In this case, the illicit narcotics contained a toxic compound known as 1-methyl-4-phenyl-1,2,3,6-tetrahydropyridine (MPTP). Later research indicated that MPTP causes selective destruction of substantia nigra neurons[38] and can invoke parkinsonism in experimental animals.[39]

The discovery of toxin-induced parkinsonism in drug addicts led to the idea that idiopathic Parkinson disease may occur when susceptible individuals are exposed to some environmental toxin.[40] For example, herbicides, insecticides, fungicides, or industrial waste may begin or accelerate the neuronal changes that ultimately result in Parkinson disease.[41,42,38,39] Environmental toxins, for example, might serve as the trigger for neuronal death in people who have genetic variations that make them vulnerable to these toxins. However, a specific environmental factor has not been identified yet.

The idea that toxins and free radicals may cause neuronal damage in Parkinson disease has also led to research in ways to delay or prevent the destructive effects of these chemicals.[33,43] For example, it has been suggested that certain medications might have neuroprotective effects if they control the production and harmful effects of endogenous toxins such as free radicals. Such medications are often referred to as *antioxidants* because they may help control oxidative stress caused by the free radicals. This idea has encouraged the development and use of agents that might delay the neurodegenerative changes seen in Parkinson disease. In particular, pharmacologists investigated the drugs used to decrease the symptoms of Parkinson disease (dopamine agonists, MAO-B inhibitors; see below) as well as antioxidants such as coenzyme Q10 and vitamin E for any possible neuroprotective effects.[33,44,45] To date, no agent has been identified that is overwhelmingly successful in delaying the neuronal changes occurring in Parkinson disease. Nonetheless, future research may continue to clarify the exact reason for the degeneration of substantia nigra neurons, and drugs that help prevent this degeneration could conceivably be developed to decrease or even eliminate the neuronal death that underlies the disease.

THERAPEUTIC AGENTS IN PARKINSONISM

The primary drug used to treat Parkinson disease is levodopa. Other agents such as dopamine agonists, anticholinergic drugs, monoamine oxidase type B inhibitors, catechol-O-methyltransferase inhibitors, and amantadine can be used alone or in conjunction with levodopa, depending on the needs of the patient. An overview of the drugs used to treat Parkinson disease is shown in Table 10-1. Each of these agents is discussed below.

Levodopa

Levodopa has been the cornerstone of anti-Parkinson drugs for over 40 years. Administration of levodopa often dramatically improves all symptoms of parkinsonism, especially bradykinesia and rigidity. The decrease in symptoms and increase in function are remarkable in patients who respond well to the drug. As with any medication, there is a portion of the population who—for unknown reasons—do not respond well or simply cannot tolerate the drug. Also, prolonged use of levodopa is associated with some rather troublesome and frustrating side effects (see "Problems and Adverse Effects of Levodopa Therapy"). However, the use of levodopa has been the most significant advancement in the management of Parkinson disease, and it remains the most effective drug in the treatment of most patients with this disorder.[46,47]

Pharmacokinetics of Levodopa

Because the underlying problem in Parkinson disease is a deficiency of dopamine in the basal ganglia, simple substitution of this chemical would seem to be a logical course of action. However, dopamine does not cross the blood-brain barrier. Administration of dopamine either orally or parenterally will therefore be

Table 10-1
OVERVIEW OF DRUG THERAPY IN PARKINSON DISEASE

Drug	Mechanism of Action	Special Comments
Levodopa (Dopar, Larodopa, Parcopa,* Sinemet*)	Resolves dopamine deficiency by being converted to dopamine after crossing blood-brain barrier.	Still the best drug for resolving parkinsonian symptoms; long-term use limited by side effects and decreased efficacy.
Carbidopa	Prevents premature conversion of levodopa to dopamine in peripheral tissues.	Given with levodopa to allow more levodopa to reach the brain intact.
Dopamine agonists (see Table 10-2)	Directly stimulates dopamine receptors in basal ganglia.	May produce fewer side effects (dyskinesias, fluctuations in response) than levodopa; early use may also delay the progression of Parkinson disease.
Anticholinergics Benztropine mesylate (Cogentin) Biperiden (Akineton) Diphenhydramine (Benadryl, others) Trihexyphenidyl (Artane)	Inhibits excessive acetylcholine influence caused by dopamine deficiency.	Use in Parkinson disease limited by frequent side effects.
Amantadine (Symmetrel)	Inhibits the effects of excitatory amino acids (glutamate) in the basal ganglia.	May be used alone during early/mild stages or added to drug regimen when levodopa loses effectiveness.
MAO-B** inhibitors Rasagiline (Azilect) Selegiline (Eldepryl, others)	Inhibits the enzyme that breaks down dopamine in the basal ganglia; enables dopamine to remain active for longer periods of time.	May improve symptoms, especially in early stages of Parkinson disease; long-term use may be neuroprotective and delay disease progression.
COMT*** inhibitors Entacapone (Comtan) Tolcapone (Tasmar)	Help prevent breakdown of dopamine in peripheral tissues; allows more levodopa to reach the brain.	Useful as an adjunct to levodopa/carbidopa administration; may improve and prolong effects of levodopa.

**Trade name for levodopa combined with carbidopa*
***MAO-B: monoamine oxidase type B*
****COMT: catechol-O-methyltransferase*

ineffective because it will be unable to cross from the systemic circulation into the brain where it is needed. Fortunately, the immediate precursor to dopamine, dihydroxyphenylalanine (dopa), crosses the blood-brain barrier quite readily (Fig. 10-2). Dopa, or more specifically levodopa (the L-isomer of dopa), can cross the brain capillary endothelium through an active transport process that is specific for this molecule and other large amino acids.[48] Upon entering the brain, levodopa is then transformed into dopamine by decarboxylation from the enzyme dopa decarboxylase (Fig. 10-3).

Levodopa is usually administered orally, and the daily dose is determined according to each patient's needs. Dosages of levodopa are also minimized by administering it with a companion drug that inhibits premature levodopa breakdown (i.e., a peripheral decarboxylase inhibitor such as carbidopa, discussed later in this section). Levodopa dosages are progressively increased until a noticeable reduction in symptoms occurs or until side effects begin to be a problem. Daily titers are usually divided into two to three doses per day, and individual doses are often given with meals to decrease gastrointestinal (GI) irritation.

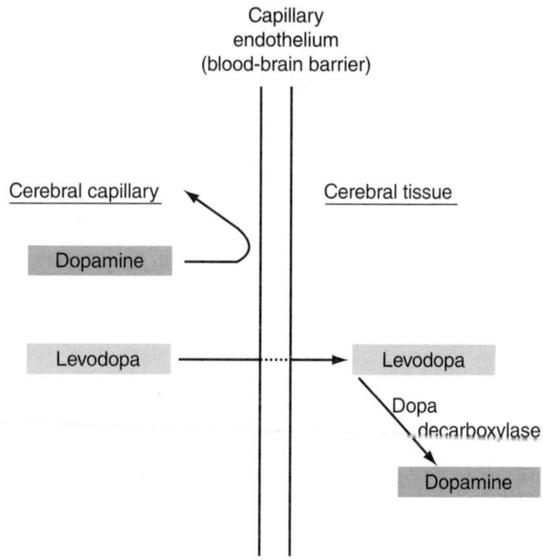

Figure ■ 10-3
Synthesis of dopamine.

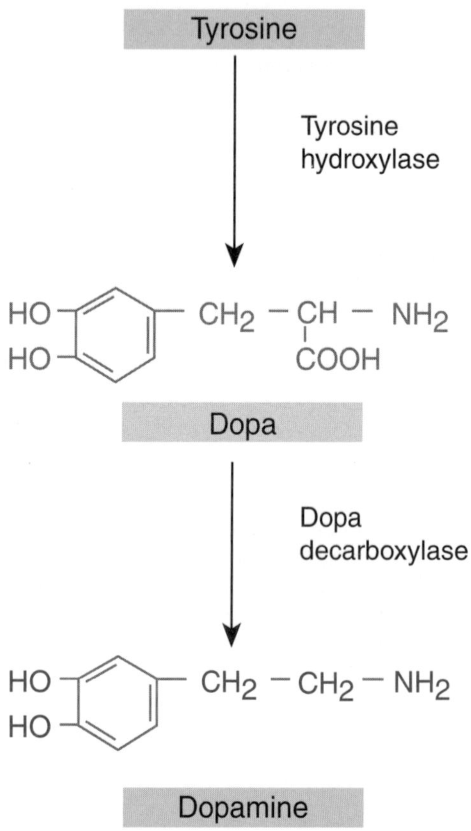

Figure ■ 10-2
Selective permeability of the blood-brain barrier to levodopa.

Following absorption from the GI tract, levodopa is rapidly converted to dopamine by the enzyme dopa decarboxylase. This enzyme is distributed extensively throughout the body and can be found in locations such as the liver, intestinal mucosa, kidneys, and skeletal muscle. Conversion of levodopa to dopamine in the periphery is rather extensive—less than 1 percent of the levodopa that is administered reaches the brain in that form.[14] This fact is significant because only levodopa will be able to cross the blood-brain barrier to be subsequently transformed into dopamine. Any levodopa that is converted prematurely to dopamine in the periphery must remain there, becoming essentially useless in alleviating parkinsonism symptoms.

Use of Peripheral Decarboxylase Inhibitors

When given alone, rather large quantities of levodopa must be administered to ensure that enough of it reaches the brain in that form. This is often undesirable because the majority of the levodopa ends up as dopamine in the peripheral circulation, and these high levels of circulating dopamine can cause some unpleasant GI and cardiovascular side effects (see the next section). An alternative method is to give levodopa in conjunction with a peripheral decarboxylase inhibitor such as carbidopa (Fig. 10-4).[14] The simultaneous use of a drug that selectively inhibits the dopa decarboxylase enzyme outside of the CNS enables more levodopa to reach the brain before being converted to dopamine. The use of carbidopa dramatically decreases the amount of levodopa needed to achieve a desired effect.[49] Another decarboxylase inhibitor known as *benserazide* is available outside of the United States; this drug can also be used to prevent peripheral conversion of levodopa to dopamine.[14]

Since levodopa is almost always administered along with carbidopa, these two drugs are often combined in the same pill and marketed under the trade name Sinemet. (Preparations of levodopa with benserazide are marketed as Madopar.) When prepared together as Sinemet, levodopa and carbidopa are usually combined in a fixed carbidopa-to-levodopa ratio of either 1:4 or 1:10.[1] The Sinemet preparation that is typically used to initiate therapy consists of tablets containing 25 mg of carbidopa and 100 mg of levodopa, administered two to three times each day. This ratio achieves a rapid and effective inhibition of the dopa decarboxylase enzyme. A 10:100- or 25:250-mg preparation of carbidopa to levodopa is usually started as the Parkinson symptoms become more pronounced and there is a need for larger relative amounts of levodopa. When administered with carbidopa, levodopa dosages typically begin at 200 to 300 mg/d and are increased periodically according to the patient's needs. Average maintenance dosages of levodopa range between 600 and 700 mg/d, and the maximum dosage is often 800 mg/d; however, these dosages are highly variable from patient to patient.

Levodopa-carbidopa is also available in a controlled-release preparation (Sinemet CR) that is absorbed more slowly and is intended to provide prolonged effects.[50] The use of this controlled-release preparation may be helpful in patients who respond well to levodopa initially but experience dyskinesias and fluctuations in response, such as end-of-dose akinesia and the on-off phenomenon.[14] Problems related to levodopa therapy are described in the next section.

Problems and Adverse Effects of Levodopa Therapy

Gastrointestinal Problems

Levodopa is often associated with nausea and vomiting. These symptoms can be quite severe, especially during the first few days of drug use. However, the incidence of this problem is greatly reduced if levodopa is given in conjunction with a peripheral decarboxylase inhibitor such as carbidopa. The reduction in nausea and vomiting when levodopa peripheral decarboxylation to dopamine is inhibited suggests that these symptoms may be caused by excessive levels of peripherally circulating dopamine.

Cardiovascular Problems

Some problems with cardiac arrhythmias may arise in a patient taking levodopa. However, these problems are usually fairly minor unless the patient has a history of cardiac irregularity. Caution should be used in cardiac patients undergoing levodopa therapy, especially during exercise.

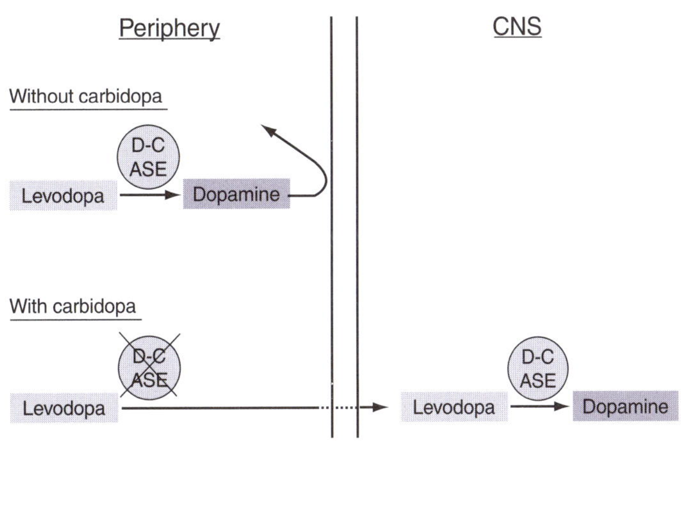

Figure ■ 10-4
Use of a carbidopa, a peripheral decarboxylase inhibitor, on levodopa absorption. Without carbidopa, most of the levodopa is converted to dopamine in the periphery, rendering it unable to cross the blood-brain barrier. Carbidopa inhibits the peripheral decarboxylase (D-Case) enzyme so that levodopa can cross the blood-brain barrier intact. Carbidopa does not cross the blood-brain barrier, so the conversion of levodopa to dopamine still occurs within the CNS.

Orthostatic hypotension (a rapid drop in blood pressure when a patient sits up or stands up suddenly) can also be an extremely troublesome problem in a patient taking levodopa. Again, this side effect is usually diminished when peripheral decarboxylation is inhibited and peripheral dopamine levels are not allowed to increase excessively. Still, patients undergoing physical therapy or similar regimens should be carefully observed during changes in posture and should be instructed to avoid sudden postural adjustments. This factor is especially true in patients beginning or resuming levodopa therapy.

Dyskinesias

A more persistent and challenging problem is the appearance of various movement disorders in patients taking levodopa for prolonged periods. Approximately 80 percent of patients receiving chronic levodopa therapy begin to exhibit various dyskinesias such as choreoathetoid movements, ballismus, dystonia, myoclonus, and various tics and tremors.[51] The specific type of movement disorder can vary from patient to patient but tends to remain constant within the individual patient. The onset of dyskinetic side effects is particularly frustrating since levodopa ameliorates one form of the movement disorder only to institute a different motor problem.

The onset of dyskinesias usually occurs after the patient has been receiving levodopa therapy for periods ranging from 3 months to several years. In some patients, these abnormal movements may simply be caused by drug-induced overstimulation of dopaminergic pathways in the basal ganglia, and a decrease in the daily dosage should help. Because levodopa has a short half-life and erratic absorption, the drug may also cause dyskinesias due to its intermittent or pulsatile stimulation of dopamine receptors.[52] That is, the sudden rapid influx of levodopa into the brain may combine with endogenous neuronal dopamine release to cause excessive stimulation that results in various dyskinesias.[14]

However, the reason for dyskinesias in some patients may be far more complex. For example, certain patients may exhibit dyskinesias when plasma levodopa levels are rising or falling or even when plasma levels are at a minimum.[14] There is evidently an intricate relationship between the basal ganglia neurons that continue to release or respond to dopamine and the pharmacological replacement of dopamine through levodopa therapy. Dyskinesias may actually be the result of functional and structural adaptations of these neurons caused by periodic fluctuations in dopamine influence supplied from exogenous sources (i.e., levodopa).[53,54] Likewise, other neurotransmitters, such as glutamate and serotonin, seem to play a role in levodopa-induced dyskinesias, and changes in the release and responsiveness to these other neurotransmitters probably contribute to the abnormal movements that occur during chronic levodopa administration.[52,55-57]

Regardless of the exact neural mechanism that underlies these dyskinesias, the goal of levodopa therapy is to find a regimen that diminishes the incapacitating parkinsonism symptoms without causing other movement disorders.[1] Strategies for minimizing dyskinesias include adjusting the dose of levodopa, using a controlled-release form of this drug, and incorporating other anti-Parkinson medications into the patient's drug regimen.[58] As indicated earlier, neurotransmitters other than dopamine may also be contributing to levodopa-induced dyskinesias, and drug strategies that help control glutamate, serotonin, and other neurochemicals may eventually emerge as therapeutic options.[52,58] Presently, however, dyskinesias remain a major problem of long-term levodopa treatment, and it may be difficult to find a dose that controls Parkinson symptoms without causing dyskinesias. Likewise, some of the parkinsonism symptoms may appear quite similar to the dyskinetic side effects, making it difficult to judge whether the levodopa dose is too high or too low. The physician, rehabilitation specialist, patient, and other individuals dealing with the patient should make careful observations to determine if adjustments in levodopa therapy are resulting in the desired effect.

Behavioral Changes

A variety of mental and behavioral side effects have been reported in patients taking levodopa. Psychotic symptoms seem especially prevalent, although depression, anxiety, confusion, impulsiveness, and other changes in behavior have also been noted.[59,60] These problems may be related directly to Parkinson disease; there is a strong prevalence of mental disorders and dementia in many patients regardless of anti-Parkinson drug treatment.[59] Nonetheless, levodopa therapy can certainly contribute to various psychological disorders given the fact that dopamine is very important in controlling mood and behavior (see Chapters 7 and 8).

Unlike the GI and vascular problems described earlier, psychotic and other behavioral symptoms appear to be exacerbated if levodopa is used in conjunction with carbidopa. This may be caused by greater quantities of levodopa crossing the blood-brain barrier before being converted to dopamine, thus generating higher quantities of dopamine within the brain. This idea seems logical, considering that increased activity in certain dopamine pathways seems to be the underlying cause of psychosis (see Chapter 8). Treatment of these symptoms is often difficult because traditional antipsychotic medications tend to increase the symptoms of Parkinson disease. However, some of the newer "atypical" antipsychotics such as clozapine (Chapter 8) may help decrease psychotic symptoms without causing an increase in parkinsonism.[61]

Diminished Response to Levodopa

One of the most serious problems in levodopa therapy is that the drug seems to become less effective in many patients when it is administered for prolonged periods. When used continually for 3 to 4 years, the ability of levodopa to relieve parkinsonism symptoms often progressively diminishes to the point where the drug is no longer effective.[51] One explanation for this is that the patient develops a tolerance to the drug. A second theory is that the decreased effectiveness of levodopa may be caused by a progressive increase in the severity of the underlying disease rather than a decrease in the drug's efficacy. These two theories have initiated a controversy as to whether levodopa therapy should be started early or late in the course of Parkinson disease (see "Clinical Course of Parkinson Disease: When to Use Specific Drugs"). Regardless of why this occurs, the loss of levodopa efficacy can be a devastating blow to the patient who had previously experienced excellent therapeutic results from this drug.

Fluctuations in Response to Levodopa

Several distinct fluctuations in the response to levodopa are fairly common in most patients.[1,62] **End-of-dose akinesia** refers to when the drug's effectiveness simply seems to wear off prior to the next dose. This condition is usually resolved by adjusting the quantity and timing of levodopa administration (i.e., smaller doses may be given more frequently) or by using a sustained release form of the drug.

A more bizarre and less understood fluctuation in response is the **on-off phenomenon**. Here, the effectiveness of levodopa may suddenly and spontaneously decrease, resulting in the abrupt worsening of parkinsonian symptoms (the "off" period). Remission of symptoms may then occur spontaneously or after taking a dose of levodopa (the "on" period). This on-off pattern may repeat itself several times during the day. Although the exact reasons for this are unclear, the off periods are directly related to diminishing plasma levels of levodopa.[14] These low levels may occur when the absorption of orally administered levodopa is delayed by poor GI motility or if levodopa must compete with large amino acids for transport across the intestinal mucosa.[63] The off periods can be eliminated by administering levodopa continuously by IV infusion, thus preventing the fall in plasma levels. However, this is not a long-term solution, and alterations in the oral dosage schedule may have to be made in an attempt to maintain plasma levels at a relatively constant level. Specifically, the drug can be taken with smaller amounts of food and meals that are relatively low in protein so that levodopa absorption is not overwhelmed by dietary amino acid absorption. As indicated earlier, use of a controlled-release formulation such as Sinemet CR can also help prevent the fluctuations in plasma levodopa by allowing a more steady, controlled release of the drug into the bloodstream.

Finally, patients may suddenly and inexplicably stop walking and appear to be frozen in an upright position. These episodes, known commonly as freezing of gait, or simply *freezing*, are poorly understood and may be related to variations in cerebral blood flow or disruptions in symmetric motor control rather than fluctuations in the response to levodopa.[64,65] Nonetheless, freezing of gait is frustrating to the patient and creates a potentially dangerous situation that can lead to falls and injury. Fortunately, there seems to be some cognitive aspects to these freezing episodes, and patients may be taught to respond to verbal or visual cues to help reinitiate steps and resume walking.[66-68] Clinicians can therefore explore ways to use these cues and other cognitive techniques, perhaps combined with motor training (treadmills, bicycles, etc.), to help patients prevent or overcome freezing episodes.[69]

Drug Holidays From Levodopa

Drug holidays are sometimes used in the patient who has become refractory to the beneficial effects of levodopa or who has had a sudden increase in adverse side effects.[51,70] During this period, the patient is gradually removed from all anti-Parkinson medication for 3 days to 3 weeks while under close medical supervision. The purpose of the holiday is to allow the body to recover from any toxicity or tolerance that may have developed because of prolonged use of levodopa at relatively high dosages. Drug holidays are done with the hope that levodopa can eventually be resumed at a lower dosage and with better results. Drug holidays do appear to be successful in some patients with Parkinson disease. Beneficial effects may be achieved at only 50 to 70 percent of the preholiday dosage, and the incidence of side effects (e.g., dyskinesias, confusion, and the on-off phenomenon) may be markedly reduced.[71]

Despite these potential benefits, drug holidays are no longer used routinely because of their potential risk to the patient. Considering that these patients are in the advanced stages of Parkinson disease, discontinuing the anti-Parkinson medications even temporarily results in severe immobility, which can lead to problems such as venous thrombosis, pulmonary embolism, pneumonia, and other impairments that could increase morbidity and mortality.[51] Consequently, drug holidays may still be used on a limited basis in a few select patients with Parkinson disease, but it is not a common intervention.

OTHER DRUGS TO TREAT PARKINSON DISEASE

Dopamine Agonists

Because the basic problem in Parkinson disease is a deficiency of striatal dopamine, it would seem logical that drugs similar in function to dopamine would be effective in treating this problem. However, many dopamine agonists have serious side effects that prevent their clinical use. Only a few dopamine agonists such as bromocriptine (Parlodel), cabergoline (Dostinex), pramipexole (Mirapex), rotigotine (Neupro), and ropinirole (Requip) are available that do not cause excessive adverse effects (Table 10-2).[72,73] These drugs are now used regularly in the long-term treatment of Parkinson disease. Another dopamine agonist, apomorphine (Apokyn), is administered by subcutaneous injection to treat severe akinetic episodes ("off" periods) in patients with advanced Parkinson disease who no longer respond to other drugs.[74]

Dopamine agonists have traditionally been used in conjunction with levodopa, especially in patients who have begun to experience a decrease in levodopa effects or in those who experience problems such as end-of-dose akinesia and the on-off effect.[75,76] Simultaneous administration of levodopa with a dopamine agonist permits optimal results with relatively smaller doses of each drug.

Table 10-2

DOPAMINE AGONISTS USED IN PARKINSON DISEASE

Generic Name	Trade Name	Dosage* (mg/d)
Apomorphine	Apokyn	2–6 mg/d
Bromocriptine	Parlodel, others	15–40 mg/d
Cabergoline	Dostinex	0.25–1 mg twice/week
Pramipexole	Mirapex	1.5–4.5 mg/d
Ropinirole	Requip	9–24 mg/d
Rotigotine	Neupro	2–6 mg/24 hr**

** Represents typical dosage range; upper limits may be exceeded in some patients.*

*** Administered by transdermal patch.*

Dopamine agonists can also be used alone in the early stages of mild-to-moderate parkinsonism, thus providing an alternative if other anti-Parkinson drugs (including levodopa) are poorly tolerated.[72,77] When used alone, dopamine agonists do not usually cause the dyskinesias and fluctuations in motor responses that occur with levodopa therapy.[73] Several of these drugs tend to have a longer half-life than levodopa and therefore produce a steadier and more prolonged effect on dopamine receptors.[78,79] One of these drugs (rotigotine [Neupro]) is also currently available in a transdermal patch; the continuous drug delivery may help prevent sudden fluctuations in plasma drug levels. Finally, dopamine agonists may be more selective than levodopa in stimulating certain dopamine receptor subtypes such as the D2 receptor, thus resulting in fewer abnormal motor responses.[80] Hence, these drugs have assumed an important role as both an adjunct to levodopa treatment and the primary drugs used to treat patients with Parkinson disease.

There is also evidence that dopamine agonists may help normalize endogenous dopamine activity, thus having a neuroprotective effect on substantia nigra neurons.[72,77] As indicated earlier, certain medications are being investigated for their potential to delay or prevent the degeneration of dopamine-producing neurons in the basal ganglia. Dopamine agonists could produce such a neuroprotective effect by providing more continuous and less pulsatile stimulation of dopamine receptors, thereby preventing the free radical–induced damage that is associated with abnormal dopamine synthesis and breakdown.[72,79] Current evidence suggests that early use of dopamine agonists can provide adequate anti-Parkinson effects while delaying the onset of side effects such as dyskinesias.[77] Long-term studies continue to clarify whether early use of dopamine agonists is successful in slowing the progression of Parkinson disease.

Dopamine agonists may produce adverse side effects such as nausea and vomiting. Orthostatic hypotension is also a problem in some patients. With prolonged use, these drugs may cause CNS-related side effects such as confusion and hallucinations.

Anticholinergic Drugs

As mentioned previously, the deficiency of striatal dopamine is also associated with increased activity in certain cholinergic pathways in the basal ganglia. Consequently, drugs that limit acetylcholine transmission can help alleviate the symptoms of Parkinson disease, especially tremors and rigidity, by blocking acetylcholine receptors in the basal ganglia.[81] When used alone, **anticholinergics** are usually only mildly to moderately successful in reducing symptoms, and they are typically administered in conjunction with levodopa or other anti-Parkinson drugs to obtain optimal results.

Antihistamine drugs with anticholinergic properties such as diphenhydramine are also used occasionally. These drugs tend to be somewhat less effective in treating parkinsonism but appear to have milder side effects than their anticholinergic counterparts.

However, anticholinergic agents are fairly nonselective, and they tend to produce a wide variety of side effects because they also block acetylcholine receptors in various tissues throughout the body. The side effects are especially prevalent in older adults and are particularly troublesome in patients with Parkinson disease.[82] CNS side effects may include mood change, confusion, hallucinations, decreased cognition, and drowsiness (see Chapter 19). In addition, cardiac irregularities, blurred vision, dry mouth, nausea/vomiting, constipation, and urinary retention are fairly common.

Given their limitations, anticholinergic drugs are used sparingly in people with Parkinson disease, and their use has diminished in favor of newer, less problematic medications.

Amantadine

Pharmacologists originally developed amantadine (Symmetrel) as an antiviral drug, and its ability to reduce parkinsonian symptoms was discovered by chance.[83] Amantadine was being used to treat influenza in a patient with Parkinson disease, and a noticeable improvement in the patient's tremor and rigidity was observed. The FDA subsequently approved amantadine for use in patients with Parkinson disease, and it is usually given along with levodopa. Amantadine has been especially helpful in reducing dyskinesias and other motor complications associated with levodopa therapy in people with advanced Parkinson disease.[77,84,85]

Amantadine's anti-Parkinson effects are probably due to its ability to block the *N*-methyl-D-aspartate (NMDA) receptor in the brain, thereby inhibiting the effects of excitatory amino acids such as glutamate.[84,85] As discussed earlier, increased glutamate activity seems to play an important role in motor complications associated with Parkinson disease.[19,20] The fact that amantadine may help reduce dyskinesias suggests that glutamate contributes to these abnormal movements and that reducing glutaminergic influence is important in improving motor function without dyskinetic side effects. Future research may discover other ways of controlling excitatory neurotransmitters such as glutamate, thus providing additional treatments for people with advanced Parkinson disease.

The primary adverse effects associated with amantadine are orthostatic hypotension, CNS disturbance (e.g., depression, confusion, hallucinations), and patches of skin discoloration on the lower extremities (livedo reticularis). However, these side effects are relatively mild compared to those of other anti-Parkinson drugs and are usually reversed by altering the drug dosage.

Monoamine Oxidase B Inhibitors

Selegiline (Deprenyl, Eldepryl) and rasagiline (Azilect) potently and selectively inhibit the monoamine oxidase type B (MAO-B) enzyme. This enzyme is responsible for breaking down dopamine in the brain. By inhibiting this enzyme, these drugs prolong the local effects of dopamine at CNS synapses. Thus, they can be used alone in the early stages of Parkinson disease to prolong the effects of endogenous dopamine produced within the basal ganglia. Early administration of selegiline and rasagiline may alleviate motor symptoms so that patients do not need to begin taking levodopa until later in the course of this disease.[86,87] These drugs can also be combined with levodopa therapy because they prolong the action of dopamine and allow the reduction of parkinsonism symptoms using a relatively low dose of levodopa.[86] Selegiline is available as a transdermal patch (Emsam), but this is currently approved to treat only major depressive disorder.[88]

It has also been suggested that selegiline and rasagiline may actually slow the progression of Parkinson disease.[86,89] Theoretically, these drugs could have neuroprotective effects because they decrease dopamine oxidation by inhibiting the MAO-B enzyme, thus preventing excessive production of harmful free radicals during dopamine breakdown.[90,91] However, the neuroprotective effects may be unrelated to their effects on dopamine metabolism.[87,92] For example, it has been suggested that MAO-B inhibitors may decrease the synthesis of proteins that ultimately lead to cell death (apoptosis) in neurons that have undergone some sort of injury.[87] Future studies will continue to clarify whether early use of MAO-B inhibitors is associated with long-term benefits in people with Parkinson disease.

Selegiline and rasagiline are relatively safe in terms of short-term adverse side effects. With some MAO inhibitors, there is frequently a sudden, large increase in blood pressure if the patient ingests foods containing tyramine (see Chapter 7). However, because they are selective for the MAO-B enzyme, selegiline and rasagiline do not appear to cause a hypertensive crisis even when such tyramine-containing foods are eaten.[93] Rasagiline is more potent than selegiline, and rasagiline is preferred in many patients because unlike selegiline, rasagiline does not cause amphetamine-like effects that could cause sleep and mood problems.[94] Other side effects of MAO-B inhibitors include dizziness, sedation, GI distress, and headache.

Catechol-O-Methyltransferase Inhibitors

Pharmacologists developed a relatively new group of drugs, including entacapone (Comtan) and tolcapone (Tasmar), to inhibit an enzyme known as **catechol-O-methyltransferase (COMT)**.[95] The enzyme converts levodopa to an inactive metabolite known as 3-O-methyldopa. The drugs, referred to as *COMT inhibitors*, prevent levodopa conversion in peripheral tissues so that more levodopa is available to reach the brain and exert beneficial effects. Hence, these drugs are used as an adjunct to levodopa therapy to provide better therapeutic effects using smaller doses of levodopa.[96] Evidence suggests that adding a COMT inhibitor to levodopa therapy may also reduce fluctuations in the response to levodopa and prolong the periods of levodopa effectiveness ("on" time) with shorter periods of unresponsiveness ("off" time).[96,97]

Likewise, a COMT inhibitor can be used with a dopa decarboxylase (e.g., carbidopa; see earlier in this chapter) to provide optimal protection for the levodopa molecule.[98,99] That is, inhibiting dopa decarboxylase and COMT prevents levodopa from being metabolized prematurely by either enzyme, thereby protecting the levodopa until it reaches the brain. Consequently, all three drug types (levodopa, a dopa decarboxylase inhibitor, and a COMT inhibitor) can be administered simultaneously for the best outcomes in some patients. In fact, Stalevo is the brand name for a product that combines levodopa, carbidopa, and entacapone in the same pill, thereby providing a convenient way to administer these drugs together.

The primary problem associated with COMT inhibitors is an initial increase in dyskinesias.[100] This could occur because the COMT inhibitor is allowing more levodopa to reach the brain, and the levodopa dosage needs to be lowered accordingly. Other side effects include nausea, diarrhea, dizziness, and muscle pain/cramps.

CLINICAL COURSE OF PARKINSON DISEASE: WHEN TO USE SPECIFIC DRUGS

Controversy exists as to when specific anti-Parkinson drugs should be administered.[1,101] Much of the debate focuses on when levodopa therapy should be initiated. Without question, levodopa is the most effective pharmacological treatment for reducing the motor symptoms of Parkinson disease. As mentioned previously, however, long-term use of levodopa poses several risks, and the effectiveness of this drug seems to diminish after several years of use. Consequently, some practitioners question whether levodopa therapy should be withheld until the parkinsonian symptoms become severe enough to truly impair motor function. In theory, this saves the levodopa for more advanced stages of this disease, when it would be needed the most.[102]

Some researchers have suggested that other drugs such as dopamine agonists or MAO-B inhibitors might be a suitable alternative to levodopa as the initial treatment of Parkinson disease.[102-104] Dopamine agonists can help resolve parkinsonian symptoms, sparing the use of levodopa until later in the course of the disease. As indicated, dopamine agonists may also have a reduced incidence of dyskinesias and may slow the degeneration of substantia nigra neurons (neuroprotective effect). Thus, early use of these medications could potentially slow the progression of Parkinson disease. Levodopa can be incorporated into the drug regimen as disability increases, along with other medications such as amantadine, anticholinergics, and COMT inhibitors.[104]

There is no clear consensus of which drugs should be used in the initial and subsequent treatment of Parkinson disease. Future research should help clarify whether it is better to begin treatment with dopamine agonists and to save levodopa and other medications until later in the disease course. Ultimately, the physician should select specific medications based on a patient's individual characteristics at each stage of the disease.[1]

NEUROSURGICAL INTERVENTIONS IN PARKINSON DISEASE

Researchers are studying several innovative approaches to try to achieve a more permanent resolution to the dopamine imbalance in Parkinson disease. One approach is to surgically implant dopamine-producing cells into the substantia nigra to replace the cells that have been destroyed by the disease process.[105,106] However, this strategy is limited by several issues, including how to get a supply of viable cells. A potential source of these cells has been from fetal mesenchymal tissues. Embryonically derived stem cells have the potential to differentiate into virtually any type of human cell, which means they could be used to repair damaged tissues in many degenerative conditions, including Parkinson disease.[105,107]

This approach has generated considerable concern about the ethical use of fetal tissues for medical research and treatment. Alternative sources such as stem cells from adult bone marrow or human chromaffin cells have also been considered, but these sources might not be as effective as cells from embryonic tissues.[108,109] Regardless of the cells' source, there are some practical limitations associated with implanting a sufficient number of these into a small area deep in the brain and then keeping these cells alive and producing dopamine. Patients who would benefit from such transplants are typically older and somewhat debilitated with a possible reduction in blood flow and oxygenation of tissues deep in the brain. These facts, combined with the presence of the original pathological process that caused Parkinson disease, may limit the transplanted tissues' chances for survival.

Hence, tissue transplants have not shown overwhelming clinical success, and the future of this technique as an effective and widely used method of treating Parkinson disease remains doubtful at present.[106,110] It may be possible that new developments, including the use of cell cultures as a source of dopamine-producing cells and the use of drugs to prolong the survival of transplanted tissues, may improve the clinical outcome of this technique. Still, it remains to be seen whether tissue transplants will ever be a practical and routine method of treating the rather large number of patients with the disease.

An alternative nonpharmacological treatment involves the use of specific surgeries (pallidotomy, thalamotomy) to produce lesions in specific neuronal pathways in patients with advanced Parkinson disease.[111,112] However, these surgical lesions have been eclipsed somewhat by the use of deep brain stimulation in these patients.[112] Deep brain stimulation consists of surgically implanting electrodes into deep brain structures such as the globus pallidus, thalamus, and subthalamic nucleus.[113,114] High-frequency stimulation of these structures may help normalize neuronal circuitry within the basal ganglia and help resolve the motor and nonmotor symptoms of advanced Parkinson disease.[115] It is beyond the scope of this chapter to review these newer surgical and electrical stimulation techniques. But these nonpharmacological interventions continue to be developed and may provide an alternative treatment for patients who have become refractory to drug therapy during the advanced stages of the disease.[116]

Special Concerns for Rehabilitation Patients

Therapists who are treating patients with Parkinson disease usually wish to coordinate the therapy session with the peak effects of drug therapy. In patients receiving levodopa, this usually occurs approximately 1 hour after a dose has been taken. If possible, scheduling the primary therapy session in elderly patients after the breakfast dose of levodopa often yields optimal effects from the standpoint of both maximal drug efficacy and low fatigue levels.

Therapists working in hospitals and other institutions are sometimes faced with the responsibility of treating patients who are on a drug holiday. The patient is placed in the hospital for several days and all anti-Parkinson medication is withdrawn so that the patient may recover from the adverse effects of prolonged levodopa administration. During the drug holiday, the goal of physical rehabilitation is to maintain as much patient mobility as possible. Obviously, without anti-Parkinson drugs, this task is often quite difficult. Many patients are well into the advanced stages of the disease, and even a few days without medication can produce profound debilitating effects. Consequently, any efforts to maintain joint range of motion and cardiovascular fitness during the drug holiday are crucial in helping the patient resume activity when medications are reinstated.

Clinicians should also be aware of the need to monitor blood pressure in patients receiving anti-Parkinson drugs. Most of these drugs cause orthostatic hypotension, especially during the first few days of treatment. Dizziness and syncope often occur because of a sudden drop in blood pressure when the patient stands up. Because patients with Parkinson disease are susceptible to falls, this problem is only increased by the chance of orthostatic hypotension. Consequently, therapists must be especially careful to guard against falls by the patient taking anti-Parkinson drugs.

Finally, rehabilitation specialists should recognize that they can have a direct and positive influence on the patient's health and need for drug treatment. There is consensus that an aggressive program of gait training, balance activities, and other appropriate exercises can be extremely helpful in promoting optimal health and function in patients with Parkinson disease.[117-120] Using physical therapy and occupational therapy interventions to maintain motor function can diminish the patient's need for anti-Parkinson drugs. The synergistic effects of physical rehabilitation and the judicious use of drugs will ultimately provide better results than either intervention used alone.

CASE STUDY

ANTI-PARKINSON DRUGS

Brief History. M.M. is a 67-year-old woman who was diagnosed with Parkinson disease 6 years ago, at which time she was treated with a dopamine receptor agonist (ropinirole, 2 mg three times per day). After approximately 2 years, the bradykinesia and the rigidity associated with this disease began to be more pronounced, so she was started on a combination of levodopa-carbidopa. The initial levodopa dosage was 400 mg/d. She was successfully maintained on levodopa for the next 3 years, with minor adjustments in the dosage. During that time, M.M. had been living at home with her husband.

CASE STUDY (Continued)

During the past 12 months, her husband noted that her ability to get around seemed to be declining, so the levodopa dosage was progressively increased to 600 mg/d. The patient was also referred to physical therapy on an outpatient basis in an attempt to maintain mobility and activities of daily living (ADL). She began attending physical therapy three times per week, and the therapist initiated a regimen designed to maintain musculoskeletal flexibility, posture, and balance.

Problem/Influence of Medication. The patient was seen by the therapist three mornings each week. After a few sessions, the therapist observed that there were certain days when the patient was able to actively and vigorously participate in the therapy program. On other days, she was essentially akinetic, and her active participation in exercise and gait activities was virtually impossible. There was no pattern to her good and bad days, and the beneficial effects of the rehabilitation program seemed limited by the rather random effects of her medication. The patient stated that these akinetic episodes sometimes occurred even on nontherapy days.

1. ***What is the likely reason for the poor response to anti-Parkinson drugs on certain days?***
2. ***What can be done to resolve this problem and improve the patient's response to drug therapy?***

See Appendix C, "Answers to Case Study Questions."

SUMMARY

The cause of Parkinson disease remains unknown. Genetic factors combined with possible environmental influences may make certain people susceptible to this disease. However, the exact factors that initiate and perpetuate Parkinson disease remain to be determined. Nonetheless, the neuronal changes that produce the symptoms associated with this movement disorder have been identified. Degeneration of dopaminergic neurons in the substantia nigra results in a deficiency of dopamine and subsequent changes in other neurotransmitters in the basal ganglia. Drugs used to treat Parkinson disease attempt to either replace the missing dopamine (levodopa, dopamine agonists), prolong the effects of dopamine (MAO-B inhibitors), or normalize the effects of other neurotransmitters such as acetylcholine and glutamate. Although no cure is currently available, drug therapy can dramatically improve the clinical picture in many patients by reducing the incapacitating symptoms of parkinsonism.

The use of levodopa and several other medications has allowed many patients with Parkinson disease to remain active despite the disease's steadily degenerative nature. Levodopa remains the most effective treatment for parkinsonism, and this drug often produces remarkable improvements in motor function in the earlier stages of this disease. However, levodopa is associated with several troublesome side effects, and its effectiveness tends to diminish with time. Other agents, such as dopamine agonists, MAO-B inhibitors, amantadine, anticholinergic drugs, and COMT inhibitors, can be used alone, in combination with levodopa, or with each other to prolong the patient's functional status. Physical therapists and other rehabilitation specialists can maximize the effectiveness of their treatments by coordinating therapy sessions with drug administration. Therapists also play a vital role in maintaining function in the patient with Parkinson disease when the efficacy of these drugs begins to diminish.

REFERENCES

1. Chen JJ, Nelson MV, Swope DM. Parkinson's disease. In: DiPiro JT, et al, eds. *Pharmacotherapy: A Pathophysiologic Approach*. 8th ed. New York: McGraw-Hill; 2011.
2. Garcia Ruiz PJ, Catalán MJ, Fernández Carril JM. Initial motor symptoms of Parkinson disease. *Neurologist*. 2011;17 (suppl 1):S18-20.

3. Parent M, Parent A. Substantia nigra and Parkinson's disease: a brief history of their long and intimate relationship. *Can J Neurol Sci.* 2010;37:313-319.
4. Ali SF, Binienda ZK, Imam SZ. Molecular aspects of dopaminergic neurodegeneration: gene-environment interaction in parkin dysfunction. *Int J Environ Res Public Health.* 2011;8:4702-4713.
5. Burbulla LF, Krüger R. Converging environmental and genetic pathways in the pathogenesis of Parkinson's disease. *J Neurol Sci.* 2011;306:1-8.
6. Gao HM, Hong JS. Gene-environment interactions: key to unraveling the mystery of Parkinson's disease. *Prog Neurobiol.* 2011;94:1-19.
7. Gelabert-Gonzalez M, Serramito-García R, Aran-Echabe E. Parkinsonism secondary to subdural haematoma. *Neurosurg Rev.* 2012;35:457-460.
8. Gupta D, Kuruvilla A. Vascular parkinsonism: what makes it different? *Postgrad Med J.* 2011;87:829-836.
9. López-Sendón JL, Mena MA, de Yébenes JG. Drug-induced parkinsonism in the elderly: incidence, management and prevention. *Drugs Aging.* 2012;29:105-118.
10. Mazokopakis EE, Koutras A, Starakis I, Panos G. Pathogens and chronic or long-term neurologic disorders. *Cardiovasc Hematol Disord Drug Targets.* 2011;11:40-52.
11. Maetzler W, Liepelt I, Berg D. Progression of Parkinson's disease in the clinical phase: potential markers. *Lancet Neurol.* 2009;8:1158-1171.
12. Xia R, Mao ZH. Progression of motor symptoms in Parkinson's disease. *Neurosci Bull.* 2012;28:39-48.
13. Hurelbrink CB, Lewis SJ. Pathological considerations in the treatment of Parkinson's disease: more than just a wiring diagram. *Clin Neurol Neurosurg.* 2011;113:1-6.
14. Standaert DG, Roberson ED. Treatment of central nervous system disorders. In: Brunton LL, et al, eds. *The Pharmacological Basis of Therapeutics.* 12th ed. New York: McGraw Hill; 2011.
15. Gerfen CR, Surmeier DJ. Modulation of striatal projection systems by dopamine. *Annu Rev Neurosci.* 2011;34:441-466.
16. Kandel ER, Scwartz JH, Jessell TM, et al. The basal ganglia. In: *Principles of Neural Science.* 5th ed. New York: McGraw-Hill; 2013:982-998.
17. Aosaki T, Miura M, Suzuki T, et al. Acetylcholine-dopamine balance hypothesis in the striatum: an update. *Geriatr Gerontol Int.* 2010;10(suppl 1):S148-157.
18. Lester DB, Rogers TD, Blaha CD. Acetylcholine-dopamine interactions in the pathophysiology and treatment of CNS disorders. *CNS Neurosci Ther.* 2010;16:137-162.
19. Girault JA. Integrating neurotransmission in striatal medium spiny neurons. *Adv Exp Med Biol.* 2012;970:407-429.
20. Jaeger D, Kita H. Functional connectivity and integrative properties of globus pallidus neurons. *Neuroscience.* 2011;198:44-53.
21. Mathur BN, Lovinger DM. Serotonergic action on dorsal striatal function. *Parkinsonism Relat Disord.* 2012;18(suppl 1):S129-131.
22. Rylander D. The serotonin system: a potential target for anti-dyskinetic treatments and biomarker discovery. *Parkinsonism Relat Disord.* 2012;18(suppl 1):S126-128.
23. Houlden H, Singleton AB. The genetics and neuropathology of Parkinson's disease. *Acta Neuropathol.* 2012;124:325-338.
24. Kumar KR, Djarmati-Westenberger A, Grünewald A. Genetics of Parkinson's disease. *Semin Neurol.* 2011;31:433-440.
25. Wan OW, Chung KK. The role of alpha-synuclein oligomerization and aggregation in cellular and animal models of Parkinson's disease. *PLoS One.* 2012;7:e38545.
26. Marques O, Outeiro TF. Alpha-synuclein: from secretion to dysfunction and death. *Cell Death Dis.* 2012;3:e350.
27. Bellucci A, Navarria L, Zaltieri M, et al. α-Synuclein synaptic pathology and its implications in the development of novel therapeutic approaches to cure Parkinson's disease. *Brain Res.* 2012;1432:95-113.
28. Schulz-Schaeffer WJ. The synaptic pathology of alpha-synuclein aggregation in dementia with Lewy bodies, Parkinson's disease and Parkinson's disease dementia. *Acta Neuropathol.* 2010;120:131-143.
29. Vekrellis K, Xilouri M, Emmanouilidou E, et al. Pathological roles of α-synuclein in neurological disorders. *Lancet Neurol.* 2011;10:1015-1025.
30. Hansen C, Li JY. Beyond α-synuclein transfer: pathology propagation in Parkinson's disease. *Trends Mol Med.* 2012;18:248-255.
31. Reale M, Pesce M, Priyadarshini M, et al. Mitochondria as an easy target to oxidative stress events in Parkinson's disease. *CNS Neurol Disord Drug Targets.* 2012;11:430-438.
32. Valko M, Leibfritz D, Moncol J, et al. Free radicals and antioxidants in normal physiological functions and human disease. *Int J Biochem Cell Biol.* 2007;39:44-84.
33. Sutachan JJ, Casas Z, Albarracin SL, et al. Cellular and molecular mechanisms of antioxidants in Parkinson's disease. *Nutr Neurosci.* 2012;15:120-126.
34. Varçin M, Bentea E, Michotte Y, Sarre S. Oxidative stress in genetic mouse models of Parkinson's disease. *Oxid Med Cell Longev.* 2012;2012:624925.
35. Khan MS, Tabrez S, Priyadarshini M, et al. Targeting Parkinson's—tyrosine hydroxylase and oxidative stress as points of interventions. *CNS Neurol Disord Drug Targets.* 2012;11:369-380.
36. Schapira AH. Mitochondrial pathology in Parkinson's disease. *Mt Sinai J Med.* 2011;78:872-881.
37. Sorce S, Krause KH, Jaquet V. Targeting NOX enzymes in the central nervous system: therapeutic opportunities. *Cell Mol Life Sci.* 2012;69:2387-2407.
38. Langston JW, Ballard P, Tetrud JW, Irwin I. Chronic parkinsonism in humans due to a product of meperidine-analog synthesis. *Science.* 1983;219:979-980.
39. Abdulwahid Arif I, Ahmad Khan H. Environmental toxins and Parkinson's disease: putative roles of impaired electron transport chain and oxidative stress. *Toxicol Ind Health.* 2010;26:121-128.
40. Vanitallie TB. Parkinson disease: primacy of age as a risk factor for mitochondrial dysfunction. *Metabolism.* 2008;57(suppl 2):S50-55.
41. Vance JM, Ali S, Bradley WG, et al. Gene-environment interactions in Parkinson's disease and other forms of parkinsonism. *Neurotoxicology.* 2010;31:598-602.
42. van der Mark M, Brouwer M, Kromhout H, et al. Is pesticide use related to Parkinson disease? Some clues to heterogeneity in study results. *Environ Health Perspect.* 2012;120:340-347.
43. Albarracin SL, Stab B, Casas Z, et al. Effects of natural antioxidants in neurodegenerative disease. *Nutr Neurosci.* 2012;15:1-9.
44. Albrecht S, Buerger E. Potential neuroprotection mechanisms in PD: focus on dopamine agonist pramipexole. *Curr Med Res Opin.* 2009;25:2977-2987.
45. Naoi M, Maruyama W. Monoamine oxidase inhibitors as neuroprotective agents in age-dependent neurodegenerative disorders. *Curr Pharm Des.* 2010;16:2799-2817.
46. Hornykiewicz O. A brief history of levodopa. *J Neurol.* 2010;257(suppl 2):S249-252.

47. Maranis S, Tsouli S, Konitsiotis S. Treatment of motor symptoms in advanced Parkinson's disease: a practical approach. *Prog Neuropsychopharmacol Biol Psychiatry.* 2011;35:1795-1807.
48. del Amo EM, Urtti A, Yliperttula M. Pharmacokinetic role of L-type amino acid transporters LAT1 and LAT2. Eur J Pharm Sci. 2008;35:161-174.
49. Seeberger LC, Hauser RA. Optimizing bioavailability in the treatment of Parkinson's disease. *Neuropharmacology.* 2007;53:791-800.
50. Koller WC, Hutton JT, Tolosa E, Capilldeo R. Immediate-release and controlled-release carbidopa/levodopa in PD: a 5-year randomized multicenter study. Carbidopa/Levodopa Study Group. *Neurology.* 1999;53:1012-1019.
51. Aminoff MJ. Pharmacologic management of parkinsonism and other movement disorders. In: Katzung BG, Masters SB, Trevor AJ, eds. *Basic and Clinical Pharmacology.* 12th ed. New York: Lange Medical Books/McGraw Hill; 2012.
52. Blandini F, Armentero MT. New pharmacological avenues for the treatment of L-DOPA-induced dyskinesias in Parkinson's disease: targeting glutamate and adenosine receptors. *Expert Opin Investig Drugs.* 2012;21:153-168.
53. Fisone G, Bezard E. Molecular mechanisms of 1-DOPA-induced dyskinesia. *Int Rev Neurobiol.* 2011;98:95-122.
54. Iravani MM, McCreary AC, Jenner P. Striatal plasticity in Parkinson's disease and L-dopa induced dyskinesia. *Parkinsonism Relat Disord.* 2012;18(suppl 1):S123-125.
55. Carta M, Bezard E. Contribution of pre-synaptic mechanisms to L-DOPA-induced dyskinesia. *Neuroscience.* 2011;198:245-251.
56. Cheshire PA, Williams DR. Serotonergic involvement in levodopa-induced dyskinesias in Parkinson's disease. *J Clin Neurosci.* 2012;19:343-348.
57. Lindgren HS, Andersson DR, Lagerkvist S, et al. L-DOPA-induced dopamine efflux in the striatum and the substantia nigra in a rat model of Parkinson's disease: temporal and quantitative relationship to the expression of dyskinesia. *J Neurochem.* 2010;112:1465-1476.
58. Iravani MM, Jenner P. Mechanisms underlying the onset and expression of levodopa-induced dyskinesia and their pharmacological manipulation. *J Neural Transm.* 2011;118:1661-1690.
59. Gallagher DA, Schrag A. Psychosis, apathy, depression and anxiety in Parkinson's disease. *Neurobiol Dis.* 2012;46:581-589.
60. Hasnain M. Psychosis in Parkinson's disease: therapeutic options. *Drugs Today.* 2011;47:353-367.
61. Frieling H, Hillemacher T, Ziegenbein M, et al. Treating dopamimetic psychosis in Parkinson's disease: structured review and meta-analysis. *Eur Neuropsychopharmacol.* 2007;17:165-171.
62. Pahwa R, Lyons KE. Levodopa-related wearing-off in Parkinson's disease: identification and management. *Curr Med Res Opin.* 2009;25:841-849.
63. Cereda E, Barichella M, Pezzoli G. Controlled-protein dietary regimens for Parkinson's disease. *Nutr Neurosci.* 2010;13:29-32.
64. Imamura K, Okayasu N, Nagatsu T. Cerebral blood flow and freezing of gait in Parkinson's disease. *Acta Neurol Scand.* 2012;126:210-218.
65. Vercruysse S, Devos H, Munks L, et al. Explaining freezing of gait in Parkinson's disease: motor and cognitive determinants. *Mov Disord.* 2012;27:1644-1651.
66. Lee SJ, Yoo JY, Ryu JS, et al. The effects of visual and auditory cues on freezing of gait in patients with Parkinson disease. *Am J Phys Med Rehabil.* 2012;91:2-11.
67. Spildooren J, Vercruysse S, Meyns P, et al. Turning and unilateral cueing in Parkinson's disease patients with and without freezing of gait. *Neuroscience.* 2012;207:298-306.
68. Velik R, Hoffmann U, Zabaleta H, et al. The effect of visual cues on the number and duration of freezing episodes in Parkinson's patients. *Conf Proc IEEE Eng Med Biol Soc.* 2012;2012:4656-4659.
69. Frazzitta G, Maestri R, Uccellini D, et al. Rehabilitation treatment of gait in patients with Parkinson's disease with freezing: a comparison between two physical therapy protocols using visual and auditory cues with or without treadmill training. *Mov Disord.* 2009;24:1139-1143.
70. Koziorowski D, Friedman A. Levodopa "drug holiday" with amantadine infusions as a treatment of complications in Parkinson's disease. *Mov Disord.* 2007;22:1033-1036.
71. Corona T, Rivera C, Otero E, Stopp L. A longitudinal study of the effects of an L-dopa drug holiday on the course of Parkinson's disease. *Clin Neuropharmacol.* 1995;18:325-332.
72. Bonuccelli U, Del Dotto P, Rascol O. Role of dopamine receptor agonists in the treatment of early Parkinson's disease. *Parkinsonism Relat Disord.* 2009;15(suppl 4):S44-53.
73. Rascol O, Lozano A, Stern M, Poewe W. Milestones in Parkinson's disease therapeutics. *Mov Disord.* 2011;26:1072-1082.
74. Ribarič S. The pharmacological properties and therapeutic use of apomorphine. *Molecules.* 2012;17:5289-5309.
75. Khan TS. Off spells and dyskinesias: pharmacologic management of motor complications. *Cleve Clin J Med.* 2012;79(suppl 2):S8-13.
76. Stowe R, Ives N, Clarke CE, et al. Evaluation of the efficacy and safety of adjuvant treatment to levodopa therapy in Parkinson's disease patients with motor complications. *Cochrane Database Syst Rev.* 2010;7:CD007166.
77. Singer C. Managing the patient with newly diagnosed Parkinson disease. *Cleve Clin J Med.* 2012;79(suppl 2):S3-7.
78. Reichmann H. Transdermal delivery of dopamine receptor agonists. *Parkinsonism Relat Disord.* 2009;15(suppl 4):S93-96.
79. Nyholm D. Pharmacokinetic optimisation in the treatment of Parkinson's disease: an update. *Clin Pharmacokinet.* 2006;45:109-136.
80. Kvernmo T, Houben J, Sylte I. Receptor-binding and pharmacokinetic properties of dopaminergic agonists. *Curr Top Med Chem.* 2008;8:1049-1067.
81. Yuan H, Zhang ZW, Liang LW, et al. Treatment strategies for Parkinson's disease. *Neurosci Bull.* 2010;26:66-76.
82. Cancelli I, Beltrame M, Gigli GL, Valente M. Drugs with anticholinergic properties: cognitive and neuropsychiatric side-effects in elderly patients. *Neurol Sci.* 2009;30:87-92.
83. Hubsher G, Haider M, Okun MS. Amantadine: the journey from fighting flu to treating Parkinson disease. *Neurology.* 2012;78:1096-1099.
84. Gottwald MD, Aminoff MJ. Therapies for dopaminergic-induced dyskinesias in Parkinson disease. *Ann Neurol.* 2011;69:919-927.
85. Paquette MA, Martinez AA, Macheda T, et al. Anti-dyskinetic mechanisms of amantadine and dextromethorphan in the 6-OHDA rat model of Parkinson's disease: role of NMDA vs. 5-HT1A receptors. *Eur J Neurosci.* 2012;36:3224-3234.
86. Fabbrini G, Abbruzzese G, Marconi S, Zappia M. Selegiline: a reappraisal of its role in Parkinson disease. *Clin Neuropharmacol.* 2012;35:134-140.
87. Magyar K. The pharmacology of selegiline. *Int Rev Neurobiol.* 2011;100:65-84.

88. Nandagopal JJ, DelBello MP. Selegiline transdermal system: a novel treatment option for major depressive disorder. *Expert Opin Pharmacother.* 2009;10:1665-1673.
89. Riederer P, Laux G. MAO-inhibitors in Parkinson's disease. *Exp Neurobiol.* 2011;20:1-17.
90. Aluf Y, Vaya J, Khatib S, et al. Selective inhibition of monoamine oxidase A or B reduces striatal oxidative stress in rats with partial depletion of the nigro-striatal dopaminergic pathway. *Neuropharmacology.* 2013;65:48-57.
91. Weinreb O, Amit T, Bar-Am O, Youdim MB. Rasagiline: a novel anti-Parkinsonian monoamine oxidase-B inhibitor with neuroprotective activity. *Prog Neurobiol.* 2010;92:330-244.
92. Mandel S, Weinreb O, Amit T, Youdim MB. Mechanism of neuroprotective action of the anti-Parkinson drug rasagiline and its derivatives. *Brain Res Brain Res Rev.* 2005;48:379-387.
93. Chen JJ, Wilkinson JR. The monoamine oxidase type B inhibitor rasagiline in the treatment of Parkinson disease: is tyramine a challenge? *J Clin Pharmacol.* 2012;52:620-628.
94. Müller T, Hoffmann JA, Dimpfel W, Oehlwein C. Switch from selegiline to rasagiline is beneficial in patients with Parkinson's disease. *J Neural Transm.* 2013;120:761-765.
95. Marsala SZ, Gioulis M, Ceravolo R, Tinazzi M. A systematic review of catechol-o-methyltransferase inhibitors: efficacy and safety in clinical practice. *Clin Neuropharmacol.* 2012;35:185-190.
96. Truong DD. Tolcapone: review of its pharmacology and use as adjunctive therapy in patients with Parkinson's disease. *Clin Interv Aging.* 2009;4:109-113.
97. Schrag A. Entacapone in the treatment of Parkinson's disease. *Lancet Neurol.* 2005;4:366-370.
98. Nissinen E. Introductory remarks: catechol-O-methyltransferase inhibition—an innovative approach to enhance L-dopa therapy in Parkinson's disease with dual enzyme inhibition. *Int Rev Neurobiol.* 2010;95:1-5.
99. Nord M, Zsigmond P, Kullman A, et al. The effect of peripheral enzyme inhibitors on levodopa concentrations in blood and CSF. *Mov Disord.* 2010;25:363-367.
100. Kaakkola S. Problems with the present inhibitors and a relevance of new and improved COMT inhibitors in Parkinson's disease. *Int Rev Neurobiol.* 2010;95:207-225.
101. Jankovic J, Poewe W. Therapies in Parkinson's disease. *Curr Opin Neurol.* 2012;25:433-447.
102. Hauser RA. Early pharmacologic treatment in Parkinson's disease. *Am J Manag Care.* 2010;16(suppl implications):S100-107.
103. Caslake R, Macleod A, Ives N, et al. Monoamine oxidase B inhibitors versus other dopaminergic agents in early Parkinson's disease. *Cochrane Database Syst Rev.* 2009;4:CD006661.
104. Lyons KE, Pahwa R. Diagnosis and initiation of treatment in Parkinson's disease. *Int J Neurosci.* 2011;121(suppl 2):27-36.
105. Bjorklund A, Kordower JH. Cell therapy for Parkinson's disease: what next? *Mov Disord.* 2013;28:110-115.
106. Politis M, Lindvall O. Clinical application of stem cell therapy in Parkinson's disease. *BMC Med.* 2012;10:1.
107. Fricker-Gates RA, Gates MA. Stem cell-derived dopamine neurons for brain repair in Parkinson's disease. *Regen Med.* 2010;5:267-278.
108. Ambriz-Tututi M, Monjaraz-Fuentes F, Drucker-Colín R. Chromaffin cell transplants: from the lab to the clinic. *Life Sci.* 2012;91:1243-1251.
109. Zhao J, Xu Q. Emerging restorative treatments for Parkinson's disease: manipulation and inducement of dopaminergic neurons from adult stem cells. *CNS Neurol Disord Drug Targets.* 2011;10:509-516.
110. Lindvall O. Developing dopaminergic cell therapy for Parkinson's disease—give up or move forward? *Mov Disord.* 2013;28:268-273.
111. Hooper AK, Okun MS, Foote KD, et al. Clinical cases where lesion therapy was chosen over deep brain stimulation. *Stereotact Funct Neurosurg.* 2008;86:147-152.
112. Gross RE. What happened to posteroventral pallidotomy for Parkinson's disease and dystonia? *Neurotherapeutics.* 2008;5:281-293.
113. Chopra A, Tye SJ, Lee KH, et al. Underlying neurobiology and clinical correlates of mania status after subthalamic nucleus deep brain stimulation in Parkinson's disease: a review of the literature. *J Neuropsychiatry Clin Neurosci.* 2012;24:102-110.
114. Follett KA, Torres-Russotto D. Deep brain stimulation of globus pallidus interna, subthalamic nucleus, and pedunculopontine nucleus for Parkinson's disease: which target? *Parkinsonism Relat Disord.* 2012;18(suppl 1):S165-167.
115. Fasano A, Daniele A, Albanese A. Treatment of motor and non-motor features of Parkinson's disease with deep brain stimulation. *Lancet Neurol.* 2012;11:429-442.
116. Sharma A, Szeto K, Desilets AR. Efficacy and safety of deep brain stimulation as an adjunct to pharmacotherapy for the treatment of Parkinson disease. *Ann Pharmacother.* 2012;46:248-254.
117. Alonso-Frech F, Sanahuja JJ, Rodriguez AM. Exercise and physical therapy in early management of Parkinson disease. *Neurologist.* 2011;17(suppl 1):S47-53.
118. Speelman AD, van de Warrenburg BP, van Nimwegen M, et al. How might physical activity benefit patients with Parkinson disease? *Nat Rev Neurol.* 2011;7:528-534.
119. Tomlinson CL, Patel S, Meek C, et al. Physiotherapy versus placebo or no intervention in Parkinson's disease. *Cochrane Database Syst Rev.* 2012;8:CD002817.
120. Uitti RJ. Treatment of Parkinson's disease: focus on quality of life issues. *Parkinsonism Relat Disord.* 2012;18(suppl 1):S34-36.

CHAPTER 11

General Anesthetics

The discovery and development of anesthetic agents has been one of the most significant contributions in the advancement of surgical technique. Before the use of anesthesia, surgery was used only as a last resort and was often performed with the patient conscious but physically restrained by several large assistants. During the past century, anesthetic drugs have allowed surgeons to perform surgery in a manner that is safer and much less traumatic to the patient and that permits lengthier and more sophisticated surgical procedures.

Anesthetics are categorized as general or local, depending on whether the patient remains conscious when the anesthetic is administered. General anesthetics are usually administered for more extensive surgical procedures. Local anesthetics are given when analgesia is needed in a relatively small, well-defined area, or when the patient needs to remain conscious during surgery. The use of general anesthesia and general anesthetic agents is presented in this chapter; local anesthetics are addressed in Chapter 12.

Most physical therapists and other rehabilitation specialists are usually not involved with patients who are under general anesthesia. However, knowledge of how these agents work will help the therapist understand some of the residual effects of anesthesia. These effects may directly influence any therapy sessions that take place during the first few days after the procedure.

REQUIREMENTS FOR GENERAL ANESTHESIA

General anesthesia is a reversible state of unconsciousness. During major surgery (e.g., laparotomy, thoracotomy, joint replacement, amputation), the patient is unconscious throughout the procedure and upon awakening has no recollection of what occurred during the surgery.[1,2] An ideal anesthetic agent must be able to produce each of the following conditions:

- Rapid onset of anesthesia (loss of consciousness and sensation)
- Skeletal muscle relaxation (this requirement is currently met with the aid of skeletal muscle blockers used in conjunction with the anesthetic [see "Neuromuscular Blockers," below])
- Inhibition of sensory and autonomic reflexes
- Easy adjustment of the anesthetic dosage during the procedure
- A minimum of toxic side effects (i.e., be relatively safe)
- Rapid, uneventful recovery after administration is terminated
- Amnesia (i.e., no recollection of what occurred during the surgery)

Current general anesthetics meet these criteria quite well, providing that the dose is high enough to produce an adequate level of anesthesia but not so high that problems occur. The relationship between dosage and level, or plane, of anesthesia is discussed in the next section

INDUCTION STAGES OF GENERAL ANESTHESIA

During general anesthesia induction, the patient goes through a series of stages as the anesthetic dosage and amount of anesthesia reaching the brain progressively increase. These four stages of anesthesia are commonly identified accordingly:[1,3]

Stage I: Analgesia. The patient begins to lose somatic sensation but is still conscious and somewhat aware of what is happening.

Stage II: Excitement (Delirium). The patient is unconscious and amnesiac but appears agitated and restless. This paradoxical increase in the level of excitation is highly undesirable because patients may injure themselves while thrashing about. Thus, an effort is made to move as quickly as possible through this stage and on to stage III.

Stage III: Surgical Anesthesia. As the name implies, this level is desirable for the surgical procedure and begins with the onset of regular, deep respiration. Some sources subdivide this stage into several planes, according to respiration rate and reflex activity.[1]

Stage IV: Medullary Paralysis. This stage is marked by the cessation of spontaneous respiration because respiratory control centers located in the medulla oblongata are inhibited by excessive anesthesia. The ability of the medullary vasomotor center to regulate blood pressure is also affected, and cardiovascular collapse ensues. If this stage is inadvertently reached during anesthesia, respiratory and circulatory support must be provided or the patient will die.[1]

Consequently, the goal of the anesthesia provider is to bring the patient to stage III as rapidly as possible and to maintain the patient at that stage for the duration of the surgical procedure. This goal is often accomplished by using both an intravenous and an inhaled anesthetic agent. Finally, the anesthetic should not be administered any longer than necessary, or recovery will be delayed. This state is often accomplished by beginning to taper off the dosage toward the end of the surgical procedure so that the patient is already emerging from anesthesia as surgery is completed.

GENERAL ANESTHETIC AGENTS: CLASSIFICATION AND USE ACCORDING TO ROUTE OF ADMINISTRATION

Specific agents are classified according to the two primary routes of administration—IV or inhaled (Table 11-1).[1] Intravenously injected anesthetics offer the advantage of a rapid onset, thus allowing the patient to pass through the first two stages of anesthesia very quickly. The primary disadvantage is that there is a relative lack of control over the level of anesthesia if too much of the drug is injected. Inhaled anesthetics provide an easier method of making adjustments in the dosage during the procedure, but it takes a relatively long time for the onset of the appropriate level of anesthesia.

Consequently, a combination of injected and inhaled agents is often used sequentially during lengthier surgical procedures.[1] The IV drug is injected first to quickly get the patient to stage III, and an inhaled agent is then administered to maintain the patient in a stage of surgical anesthesia. In addition, IV and inhaled agents can be used in various combinations throughout surgery to provide optimal anesthetic effects with minimal side effects, an idea known commonly as *balanced anesthesia*. Ultimately, the selection of exactly which agents to use depends on the type and length of the surgical procedure, the surgeon's preference, the patient's condition, coexisting diseases, any possible interactions with other anesthetics, and even the patient's position during the procedure. We will look at the inhaled anesthetics first.

Inhalation Anesthetics

Inhaled anesthetics exist either as gases or as volatile liquids that can be easily mixed with air or oxygen and then inhaled by a patient.[4] A system of tubing and valves is usually employed to deliver the anesthetic directly to the patient through an endotracheal tube or a mask over the face (Fig. 11-1). This delivery system offers the obvious benefit of focusing the drug on the patient without anesthetizing everyone else in the room. These systems also allow for easy adjustment of the rate of delivery and concentration of the inhaled

Table 11-1
GENERAL ANESTHETICS

Anesthetic	Representative Structure
Inhaled Anesthetics	
Volatile liquids Desflurane (Suprane) Enflurane (Ethrane) Halothane (Fluothane) Isoflurane (Forane) Sevoflurane (Ultane)	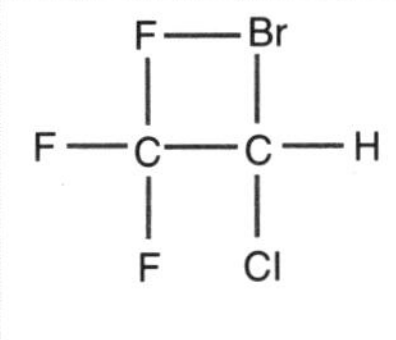 Halothane
Gas Nitrous oxide (nitrogen monoxide)	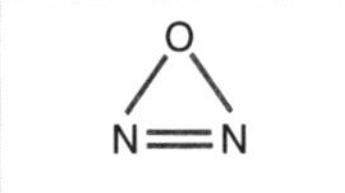 Nitrous oxide
Intravenous Anesthetics	
Barbiturates Methohexital (Brevital sodium) Thiopental (Pentothal)	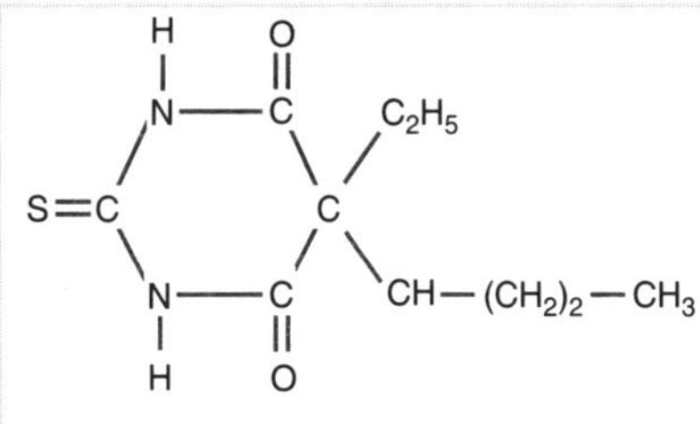 Thiopental
Benzodiazepines Diazepam (Valium) Lorazepam (Ativan) Midazolam (Versed)	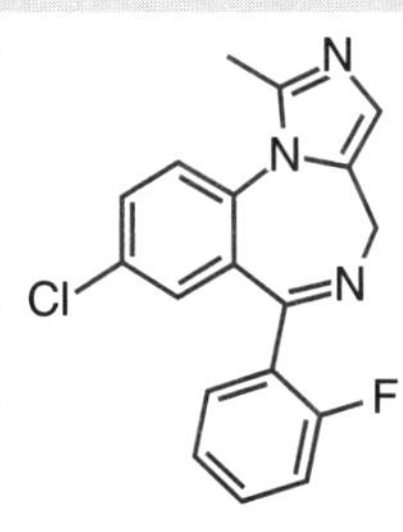 Midazolam
Opioids Butorphanol (Stadol) Fentanyl derivatives (Sublimaze, others) Meperidine (Demerol) Nalbuphine (Nubain) Oxymorphone (Opana) Pentazocine (Talwin)	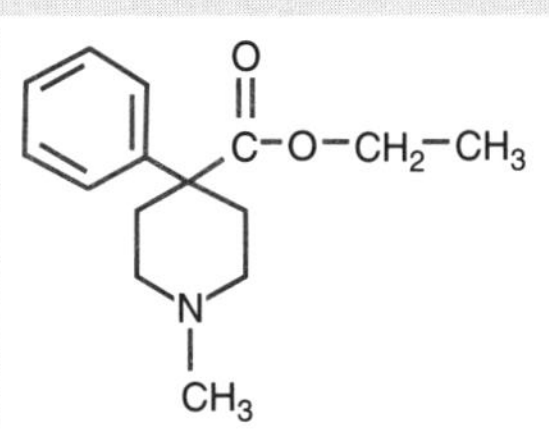 Meperidine

Continued

Table 11-1
GENERAL ANESTHETICS—cont'd

Anesthetic	Representative Structure
Dexmedetomidine (Precedex)	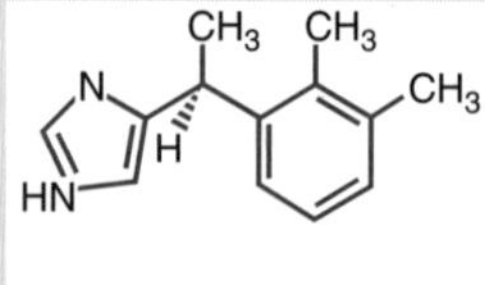 Dexmedetomidine
Etomidate (Amidate)	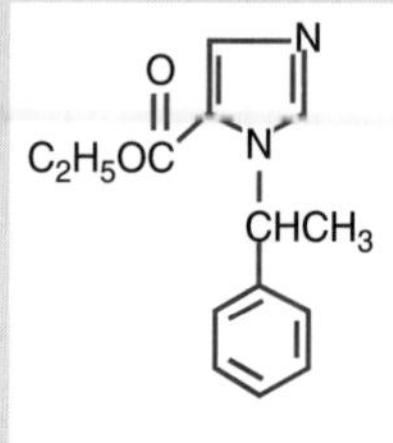 Etomidate
Ketamine (Ketalar)	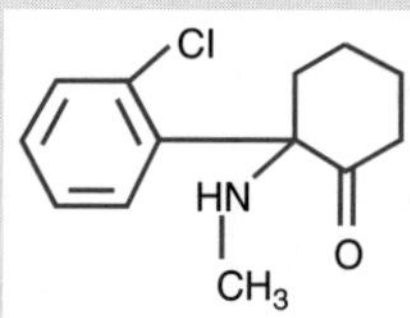 Ketamine
Fospropofol (Lusedra)	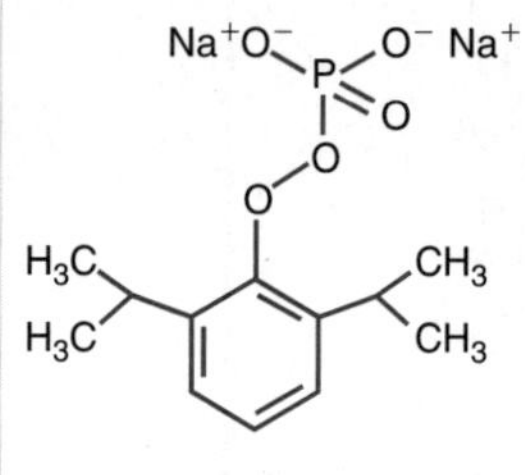 Fospropofol
Propofol (Diprivan)	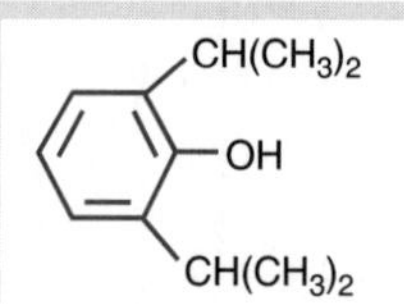 Propofol

drug. Some of these delivery systems have become very sophisticated, incorporating computerized feedback systems and other technological advancements that help monitor the depth of anesthesia and adjust anesthetic delivery throughout surgery.[5]

Inhaled anesthetics currently in use include halogenated volatile liquids such as enflurane, halothane, isoflurane, and the newer agents desflurane and sevoflurane. They are all chemically similar, but desflurane and sevoflurane are often preferred because they

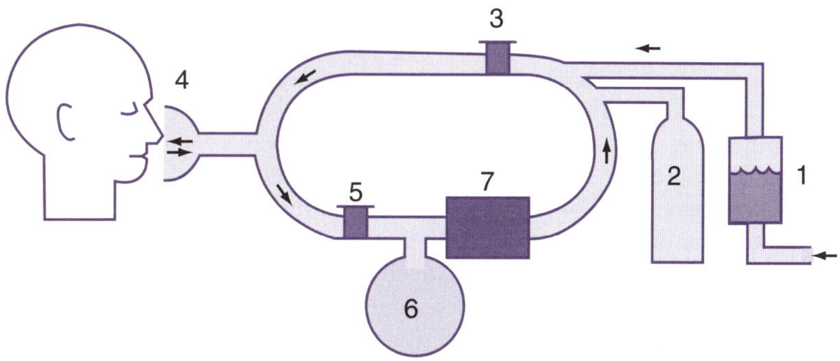

Figure ■ 11-1
Schematic diagram of a basic closed anesthesia system. **1.** Vaporizer for volatile liquid anesthetics. **2.** Compressed gas source. **3.** Inhalation unidirectional valve. **4.** Mask. **5.** Unidirectional exhalation valve. **6.** Rebreathing bag. **7.** Carbon dioxide absorption chamber.

permit a more rapid onset, a faster recovery, and better control during anesthesia compared to older agents such as halothane.[6-8] These volatile liquids represent the primary form of inhaled anesthetics. The only gaseous anesthetic currently in widespread use is nitrous oxide, which is usually reserved for relatively short-term procedures (e.g., tooth extractions). Earlier inhaled anesthetics, such as ether, chloroform, and cyclopropane, are not currently used because they are explosive in nature or produce toxic effects that do not occur with the more modern anesthetic agents.

Intravenous Anesthetics

When given in appropriate doses, several categories of central nervous system (CNS) depressants can be injected intravenously to provide general anesthesia (see Table 11-1).[9,10] Barbiturate drugs such as thiopental and methohexital have been used to induce anesthesia in many situations. Barbiturates are noted for their fast onset (when administered intravenously) and relative safety when used appropriately. However, use of barbiturates to induce anesthesia has declined somewhat in favor of newer agents such as propofol (discussed shortly).

Several other types of drugs, including benzodiazepines (e.g., diazepam, lorazepam, midazolam) and opioid analgesics (e.g., fentanyl, meperidine, others), have also been used to induce or help maintain general anesthesia. Although these other agents are often used as preoperative sedatives, larger doses can be used alone or in combination with other general anesthetics to produce anesthesia in short surgical or diagnostic procedures, or where other general anesthetics may be contraindicated (e.g., cardiovascular disease).

Another IV general anesthetic is ketamine (Ketalar).[11] This agent produces a somewhat different type of condition known as *dissociative anesthesia*.[1] This term is used because of the clinical observation that the patient appears detached or dissociated from the surrounding environment. The patient appears awake but is sedated and usually unable to recall events that occurred when the ketamine was in effect. Dissociative anesthesia using ketamine has certain drawbacks, including hallucinations, strange dreams, delusions, and other psychotropic reactions that can occur as the patient recovers from the anesthesia. On the other hand, ketamine does not cause respiratory problems or cardiac dysfunction to the same degree as traditional general anesthetics. Ketamine is therefore useful during relatively short diagnostic or surgical procedures (e.g., endoscopy) and during invasive procedures in children or certain high-risk patients—for example, in some older adults or people with low blood pressure or bronchospastic disease.[12,13]

In the past, combining the opioid fentanyl with the antipsychotic drug droperidol produced a similar type of dissociative anesthesia. The combination of these two agents produced a condition known as *neuroleptanesthesia*, which was also characterized by a dissociation from what was happening around the patient, with or without loss of consciousness.[14,15] Neuroleptanesthesia was typically used for short surgical procedures, including endoscopy or burn dressings or for patients who were seriously ill and might not tolerate general anesthesia using more conventional methods. However, neuroleptanesthesia is no longer used routinely due to the development of safer regimens using fast-acting anesthetics or by combining opioids with propofol or midazolam (a benzodiazepine).[14] At present, droperidol is used primarily as an antiemetic to prevent vomiting during and after surgery.

Propofol (Diprivan) is a short-acting hypnotic that takes effect rapidly and is often the drug of choice for inducing general anesthesia. This drug is also useful as a general anesthetic in some short invasive procedures or to maintain anesthesia in longer procedures.[16] Recovery from propofol may also be more rapid than with other anesthetics, making this drug useful when early mobilization of the patient is desirable.[2] Anesthesia providers can use continuous propofol infusion to sedate patients in the intensive care unit (ICU) who are critically ill and maintained on mechanical ventilation. Continuous infusion, however, may produce propofol infusion syndrome, which is a rare but potentially fatal syndrome characterized by bradycardia, metabolic acidosis, hyperlipidemia, rhabdomyolysis, and liver enlargement.[17]

Other IV anesthetics include etomidate (Amidate) and fospropofol (Lusedra). Etomidate is a hypnotic-like drug that causes a rapid onset of general anesthesia with a minimum of cardiopulmonary side effects. Hence, this drug may be useful in patients with compromised cardiovascular or respiratory function. Fospropofol is converted to propofol within the body. It is used primarily as an alternative to propofol during minor surgeries and diagnostic procedures (e.g., bronchoscopy, colonoscopy).

Finally, dexmedetomidine (Precedex) is a newer anesthetic used primarily for short-term (less than 24 hours) sedation in mechanically ventilated patients in the ICU.[18] Anesthesia providers can administer this drug as an adjunct during surgery to provide adequate anesthesia using relatively lower doses of the primary anesthetics. Dexmedetomidine differs chemically and functionally from more traditional anesthetics in that this drug stimulates certain alpha receptors in the brain; details about the mechanisms of general anesthetics are addressed later in this chapter.

PHARMACOKINETICS

Following either injection or inhalation administration, general anesthetics become widely and uniformly distributed throughout the body. The uniform distribution is largely due to their high degree of lipid solubility. As a result, a great deal of the anesthetic may become temporarily stored in adipose tissues and slowly washed out when the patient is recovering from surgery. If the person was anesthetized for an extended period of time and has large deposits of fat, this washout may take quite some time.[19] During this period, symptoms such as confusion, disorientation, and lethargy may occur, presumably because the drug is being redistributed to the CNS. The patient's age also influences anesthetic requirements and distribution. Because older people need smaller concentrations of anesthetic, there is a greater chance that too much anesthetic will be administered during surgery and recovery will be somewhat delayed.[20] Likewise, use of anesthetics in neonates is complicated; very young children have small body mass and their organ function is immature but changes rapidly as the child ages.[21] Hence, anesthetic dosages must be adjusted carefully, depending on the child's age and current level of function in the liver, kidneys, and other organ systems.

Depending on the individual drug, elimination occurs primarily through excretion from the lungs, biotransformation in the liver, or a combination of these two methods.[1] If the patient has any pulmonary or hepatic dysfunction, elimination of the anesthetic will be further delayed.

MECHANISM OF ACTION

Although general anesthetics have been used extensively for over 150 years, debate still exists as to exactly how these drugs work. Clearly they inhibit the neuronal activity throughout the CNS. It also appears that they can decrease activity of neurons in the reticular activating system in the brain, which explains their ability to produce sedation, hypnosis, and amnesia during surgery.[4] General anesthetics likewise inhibit neuronal function in the spinal cord, and this action produces immobility and inhibits motor responses to painful stimuli.[4]

The exact way in which these drugs affect these neurons remains somewhat speculative. In the past, it was believed that all general anesthetics shared a common mechanism of action involving the lipid bilayer of CNS neurons. This so-called unitary or general perturbation theory was based on the premise that general anesthetic molecules dissolve directly in the nerve membrane's lipid bilayer. Once the molecules are dissolved, they serve to generally perturb membrane function by increasing membrane fluidity and disrupting the phospholipid environment that surrounds the protein channel.[4,22] Membrane excitability would be decreased because ion channels, including sodium channels, are unable to open and allow the influx of sodium needed to initiate an action potential. The primary support for the membrane perturbation theory was the direct correlation between anesthetic potency and lipid solubility,[4] meaning that the more easily the drug dissolves in the bilayer, the less is needed to achieve a given level of anesthesia. This theory was further supported by the fact that general anesthetics all produce a similar effect, even though they have quite diverse chemical structures (see Table 11-1). Presumably, if drugs bind to a certain type of receptor, they should share some structural similarities.

However, more recent evidence suggests that general anesthetics bind to specific receptors located on the outer surface of CNS neurons (Fig. 11-2).[4,22] In particular, many general anesthetics bind to CNS receptors that are specific for gamma-aminobutyric acid (GABA). As discussed in Chapter 6, GABA receptors contain a chloride ion channel that, when activated by GABA, increases influx of chloride ions into the neuron, thereby inhibiting that neuron. By binding to the $GABA_A$ subtype receptors in the brain and cord, IV anesthetics such as barbiturates, benzodiazepines, and propofol, as well as the typical inhaled forms such as enflurane, halothane, and sevoflurane, increase the effects of GABA, thus enhancing CNS inhibition throughout the CNS.[23-25] This widespread CNS inhibition ultimately leads to a state of general anesthesia.

But some of the anesthetic effects might also be mediated by other receptors. For example, many general anesthetics also affect a glycine receptor that is structurally and functionally similar to the $GABA_A$ receptor—that is, when the anesthetic binds to this receptor, glycine (an inhibitory amino acid) is able to increase chloride entry to a greater extent, resulting in increased inhibition of the synapse.[2]

Halothane and similar inhaled general anesthetics may also activate specific pre- and postsynaptic potassium channels at excitatory synapses, thus increasing potassium exit from the cell and causing hyperpolarization and inhibition of these neurons.[2] These inhaled agents also bind to excitatory acetylcholine receptors on CNS neurons and inhibit the function of these receptors. This combination of increased inhibition (through GABA receptors and glycine receptors) and decreased excitation (through potassium channels and acetylcholine receptors) would certainly explain why these drugs are so effective in reducing the level of consciousness and excitability throughout the brain and cord.[26]

In addition to GABA and acetylcholine receptors, other CNS receptors have been implicated in mediating the effects of specific general anesthetics (see Fig. 11-2). In particular, researchers identified the *N*-methyl-D-aspartate (NMDA) receptor in the brain as an important site of action for certain agents. This receptor is normally stimulated by excitatory amino acids such as glutamate. Anesthetics like ketamine and nitrous oxide block this receptor, thus reducing excitation

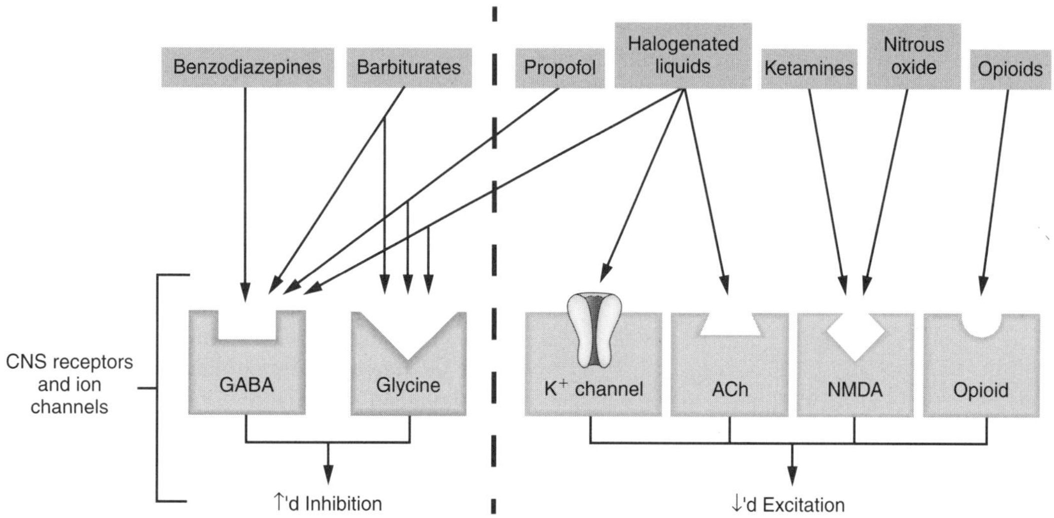

Figure ■ 11-2
General anesthetic effects on protein receptors and ion channels in the CNS. Specific agents produce anesthesia by increasing inhibitory receptor/channel activity, decreasing excitatory receptor/channel activity, or by a combination of these two mechanisms. Abbreviations: GABA = gamma-aminobutyric acid; K^+ = potassium; ACh = acetylcholine; NMDA = *N*-methyl-D-aspartate.

at these synapses.[22] Opioids likewise decrease transmission in nociceptive pathways by binding to specific presynaptic and postsynaptic opioid receptors in the brain and spinal cord (see Chapter 14). Other potential cellular targets for general anesthetics include serotonin receptors and neuronal ion channels, such as sodium and calcium channels.[23,27,28] However, the response of these other targets to currently available drugs remains to be clarified.

Finally, dexmedetomidine has a unique mechanism of action because it is an alpha-2 receptor agonist—that is, it stimulates alpha-2 receptors in the CNS.[18] Alpha-2 receptors are located presynaptically in specific CNS pathways, and activation of these receptors generally causes inhibition of neuronal activity in these pathways (see Chapter 20). Hence, it seems that dexmedetomidine produces analgesia by stimulating alpha-2 receptors in the spinal cord and causes hypnosis via an effect on these receptors in the locus coeruleus area of the brain.[1] It will be interesting to see if other alpha-2 agonists with anesthetic properties are developed in the future.

It is therefore believed that general anesthetics exert most, if not all, of their effects by binding to one or more neuronal receptors in the CNS. This idea is a departure from the lipid-based general perturbation theory described earlier—that anesthetics affected the lipid bilayer rather than a specific protein. By affecting specific neuronal protein receptors, general anesthetics can increase the inhibitory effects of neurotransmitters such as GABA and glycine, decrease the excitatory effects of neurotransmitters such as glutamate and acetylcholine, or directly affect the movements of other ions across neuronal membranes. These effects share the common goal of decreasing excitability in neurons throughout the CNS that affect consciousness. Researchers will continue to clarify the mechanism of these drugs, and future studies may lead to more agents that produce selective anesthetic effects by acting at specific receptor sites in the brain and spinal cord.

ADJUVANTS IN GENERAL ANESTHESIA

The general anesthetic drug cannot always provide all the effects needed for optimal patient comfort and safety throughout a surgical procedure. Hence, other drugs can be administered as adjuvants to balance the effects of the general anesthetic. Such adjuvant drugs include preoperative medications and neuromuscular blockers.

Preoperative Medications

Frequently, a preoperative sedative is given to a patient 1 to 2 hours before the administration of general anesthesia.[29] Sedatives are usually administered orally or by intramuscular injection and are often given while the patient is still in his or her hospital room or a preoperative preparatory area. This approach serves to relax the patient and reduce anxiety when arriving at the operating room. Some sedatives also decrease the patient's ability to remember what happened during certain procedures such as colonoscopy (amnesiac effect). Commonly used preoperative sedatives include barbiturates, opioids, and benzodiazepines (Table 11-2). Different sedatives are selected depending on the patient, the type of general anesthesia used, and the physician's preference. Likewise, analgesics and other preoperative sedatives may be continued during and after the surgery to supplement the effects of the primary anesthetic(s) and help the patient recover from surgery. A number of other medications can be used preoperatively to achieve various goals (see Table 11-2).[1,30]

Antihistamines (e.g., promethazine, hydroxyzine) offer the dual advantage of producing sedation and reducing vomiting (antiemesis) during and after surgery. Drugs that decrease stomach acidity, such as the histamine type 2 receptor blockers cimetidine (Tagamet) and ranitidine (Zantac) (see Chapter 27), can be administered preoperatively to reduce the risk of serious lung damage if gastric fluid is aspirated during general surgery.[31,32] Preoperative administration of an anti-inflammatory steroid such as dexamethasone (see Chapter 29) can help control postoperative symptoms such as pain and vomiting.[33,34]

Likewise, drugs such as ondansetron (Zofran) and granisetron (Kytril) also decrease postoperative nausea and vomiting via their ability to block certain CNS 5-HT_3 (serotonin) receptors associated with GI function. Anticholinergics such as atropine and scopolamine (Chapter19) can also help decrease postoperative nausea and vomiting. In the past, anticholinergics were commonly used to reduce bronchial secretions and aid in airway intubation. However, modern anesthetics do not produce excessive airway secretions (as did prior agents), so the preoperative use of anticholinergics to decrease airway secretions is no longer critical.[29]

Table 11-2
COMMON PREOPERATIVE MEDICATIONS: DRUGS AND DOSES USED

Preoperative Indication	Drug	Method of Administration*
Barbiturates		
Decrease anxiety; facilitate induction of anesthesia	Amobarbital	Oral: 200 mg 1 to 2 hours before surgery
	Pentobarbital	Oral: 100 mg IM: 150–200 mg
	Phenobarbital	IM: 100–200 mg 60 to 90 minutes before surgery
	Secobarbital	Oral: 200–300 mg 1 to 2 hours before surgery
Opioids**		
Provide analgesic, antianxiety, and sedative effects	Butorphanol	IV: 2 mg 60–90 minutes before surgery
	Fentanyl	IM or IV: 0.05-.10 mg 30-60 minutes before surgery
	Meperidine	IM or SC: 50-100 mg 30 to 90 minutes before surgery
Benzodiazepines		
Decrease anxiety and tension; provide sedation and amnesia	Diazepam	IM: 5–10 mg 30 minutes prior to surgery IV: 2.5-20 mg 30 minutes prior to surgery
	Lorazepam	IM: 0.05 mg/kg body weight (4 mg maximum) 2 hours before surgery IV: 0.044 mg/kg body weight (2 mg maximum) 15 to 20 minutes before surgery
	Midazolam	IM: 0.07-0.08 mg/kg (usual total dose 5 mg) 60 minutes before surgery
Antihistamines		
Provide sedative-hypnotic effects. Reduces vomiting.	Hydroxyzine	Oral: 50–100 mg
	Promethazine	IM or IV: 25-50 mg before surgery
Anticholinergics		
Prevent excessive salivation and respiratory tract secretions; reduce postoperative nausea and vomiting	Atropine	Oral: 2 mg IM, IV, or SC: 0.4–0.6 mg 30 to 60 minutes before surgery
	Glycopyrrolate	IM: 0.0044 mg/kg body weight 30 to 60 minutes before induction of anesthesia (0.1 mg maximum)
	Scopolamine	IM, IV, or SC: 0.2–0.6 mg 30 to 60 minutes before induction of anesthesia
H2 Receptor Blockers		
Reduce gastric acidity; help prevent aspiration pneumonitis	Cimetidine	IM: 300 mg 1 hour before induction of anesthesia; 300 mg every 4 hours until patient regains consciousness
	Ranitidine	IM: 50 mg 45 to 60 minutes before induction of anesthesia
5-HT$_3$ (Serotonin) Receptor Antagonists		
Reduce postoperative nausea and vomiting	Granisetron	IV: 1 mg prior to induction of anesthesia or just prior to reversal of anesthesia
	Ondansetron	IM or IV: 4 mg before induction of anesthesia or postoperatively

* *Typical adult doses. IV, intravenous; IM, intramuscular; SC, subcutaneous.*
** *Virtually all opioids can be used as a preoperative medication. Selection of a specific type and dose can be individualized based on the needs of each patient.*

Neuromuscular Blockers

Skeletal muscle paralysis is essential during surgical procedures. The patient must be relaxed to allow proper positioning on the operating table and to prevent spontaneous muscle contractions from hampering the surgery.[1,35] Imagine the disastrous effects that a muscular spasm in the arm would have on a delicate procedure such as nerve repair or limb reattachment. Neuromuscular paralysis also makes it easier for the patient to be ventilated mechanically because the thoracic wall is more compliant and does not offer as much resistance to mechanical inflation and deflation of the chest cavity. Hence, these drugs are used as an adjunct to general anesthesia and in other situations that require mechanical ventilation (e.g., ICUs).

Most currently used general anesthetics also produce skeletal muscle relaxation. However, to produce adequate muscular relaxation requires more anesthetic than is needed to produce unconsciousness and amnesia. The patient must be well into stage III and almost into stage IV of anesthesia before muscle paralysis is complete. Consequently, a drug that ensures skeletal muscle paralysis is given in conjunction with a general anesthetic to allow the use of a lower dose of anesthetic. These drugs work by blocking the postsynaptic acetylcholine receptor located at the skeletal neuromuscular junction.

Several different neuromuscular blockers are currently available, and the choice of agent depends primarily on the desired length of action and the drug's potential side effects (Table 11-3).[36,37] Possible side effects include cardiovascular problems (tachycardia), increased histamine release, increased plasma potassium levels (hyperkalemia), residual muscle pain and weakness, and immunological reactions (anaphylaxis).[36] For example, a drug that produces relatively little cardiovascular effects would be selected for a patient with cardiovascular disease.

Efforts are also made to use small doses of relatively short-acting agents so that the length of muscle paralysis is minimized.[35] The paralytic effects of these agents should disappear by the end of the surgical procedure. If necessary, drugs such as neostigmine or edrophonium can also be administered to help reverse the effects of neuromuscular blockade.[38,39] These drugs inhibit acetylcholinesterase, the enzyme that breaks down acetylcholine, thereby prolonging the effects of acetylcholine and hastening recovery of motor function. The pharmacology of acetylcholinesterase inhibitors is addressed in more detail in Chapter 19. Likewise, an agent called *sugammedex* rapidly inactivates two common neuromuscular blockers (rocuronium, vecuronium) by encapsulating them and terminating their ability to block the neuromuscular junction.[40,41] Sugammedex appears to work faster and

Table 11-3
NEUROMUSCULAR JUNCTION BLOCKERS

Generic Name	Trade Name	Onset*	Peak	Duration
Depolarizing Blocker				
Succinylcholine	Anectine, Quelicin	0.5–1.0 min	1–2 min	4–10 min
Nondepolarizing Blockers				
Atracurium	Tracrium	1–4 min	3–5 min	20–35 min
Cisatracurium	Nimbex	2–3 min	3–5 min	28–50 min
Doxacurium	Nuromax	5–11 min	Unknown	12–54 min
Gallamine	Flaxedil	1–2 min	3–5 min	15–30 min
Metocurine	Metubine	Within min	6 min	25–90 min‡
Mivacurium	Mivacron	1–3 min	3.3 min	26 min
Pancuronium	Pavulon	30–45 sec	2–3 min	40–60 min
Pipecuronium	Arduan	2.5–3 min	5 min	1–2 hr
Rocuronium	Zemuron	1 min	3.7 min	26–40 min
Tubocurarine	Tubarine	1 min	2–5 min	2–90 min
Vecuronium	Norcuron	1–3 min	3–5 min	30–40 min

**Reflects usual adult intravenous dose.*
‡Total recovery of function may take several hours.
Source: Ciccone CD: Davis's Drug Guide for Rehabilitation Professionals. *Philadelphia: FA Davis; 2013.*

may be associated with fewer side effects than more traditional acetylcholinesterase inhibitors.[40,42] At the time of this writing, sugammedex is available in other countries and is currently awaiting approval in the United States.

Clinicians should be aware that the residual effects of the neuromuscular blocker can persist in some patients long after surgery is complete.[35] The most serious complication is residual paralysis—that is, skeletal muscle contraction remains depressed for several hours after the drug should have worn off.[43,44] In extreme cases, this residual paralysis necessitates that the patient remain in intensive care with a mechanical ventilator to provide respiratory support.

It is not always clear why certain patients do not recover adequately from neuromuscular blockade. In some cases, the residual effects are attributed to genetic differences in the enzymes responsible for metabolizing the neuromuscular blocker.[36] If these enzymes are deficient or absent, the patient cannot adequately metabolize the blocker, hence paralysis continues for days or even weeks. In other patients, residual effects may occur if the patient has impaired liver and kidney function that results in decreased ability to metabolize and excrete the drugs.[36,45]

Anesthesia providers tend to use these drugs carefully and must verify that their effects have worn off before the patient leaves the operating room. In fact, electric stimulation of a peripheral nerve (e.g., ulnar nerve) can be used to objectively determine if there is residual muscle paralysis.[43] The muscles supplied by the nerve must show an appropriate twitch response to a given electric stimulus to ensure the patient has recovered adequately from the neuromuscular blocking drug.[43,46]

It should also be realized that neuromuscular junction blockers are an adjunct to general anesthesia; these blockers do not cause anesthesia or analgesia when used alone.[2] The anesthesia provider must give the patient an adequate amount of the general anesthetic throughout the surgery when a neuromuscular junction blocker is used. This idea is critical considering that the patient will be paralyzed by the neuromuscular junction blocker and unable to respond to painful stimuli if the anesthesia is inadequate. Failure to provide adequate anesthesia has resulted in some harrowing reports from patients who were apparently fully awake during surgery but unable to move or cry out.[47,48]

There are two general types of neuromuscular blockers. The types are classified according to those that depolarize the skeletal muscle cell when binding to the cholinergic receptor and those that do not.[49]

Nondepolarizing Blockers

These drugs act as competitive antagonists of the postsynaptic receptor; they bind to the receptor but do not activate it (see Chapter 4). This binding prevents the agonist (acetylcholine) from binding to the receptor; the result is paralysis of the muscle cell. These drugs all share a structural similarity to curare (the first neuromuscular blocker), which explains their affinity and relative selectivity for the cholinergic receptor at the skeletal neuromuscular junction. Specific agents, their onset, and duration of action are listed in Table 11-3.

Depolarizing Blocker

Although these drugs also inhibit transmission at the skeletal neuromuscular junction, their mechanism is different from that of the nondepolarizing agents. These drugs initially act like acetylcholine by binding to and stimulating the receptor, resulting in depolarization of the muscle cell. However, the enzymatic degradation of the drug is not as rapid as the destruction of acetylcholine, so the muscle cell remains depolarized for a prolonged period. While depolarized, the muscle is unresponsive to further stimulation. The cell must become repolarized, or reprimed, before the cell will respond to a second stimulus. This event is often referred to as *phase I blockade*.[49]

If the depolarizing blocker remains at the synapse, the muscle cell eventually repolarizes, but it will remain unresponsive to stimulation by acetylcholine. This occurrence is referred to as *phase II blockade* and is believed to occur because the drug modifies the receptor in some way. This modification could be in the form of a temporary change in the receptor's shape. Clinically, when these drugs are first administered, they are often associated with a variable amount of muscle tremor and fasciculation (because of the initial depolarization), but this is followed by a period of flaccid paralysis. Although several drugs can act as depolarizing blockers, the only agent currently in clinical use is succinylcholine (see Table 11-3).[49]

Special Concerns for Rehabilitation Patients

A rehabilitation specialist is most likely to encounter major problems when the patient is not quite over the effects of the anesthesia. Dealing with a patient the day after surgery or even on the same day might be difficult because he or she is woozy. Some anesthetics may produce confusion or psychotic-like behavior (delirium) during the recovery period, especially in older adults and after certain procedures such as cardiac surgery or joint replacement.[50,51] Muscle weakness may also occur for a variable amount of time, especially if a neuromuscular blocker was used during the surgical procedure. Of course, patients who are in relatively good health and who have had relatively short or minor surgeries will have minimal residual effects. However, patients who are debilitated or who have other medical problems impairing drug elimination may continue to show some anesthesia aftereffects for several days.[2] These problems should disappear with time, so clinicians must plan activities accordingly until recovery from the anesthetic is complete.

Another problem that therapists frequently deal with is the tendency for bronchial secretions to accumulate in the lungs of patients recovering from general anesthesia. General anesthetics depress mucociliary clearance in the airway, leading to a pooling of mucus, which may produce respiratory infections and atelectasis. Therapists play an important role in preventing this accumulation by encouraging the patient's early mobilization and by implementing respiratory hygiene protocols (i.e., breathing exercises and postural drainage).

Finally, there is concern that general anesthesia may cause long-term detrimental effects on memory, attention, and other aspects of cognition.[52,53] In particular, there may be a subtle but progressive decrease in cognition that occurs during the weeks and months after surgery. Postoperative cognitive decline may be especially prevalent in older adults and patients who already had some degree of cognitive dysfunction before surgery.[54,55] Likewise, patients with delirium immediately after surgery may be more susceptible to changes in cognition within the first postoperative year.[51,56] The exact reasons for this cognitive decline are not clear but may be related to several factors, including the type of surgery, the anesthetic used, the duration the anesthetic was administered, and how deeply the patient was anesthetized during the surgery. Hence, clinicians should be alert for any changes in the patient's cognition, intellect, or memory that may occur following use of general anesthesia. Evidence of cognitive decline should be documented and reported to the physician.

CASE STUDY

GENERAL ANESTHETICS

Brief History. B.W., a 75-year-old woman, fell at home and experienced a sudden sharp pain in her left hip. She was unable to walk and was taken to a nearby hospital where x-ray examination showed an impacted fracture of the left hip. The patient was alert and oriented at the time of admission. She had a history of arteriosclerotic cardiovascular disease and diabetes mellitus, which were managed successfully by various medications. The patient was relatively obese, and a considerable amount of osteoarthritis was present in both hips. Two days after admission, a total hip arthroplasty was performed under general anesthesia. Meperidine (Demerol) was given intramuscularly as a preoperative

CASE STUDY (Continued)

sedative. General anesthesia was induced by IV administration of thiopental (Pentothal) and sustained by inhalation of sevoflurane (Ultane). The surgery was completed successfully, and physical therapy was initiated at the patient's bedside on the subsequent day.

Problem/Influence of Medication. At the initial therapy session, the therapist found the patient to be extremely lethargic and disoriented. She appeared confused about recent events and was unable to follow most commands. Apparently, she was experiencing some residual effects of the general anesthesia.

1. ***How can the therapist safely begin rehabilitation given this patient's confusion?***
2. ***Can any interventions help the patient overcome the residual anesthetic effects?***

See Appendix C, "Answers to Case Study Questions."

SUMMARY

General anesthesia has been used for some time to permit surgical procedures of various types and durations. Several different effective agents are currently available and are relatively safe in producing a suitable anesthetic condition in the patient. General anesthetics are classified according to their two primary routes of administration: inhalation and IV infusion. There is still considerable debate about exactly how these drugs cause general anesthesia, but it is clear that at least some of the anesthetic effects of inhaled and IV agents are mediated by specific receptors located on CNS neurons. These drugs are also highly lipid soluble and can be stored temporarily in adipose tissues. Release from these storage sites may help account for prolonged sedative-like effects when the patient is recovering from a lengthy surgical procedure.

Specific anesthetic agents and anesthetic adjuvants (e.g., preoperative sedatives, neuromuscular blockers, etc.) are selected according to many factors, including the type of surgical procedure being performed, the surgeon's preference, and the patient's overall condition. Several different anesthetics and anesthetic adjuvants are often combined to provide optimal results during surgery and provide balanced anesthesia. Health professionals should be cognizant of the fact that their patients may take some time to fully recover from the effects of general anesthesia and should adjust their postoperative care accordingly.

REFERENCES

1. Eilers H, Yost S. General anesthetics. In: Katzung BG, Masters SB, Trevor AJ, eds. *Basic and Clinical Pharmacology.* 12th ed. New York: Lange Medical Books/McGraw Hill; 2012:429-447.
2. Patel PM, Patel HH, Roth DM. General anesthetics and therapeutic gases. In: Brunton LL, et al, eds. *The Pharmacological Basis of Therapeutics.* 12th ed. New York: McGraw Hill; 2011:527-564.
3. Prielipp RC. An anesthesiologist's perspective on inhaled anesthesia decision-making. *Am J Health Syst Pharm.* 2010;67 (suppl 4):S13-20.
4. Perouansky M, Pearce RA, Hemmings HC. Inhaled anesthetics: mechanisms of action. In: Miller RD, et al, eds. *Miller's Anesthesia.* Vol 1. 7th ed. Philadelphia, PA: Churchill Livingstone Elsevier; 2010:515-538.
5. Brockwell RC, Andrews JJ. Inhaled anesthetic delivery systems. In: Miller RD, et al, eds. *Miller's Anesthesia.* Vol 1. 7th ed. Philadelphia, PA: Churchill Livingstone Elsevier; 2010: 667-718.
6. Jakobsson J. Desflurane: a clinical update of a third-generation inhaled anaesthetic. *Acta Anaesthesiol Scand.* 2012;56: 420-432.
7. Michel F, Constantin JM. Sevoflurane inside and outside the operating room. *Expert Opin Pharmacother.* 2009;10:861-873.
8. Torri G. Inhalation anesthetics: a review. *Minerva Anestesiol.* 2010;76:215-228.
9. Reves JG, Glass PSA, Lubarsky DA, et al. Intravenous anesthetics. In: Miller RD, et al, eds. *Miller's Anesthesia.* Vol 1. 7th ed. Philadelphia, PA: Churchill Livingstone Elsevier; 2010:719-768.
10. Sneyd JR, Rigby-Jones AE. New drugs and technologies, intravenous anaesthesia is on the move (again). *Br J Anaesth.* 2010; 105:246-254.
11. Berti M, Baciarello M, Troglio R, Fanelli G. Clinical uses of low-dose ketamine in patients undergoing surgery. *Curr Drug Targets.* 2009;10:707-715.

12. Jamora C, Iravani M. Unique clinical situations in pediatric patients where ketamine may be the anesthetic agent of choice. *Am J Ther.* 2010;17:511-515.
13. Strayer RJ, Nelson LS. Adverse events associated with ketamine for procedural sedation in adults. *Am J Emerg Med.* 2008;26:985-1028.
14. Bissonnette B, Swan H, Ravussin P, Un V. Neuroleptanesthesia: current status. *Can J Anaesth.* 1999;46:154-168.
15. Meltzer H. Antipsychotic agents and lithium. In: Katzung BG, Masters SB, Trevor AJ, eds. *Basic and Clinical Pharmacology.* 12th ed. New York: Lange Medical Books/McGraw Hill; 2012: 501-520.
16. Ellett ML. Review of propofol and auxiliary medications used for sedation. *Gastroenterol Nurs.* 2010;33:284-295; quiz 296-297.
17. Wong JM. Propofol infusion syndrome. *Am J Ther.* 2010;17: 487-491.
18. Hoy SM, Keating GM. Dexmedetomidine: a review of its use for sedation in mechanically ventilated patients in an intensive care setting and for procedural sedation. *Drugs.* 2011;71: 1481-1501.
19. Leykin Y, Miotto L, Pellis T. Pharmacokinetic considerations in the obese. *Best Pract Res Clin Anaesthesiol.* 2011;25:27-36.
20. Kruijt Spanjer MR, Bakker NA, Absalom AR. Pharmacology in the elderly and newer anaesthesia drugs. *Best Pract Res Clin Anaesthesiol.* 2011;25:355-365.
21. Anderson BJ. Pharmacology in the very young: anaesthetic implications. *Eur J Anaesthesiol.* 2012;29:261-270.
22. Chau PL. New insights into the molecular mechanisms of general anaesthetics. *Br J Pharmacol.* 2010;161:288-307.
23. Forman SA, Miller KW. Anesthetic sites and allosteric mechanisms of action on Cys-loop ligand-gated ion channels. *Can J Anaesth.* 2011;58:191-205.
24. Olsen RW, Li GD. GABA(A) receptors as molecular targets of general anesthetics: identification of binding sites provides clues to allosteric modulation. *Can J Anaesth.* 2011;58: 206-215.
25. Akk G, Steinbach JH. Structural studies of the actions of anesthetic drugs on the γ-aminobutyric acid type A receptor. *Anesthesiology.* 2011;115:1338-1348.
26. Rossman AC. The physiology of the nicotinic acetylcholine receptor and its importance in the administration of anesthesia. *AANA J.* 2011;79:433-440.
27. Hemmings HC Jr. Sodium channels and the synaptic mechanisms of inhaled anaesthetics. *Br J Anaesth.* 2009;103: 61-69.
28. Orestes P, Todorovic SM. Are neuronal voltage-gated calcium channels valid cellular targets for general anesthetics? *Channels.* 2010;4:518-522.
29. White PF, Eng MR. Ambulatory (outpatient) anesthesia. In: Miller RD et al, eds. *Miller's Anesthesia.* Vol 1. 7th ed. Philadelphia, PA: Churchill Livingstone Elsevier; 2010:667-718.
30. van den Berg AA. Premedications and peribulbar analgesia—a prospective audit. *Middle East J Anesthesiol.* 2004;17:875-890.
31. Pisegna JR, Martindale RG. Acid suppression in the perioperative period. *J Clin Gastroenterol.* 2005;39:10-16.
32. Puig I, Calzado S, Suárez D, et al. Meta-analysis: comparative efficacy of H2-receptor antagonists and proton pump inhibitors for reducing aspiration risk during anaesthesia depending on the administration route and schedule. *Pharmacol Res.* 2012;65: 480-490.
33. Chen CC, Siddiqui FJ, Chen TL, et al. Dexamethasone for prevention of postoperative nausea and vomiting in patients undergoing thyroidectomy: meta-analysis of randomized controlled trials. *World J Surg.* 2012;36:61-68.
34. De Oliveira GS Jr, Castro-Alves LJ, Ahmad S, et al. Dexamethasone to prevent postoperative nausea and vomiting: an updated meta-analysis of randomized controlled trials. *Anesth Analg.* 2013;116:58-74.
35. Lien CA. Development and potential clinical impairment of ultra-short-acting neuromuscular blocking agents. *Br J Anaesth.* 2011;107(suppl 1):i60-71.
36. Hibbs RE, Zambon AC. Agents acting at the neuromuscular junction and autonomic ganglia. In: Brunton LL, et al, eds. *The Pharmacological Basis of Therapeutics.* 12th ed. New York: McGraw Hill; 2011:255-276.
37. Lee C, Katz RL. Clinical implications of new neuromuscular concepts and agents: so long, neostigmine! So long, sux! *J Crit Care.* 2009;24:43-49.
38. Illman HL, Laurila P, Antila H, et al. The duration of residual neuromuscular block after administration of neostigmine or sugammadex at two visible twitches during train-of-four monitoring. *Anesth Analg.* 2011;112:63-68.
39. Srivastava A, Hunter JM. Reversal of neuromuscular block. *Br J Anaesth.* 2009;103:115-129.
40. Aniskevich S, Leone BJ, Brull SJ. Sugammadex: a novel approach to reversal of neuromuscular blockade. *Expert Rev Neurother.* 2011;11:185-198.
41. Makri I, Papadima A, Lafioniati A, et al. Sugammadex, a promising reversal drug. A review of clinical trials. *Rev Recent Clin Trials.* 2011;6:250-255.
42. Khuenl-Brady KS, Wattwil M, Vanacker BF, et al. Sugammadex provides faster reversal of vecuronium-induced neuromuscular blockade compared with neostigmine: a multicenter, randomized, controlled trial. *Anesth Analg.* 2010;110:64-73.
43. Brull SJ, Murphy GS. Residual neuromuscular block: lessons unlearned. Part II: methods to reduce the risk of residual weakness. *Anesth Analg.* 2010;111(1):129-140.
44. Murphy GS, Brull SJ. Residual neuromuscular block: lessons unlearned. Part I: definitions, incidence, and adverse physiologic effects of residual neuromuscular block. *Anesth Analg.* 2010;111:120-128.
45. Craig RG, Hunter JM. Neuromuscular blocking drugs and their antagonists in patients with organ disease. *Anaesthesia.* 2009;64(suppl 1):55-65.
46. Kopman AF. Neuromuscular monitoring: old issues, new controversies. *J Crit Care.* 2009;24:11-20.
47. Mashour GA, Orser BA, Avidan MS. Intraoperative awareness: from neurobiology to clinical practice. *Anesthesiology.* 2011;114:1218-1233.
48. Radovanovic D, Radovanovic Z. Awareness during general anaesthesia—implications of explicit intraoperative recall. *Eur Rev Med Pharmacol Sci.* 2011;15:1085-1089.
49. Kruidering-Hall M, Campbell L. Skeletal muscle relaxants. In: Katzung BG, Masters SB, Trevor AJ, eds. *Basic and Clinical Pharmacology.* 12th ed. New York: Lange Medical Books/ McGraw Hill; 2012:465-482.
50. Guenther U, Radtke FM. Delirium in the postanaesthesia period. *Curr Opin Anaesthesiol.* 2011;24:670-675.
51. Saczynski JS, Marcantonio ER, Quach L, et al. Cognitive trajectories after postoperative delirium. *N Engl J Med.* 2012;367:30-39.

52. Ghoneim MM, Block RI. Clinical, methodological and theoretical issues in the assessment of cognition after anaesthesia and surgery: a review. *Eur J Anaesthesiol.* 2012;29:409-422.
53. Monk TG, Price CC. Postoperative cognitive disorders. *Curr Opin Crit Care.* 2011;17:376-381.
54. Bekker A, Lee C, de Santi S, et al. Does mild cognitive impairment increase the risk of developing postoperative cognitive dysfunction? *Am J Surg.* 2010;199:782-788.
55. Hartholt KA, van der Cammen TJ, Klimek M. Postoperative cognitive dysfunction in geriatric patients. *Z Gerontol Geriatr.* 2012;45:411-416.
56. Quinlan N, Rudolph JL. Postoperative delirium and functional decline after noncardiac surgery. J Am Geriatr Soc. 2011;59 (suppl 2):S301-S304.

CHAPTER 12

Local Anesthetics

Local anesthesia produces a loss of sensation in a specific body part or region. Medical practitioners use it to perform relatively minor surgical procedures. The approach involves introducing an anesthetic drug near the peripheral nerve that innervates the desired area. The basic goal is to block afferent neural transmission along the peripheral nerve so that the procedure is painless. When a local anesthetic is introduced in the vicinity of the spinal cord, transmission of impulses may be effectively blocked at a specific level of the cord, allowing for more extensive surgical procedures (e.g., cesarean delivery) because a larger region of the body is being anesthetized. This approach is still considered a local anesthetic because the drug acts locally at the spinal cord and the patient remains conscious during the surgical procedure.

Using a local anesthetic during a surgical procedure offers several advantages over the use of general anesthesia, including a relatively rapid recovery and lack of residual effects.[1,2] There is a virtual absence of the postoperative confusion and lethargy often seen after general anesthesia. In most cases of minor surgery, patients are able to leave the practitioner's office or hospital almost as soon as the procedure is completed. In more extensive procedures, local anesthesia offers the advantage of not interfering with cardiovascular, respiratory, and renal functioning. This fact can be important in patients with problems in these physiological systems. During childbirth, local (spinal) anesthesia imposes a lesser risk to the mother and neonate than general anesthesia.[3]

The primary disadvantages of local anesthesia are the length of time required to establish an anesthetic effect and the risk that analgesia will be incomplete or insufficient for the procedure.[4] The latter problem can usually be resolved by administering more local anesthesia if the procedure is relatively minor or by switching to a general anesthetic during a major procedure if an emergency arises during surgery.

In nonsurgical situations, local anesthetics are sometimes used to provide analgesia. These drugs may be used for short-term pain relief in conditions such as musculoskeletal and joint pain (e.g., bursitis, tendinitis) or in more long-term situations such as pain relief in cancer or treatment of chronic pain. In addition, local anesthetics may be used to block efferent sympathetic activity in conditions such as complex regional pain syndrome.

During these nonsurgical applications, you will often be directly involved in treating the patient while the local anesthetic is in effect. Physical therapists may actually administer the local anesthetic via phonophoresis or iontophoresis (if prescribed by a physician). Consequently, you should have adequate knowledge of the pharmacology of local anesthetics.

TYPES OF LOCAL ANESTHETICS

Commonly used local anesthetics are listed in Table 12-1. Most of these drugs share a common chemical strategy consisting of both a lipophilic and hydrophilic group connected by an intermediate chain (Fig. 12-1). A local anesthetic is chosen depending on

Table 12-1
COMMON LOCAL ANESTHETICS

Generic Name	Trade Name(s)	Onset of Action	Duration of Action	Principle Use(s)
Articaine	Septocaine	Rapid	Intermediate	Peripheral nerve block
Benzocaine	Americaine, others	—	—	Topical
Bupivacaine	Marcaine, Sensorcaine	Slow to intermediate	Long	Infiltration; peripheral nerve block; epidural; spinal; sympathetic block
Butamben	Butesin Picrate	—	—	Topical
Chloroprocaine	Nesacaine	Rapid	Short	Infiltration; peripheral nerve block; epidural; intravenous regional block
Dibucaine	Nupercainal	—	—	Topical
Etidocaine	Duranest	Rapid	Long	Infiltration; peripheral nerve block; epidural
Levobupivacaine	Chirocaine	Slow to intermediate	Short to long	Infiltration; peripheral nerve block; epidural
Lidocaine	Xylocaine	Rapid	Intermediate	Infiltration; peripheral nerve block; epidural; spinal; transdermal; topical; sympathetic block; intravenous regional block
Mepivacaine	Carbocaine, Polocaine	Intermediate to rapid	Intermediate	Infiltration; peripheral nerve block; epidural; intravenous regional block
Pramoxine	Prax, Tronolane	—	—	Topical
Prilocaine	Citanest	Rapid	Intermediate	Infiltration; peripheral nerve block
Procaine	Novocain	Intermediate	Short	Infiltration; peripheral nerve block; spinal
Tetracaine	Pontocaine	Rapid	Intermediate to long	Topical; spinal

**Values for onset and duration of action refer to use during injection. Relative durations of action are as follows: short = 30–60 min, intermediate = 1–3 hr, and long = 3–10 hr of action.*

Source: USP DI. 25th ed. Copyright 2005. Thomson MICROMEDEX. Permission granted.

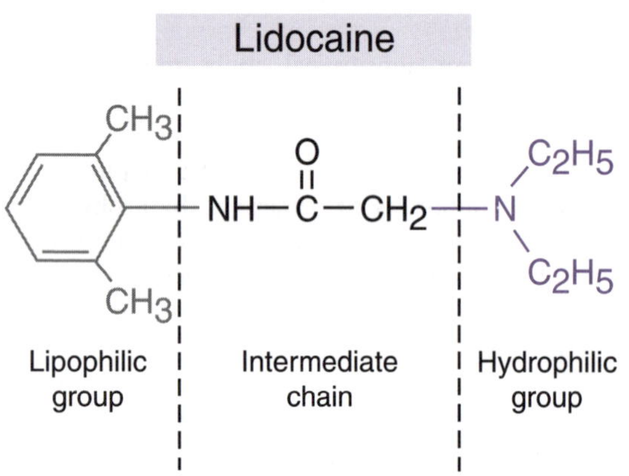

Figure 12-1
Structure of lidocaine. The basic structure of a lipophilic and hydrophilic group connected by an intermediate chain is common to most local anesthetics.

factors such as the operative site and nature of the procedure, the type of regional anesthesia desired (e.g., single peripheral nerve block or spinal anesthesia), the patient's size and general health, and the anesthetic's duration of action.[4,5]

The *-caine* suffix (e.g., lidocaine, procaine, etc.) usually identifies local anesthetics. The first clinically useful local anesthetic identified was cocaine in 1884. However, its tendency for abuse and its high incidence of addiction and systemic toxicity initiated the search for safer local anesthetics, such as those in Table 12-1. Cocaine abuse grew because of its effects on the brain, not for its local anesthetic effects. This drug produces intense feelings of euphoria and excitement through increased synaptic transmission in the brain. This explains why cocaine abusers either inject this drug or "snort" it through the nose. It absorbs through those mucous membranes and into systemic circulation, where it ultimately reaches the brain.

PHARMACOKINETICS

Local anesthetics are administered through a variety of routes and techniques, depending on the specific clinical situation (see "Clinical Use of Local Anesthetics" later in this chapter). In local anesthesia, the drug should remain at the site of administration. For instance, injecting procaine (Novocain) into the trigeminal nerve area during a dental procedure will be more effective if it is not washed away from the administration site by blood flow through that region. Likewise, injection of a local anesthetic into the area surrounding the spinal cord (e.g., epidural or spinal injection; see next section) will be more effective if the drug remains near the administration site.[6] Consequently, a vasoconstricting agent (e.g., epinephrine) is often administered simultaneously to help prevent washout from the desired site.[7] Preventing the anesthetic from reaching the bloodstream is also beneficial because local anesthetics can cause toxic side effects when sufficient amounts reach the systemic circulation (see "Systemic Effects of Local Anesthetics"). This occurrence is usually not a problem if a single, small dose of regional anesthesia is administered properly, but the buildup of the drug in the bloodstream should be monitored if larger doses are administered repeatedly or continuously to treat acute or chronic pain.[8,9]

Local anesthetics are usually eliminated by hydrolyzing or breaking apart the drug molecule. This metabolic hydrolysis is catalyzed by hepatic enzymes or enzymes circulating in the plasma (e.g., the plasma cholinesterase). Once the drug is metabolized, the kidneys excrete the polar metabolites.

CLINICAL USE OF LOCAL ANESTHETICS

Local anesthetics all basically work the same way, but their clinical effects depend largely on how they are administered. For example, administering a local anesthetic to a small patch of skin or near a single nerve will produce a limited area of anesthesia, while the same agent administered near a nerve plexus or near the spinal cord might affect a much larger part of the body or both lower extremities. The primary clinical uses of local anesthetics and their method of administration and specific indications are presented here.

Topical Administration

Local anesthetics can be applied directly to the surface of the skin, mucous membranes, cornea, and other regions to produce analgesia. This is usually done for the symptomatic relief of minor surface irritation and injury (e.g., minor burns, abrasions, inflammation). Local anesthetics can also be applied topically to reduce pain prior to minor surgical procedures such as wound cleansing, myringotomy, circumcision, and cataract surgery.[10-13] A topical anesthesia can be made by applying a single agent or a mixture of two or more local anesthetics (e.g., lidocaine and prilocaine).[10,14]

Preliminary studies suggest that topical anesthesia can be used to improve motor function in some patients with skeletal muscle hypertonicity resulting from a cerebrovascular accident (CVA) or head trauma.[15] In this situation, a local anesthetic (e.g., 20 percent benzocaine) is sprayed on the skin overlying hypertonic muscles, and then various exercises and facilitation techniques can be performed to increase and improve mobility in the affected limbs. The rationale of this treatment is to temporarily decrease abnormal or excessive excitatory feedback of cutaneous receptors on efferent motor pathways so that normal integration and control of motor function can be reestablished. However, additional studies on this technique have not been forthcoming, and this intervention does not currently appear to be used routinely in clinical practice.

Transdermal Administration

To administer anesthetic transdermally, the drug is applied to the surface of the skin or other tissues, where the drug then absorbs into underlying tissues. Transdermal administration of some local anesthetics may be enhanced by the use of electrical current (iontophoresis) or ultrasound (phonophoresis; see Appendix A).[16-18] Moreover, iontophoresis and phonophoresis offer the advantage of anesthetizing a region of the skin before treating painful subcutaneous structures (e.g., bursae, tendons, other soft tissues) without breaking the skin. Physical therapists can therefore use iontophoresis and phonophoresis to administer local anesthetics, such as lidocaine, for treating certain musculoskeletal injuries. However, a comprehensive discussion of the efficacy of these techniques in physical therapist practice is beyond the scope of this chapter. The references at the end of this chapter provide several sources that address this topic in more detail.[16,19,20]

Medical practitioners may also administer local anesthetics via iontophoresis to produce topical anesthesia prior to certain dermatologic procedures. For example, lidocaine iontophoresis is applied to a small patch of skin before performing minor surgical procedures such as placement of an IV catheter, lumbar puncture, use of needle electromyography, and similar invasive procedures.[21-23] Iontophoresis of local anesthetics may offer a relatively noninvasive way to decrease skin sensation and reduce pain associated with needles and other dermatologic procedures.

Finally, local anesthetics can be administered via a transdermal patch.[24] In particular, medical practitioners prescribe transdermal patches containing 5 percent lidocaine to treat localized pain in musculoskeletal conditions (e.g., osteoarthritis, low back pain, myofascial pain, fractures)[25-28] and various types of neuropathic pain (e.g., postherpetic neuralgia, diabetic neuropathy).[29-31] As indicated in Chapter 2, transdermal patches provide a convenient and predictable method for administering drugs to a given anatomical site, and patients can use lidocaine patches to provide symptomatic relief in many conditions involving fairly localized pain.

Infiltration Anesthesia

With this method, the drug is injected directly into the selected tissue, allowing it to diffuse to sensory nerve endings within that tissue. This technique saturates an area such as a skin laceration for performing surgical repair (suturing).

Peripheral Nerve Block

In a peripheral nerve block, the anesthetic is injected close to the nerve trunk so that transmission along the peripheral nerve is interrupted.[32] This type of local anesthesia is common in dental procedures for tooth extractions and can also be used to block other peripheral nerves to allow certain surgical procedures of the hand, foot, shoulder, and so forth.[32,33] Injection near larger nerves (femoral, sciatic) or around a nerve plexus (brachial plexus) anesthetizes larger areas of an upper or lower extremity.[34-36] Nerve blocks can be classified as minor when only one distinct nerve (e.g., ulnar, median) is blocked, or major, when several peripheral nerves or a nerve plexus (brachial, lumbosacral) are involved. In certain procedures, a medical practitioner will use diagnostic ultrasound to guide needle placement so the local anesthetic is injected as close as possible to a specific nerve without the needle penetrating the nerve and causing neural damage.[32]

Nerve blocks can also be continued after the completion of the surgery to provide optimal pain management.[37,38] In this situation, a small catheter is left implanted near the nerve(s) so that small dosages of the local anesthetic are administered continuously for the first 24 hours or so after surgery. Anesthesia providers routinely use continuous peripheral nerve blocks after joint replacements, ligament reconstruction, and various other orthopedic and nonorthopedic surgeries.[38-40] However, prolonged administration of local anesthetics within skeletal muscle can produce localized muscle pain and necrosis.[9] Likewise, the patient's ability to feel and move the affected area will be decreased while the anesthetic block is in effect. For example, a patient may not be able to voluntarily control his or her quadriceps during a femoral nerve block, and the knee could buckle when the patient tries to stand on the affected leg.[41] Hence, clinicians should use extra caution to protect the involved limb when the block is in effect and should report any muscle pain or signs of infection following the use of continuous peripheral nerve blocks.

Central Neural Blockade

The anesthetic for a central neural blockade is injected within the spaces surrounding the spinal cord[42-44] (Fig.12-2). Specifically, the term **epidural nerve blockade** refers to injection of the drug into the epidural space—that is, the space between the bony vertebral column and the dura mater. Anesthesia providers sometimes perform a variation of epidural administration, known as a *caudal block*, by injecting the local anesthetic into the lumbar epidural space via the sacral hiatus (see Fig. 12-2). **Spinal nerve blockade** refers to injection within the subarachnoid space—that is, the space between the arachnoid membrane and the pia mater. Spinal blockade is also referred to as *intrathecal anesthesia* because the drug is injected within the tissue sheaths surrounding the spinal cord (*intrathecal* means "within a sheath"; see Chapter 2).

In theory, epidural and spinal blocks can be done at any level of the cord, but they are usually administered

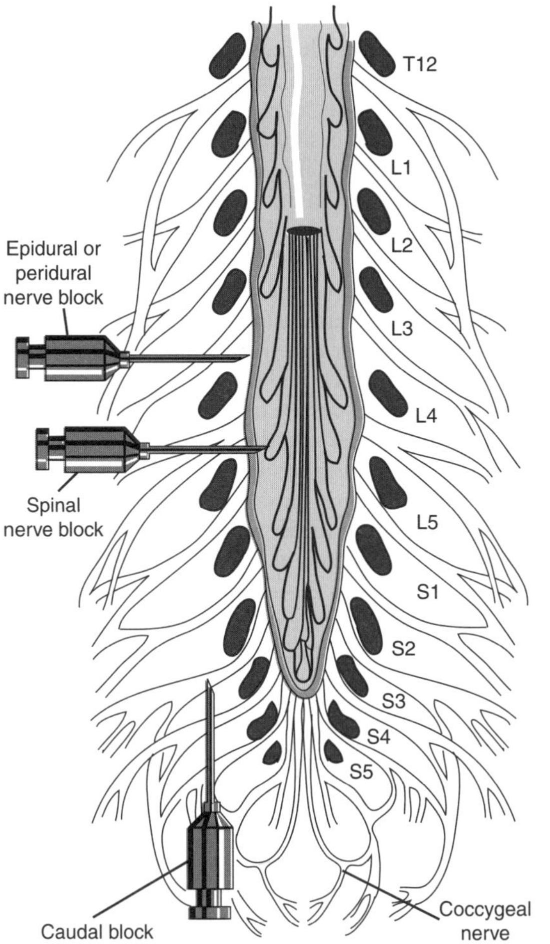

Figure ■ 12-2
Sites of epidural and spinal administration of a local anesthetic. Caudal block represents epidural administration via the sacral hiatus. *(From Clark JB, Queener SF, Karb VB.* Pharmacological Basis of Nursing Practice. *4th ed. St Louis: CV Mosby; 1993:688. Adapted with permission.)*

at the L3-4 or L4-5 vertebral interspace (i.e., caudal to the L-2 vertebral body, which is the point where the spinal cord ends). Epidural anesthesia is somewhat easier to perform than spinal blockade because the epidural space is larger and more accessible than the subarachnoid space. However, spinal anesthesia is more rapid and usually creates a more effective or solid block using a smaller amount of the local anesthetic.[1,45] The drawback, of course, is that higher concentrations of the drug are administered in close proximity to neural structures during spinal anesthesia. Local anesthetics are neurotoxic when administered in high concentrations.[4] Spinal anesthesia carries a somewhat higher risk for neurotoxicity because a relatively large amount of the local anesthetic is being introduced fairly close to the spinal cord and related neural structures (cauda equina). Any physical damage from the injection technique or neurotoxicity from the drugs will therefore be more problematic during spinal administration compared to the epidural route.

Anesthesia providers use central neural blockade whenever analgesia is needed in a large region. For example, they frequently use epidural and spinal routes to administer local anesthetics during obstetric procedures (including cesarean delivery).[46,47] These routes can also be used as an alternative to general anesthesia for other surgical procedures, including lumbar spine surgery and hip and knee arthroplasty.[48,49] Medical practitioners may also use the epidural and intrathecal routes to administer anesthetics and narcotic analgesics for relief of acute and chronic pain.[50] In these instances, an indwelling catheter is often left implanted in the epidural or subarachnoid space to allow repeated or continuous delivery of the anesthetic to the patient. The use of implanted drug delivery systems in managing chronic and severe pain is discussed further in Chapters 14 and 17.

Sympathetic Blockade

Although blockade of sympathetic function usually occurs during peripheral and central nerve blocks, sometimes the selective interruption of sympathetic efferent discharge is desirable. This intervention is especially useful in cases of complex regional pain syndrome (CRPS). This syndrome, also known as *reflex sympathetic dystrophy syndrome* (RSDS) and *causalgia*, involves increased sympathetic discharge to an upper or lower extremity, often causing severe pain and dysfunction in the distal part of the extremity. As part of the treatment, a local anesthetic can be administered to interrupt sympathetic discharge to the affected extremity.[51,52] One approach is to inject the local anesthetic into the area surrounding the sympathetic chain ganglion that innervates the affected limb. For example, the injection is near the stellate ganglion when the upper extremity is involved, and the injection is around the sympathetic ganglion at the L-2 vertebral level for lower-extremity CRPS.[53,54] Usually a series of five injections on alternate days is necessary to attenuate the sympathetic discharge and to provide remission from the CRPS episode. Alternatively, the local anesthetic can be administered subcutaneously to an affected area[55] or injected intravenously into the affected limb using regional IV block techniques.[56] Hence, several techniques are currently being used to promote sympathetic blockade using local anesthetic drugs. With these techniques, the goal is not to provide analgesia, but rather to reduce excessive sympathetic outflow to the affected extremity.

Intravenous Regional Anesthesia (Bier Block)

During IV regional anesthesia (also known as *Bier block*), the anesthetic is injected into a peripheral vein located in a selected arm or leg.[1,57] The local vasculature can then carry the anesthetic to the nerves in that extremity, thereby producing anesthesia in the limb. A tourniquet must be applied proximally on the limb to localize the drug temporarily within the extremity and to prevent the anesthetic from reaching the systemic circulation where it would cause toxic effects on the heart and CNS. This technique is somewhat difficult to use because the tourniquet can cause pain or increase the risk of ischemic neuropathy if left in place for more than 2 hours.[58] The IV regional block, however, anesthetizes the forearm–hand or distal leg–ankle–foot for short periods to allow certain surgical procedures or to treat conditions such as CRPS.[56,59]

MECHANISM OF ACTION

Local anesthetics inhibit the opening of sodium channels located on nerve membranes, thus blocking action potential propagation along neuronal axons (Fig.12-3).[60,61] The sudden influx of sodium into the neuron through open (activated) ion channels depolarizes the neuron during impulse propagation. If the sodium ion channels are inhibited from opening along a portion of the axon, the action potential will not be propagated past that point. If the neuron is sensory in nature, this information will not reach the brain and will result in anesthesia of the area innervated by that neuron. At higher concentrations, local anesthetics may also affect several other cellular components, including potassium channels.[1] Nonetheless, at the dosages used clinically, these drugs exert anesthetic effects because they rapidly and effectively block sodium channels and thus stop action potential propagation along sensory neurons.

Exactly how local anesthetics inhibit the sodium channel from opening has been the subject of much debate. The current consensus is that local anesthetics temporarily attach to a binding site located within the sodium channel.[62,63] This binding site controls the opening of the channel, and when bound by the anesthetic molecule, the sodium channel is maintained in a closed, inactivated position. The most likely location of this binding site is within the lumen or pore of the channel itself, probably near the inner, cytoplasmic opening of the channel (Fig. 12-3).[62,64] When bound by the anesthetic molecule, this site effectively locks the sodium channel shut, much in the same way that the correct key fitting into a keyhole is able to lock a door. Local anesthetics probably reach this site via different pathways, depending on the chemical properties of each drug—that is, charged, hydrophilic agents can reach this binding site through the open, activated channel, while neutral, lipophilic agents probably reach this site by first diffusing through the lipid bilayer and then approaching the site from the inner opening of the channel. Likewise, affinity of the local anesthetic for the binding site depends on the

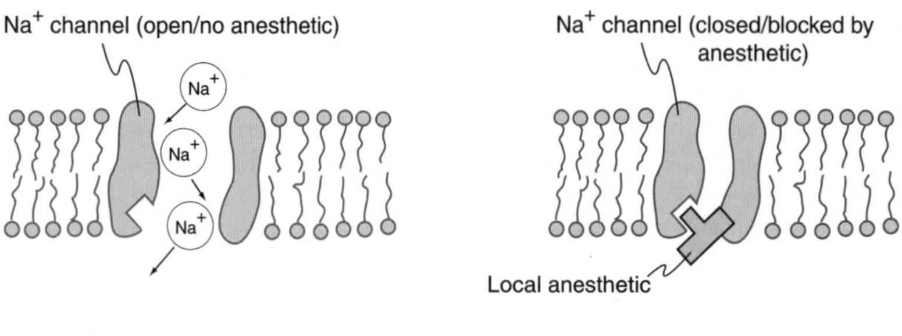

Figure ■ 12-3
Schematic diagram showing mechanism of action of local anesthetics on the nerve membrane. Local anesthetics appear to bind directly to a site within the sodium channel, thereby locking the channel in a closed position, thus preventing sodium entry and action potential propagation.

channel's activity. These drugs tend to bind more readily if the channel is open and activated or closed and inactivated, rather than in a resting state where the channel is closed but can be activated (opened) by an appropriate stimulus.[1]

Consequently, local anesthetics exert their primary effects by binding directly to sodium channels on the nerve axon. By keeping these channels in a closed, inactivated state, the anesthetic prevents action potential propagation along the affected portion of the axon. Likewise, only a relatively short portion of the axon (e.g., the length of two to three nodes of Ranvier in a myelinated neuron) needs to be affected by the anesthetic to block action potential propogation.[5] That is, the anesthetic does not need to affect the entire length of the axon but must block only one specific segment of the axon to completely prevent sensory or motor information from being transmitted past the point of the blockade.

DIFFERENTIAL NERVE BLOCK

Differential nerve block refers to the ability of a local anesthetic dose to block specific nerve fiber groups depending on the size (diameter) of the fibers.[5] In intact nerves, smaller diameter fibers seem to be the most sensitive to anesthetic effects, with progressively larger fibers being affected as anesthetic concentration increases.[1] This point is significant because different diameter fibers transmit different types of information (Table 12-2). Thus, information transmitted by the smallest fibers will be lost first, with other types of transmission being successively lost as the local anesthetic effect increases. The smallest diameter (type C) fibers that transmit pain are usually the first sensory information blocked as the anesthetic takes effect. Type C fibers also transmit postganglionic autonomic information, including sympathetic vasomotor control of the peripheral vasculature, and are therefore the most susceptible efferent fibers to blockade by local anesthetics. Other sensory information—such as temperature, touch, and proprioception—is successively lost as the concentration and effect of the anesthetic increases. Skeletal motor function is usually last to disappear because efferent impulses to the skeletal muscle are transmitted over the large type A alpha fibers.

The exact reason for the differential susceptibility of nerve fibers to local anesthetics is not known, but this effect does not seem to be related directly to the axon's diameter. A neuron in an intact nerve is not more sensitive to local anesthetics simply

Table 12-2

RELATIVE SIZE OF NERVE FIBER TYPES AND THEIR SUSCEPTIBILITY TO DIFFERENTIAL NERVE BLOCK

Fiber Type*	Function	Diameter (μm)	Myelination	Conduction Velocity (m/s)	Sensitivity to Block
Type A					
Alpha	Proprioception, motor	12–20	Heavy	70–120	+
Beta	Touch, pressure	5–12	Heavy	30–70	++
Gamma	Muscle spindles	3–6	Heavy	15–30	++
Delta	Pain, temperature	2–5	Heavy	5–25	+++
Type B	Preganglionic, autonomic	< 3	Light	3–15	++++
Type C					
Dorsal root	Pain	0.4–1.2	None	0.5–2.3	++++
Sympathetic	Postganglionic	0.3–1.3	None	0.7–2.3	++++

**Fiber types are classified according to the system established by Gasser and Erlanger. Am J Physiol. 1929;88:581.*

Reproduced with permission from Drasner: Local anesthetics. In: Katzung BG, et al, eds. Basic and Clinical Pharmacology. 12th ed. New York: Lange Medical Books/McGraw Hill; 2012.

because the diameter of its axon is smaller than other neurons in the nerve. An alternative explanation is that the anesthetic is able to affect a critical length of the axon more quickly in small unmyelinated fibers or small myelinated neurons with nodes of Ranvier that are spaced closely together compared to larger fibers where the nodes are farther apart.[1] As indicated earlier, a specific length of the axon must be affected by the anesthetic so that action potentials cannot be transmitted past the point of blockade. Other factors such as the firing rate of each axon or the position of the axon in the nerve bundle (e.g., in the outer part of the bundle versus buried toward the center of the nerve) may also affect susceptibility to local anesthesia.[1] In any event, from a clinical perspective, the smaller-diameter fibers appear to be affected first.

The clinical importance of a differential nerve block is that certain sensory modalities may be blocked without the loss of motor function. Fortunately, the most susceptible modality is pain because analgesia is usually the desired effect. If the dosage and administration of the anesthetic is optimal, it will produce analgesia without any significant loss of skeletal muscle function. This fact may be advantageous if motor function is beneficial, such as allowing expectant mothers to continue to ambulate during earlier stages of labor while receiving epidural anesthesia to control pain.[65] If local anesthetics are used to produce sympathetic blockade, postganglionic type C fibers are the first to be blocked, thus producing the desired effect at the lowest anesthetic concentration.

SYSTEMIC EFFECTS OF LOCAL ANESTHETICS

The intent of administering a local anesthetic is to produce a regional effect on specific neurons. However, these drugs may occasionally be absorbed into the general circulation and exert toxic effects on other organs and tissues. This problem is known commonly as *local anesthetic systemic toxicity* (LAST). Local anesthetics can inhibit action potential initiation and propagation in all excitable tissues, but the most important systemic effects involve the CNS and cardiovascular system.[66,67] That is, local anesthetics can inadvertently disrupt the excitability of the CNS and cardiac tissues if meaningful amounts of these drugs reach the systemic circulation.

Virtually all local anesthetics stimulate the brain initially, and symptoms such as somnolence, confusion, agitation, excitation, and seizures can occur if sufficient amounts reach the brain via the bloodstream.[68,69] Central excitation is usually followed by a period of CNS depression. This depression may result in impaired respiratory function and may cause death.[68] The primary cardiovascular effects associated with local anesthetics include decreased cardiac excitation, heart rate, and force of contraction.[69,70] Again, this general inhibitory effect on the myocardium may produce serious consequences if sufficient amounts of the local anesthetic reach the general circulation.[5]

LAST is more likely to occur if an excessive dose is used, if absorption into the bloodstream is accelerated for some reason, or if the drug is accidentally injected into the systemic circulation rather than into extravascular tissues.[5,71] Other factors that can predispose a patient to systemic effects include the type of local anesthetic administered and the route and method of administration.[4] Therapists and other health-care professionals should always be alert for signs of the systemic effects of local anesthetics in patients. Early symptoms of CNS toxicity typically include ringing/buzzing in the ears (tinnitus), agitation, restlessness, and decreased sensation in the tongue, around the mouth, or other areas of the skin.[5] Changes in heart rate (bradycardia), electrocardiogram (ECG) abnormalities, or clinical signs of cardiac depression (fatigue, dizziness) may indicate cardiotoxicity. Again, early recognition of these CNS and cardiac abnormalities is essential to help avert fatalities due to the drug's systemic effects.

Fortunately, a strategy known as *lipid rescue* or *lipid resuscitation* can treat LAST.[72,73] This strategy involves IV administration of an emulsion of lipid compounds that basically soak up the lipophilic local anesthetic molecules so that they cannot bind to sodium channels in the CNS, myocardium, and other tissues. Lipid rescue can therefore be a life-saving intervention if LAST is recognized early and the lipid emulsion is administered soon after toxic symptoms appear.[72,74]

Special Concerns for Rehabilitation Patients

Clinicians may encounter the use of local anesthetics in several patient situations related to the clinical applications of these drugs. For example, therapists may be involved directly in the topical or transdermal administration of local anesthetics to treat certain types of musculoskeletal pain. In these situations, therapists can administer local anesthetics transdermally, using the techniques of iontophoresis and phonophoresis. Agents such as lidocaine can be administered through this method to treat, for example, acute inflammation in bursitis or tendinitis.

Clinicians should also be alert for any patients wearing transdermal patches to administer local anesthetics such as lidocaine. These patches are intended to deliver the drug in a slow, controlled fashion, and care must be taken to not disturb the patch during exercise, manual therapy, or other therapeutic interventions. Moreover, heating modalities should never be applied on or near the patch because the heat will accelerate absorption of the drug, which could result in systemic absorption and toxic effects. Clinicians should likewise educate the patient and his or her family about the proper use of the patch, and make sure everyone understands that heat should not be applied on or near the patch.

As indicated earlier, continuous nerve blocks have become a popular way to provide analgesia following joint replacement, ligament reconstruction, and other surgeries. These techniques are often very effective in controlling postoperative pain, but the patient will lack sensation in the affected area and may also lack motor control if the block affects the large type A alpha fibers in the nerve. Hence, care must be taken when exercising joints because the patient will not feel any pain if the joint tissues are being overstressed during exercise. Likewise, the knee may need to be supported by a brace to prevent buckling when attempting ambulation during, or immediately after, lower extremity nerve blocks.

Clinicians may also work with patients who are receiving local anesthetic injections for the treatment of CRPS/RSDS. Because these patients often receive a series of anesthetic injections, therapists may want to schedule the rehabilitation session immediately after each injection so that they can perform exercises and other rehabilitation techniques while the anesthetic is still in effect. This strategy may help reestablish normal sympathetic function and blood flow to the affected extremity so that optimal results are obtained from the sympathetic blockade.

Finally, therapists may work with patients who are receiving central neural blockade in the form of an epidural or spinal injection. These procedures are common during natural and cesarean childbirth and in some other surgical procedures. Administration of local anesthetics into the spaces around the spinal cord are also used to treat individuals with severe and chronic pain, such as those recovering from extensive surgery, patients who have cancer, or patients with other types of intractable pain. In these situations, the patient may have an indwelling catheter in the epidural or subarachnoid space to allow repeated or sustained administration of the spinal anesthesia.

When central neural blockade is used, therapists should be especially aware that sensation might be diminished below the level of epidural or spinal administration. Decreased sensation to thermal agents and electrical stimulation will occur when the central block is in effect.[42] Likewise, motor function may be affected in the lower extremities when local anesthetics are administered spinally or epidurally.[42] Hence, therapists should test sensation and motor strength before applying any physical agents or attempting ambulation with patients who have received some type of central neural blockade using a local anesthetic.

CASE STUDY

LOCAL ANESTHETICS

Brief History. A.T. is a 61-year-old woman with a history of chronic obstructive pulmonary disease. Her respiratory condition is managed pharmacologically by inhaling a combination of a long-acting bronchodilator (salmeterol) and an anti-inflammatory steroid (fluticasone). She is also being seen in her home by a physical therapist to improve respiratory function, reduce fatigue, and increase functional ability. She recently developed a painful, blistering rash over her lateral thorax that was diagnosed as herpes zoster (shingles). A.T. had chickenpox as a child, and this episode of shingles was attributed to a flare-up of the varicella zoster virus that remained in her body. The rash gradually diminished, but she continued to experience sharp, stabbing pain due to post-herpetic neuralgia. She consulted her physician, who prescribed a Lidoderm patch containing 5 percent lidocaine. This patch was applied to the skin over the painful area.

Problem/Influence of Medication. A.T. asked the therapist if she could also apply a heating pad over the painful area to help provide analgesia. She had been leaving the patch on continuously and only taking the old patch off when it was time to apply a new one.

1. ***What should the therapist tell this patient about applying heat over the lidocaine patch?***
2. ***What are the typical recommendations for applying and changing the patch?***

See Appendix C, "Answers to Case Study Questions."

SUMMARY

Local anesthetics are used frequently when a limited, well-defined area of anesthesia is required, as is the case for most minor surgical procedures. Depending on the method of administration, local anesthetics can be used to temporarily block transmission in the area of peripheral nerve endings, along the trunk of a single peripheral nerve, along several peripheral nerves or plexuses, or at the level of the spinal cord. Local anesthetics may also be used to block efferent sympathetic activity. These drugs appear to block transmission along nerve axons by binding to membrane sodium channels and by preventing the channels from opening during neuronal excitation. Physical therapists may frequently encounter patients using these agents for both short- and long-term pain control and to manage sympathetic hyperactivity.

REFERENCES

1. Catterall WA, Mackie K. Local anesthetics. In: Brunton LL, et al, eds. *The Pharmacological Basis of Therapeutics.* 12th ed. New York: McGraw Hill; 2011:565-582.
2. O'Donnell BD, Iohom G. Regional anesthesia techniques for ambulatory orthopedic surgery. *Curr Opin Anaesthesiol.* 2008;21:723-728.
3. Beckmann M, Calderbank S. Mode of anaesthetic for category 1 caesarean sections and neonatal outcomes. *Aust N Z J Obstet Gynaecol.* 2012;52:316-320.
4. Berde CB, Strichartz GR. Local anesthetics. In: Miller RD et al, eds. *Miller's Anesthesia.* Vol 1. 7th ed. Philadelphia, PA: Churchill Livingstone Elsevier; 2010:913-939.
5. Drasner K. Local anesthetics. In: Katzung BG, Masters SB, Trevor AJ, eds. *Basic and Clinical Pharmacology.* 12th ed. New York: Lange Medical Books/McGraw Hill; 2012:449-464.
6. Hermanides J, Hollmann MW, Stevens MF, Lirk P. Failed epidural: causes and management. *Br J Anaesth.* 2012;109:144-154.
7. Wahl MJ, Brown RS. Dentistry's wonder drugs: local anesthetics and vasoconstrictors. *Gen Dent.* 2010;58:114-123.

8. Fagenholz PJ, Bowler GM, Carnochan FM, Walker WS. Systemic local anaesthetic toxicity from continuous thoracic paravertebral block. *Br J Anaesth*. 2012;109:260-262.
9. Jeng CL, Torrillo TM, Rosenblatt MA. Complications of peripheral nerve blocks. *Br J Anaesth*. 2010;105(suppl 1):97-107.
10. Briggs M, Nelson EA, Martyn-St James M. Topical agents or dressings for pain in venous leg ulcers. *Cochrane Database Syst Rev.* 2012;11:CD001177.
11. Eidelman A, Weiss JM, Baldwin CL, et al. Topical anaesthetics for repair of dermal laceration. *Cochrane Database Syst Rev.* 2011;6:CD005364.
12. Kumar R, Banerjee A. Myringotomy and ventilation tube insertion with minims tetracaine drops. *Eur Arch Otorhinolaryngol.* 2011;268:1533-1534.
13. Zhao LQ, Zhu H, Zhao PQ, et al. Topical anesthesia versus regional anesthesia for cataract surgery: a meta-analysis of randomized controlled trials. *Ophthalmology*. 2012;119:659-667.
14. Purcell A, Marshall A, King J, Buckley T. Eutectic mixture of local anaesthetics (EMLA) 5% cream as a primary dressing on a painful lower leg ulcer. *J Wound Care*. 2012;21:309-314.
15. Sabbahi MA, De Luca CJ. Topical anesthetic-induced improvements in the mobility of patients with muscular hypertonicity: preliminary results. *J Electromyogr Kinesiol.* 1991;1:41-46.
16. Ciccone CD. Electrical stimulation for delivery of medications: iontophoresis. In: Robinson AJ, Snyder-Mackler L, eds. *Clinical Electrophysiology: Electrotherapy and Electrophysiologic Testing.* 3rd ed. Baltimore, MD: Lippincott, Williams & Wilkins; 2007.
17. Coglianese M, Draper DO, Shurtz J, Mark G. Microdialysis and delivery of iontophoresis-driven lidocaine into the human gastrocnemius muscle. *J Athl Train.* 2011;46:270-276.
18. Glaviano NR, Selkow NM, Saliba E, et al. No difference between doses in skin anesthesia after lidocaine delivered via iontophoresis. *J Sport Rehabil.* 2011;20:187-197.
19. Guy RH. Transdermal drug delivery. *Handb Exp Pharmacol.* 2010;197:399-410.
20. Sieg A, Wascotte V. Diagnostic and therapeutic applications of iontophoresis. *J Drug Target.* 2009;17:690-700.
21. Annaswamy TM, Morchower AH. Effect of lidocaine iontophoresis on pain during needle electromyography. *Am J Phys Med Rehabil.* 2011;90:961-968.
22. Strout TD, Schultz AA, Baumann MR, et al. Reducing pain in ED patients during lumbar puncture: the efficacy and feasibility of iontophoresis, collaborative approach. *J Emerg Nurs.* 2004;30:423-430.
23. Zempsky WT. Pharmacologic approaches for reducing venous access pain in children. *Pediatrics*. 2008;122(suppl 3):S140-153.
24. Neafsey PJ. Patching pain with lidocaine: new uses for the lidocaine 5% patch. *Home Healthc Nurse*. 2004;22:562-564.
25. Affaitati G, Fabrizio A, Savini A, et al. A randomized, controlled study comparing a lidocaine patch, a placebo patch, and anesthetic injection for treatment of trigger points in patients with myofascial pain syndrome: evaluation of pain and somatic pain thresholds. *Clin Ther.* 2009;31:705-720.
26. Kivitz A, Fairfax M, Sheldon EA, et al. Comparison of the effectiveness and tolerability of lidocaine patch 5% versus celecoxib for osteoarthritis-related knee pain: post hoc analysis of a 12 week, prospective, randomized, active-controlled, open-label, parallel-group trial in adults. *Clin Ther.* 2008;30:2366-2377.
27. Lin YC, Kuan TS, Hsieh PC, et al. Therapeutic effects of lidocaine patch on myofascial pain syndrome of the upper trapezius: a randomized, double-blind, placebo-controlled study. *Am J Phys Med Rehabil.* 2012;91:871-882.
28. Zink KA, Mayberry JC, Peck EG, Schreiber MA. Lidocaine patches reduce pain in trauma patients with rib fractures. *Am Surg.* 2011;77:438-442.
29. Dworkin RH, O'Connor AB, Audette J, et al. Recommendations for the pharmacological management of neuropathic pain: an overview and literature update. *Mayo Clin Proc.* 2010;85(suppl):S3-14.
30. Fleming JA, O'Connor BD. Use of lidocaine patches for neuropathic pain in a comprehensive cancer centre. *Pain Res Manag.* 2009;14:381-388.
31. Spallone V, Lacerenza M, Rossi A, et al. Painful diabetic polyneuropathy: approach to diagnosis and management. *Clin J Pain.* 2012;28:726-743.
32. Choquet O, Morau D, Biboulet P, Capdevila X. Where should the tip of the needle be located in ultrasound-guided peripheral nerve blocks? *Curr Opin Anaesthesiol.* 2012;25:596-602.
33. Ogle OE, Mahjoubi G. Local anesthesia: agents, techniques, and complications. *Dent Clin North Am.* 2012;56:133-148.
34. Chin KJ, Singh M, Velayutham V, Chee V. Infraclavicular brachial plexus block for regional anaesthesia of the lower arm. *Anesth Analg.* 2010;111:1072.
35. Maga JM, Cooper L, Gebhard RE. Outpatient regional anesthesia for upper extremity surgery update (2005 to present) distal to shoulder. *Int Anesthesiol Clin.* 2012;50:47-55.
36. Vermeylen K, Engelen S, Sermeus L, et al. Supraclavicular brachial plexus blocks: review and current practice. *Acta Anaesthesiol Belg.* 2012;63:15-21.
37. Ilfeld BM. Continuous peripheral nerve blocks in the hospital and at home. *Anesthesiol Clin.* 2011;29:193-211.
38. Stein BE, Srikumaran U, Tan EW, et al. Lower-extremity peripheral nerve blocks in the perioperative pain management of orthopaedic patients: AAOS exhibit selection. *J Bone Joint Surg Am.* 2012;94:e167.
39. Chelly JE, Ghisi D, Fanelli A. Continuous peripheral nerve blocks in acute pain management. *Br J Anaesth.* 2010;105(suppl 1): i86-96.
40. Ilfeld BM. Continuous peripheral nerve blocks: a review of the published evidence. *Anesth Analg.* 2011;113:904-925.
41. Ganapathy S. Wound/intra-articular infiltration or peripheral nerve blocks for orthopedic joint surgery: efficacy and safety issues. *Curr Opin Anaesthesiol.* 2012;25:615-620.
42. Brown DL. Spinal, epidural, and caudal anesthesia. In: Miller RD et al, eds. *Miller's Anesthesia*. Vol 1. 7th ed. Philadelphia, PA: Churchill Livingstone Elsevier; 2010:913-939.
43. Cwik J. Postoperative considerations of neuraxial anesthesia. *Anesthesiol Clin.* 2012;30:433-443.
44. Kokki H. Spinal blocks. *Paediatr Anaesth.* 2012;22:56-64.
45. Ng K, Parsons J, Cyna AM, Middleton P. Spinal versus epidural anaesthesia for caesarean section. *Cochrane Database Syst Rev.* 2004;2:CD003765.
46. Afolabi BB, Lesi FE. Regional versus general anaesthesia for caesarean section. *Cochrane Database Syst Rev*. 2012;10:CD004350.
47. Loubert C, Hinova A, Fernando R. Update on modern neuraxial analgesia in labour: a review of the literature of the last 5 years. *Anaesthesia*. 2011;66:191-212.

48. Nader A, Kendall MC, Wixson RL, et al. A randomized trial of epidural analgesia followed by continuous femoral analgesia compared with oral opioid analgesia on short- and long-term functional recovery after total knee replacement. *Pain Med.* 2012;13:937-947.
49. Vercauteren M, Waets P, Pitkänen M, Förster J. Neuraxial techniques in patients with pre-existing back impairment or prior spine interventions: a topical review with special reference to obstetrics. *Acta Anaesthesiol Scand.* 2011;55:910-917.
50. Moore JM. Continuous spinal anesthesia. *Am J Ther.* 2009; 16:289-294.
51. Hsu ES. Practical management of complex regional pain syndrome. *Am J Ther.* 2009;16:147-154.
52. Tran de QH, Duong S, Bertini P, Finlayson RJ. Treatment of complex regional pain syndrome: a review of the evidence. *Can J Anaesth.* 2010;57:149-166.
53. Hong JH, Kim AR, Lee MY, et al. A prospective evaluation of psoas muscle and intravascular injection in lumbar sympathetic ganglion block. *Anesth Analg.* 2010;111:802-807.
54. Siegenthaler A, Mlekusch S, Schliessbach J, et al. Ultrasound imaging to estimate risk of esophageal and vascular puncture after conventional stellate ganglion block. *Reg Anesth Pain Med.* 2012;37:224-227.
55. Linchitz RM, Raheb JC. Subcutaneous infusion of lidocaine provides effective pain relief for CRPS patients. *Clin J Pain.* 1999;15:67-72.
56. Mohr B. Safety and effectiveness of intravenous regional anesthesia (Bier block) for outpatient management of forearm trauma. *CJEM.* 2006;8:247-250.
57. Horn JL, Cordo P, Künster D, et al. Progression of forearm intravenous regional anesthesia with ropivacaine. *Reg Anesth Pain Med.* 2011;36:177-180.
58. Frank R, Cowan BJ, Lang S, et al. Modification of the forearm tourniquet techniques of intravenous regional anaesthesia for operations on the distal forearm and hand. *Scand J Plast Reconstr Surg Hand Surg.* 2009;43:102-108.
59. Fishman SM. Biofeedback in pain management: Bier blocks for complex regional pain syndrome. *J Pain Palliat Care Pharmacother.* 2008;22:61-63.
60. Docherty RJ, Farmer CE. The pharmacology of voltage-gated sodium channels in sensory neurones. *Handb Exp Pharmacol.* 2009;194:519-561.
61. Mazoit JX. Local anesthetics and their adjuncts. *Paediatr Anaesth.* 2012;22:31-38.
62. Lee S, Goodchild SJ, Ahern CA. Local anesthetic inhibition of a bacterial sodium channel. *J Gen Physiol.* 2012;139: 507-516.
63. Yanagidate F, Strichartz GR. Local anesthetics. *Handb Exp Pharmacol.* 2007;177:95-127.
64. Ahern CA, Eastwood AL, Dougherty DA, Horn R. New insights into the therapeutic inhibition of voltage-gated sodium channels. *Channels.* 2008;2:1-3.
65. Stewart A, Fernando R. Maternal ambulation during labor. *Curr Opin Anaesthesiol.* 2011;24:268-273.
66. Mercado P, Weinberg GL. Local anesthetic systemic toxicity: prevention and treatment. *Anesthesiol Clin.* 2011;29: 233-242.
67. Wolfe JW, Butterworth JF. Local anesthetic systemic toxicity: update on mechanisms and treatment. *Curr Opin Anaesthesiol.* 2011;24:561-566.
68. Di Gregorio G, Neal JM, Rosenquist RW, Weinberg GL. Clinical presentation of local anesthetic systemic toxicity: a review of published cases, 1979 to 2009. *Reg Anesth Pain Med.* 2010;35:181-187.
69. Dillane D, Finucane BT. Local anesthetic systemic toxicity. *Can J Anaesth.* 2010;57:368-380.
70. Drasner K. Local anesthetic systemic toxicity: a historical perspective. *Reg Anesth Pain Med.* 2010;35:162-166.
71. Dudley MH, Fleming SW, Garg U, Edwards JM. Fatality involving complications of bupivacaine toxicity and hypersensitivity reaction. *J Forensic Sci.* 2011;56:1376-1379.
72. Ciechanowicz S, Patil V. Lipid emulsion for local anesthetic systemic toxicity. *Anesthesiol Res Pract.* 2012;2012:131784.
73. Manavi MV. Lipid infusion as a treatment for local anesthetic toxicity: a literature review. *AANA J.* 2010;78:69-78.
74. Bern S, Akpa BS, Kuo I, Weinberg G. Lipid resuscitation: a life-saving antidote for local anesthetic toxicity. *Curr Pharm Biotechnol.* 2011;12:313-319.

SECTION

3

Drugs Affecting Skeletal Muscle

CHAPTER 13

Skeletal Muscle Relaxants

Skeletal muscle relaxants are used to treat conditions associated with hyperexcitable skeletal muscle—specifically, spasticity and muscle spasms. Although these two terms are often used interchangeably, spasticity and muscle spasms represent two distinct abnormalities. However, the use of relaxant drugs is similar in each condition because the ultimate goal is to normalize muscle excitability without a profound decrease in muscle function.

Skeletal muscle relaxants are important when one considers the large number of rehabilitation patients with muscle hyperexcitability that is associated with either spasm or spasticity. Likewise, certain rehabilitation interventions complement the actions of muscle relaxant drugs. For example, therapists often use therapeutic exercise, physical agents, and other techniques to help reduce muscle spasms and spasticity. These interventions can supplement drug effects, thus enhancing muscle relaxation and enabling the patient to engage more actively in physical rehabilitation. You should therefore understand the actions and effects of skeletal muscle relaxants to take advantage of the synergy between drug therapy and physical interventions.

The drugs discussed in this chapter decrease muscle excitability and contraction by acting at the spinal cord level, at the neuromuscular junction, or within the muscle cell itself. Some texts also classify neuromuscular junction blockers such as curare derivatives and succinylcholine as skeletal muscle relaxants. However, these drugs are more appropriately classified as skeletal muscle paralytics because they eliminate muscle contraction by blocking transmission at the myoneural synapse. This type of skeletal muscle paralysis is used primarily during general anesthesia (see Chapter 11). Skeletal muscle relaxants do not typically prevent muscle contraction; they only attempt to normalize muscle excitability to decrease pain and improve motor function.

INCREASED MUSCLE TONE: SPASTICITY VERSUS MUSCLE SPASMS

Much confusion and consternation often arise from the erroneous use of the terms *spasticity* and *spasm*. For the purpose of this text, these terms will be used to describe two different types of increased excitability, which result from different underlying pathologies.

Spasticity occurs in many patients following an injury to the central nervous system (CNS), including cord-related problems (e.g., multiple sclerosis, spinal cord transection) and injuries to the brain (e.g., cerebrovascular accident [CVA], cerebral palsy, acquired brain injury). Although there is considerable controversy about the exact changes in motor control, most clinicians agree that spasticity is characterized primarily by an exaggerated muscle stretch reflex (Fig. 13-1).[1,2] This abnormal reflex activity is velocity-dependent, with a rapid lengthening of the muscle invoking a strong contraction in the stretched muscle.

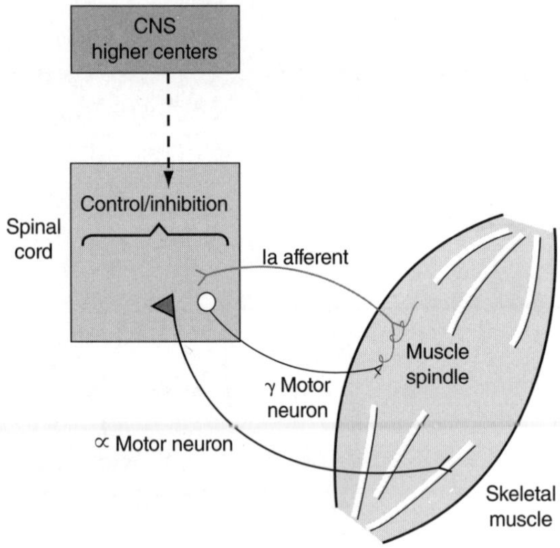

Figure ■ 13-1
Schematic illustration of the basic components of the stretch reflex. Normally, higher CNS centers control the sensitivity of this reflex by inhibiting synaptic connections within the spinal cord. Spasticity is thought to occur when this higher center influence is lost because of cerebral trauma or damage to descending pathways in the spinal cord.

The neurophysiological mechanisms underlying spasticity are complex, but this phenomenon occurs when supraspinal inhibition or control is lost because of a lesion in the spinal cord or brain.[2,3] Presumably, specific upper motor neuron lesions interrupt the cortical control of stretch reflex and alpha motor neuron excitability. Spasticity, therefore, is not in itself a disease but rather the motor sequela to the pathologies such as CVA, cerebral palsy, multiple sclerosis (MS), and traumatic lesions to the brain and spinal cord (including quadriplegia and paraplegia).

Spasms of skeletal muscle describe the increased tension often seen in skeletal muscle after certain musculoskeletal injuries and inflammation, such as muscle strains or nerve root impingements.[4] This tension is involuntary, so the patient is unable to relax the muscle. Spasms differ from spasticity because they typically arise from an orthopedic injury to a musculoskeletal structure or peripheral nerve root rather than an injury to the CNS. Likewise, muscle spasms are often a continuous, tonic contraction of specific muscles rather than the velocity-dependent increase in stretch reflex activity commonly associated with spasticity. The exact reasons for muscle spasms are poorly understood. According to some authorities, muscle spasms occur because a vicious cycle is created when the initial injury causes muscular pain and spasm, which increases afferent nociceptive input to the spinal cord, which further excites the alpha motor neuron to cause more spasms, and so on.[5] Other experts believe that muscle spasms occur because of a complex protective mechanism, whereby muscular contractions are intended to support an injured vertebral structure or peripheral joint.[4,6] Regardless of the exact reason, tonic contraction of the affected muscle is often quite painful because of the buildup of pain-mediating metabolites (e.g., lactate).

Consequently, various skeletal muscle relaxants attempt to decrease skeletal muscle excitation and contraction in cases of spasticity and spasm. The relaxants are categorized in this chapter according to their primary clinical application: agents used to decrease spasms and agents used to decrease spasticity. One agent, diazepam (Valium), is indicated for both conditions and will appear in both categories. Finally, the use of botulinum toxin (Botox) as an alternative strategy for reducing focal spasms or spasticity will be addressed.

ANTISPASM DRUGS

Diazepam

The effects of diazepam on the CNS and its use as an antianxiety drug are discussed in Chapter 6. Basically, diazepam and other benzodiazepines work by increasing the central inhibitory effects of gamma-aminobutyric acid (GABA)—that is, diazepam binds to receptors located at GABAergic synapses and increases the GABA-induced inhibition at that synapse. Diazepam appears to work as a muscle relaxant through this mechanism, potentiating the inhibitory effect of GABA on alpha motor neuron activity in the spinal cord.[7,8] The drug also exerts some supraspinal sedative effects; in fact, some of its muscle relaxant properties may derive from the drug's ability to produce a more generalized state of sedation.[9]

Uses

Diazepam is one of the oldest medications for treating muscle spasms. It has been used extensively in treating spasms associated with musculoskeletal injuries such as acute low-back strains. Diazepam has also been used to control muscle spasms associated with tetanus toxin; Valium's ability to inhibit spasms of the larynx and other muscles in this situation can be lifesaving.[10]

Adverse Effects

The primary side effect with diazepam is that dosages successful in relaxing skeletal muscle also produce sedation and a general reduction in psychomotor ability.[10,11] However, this effect may actually be advantageous for the patient recovering from an acute musculoskeletal injury. For example, a patient with an acute lumbosacral strain may benefit from the sedative properties because he or she will remain fairly inactive, thereby allowing better healing during the first few days after the injury. Continued use, however, may be problematic because of diazepam's sedative effects. The drug can also produce tolerance and physical dependence, and sudden withdrawal after prolonged use can cause seizures, anxiety, agitation, tachycardia, and even death.[12,13] Likewise, an overdose of diazepam can result in coma or death.[12] Hence, this drug might be beneficial for the short-term management of acute muscle spasms, but long-term use should be discouraged.

Centrally Acting Antispasm Drugs

Medical practitioners can use a variety of centrally acting compounds in an attempt to enhance muscle relaxation and decrease muscle spasms. Some common examples include cyclobenzaprine (Flexeril), carisoprodol (Soma), and the other drugs listed in Table 13-1. These drugs' mechanism of action is not well defined.[14] Research in animals has suggested that they may decrease polysynaptic reflex activity in the spinal cord; hence the term *polysynaptic inhibitors* is sometimes used to describe these agents. A polysynaptic reflex arc in the spinal cord is comprised of several small interneurons that link incoming (afferent) input into the dorsal horn with outgoing (efferent) outflow onto the alpha motor neuron. By inhibiting the neurons in the polysynaptic pathways, these drugs could decrease alpha motor neuron excitability and therefore cause relaxation of skeletal muscle.

However, it is not clear whether these drugs actually inhibit neurons involved in the polysynaptic pathways. For example, carisoprodol, or its primary metabolite meprobamate (see "Adverse Effects" below), may affect $GABA_A$ receptors, thus producing sedation in a manner similar to diazepam and other benzodiazepines.[15,16] On the other hand, cyclobenzaprine might increase serotonin activity at the brainstem level, thereby increasing the inhibitory influence of serotonin on alpha motor neuron activity.[17] This idea is based primarily on the fact that cyclobenzaprine is structurally similar to tricyclic antidepressants, which increase serotonin activity, and the observation that cyclobenzaprine may contribute to serotonin syndrome when used with other drugs that enhance serotonin effects in the CNS (see Chapter 7 for details about antidepressants and serotonin syndrome).

Table 13-1
DRUGS COMMONLY USED TO TREAT SKELETAL MUSCLE SPASMS

Drug	Usual Adult Oral Dosage (mg)	Onset of Action (min)	Peak (hr)	Duration of Action (hr)
Carisoprodol (Soma, Vanadom)	250–350 tid or qid, for no more than 2–3 wks	30	Unknown	4–6
Chlorzoxazone (Paraflex, Parafon Forte, others)	250–750 tid or qid	Within 60	1–2	3–4
Cyclobenzaprine (Amrix, Flexeril)	10 tid	Within 60	3–8	12–24
Diazepam (Valium, others)	2–10 tid or qid	30–60	1–2	Up to 24
Metaxalone (Skelaxin)	800 tid or qid	60	2	4–6
Methocarbamol (Carbacot, Robaxin)	1,500 qid for first 2–3 d; adjust as needed to maintenance dose of 750 q 4 hr or 1,500 tid	Within 30	2	Unknown
Orphenadrine citrate (Antiflex, Norflex, others)	100 BID	Within 60	6–8	12

Source: Ciccone, CD: Davis's Drug Guide for Rehabilitation Professionals. *Philadelphia: FA Davis; 2013.*

Hence, the effects of specific muscle relaxants on CNS neurochemicals may vary, depending on the drug. Nonetheless, these drugs may all share a common mechanism in that they increase sedation in the CNS—that is, they cause a global decrease in CNS excitability that results in generalized sedation, which in turn leads to skeletal muscle relaxation. It therefore seems possible that some of their muscle relaxant effects are caused by their sedative powers rather than a selective effect on specific neuronal reflex pathways.[16] This doesn't mean they are ineffective, because clinical research has shown that these drugs can be superior to a placebo in producing subjective muscle relaxation.[18,19] However, the specific ability of these drugs to relax skeletal muscle remains doubtful, and it is generally believed that their muscle relaxant properties are secondary to a nonspecific CNS sedation.

Uses

These drugs are typically used as adjuncts to rest and physical therapy for the short-term relief of muscle spasms associated with acute, painful musculoskeletal injuries.[20,21] When used to treat spasms, these compounds are often given with NSAIDs (see Chapter 15) or sometimes incorporated into the same tablet with an analgesic such as acetaminophen or aspirin. For instance, Norgesic is one of the brand names for orphenadrine combined with aspirin and caffeine. Such combinations are reportedly more effective than the individual components given separately.[22]

Adverse Effects

Because of their sedative properties, the primary side effects of these drugs are drowsiness and dizziness (Table 13-2). A variety of additional adverse effects, including nausea, light-headedness, vertigo, ataxia, and headache, may occur, depending on the patient and the specific drug administered (see Table 13-2). Cases of fatal overdose have also been documented for several of these drugs, including cyclobenzaprine and metaxolone.[23,24] Likewise, cyclobenzaprine has been associated with severe skeletal muscle pain and inflammation (rhabdomyolysis) in certain patients.[25]

Long-term or excessive use of these medications may also cause tolerance and physical dependence.[18] In particular, carisoprodol must be used cautiously because it is metabolized in the body to form meprobamate, a drug that has sedative/anxiolytic properties but is not used extensively because it has strong potential for abuse.[26] In fact, carisoprodol and meprobamate are now both classified as Schedule IV controlled substances (see Chapter 1 for a description of controlled substances). Hence, use of carisoprodol represents a rather unique situation where the drug and its metabolic by-product (meprobamate) can produce effects and side effects that lead to addiction and abuse, especially in people with a history of substance abuse.[26] Likewise, discontinuing carisoprodol suddenly after long-term use can lead to withdrawal symptoms such as anxiety, tremors, muscle twitching, and hallucinations.[26,27]

Consequently, centrally acting antispasm drugs can help provide short-term relief for muscle spasms associated with certain musculoskeletal conditions, and they may work synergistically with physical therapy and other interventions during acute episodes of back pain, neck pain, and so forth. Nonetheless, they have some rather serious side effects and potential for abuse, and the long-term use of these drugs should be discouraged.

Table 13-2
RELATIVE SIDE EFFECTS OF CENTRALLY ACTING DRUGS USED AS ANTISPASM AGENTS

Drug	Drowsiness	Dizziness or Light-Headedness	Nausea and Headache	Vomiting
Carisoprodol	M	L	L	L
Chlorzoxazone	M	M	L	L
Cyclobenzaprine	M	M	L	L
Metaxalone	M	M	M	M
Methocarbamol	M	M	L	L
Orphenadrine citrate	L	L	L	L

Relative incidence of side effects: M = more frequent; L = less frequent.
Taken from USP DI. 25th ed. Copyright 2005.Thompson MICROMEDEX.

ANTISPASTICITY DRUGS

Agents traditionally used in the treatment of spasticity include baclofen, dantrolene sodium, diazepam, gabapentin, and tizanidine (Table 13-3). Botulinum toxin can also be administered locally to treat spasticity in specific muscles.

Baclofen

The chemical name of baclofen is beta-(*p*-chlorophenyl)-GABA. As this name suggests, baclofen is a derivative of the central inhibitory neurotransmitter GABA. However, there appears to be some differences between baclofen and GABA. Baclofen seems to bind preferentially to certain GABA receptors, which have been classified as $GABA_B$ receptors (as opposed to $GABA_A$ receptors).[11,28] Preferential binding to $GABA_B$ receptors enables baclofen to act as a GABA agonist, inhibiting transmission within the spinal cord at specific synapses.[29,30] To put this in the context of its use as a muscle relaxant, baclofen appears to have an inhibitory effect on alpha motor neuron activity within the spinal cord. This inhibition apparently occurs by inhibiting excitatory neurons that synapse with the alpha motor neuron (presynaptic inhibition) and by directly affecting the alpha motor neuron itself (postsynaptic inhibition).[11,31] The result is decreased firing of the alpha motor neuron, with a subsequent relaxation of the skeletal muscle.

Uses

Baclofen is administered orally to treat spasticity associated with lesions of the spinal cord, including traumatic injuries resulting in paraplegia or quadriplegia and spinal cord demyelination resulting in MS.[32,33]

Table 13-3
ANTISPASTICITY DRUGS

Drug	Oral Dosage	Comments
Baclofen (Lioresal, Kemstro)	Adult: 5 mg tid initially; increase by 5 mg at 3-day intervals as required; maximum recommended dosage is 80 mg/day. Children: No specific pediatric dosage is listed; the adult dose must be decreased according to the size and age of the child.	More effective in treating spasticity resulting from spinal cord lesions (versus cerebral lesions).
Dantrolene sodium (Dantrium)	Adult: 25 mg/d initially; increase by 25 mg/d every 4–7 d until desired response is observed; maximum recommended dose is 400 mg/day in 4 divided doses. Children (older than 5 yr of age): initially, 0.5 mg/kg body weight bid; increase total daily dosage by 0.5 mg/kg every 4–7 days as needed, and give total daily amount in 4 divided dosages; maximum recommended dose is 400 mg/d.	Exerts an effect directly on the muscle cell; may cause generalized weakness in all skeletal musculature.
Diazepam (Valium, others)	Adult: 2–10 mg tid or qid. Children (older than 6 mo of age): 1–2.5 mg tid or qid (in both adults and children, begin at lower end of dosage range and increase gradually as tolerated and needed).	Produces sedation at dosages that decrease spasticity.
Gabapentin (Neurontin)	Adult:* initially, 300 mg tid. Can be gradually increased up to 3,600 mg/d based on desired response. Children* (3–12 years of age): Initially, 10–15 mg/kg body weight in 3 divided dosages; increase over 3 days until desired effect or a maximum of 50 mg/kg/d.	Developed originally as an anticonvulsant; may also be helpful as an adjunct to other drugs in treating spasticity associated with spinal cord injury and multiple sclerosis.
Tizanidine (Zanaflex)	Adult: 4 mg every 6–8 hours initially (no more than 3 doses per 24 hr); increase by 2–4 mg/dose up to 8 mg/dose or 24 mg/d. Children: The safety and efficacy of this drug in treating spasticity in children have not been established.	May reduce spasticity in spinal cord disorders while producing fewer side effects and less generalized muscle weakness than other agents (e.g., oral baclofen, diazepam).

**Anticonvulsant dose*

Baclofen is often the drug of choice in reducing the muscle spasticity associated with MS because it produces beneficial effects with a remarkable lack of adverse side effects.[34] Baclofen treatment also causes less generalized muscle weakness than direct-acting relaxants, such as dantrolene, which can be a major advantage for many patients with MS.[11] Baclofen also appears to produce fewer side effects when used appropriately to reduce spasticity secondary to traumatic spinal cord lesions, thus providing a relatively safe and effective form of treatment.[35] When administered systemically, baclofen is less effective in treating spasticity associated with supraspinal lesions (stroke, cerebral palsy), because these patients are more prone to the adverse side effects of this drug and because baclofen does not readily penetrate the blood-brain barrier.[30,35]

Oral baclofen has been used to reduce alcohol consumption in people who chronically abuse alcohol.[36,37] Apparently, baclofen can reduce the cravings and desire for alcohol consumption via the effects it has on CNS GABA receptors.[38,39] This effect seems to be dose related, and some successful studies report using baclofen doses well above those needed to reduce spasticity.[36] Research on this topic continues to clarify exactly how baclofen suppresses alcohol dependence and whether it might also be used to treat other drug addictions.

Adverse Effects

When initiating baclofen therapy, the most common side effect is transient drowsiness, which usually disappears within a few days.[32] When given to patients with spinal cord lesions, there are usually few other adverse effects. When given to patients who have had a CVA or to elderly individuals, there is sometimes a problem with confusion and hallucinations. Other side effects, occurring on an individual basis, include fatigue, nausea, dizziness, muscle weakness, and headache. Abrupt discontinuation of baclofen may also cause withdrawal symptoms such as hyperthermia, hallucinations, and seizures.[32,40] Increased seizure activity and coma have also been reported following baclofen overdose and in selected patient populations, such as certain children with cerebral palsy and certain adults with multiple sclerosis.[41-43]

Intrathecal Baclofen

Although baclofen is administered orally in most patients, it can also be administered intrathecally in patients with severe, intractable spasticity.[44,45] Intrathecal administration is the delivery of a drug directly into the subarachnoid space surrounding a specific level of the spinal cord. This places the drug very close to the spinal cord, thus allowing increased drug effectiveness with much smaller drug doses. Likewise, fewer systemic side effects occur because the drug tends to remain in the area of the cord rather than circulating in the bloodstream and causing adverse effects on other tissues.

When baclofen is administered intrathecally for the long-term treatment of spasticity, a small catheter is usually implanted surgically so that the open end of the catheter is located in the subarachnoid space and the other end is attached to a programmable pump (Fig. 13-2). The pump is implanted subcutaneously in the abdominal wall and is adjusted to deliver the drug at a slow, continuous rate. The rate of infusion is adjusted over time to achieve the best clinical reduction in spasticity.

Uses for Intrathecal Baclofen Delivery

Intrathecal baclofen delivery using implantable pumps is used in patients with spasticity of spinal origin (e.g., spinal cord injury, multiple sclerosis)[32,46] and in patients with spasticity resulting from supraspinal

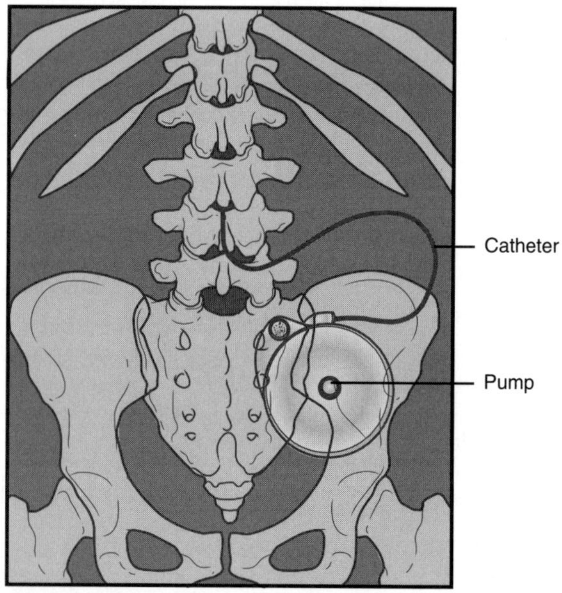

Figure ■ 13-2
Location of an intrathecal baclofen pump. The pump is typically placed in the lower abdominal wall, and the catheter leads from the pump to the subarachnoid space in the lumbar vertebral column.

(cerebral) injury, including cerebral palsy, CVA, and traumatic brain injury.[46-49] Studies involving these patients have typically noted a substantial decrease in rigidity (as indicated by decreased Ashworth scores, decreased reflex activity, etc.).[45,48] Patient satisfaction is generally favorable, and caregivers for younger children report ease of care following implantation of intrathecal baclofen pumps.[49,50] There is growing evidence that intrathecal baclofen can also reduce pain of central origin in some people with spasticity—that is, continuous baclofen administration to the subarachnoid space may inhibit the neural circuitry that induces chronic pain in people with multiple sclerosis, stroke, and other CNS injuries.[51,52]

Intrathecal baclofen intervention can also result in functional improvements, especially in cases where voluntary motor control was being masked by spasticity.[49,53] For example, ambulatory patients with spasticity resulting from a CVA may be able to increase their walking speed and their functional mobility after intrathecal baclofen therapy.[49,54] However, there may be a small margin between the baclofen dose that reduces spasticity and the dose that inhibits useful voluntary motor function.[53] Clinicians will often need to work closely with the patient, physician, and caregivers to find the optimal dose of intrathecal baclofen that reduces spasticity without impairing voluntary movements.

Functional improvements may not occur in all types of spasticity. Patients with severe spasticity of spinal origin, for example, may not experience improvements in mobility or decreased disability.[55] If these patients do not have adequate voluntary motor function, there is simply not enough residual motor ability to perform functional tasks after spasticity is reduced. Nonetheless, patients with severe spasticity from spinal and supraspinal causes often still benefit from intrathecal baclofen because of decreased rigidity and pain, which can result in improved self-care and the ability to perform daily living activities.[49,54,56]

Adverse Effects

Despite these benefits, intrathecal baclofen is associated with several potential complications. Primary among these is a possible disruption in the delivery system—that is, a pump malfunction or a problem with the delivery catheter can occur.[57,58] In particular, the catheter can become obstructed, or its tip can become displaced so that baclofen is not delivered into the correct area of the subarachnoid space. Increased drug delivery due to a pump malfunction could cause overdose and lead to respiratory depression, decreased cardiac function, and coma.[59,60] Conversely, abruptly stopping the drug due to pump failure, pump removal, or catheter displacement/blockage may cause a withdrawal syndrome that includes fever, confusion, delirium, and seizures.[59,60]

A second major concern is the possibility that tolerance could develop with long-term, continuous baclofen administration. Tolerance is the need for more of a drug to achieve its beneficial effects when used for prolonged periods. Several studies have reported that dosage must indeed be increased progressively in some patients when intrathecal baclofen systems are used for periods of several months to several years.[61,62] Tolerance to intrathecal baclofen, however, can usually be dealt with by periodic adjustments in dosage, and tolerance does not usually develop to such an extent that intrathecal baclofen must be discontinued.

Hence, intrathecal baclofen offers a means of treating certain patients with severe spasticity who have not responded to more conventional treatments, including oral baclofen. Additional research will help determine optimal ways that this intervention can be used to decrease spasticity. Further improvements in the technological and mechanical aspects of intrathecal delivery, including better pumps and catheter systems, will also make this a safer and more practical method of treating these patients.

Dantrolene Sodium

The only muscle relaxant available that exerts its effect directly on the skeletal muscle cell is dantrolene sodium (Dantrium).[63] This drug works by binding to the ryanodine type 1 receptor, located on calcium channels in skeletal muscle sarcoplasmic reticulum.[64,65] By binding to this receptor, dantrolene inhibits channel opening and subsequent release of calcium from the sarcoplasmic reticulum within the muscle cell during excitation (Fig. 13-3). In response to an action potential, the release of calcium from sarcoplasmic storage sites normally initiates myofilament cross-bridging and subsequent muscle contraction. By inhibiting calcium release, dantrolene attenuates muscle contraction and therefore enhances relaxation.

Uses

Dantrolene is often effective in treating severe spasticity, regardless of the underlying pathology.[63,66]

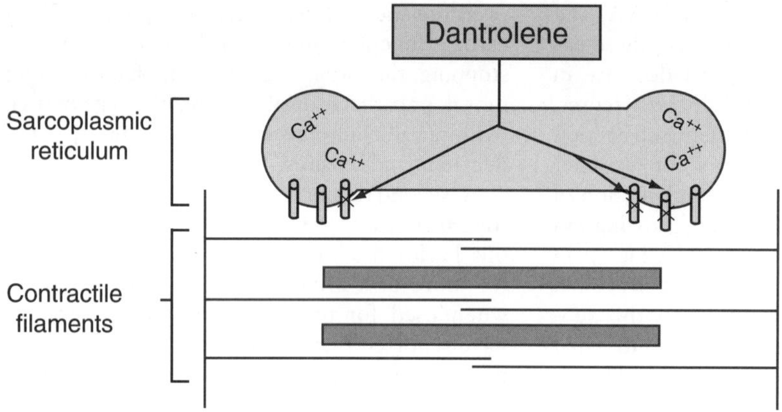

Figure ■ 13-3
Possible mechanism of action of dantrolene sodium (Dantrium). Dantrolene blocks channels in the sarcoplasmic reticulum, thus interfering with calcium release onto the contractile (actin, myosin) filaments. Muscle contraction is reduced because less calcium is available to initiate cross-bridge formation between actin and myosin filaments.

It can reduce spasticity in patients with traumatic cord lesions, advanced MS, cerebral palsy, or CVAs. This drug is also invaluable in treating malignant hyperthermia, which is a potentially life-threatening reaction occurring in susceptible individuals following exposure to general anesthesia, muscle paralytics used during surgery, or certain antipsychotic medications (a condition also called *neuroleptic malignant syndrome*; see Chapter 8).[67,68] In this situation, dantrolene inhibits skeletal muscle contraction throughout the body, thereby limiting the rise in body temperature generated by strong, repetitive skeletal muscle contractions.[67] Dantrolene is not prescribed to treat muscle spasms caused by musculoskeletal injury.

Adverse Effects

The most common side effect of dantrolene is generalized muscle weakness; this makes sense considering that dantrolene impairs sarcoplasmic calcium release in skeletal muscles throughout the body, not just in the hyperexcitable tissues. Thus, the use of dantrolene is sometimes counterproductive because the increased motor function that occurs when spasticity is reduced may be offset by generalized motor weakness. This drug may also cause severe hepatotoxicity, and cases of fatal hepatitis have been reported.[35,69] The risk of toxic effects on the liver seems to be greater in women over 35 years of age and in individuals receiving higher doses of this drug (over 300 mg).[35,69,70] Other, less serious side effects that sometimes occur during the first few days of therapy include drowsiness, dizziness, nausea, and diarrhea, but these problems are usually transient.

Diazepam

As indicated earlier, diazepam is effective in reducing spasticity as well as muscle spasms because it increases the inhibitory effects of GABA in the CNS.

Uses

Diazepam is used in patients with spasticity resulting from cord lesions and is sometimes effective in patients with cerebral palsy.

Adverse Effects

Use of diazepam as an antispasticity agent is limited by its sedative effects—that is, patients with spasticity who do not want a decrease in mental alertness will not tolerate diazepam therapy very well, especially at higher doses. Prolonged use of the drug can also cause tolerance and physical dependence. Nonetheless, diazepam may be an option for some patients with mild spasticity or as an adjunct to other antispasticity drugs.[71]

Gabapentin

Developed originally as an antiseizure drug (see Chapter 9), gabapentin (Neurontin) has also shown some promise in treating spasticity.[63] This drug was originally thought to cause inhibition in the spinal cord by affecting GABA receptors, but gabapentin probably works by inhibiting calcium entry into presynaptic nerve terminals that release glutamate and other excitatory neurotransmitters.[72,73] Calcium entry into presynaptic terminals normally facilitates the release of neurotransmitters at chemical synapses. By inhibiting calcium influx, gabapentin reduces the presynaptic release of excitatory neurotransmitters, thus decreasing the level of excitation in the CNS. It is believed that this general decrease in excitation reduces activity of the alpha motor neuron with subsequent skeletal muscle relaxation.[74] However, the exact way this drug exerts its antispasticity effects remains under investigation.

Uses

Gabapentin is effective in decreasing the spasticity associated with spinal cord injury and multiple sclerosis.[63] As indicated in Chapter 9, gabapentin is also helpful in treating various types of neuropathic pain. Hence, this drug may provide dual benefit in patients with neurological injuries that cause spasticity and chronic neuropathic pain.[75,76] Additional research should clarify how this drug can be used alone or with other agents to provide optimal benefits in spasticity resulting from various spinal, and possibly cerebral, injuries.

Adverse effects

The primary side effects of this drug are sedation, fatigue, dizziness, and ataxia.

Tizanidine

Tizanidine (Zanaflex) is classified as an alpha-2 adrenergic agonist, meaning that it binds selectively to the alpha-2 receptors in the CNS and stimulates them. Alpha-2 receptors are found at various locations in the brain and spinal cord, including the presynaptic and postsynaptic membranes of spinal interneurons that control alpha motor neuron excitability. Stimulation of these alpha-2 receptors inhibits the firing of interneurons that relay information to the alpha motor neuron—that is, interneurons that comprise polysynaptic reflex arcs within the spinal cord.[77] Tizanidine therefore appears to exert its antispasticity effects by stimulating alpha-2 receptors on pre- and postsynaptic terminals of spinal interneurons. This stimulation decreases the release of excitatory neurotransmitters from their presynaptic terminals (presynaptic inhibition) and decreases the excitability of the postsynaptic neuron (postsynaptic inhibition).[78] Inhibition of spinal interneurons results in decreased excitatory input onto the alpha motor neuron, with a subsequent decrease in spasticity of the skeletal muscle supplied by that neuron.

Uses

Tizanidine is used primarily to control spasticity resulting from spinal lesions (e.g., multiple sclerosis, spinal cord injury),[79,80] and this drug may also be effective in treating spasticity in people with cerebral lesions (e.g., CVA, acquired brain injury).[79,81] There is some concern, however, that tizanidine might slow neuronal recovery following brain injury, so some practitioners are reluctant to use this drug during the acute phase of stroke or traumatic brain injury.[35] Because it may inhibit pain pathways in the spinal cord, tizanidine has also been used to treat chronic headaches and other types of chronic pain (e.g., fibromyalgia, chronic regional pain syndromes, etc.).[81]

As an antispasticity drug, tizanidine appears to be as effective as orally administered baclofen or diazepam, but tizanidine generally has milder side effects and produces less generalized muscle weakness than these other agents.[79] Tizanidine is also superior to other alpha-2 agonists such as clonidine (Catapres) because it does not cause as much hypotension and other cardiovascular side effects. Clonidine exerts antispasticity as well as antihypertensive effects because it stimulates alpha-2 receptors in the cord and brainstem, respectively.[82] Use of clonidine in treating spasticity is limited because of the cardiovascular side effects; it is used primarily for treating hypertension (see Chapter 21).

Adverse Effects

The most common side effects associated with tizanidine include sedation, dizziness, and dry mouth.[11] As indicated, however, tizanidine tends to have a more favorable side effect profile than other alpha-2 agonists, and it produces less generalized weakness than oral baclofen or diazepam. Tizanidine may therefore be a better alternative to these other agents in patients who need to reduce spasticity while maintaining adequate muscle strength for ambulation, transfers, and so forth.

USE OF BOTULINUM TOXIN AS A MUSCLE RELAXANT

The injection of botulinum toxin is a rather innovative way to control localized muscle hyperexcitability. Botulinum toxin is a purified version of the toxin that causes botulism. Systemic doses of this toxin can be extremely dangerous or fatal because it inhibits the release of acetylcholine from presynaptic terminals at the skeletal neuromuscular junction. Loss of presynaptic acetylcholine release results in paralysis of the muscle fiber supplied by that terminal. Systemic dissemination of botulinum toxin can therefore cause widespread paralysis, including loss of respiratory muscle function. Injection into specific muscles, however, can sequester the toxin within these muscles, thus producing localized effects that are beneficial in certain forms of muscle hyperexcitability.

Mechanism of Action

The botulinum toxin is attracted to glycoproteins located on the surface of the presynaptic terminal at the skeletal neuromuscular junction.[83] Once attached to the membrane, the toxin enters the presynaptic terminal and inhibits fusion proteins that are needed for acetylcholine release (Fig. 13-4).[84] Specifically, the soluble NSF attachment protein receptor (SNARE) is normally responsible for directing presynaptic vesicles to fuse with the inner surface of the presynaptic terminal, thereby allowing the vesicles to release acetylcholine via exocytosis. Botulinum toxin cleaves and destroys these fusion proteins, thus making it impossible for the neuron to release acetylcholine into the synaptic cleft.[84,85] Local injection of botulinum toxin into specific muscles will therefore decrease muscle excitation by disrupting synaptic transmission at the neuromuscular junction. The affected muscle will invariably undergo some degree of paresis and subsequent relaxation because the toxin prevents the release of acetylcholine.

It has been suggested that botulinum toxin might have other effects on neuronal excitability. For example, this toxin might inhibit contraction of intrafusal muscle fibers that are located within skeletal muscle and help control sensitivity of the stretch reflex.[86] Inhibiting these intrafusal fibers would diminish activity in the afferent limb of the stretch reflex, thereby contributing to the antispasticity effects of this intervention.[86,87]

Through its direct action on muscle excitability, botulinum toxin may also have other neurophysiological effects at the spinal cord level—that is, reducing spasticity might result in complex neurophysiological changes at the spinal cord, ultimately resulting in more normal control of motor function in both the injected muscle and its antagonist.[88] In other words, reduction of excessive afferent discharge from the spastic muscle might help reestablish a more reasonable level of excitation at the cord level, thus improving efferent discharge to the injected muscle and its antagonist.[87]

In addition, research from animal models suggests that when botulinum toxin is injected into skeletal muscles, it may ultimately reach the CNS via transport within motor neurons. The botulinum toxin that enters the presynaptic terminal at the neuromuscular junction can be carried within motor neurons back to

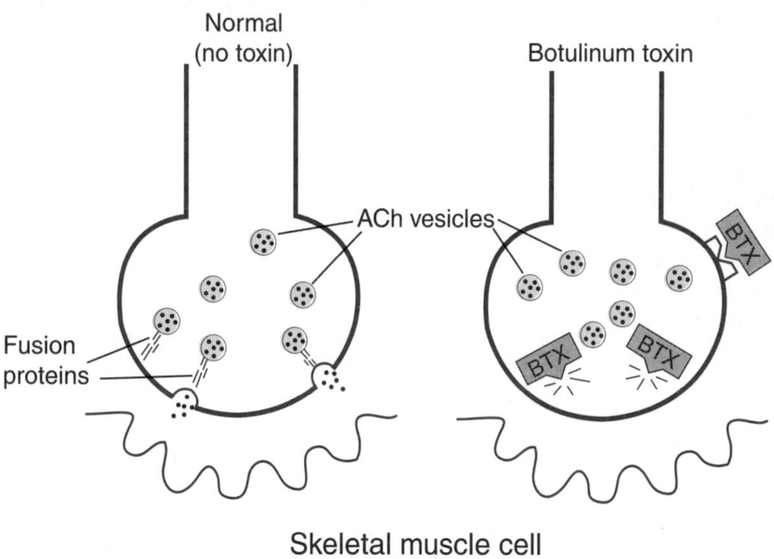

Figure ■ 13-4
Mechanism of action of botulinum toxin at the skeletal neuromuscular junction. At a normal synapse (shown on left), fusion proteins connect acetylcholine (ACh) vesicles with the presynaptic membrane, and ACh is released via exocytosis. Botulinum toxin (represented by "BTX" on the right) binds to the presynaptic terminal and enters the terminal where it destroys the fusion proteins so that ACh cannot be released.

the spinal cord via a process known as *retrograde axonal transport*.[89,90] Botulinum toxin might even be transferred from motor neurons to other neurons within the spinal cord and transported to higher CNS structures by afferent pathways within the cord.[91] These findings suggest that botulinum toxin may not just affect transmission at the skeletal neuromuscular junction, but might also alter neurotransmission within the CNS.[90,92] For example, botulinum toxin's analgesic effects in migraine headache and other pain syndromes might be explained by this toxin's ability to reach the CNS via axonal transport and then moderate the activity in central pain pathways.[93,94] More research is needed to clarify how peripheral administration of botulinum toxin might ultimately affect the spinal cord and brain and whether these neurophysiological effects have clinical significance.

Clinical Use of Botulinum Toxin

Seven strains (serotypes) of botulinum toxin have been identified, but only two types are currently available for clinical use: botulinum toxin types A and B.[95,96] These types differ somewhat in their chemistry, duration of action, and so forth. The most commonly used therapeutic type is botulinum toxin type A; this agent is marketed commercially under trade names such as Botox and Dysport. Botulinum toxin type B (Myobloc) is also available and can be useful in patients who develop immunity to the type A form of this toxin (discussed later). Likewise, a form of botulinum toxin type A known as *incobotulinumtoxinA* (Xeomin) was approved recently. Unlike more traditional preparations, incobotulinumtoxinA does not contain certain complexing proteins that may increase the chance of an immune reaction.[97] Hence, this newer type of botulinum toxin may be helpful in treating localized muscle hypertonicity with less chance of stimulating antibody production against this toxin.

Botulinum toxin has been used for some time to control localized muscle dystonias, including conditions such as spasmodic torticollis, blepharospasm, laryngeal dystonia, strabismus, and several other types of focal dystonias.[98-101] When used therapeutically, small amounts of this toxin are injected directly into the dystonic muscles, which begin to relax within a few days to 1 week. This technique appears to be fairly safe and effective in many patients, but relief may only be temporary. Symptoms often return within 3 months after each injection, necessitating additional treatments.[102] Still, this technique represents a method for treating patients with severe, incapacitating conditions marked by focal dystonias and spasms.

There is considerable interest in using botulinum toxin to reduce spasticity in specific muscles or muscle groups resulting from various disorders, including cerebral palsy,[103-105] traumatic brain injury,[106,107] CVA,[108-110] and spinal cord injury.[111] As with treatment of focal dystonias, the toxin is injected directly into selected muscles. If necessary, the medical practitioner can use electromyography or ultrasonography to identify specific muscles and guide the injection to the desired site within the muscle belly (e.g., the motor point of the muscle).[112] There is also some evidence that electrical stimulation of the nerve supplying the muscle for the first few days following injection may help increase the efficacy of the toxin, presumably by enhancing its uptake by the presynaptic nerve terminals.[113]

Intervention with botulinum toxin injection can help remove spastic dominance in certain patients to facilitate volitional motor function. For example, judicious administration of botulinum toxin can result in improved gait and other functional activities in selected patients with cerebral palsy, stroke, or traumatic brain injury.[105,114-116] Even if voluntary motor function is not improved dramatically, reducing spasticity in severely affected muscles may produce other musculoskeletal benefits. For example, injection of botulinum toxin can reduce spasticity so that muscles can be stretched or casted more effectively, thus helping to prevent joint contractures and decreasing the need for surgical procedures such as heel-cord lengthening and adductor release.[117-119]

These injections can likewise enable patients to wear and use orthotic devices more effectively. Injection into the triceps surae musculature can improve the fit and function of an ankle-foot orthosis by preventing excessive plantar flexor spasticity from "pistoning" the foot out of the orthosis.[120] Injections into severely spastic muscles can also increase patient comfort and ability to perform activities of daily living (ADL) and hygiene activities. Consider, for example, the patient with severe upper extremity flexor spasticity following a CVA. Local injection of botulinum toxin into the affected muscles may permit active or passive extension of the elbow, wrist, and fingers, thereby allowing better hand cleansing, ability to dress, decreased pain, and so forth.[121]

Finally, local botulinum toxin administration has been advocated as a way to control muscle hyperexcitability in other clinical situations. There has, of course, been considerable interest in using this toxin for cosmetic reasons. Injection of botulinum toxin into specific facial muscles can paralyze these muscles, thereby reducing the appearance of wrinkles around the eyes, mouth, and so forth.[122] Patients undergoing physical rehabilitation may also benefit from uses of this toxin. For example, patients with hyperactive (neurogenic) bladder following spinal cord injury can be treated by injecting botulinum toxin directly into the bladder detrusor muscle or external urethral sphincter.[123,124] This intervention may help normalize bladder function and allow more effective voiding or intermittent catheterization.[125,126] Likewise, injection of botulinum toxin into the bladder detrusor muscle can help reduce the incidence of stress urinary incontinence in people with idiopathic overactive bladder syndrome that is resistant to oral drug therapy and other interventions.[127,128] Botulinum toxin is also used to treat patients with chronic pain syndromes, including chronic headache, migraine, neuropathic pain, and various musculoskeletal disorders (e.g., back pain, whiplash injuries, etc.).[129-131] The use of this intervention has many potential benefits in many different clinical situations, and additional research will be needed to document how botulinum toxin can be used to reduce muscle hyperexcitability and improve function in various patient populations.

Limitations and Adverse Effects

Botulinum toxin does not cure spasticity, and there are several limitations to its use. In particular, only a limited amount of botulinum toxin can be administered during each set of injections. The total amount of botulinum toxin type A injected during each treatment session is typically between 200 and 300 units in adults, with proportionally smaller amounts used in children, depending on the child's size and age.[132] The typical dose of the type B form is 2,500 to 5,000 units. These doses are usually low enough to remain localized within the injected muscle and do not spread too far from the administration site. Moreover, higher doses of traditional botulinum toxin preparations may cause an immune response whereby antibodies are synthesized against the toxin. Subsequent treatments are ineffective because the patient's immune system will recognize and inactivate the toxin.[95,102]

However, the risk of an immune response may be negligible when administering a newer type of botulinum toxin type A known as incobotulinumtoxinA (Xeomin).[97,133] As indicated earlier, this newer preparation does not contain certain chemical constituents (complexing proteins) that can cause an immune reaction. It can therefore reduce the chance that antibodies will be produced against the toxin, thus allowing more long-term use with less treatment failure.[97,133]

Because only a relatively small amount of botulinum toxin can be injected safely at one time, the number of muscles that can be treated is typically limited to one or two muscle groups. For example, a treatment session might involve injection of the elbow and wrist flexors in one upper extremity of an adult or the bilateral triceps surae musculature of a child. Hence, decisions about injecting specific muscles should be considered carefully in each patient in order to use each dose most effectively and achieve optimal outcomes for that patient.

In addition, the relaxant effects of the toxin are often temporary and typically diminish within 2 to 3 months after injection.[102] The effects apparently wear off because a new presynaptic terminal "sprouts" from the axon that contains the originally affected presynaptic terminal. This new terminal grows downward, reattaching to the skeletal muscle and creating a new motor end plate with a new source of acetylcholine. The effects of the previous injection are overcome when this new presynaptic terminal begins to function. Another injection will be needed to block the release from this new presynaptic terminal, thus allowing another 2 to 3 months of antispasticity effects. This fact raises the question of how many times the injection cycle can be repeated safely and effectively. At the present time, there is no clear limit to the number of times a muscle can be injected, providing, of course, that sufficient time has elapsed between each series of injections.[102] One study reported that a group of patients with focal hand dystonias received botulinum toxin injections repeatedly for over 10 years with no adverse effects.[134] Additional studies will be needed to determine if there are any detrimental effects of long-term use of this intervention in other clinical situations.

Consequently, botulinum toxin represents a strategy for dealing with spasticity that is especially problematic in specific muscles or groups of muscles. Despite the rather ominous prospect of injecting a potentially lethal toxin into skeletal muscles, this intervention has a remarkably small incidence of severe adverse effects when administered correctly at therapeutic doses.[108,135] Nonetheless, severe adverse effects and death can occur if this drug is administered improperly or if the toxin accidentally enters the skeletal muscle vasculature and is carried into the systemic circulation. Clinicians should therefore be alert for signs that botulinum toxin is not being retained at the injection site and may be causing systemic effects. Such effects include generalized muscle weakness, difficulty speaking or swallowing, and respiratory distress.

Although rare, botulinum toxin can also cause a systemic allergic reaction, as indicated by pulmonary symptoms (e.g., laryngeal edema, wheezing, cough, dyspnea) or skin reactions (e.g., rash, pruritus, urticaria). Hence, botulinum toxin can be used as part of a comprehensive rehabilitation program, but clinicians should watch for any untoward responses and seek emergency medical assistance if signs of systemic toxicity are present.

PHARMACOKINETICS

Most muscle relaxants are absorbed fairly easily from the gastrointestinal tract, and the oral route is the most frequent method of drug administration. In cases of severe spasms, certain drugs such as methocarbamol and orphenadrine can be injected intramuscularly or intravenously to permit a more rapid effect. Likewise, diazepam and dantrolene can be injected to treat spasticity if the situation warrants a faster onset. As discussed earlier, continuous intrathecal baclofen administration may be used in certain patients with severe spasticity, and local injection of botulinum toxin is a possible strategy for treating focal dystonias and spasticity. Metabolism of muscle relaxants is usually accomplished by hepatic microsomal enzymes, and the metabolite or intact drug is excreted through the kidneys.

Special Concerns for Rehabilitation Patients

Because of the very nature of their use, skeletal muscle relaxants are prescribed for many patients involved in rehabilitation programs. Physical therapists and other rehabilitation professionals will encounter these drugs applied as both antispasm and antispasticity agents. When used to reduce muscle spasms following nerve root impingements, muscle strains, and the like, these drugs will complement the physical therapy interventions. Concomitant use of muscle relaxants with thermal, electrotherapeutic, and manual techniques can produce optimal benefits during the acute phase of musculoskeletal injuries causing spasms. Of course, the long-term use of antispasm agents is not practical because these drugs often cause sedation, and they can have addictive properties that lead to tolerance and physical dependence. This fact further emphasizes the need for aggressive physical therapy so that the drugs can be discontinued as soon as possible. Physical therapists and occupational therapists can also help prevent reinjury and recurrence of spasms by improving the patient's muscle strength, flexibility, and posture and by teaching proper body mechanics and lifting techniques. These interventions may help decrease the incidence of spasms and the need for drugs used to treat them.

The pharmacological reduction of spasticity is also an important goal in patients receiving physical therapy and occupational therapy. As indicated earlier, decreased spasticity can result in increased motor function, easier self-care or nursing care, and decreased painful and harmful effects of strong spastic contractions. Drug treatment is

Continued on following page

Special Concerns for Rehabilitation Patients (Continued)

likewise synergistic with rehabilitation; antispasticity agents can allow more effective passive range-of-motion and stretching activities and can permit more effective use of neuromuscular facilitation techniques, orthotic devices, and other interventions designed to reduce spasticity and improve function.

Rehabilitation specialists also play a critical role in helping patients adapt to sudden changes in muscle excitability caused by antispasticity drugs. Reducing spasticity may, in fact, adversely affect the individual relying on increased muscle tone to assist in functional activities such as ambulation. For example, patients who have had a CVA and use extensor spasticity in the lower extremity to support themselves when walking may begin to fall if this spasticity is suddenly reduced by drugs. This loss of support from the hypertonic muscles will hopefully be replaced by a more normal form of motor function.

Therapists can therefore play a vital role in facilitating the substitution of normal physiological motor control for the previously used spastic tone. This idea seems especially true when one of the parenteral antispasticity techniques is used, such as intrathecal baclofen or botulinum toxin injections. For example, patients who receive intrathecal baclofen through programmable pump systems often require a period of intensive rehabilitation to enable the benefits from decreased spasticity and increased voluntary motor function to occur. Therapists must be ready to use aggressive rehabilitation techniques to help patients adapt to the relatively rapid and dramatic decrease in muscle tone that is often associated with antispasticity drug therapy.

Rehabilitation specialists can also play a critical role in determining which patients might benefit from specific antispasticity drugs. In particular, therapists can help identify patients who are suitable candidates for botulinum toxin injections and help evaluate these patients pre- and postinjection to determine if they achieved the desired outcomes. Rehabilitation specialists are often in the best position to evaluate the effects of all antispasticity drugs. By working closely with the patient, the patient's family, and the physician, therapists can provide valuable feedback about the efficacy of antispasticity drugs and whether they are helping to improve the patient's function and well-being.

Finally, therapists may have to deal with the side effects of these drugs. Depending on the drug, problems with sedation, generalized muscle weakness, and hepatotoxicity can negate any beneficial effects from a reduction in muscle tone. Sedation, which may occur to a variable degree with all systemic skeletal muscle relaxants, must sometimes be accommodated in the rehabilitation program. If the patient needs to be awake and alert, treatments may have to be scheduled at a time of day when the sedative effects are minimal.

In situations of generalized muscle weakness (e.g., during the use of dantrolene sodium or oral baclofen), there is often little that the physical therapist can do to resolve this problem. For instance, the patient with paraplegia who requires adequate upper extremity strength to perform transfers, wheelchair mobility, and ambulation with crutches and braces may find his or her ability to perform these activities compromised by the antispasticity drug. The therapist's role in this situation may simply be to advise the patient that voluntary muscular power is limited and that some upper extremity strength deficits can be expected. The therapist may also work closely with the physician in trying to find the minimum acceptable dose for that patient or in attempting to find a better drug (e.g., switching from dantrolene to tizanidine).

CASE STUDY

MUSCLE RELAXANTS

Brief History. F.D. is a 28-year-old man who sustained complete paraplegia below the L-2 spinal level during an automobile accident. Through the course of rehabilitation, he was becoming independent in self-care, and he had begun to ambulate in the parallel bars and with crutches while wearing temporary long leg braces. He was highly motivated to continue this progress and was eventually fitted with permanent leg orthoses. During this period, spasticity had increased in his lower extremities to the point where dressing and self-care were often difficult. Also, the ability of the patient to put his leg braces on was often compromised by lower extremity spasticity. The patient was started on oral baclofen (Lioresal) at an initial oral dosage of 15 mg/day. The daily dosage of baclofen was gradually increased until he was receiving 60 mg/day. Despite the higher dose, F.D.'s spasticity was only partially controlled, and he still had problems when he was trying to sleep or during ADLs such as bathing and dressing.

Problem/Influence of Medication. The physician wanted to further increase the oral dose to 80 mg/day, but the therapist was concerned that this would create sedation and cognitive impairments. Moreover, F.D. had already noticed some weakness in his arms and upper torso due to the effects of baclofen on his nonspastic muscles. A higher dose would probably cause additional motor impairment to the point where his ability to transfer and ambulate would be compromised.

1. ***How does baclofen work, and why does oral baclofen affect F.D.'s nonspastic muscles?***
2. ***Is there an alternative way to administer this drug to better focus its effects on the spastic lower extremity muscles with less effect on F.D.'s trunk and upper extremities?***
3. ***How can the therapist address alternative administration methods with the physician and patient?***

See Appendix C, "Answers to Case Study Questions."

SUMMARY

Skeletal muscle relaxants are used to treat the muscle spasms that result from musculoskeletal injuries or spasticity that occurs following lesions in the CNS. Depending on the specific agent, these drugs reduce muscle excitability by acting on the spinal cord, at the neuromuscular junction, or directly within the skeletal muscle fiber. Diazepam and other centrally acting antispasm drugs are used in the treatment of muscle spasms, but their effectiveness as muscle relaxants may be because of their nonspecific sedative properties. Agents used to treat spasticity include baclofen, dantrolene, diazepam, gabapentin, and tizanidine. Each drug works by a somewhat different mechanism, and the selection of a specific antispasticity agent depends on the patient and the underlying CNS lesion (e.g., stroke, MS, spinal cord injury, etc.). Local injection of botulinum toxin can also be used to treat focal dystonias and spasticity, and this technique may help control spasms and spasticity in specific muscles or muscle groups. Physical therapists and other rehabilitation personnel will frequently work with patients taking these drugs for the treatment of either spasticity or spasms. Although there are some troublesome side effects, these drugs generally facilitate the rehabilitation program by directly providing benefits (i.e., muscle relaxation) that are congruent with the major rehabilitation goals.

REFERENCES

1. Nielsen JB, Crone C, Hultborn H. The spinal pathophysiology of spasticity—from a basic science point of view. *Acta Physiol (Oxf)*. 2007;189:171-180.
2. Sheean G, McGuire JR. Spastic hypertonia and movement disorders: pathophysiology, clinical presentation, and quantification. *PM R*. 2009;1:827-833.
3. Kandel ER, Scwartz JH, Jessell TM, et al. Spinal reflexes. In: *Principles of Neural Science*. 5th ed. New York: McGraw-Hill; 2013:790-811.
4. Hertling D, Kessler RM. *Management of Common Musculoskeletal Disorders*. 4th ed. Philadelphia: Lippincott Williams and Wilkins; 2006:152-153.
5. Clark BC, Thomas JS, Walkowski SA, Howell JN. The biology of manual therapies. *J Am Osteopath Assoc*. 2012;112:617-629.
6. Fryer G, Morris T, Gibbons P. Paraspinal muscles and intervertebral dysfunction: part two. *J Manipulative Physiol Ther*. 2004;27:348-357.
7. Gajcy K, Lochy_ski S, Librowski T. A role of GABA analogues in the treatment of neurological diseases. *Curr Med Chem*. 2010;17:2338-2347.
8. Trincavelli ML, Da Pozzo E, Daniele S, Martini C. The GABAA-BZR complex as target for the development of anxiolytic drugs. *Curr Top Med Chem*. 2012;12:254-269.
9. Chou R. Pharmacological management of low back pain. *Drugs*. 2010;70:387-402.
10. Ismoedijanto, Nassiruddin M, Prajitno BW. Case report: Diazepam in severe tetanus treatment. *Southeast Asian J Trop Med Public Health*. 2004;35:175-180.
11. Kruidering-Hall M, Campbell L. Skeletal muscle relaxants. In: Katzung BG, Masters SB, Trevor AJ, eds. *Basic and Clinical Pharmacology*. 12th ed. New York: Lange Medical Books/McGraw Hill; 2012:465-482.
12. Lader M. Benzodiazepine harm: how can it be reduced? *Br J Clin Pharmacol*. 2014:77:295-301.
13. Lader M, Tylee A, Donoghue J. Withdrawing benzodiazepines in primary care. *CNS Drugs*. 2009;23:19-34.
14. Gregori-Puigjané E, Setola V, Hert J, et al. Identifying mechanism-of-action targets for drugs and probes. *Proc Natl Acad Sci USA*. 2012;109:11178-11183.
15. Bramness JG, Skurtveit S, Mørland J. Impairment due to intake of carisoprodol. *Drug Alcohol Depend*. 2004;74:311-318.
16. Gonzalez LA, Gatch MB, Taylor CM, et al. Carisoprodol-mediated modulation of GABAA receptors: in vitro and in vivo studies. *J Pharmacol Exp Ther*. 2009;329:827-837.
17. Mestres J, Seifert SA, Oprea TI. Linking pharmacology to clinical reports: cyclobenzaprine and its possible association with serotonin syndrome. *Clin Pharmacol Ther*. 2011;90:662-665.
18. Toth PP, Urtis J. Commonly used muscle relaxant therapies for acute low back pain: a review of carisoprodol, cyclobenzaprine hydrochloride, and metaxalone. *Clin Ther*. 2004;26:1355-1367.
19. van Tulder MW, Touray T, Furlan AD, et al. Muscle relaxants for non-specific low back pain. *Cochrane Database Syst Rev*. 2003;2:CD004252.
20. Chou R, Huffman LH; American Pain Society; American College of Physicians. Medications for acute and chronic low back pain: a review of the evidence for an American Pain Society/American College of Physicians clinical practice guideline. *Ann Intern Med*. 2007;147:505-514.
21. See S, Ginzburg R. Choosing a skeletal muscle relaxant. *Am Fam Physician*. 2008;78:365-370.
22. Beebe FA, Barkin RL, Barkin S. A clinical and pharmacologic review of skeletal muscle relaxants for musculoskeletal conditions. *Am J Ther*. 2005;12:151-171.
23. Poklis JL, Ropero-Miller JD, Garside D, Winecker RE. Metaxalone (Skelaxin)-related death. *J Anal Toxicol*. 2004;28:537-541.
24. Spiller HA, Cutino L. Fatal cyclobenzaprine overdose with postmortem values. *J Forensic Sci*. 2003;48:883-884.
25. Chabria SB. Rhabdomyolysis: a manifestation of cyclobenzaprine toxicity. *J Occup Med Toxicol*. 2006;1:16.
26. Reeves RR, Burke RS, Kose S. Carisoprodol: update on abuse potential and legal status. *South Med J*. 2012;105:619-623.
27. Eleid MF, Krahn LE, Agrwal N, Goodman BP. Carisoprodol withdrawal after Internet purchase. *Neurologist*. 2010;16:262-264.
28. Brown JT, Davies CH, Randall AD. Synaptic activation of GABA(B) receptors regulates neuronal network activity and entrainment. *Eur J Neurosci*. 2007;25:2982-2990.
29. Hori K, Hoshino M. GABAergic neuron specification in the spinal cord, the cerebellum, and the cochlear nucleus. *Neural Plast*. 2012;2012:921732.
30. Taira T. Intrathecal administration of GABA agonists in the vegetative state. *Prog Brain Res*. 2009;177:317-328.
31. Gaiarsa JL, Kuczewski N, Porcher C. Contribution of metabotropic GABA(B) receptors to neuronal network construction. *Pharmacol Ther*. 2011;132:170-179.
32. Dario A, Tomei G. A benefit-risk assessment of baclofen in severe spinal spasticity. *Drug Saf*. 2004;27:799-818.
33. Rekand T. Clinical assessment and management of spasticity: a review. *Acta Neurol Scand Suppl*. 2010;190:62-66.
34. Bainbridge JL, Corboy JR. Multiple sclerosis. In: DiPiro JT, et al, eds. *Pharmacotherapy: A Pathophysiologic Approach*. 8th ed. New York: McGraw-Hill; 2011:963-978.
35. Zafonte R, Lombard L, Elovic E. Antispasticity medications: uses and limitations of enteral therapy. *Am J Phys Med Rehabil*. 2004;83(suppl):S50-58.
36. de Beaurepaire R. Suppression of alcohol dependence using baclofen: a 2-year observational study of 100 patients. *Front Psychiatry*. 2012;3:103.
37. Howland RH. Baclofen for the treatment of alcohol dependence. *J Psychosoc Nurs Ment Health Serv*. 2012;50:11-14.
38. Agabio R, Maccioni P, Carai MA, et al. The development of medications for alcohol-use disorders targeting the GABAB receptor system. *Recent Pat CNS Drug Discov*. 2012;7:113-128.
39. Leggio L, Zywiak WH, McGeary JE, et al. A human laboratory pilot study with baclofen in alcoholic individuals. *Pharmacol Biochem Behav*. 2013;103:784-791.
40. Ross JC, Cook AM, Stewart GL, Fahy BG. Acute intrathecal baclofen withdrawal: a brief review of treatment options. *Neurocrit Care*. 2011;14:103-108.
41. De Rinaldis M, Losito L, Gennaro L, Trabacca A. Long-term oral baclofen treatment in a child with cerebral palsy: electroencephalographic changes and clinical adverse effects. *J Child Neurol*. 2010;25:1272-1274.
42. Leung NY, Whyte IM, Isbister GK. Baclofen overdose: defining the spectrum of toxicity. *Emerg Med Australas*. 2006;18:77-82.
43. Schuele SU, Kellinghaus C, Shook SJ, et al. Incidence of seizures in patients with multiple sclerosis treated with intrathecal baclofen. *Neurology*. 2005;64:1086-1087.

44. Ammar A, Ughratdar I, Sivakumar G, Vloeberghs MH. Intrathecal baclofen therapy—how we do it. *J Neurosurg Pediatr.* 2012;10:439-444.
45. Natale M, Mirone G, Rotondo M, Moraci A. Intrathecal baclofen therapy for severe spasticity: analysis on a series of 112 consecutive patients and future prospectives. *Clin Neurol Neurosurg.* 2012;114:321-325.
46. Saval A, Chiodo AE. Intrathecal baclofen for spasticity management: a comparative analysis of spasticity of spinal vs cortical origin. *J Spinal Cord Med.* 2010;33:16-21.
47. Francisco GE. Intrathecal baclofen in the management of poststroke hypertonia: current applications and future directions. *Acta Neurochir Suppl.* 2007;97:219-226.
48. Motta F, Antonello CE, Stignani C. Intrathecal baclofen and motor function in cerebral palsy. *Dev Med Child Neurol.* 2011;53:443-448.
49. Schiess MC, Oh IJ, Stimming EF, et al. Prospective 12-month study of intrathecal baclofen therapy for poststroke spastic upper and lower extremity motor control and functional improvement. *Neuromodulation.* 2011;14:38-45.
50. Morton RE, Gray N, Vloeberghs M. Controlled study of the effects of continuous intrathecal baclofen infusion in non-ambulant children with cerebral palsy. *Dev Med Child Neurol.* 2011;53:736-741.
51. Pöllmann W, Feneberg W. Current management of pain associated with multiple sclerosis. *CNS Drugs.* 2008;22:291-324.
52. Taira T, Hori T. Intrathecal baclofen in the treatment of poststroke central pain, dystonia, and persistent vegetative state. *Acta Neurochir Suppl.* 2007;97:227-229.
53. Kofler M, Quirbach E, Schauer R, et al. Limitations of intrathecal baclofen for spastic hemiparesis following stroke. *Neurorehabil Neural Repair.* 2009;23:26-31.
54. Francisco GE, Latorre JM, Ivanhoe CB. Intrathecal baclofen therapy for spastic hypertonia in chronic traumatic brain injury. *Brain Inj.* 2007;21:335-338.
55. Zahavi A, Geertzen JH, Middel B, et al. Long term effect (more than five years) of intrathecal baclofen on impairment, disability, and quality of life in patients with severe spasticity of spinal origin. *J Neurol Neurosurg Psychiatry.* 2004;75:1553-1557.
56. Staal C, Arends A, Ho S. A self-report of quality of life of patients receiving intrathecal baclofen therapy. *Rehabil Nurs.* 2003;28:159-163.
57. Sgouros S, Charalambides C, Matsota P, et al. Malfunction of SynchroMed II baclofen pump delivers a near-lethal baclofen overdose. *Pediatr Neurosurg.* 2010;46:62-65.
58. Dvorak EM, McGuire JR, Nelson ME. Incidence and identification of intrathecal baclofen catheter malfunction. *PM R.* 2010;2:751-756.
59. Shirley KW, Kothare S, Piatt JH Jr, Adirim TA. Intrathecal baclofen overdose and withdrawal. *Pediatr Emerg Care.* 2006;22:258-261.
60. Watve SV, Sivan M, Raza WA, Jamil FF. Management of acute overdose or withdrawal state in intrathecal baclofen therapy. *Spinal Cord.* 2012;50:107-111.
61. Dones I, Broggi G. A case of very long-term appearing drug tolerance to intrathecal baclofen. *J Neurosurg Sci.* 2010;54:77-78.
62. Heetla HW, Staal MJ, Kliphuis C, van Laar T. The incidence and management of tolerance in intrathecal baclofen therapy. *Spinal Cord.* 2009;47:751-756.
63. Lapeyre E, Kuks JB, Meijler WJ. Spasticity: revisiting the role and the individual value of several pharmacological treatments. *NeuroRehabilitation.* 2010;27:193-200.
64. Dulhunty AF, Casarotto MG, Beard NA. The ryanodine receptor: a pivotal Ca2+ regulatory protein and potential therapeutic drug target. *Curr Drug Targets.* 2011;12:709-723.
65. Inan S, Wei H. The cytoprotective effects of dantrolene: a ryanodine receptor antagonist. *Anesth Analg.* 2010;111:1400-1410.
66. Kheder A, Nair KP. Spasticity: pathophysiology, evaluation and management. *Pract Neurol.* 2012;12:289-298.
67. Krause T, Gerbershagen MU, Fiege M, et al. Dantrolene—a review of its pharmacology, therapeutic use and new developments. *Anaesthesia.* 2004;59:364-373.
68. Rosenberg H, Davis M, James D, et al. Malignant hyperthermia. *Orphanet J Rare Dis.* 2007;2:21.
69. Chan CH. Dantrolene sodium and hepatic injury. *Neurology.* 1990;40:1427-1432.
70. Kim JY, Chun S, Bang MS, et al. Safety of low-dose oral dantrolene sodium on hepatic function. *Arch Phys Med Rehabil.* 2011;92:1359-1363.
71. Quality Standards Subcommittee of the American Academy of Neurology and the Practice Committee of the Child Neurology Society; Delgado MR, Hirtz D, Aisen M, et al. Practice parameter: pharmacologic treatment of spasticity in children and adolescents with cerebral palsy (an evidence-based review): report of the Quality Standards Subcommittee of the American Academy of Neurology and the Practice Committee of the Child Neurology Society. *Neurology.* 2010;74:336-343.
72. Bockbrader HN, Wesche D, Miller R, et al. A comparison of the pharmacokinetics and pharmacodynamics of pregabalin and gabapentin. *Clin Pharmacokinet.* 2010;49:661-669.
73. Striano P, Striano S. Gabapentin: a Ca2+ channel alpha 2-delta ligand far beyond epilepsy therapy. *Drugs Today.* 2008;44:353-368.
74. Kitzman PH, Uhl TL, Dwyer MK. Gabapentin suppresses spasticity in the spinal cord-injured rat. *Neuroscience.* 2007;149:813-821.
75. Attal N, Mazaltarine G, Perrouin-Verbe B, Albert T; SOFMER French Society for Physical Medicine and Rehabilitation. Chronic neuropathic pain management in spinal cord injury patients. What is the efficacy of pharmacological treatments with a general mode of administration? (oral, transdermal, intravenous). *Ann Phys Rehabil Med.* 2009;52:124-141.
76. Solaro C, Messmer Uccelli M. Pharmacological management of pain in patients with multiple sclerosis. *Drugs.* 2010;70:1245-1254.
77. Rank MM, Murray KC, Stephens MJ, et al. Adrenergic receptors modulate motoneuron excitability, sensory synaptic transmission and muscle spasms after chronic spinal cord injury. *J Neurophysiol.* 2011;105:410-422.
78. Mirbagheri MM, Chen D, Rymer WZ. Quantification of the effects of an alpha-2 adrenergic agonist on reflex properties in spinal cord injury using a system identification technique. *J Neuroeng Rehabil.* 2010;7:29.
79. Kamen L, Henney HR 3rd, Runyan JD. A practical overview of tizanidine use for spasticity secondary to multiple sclerosis, stroke, and spinal cord injury. *Curr Med Res Opin.* 2008;24:425-439.
80. Vakhapova V, Auriel E, Karni A. Nightly sublingual tizanidine HCl in multiple sclerosis: clinical efficacy and safety. *Clin Neuropharmacol.* 2010;33:151-154.

81. Malanga G, Reiter RD, Garay E. Update on tizanidine for muscle spasticity and emerging indications. *Expert Opin Pharmacother.* 2008;9:2209-2215.
82. Crassous PA, Denis C, Paris H, Sénard JM. Interest of alpha2-adrenergic agonists and antagonists in clinical practice: background, facts and perspectives. *Curr Top Med Chem.* 2007;7: 187-194.
83. Blum FC, Chen C, Kroken AR, Barbieri JT. Tetanus toxin and botulinum toxin a utilize unique mechanisms to enter neurons of the central nervous system. *Infect Immun.* 2012;80: 1662-1669.
84. Montal M. Botulinum neurotoxin: a marvel of protein design. *Annu Rev Biochem.* 2010;79:591-617.
85. Baldwin MR, Barbieri JT. Association of botulinum neurotoxins with synaptic vesicle protein complexes. *Toxicon.* 2009;54: 570-574.
86. Phadke CP, On AY, Kirazli Y, et al. Intrafusal effects of botulinum toxin injections for spasticity: revisiting a previous paper. *Neurosci Lett.* 2013;541:20-23.
87. Frascarelli F, Di Rosa G, Bisozzi E, et al. Neurophysiological changes induced by the botulinum toxin type A injection in children with cerebral palsy. *Eur J Paediatr Neurol.* 2011; 15:59-64.
88. Vinti M, Costantino F, Bayle N, et al. Spastic cocontraction in hemiparesis: effects of botulinum toxin. *Muscle Nerve.* 2012;46:926-931.
89. Matak I, Riederer P, Lacković Z. Botulinum toxin's axonal transport from periphery to the spinal cord. *Neurochem Int.* 2012;61:236-239.
90. Restani L, Giribaldi F, Manich M, et al. Botulinum neurotoxins A and E undergo retrograde axonal transport in primary motor neurons. *PLoS Pathog.* 2012;8:e1003087.
91. Currà A, Berardelli A. Do the unintended actions of botulinum toxin at distant sites have clinical implications? *Neurology.* 2009;72:1095-1099.
92. Akaike N, Shin MC, Wakita M, et al. Transsynaptic inhibition of spinal transmission by A2 botulinum toxin. *J Physiol.* 2013;591:1031-1043.
93. Filipović B, Matak I, Bach-Rojecky L, Lacković Z. Central action of peripherally applied botulinum toxin type A on pain and dural protein extravasation in rat model of trigeminal neuropathy. *PLoS One.* 2012;7:e29803.
94. Marinelli S, Vacca V, Ricordy R, et al. The analgesic effect on neuropathic pain of retrogradely transported botulinum neurotoxin A involves Schwann cells and astrocytes. *PLoS One.* 2012;7:e47977.
95. Bigalke H. Botulinum toxin: application, safety, and limitations. *Curr Top Microbiol Immunol.* 2013;364:307-317.
96. Wheeler A, Smith HS. Botulinum toxins: mechanisms of action, antinociception and clinical applications. *Toxicology.* 2013;306: 124-146.
97. Dressler D. Five-year experience with incobotulinumtoxinA (Xeomin): the first botulinum toxin drug free of complexing proteins. *Eur J Neurol.* 2012;19:385-389.
98. Chen S. Clinical uses of botulinum neurotoxins: current indications, limitations and future developments. *Toxins (Basel).* 2012;4:913-939.
99. Lee RM, Chowdhury HR, Hyer JN, et al. Patient-reported benefit from botulinum toxin treatment for essential blepharospasm: using 2 assessment scales. *Ophthal Plast Reconstr Surg.* 2013;29:196-197.
100. Patel S, Martino D. Cervical dystonia: from pathophysiology to pharmacotherapy. *Behav Neurol.* 2012. [Epub ahead of print]
101. Truong D. Botulinum toxins in the treatment of primary focal dystonias. *J Neurol Sci.* 2012;316:9-14.
102. Benecke R. Clinical relevance of botulinum toxin immunogenicity. *BioDrugs.* 2012;26:e1-9.
103. Love SC, Novak I, Kentish M, et al. Botulinum toxin assessment, intervention, and after-care for lower limb spasticity in children with cerebral palsy: international consensus statement. *Eur J Neurol.* 2010;17(suppl 2):9-37.
104. Lukban MB, Rosales RL, Dressler D. Effectiveness of botulinum toxin A for upper and lower limb spasticity in children with cerebral palsy: a summary of evidence. *J Neural Transm.* 2009;116:319-331.
105. Ryll U, Bastiaenen C, De Bie R, Staal B. Effects of leg muscle botulinum toxin A injections on walking in children with spasticity-related cerebral palsy: a systematic review. *Dev Med Child Neurol.* 2011;53:210-216.
106. Clemenzi A, Formisano R, Matteis M, et al. Care management of spasticity with botulinum toxin-A in patients with severe acquired brain injury: a 1-year follow-up prospective study. *Brain Inj.* 2012;26:979-983.
107. Guettard E, Roze E, Abada G, et al. Management of spasticity and dystonia in children with acquired brain injury with rehabilitation and botulinum toxin A. *Dev Neurorehabil.* 2009;12:128-138.
108. Rosales RL, Chua-Yap AS. Evidence-based systematic review on the efficacy and safety of botulinum toxin-A therapy in post-stroke spasticity. *J Neural Transm.* 2008;115:617-623.
109. Shaw L, Rodgers H. Botulinum toxin type A for upper limb spasticity after stroke. *Expert Rev Neurother.* 2009;9:1713-1725.
110. Teasell R, Foley N, Pereira S, et al. Evidence to practice: botulinum toxin in the treatment of spasticity post stroke. *Top Stroke Rehabil.* 2012;19:115-121.
111. Ward AB. Spasticity treatment with botulinum toxins. *J Neural Transm.* 2008;115:607-616.
112. Lim EC, Quek AM, Seet RC. Accurate targeting of botulinum toxin injections: how to and why. *Parkinsonism Relat Disord.* 2011;17(suppl 1):S34-39.
113. Frasson E, Priori A, Ruzzante B, et al. Nerve stimulation boosts botulinum toxin action in spasticity. *Mov Disord.* 2005;20: 624-629.
114. Balaban B, Tok F, Tan AK, Matthews DJ. Botulinum toxin a treatment in children with cerebral palsy: its effects on walking and energy expenditure. *Am J Phys Med Rehabil.* 2012;91: 53-64.
115. Fock J, Galea MP, Stillman BC, et al. Functional outcome following botulinum toxin A injection to reduce spastic equinus in adults with traumatic brain injury. *Brain Inj.* 2004;18: 57-63.
116. Tok F, Balaban B, Ya_ar E, et al. The effects of onabotulinum toxin A injection into rectus femoris muscle in hemiplegic stroke patients with stiff-knee gait: a placebo-controlled, nonrandomized trial. *Am J Phys Med Rehabil.* 2012;91:321-326.
117. Carda S, Invernizzi M, Baricich A, Cisari C. Casting, taping or stretching after botulinum toxin type A for spastic equinus foot: a single-blind randomized trial on adult stroke patients. *Clin Rehabil.* 2011;25:1119-1127.
118. Farina S, Migliorini C, Gandolfi M, et al. Combined effects of botulinum toxin and casting treatments on lower limb spasticity after stroke. *Funct Neurol.* 2008;23:87-91.

119. Park ES, Rha DW, Yoo JK, et al. Short-term effects of combined serial casting and botulinum toxin injection for spastic equinus in ambulatory children with cerebral palsy. *Yonsei Med J.* 2010;51:579-584.
120. Molenaers G, Van Campenhout A, Fagard K, et al. The use of botulinum toxin A in children with cerebral palsy, with a focus on the lower limb. *J Child Orthop.* 2010;4:183-195.
121. Shaw LC, Price CI, van Wijck FM, et al. Botulinum Toxin for the Upper Limb after Stroke (BoTULS) Trial: effect on impairment, activity limitation, and pain. *Stroke.* 2011;42: 1371-1379.
122. Flynn TC. Advances in the use of botulinum neurotoxins in facial esthetics. *J Cosmet Dermatol.* 2012;11:42-50.
123. Alvares RA, Silva JA, Barboza AL, Monteiro RT. Botulinum toxin A in the treatment of spinal cord injury patients with refractory neurogenic detrusor overactivity. *Int Braz J Urol.* 2010;36:732-737.
124. Goessaert AS, Everaert KC. Onabotulinum toxin A for the treatment of neurogenic detrusor overactivity due to spinal cord injury or multiple sclerosis. *Expert Rev Neurother.* 2012;12:763-775.
125. Chen G, Liao L. Injections of botulinum toxin A into the detrusor to treat neurogenic detrusor overactivity secondary to spinal cord injury. *Int Urol Nephrol.* 2011;43:655-662.
126. Mehta S, Hill D, Foley N, et al. A meta-analysis of botulinum toxin sphincteric injections in the treatment of incomplete voiding after spinal cord injury. *Arch Phys Med Rehabil.* 2012;93:597-603.
127. Duthie JB, Vincent M, Herbison GP, et al. Botulinum toxin injections for adults with overactive bladder syndrome. *Cochrane Database Syst Rev.* 2011;12:CD005493.
128. Ellsworth P. Treatment of overactive bladder symptoms beyond antimuscarinics: current and future therapies. *Postgrad Med.* 2012;124:16-27.
129. Frampton JE. OnabotulinumtoxinA (BOTOX): a review of its use in the prophylaxis of headaches in adults with chronic migraine. *Drugs.* 2012;72:825-845.
130. Francisco GE, Tan H, Green M. Do botulinum toxins have a role in the management of neuropathic pain?: a focused review. *Am J Phys Med Rehabil.* 2012;91:899-909.
131. Jabbari B, Machado D. Treatment of refractory pain with botulinum toxins—an evidence-based review. *Pain Med.* 2011;12:1594-1606.
132. Gallichio JE. Pharmacologic management of spasticity following stroke. *Phys Ther.* 2004;84:973-981.
133. Pagan FL, Harrison A. A guide to dosing in the treatment of cervical dystonia and blepharospasm with Xeomin: a new botulinum neurotoxin A. *Parkinsonism Relat Disord.* 2012;18: 441-445.
134. Lungu C, Karp BI, Alter K, et al. Long-term follow-up of botulinum toxin therapy for focal hand dystonia: outcome at 10 years or more. *Mov Disord.* 2011;26:750-753.
135. Albavera-Hernández C, Rodríguez JM, Idrovo AJ. Safety of botulinum toxin type A among children with spasticity secondary to cerebral palsy: a systematic review of randomized clinical trials. *Clin Rehabil.* 2009;23:394-407.

SECTION

4

Drugs Used to Treat Pain and Inflammation

CHAPTER 14

Opioid Analgesics

Analgesic drug therapy and certain rehabilitation interventions share a common goal: pain relief. Consequently, analgesics are among the drugs most frequently taken by patients who are treated in a rehabilitation setting. The vast array of drugs that are used to treat pain can be roughly divided into two categories: opioid and nonopioid analgesics. Nonopioid analgesics are composed of drugs such as acetaminophen, aspirin, ibuprofen, and similar agents. These drugs are discussed in Chapter 15.

Opioid analgesics are a group of naturally occurring, semisynthetic, and synthetic agents that are characterized by their ability to relieve moderate-to-severe pain. These drugs exert their effects by binding to specific neuronal receptors that are located primarily in the central nervous system (CNS). Opioid analgesics are also characterized by their potential ability to produce physical dependence and are classified as controlled substances in the United States because of their potential for abuse (see Chapter 1 for a description of controlled substance classification). Morphine is considered the prototypical opioid analgesic, and other drugs of this type are often compared to morphine in terms of efficacy and potency (Fig. 14-1).[1]

In the past, the term *narcotic* was often applied to these compounds because when taken, they tend to have sedative or sleep-inducing side effects, and high doses can produce a state of unresponsiveness and stupor. However, *narcotic* is a misleading name, because it describes a side effect rather than the principal therapeutic effect.

Likewise, these drugs are frequently referred to as *opiate analgesics* because some of these compounds are derived from opium. More recently, the term **opioid** has also been instituted to represent all types of narcotic analgesiclike agents, regardless of their origin.[2] Consequently, most sources preferentially use the term *opioid* to describe these drugs, and clinicians should recognize that this term represents all of the morphinelike medications.

You will frequently encounter patients taking opioids for acute pain after surgery and trauma and for more long-term conditions such as chronic severe musculoskeletal pain. These drugs are also a mainstay in reducing pain and improving quality of life in patients with advanced cancer. Opioids are often very helpful in reducing pain and in helping the patient be more active and engaged in exercise and other rehabilitation interventions. But these drugs are notorious for producing serious side effects, and their addictive potential often raises concerns in patients and medical practitioners. Hence, this chapter will introduce you to the actions and beneficial effects of opioid analgesics, their potential side effects, and how these drugs can have positive and negative effects on physical rehabilitation.

SOURCES OF OPIOID ANALGESICS

As mentioned previously, opioid analgesics can be obtained from natural, synthetic, or semisynthetic sources. Synthetic agents, as the designation implies, are simply formulated from basic chemical components

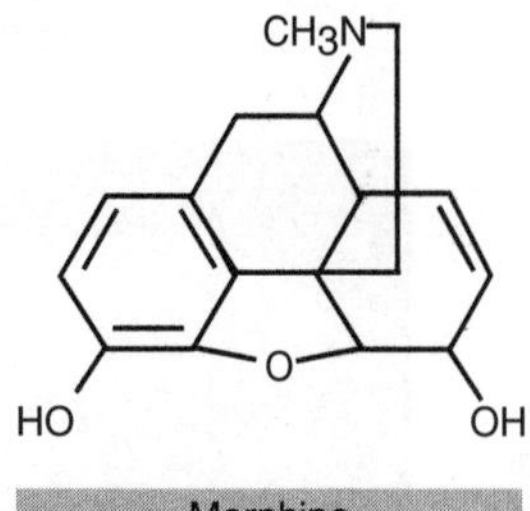

Figure ■ 14-1
Structure of morphine.

in the laboratory. The source of naturally occurring and semisynthetic narcotic analgesics is from the opium poppy.[2] When the extract from the seeds of this flower is allowed to dry and harden, the resulting substance is opium. Opium contains about 20 biologically active compounds, including morphine and codeine. Other derivatives from opium can also directly produce analgesia in varying degrees or can serve as precursors for analgesic drugs. The most notable of these precursors is thebaine, which can be modified chemically to yield compounds such as heroin. Likewise, semisynthetic narcotic analgesics are derived from these precursors. Semisynthetic opioids can also be formulated by modifying one of the other naturally occurring narcotic drugs, such as morphine.

In addition to analgesic drugs and their precursors, opium also contains compounds that do not have any analgesic properties. These compounds can actually antagonize the analgesic effects of opioid agonists such as morphine. (As defined in Chapter 4, an *agonist* stimulates its respective receptor and exerts a physiological response, whereas an *antagonist* blocks the receptor, thus preventing the response.) The role of these opioid antagonists is discussed in "Classification of Specific Agents," later in this chapter.

ENDOGENOUS OPIOID PEPTIDES AND OPIOID RECEPTORS

Endogenous Opioids

Neurons at specific locations within the CNS and some peripheral tissues have been identified as having receptors that serve as binding sites for morphine and other similar exogenous substances.[3] Exogenous opioids exert their effects by binding to these receptors; the proposed mechanisms of these drug-receptor interactions are discussed later in "Mechanism of Action." The discovery of these opioid receptors also suggested the existence of an endogenous opioidlike substance. Rather than isolating one such compound, the search for an "endogenous morphine" has actually revealed several groups of peptides with analgesic and other pharmacological properties. It is now recognized that three distinct families of endogenous opioids exist: the endorphins, enkephalins, and dynorphins.[2,4] The body manufactures and releases these peptides to control pain and inflammation under specific conditions.[5,6] Endogenous opioids may also help regulate the immune system, gastrointestinal (GI) function, cardiovascular responses, and many other physiological systems.[7-10] Endogenous opioids also are involved in many aspects of behavior, including response to physical and psychological stress, eating and drinking behaviors, and physiological addiction to exogenous opioids and other drugs.[5,11,12]

This chapter is not intended to elucidate all of the known details of the endogenous opioid peptide system or to illustrate how these endogenous compounds can be influenced by opioid drugs. However, the endogenous compounds described do exert their effects via the same receptors as the exogenous opioid drugs. Obviously, there is the possibility for a great deal of interaction between the endogenous and exogenous opioids, and researchers continue to investigate how exogenous drugs influence the function of the endogenous peptides, and vice versa.[4,13]

Opioid Receptors

Since their discovery, the opioid receptors have been examined in considerable detail. Studies in animals have suggested that rather than only one homogeneous opioid receptor, there are at least three primary classes known as *mu*, *kappa*, and *delta receptors*[2,14] (Table 14-1). A fourth class known as the *nociceptin/orphanin FQ peptide* (NOP) *receptor* has also been identified, but the relevance of the receptor remains unclear because no pharmacological agents have yet been identified that specifically affect this receptor.[15] Hence, most opioid drugs are characterized by their ability to affect the mu, kappa, and delta opioid receptors. Studies from experimental animal models also suggest that each primary receptor class can be categorized into two or three subclasses (i.e., $mu_{1\text{-}3}$, $delta_{1,2}$ and $kappa_{1\text{-}3}$) based on how well various opioids affect these receptors.[16]

Table 14-1
OPIOID RECEPTORS

Receptor Class	Primary Therapeutic Effect(s)	Other Effects
Mu (μ)	Spinal and supraspinal analgesia	Sedation; respiratory depression; constipation; inhibits neurotransmitter release (acetylcholine, dopamine); increases hormonal release (prolactin; growth hormone)
Kappa (κ)	Spinal and supraspinal analgesia	Sedation; constipation; psychotic effects
Delta (δ)	Spinal and supraspinal analgesia	Increases hormonal release (growth hormone); inhibits neurotransmitter release (dopamine)

Adapted from Schumacher et al. Opioid analgesics and antagonists. In: Katzung BG, et al, eds. Basic and Clinical Pharmacology. 12th ed. New York: Lange McGraw-Hill; 2012:544.

The significance of these subclasses has been questioned somewhat based on studies using opioid receptors that were cloned from rodent cell lines.[3,16] It is not clear at the present time if there are really physical differences within each primary class (i.e., is mu_1 structurally different from mu_2, and so forth). The apparent differences within each class may instead be due to functional differences related to the local environment surrounding the receptor, control by other chemicals (allosteric modulators), and other factors that control how each primary class responds to specific opioid drugs.[3] Nonetheless, mu opioid receptors are somewhat distinct from kappa receptors, and kappa receptors are distinct from delta receptors, and so on. Some specialization regarding both the location and the response of specific primary classes of opioid receptors does appear to exist (see Table 14-1).

Stimulation of all three classes of opioid receptors causes analgesia. However, the mu receptors, located in the brain and spinal cord, seem to be the most important in mediating the analgesic effects of many opioids, including morphine.[4,17,18] Opioids that are used clinically to reduce pain typically have a fairly high affinity for the mu receptors.[2] Unfortunately, some of the more problematic side effects of opioid drugs may also be mediated by stimulation of mu receptors. For example, stimulation of mu receptors may cause respiratory depression and constipation, and repeated stimulation of mu opioid receptors has been associated with the cellular changes that may lead to opioid abuse and addiction.[19-21]

The existence of the other classes of opioid receptors has therefore led to the development of drugs that are somewhat more selective in the receptor class or subclass that they stimulate while still providing sufficient analgesia. For example, certain opioid drugs stimulate kappa receptors while avoiding or blocking the mu receptors. As a result, drugs that selectively stimulate kappa or delta receptors will be less likely to provoke problems like respiratory depression and opioid abuse. These agents are known as *mixed agonist–antagonist opioids*, and their clinical significance is addressed in the next section, "Classification of Specific Agents."

The discovery of several classes of opioid receptors that cause different effects and side effects has important pharmacological implications. Research in this area continues to expand our knowledge about the structural and functional aspects of these receptor classes. Drug developers will hopefully capitalize on the unique aspects of opioid receptor classes and produce new agents that are even more specific in relieving pain without provoking excessive side effects.

CLASSIFICATION OF SPECIFIC AGENTS

Opioid analgesics are classified as strong agonists, mild-to-moderate agonists, mixed agonist–antagonists, and antagonists according to their interaction with opioid receptors. Some of the opioids in these categories are listed in Table 14-2. The basic characteristics of each category and clinically relevant examples are discussed next.

Strong Agonists

Strong agonist agents are used to treat severe pain. These drugs have a high affinity for certain receptors and are believed to interact primarily with mu opioid receptors in the CNS. The best-known member of this group is morphine—the other strong agonists are

Table 14-2
OPIOID ANALGESICS

Drug	Route of Administration*	Onset of Action (min)**	Peak Effects (min)	Duration of Action (hr)
Strong Agonists				
Alfentanil (Alfenta, Rapifen)	IV	Immediate	1–1.5	0.08–0.17
Fentanyl (Sublimaze, other trade names depend on administration route)	IM	7–15	20–30	1–2
	IV	1–2	3–5	0.5–1
	Sublingual	Within 30	30–60	2–4
	Oral transmucosal	Rapid	15–30	Several hr
	Buccal	15	40–60	1
	Buccal soluble film	15–30	60	2–6
	Iontophoretic transdermal system	Within minutes	5	0.17
Hydromorphone (Hydrostat, Dilaudid)	Oral	30	30–90	4–5
	IM	15	30–60	4–5
	IV	10–15	15–30	2–3
	Sub-Q	15	30–90	4–5
	Rectal	15–30	30–90	4–5
Levorphanol (Levo-Dromoran, Levorphan)	Oral	10–60	90–120	4–5
	IV	Unknown	Within 20	4–5
	Sub-Q	Unknown	60–90	4–5
Meperidine (Demerol, Pethidine)	Oral	15	60	2–4
	IM	10–15	30–50	2–4
	IV	Immediate	5–7	2–3
	Sub-Q	10–15	40–60	2–4
Methadone (Methadose)	Oral	30–60	90–120	4–12
	IM	10–20	60–120	4–6
	Sub-Q	10–20	60–120	4–6
Morphine (many trade names)	Oral	Unknown	60	4–5
	IM	10–30	30–60	4–5
	IV	Rapid	20	4–5
	Sub-Q	20	50–90	4–5
	Epidural	6–30	60	Up to 24
	Intrathecal	Rapid	Unknown	Up to 24
	Rectal	Unknown	20–60	3–7
Oxymorphone (Opana)	Oral	Unknown	Unknown	4–6
	IM	10–15	30–90	3–6
	IV	5–10	15–30	3–6
	Sub-Q	10–20	Unknown	3–4

Table 14-2
OPIOID ANALGESICS—cont'd

Drug	Route of Administration*	Onset of Action (min)**	Peak Effects (min)	Duration of Action (hr)
Remifentanil (Ultiva)	IV	Rapid	3–5	0.08–0.17
Sufentanil (Sufenta)	IV	Within 1	Unknown	0.08
	Epidural	Unknown	Unknown	1.17–1.5
Tapentadol (Nucynta)	Oral	Unknown	60	4–6
Tramadol (Ralivia, Ultram)	Oral	60	120–180	4–6
Mild-to-Moderate Agonists				
Codeine (Paveral)	Oral	30–45	60–120	4
	IM	10–30	30–60	4
	Sub–Q	10–30	Unknown	4
Hydrocodone (Hycodan)	Oral	10–30	30–60	4–6
Oxycodone (OxyContin, Roxicodone, others)	Oral	10–15	60–90	3–6
Propoxyphene (Darvon)	Oral	15–60	120–180	4–6
Mixed Agonist-Antagonist				
Buprenorphine (Buprenex)	IM	15	60	6
	IV	Rapid	Within 60	6
Butorphanol (Stadol)	IM	Within 15	30–60	3–4
	IV	Within minutes	4–5	2–4
	Intranasal	Within 15	60–120	4–5
Nalbuphine (Nubain)	IM	Within 15	60	3–6
	IV	2–3	30	3–6
	Sub–Q	Within 15	Unknown	3–6
Pentazocine (Talwin)	Oral	15–30	60–90	3
	IM	15–20	30–60	2–3
	IV	2–3	15–30	2–3
	Sub–Q	15–20	30–60	2–3

**IM= intramuscular; IV = intravenous; Sub–Q = subcutaneous*

***Times for drug onset, peak, and duration reflect regular formulations administered to young adults. Times will be longer for extended release preparations and may also differ in children, older adults, or patients with various diseases and organ dysfunction.*

pharmacologically similar. Examples of strong opioid agonists include the following:

- Fentanyl (Actiq, Duragesic, Sublimaze)
- Hydromorphone (Hydrostat, Dilaudid)
- Levorphanol (Levo-Dromoran)
- Meperidine (Demerol)
- Methadone (Dolophine, Methadose)
- Morphine (MS Contin, Roxanol, Statex, others)
- Oxymorphone (Numorphan)

Mild-to-Moderate Agonists

These drugs are still considered agonists that stimulate opioid receptors, but they do not have as high an affinity or efficacy as the drugs listed previously. These drugs are more effective in treating moderate pain. Examples include the following:

- Codeine
- Hydrocodone (Hycodan)

- Oxycodone (OxyContin, Roxicodone)
- Propoxyphene (Darvon)

Mixed Agonist–Antagonists

Mixed agonist–antagonist drugs exhibit some agonist and antagonistlike activity at the same time because the drugs have the ability to act differently at specific classes of opioid receptors. For instance, certain drugs in this category (e.g., butorphanol, nalbuphine, pentazocine) cause analgesia because they bind to and activate kappa receptors; they are kappa receptor agonists. At the same time, these drugs block or only partially activate mu receptors, thus acting as mu receptor antagonists or partial agonists, respectively[2] (the effects of partial agonists are described in more detail in Chapter 4).

Mixed agonist–antagonist opioids appear to have the advantage of producing adequate analgesia with less risk of the side effects associated with mu receptors, including respiratory depression. The drugs therefore have a reduced risk of fatal overdose, and they may have fewer addictive qualities than strong mu receptor agonists such as morphine.[2,22] However, mixed agonist–antagonists may produce more psychotropic effects (e.g., hallucinations, vivid dreams), and their maximal analgesic effect may not be as great as strong mu agonists.[2] Consequently, these drugs are not used extensively, but they do offer an alternative to strong-to-moderate opioid agonists in certain patients.

A relatively new addition to this category is buprenorphine (Buprenex). This drug partially activates mu receptors but is an antagonist at kappa receptors. Because of these selective effects, buprenorphine has been advocated not only as an analgesic, but also as a treatment for opioid dependence and withdrawal.[23-25] The use of this drug in treating opioid addiction is discussed in more detail later in this chapter.

Examples of mixed agonist–antagonists include the following:

- Butorphanol (Stadol)
- Buprenorphine (Buprenex)
- Nalbuphine (Nubain)
- Pentazocine (Talwin)

Antagonists

Antagonists block all opioid receptors, with a particular affinity for the mu variety. Because of their antagonistic properties, these agents will not produce analgesia but will displace opioid agonists from the opioid receptors and block any further effects of the agonist molecules. Consequently, antagonists are used primarily to treat opioid overdoses and addiction. The primary agent currently used in the United States to treat opioid overdose is naloxone. When administered in emergency situations, this drug can rapidly (within 1 to 2 minutes) and dramatically reverse the respiratory depression that is usually the cause of death in excessive opioid ingestion. Naltrexone is also commonly used in conjunction with behavioral therapy to maintain an opioid-free state in individuals recovering from opioid addiction. This drug may also be useful in treating alcohol dependence. The primary agents used clinically as opioid antagonists are naloxone (Narcan) and naltrexone (ReVia, Vivitrol).

PHARMACOKINETICS

Some opioid analgesics can be given orally, a preferred route of administration in terms of convenience and safety. Several of these enteral drugs also come in suppository form, permitting rectal administration if nausea and vomiting prohibit the oral route. Some opioids—including morphine—are now available in longer-acting formulations, as indicated by the sustained-, extended-, or controlled-release term on the drug label. These formulations tend to provide more prolonged effects and allow longer intervals between doses.[26] Other agents must be administered parenterally, usually through subcutaneous or intramuscular injection, because of poor intestinal absorption or significant first-pass inactivation.

IV administration must be done slowly and cautiously. The narcotic is frequently diluted, and an infusion pump allows slow, controlled administration. The IV route or other parenteral routes (e.g., epidural and intrathecal infusion) can also be used to administer opioids during patient-controlled analgesia; this concept is addressed in Chapter 17.

Transdermal patches can administer opioids such as fentanyl (Duragesic) and buprenorphine (Butrans).[27,28] These patches provide a convenient method for the steady, prolonged administration of opioids into the systemic circulation. Transdermal patches also avoid directly administering the drug to the GI tract, which may help reduce GI problems such as constipation.[29]

Iontophoresis techniques (i.e., the use of electric current to facilitate transdermal delivery) have also been advocated as a way to enhance transdermal opioid delivery to the systemic circulation.[30] By varying the amount of electric current, iontophoresis may ultimately allow the patient to control the rate of transdermal administration of the opioid.[31] Finally, certain opioids such as fentanyl can be administered systemically via lozenges or a "lollipop" that dissolves in the mouth (transmucosal delivery) or via nasal spray (intranasal administration).[32] It will be interesting to see if other innovative techniques will be developed in the future to provide alternative methods for opioid administration.

Because of differing degrees of solubility, the distribution and subsequent onset of action of specific agents varies (see Table 14-2). Opioids are ultimately distributed throughout all tissues, and these agents probably exert their principal analgesic effects after they reach the CNS. Some opioid effects may also be mediated by peripheral receptors located at the site of painful inflammation (see "Mechanism of Action" below). Metabolic inactivation of these drugs takes place primarily in the liver, although some degree of metabolism also occurs in other tissues such as the kidneys, lungs, and CNS. The kidneys excrete the drug metabolite and—to a lesser extent—the intact drug in the urine.

MECHANISM OF ACTION

Sites of Opioid Effects

As discussed earlier, opioids act on neuronal receptors in the spinal cord, brain, and peripheral tissues. The opioids exert their analgesic effects by modifying synaptic activity at these locations.

Spinal Effects

Opioid receptors in the spinal cord are concentrated primarily on neurons in the dorsal horn and inhibit synapses responsible for transmitting nociceptive input to higher (supraspinal) levels.[3] That is, opioids act at the spinal cord to inhibit painful impulses from being sent from the periphery to the brain. This inhibitory effect is mediated by opioid receptors that are located on both presynaptic and postsynaptic membranes of pain-mediating synapses (Fig. 14-2). Specifically, receptors are located on the presynaptic terminals of specific primary (first-order) nociceptive afferents, and when bound

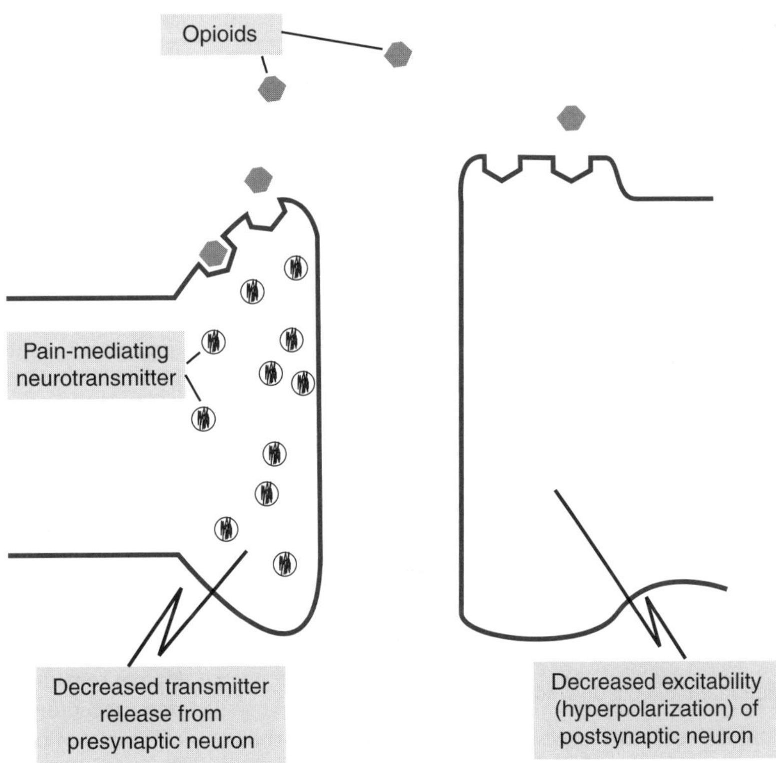

Figure ■ 14-2
Schematic representation of opioid effects at the spinal cord. Opioids bind to specific receptors on the presynaptic and postsynaptic membranes of pain-transmitting synapses in the dorsal horn. Decreased neurotransmitter release (presynaptic effect) and decreased excitability (postsynaptic effect) impair the ability of the synapse to transmit painful impulses to the brain.

by opioids, they directly decrease the release of pain-mediating transmitters such as substance P.[33]

Opioid drug-receptor interactions also take place on the postsynaptic membrane of the secondary afferent neuron—the second-order nociceptive afferent neuron in the spinal cord.[34] When stimulated, these receptors also inhibit pain transmission by hyperpolarizing the postsynaptic neuron.[34] Thus, the synapse is not as effective in relaying the painful sensation to the brain because less neurotransmitter is released (presynaptic effect) and because the postsynaptic neuron is hyperpolarized and therefore less excitable (postsynaptic effect). How opioids exert these effects on synapses is addressed later in "Effects of Opioids on Synaptic Activity."

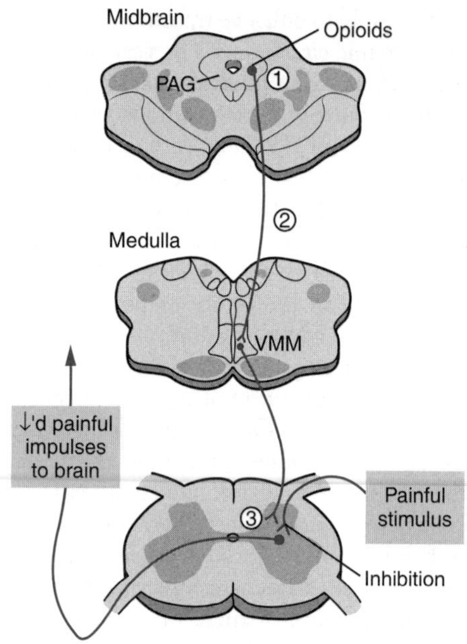

Figure ■ 14-3
Effects of opioids on supraspinal pathways: (1) Opioids bind to specific receptors in the midbrain periaqueductal gray matter (PAG) and remove inhibition of descending pathways that decrease pain. (2) Increased activity of descending pathways travels through the ventromedial medulla (VMM) to reach the dorsal horn of the spinal cord. (3) Neurons in descending pathways release serotonin and norepinephrine onto dorsal horn synapses and inhibit the ability of these synapses to transmit painful impulses to the brain.

Supraspinal (Brain) Effects

Opioid receptors have been identified in several locations in the brain (i.e., supraspinal sites) that are associated with pain transmission and interpretation. It is also believed that opioids exert some of their analgesic effects by binding to these supraspinal receptors and activating *descending* pain pathways (Fig. 14-3).[35] In particular, opioids affect the periaqueductal gray matter in the midbrain to influence descending (efferent) pathways that influence pain.[2,36] This effect probably occurs because opioids inhibit interneurons that normally inhibit the ability of these descending pathways to moderate painful stimuli. This effect, known as *disinhibition*, results in *increased* activity of descending pathways that project from the periaqueductal gray matter to the ventromedial medulla and ultimately to the dorsal horn of the spinal cord.

Upon reaching the dorsal horn, these descending neurons release norepinephrine and 5-hydroxytryptamine (serotonin).[2] These neurotransmitters inhibit activity at synapses that transmit painful sensations to the brain. Hence, the supraspinal effects of opioids complement their spinal effects—that is, opioids in the spinal cord directly inhibit activity of pain-transmitting synapses in the dorsal horn, whereas opioids in the brain activate descending pathways that release neurotransmitters that also inhibit these synapses in the cord. Opioids therefore exert analgesic effects through their ability to decrease ascending (afferent) pain transmission, combined with their ability to activate descending (efferent) pathways that reduce pain.

Peripheral Effects of Opioids

Opioid receptors exist outside the CNS, and some of the analgesic effects of opioids may be mediated at peripheral sites.[37,38] Opioid receptors have been identified on the distal (peripheral) ends of primary afferent (sensory) neurons.[39,40] Binding opioid agents to these peripheral receptors will provide an analgesic effect by decreasing the excitability of these sensory neurons (Fig. 14-4). This idea is supported by the fact that endogenous opioids (endorphins, enkephalins) are often produced by leukocytes in peripheral tissues during certain types of painful inflammation, and these endogenous substances seem to act locally on the peripheral sensory nerve terminals.[39,41] Likewise, results from some studies in animals and humans suggest that exogenous opioids can be administered directly into peripheral tissues (e.g., injected into an inflamed joint) and these agents exert analgesic effects even though the drug never reaches the CNS.[42]

The clinical significance of these peripheral opioid effects remains to be fully determined. For instance, these receptors may play a role in mediating only certain types of pain, such as the pain associated with inflammation.[43,44] Nonetheless, the fact that certain types

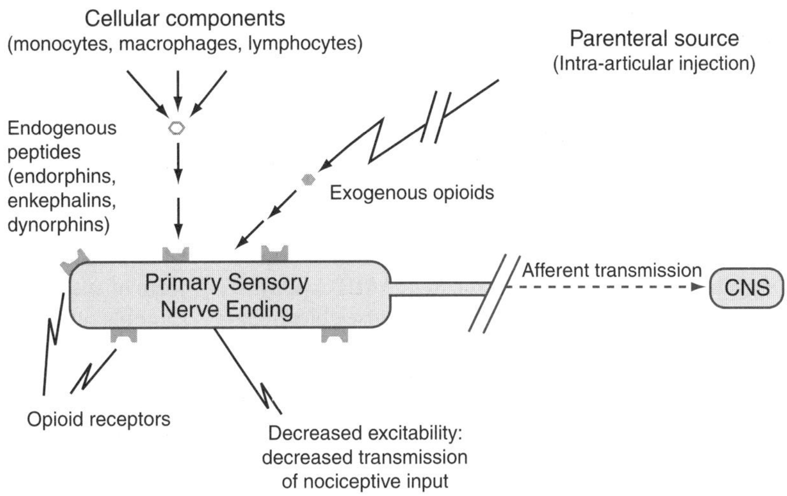

Figure ■ 14-4
Putative mechanism of opioid action on peripheral nerve terminals.

of pain might be controlled by peripherally acting opioids has important pharmacological implications. For instance, opioids that work exclusively in the periphery would not cause CNS-mediated side effects such as sedation, respiratory depression, and tolerance.[44,45] Peripheral-acting opioids could be developed by creating lipophobic compounds that are unable to cross the blood-brain barrier.[46] Currently, the use of these peripheral-acting drugs remains fairly experimental, and additional clinical trials are needed to determine whether this becomes a viable means of treating certain types of pain.

Effects of Opioids on Synaptic Activity

In the CNS, opioids inhibit synaptic transmission by decreasing neurotransmitter release from the presynaptic terminal and by decreasing excitability (hyperpolarizing) in postsynaptic neurons within key pain pathways in the spinal cord and brain. Again, these synaptic effects can either limit the transmission of painful stimuli in ascending pain pathways, or they can activate descending antinociceptive pathways by inhibiting interneurons that control these pathways. At peripheral sensory nerve endings, opioids decrease excitability of the neuron and inhibit the neuron from initiating transmission of painful stimuli toward the spinal cord. All of these effects appear to be mediated through opioid receptors that are located on the membrane of these neurons but are linked to the internal chemistry on the neurons through regulatory G proteins.[47,48]

As described in Chapter 4, regulatory G proteins act as an intermediate link between receptor activation and the intracellular effector mechanism that ultimately causes a change in cellular activity. In the case of opioid receptors, these G proteins interact with three primary cellular effectors: calcium channels, potassium channels, and intracellular signaling pathways such as those regulated by the adenyl cyclase enzyme.[3] At presynaptic terminals, stimulation of opioid receptors activates G proteins, which in turn inhibit the opening of calcium channels on the nerve membrane.[33] Decreased calcium entry into the presynaptic terminal causes decreased neurotransmitter release because calcium influx mediates transmitter release at a chemical synapse. At postsynaptic neurons, opioid receptors are linked via G proteins to potassium channels, and activation of the receptor leads to an opening of these channels and a loss of potassium from the postsynaptic neuron.[34] A relative loss of potassium from the postsynaptic neuron causes hyperpolarization because efflux of potassium (a cation) results in a relative increase in the negative intracellular electric potential. The postsynaptic neuron is therefore more difficult to excite because the interior of the cell is more negative.

The electrophysiological effects of opioids on peripheral sensory nerve endings are less clear. Stimulation of these receptors decreases excitability of the primary afferent neuron, probably because the receptors are linked to G proteins that inhibit adenyl cyclase activity (see below) and ultimately control calcium ion channels and other ion channels in the nerve membrane.[41] Regardless of their exact mechanism, binding of opioids to receptors on peripheral sensory nerve endings decreases the excitability of the neuron and thus inhibits the initiation of painful impulses that are transmitted toward the spinal cord.

Finally, opioid receptors are linked via G proteins to signaling pathways within the neuron. The primary pathway involves the adenyl cyclase enzyme-cyclic AMP system. Opioid stimulation of the receptor leads to inhibition of this enzyme and decreased synthesis of cyclic adenosine monophosphate (cAMP). cAMP is an important second messenger that causes biochemical changes in the neuron that lowers the neuronal firing threshold and increases excitability of neurons that transmit painful impulses to the brain.[49] Opioid-mediated inhibition of this second messenger system helps to explain how these drugs alter pain transmission. Likewise, G protein–linked opioid receptors may affect other intracellular signaling pathways such as protein kinase C, mitogen activated protein kinases, and other extracellular signal-related kinases.[3] These pathways may also affect neuronal function and excitability, and activation or inhibition of these other pathways seems to be related to how specific opioids affect mu, kappa, and delta receptors found on specific neurons.[50,51]

In summary, opioid drugs exert their therapeutic (analgesic) effects by interacting with receptors that are linked to G proteins that control several intracellular effector mechanisms. These effector mechanisms ultimately lead to decreased neuronal excitability and altered synaptic transmission in specific pain pathways.

CLINICAL APPLICATIONS

Treatment of Pain

Opioid analgesics are most effective in treating moderate-to-severe pain that is more or less constant in duration. These drugs are not as effective in treating sharp, intermittent pain—although higher dosages will relieve this type of pain as well. Some examples of the clinical usage of opioid analgesics include the treatment of acute pain following surgery, trauma, and myocardial infarction, as well as the treatment of chronic pain in patients with conditions such as cancer. Because of the potential for serious side effects (see "Problems and Adverse Effects" below), these drugs should be used only when necessary, and the dose should be titrated according to the patient's pain. Generally, oral administration of a mild-to-moderate opioid agonist should be used first, with stronger agonists being instituted orally and then parenterally if needed. In cases of chronic pain, nonopioid drugs should be attempted first. However, opioid analgesics should be instituted when the improvement in the quality of life offered to the patient with chronic pain clearly outweighs the potential risks of these drugs.[52,53]

Opioid analgesics often produce a rather unique form of analgesia as compared to the nonopioid agents. Opioids often alter the perception of pain rather than eliminating the painful sensation entirely. The patient may still be aware of the pain but it is no longer the primary focus of his or her attention. In a sense, the patient is no longer preoccupied by the pain. This type of analgesia is also often associated with euphoria and a sensation of floating. These sensations may be caused by the stimulation of specific types of opiate receptors within the limbic system (i.e., delta receptors).

The route of opioid administration appears to be important in providing safe and effective pain relief.[1,54] Although the oral route is the easiest and most convenient, parenteral routes may be more effective in chronic or severe, intractable pain. In particular, administration directly into the epidural or intrathecal space has been suggested as being optimal in relieving pain following certain types of surgery or in various types of acute or chronic pain.[55-58] Because it is impractical to reinsert a needle every time the drug is needed, indwelling catheters are often implanted surgically so that the tip of the catheter lies in the epidural or intrathecal space. The free end of the catheter can be brought out through the patient's skin and used to administer the opioid directly into the area surrounding the spinal cord. Alternatively, the catheter can be connected to some sort of a drug reservoir or pump that contains the opioid drug. Such devices can be located outside the patient's body or implanted surgically beneath the patient's skin (e.g., in the abdominal wall) and are programmed to deliver the drug at a fixed rate into the indwelling catheter.[59] Although these programmable drug-delivery systems do have some risks, they appear to be an effective way of treating patients with severe, chronic pain from malignant and nonmalignant sources.[59]

The effectiveness of opioid analgesics also appears to be influenced by the dosing schedule. The current consensus is that orally administered opioids are more effective when given at regularly scheduled intervals rather than when the patient feels the need for them.[60] This may be because with regularly scheduled dosages, plasma concentrations may be maintained within a therapeutic range, rather than allowing the large plasma fluctuations that may occur if the drugs are given at sporadic intervals. On the other hand, it may simply be easier to control pain in its earlier stages before the pain can reach full intensity.[60] Consistent with these hypotheses is the finding that continuous infusion of the opioid into the epidural or intrathecal space provides optimal pain relief postoperatively or in cases of chronic, intractable pain.[55,58] Continuous infusion is associated with certain side effects, especially nausea and constipation, as well as the potential for disruption of the drug delivery system.[59,61] Problems with tolerance have also been reported during continuous administration,[62] but it is somewhat controversial whether tolerance really develops when these drugs are used appropriately in the clinical management of pain (see "Concepts of Addiction, Tolerance, and Physical Dependence"). Nevertheless, the benefit-to-risk ratio for continuous epidural or intrathecal infusion is often acceptable in patients with severe pain, and this method of opioid administration continues to gain acceptance.[55,58]

Use of Opioids in Patient-Controlled Analgesia

Finally, techniques have been developed that enable the patient to control the delivery of the analgesic.[63,64] These techniques are collectively known as **patient-controlled analgesia (PCA)** because the patient is able to periodically administer a specific dose of the drug by pushing a button or some other device. PCA systems have some distinct advantages over conventional administration, and PCAs are often used following various types of surgery and in the treatment of certain types of chronic pain and cancer-related pain.[65-67] The use of opioids and other drugs in PCA systems is discussed in Chapter 17.

Other Opioid Uses

Opioids have several other clinical applications. These agents can be used as an anesthetic premedication or as an adjunct in general anesthesia. Opioids are effective in cough suppression, and the short-term use of codeine and codeinelike agents in this regard is quite common. Opioid agonists decrease GI motility and can be used to control cases of severe diarrhea. This effect is probably mediated indirectly through an effect on the CNS and through a direct effect on the intestine. Finally, opioid agonists are used as an adjunct in cases of acute pulmonary edema. These drugs probably do not directly improve ventilatory capacity, but they do reduce feelings of intense panic and anxiety associated with the dyspnea inherent to this disorder. Patients feel they can breathe more easily following opioid administration.

PROBLEMS AND ADVERSE EFFECTS

Opioid analgesics produce several central and peripheral side effects.[68,69] Virtually all of these drugs have sedative properties and induce some degree of mental slowing and drowsiness. Patients taking opioids for the relief of pain may also become somewhat euphoric, although the manner and degree of such mood changes varies from individual to individual.

One of the more potentially serious side effects is the respiratory depression often seen after narcotic administration.[70,71] Within a few minutes after administration, these drugs slow the breathing rate, which can last for several hours. Although not usually a major problem when therapeutic doses are given to relatively healthy individuals, respiratory depression can be severe or even fatal in seriously ill patients, in patients with preexisting pulmonary problems, or in cases of overdose. Some cardiovascular problems such as orthostatic hypotension may also occur immediately after opioids are administered, especially when parenteral routes are used.

GI distress in the form of nausea and vomiting is quite common with many of the narcotic analgesics. Because of their antiperistaltic action, these drugs can also cause constipation, which can be severe.[68,70,72] Therefore, laxatives and stool softeners (see Chapter 27) can be used to prevent opioid-induced constipation in certain people, such as patients who are at risk for fecal impaction (e.g., people with spinal cord injuries) or with people who are taking opioids for an extended period of time (e.g., patients receiving opioids for treatment of cancer-related pain).[72,73]

CONCEPTS OF ADDICTION, TOLERANCE, AND PHYSICAL DEPENDENCE

When used inappropriately, opioid drugs can produce addiction. The term *addiction* typically refers to when an individual repeatedly ingests certain substances for mood-altering and pleasurable experiences, such as the heroin addict who takes the drug illicitly to achieve an opioid "high." In this sense, addiction is a very complex phenomenon that has strong psychological implications regarding why certain chemicals cause this behavior in certain people. This concept of addiction is often separated from the physiological changes that can accompany prolonged opioid use, namely tolerance and physical dependence. Tolerance and physical dependence are also rather complex phenomena, and a complete discussion of the factors involved in producing these occurrences is not possible in this chapter. However, the primary characteristics of tolerance and physical dependence will be briefly discussed here as they relate to opioid usage.

Tolerance

Tolerance is defined as the need to progressively increase the dosage of a drug to achieve a therapeutic effect when the drug is used for prolonged periods.[4] When used for the treatment of pain in some patients, the dosage of the opioid may need to be increased periodically to continue to provide adequate relief. The physiological reasons for tolerance are complex and probably involve several changes in the intracellular response to repeated stimulation of opioid receptors. Prolonged exposure to opioids can, for example, cause a decrease in the number and sensitivity of the opioid receptors—a phenomenon known as *receptor downregulation* and *desensitization* (see Chapter 4).[74,75] Likewise, prolonged opioid exposure can cause the cell to remove opioid receptors from its surface by endocytosis, store these receptors temporarily inside itself, and then recycle them back to its surface. However, these changes in the quantity, sensitivity, and location of opioid receptors do not seem to fully explain why opioid tolerance occurs in clinical situations.[75]

Other changes associated with opioid tolerance involve a loss of communication between the opioid receptor and the G protein that transmits information to the cell's interior.[4,47] As described earlier, opioid receptors mediate their effects through regulatory G proteins that are linked to intracellular effectors, including the adenyl cyclase enzyme. Tolerance to opioid drugs may be caused by a disruption in the link between the opioid receptor and its regulatory G protein—that is, the receptor may become uncoupled from the G protein and therefore fail to exert an effect on the adenyl cyclase enzyme and other signaling pathways that affect neuronal function.[3] Opioid tolerance might also involve activation of neurochemical pathways that promote pain.[75,76] In this case, the ability of opioids to control activity in certain pain pathways may be counterbalanced by increased activity in other (nociceptive) pathways the mediate painful responses. The activation of these nociceptive pathways may also be important in producing increased pain sensitivity (hyperalgesia) in certain patients receiving opioids. This phenomenon is discussed in more detail later in "Opioid-Induced Hyperalgesia."

Opioid tolerance typically follows a predictable time course. Tolerance begins after the first dose of the narcotic, but the need for increased amounts of the drug usually becomes obvious after 2 to 3 weeks of administration. Tolerance seems to last approximately 1 to 2 weeks after the drug is removed. This does not mean that the patient no longer has any desire for the drug; rather, the patient will again respond to the initial dosage after 14 days or so. Other factors, such as physical dependence, may influence the individual's desire for the drug long after any physiological effects have disappeared.

Physical Dependence

Physical dependence is usually defined as the onset of withdrawal symptoms when the drug is abruptly removed. Withdrawal syndrome from opioid dependence is associated with several unpleasant symptoms (Table 14-3). In severe dependence, withdrawal symptoms become evident within 6 to 10 hours after the last dose of the drug, and symptoms reach their peak in the second or third day after the drug has been stopped.

Table 14-3
ABSTINENCE SYNDROMES: SYMPTOMS OF NARCOTIC WITHDRAWAL

Body aches	Runny nose
Diarrhea	Shivering
Fever	Sneezing
Gooseflesh	Stomach cramps
Insomnia	Sweating
Irritability	Tachycardia
Loss of appetite	Uncontrollable yawning
Nausea/vomiting	Weakness/fatigue

Withdrawal symptoms last approximately 5 days. This does not necessarily mean that the individual no longer desires the drug, only that the physical symptoms of withdrawal have ceased. Indeed, an addict may continue to crave the drug after months or years of abstinence.

Physical dependence must therefore be differentiated from the more intangible concepts of addiction and psychological dependence. Psychological dependence seems to be related to pleasurable changes in mood and behavior evoked by the drug. The individual is motivated to continually reproduce these pleasurable sensations because of the feelings of well-being, relaxation, and so on. Psychological dependence seems to create the drug-seeking behavior that causes the addict to relapse long after the physiological effects have disappeared.

Tolerance and Dependence During Therapeutic Opioid Use

Although tolerance and dependence can occur whenever opioid drugs are used indiscriminately for prolonged periods, there is some debate as to whether these phenomena must always accompany the therapeutic use of opioid drugs for the treatment of chronic pain. There is growing evidence that the risk of tolerance and dependence is actually very low when opioid drugs are used appropriately to treat chronic pain.[77,78] For example, there appear to be relatively few problems with long-term opioid use when these drugs are administered to treat pain in patients who do not have a history of substance abuse, who adhere to the prescribed opioid regimen, and who have pain from physiological rather than psychological causes.[77,78]

Some experts also feel that tolerance and physical dependence will not occur in most patients if the dosage is carefully adjusted to meet the patient's needs.[79,80] It is believed that when the opioid dose exactly matches the patient's need for pain control, there is no excess drug to stimulate the drug-seeking behavior commonly associated with opioid addiction. The opioid is essentially absorbed by the patient's pain. Of course, patients with chronic pain may still need to have the dosage increased periodically, possibly because the pain has increased or the patient's condition has worsened (e.g., the cancer has increased), rather than because the patient developed pharmacological tolerance to the drug.[52,81] Thus, many practitioners feel that problems with addiction, tolerance, and dependence are minimized when opioid drugs are used therapeutically in patients who do not have a history of substance abuse. These agents are essentially being used for a specific reason—the treatment of pain—rather than for the pleasure-seeking purpose associated with the recreational use of these drugs. These drugs must, of course, be used carefully and with strict regard to using the lowest effective dose. Hence, most practitioners feel that opioids are very effective and important analgesic agents and should be used under appropriate therapeutic conditions without excessive fear of the patient developing addiction or becoming especially tolerant to the drug's effects.[80,82]

Opioid-Induced Hyperalgesia

As indicated earlier, certain patients may fail to respond to opioids or may report increased pain (hyperalgesia) when administered opioid drugs.[83] The reasons for opioid-induced hyperalgesia are not fully understood and may involve genetic factors that predispose certain patients to increased activity in nociceptive pathways.[84] In particular, opioid administration may cause a compensatory increase in the activity of glutamate pathways in certain patients. Glutamate is an excitatory neurotransmitter that promotes painful responses in the CNS by stimulating the N-methyl-d-aspartate (NMDA) receptor.[75,76] In other words, administration of opioids to certain patients may turn on nociceptive pathways that use glutamate. This effect may be caused by increased glutamate release, decreased glutamate breakdown, increased sensitivity of the NMDA receptor, and other complex changes in these nociceptive pathways.

Regardless of the exact cause, there is increasing awareness that some patients may simply not respond to opioids even before tolerance develops, and these individuals may be exhibiting opioid-induced hyperalgesia. Clinicians should be alert whenever a patient taking opioids fails to respond to the drug or seems to have increased pain. These patients should be observed closely to see if pain worsens when the opioid drugs are reaching peak effects, or if pain is reduced when drug effects are minimal or the dosage is reduced. It may be difficult to discern changes in pain considering that the patient is probably in moderate to severe pain even before the opioid is administered. Hence, careful baseline pain measurements will be needed to see if pain increases when the opioid drug begins to take effect. Likewise, opioid-induced hyperalgesia should be considered if pain remains unchanged or increases even after a higher dose. Clinicians should notify the physician whenever opioids fail to produce a therapeutic analgesic effect, and alternative analgesics should be considered.[84,85]

Pharmacological Treatment of Opioid Addiction

The inappropriate or illegal use and abuse of narcotics such as heroin is a major problem in many countries. As a result, practitioners employ various strategies to treat people who are addicted to heroin and other opioids. Methadone is the primary pharmacological intervention used to treat opioid addiction.[86] This is a strong opioid agonist, similar in potency and efficacy to morphine. While giving an opioid to treat an opioid addiction may at first appear odd, methadone offers several advantages, such as milder withdrawal symptoms. Methadone is essentially substituted for the abused opioid (e.g., heroin) and is then slowly withdrawn as various methods of counseling are employed to discourage further drug abuse.[87,88] Use of methadone is controversial because of its rather low success rate and the tendency for many patients to relapse and return to opioid abuse.[87] Still, methadone maintenance programs are more successful than using no pharmacological intervention.[89]

Recently, medical researchers have been advocating buprenorphine as an alternative pharmacological method for treating opioid addiction.[23,87] As indicated earlier, buprenorphine is a mixed agonist–antagonist that partially stimulates mu opioid receptors while acting as a strong antagonist at kappa opioid receptors. By weakly stimulating the mu receptors, this drug can sustain the opioid effects and prevent sudden withdrawal. At the same time, buprenorphine can block kappa receptors, thereby affecting some of the cellular changes that seem to promote opioid addiction. Buprenorphine can be used alone or combined with naloxone (an opioid antagonist).[90] Combining these two drugs may decrease the potential for abusing buprenorphine and other opioids during maintenance programs because naloxone will block the opioid effects and hopefully decrease the chance of relapse.[91]

Efforts continue to provide more effective pharmacological and nonpharmacological interventions for treating opioid addiction.[92] The ultimate goal is to eventually wean the patient from all opioid drugs.[88] As more information is gained about the cellular and subcellular mechanisms that cause addiction, we may see other agents being used to specifically treat these changes.

Special Concerns for Rehabilitation Patients

Opioid analgesics are commonly administered to patients undergoing physical rehabilitation, and these drugs can have positive and negative effects that influence physical therapy and occupational therapy. For example, side effects such as sedation and GI discomfort may be bothersome during some of the therapy sessions. However, the relief of pain afforded by these drugs may be helpful in allowing a relatively more vigorous and comprehensive rehabilitation regimen. The benefits of pain relief usually outweigh side effects such as sedation. Scheduling therapy when these drugs reach their peak effects may be advantageous (see Table 14-2).

The tendency of these drugs to produce respiratory depression should be taken into account during therapy. Opioids tend to make the medullary chemoreceptors less responsive to carbon dioxide, thus slowing down the respiratory rate and inducing a

Special Concerns for Rehabilitation Patients (Continued)

relative hypoxia and hypercapnia.[71] As a result, the respiratory response to any rehabilitation exercise may be blunted.

The tendency for these drugs to produce constipation is another side effect that could have important implications for patients receiving physical rehabilitation. Opioid-induced constipation is especially problematic in patients with spinal cord injuries or other conditions that decrease GI motility. In such patients, opioids are often administered along with laxatives and GI stimulants (see Chapter 27) to minimize the constipating effects and risk of fecal impaction. Therapists should therefore be aware of these constipating effects and help educate patients and their families so that these effects do not result in serious problems.

Therapists may also be working with patients who are experiencing withdrawal symptoms from opioid drugs. Such patients may be in the process of being weaned off the therapeutic use of these agents, or they may be heroin addicts who have been hospitalized for other reasons (e.g., trauma, surgery). If not on some type of methadone maintenance or similar intervention, the addict may be experiencing a wide variety of physical symptoms, including diffuse muscle aches. The therapist should be aware that these aches and pains may be caused by opioid withdrawal rather than an actual somatic disorder. Therapists may help the patient cope with the physical symptoms of opioid withdrawal by using various physical agents (e.g., heat, electrotherapy) and manual techniques (e.g., massage, relaxation techniques).

CASE STUDY

OPIOID ANALGESICS

Brief History. N.P., a 45-year-old woman, was involved in an automobile accident approximately 6 months ago. She received multiple contusions from the accident, but no major injuries were sustained. Two months later, she began to develop pain in the right shoulder. This pain progressively increased, and she was treated for bursitis using anti-inflammatory drugs. Her shoulder motion became progressively more limited; however, any movement of her glenohumeral joint caused rather severe pain. She was reevaluated and a diagnosis of adhesive capsulitis was made. The patient was admitted to the hospital, and while she was under general anesthesia, a closed manipulation of the shoulder was performed. When the patient recovered from the anesthesia, meperidine (Demerol) was prescribed for pain relief. This drug was given orally at a dosage of 75 mg every 4 hours. Physical therapy was also initiated the afternoon following the closed manipulation. Passive range-of-motion exercises were used to maintain the increased joint mobility achieved during the manipulative procedure.

1. ***When should the therapist schedule the treatment session so that meperidine is reaching peak effects?***
2. ***What precautions should the therapist use during the initial treatments given the potential side effects of this drug?***

See Appendix C, "Answers to Case Study Questions."

SUMMARY

Opioid analgesics represent some of the most effective methods of treating moderate-to-severe pain. When used properly, these agents can alleviate acute and chronic pain in a variety of situations. The use of these drugs is sometimes tempered with their tendency to produce tolerance and physical dependence, but their potential for abuse seems relatively low when they are used appropriately to treat pain. Opioid drugs therefore represent the most effective pharmacological means of helping patients deal with acute and chronic pain. The analgesic properties of these drugs often provide a substantial benefit in patients involved in rehabilitation. Clinicians should be aware of side effects such as sedation and respiratory depression and should be cognizant of the impact of these effects during the rehabilitation session.

REFERENCES

1. Schug SA, Gandham N. Opioids: clinical use. In: McMahon SB, Koltzenberg M, eds. *Wall and Melzack's Textbook of Pain*. 5th ed. New York: Elsevier/Churchill Livingstone; 2005: 443-458.
2. Yaksh TL, Wallace MS. Opioids, analgesia, and pain management. In: Brunton LL, et al, eds. *The Pharmacological Basis of Therapeutics*. 12th ed. New York: McGraw Hill; 2011.
3. Dickenson AH, Kieffer B. Opioids: basic mechanisms. In: McMahon SB, Koltzenberg M, eds. *Wall and Melzack's Textbook of Pain*. 5th ed. New York: Elsevier/Churchill Livingstone; 2005: 427-442.
4. Schumacher MA, Basbaum AI, Way WL. Opioid analgesics and antagonists. In: Katzung BG, Masters SB, Trevor AJ, eds. *Basic and Clinical Pharmacology*. 12th ed. New York: Lange Medical Books/McGraw Hill; 2012.
5. Bodnar RJ. Endogenous opiates and behavior: 2010. *Peptides*. 2011;32:2522-2552.
6. Roques BP, Fournié-Zaluski MC, Wurm M. Inhibiting the breakdown of endogenous opioids and cannabinoids to alleviate pain. *Nat Rev Drug Discov*. 2012;11:292-310.
7. Beard TL, Leslie JB, Nemeth J. The opioid component of delayed gastrointestinal recovery after bowel resection. *J Gastrointest Surg*. 2011;15:1259-1268.
8. Headrick JP, Pepe S, Peart JN. Non-analgesic effects of opioids: cardiovascular effects of opioids and their receptor systems. *Curr Pharm Des*. 2012;18:6090-6100.
9. Krazinski BE, Koziorowski M, Brzuzan P, Okrasa S. The expression of genes encoding opioid precursors and the influence of opioid receptor agonists on steroidogenesis in porcine adrenocortical cells in vitro. *J Physiol Pharmacol*. 2011;62: 461-468.
10. Sacerdote P, Franchi S, Panerai AE. Non-analgesic effects of opioids: mechanisms and potential clinical relevance of opioid-induced immunodepression. *Curr Pharm Des*. 2012;18: 6034-6042.
11. Chavkin C. Dynorphin—still an extraordinarily potent opioid peptide. *Mol Pharmacol*. 2013;83:729-736.
12. D'Amato FR, Pavone F. Modulation of nociception by social factors in rodents: contribution of the opioid system. *Psychopharmacology*. 2012;224:189-200.
13. Chen TC, Cheng YY, Sun WZ, Shyu BC. Differential regulation of morphine antinociceptive effects by endogenous enkephalinergic system in the forebrain of mice. *Mol Pain*. 2008;4:41.
14. Feng Y, He X, Yang Y, et al. Current research on opioid receptor function. *Curr Drug Targets*. 2012;13:230-246.
15. Donica CL, Awwad HO, Thakker DR, Standifer KM. Cellular mechanisms of nociceptin/orphanin FQ (N/OFQ) peptide (NOP) receptor regulation and heterologous regulation by N/OFQ. *Mol Pharmacol*. 2013;83:907-918.
16. Dietis N, Rowbotham DJ, Lambert DG. Opioid receptor subtypes: fact or artifact? *Br J Anaesth*. 2011;107:8-18.
17. Mizoguchi H, Watanabe C, Sakurada T, Sakurada S. New vistas in opioid control of pain. *Curr Opin Pharmacol*. 2012;12:87-91.
18. Spetea M, Asim MF, Wolber G, Schmidhammer H. The μ opioid receptor and ligands acting at the μ opioid receptor, as therapeutics and potential therapeutics. *Curr Pharm Des*. 2013;19:7415-7434. [Epub ahead of print]
19. Diego L, Atayee R, Helmons P, et al. Novel opioid antagonists for opioid-induced bowel dysfunction. *Expert Opin Investig Drugs*. 2011;20:1047-1056.
20. Lalley PM. Opioidergic and dopaminergic modulation of respiration. *Respir Physiol Neurobiol*. 2008;164:160-167.
21. Terenius L, Johansson B. The opioid systems—panacea and nemesis. *Biochem Biophys Res Commun*. 2010;396:140-142.
22. Schiller PW. Bi- or multifunctional opioid peptide drugs. *Life Sci*. 2010;86:598-603.
23. Bonhomme J, Shim RS, Gooden R, Tyus D, Rust G. Opioid addiction and abuse in primary care practice: a comparison of methadone and buprenorphine as treatment options. *J Natl Med Assoc*. 2012;104:342-350.
24. Davis MP. Twelve reasons for considering buprenorphine as a frontline analgesic in the management of pain. *J Support Oncol*. 2012;10:209-219.
25. Ling W. Buprenorphine for opioid dependence. *Expert Rev Neurother*. 2009;9:609-616.
26. Rauck RL. What is the case for prescribing long-acting opioids over short-acting opioids for patients with chronic pain? A critical review. *Pain Pract*. 2009;9:468-479.
27. Paech MJ, Bloor M, Schug SA. New formulations of fentanyl for acute pain management. *Drugs Today*. 2012;48:119-132.
28. Plosker GL, Lyseng-Williamson KA. Buprenorphine 5, 10 and 20 μg/h transdermal patch: a guide to its use in chronic non-malignant pain. *CNS Drugs*. 2012;26:367-373.
29. Tassinari D, Sartori S, Tamburini E, et al. Transdermal fentanyl as a front-line approach to moderate-severe pain: a meta-analysis of randomized clinical trials. *J Palliat Care*. 2009;25:172-180.
30. Herwadkar A, Banga AK. An update on the application of physical technologies to enhance intradermal and transdermal drug delivery. *Ther Deliv*. 2012;3:339-355.
31. Herndon CM. Iontophoretic drug delivery system: focus on fentanyl. *Pharmacotherapy*. 2007;27:745-754.

32. Leppert W, Krajnik M, Wordliczek J. Delivery systems of opioid analgesics for pain relief: a review. *Curr Pharm Des.* 2013;19:7271-7293.
33. Heinke B, Gingl E, Sandkühler J. Multiple targets of μ-opioid receptor-mediated presynaptic inhibition at primary afferent Aδ- and C-fibers. *J Neurosci.* 2011;31:1313-1322.
34. Honda H, Kawasaki Y, Baba H, Kohno T. The mu opioid receptor modulates neurotransmission in the rat spinal ventral horn. *Anesth Analg.* 2012;115:703-712.
35. Heinricher MM, Tavares I, Leith JL, Lumb BM. Descending control of nociception: specificity, recruitment and plasticity. *Brain Res Rev.* 2009;60:214-225.
36. Kandel ER, Scwartz JH, Jessell TM, et al. Pain. In: *Principles of Neural Science.* 5th ed. New York: McGraw-Hill; 2013:530-555.
37. Khalefa BI, Shaqura M, Al-Khrasani M, Fürst S, Mousa SA, Schäfer M. Relative contributions of peripheral versus supraspinal or spinal opioid receptors to the antinociception of systemic opioids. *Eur J Pain.* 2012;16:690-705.
38. Labuz D, Mousa SA, Schäfer M, et al. Relative contribution of peripheral versus central opioid receptors to antinociception. *Brain Res.* 2007;1160:30-38.
39. Stein C, Machelska H. Modulation of peripheral sensory neurons by the immune system: implications for pain therapy. *Pharmacol Rev.* 2011;63:860-881.
40. Vadivelu N, Mitra S, Hines RL. Peripheral opioid receptor agonists for analgesia: a comprehensive review. *J Opioid Manag.* 2011;7:55-68.
41. Stein C, Lang LJ. Peripheral mechanisms of opioid analgesia. *Curr Opin Pharmacol.* 2009;9:3-8.
42. Sehgal N, Smith HS, Manchikanti L. Peripherally acting opioids and clinical implications for pain control. *Pain Physician.* 2011;14:249-258.
43. Alves DP, da Motta PG, Lima PP, et al. Inflammation mobilizes local resources to control hyperalgesia: the role of endogenous opioid peptides. *Pharmacology.* 2012;89:22-28.
44. Smith HS. Peripherally-acting opioids. *Pain Physician.* 2008; 11(suppl):S121-132.
45. Varamini P, Goh WH, Mansfeld FM, et al. Peripherally acting novel lipo-endomorphin-1 peptides in neuropathic pain without producing constipation. *Bioorg Med Chem.* 2013;21: 1898-1904.
46. Rachinger-Adam B, Conzen P, Azad SC. Pharmacology of peripheral opioid receptors. *Curr Opin Anaesthesiol.* 2011;24: 408-413.
47. Al-Hasani R, Bruchas MR. Molecular mechanisms of opioid receptor-dependent signaling and behavior. *Anesthesiology.* 2011;115:1363-1381.
48. Traynor J. μ-Opioid receptors and regulators of G protein signaling (RGS) proteins: from a symposium on new concepts in mu-opioid pharmacology. *Drug Alcohol Depend.* 2012;121: 173-180.
49. Cao JL, Vialou VF, Lobo MK, et al. Essential role of the cAMP-cAMP response-element binding protein pathway in opiate-induced homeostatic adaptations of locus coeruleus neurons. *Proc Natl Acad Sci USA.* 2010;107:17011-17016.
50. Bruchas MR, Chavkin C. Kinase cascades and ligand-directed signaling at the kappa opioid receptor. *Psychopharmacology.* 2010; 210:137-147.
51. Wang Q, Traynor JR. Modulation of μ-opioid receptor signaling by RGS19 in SH-SY5Y cells. *Mol Pharmacol.* 2013;83: 512-520.
52. Sarzi-Puttini P, Vellucci R, Zuccaro SM, et al. The appropriate treatment of chronic pain. *Clin Drug Investig.* 2012;32 (suppl 1):21-33.
53. Watson CP. Opioids in chronic noncancer pain: more faces from the crowd. *Pain Res Manag.* 2012;17:263-275.
54. Heitz JW, Witkowski TA, Viscusi ER. New and emerging analgesics and analgesic technologies for acute pain management. *Curr Opin Anaesthesiol.* 2009;22:608-617.
55. Bujedo BM, Santos SG, Azpiazu AU. A review of epidural and intrathecal opioids used in the management of postoperative pain. *J Opioid Manag.* 2012;8:177-192.
56. Grider JS, Harned ME, Etscheidt MA. Patient selection and outcomes using a low-dose intrathecal opioid trialing method for chronic nonmalignant pain. *Pain Physician.* 2011;14: 343-351.
57. Krames ES. A history of intraspinal analgesia, a small and personal journey. *Neuromodulation.* 2012;15:172-193.
58. Upadhyay SP, Mallick PN. Intrathecal drug delivery system (IDDS) for cancer pain management: a review and updates. *Am J Hosp Palliat Care.* 2012;29:388-398.
59. Lawson EF, Wallace MS. Advances in intrathecal drug delivery. *Curr Opin Anaesthesiol.* 2012;25:572-576.
60. Baumann TL, Strickland JM, Herndon CM. Pain management. In: DiPiro JT, et al, eds. *Pharmacotherapy: A Pathophysiologic Approach.* 8th ed. New York: McGraw-Hill; 2011:1045-1059.
61. Ruan X. Drug-related side effects of long-term intrathecal morphine therapy. *Pain Physician.* 2007;10:357-366.
62. Duarte RV, Raphael JH, Haque MS, et al. A predictive model for intrathecal opioid dose escalation for chronic non-cancer pain. *Pain Physician.* 2012;15:363-369.
63. Hudcova J, McNicol E, Quah C, et al. Patient controlled opioid analgesia versus conventional opioid analgesia for postoperative pain. *Cochrane Database Syst Rev.* 2006;4:CD003348.
64. Palmer PP, Miller RD. Current and developing methods of patient-controlled analgesia. *Anesthesiol Clin.* 2010;28:587-599.
65. Brogan SE, Winter NB. Patient-controlled intrathecal analgesia for the management of breakthrough cancer pain: a retrospective review and commentary. *Pain Med.* 2011;12:1758-1768.
66. Liu SS, Bieltz M, Wukovits B, John RS. Prospective survey of patient-controlled epidural analgesia with bupivacaine and hydromorphone in 3736 postoperative orthopedic patients. *Reg Anesth Pain Med.* 2010;35:351-354.
67. Mercadante S. Intravenous patient-controlled analgesia and management of pain in post-surgical elderly with cancer. *Surg Oncol.* 2010;19:173-177.
68. Ahlbeck K. Opioids: a two-faced Janus. *Curr Med Res Opin.* 2011;27:439-448.
69. Mercadante S. Prospects and challenges in opioid analgesia for pain management. *Curr Med Res Opin.* 2011;27:1741-1743.
70. Barletta JF. Clinical and economic burden of opioid use for postsurgical pain: focus on ventilatory impairment and ileus. *Pharmacotherapy.* 2012;32(suppl):12S-18S.
71. Macintyre PE, Loadsman JA, Scott DA. Opioids, ventilation and acute pain management. *Anaesth Intensive Care.* 2011;39: 545-558.
72. Brock C, Olesen SS, Olesen AE, et al. Opioid-induced bowel dysfunction: pathophysiology and management. *Drugs.* 2012;72: 1847-1865.
73. Walters JB, Montagnini M. Current concepts in the management of opioid-induced constipation. *J Opioid Manag.* 2010;6: 435-444.

74. Dang VC, Christie MJ. Mechanisms of rapid opioid receptor desensitization, resensitization and tolerance in brain neurons. *Br J Pharmacol.* 2012;165:1704-1716.
75. Ueda H, Ueda M. Mechanisms underlying morphine analgesic tolerance and dependence. *Front Biosci.* 2009;14:5260-5272.
76. Raith K, Hochhaus G. Drugs used in the treatment of opioid tolerance and physical dependence: a review. *Int J Clin Pharmacol Ther.* 2004;42:191-203.
77. Cheatle MD, O'Brien CP. Opioid therapy in patients with chronic noncancer pain: diagnostic and clinical challenges. *Adv Psychosom Med.* 2011;30:61-91.
78. Fishbain DA, Cole B, Lewis J, et al. What percentage of chronic nonmalignant pain patients exposed to chronic opioid analgesic therapy develop abuse/addiction and/or aberrant drug-related behaviors? A structured evidence-based review. *Pain Med.* 2008;9:444-459.
79. Geppetti P, Benemei S. Pain treatment with opioids: achieving the minimal effective and the minimal interacting dose. *Clin Drug Investig.* 2009;29(suppl 1):3-16.
80. Zorba Paster R. Chronic pain management issues in the primary care setting and the utility of long-acting opioids. *Expert Opin Pharmacother.* 2010;11:1823-1833.
81. Chou R, Fanciullo GJ, Fine PG, et al. Clinical guidelines for the use of chronic opioid therapy in chronic noncancer pain. *J Pain.* 2009;10:113-130.
82. Cherubino P, Sarzi-Puttini P, Zuccaro SM, Labianca R. The management of chronic pain in important patient subgroups. *Clin Drug Investig.* 2012;32(suppl 1):35-44.
83. Bekhit MH. Opioid-induced hyperalgesia and tolerance. *Am J Ther.* 2010;17:498-510.
84. Lee M, Silverman SM, Hansen H, et al. A comprehensive review of opioid-induced hyperalgesia. *Pain Physician.* 2011;14:145-161.
85. Raffa RB, Pergolizzi JV Jr. Multi-mechanistic analgesia for opioid-induced hyperalgesia. *J Clin Pharm Ther.* 2012;37:125-127.
86. Lobmaier P, Gossop M, Waal H, Bramness J. The pharmacological treatment of opioid addiction—a clinical perspective. *Eur J Clin Pharmacol.* 2010;66:537-545.
87. Bart G. Maintenance medication for opiate addiction: the foundation of recovery. *J Addict Dis.* 2012;31:207-225.
88. Veilleux JC, Colvin PJ, Anderson J, York C, Heinz AJ. A review of opioid dependence treatment: pharmacological and psychosocial interventions to treat opioid addiction. *Clin Psychol Rev.* 2010;30:155-166.
89. Mattick RP, Breen C, Kimber J, Davoli M. Methadone maintenance therapy versus no opioid replacement therapy for opioid dependence. *Cochrane Database Syst Rev.* 2009;3:CD002209.
90. Orman JS, Keating GM. Spotlight on buprenorphine/naloxone in the treatment of opioid dependence. *CNS Drugs.* 2009;23:899-902.
91. Wesson DR, Smith DE. Buprenorphine in the treatment of opiate dependence. *J Psychoactive Drugs.* 2010;42:161-175.
92. Tetrault JM, Fiellin DA. Current and potential pharmacological treatment options for maintenance therapy in opioid-dependent individuals. *Drugs.* 2012;72:217-222.

CHAPTER 15

Nonsteroidal Anti-Inflammatory Drugs

This chapter discusses a chemically diverse group of substances that exert several distinct pharmacological properties: (1) the ability to decrease inflammation, (2) the ability to relieve mild-to-moderate pain (analgesia), (3) the ability to decrease elevated body temperature associated with fever (antipyresis), and (4) the ability to decrease blood clotting by inhibiting platelet aggregation (anticoagulation). These drugs are commonly referred to as *nonsteroidal anti-inflammatory drugs* (NSAIDs) to distinguish them from the glucocorticoids (i.e., the other main group of drugs used to treat inflammation). Obviously, the term *NSAID* does not fully describe the pharmacological actions of these drugs; a more inclusive terminology should also mention the analgesic, antipyretic, and anticoagulant effects. However, NSAIDs is the accepted term, and it is used throughout this chapter.

Because of these drugs' analgesic and anti-inflammatory effects, patients receiving physical rehabilitation often take NSAIDs for any number of problems. These drugs are a mainstay in the treatment of many types of mild-to-moderate pain, and NSAIDs are especially useful in treating pain and inflammation occurring in acute and chronic musculoskeletal disorders. Other patients are given NSAIDs to treat fever or to prevent excessive blood clotting. Consequently, you will notice that these drugs are used quite frequently in various patient populations, with the specific therapeutic goal related to each patient's individual needs. You should therefore understand the mechanism of action, applications, and effects of aspirin, acetaminophen, and other NSAIDs.

ASPIRIN AND OTHER NSAIDS: GENERAL ASPECTS

Aspirin (acetylsalicylic acid) is usually considered the original NSAID (Fig. 15-1). Newer NSAIDs are often compared to aspirin in terms of efficacy and safety. Acetaminophen is similar to aspirin and other NSAIDs in its ability to decrease pain and fever, but it is not considered an NSAID because it lacks anti-inflammatory and anticoagulant properties. Other differences between aspirin, other NSAIDs, and acetaminophen are addressed later in this chapter.

For years, it was a mystery how a drug like aspirin could exert such a diverse range of therapeutic effects. How could one drug influence so many different systems—effectively alleviating pain and inflammation, decreasing fever, and even affecting blood clotting? This issue was essentially resolved in the early 1970s, when researchers found that aspirin and the other NSAIDs exert most, if not all, of their therapeutic effects by interfering with the biosynthesis of a group of endogenous compounds known collectively as the *prostaglandins*.[1,2] The next section presents a brief discussion of prostaglandins and similar endogenously produced substances to help you understand how these drugs work.

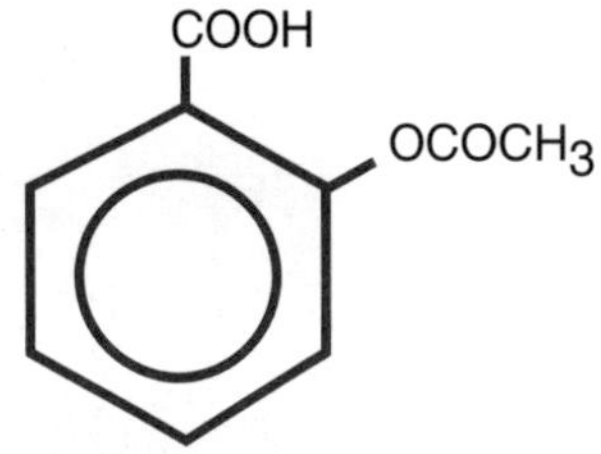

Aspirin
(acetylsalicylic acid)

Figure ■ 15-1
Structure of aspirin.

PROSTAGLANDINS, THROMBOXANES, AND LEUKOTRIENES

Prostaglandins are a group of lipidlike compounds that exhibit a wide range of physiological activities.[2-5] With the exception of the red blood cell, virtually every type of living cell in the human body is able to produce prostaglandins. These compounds appear to be hormones that act locally to help regulate cell function under normal and pathological conditions. Other biologically active compounds known as the **thromboxanes** and *leukotrienes* are derived from the same precursor as the prostaglandins.[6] Together, the prostaglandins, thromboxanes, and leukotrienes are often referred to as *eicosanoids* because they all are derived from 20-carbon fatty acids that contain several double bonds.[7,8] (The term *eicosanoid* is derived from *eicosa*, meaning "20-carbon," and *enoic*, meaning "containing double bonds.") The term *prostanoid* is also often used to describe specific eicosanoids, including the prostaglandins, thromboxanes, and prostacyclins.[9]

Eicosanoid Biosynthesis

The biosynthetic pathway of prostaglandins and other eicosanoids is outlined in Figure 15-2. Basically, these compounds are derived from a 20-carbon essential fatty acid. In humans, this fatty acid is usually arachidonic acid,[8,10] which is ingested in the diet and stored as a phospholipid in the cell membrane. Thus, the cell has an abundant and easily accessible supply of this precursor. When needed, arachidonic acid is cleaved from the cell membrane by a phospholipase enzyme (i.e., phospholipase A_2). The 20-carbon fatty acid can then be metabolized by several enzyme systems to generate a variety of biologically active compounds. One of the primary enzyme systems involves the cyclooxygenase (COX) enzyme, and a second system involves the lipoxygenase (LOX) enzyme. The prostaglandins and thromboxanes are synthesized from the cyclooxygenase pathway, and the leukotrienes come from the lipoxygenase system (see Fig. 15-2).[11]

Exactly which pathway is used in any particular cell depends on the type and quantity of enzymes in that cell and its physiological status. The end products within a given pathway (i.e., prostaglandins, thromboxanes, or leukotrienes) also depend on the individual cell. Any drug inhibiting COX or LOX will also inhibit the formation of all of the subsequent products of that particular pathway. For example, a drug that blocks cyclooxygenase will essentially eliminate all prostaglandin and thromboxane synthesis in that cell. Therefore, aspirin and other NSAIDs are ultimately cyclooxygenase inhibitors.

Aspirin and other NSAIDs do not inhibit the lipoxygenase enzyme and thus do not appreciably decrease leukotriene synthesis.[8] Like the prostaglandins, leukotrienes are pro-inflammatory but seem to be more important in mediating airway inflammation in conditions such as asthma and allergic rhinitis.[12,13] Drugs have therefore been developed to reduce leukotriene-mediated inflammation by either inhibiting the lipoxygenase enzyme (e.g., zileuton) or by blocking leukotriene receptors on respiratory tissues (e.g., montelukast and zafirlukast).[14] These antileukotriene drugs will be discussed in more detail in Chapter 26. The remainder of this chapter will focus on drugs that inhibit prostaglandin and thromboxane production by selectively inhibiting the cyclooxygenase enzyme.

Role of Eicosanoids in Health and Disease

The prostaglandins and thromboxanes have been shown to have a variety of effects on virtually every major physiological system. Studies have indicated that these compounds can influence cardiovascular, respiratory, renal, gastrointestinal (GI), nervous, and reproductive function.[8,9] The biological effects of the various eicosanoids cannot be generalized. Different classes of eicosanoids, and even different members within the same class, can exert various effects on the same system. For instance, certain prostaglandins such

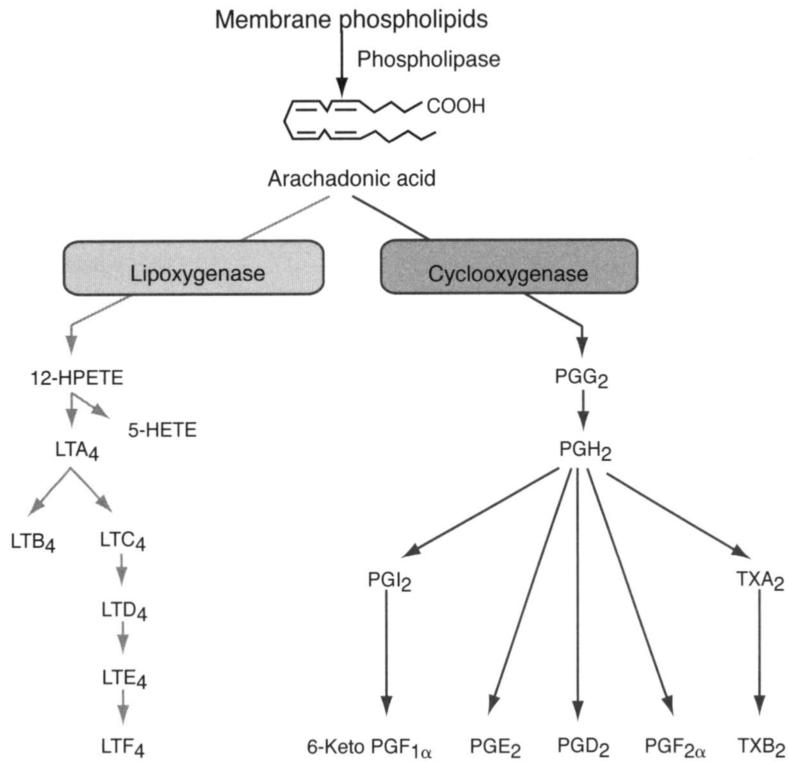

Figure 15-2
Eicosanoid biosynthesis. PG = prostaglandin; TX = thromboxane; LT = leukotriene.

as the PGIs and PGEs tend to produce vasodilation in most vascular beds, whereas other prostaglandins (e.g., $PGF_{2\alpha}$) and the thromboxanes are often vasoconstrictors.[8,15] Some of the major effects of the eicosanoids are summarized in Table 15-1.

All the effects of different prostaglandins and thromboxanes on various systems in the body cannot be reviewed in this chapter; this issue has been addressed extensively elsewhere.[8,9,16] Of greater interest is the role of prostaglandins and related substances in pathological conditions. In general, cells that are subjected to various types of trauma or disturbances in homeostasis tend to increase the production of prostaglandins.[8] This finding suggests that prostaglandins

Table 15-1
PRIMARY PHYSIOLOGICAL EFFECTS OF THE MAJOR CLASSES OF PROSTAGLANDINS, THROMBOXANES, AND LEUKOTRIENES

Class	Vascular Smooth Muscle	Airway Smooth Muscle	Gastrointestinal Smooth Muscle	Gastrointestinal Secretions	Uterine Muscle (Nonpregnant)	Platelet Aggregation
PGAs	Vasodilation	—	—	Decrease	Relaxation	—
PGEs	Vasodilation	Bronchodilation	Contraction	Decrease	Relaxation	Variable
PGIs	Vasodilation	—	Relaxation	Decrease	—	Decrease
PGFs	Variable	Bronchoconstriction	Contraction	—	Contraction	—
TXA_2	Vasoconstriction	Bronchoconstriction	—	—	—	Increase
LTs	Vasoconstriction	Bronchoconstriction	Contraction	—	—	—

PGs = prostaglandins, TXs = thromboxanes, LTs = leukotrienes.

and other eicosanoids may be important in the protective response to cellular injury.

In addition, prostaglandins are important in mediating some of the painful effects of injury and inflammation and the symptoms of other pathological conditions. Some of the better-documented conditions associated with excessive prostaglandin synthesis include the following:

Inflammation. Increased prostaglandin synthesis is usually detected at the site of acute inflammation.[17-19] Certain prostaglandins, such as PGE2, are thought to help mediate the local erythema and edema associated with inflammation in certain tissues by increasing local blood flow and capillary permeability and potentiating the permeability effects of histamine and bradykinin.[4,20] Leukotrienes, particularly LTB4, also contribute to the inflammatory response by increasing vascular permeability, and LTB4 has a potent chemotactic effect on polymorphonuclear leukocytes.[21] However, the role of prostaglandins and other eicosanoids during inflammation is complex. In fact, certain prostaglandins may actually help decrease inflammation, especially during the resolution phase of an acute inflammatory response.[22] Regardless, prostaglandins clearly play a key role in regulating inflammation, and inhibition of prostaglandin synthesis is important in treating specific stages of acute and chronic inflammation.

Pain. Prostaglandins appear to help mediate painful stimuli in a variety of conditions (including inflammation). The compounds do not usually produce pain directly but are believed to increase the sensitivity of pain receptors to mechanical pressure and the effects of other pain-producing substances such as bradykinin.[23]

Fever. Prostaglandins appear to be pyretogenic—that is, they play a role in promoting fever associated with systemic infection and other pyretogenic disorders.[24] It seems that prostaglandins produced locally by brain endothelial cells promote fever by altering the thermoregulatory set-point within the hypothalamus so that body temperature is maintained at a higher level.[24,25] Prostaglandins produced in peripheral tissues can also promote fever by traveling to the hypothalamus via the cerebral blood vessels.[26]

Dysmenorrhea. The painful cramps that accompany menstruation in some women have been attributed at least in part to increased prostaglandin production in the endometrium of the uterus.[27,28]

Thrombus formation. The thromboxanes, especially TXA_2, cause platelet aggregations that result in blood clot formation.[29] It is unclear whether excessive **thrombus** formation (as in deep vein thrombosis or coronary artery occlusion) is initiated by abnormal thromboxane production. Certainly, inhibition of thromboxane synthesis will help prevent platelet-induced thrombus formation in individuals who are prone to specific types of excessive blood clotting.[30]

Other pathologies. Because of their many varied physiological effects, the eicosanoids are involved in several other pathological conditions. Prostaglandins have been implicated in cardiovascular disorders (hypertension), neoplasms (colon cancer), respiratory dysfunction (asthma), neurological disorders (multiple sclerosis, allergic encephalomyelitis, affective disorders), endocrine dysfunction (Bartter syndrome, diabetes mellitus), and a variety of other problems.[5,8,9,19,31]

Although the role of these compounds in health and disease has become clearer with ongoing research, the exact role of prostaglandins and the other eicosanoids in various diseases continues to be evaluated.

MECHANISM OF NSAID ACTION: INHIBITION OF PROSTAGLANDIN AND THROMBOXANE SYNTHESIS

Aspirin and the other NSAIDs are all potent inhibitors of the cyclooxygenase enzyme.[1,8] Because cyclooxygenase represents the first step in the synthesis of prostaglandins and thromboxanes, drugs that inhibit this enzyme in any given cell will block the production of all prostaglandins and thromboxanes in that cell. Considering that prostaglandins and thromboxanes are implicated in producing pain, inflammation, fever, excessive blood clotting, and other pathological conditions, virtually all of the therapeutic effects of aspirin and similar drugs can be explained by their ability to inhibit the synthesis of these two eicosanoid classes.[8]

The **cyclooxygenase** or COX enzyme system is therefore the key site of NSAID action within the cell. It is now realized that there are at least two primary subtypes (isozymes) of the COX enzyme: COX-1 and COX-2.[32-34] In general, prostaglandins synthesized by

COX-1 help regulate normal cell activity and maintain cellular homeostasis. For example, COX-1 enzymes located in the stomach mucosa synthesize prostaglandins that help protect the stomach lining from gastric acid, and COX-1 enzymes in the kidneys produce beneficial prostaglandins that help maintain renal function, especially when kidney function is compromised.[8,35] COX-1 is also the enzyme responsible for synthesizing prostaglandins and thromboxanes regulating normal platelet activity.[36]

The COX-2 enzyme, however, seems to be produced primarily in injured cells—that is, other chemical mediators (**cytokines**, growth factors) induce the injured cell to synthesize the COX-2 enzyme, and this enzyme then produces prostaglandins that mediate pain and other aspects of the inflammatory response.[8] There is also considerable evidence that the COX-2 form is responsible for producing prostaglandins in other pathological conditions such as colorectal cancer.[37]

Hence, the primary roles of COX-1 and COX-2 enzymes seem somewhat different. In some tissues, the COX-1 enzyme is a "normal" cell component that synthesizes prostaglandins to help regulate and maintain cell activity. COX-2 often represents an "emergency" enzyme that synthesizes prostaglandins in response to cell injury (i.e., pain and inflammation). However, recent evidence suggests that prostaglandins produced by COX-1 are not always beneficial, and COX-2-induced prostaglandins are not always harmful.[38] Certain prostaglandins produced by the COX-2 enzyme, for example, may help lower blood pressure and prevent arterial thrombosis that would otherwise cause heart attack and stroke in susceptible individuals.[8] There seems to be considerable overlap in how the two forms of the COX enzyme affect cell function, depending on the specific tissue and circumstances affecting that tissue. Nonetheless, it is still generally accepted that the best clinical effects are achieved by inhibiting the harmful prostaglandins produced primarily by the COX-2 enzyme, while sparing the production of the beneficial prostaglandins produced primarily by the COX-1 enzyme.

NSAIDs are therefore often classified according to whether they affect both COX forms or whether they are selective for only the COX-2 enzyme. Aspirin and most of the traditional NSAIDs are nonselective—they inhibit both enzymes. These nonselective NSAIDs cause primary beneficial effects (decreased pain and inflammation) by inhibiting the COX-2 enzyme. Because these drugs also inhibit the COX-1 enzyme, they decrease the production of the beneficial and protective prostaglandins. It is the loss of these beneficial prostaglandins that accounts for the primary side effects of NSAIDs—that is, loss of protective prostaglandins in the stomach and kidneys result in gastric damage and decreased renal function, respectively.

It follows that drugs selectively inhibiting the COX-2 enzyme offer certain advantages over aspirin and nonselective NSAIDs. Selective COX-2 inhibitors should decrease the production of prostaglandins that mediate pain and inflammation while sparing the synthesis of protective prostaglandins that are synthesized by COX-1. Such COX-2 selective drugs are currently available, and their pharmacology is addressed later in this chapter.

ASPIRIN: THE PROTOTYPICAL NSAID

Acetylsalicylic acid, or aspirin, represents the major form of a group of drugs known as the *salicylates* (see Fig. 15-1). Other salicylates (sodium salicylate, choline salicylate) are used clinically, but aspirin is the most frequently used and appears to have the widest range of therapeutic effects. Because aspirin has been used clinically for more than 100 years, is inexpensive, and is readily available without prescription, many individuals may be under the impression that this drug is only a marginally effective therapeutic agent. On the contrary, aspirin is a very powerful and effective drug that should be considered a major medicine.[1] As discussed previously, aspirin is a potent inhibitor of all cyclooxygenase activity (COX-1 and COX-2), and thus it has the potential to affect several conditions involving excessive prostaglandin and thromboxane production. Aspirin is the oldest NSAID, and other NSAIDs are often compared with aspirin in terms of efficacy and safety.

Over the last few decades, newer NSAIDs have received considerably more attention for treating pain and inflammation. Nonetheless, aspirin continues to be used extensively for musculoskeletal disorders, and it has emerged as an important medication for preventing thromboembolic conditions (e.g., heart attack, stroke) and possibly preventing certain forms of cancer. Hence, this discussion focuses primarily on the clinical applications of aspirin and the problems typically associated with it. For the most part, clinical use and problems can also be applied to most nonaspirin NSAIDs. The major similarities and differences between aspirin and the other NSAIDs are discussed in "Comparison of Aspirin with Other NSAIDs."

CLINICAL APPLICATIONS OF ASPIRINLIKE DRUGS

Treatment of Pain and Inflammation

Aspirin and other NSAIDs are effective in treating mild-to-moderate pain of various origins, including headache, toothache, and diffuse muscular aches and soreness. Aspirin appears to be especially useful in treating pain and inflammation in musculoskeletal and joint disorders.[39,40] The safe and effective use of aspirin in both rheumatoid arthritis and osteoarthritis is well documented (see Chapter 16).[33,41,42] Aspirin is also recommended for treating the pain and cramping associated with primary dysmenorrhea.[43]

Aspirin and aspirinlike drugs are also used to manage pain following certain types of surgery, including arthroscopic surgery.[44,45] These drugs can serve as the primary analgesic following other types of minor or intermediate surgeries, and they can be used after extensive surgery to decrease the need for high doses of other drugs such as opioids.[46,47] For example, ketorolac tromethamine (Toradol) is a relatively new NSAID that has shown exceptional promise in treating postoperative pain. This drug can be given orally or by intramuscular injection, and it is reported to provide analgesic effects similar to opioid drugs (e.g., morphine) but without the harmful or undesirable opioid side effects (i.e., sedation, nausea, respiratory depression).[48-50]

Treatment of Fever

Although the use of aspirin in treating fever in children is contraindicated (because of the association with Reye syndrome; see "Problems and Adverse Effects of Aspirinlike Drugs"), aspirin remains the primary NSAID used in treating fever in adults.[51] Ibuprofen is also used frequently as a nonprescription antipyretic NSAID in both adults and children.

Treatment of Vascular Disorders

As discussed previously, aspirin inhibits platelet-induced thrombus formation through its ability to inhibit thromboxane biosynthesis. Aspirin has therefore been used to help prevent the onset or recurrence of heart attacks in some individuals by inhibiting thrombus formation in the coronary arteries.[52,53] Similarly, daily aspirin use may help prevent transient ischemic attacks and stroke by preventing cerebral infarction in certain patients.[53,54] The role of aspirin in treating coagulation disorders is discussed in more detail in Chapter 25.

Prevention of Cancer

There is now considerable evidence that regular aspirin use decreases the risk of colorectal cancer.[55-57] It has been estimated that people who use aspirin on a regular basis have more than a 50 percent lower risk of fatal colon cancer as compared with people who do not use aspirin.[58] To a lesser extent, aspirin might also help prevent other types of GI cancers (stomach, esophageal) and non-GI cancers (e.g., bladder, breast, prostate cancers).[59,60] It is hypothesized that aspirin may help prevent tumor growth by directly inhibiting the COX-2 enzyme in susceptible tissues and inhibiting the synthesis of prostaglandins that would otherwise cause abnormal cell division in these tissues.[8]

Likewise, aspirin may prevent certain cancers through its antiplatelet effects. Activated platelets may help promote abnormal cell proliferation by releasing chemical mediators that induce specific cells to generate COX-2 enzymes that in turn synthesize prostaglandins that promote abnormal cell division.[61] Aspirin and similar agents inhibit platelet activation, thus preventing the platelets from generating signals that might cause other tissues to undergo abnormal cell proliferation and tumor formation.[58,61] Hence, aspirin continues to gain acceptance as an anticancer drug, especially in individuals who are at an increased risk for developing colorectal cancer and possibly other forms of cancer.

PROBLEMS AND ADVERSE EFFECTS OF ASPIRINLIKE DRUGS

Gastrointestinal Problems

The primary problem with all NSAIDs, including aspirin, is GI damage. Problems ranging from minor stomach discomfort to variable amounts of upper GI hemorrhage and ulceration are fairly common.[62,63] These effects are most likely caused by the loss of protective prostaglandins from the mucosal lining. Certain prostaglandins such as PGI_2 and PGE_2 are produced locally in the stomach, and these prostaglandins help protect the gastric mucosa by inhibiting gastric acid secretion, increasing the production of mucus in the stomach lining, and maintaining blood flow to the gastric mucosa.[8] By inhibiting the formation of these protective prostaglandins, aspirin and most traditional NSAIDs render the stomach more susceptible to damage from acidic gastric juices.[62]

Certain patients are more susceptible to GI injury from aspirinlike drugs. Factors such as advanced age, a history of ulcers, use of multiple NSAIDs, use of high doses of an NSAID, and use of other agents (e.g., anti-inflammatory steroids, anticoagulants) appear to increase the risk of serious GI damage.[35,64] *Helicobacter pylori*, a bacterium that is sometimes present in the stomach (see Chapter 27), can also contribute to the increased risk of gastric irritation associated with NSAIDs.[65]

Pharmacologists employ different strategies to manage GI problems associated with aspirinlike drugs. Enteric-coated aspirin tablets delay dissolution and release of the drug until it reaches the small intestine. These coated forms of aspirin spare the stomach from irritation, but the duodenum and upper small intestine may still be subjected to damage.[66] Enteric-coated aspirin also has the disadvantage of delaying the onset of analgesic effects to relieve acute pain. The buffered aspirin tablet is also available to help decrease stomach irritation. The rationale is that including a chemical buffer helps blunt the acidic effects of the aspirin molecule on the stomach mucosa. But it is questionable whether sufficient buffer is added to commercial aspirin preparations to actually make a difference in stomach irritation.

During chronic aspirin therapy (e.g., treatment of arthritis), taking aspirin with meals may help decrease GI irritation because the food in the stomach will offer some direct protection of the gastric mucosa. However, the presence of food will also delay drug absorption, which may decrease the peak levels of drug that reach the bloodstream.

The use of other drugs in conjunction with aspirin and the other NSAIDs can prevent or treat the GI side effects. Misoprostol (Cytotec) is a prostaglandin E_1 analog that inhibits gastric acid secretion and prevents gastric damage.[67,68] This drug has been beneficial in decreasing aspirin-induced irritation, but the clinical use of misoprostol is limited by side effects such as diarrhea.[68] Omeprazole (Prilosec), esomeprazole (Nexium), and lansoprazole (Prevacid) inhibit the "proton pump" that is ultimately responsible for secreting gastric acid from mucosal cells into the lumen of the stomach (see Chapter 27). These proton pump inhibitors have therefore been used successfully to increase healing and decrease NSAID-induced ulcers.[69,70] Drugs that antagonize certain histamine receptors—that is, the histamine receptor (H_2) blockers—can also decrease GI damage.[71] H_2 blockers such as cimetidine (Tagamet) and ranitidine (Zantac) inhibit gastric acid secretion by antagonizing histamine receptors in the gastric mucosa (see Chapter 27). These drugs are tolerated quite well but are generally not as effective in controlling NSAID-induced ulceration as other drugs, such as misoprostol and proton pump inhibitors.[71]

Drugs such as misoprostol, proton pump inhibitors, and H_2 receptor blockers are not usually prescribed to every person taking aspirinlike drugs. They are typically reserved for people who exhibit symptoms of GI irritation or who are at risk for developing ulceration while undergoing NSAID therapy.[64]

Finally, COX-2 selective drugs comprise an alternative strategy for reducing the risk of gastric irritation in patients who require NSAID-type drugs.[72-76] This strategy is addressed in more detail later in this chapter.

Cardiovascular Problems

As addressed earlier, aspirin and aspirinlike drugs inhibit the production of thromboxanes, which can decrease platelet activity and reduce the risk of platelet-induced clots that cause heart attack and ischemic stroke. However, these drugs can also increase blood pressure and increase the chance of thrombotic events through an effect on other prostaglandins such as PGI_2 (known also as *prostacyclin*) and PGE_2.[77-80] These prostaglandins are vasoactive and help regulate vascular tone. In particular, they tend to relax the vasculature and inhibit the effects of other factors that cause arterial thrombus (clot) formation. Loss of these vasoactive prostaglandins can therefore result in increased blood pressure and increased clotting activity that can lead to myocardial infarction and stroke in susceptible individuals. This increase, for example, is modest in normotensive individuals but can be especially problematic in people with hypertension or other cardiac risk factors.

The possibility of serious cardiac complications was widely publicized with certain COX-2 selective drugs, such as rofecoxib and valdecoxib (see "COX-2 Drugs and the Risk of Heart Attack and Stroke"). It is now realized that all NSAIDs can cause cardiovascular problems because they affect the COX-2 enzyme and its synthesis of vasoactive prostaglandins.

The risk of cardiovascular problems appears to vary according to which NSAID is administered. Studies suggest that the risk of cardiovascular problems increases if the drug is more selective for the COX-2 isoenzyme.[77,80] This increased risk may be due to the fact that prostaglandins produced by the COX-2 form of the enzyme predominately cause vasodilation, and the likelihood of cardiovascular problems will increase if the drug selectively inhibits these vasodilating prostaglandins. In other words, a COX-2 selective drug will alter the balance of prostaglandin production in favor of increased COX-1 prostaglandins that cause vasoconstriction and subsequent cardiovascular problems. A nonselective NSAID will decrease the production of prostaglandins from both forms of the enzyme, thus maintaining the balance between vasodilation and vasoconstriction. Hence, the cardiovascular risk appears lowest with nonselective NSAIDs, such as ibuprofen and naproxen, but is considerably higher with diclofenac (a traditional NSAID that is fairly COX-2 specific) and probably highest with COX-2 selective drugs, such as celecoxib [77,80]

Nonetheless, cardiovascular risks should be considered whenever NSAIDs are administered, even if the individual is relatively healthy and has normal blood pressure.[77] Likewise, people with hypertension, coronary artery disease, and other cardiovascular problems may be especially at risk for heart attack and stroke when taking NSAIDs, especially the COX-2 selective drugs.[81] Hence, NSAIDs should be used sparingly and cautiously in these individuals or avoided entirely in certain high-risk cardiovascular patients.

Other Side Effects

Aspirin and other NSAIDs can cause toxic side effects if used improperly or if taken by patients who have preexisting diseases. For instance, serious hepatotoxicity is relatively rare in most patients, but aspirinlike drugs can produce adverse changes in hepatic function in patients with liver disease, when taken in excessive doses, and in people who may have genetic susceptibility to drug-induced liver damage.[82,83] On the other hand, aspirin and other NSAIDs do not seem to cause renal disease in an individual with normal kidneys,[84] but problems such as nephrotic syndrome, acute interstitial nephritis, and even acute renal failure have been observed when these drugs are given to patients with impaired renal function, diabetes mellitus, heart failure, or people with decreased body water (volume depletion).[84]

Aspirinlike drugs cause renal and hepatic problems by inhibiting the synthesis of prostaglandins that serve a protective role in maintaining blood flow and function in the liver and kidneys,[85-87] especially when blood flow and perfusion pressure to these organs becomes compromised. Consequently, aspirin and other NSAIDs may create problems in patients with conditions such as hypovolemia, hepatic cirrhosis, congestive heart failure, and hypertension.[63,81,86]

In cases of aspirin overdose, a condition known as *aspirin intoxication* or *poisoning* may occur. This is usually identified by several symptoms, including headache, tinnitus, difficulty hearing, confusion, and GI distress. More severe cases also result in metabolic acidosis and dehydration, which can be life-threatening. In adults, a dose of 10 to 30 g of aspirin is sometimes fatal, although much higher doses (130 g in one documented case) have been ingested without causing death.[2] Of course, much smaller doses can produce fatalities in children.

Evidence has suggested that aspirin may also be associated with a relatively rare condition known as Reye syndrome.[88] This condition occurs in children and teenagers, usually following a bout of influenza or chicken pox. Reye syndrome is marked by a high fever, vomiting, liver dysfunction, and increasing unresponsiveness, often progressing rapidly and leading to delirium, convulsions, coma, and possibly death. Because aspirin is one factor that may contribute to Reye syndrome, physicians recommend that aspirin and other aspirinlike drugs not be used to treat fever in children and teenagers.[88,89] Non-aspirin antipyretics such as acetaminophen and ibuprofen are not associated with Reye syndrome, so products containing these drugs are preferred for treating fever.[2]

Approximately 1 percent of the general population will exhibit aspirin intolerance or hypersensitivity,[90] but the incidence is considerably higher (10 to 25 percent) in people with asthma or other hypersensitivity reactions.[2] People with aspirin intolerance will display allergic-type reactions, including acute bronchospasm, urticaria, and severe rhinitis, within a few hours after taking aspirin and aspirinlike NSAIDs.[91] These reactions may be quite severe, and cardiovascular shock may occur. Sensitivity to aspirin often indicates a concomitant sensitivity to other nonselective NSAIDs.[91] Consequently, the use of aspirin and all nonselective NSAIDs is usually contraindicated in these individuals.[2] Some studies suggest that COX-2 selective drugs may greatly reduce, but not totally eliminate, the chance of an allergic reaction in aspirin-hypersensitive patients.[91] In cases where aspirin therapy would be extremely beneficial (e.g., patients with coronary artery disease), attempts may be made to gradually introduce low aspirin doses and allow the body to become desensitized.[90-92] This action must be done cautiously under close medical supervision.

Finally, there is evidence that aspirin and other commonly used NSAIDs may inhibit healing of certain tissues. In particular, it has been suggested that these drugs may inhibit bone healing after fracture and certain types of surgery (spinal fusion),[93,94] because certain prostaglandins may be important in stimulating the early stages of bone formation following fracture or bone surgery.[95] By inhibiting the synthesis of these prostaglandins, NSAIDS may retard bone healing and delay the formation of new bone.[96] However, much of this evidence is based on laboratory studies on animal models, and a definitive link between NSAIDs (including COX-2 selective drugs) and delayed bone healing in humans remains under investigation.[93,94] Still, some experts feel that it might be prudent to avoid the use of NSAIDs immediately following fracture or bone surgery.[97,98]

The effect of NSAIDs on soft tissue healing is also a topic of concern. In particular, it has been debated whether NSAIDs can affect articular cartilage health in conditions such as osteoarthritis. This question is important because NSAIDs are often used to treat pain and inflammation in patients with osteoarthritis and other joint diseases. Although it was originally believed that NSAIDs may impair articular cartilage growth, studies suggest that COX-2 selective NSAIDs such as celecoxib may actually facilitate the incorporation of proteoglycans, hyaluronan, and other components into articular cartilage.[99,100] Moreover, COX-2 selective drugs may enhance chondrocyte survival in animal models of osteoarthritis, thus having a potential beneficial effect on cartilage health.[101] As such, these NSAIDs may improve cartilage healing in osteoarthritis and perhaps other soft tissue injuries.[97] Once again, much of this evidence was obtained from animal and in vitro studies. Additional research will be needed to clarify whether these benefits occur in humans and whether these effects are limited to only COX-2 selective drugs or if aspirin and other nonselective NSAIDs can also improve cartilage health in conditions such as osteoarthritis.

COMPARISON OF ASPIRIN WITH OTHER NSAIDS

Over the past several decades, pharmacologists have developed numerous drugs that bear a functional similarity to aspirin. A comprehensive list of currently available NSAIDs is shown in Table 15-2. Other NSAIDs are like aspirin in that they exert their therapeutic effects by inhibiting prostaglandin and thromboxane synthesis. Although specifically approved uses of individual

Table 15-2
COMMON NONSTEROIDAL ANTI-INFLAMMATORY DRUGS

Generic Name	Trade Name(s)	Specific Comments—Comparison to Other NSAIDs
Aspirin	Many trade names	The original NSAID used for analgesic and anti-inflammatory effects Also used frequently for antipyretic and anticoagulant effects
Celecoxib	Celebrex	Classified as a COX-2 inhibitor May cause less gastric irritation than traditional NSAIDs but may also cause serious cardiovascular problems (heart attack, stroke)
Diclofenac	Voltaren	Substantially more potent than naproxen and several other NSAIDs Has affinity for the COX-2 isoenzyme similar to celecoxib; adverse side effects occur in about 20% of patients
Diflunisal	Dolobid	Has potency 3–4 times greater than aspirin in terms of analgesic and anti-inflammatory effects but lacks antipyretic activity
Etodolac	Lodine	Effective as analgesic/anti-inflammatory agent with fewer side effects than most NSAIDs Relatively selective for COX-2 isoenzyme; may have gastric-sparing properties
Fenoprofen	Nalfon	GI side effects fairly common but usually less intense than those occurring with similar doses of aspirin

Continued

Table 15-2
COMMON NONSTEROIDAL ANTI-INFLAMMATORY DRUGS—cont'd

Generic Name	Trade Name(s)	Specific Comments—Comparison to Other NSAIDs
Flurbiprofen	Ansaid	Similar to aspirin's benefits and side effects Also available as topical ophthalmic preparation (Ocufen)
Ibuprofen	Motrin, many others	First nonaspirin NSAID also available in nonprescription form Fewer GI side effects than aspirin but GI effects still occur in 5%–15% of patients
Indomethacin	Indocin	Relative high incidence of dose-related side effects Problems occur in 25%–50% of patients
Ketoprofen	Orudis, Oruvail, others	Similar to aspirin's benefits and side effects but has relatively short half-life (1–2 hours)
Ketorolac	Toradol	Can be administered orally or by intramuscular injection Parenteral doses provide postoperative analgesia equivalent to opioids
Meclofenamate	Meclomen	No apparent advantages or disadvantages compared to aspirin and other NSAIDs
Meloxicam	Mobic	Relatively fewer gastric side effects than piroxicam Tends to be somewhat more selective for COX-2 isoenzyme compared to older, more traditional NSAIDs
Nabumetone	Relafen	Effective as analgesic/anti-inflammatory agent with fewer side effects than most NSAIDs
Naproxen	Anaprox, Naprosyn, others	Similar to ibuprofen in terms of benefits and adverse effects
Oxaprozin	Daypro	Analgesic and anti-inflammatory effects similar to aspirin May produce fewer side effects than other NSAIDs
Piroxicam	Feldene	Long half-life (45 hours) allows once-daily dosing May be somewhat better tolerated than aspirin
Sulindac	Clinoril	Relatively little effect on kidneys (renal-sparing) May produce more GI side effects than aspirin
Tolmetin	Tolectin	Similar to aspirin's benefits and side effects but must be given frequently (qid) because of short half-life (1 hour)

members of this group vary, NSAIDs are used in much the same way as aspirin; they are administered primarily for their analgesic and anti-inflammatory effects, with some also being used as antipyretic and anticoagulant agents. Dosages commonly used to achieve analgesic or anti-inflammatory effects with some of the more common NSAIDs are listed in Table 15-3.

With respect to therapeutic effects, there is no clear evidence that any of the commonly used NSAIDs are markedly better than aspirin as anti-inflammatory analgesics.[102] The primary differences between aspirin and other NSAIDs are related to the side effects and safety profile of each agent (see Table 15-2).[2] As a group, the nonaspirin NSAIDs tend to be associated with less GI discomfort than plain aspirin, but most of these NSAIDs (with the possible exception of the COX-2 drugs, see the next section) are still associated with some degree of stomach irritation.[102,103] Certain NSAIDs may offer an advantage over aspirin or other aspirinlike drugs because they are less toxic to other organs such as the liver and kidneys. However, the effect on these other organs seems to be related more to the status of each patient rather than the drug—that is, all NSAIDs, including aspirin, are relatively safe in people with normal liver and kidney function when administered at moderate dosages for a short period of time.[2] A specific patient may also respond more favorably to a particular NSAID in terms of therapeutic effects (e.g., decreased pain, inflammation), but these responses are due to patient variability rather than a unique characteristic of the drug.[104] Hence, it cannot be generalized that the nonaspirin NSAIDs are significantly better or worse than aspirin in terms of either therapeutic or adverse effects.[2]

Another important difference between aspirin and other NSAIDs is cost. Most of the NSAIDs still require a physician's prescription. The cost of prescription NSAIDs can be anywhere from 10 to 20 times more expensive than an equivalent supply of aspirin. NSAIDs

Table 15-3
DOSAGES OF COMMON ORAL NSAIDS (ACCORDING TO DESIRED EFFECT)*

Drug	Analgesia	Anti-inflammation**
Aspirin (many trade names)	325–1,000 mg every 4–6 hr	3.6–5.4 g/d in divided doses
Celecoxib (Celebrex)	200–400 mg/day	200–400 mg/day
Diclofenac (Voltaren)	Up to 100 mg for the first dose; then up to 50 mg tid thereafter	Initially: 150–200 mg/d in 3–4 divided doses; try to reduce to 75–100 mg/d in 3–4 divided doses
Diflunisal (Dolobid)	500–1,000 mg initially; 500 mg every 8–12 hr as needed	250–500 mg BID
Etodolac (Lodine)	200–400 mg every 6–8 hours as needed	400 mg bid or tid or 300 mg tid or qid; total daily dose is typically between 600–1,200 mg/d
Fenoprofen (Nalfon)	200 mg every 4–6 hr	300–600 mg tid or qid
Flurbiprofen (Ansaid)	50 mg every 4–6 hr as needed	200–300 mg/d in 2–4 divided doses
Ibuprofen (Advil, Motrin, Nuprin, others)	200–400 mg every 4–6 hr as needed	400–800 mg tid or qid
Indomethacin (Indocin)	—	25–50 mg 2–4 times each day initially. Can be increased up to 200 mg/d as tolerated.
Ketoprofen (Orudis)	25–50 mg every 6–8 hr	150–300 mg/d in 3–4 divided doses
Meclofenamate (Meclomen)	50–100 mg every 4–6 hr	200–400 mg/d in 3–4 divided doses
Meloxicam (Mobic)	7.5–15 mg/day	7.5–15 mg/day
Nabumetone (Relafen)	—	Initially: 1,000 mg/d in a single dose or 2 divided doses. Can be increased up to 2,000 mg/d if needed
Naproxen (Naprosyn)	250–500 mg bid	250–500 mg bid
Naproxen sodium (Aleve, Anaprox, others)	275–550 mg bid	275–550 mg bid
Oxaprozin (Daypro)	—	Initially: 1,200 mg/d, then adjust to patient tolerance
Piroxicam (Feldene)	—	20 mg/d single dose; or 10 mg bid
Sulindac (Clinoril)	—	150 or 200 mg bid
Tolmetin (Tolectin)	—	200–600 mg bid or tid

**Doses refer to use of standard release preparations in adults.*
***Includes chronic inflammatory conditions, such as rheumatoid arthritis.*

that are available in nonprescription form (e.g., ibuprofen) can still cost up to five times as much as aspirin. If a patient responds equally well to a variety of NSAIDs, efforts should be made to use the NSAID that will produce adequate therapeutic effects at a minimal cost.[105]

COX-2 SELECTIVE DRUGS

As discussed earlier, the cyclooxygenase enzyme that synthesizes prostaglandins exists in at least two forms: COX-1 and COX-2.[32,33] Aspirin and most other NSAIDs are nonselective cyclooxygenase inhibitors—that is, they inhibit both the COX-1 and COX-2 forms of the cyclooxygenase. This nonselective inhibition results in decreased synthesis of prostaglandins that cause pain and inflammation (COX-2 prostaglandins) and the loss of prostaglandins that are protective and beneficial to tissues such as the stomach lining and kidneys (COX-1 prostaglandins). Pharmacologists have therefore developed drugs that are relatively selective for the COX-2 isoenzyme. These drugs are known collectively as *COX-2 inhibitors* or *coxibs* to differentiate them from the more traditional NSAIDs.

COX-2 drugs represent an important addition to the NSAID armamentarium. COX-2 inhibitors such as celecoxib (Celebrex) have the potential to inhibit synthesis of inflammatory prostaglandins produced by COX-2, while sparing the production of beneficial COX-1 prostaglandins that help regulate normal physiological function.[76,106] It should be noted that certain non-coxib NSAIDs such as diclofenac, etodolac, and meloxicam are also relatively selective for the COX-2 enzyme (see Table 15-2). These traditional NSAIDs may therefore be similar to the coxib drugs with regard to their beneficial and adverse side effects. However, drugs classified specifically as COX-2 inhibitors typically consist of drugs with a *–coxib* suffix that are similar structurally and functionally to celecoxib.

COX-2 selective inhibitors are not necessarily more effective in reducing pain and inflammation than aspirin and traditional NSAIDs. However, because of their relative selectivity, they have a much lower incidence of gastric irritation than aspirinlike drugs.[106,107] Likewise, COX-2 drugs may be preferred in patients who are at risk for the prolonged bleeding and bruising that can occur with aspirin and other NSAIDs. This type of bleeding typically occurs when aspirin and traditional NSAIDs reduce platelet activity by inhibiting thromboxane synthesis from the COX-1 enzyme. COX-2 drugs spare the production of thromboxanes, thus allowing normal platelet activity and less chance of excessive bleeding.

The COX-2 drugs are not devoid of side effects, of course, and they may increase the risk of upper respiratory tract infections. Even though these drugs are purportedly easier on the stomach than traditional NSAIDs, certain patients may still experience GI problems such as diarrhea, heartburn, stomach cramps, and upper GI bleeding. Nonetheless, COX-2 drugs offer an alternative to more traditional NSAIDs, and COX-2 agents may be especially useful to patients who cannot tolerate aspirin or other NSAIDs because of gastric irritation or other side effects typically associated with aspirin and the more traditional NSAIDs.[106]

COX-2 Drugs and the Risk of Heart Attack and Stroke

The primary concern about COX-2 drugs is that they may increase the risk of serious cardiovascular events such as heart attack and stroke,[108,109] especially if patients have other cardiovascular risk factors such as hypertension and atherosclerotic heart disease. As discussed earlier, these drugs inhibit the synthesis of vasoactive prostaglandins such as PGE_2 and PGI_2 (prostacyclin). These prostaglandins normally promote vasodilation and inhibit platelet-induced occlusion in the coronary and carotid arteries.[8,109] Loss of these protective prostaglandins increases the chance of arterial thrombus formation, which can lead to myocardial infarction and stroke.

Granted, these problems can occur with all NSAIDs, but the risk of infarction is greater with drugs that are more selective for the COX-2 enzyme—that is, COX-2 inhibition may cause a selective loss of prostaglandins that cause vasodilation and prevent thrombosis, thus allowing the prothrombotic prostaglandins to predominate. COX-2 drugs, for example, do not inhibit the production of thromboxane from the COX-1 enzyme, and thromboxane is a prostaglandin that facilitates platelet aggregation and clot formation.[8] The balance of prostaglandin production is therefore shifted to favor increased platelet activity and an increased risk of clots in the coronary and carotid arteries in susceptible individuals.[106] Nonselective COX inhibitors such as the traditional NSAIDs inhibit both anti- and proclotting prostaglandins, thus keeping the relative balance intact between these two opposing factors.

The fact that certain people taking COX-2 selective inhibitors may be at risk for heart attack or ischemic stroke was the primary reason that certain COX-2 drugs such as rofecoxib (Vioxx) and valdecoxib (Bextra) were taken off the market. On the other hand, the risk of heart attack and stroke may be acceptable if COX-2 drugs are used appropriately.[108] Patients must be screened carefully to determine individuals who are at risk for coronary or carotid ischemia.[110,111] Dosages must likewise be kept to a minimum to prevent untoward cardiovascular events.

At the time of this writing, celecoxib (Celebrex) is the only COX-2 selective drug that is still available. It will be interesting to see if new COX-2 drugs can be developed that have an acceptable cardiovascular risk profile.

ACETAMINOPHEN

Acetaminophen (known also as *paracetamol*) has several distinct differences from aspirin and the other

NSAIDs. Acetaminophen is often equal to aspirin and NSAIDs in terms of analgesic and antipyretic effects, but it does not have any appreciable anti-inflammatory or anticoagulant effects.[112] One major advantage of acetaminophen is that it is not associated with upper GI tract irritation.[113] Consequently, acetaminophen has been used widely in the treatment of noninflammatory conditions associated with mild-to-moderate pain and in patients who have a history of gastric damage (such as ulcers). Acetaminophen is often the first drug used to control pain in the early stages of osteoarthritis and other musculoskeletal conditions that do not have an inflammatory component.[114,115] In addition, Reye syndrome has not been implicated with acetaminophen use, so this drug is often given to children and teenagers to treat fever.[2]

The mechanism of action of acetaminophen is not fully understood. It does inhibit the cyclooxygenase enzyme, and its analgesic and antipyretic effects are probably mediated through prostaglandin inhibition. Why acetaminophen fails to exert anti-inflammatory and anticoagulant effects is unclear. One explanation is that this drug preferentially inhibits central nervous system (CNS) prostaglandin production but has little effect on peripheral cyclooxygenase activity.[112] This specific effect on central prostaglandins has generated the theory that a third subset of cyclooxygenase enzymes known as the COX-3 variant exists in the CNS and that acetaminophen may be somewhat selective for this COX-3 subtype.[112] The existence and functional role of such a COX-3 enzyme remains to be fully determined.

Researchers have also suggested that acetaminophen can inhibit peripheral COX enzymes, but this drug may have preferential effects on the COX-2 isoform.[116] That is, acetaminophen may act more like a COX-2 selective inhibitor, hence its ability to spare the production of COX-1 prostaglandins that help protect the stomach and help regulate normal platelet activity. This theory, however, fails to account for why acetaminophen is not an anti-inflammatory drug. If acetaminophen inhibits the COX-2 isoform, one would expect it to reduce inflammation because proinflammatory prostaglandins are typically produced by the COX-2 isoform. It remains to be determined why this drug does not have an appreciable effect on tissue inflammation and platelet aggregation.

Regardless of its exact mechanism, acetaminophen is a very important and useful medication in the treatment of fever and mild to moderate pain. However, the fact that it does not cause gastric irritation might give users the false impression that it is an innocuous drug devoid of all adverse effects. On the contrary, high doses of acetaminophen (e.g., 15 g) can be especially toxic to the liver and may be fatal because of hepatic necrosis.[117] Normally, acetaminophen is metabolized in the liver via a series of reactions illustrated in Figure 15-3. In the liver, acetaminophen is converted initially into a highly reactive intermediate by-product known as N-acetyl-p-benzoquinone imine (NAPQI). This intermediate by-product is quickly detoxified by coupling it with glutathione (GHS) to create a final, nonreactive by-product (mercapturic acid) that is sent to the kidneys for excretion. At moderate doses, these reactions occur rapidly so that NAPQI does not accumulate within the liver. At high doses, however,

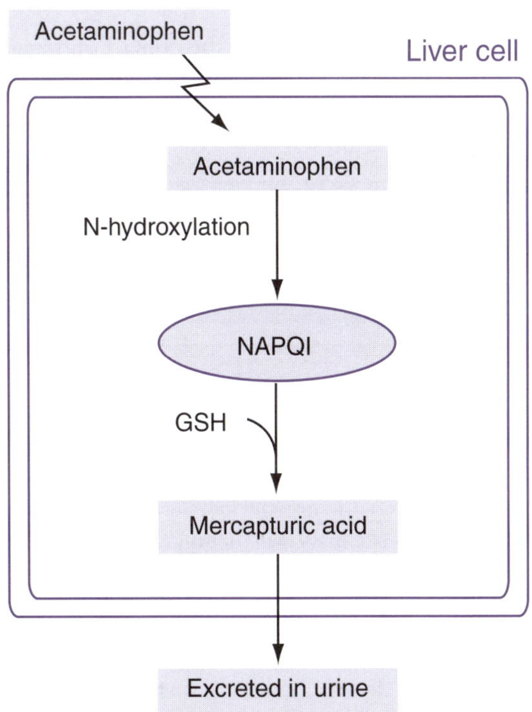

Figure 15-3
Acetaminophen metabolism. In the liver, acetaminophen is metabolized to a toxic intermediate N-acetyl-p-benzoquinone imine (NAPQI). NAPQI is quickly detoxified by conjugation with glutathione (GSH), forming mercapturic acid, which is eliminated via the urine. High doses of acetaminophen or liver dysfunction can result in accumulation of NAPQI and subsequent toxicity to liver proteins.

the conversion of NAPQI to mercapturic acid is delayed, resulting in the accumulation of NAPQI. In sufficient amounts, this metabolite induces hepatic necrosis by binding to and inactivating certain liver proteins.[117] These changes are also associated with the formation of reactive oxygen species, oxidative stress, and mitochondrial dysfunction that trigger additional destruction and death of hepatic tissues.[117,118] Likewise, previous damage to the liver may impair the ability of this organ to convert NAPQI to mercapturic acid, thus resulting in accumulation and damage even at relatively low doses. Hence, people with preexisting liver disease or individuals who are chronic alcohol abusers may be particularly susceptible to liver damage caused by acetaminophen.[119]

PHARMACOKINETICS OF NSAIDS AND ACETAMINOPHEN

Aspirin is absorbed readily from the stomach and small intestine. Approximately 80 to 90 percent of aspirin remains bound to plasma proteins such as albumin. The remaining 10 to 20 percent is widely distributed throughout the body. The unbound or free drug exerts the therapeutic effects. Aspirin itself (acetylsalicylic acid) is hydrolyzed to an active metabolite—salicylic acid. This biotransformation occurs primarily in the bloodstream, and the salicylic acid is further metabolized by oxidation or conjugation in the liver. Excretion of salicylic acid and its metabolites occurs through the kidneys. Although there is some pharmacokinetic variability within the nonaspirin NSAIDs, these drugs generally follow a pattern of absorption, protein binding, metabolism, and excretion similar to that of aspirin.

Acetaminophen is also absorbed rapidly and completely from the upper GI tract. Plasma protein binding with acetaminophen is highly variable (20 to 50 percent) but is considerably less than with aspirin. As indicated earlier in this chapter, metabolism of acetaminophen occurs in the liver via conjugation with an endogenous substrate (glutathione), and the conjugated metabolites are excreted through the kidneys.

Special Concerns for Rehabilitation Patients

Aspirin and the other NSAIDs are among the most frequently used drugs in the rehabilitation population. Aside from the possibility of stomach discomfort, these drugs have a remarkable lack of adverse effects that could directly interfere with physical therapy and occupational therapy. When used for various types of musculoskeletal pain and inflammation, these drugs can often provide analgesia without sedation and psychomimetic (e.g., hallucinogenic, etc.) effects that are associated with opioid (narcotic) analgesics. Thus, the therapy session can be conducted with the benefit of pain relief but without the loss of patient attentiveness and concentration. In inflammatory conditions, NSAIDs can be used for prolonged periods without the serious side effects associated with steroidal drugs (see Chapters 16 and 29). Of course, NSAIDs are limited in that they may not be as effective in moderate-to-severe pain or in severe, progressive inflammation. Still, these agents are a beneficial adjunct in many painful conditions and can usually help facilitate physical rehabilitation. These drugs may also be given to patients for other clinical uses, such as antipyresis and anticoagulation, and these effects are usually achieved with a minimum of adverse effects.

Acetaminophen is also frequently employed for pain relief in many physical rehabilitation patients. Remember that this drug is often equal to an NSAID in analgesic properties but lacks anti-inflammatory effects. Because both aspirin and acetaminophen are available without a prescription, a patient may inquire about the differences between these two drugs. Clinicians should be able to provide an adequate explanation of the differential effects of aspirin and acetaminophen, but the suggested use of these agents should ultimately come from a physician.

CASE STUDY

NONSTEROIDAL ANTI-INFLAMMATORY DRUGS

Brief History. D.B., a 38-year-old man, began to develop pain in his right shoulder. He was employed as a carpenter and had recently been working long hours building a new house. The increasing pain required medical attention. A physician evaluated the patient and diagnosed subacromial bursitis. The patient was referred to physical therapy, and a program of heat, ultrasound, and exercise was initiated to help resolve this condition.

Problem/Influence of Medication. During the initial physical therapy evaluation, the therapist asked if the patient was taking any medication for the bursitis. The patient said the physician advised him to take aspirin or ibuprofen as needed to help relieve the pain. When asked if he had done this, the patient said that he had taken some aspirin once or twice, especially when his shoulder pain kept him awake at night. When he was asked specifically what type of analgesic he had taken, he named a commercial acetaminophen preparation.

Questions to Consider

1. ***How does acetaminophen differ from NSAIDs such as aspirin and ibuprofen, and why is this difference important in this case?***
2. ***What should the therapist tell D.B. about taking over-the-counter pain medications?***

See Appendix C, "Answers to Case Study Questions."

SUMMARY

Aspirin and similarly acting drugs comprise a group of therapeutic agents that are usually referred to as NSAIDs. In addition to their anti-inflammatory effects, these drugs are also known for their ability to decrease mild-to-moderate pain (analgesia), alleviate fever (antipyresis), and inhibit platelet aggregation (anticoagulation). These drugs seem to exert all of their therapeutic effects by inhibiting the function of the cellular cyclooxygenase enzyme, which results in decreased prostaglandin and thromboxane synthesis. Aspirin is the prototypical NSAID, and newer prescription and nonprescription drugs appear to be similar in terms of pharmacological effects and therapeutic efficacy.

Newer drugs known as COX-2 inhibitors inhibit prostaglandins that cause pain and inflammation while sparing the production of beneficial prostaglandins that protect the stomach and other organs. These COX-2 drugs have the potential to produce therapeutic effects with less gastritis, but their status remains controversial because COX-2 agents may increase the risk of heart attack and stroke. Acetaminophen also seems to be similar to aspirin in analgesic and antipyretic effects, but acetaminophen lacks anti-inflammatory and anticoagulant properties. Patients requiring physical rehabilitation use aspirin, other NSAIDs, and COX-2 inhibitors frequently, which usually provides beneficial effects (e.g., analgesia, decreased inflammation, etc.) without producing cognitive side effects (e.g., sedation, mood changes) that can interfere with the rehabilitation program.

REFERENCES

1. Botting RM. Vane's discovery of the mechanism of action of aspirin changed our understanding of its clinical pharmacology. *Pharmacol Rep.* 2010;62:518-525.
2. Grosser T, Smyth E, FitzGerald GA. Anti-inflammatory, antipyretic, and analgesic agents: pharmacotherapy of gout. In: Brunton LL, et al, eds. *The Pharmacological Basis of Therapeutics.* 12th ed. New York: McGraw Hill; 2011.
3. Hirata T, Narumiya S. Prostanoids as regulators of innate and adaptive immunity. *Adv Immunol.* 2012;116:143-174.
4. Ricciotti E, FitzGerald GA. Prostaglandins and inflammation. *Arterioscler Thromb Vasc Biol.* 2011;31:986-1000.

5. Suzuki J, Ogawa M, Watanabe R, et al. Roles of prostaglandin E2 in cardiovascular diseases. *Int Heart J.* 2011;52:266-269.
6. Haeggström JZ, Rinaldo-Matthis A, Wheelock CE, Wetterholm A. Advances in eicosanoid research, novel therapeutic implications. *Biochem Biophys Res Commun.* 2010;396:135-139.
7. Gleim S, Stitham J, Tang WH, et al. An eicosanoid-centric view of atherothrombotic risk factors. *Cell Mol Life Sci.* 2012;69:3361-3380.
8. Smyth E, Grosser T, FitzGerald GA. Lipid-derived autocoids: eicosanoids and platelet-activating factor. In: Brunton LL, et al, eds. *The Pharmacological Basis of Therapeutics.* 12th ed. New York: McGraw Hill; 2011.
9. Smyth EM, Grosser T, Wang M, et al. Prostanoids in health and disease. *J Lipid Res.* 2009;50(suppl):S423-428.
10. Bozza PT, Bakker-Abreu I, Navarro-Xavier RA, Bandeira-Melo C. Lipid body function in eicosanoid synthesis: an update. *Prostaglandins Leukot Essent Fatty Acids.* 2011;85:205-213.
11. Jenkins CM, Cedars A, Gross RW. Eicosanoid signaling pathways in the heart. *Cardiovasc Res.* 2009;82:240-249.
12. Hallstrand TS, Henderson WR Jr. An update on the role of leukotrienes in asthma. *Curr Opin Allergy Clin Immunol.* 2010; 10:60-66.
13. Okunishi K, Peters-Golden M. Leukotrienes and airway inflammation. Biochim Biophys Acta. 2011;1810:1096-1102.
14. Montuschi P, Peters-Golden ML. Leukotriene modifiers for asthma treatment. *Clin Exp Allergy.* 2010;40:1732-1741.
15. Wong SL, Wong WT, Tian XY, et al. Prostaglandins in action indispensable roles of cyclooxygenase-1 and -2 in endothelium-dependent contractions. *Adv Pharmacol.* 2010;60:61-83.
16. Goodwin GM. *Prostaglandins: Biochemistry, Functions, Types and Roles.* Hauppauge NY: Nova Science Publishers; 2010.
17. Aoki T, Narumiya S. Prostaglandins and chronic inflammation. *Trends Pharmacol Sci.* 2012;33:304-311.
18. Khanapure SP, Garvey DS, Janero DR, Letts LG. Eicosanoids in inflammation: biosynthesis, pharmacology, and therapeutic frontiers. *Curr Top Med Chem.* 2007;7:311-340.
19. Lima IV, Bastos LF, Limborço-Filho M, et al. Role of prostaglandins in neuroinflammatory and neurodegenerative diseases. *Mediators Inflamm.* 2012;2012:946813.
20. Erol K, Sirmagul B, Kilic FS, et al. The role of inflammation and COX-derived prostanoids in the effects of bradykinin on isolated rat aorta and urinary bladder. *Inflammation.* 2012;35:420-428.
21. Yousefi B, Jadidi-Niaragh F, Azizi G, et al. The role of leukotrienes in immunopathogenesis of rheumatoid arthritis. *Mod Rheumatol.* 2014;24:225-235.
22. Scher JU, Pillinger MH. The anti-inflammatory effects of prostaglandins. *J Investig Med.* 2009;57:703-708.
23. Mizumura K, Sugiura T, Katanosaka K, et al. Excitation and sensitization of nociceptors by bradykinin: what do we know? *Exp Brain Res.* 2009;196:53-65.
24. Engström L, Ruud J, Eskilsson A, et al. Lipopolysaccharide-induced fever depends on prostaglandin E2 production specifically in brain endothelial cells. *Endocrinology.* 2012;153:4849-4861.
25. Gaetano L, Watanabe K, Barogi S, Coceani F. Cyclooxygenase-2/microsomal prostaglandin E synthase-1 complex in the preoptic-anterior hypothalamus of the mouse: involvement through fever to intravenous lipopolysaccharide. *Acta Physiol.* 2010;200: 315-324.
26. Ootsuka Y, Blessing WW, Steiner AA, Romanovsky AA. Fever response to intravenous prostaglandin E2 is mediated by the brain but does not require afferent vagal signaling. *Am J Physiol Regul Integr Comp Physiol.* 2008;294:R1294-1303.
27. Harel Z. Dysmenorrhea in adolescents and young adults: an update on pharmacological treatments and management strategies. *Expert Opin Pharmacother.* 2012;13:2157-2170.
28. Sultan C, Gaspari L, Paris F. Adolescent dysmenorrhea. *Endocr Dev.* 2012;22:171-180.
29. Angiolillo DJ, Ueno M, Goto S. Basic principles of platelet biology and clinical implications. *Circ J.* 2010;74:597-607.
30. Ueno M, Kodali M, Tello-Montoliu A, Angiolillo DJ. Role of platelets and antiplatelet therapy in cardiovascular disease. *J Atheroscler Thromb.* 2011;18:431-442.
31. Allaj V, Guo C, Nie D. Non-steroid anti-inflammatory drugs, prostaglandins, and cancer. *Cell Biosci.* 2013;3:8.
32. Chakraborti AK, Garg SK, Kumar R, et al. Progress in COX-2 inhibitors: a journey so far. *Curr Med Chem.* 2010;17: 1563-1593.
33. Rao P, Knaus EE. Evolution of nonsteroidal anti-inflammatory drugs (NSAIDs): cyclooxygenase (COX) inhibition and beyond. *J Pharm Pharm Sci.* 2008;11:81s-110s.
34. Rouzer CA, Marnett LJ. Cyclooxygenases: structural and functional insights. *J Lipid Res.* 2009;50(suppl):S29-34.
35. Sostres C, Gargallo CJ, Arroyo MT, Lanas A. Adverse effects of non-steroidal anti-inflammatory drugs (NSAIDs, aspirin and coxibs) on upper gastrointestinal tract. *Best Pract Res Clin Gastroenterol.* 2010;24:121-132.
36. Patrono C, Rocca B. Aspirin and other COX-1 inhibitors. *Handb Exp Pharmacol.* 2012;210:137-164.
37. Dixon DA, Blanco FF, Bruno A, Patrignani P. Mechanistic aspects of COX-2 expression in colorectal neoplasia. *Recent Results Cancer Res.* 2013;191:7-37.
38. Perrone MG, Scilimati A, Simone L, Vitale P. Selective COX-1 inhibition: a therapeutic target to be reconsidered. *Curr Med Chem.* 2010;17:3769-3805.
39. Ekman EF, Koman LA. Acute pain following musculoskeletal injuries and orthopaedic surgery: mechanisms and management. *Instr Course Lect.* 2005;54:21-33.
40. Weaver AL. Current and emerging treatments for mild/ moderate acute ambulatory pain. *Am J Ther.* 2008;15(suppl 10): S12-16.
41. Adebajo A. Non-steroidal anti-inflammatory drugs for the treatment of pain and immobility-associated osteoarthritis: consensus guidance for primary care. *BMC Fam Pract.* 2012;13:23.
42. Feeley BT, Gallo RA, Sherman S, Williams RJ. Management of osteoarthritis of the knee in the active patient. *J Am Acad Orthop Surg.* 2010;18:406-416.
43. Marjoribanks J, Proctor M, Farquhar C, Derks RS. Nonsteroidal anti-inflammatory drugs for dysmenorrhoea. *Cochrane Database Syst Rev.* 2010;1:CD001751.
44. Brattwall M, Jacobson E, Forssblad M, Jakobsson J. Knee arthroscopy routines and practice. *Knee Surg Sports Traumatol Arthrosc.* 2010;18:1656-1660.
45. Moore RA, Derry S, McQuay HJ, Wiffen PJ. Single dose oral analgesics for acute postoperative pain in adults. *Cochrane Database Syst Rev.* 2011;9:CD008659.
46. Michelet D, Andreu-Gallien J, Bensalah T, et al. A meta-analysis of the use of nonsteroidal antiinflammatory drugs for pediatric postoperative pain. *Anesth Analg.* 2012;114:393-406.
47. Southworth S, Peters J, Rock A, Pavliv L. A multicenter, randomized, double-blind, placebo-controlled trial of intravenous ibuprofen 400 and 800 mg every 6 hours in the management of postoperative pain. *Clin Ther.* 2009;31:1922-1935.

48. Cassinelli EH, Dean CL, Garcia RM, et al. Ketorolac use for postoperative pain management following lumbar decompression surgery: a prospective, randomized, double-blinded, placebo-controlled trial. *Spine*. 2008;33:1313-1317.
49. Russo A, Di Stasio E, Bevilacqua F, et al. Efficacy of scheduled time ketorolac administration compared to continuous infusion for post-operative pain after abdominal surgery. *Eur Rev Med Pharmacol Sci*. 2012;16:1675-1679.
50. De Oliveira GS Jr, Agarwal D, Benzon HT. Perioperative single dose ketorolac to prevent postoperative pain: a meta-analysis of randomized trials. *Anesth Analg*. 2012;114:424-433.
51. Bartfai T, Conti B. Fever. *ScientificWorldJournal*. 2010;10: 490-503.
52. Angiolillo DJ. The evolution of antiplatelet therapy in the treatment of acute coronary syndromes: from aspirin to the present day. *Drugs*. 2012;72:2087-2116.
53. Tanguay JF. Antiplatelet therapy in acute coronary syndrome and atrial fibrillation: aspirin. *Adv Cardiol*. 2012;47:20-30.
54. Weber R, Brenck J, Diener HC. Antiplatelet therapy in cerebrovascular disorders. *Handb Exp Pharmacol*. 2012;210:519-546.
55. Chan AT, Arber N, Burn J, et al. Aspirin in the chemoprevention of colorectal neoplasia: an overview. *Cancer Prev Res*. 2012; 5:164-178.
56. Ferrández A, Piazuelo E, Castells A. Aspirin and the prevention of colorectal cancer. *Best Pract Res Clin Gastroenterol*. 2012;26:185-195.
57. Rothwell PM. Aspirin in prevention of sporadic colorectal cancer: current clinical evidence and overall balance of risks and benefits. *Recent Results Cancer Res*. 2013;191:121-142.
58. Bruno A, Dovizio M, Tacconelli S, Patrignani P. Mechanisms of the antitumoural effects of aspirin in the gastrointestinal tract. *Best Pract Res Clin Gastroenterol*. 2012;26:e1-e13.
59. Bosetti C, Rosato V, Gallus S, et al. Aspirin and cancer risk: a quantitative review to 2011. *Ann Oncol*. 2012;23:1403-1415.
60. Bosetti C, Rosato V, Gallus S, La Vecchia C. Aspirin and urologic cancer risk: an update. *Nat Rev Urol*. 2012;9:102-110.
61. Dovizio M, Bruno A, Tacconelli S, Patrignani P. Mode of action of aspirin as a chemopreventive agent. *Recent Results Cancer Res*. 2013;191:39-65.
62. Thiagarajan P, Jankowski JA. Aspirin and NSAIDs; benefits and harms for the gut. *Best Pract Res Clin Gastroenterol*. 2012;26: 197-206.
63. Vonkeman HE, van de Laar MA. Nonsteroidal anti-inflammatory drugs: adverse effects and their prevention. *Semin Arthritis Rheum*. 2010;39:294-312.
64. Scheiman JM, Hindley CE. Strategies to optimize treatment with NSAIDs in patients at risk for gastrointestinal and cardiovascular adverse events. *Clin Ther*. 2010;32:667-677.
65. Chan FK, Ching JY, Suen BY, et al. Effects of *Helicobacter pylori* infection on long-term risk of peptic ulcer bleeding in low-dose aspirin users. *Gastroenterology*. 2013;144:528-535.
66. Endo H, Sakai E, Higurashi T, et al. Differences in the severity of small bowel mucosal injury based on the type of aspirin as evaluated by capsule endoscopy. *Dig Liver Dis*. 2012;44:833-838.
67. Coté GA, Norvell JP, Rice JP, et al. Use of gastroprotection in patients discharged from hospital on nonsteroidal anti-inflammatory drugs. *Am J Ther*. 2008;15:444-449.
68. Lee KN, Lee OY, Choi MG, et al. Prevention of NSAID-associated gastroduodenal injury in healthy volunteers-a randomized, double-blind, multicenter study comparing DA-9601 with misoprostol. *J Korean Med Sci*. 2011;26:1074-1080.
69. Gigante A, Tagarro I. Non-steroidal anti-inflammatory drugs and gastroprotection with proton pump inhibitors: a focus on ketoprofen/omeprazole. *Clin Drug Investig*. 2012;32:221-233.
70. Lazzaroni M, Porro GB. Management of NSAID-induced gastrointestinal toxicity: focus on proton pump inhibitors. *Drugs*. 2009;69:51-69.
71. Scheiman JM. Prevention of damage induced by aspirin in the GI tract. *Best Pract Res Clin Gastroenterol*. 2012;26:153-162.
72. Coruzzi G, Venturi N, Spaggiari S. Gastrointestinal safety of novel nonsteroidal antiinflammatory drugs: selective COX-2 inhibitors and beyond. *Acta Biomed*. 2007;78:96-110.
73. Shi S, Klotz U. Clinical use and pharmacological properties of selective COX-2 inhibitors. *Eur J Clin Pharmacol*. 2008;64:233-252.
74. Wallace JL, Vong L. NSAID-induced gastrointestinal damage and the design of GI-sparing NSAIDs. *Curr Opin Investig Drugs*. 2008;9:1151-1156.
75. Frampton JE, Keating GM. Celecoxib: a review of its use in the management of arthritis and acute pain. *Drugs*. 2007;67: 2433-2472.
76. McCormack PL. Celecoxib: a review of its use for symptomatic relief in the treatment of osteoarthritis, rheumatoid arthritis and ankylosing spondylitis. *Drugs*. 2011;71:2457-2489.
77. Fosbøl EL, Køber L, Torp-Pedersen C, Gislason GH. Cardiovascular safety of non-steroidal anti-inflammatory drugs among healthy individuals. *Expert Opin Drug Saf*. 2010;9:893-903.
78. García Rodríguez LA, González-Pérez A, Bueno H, Hwa J. NSAID use selectively increases the risk of non-fatal myocardial infarction: a systematic review of randomised trials and observational studies. *PLoS One*. 2011;6:e16780.
79. Sudano I, Flammer AJ, Roas S, et al. Nonsteroidal antiinflammatory drugs, acetaminophen, and hypertension. *Curr Hypertens Rep*. 2012;14:304-309.
80. Trelle S, Reichenbach S, Wandel S, et al. Cardiovascular safety of non-steroidal anti-inflammatory drugs: network meta-analysis. *BMJ*. 2011;342:c7086.
81. Amer M, Bead VR, Bathon J, et al. Use of nonsteroidal anti-inflammatory drugs in patients with cardiovascular disease: a cautionary tale. *Cardiol Rev*. 2010;18:204-212.
82. Agúndez JA, Lucena MI, Martínez C, et al. Assessment of nonsteroidal anti-inflammatory drug-induced hepatotoxicity. *Expert Opin Drug Metab Toxicol*. 2011;7:817-828.
83. Teoh NC, Farrell GC. Hepatotoxicity associated with non-steroidal anti-inflammatory drugs. *Clin Liver Dis*. 2003;7:401-413.
84. Harirforoosh S, Jamali F. Renal adverse effects of nonsteroidal anti-inflammatory drugs. *Expert Opin Drug Saf*. 2009;8:669-681.
85. Knights KM, Tsoutsikos P, Miners JO. Novel mechanisms of nonsteroidal anti-inflammatory drug-induced renal toxicity. *Expert Opin Drug Metab Toxicol*. 2005;1:399-408.
86. Musu M, Finco G, Antonucci R, et al. Acute nephrotoxicity of NSAID from the foetus to the adult. *Eur Rev Med Pharmacol Sci*. 2011;15:1461-1472.
87. Zardi EM, Dobrina A, Amoroso A, Afeltra A. Prostacyclin in liver disease: a potential therapeutic option. *Expert Opin Biol Ther*. 2007;7:785-790.
88. Pugliese A, Beltramo T, Torre D. Reye's and Reye's-like syndromes. *Cell Biochem Funct*. 2008;26:741-746.
89. Bennett CL, Starko KM, Thomsen HS, et al. Linking drugs to obscure illnesses: lessons from pure red cell aplasia, nephrogenic systemic fibrosis, and Reye's syndrome. A report from the Southern Network on Adverse Reactions (SONAR). *J Gen Intern Med*. 2012;27:1697-1703.

90. Kong JS, Teuber SS, Gershwin ME. Aspirin and nonsteroidal anti-inflammatory drug hypersensitivity. *Clin Rev Allergy Immunol.* 2007;32:97-110.
91. Knowles SR, Drucker AM, Weber EA, Shear NH. Management options for patients with aspirin and nonsteroidal anti-inflammatory drug sensitivity. *Ann Pharmacother.* 2007;41:1191-1200.
92. McMullan KL, Wedner HJ. Safety of aspirin desensitization in patients with reported aspirin allergy and cardiovascular disease. *Clin Cardiol.* 2013;36:25-30.
93. Lack WD, Fredericks D, Petersen E, et al. Effect of aspirin on bone healing in a rabbit ulnar osteotomy model. *J Bone Joint Surg Am.* 2013;95:488-496.
94. O'Connor JP, Capo JT, Tan V, et al. A comparison of the effects of ibuprofen and rofecoxib on rabbit fibula osteotomy healing. *Acta Orthop.* 2009;80:597-605.
95. Vuolteenaho K, Moilanen T, Moilanen E. Non-steroidal anti-inflammatory drugs, cyclooxygenase-2 and the bone healing process. *Basic Clin Pharmacol Toxicol.* 2008;102:10-14.
96. Harder AT, An YH. The mechanisms of the inhibitory effects of nonsteroidal anti-inflammatory drugs on bone healing: a concise review. *J Clin Pharmacol.* 2003;43:807-815.
97. Chen MR, Dragoo JL. The effect of nonsteroidal anti-inflammatory drugs on tissue healing. *Knee Surg Sports Traumatol Arthrosc.* 2013;21:540-549.
98. Thaller J, Walker M, Kline AJ, Anderson DG. The effect of nonsteroidal anti-inflammatory agents on spinal fusion. *Orthopedics.* 2005;28:299-303.
99. El Hajjaji H, Marcelis A, Devogelaer JP, Manicourt DH. Celecoxib has a positive effect on the overall metabolism of hyaluronan and proteoglycans in human osteoarthritic cartilage. *J Rheumatol.* 2003;30:2444-2451.
100. Mastbergen SC, Bijlsma JW, Lafeber FP. Selective COX-2 inhibition is favorable to human early and late-stage osteoarthritic cartilage: a human in vitro study. *Osteoarthritis Cartilage.* 2005;13:519-526.
101. Ou Y, Tan C, An H, et al. Selective COX-2 inhibitor ameliorates osteoarthritis by repressing apoptosis of chondrocyte. *Med Sci Monit.* 2012;18:BR247-252.
102. Sachs CJ. Oral analgesics for acute nonspecific pain. *Am Fam Physician.* 2005;71:913-918.
103. Roth SH. Nonsteroidal anti-inflammatory drug gastropathy: new avenues for safety. *Clin Interv Aging.* 2011;6:125-131.
104. Grosser T. Variability in the response to cyclooxygenase inhibitors: toward the individualization of nonsteroidal anti-inflammatory drug therapy. *J Investig Med.* 2009;57:709-716.
105. Fish L, Nicholson BD. The payer side: patient outcomes and cost. *Am J Ther.* 2008;15(suppl 10):S20-22.
106. Gatti D, Adami S. Coxibs: a significant therapeutic opportunity. *Acta Biomed.* 2010;81:217-224.
107. Mallen SR, Essex MN, Zhang R. Gastrointestinal tolerability of NSAIDs in elderly patients: a pooled analysis of 21 randomized clinical trials with celecoxib and nonselective NSAIDs. *Curr Med Res Opin.* 2011;27:1359-1366.
108. Khan M, Fraser A. Cox-2 inhibitors and the risk of cardiovascular thrombotic events. *Ir Med J.* 2012;105:119-121.
109. Martínez-González J, Badimon L. Mechanisms underlying the cardiovascular effects of COX-inhibition: benefits and risks. *Curr Pharm Des.* 2007;13:2215-2227.
110. Conaghan PG. A turbulent decade for NSAIDs: update on current concepts of classification, epidemiology, comparative efficacy, and toxicity. *Rheumatol Int.* 2012;32:1491-1502.
111. Moodley I. Review of the cardiovascular safety of COXIBs compared to NSAIDS. *Cardiovasc J Afr.* 2008;19:102-107.
112. Toussaint K, Yang XC, Zielinski MA, et al. What do we (not) know about how paracetamol (acetaminophen) works? *J Clin Pharm Ther.* 2010;35:617-638.
113. Klotz U. Paracetamol (acetaminophen)—a popular and widely used nonopioid analgesic. *Arzneimittelforschung.* 2012;62:355-359.
114. Seed SM, Dunican KC, Lynch AM. Osteoarthritis: a review of treatment options. *Geriatrics.* 2009;64:20-29.
115. Sinusas K. Osteoarthritis: diagnosis and treatment. *Am Fam Physician.* 2012;85:49-56.
116. Hinz B, Brune K. Paracetamol and cyclooxygenase inhibition: is there a cause for concern? *Ann Rheum Dis.* 2012;71:20-25.
117. Hinson JA, Roberts DW, James LP. Mechanisms of acetaminophen-induced liver necrosis. *Handb Exp Pharmacol.* 2010;196:369-405.
118. McGill MR, Williams CD, Xie Y, et al. Acetaminophen-induced liver injury in rats and mice: comparison of protein adducts, mitochondrial dysfunction, and oxidative stress in the mechanism of toxicity. *Toxicol Appl Pharmacol.* 2012;264:387-394.
119. Myers RP, Shaheen AA, Li B, et al. Impact of liver disease, alcohol abuse, and unintentional ingestions on the outcomes of acetaminophen overdose. *Clin Gastroenterol Hepatol.* 2008;6:918-925.

CHAPTER 16

Pharmacological Management of Rheumatoid Arthritis and Osteoarthritis

Rheumatoid arthritis and osteoarthritis represent the two primary pathological conditions that affect the joints and periarticular structures. Although the causes underlying these conditions are quite different from one another, both conditions can cause severe pain and deformity in various joints in the body. Pharmacological management plays an important role in the treatment of each disorder. Because physical therapists and other rehabilitation specialists often work with patients who have rheumatoid arthritis or osteoarthritis, an understanding of the types of drugs used to treat these diseases is important.

This chapter begins by describing the etiology of rheumatoid joint disease and the pharmacological treatment of rheumatoid arthritis. An analogous discussion of osteoarthritis follows. These descriptions should clarify drug therapy's role in arthritis and the impact drugs can have on patients receiving physical therapy and occupational therapy.

RHEUMATOID ARTHRITIS

Rheumatoid arthritis (RA) is a chronic, systemic disorder that affects many different tissues in the body but is primarily characterized by synovitis and the destruction of articular tissue.[1-3] This disease is associated with pain, stiffness, and inflammation in the small synovial joints of the hands and feet and in larger joints such as the knee. Although marked by periods of exacerbation and remission, RA is often progressive in nature, with advanced stages leading to severe joint destruction and bone erosion. Specific criteria for the diagnosis of RA in adults are listed in Table 16-1.

There is also a form of arthritis that occurs in children, known commonly as *juvenile rheumatoid arthritis* or, more recently, *juvenile idiopathic arthritis* (JIA). The age of onset (younger than 16 years) and other criteria help to differentiate adult and juvenile types of rheumatoid joint disease.[4,5] Drug treatment of adult and juvenile RA is fairly similar, especially with regard to the use of the newer biological agents to modify disease progression.[6] Consequently, in this chapter most of the discussion of the management of RA is directed toward the adult form.

RA affects approximately 0.5 to 1 percent of the population worldwide.[1,3] It occurs three times more often in women than in men, with the prevalence of RA also increasing in older adults.[7,8] Joint damage from RA is often the cause of severe pain and suffering, resulting in significant disability and reduced quality of life.[9] This condition is also associated with an increased incidence of cardiovascular disease and several other comorbidities.[10,11] The economic impact of this disease is also staggering; direct medical costs combined with indirect costs due to loss of productivity approach $20 billion annually in the United States.[12] Consequently, RA is a formidable and serious problem in contemporary health care.

Table 16-1

THE 2010 ACR-EULAR* CLASSIFICATION CRITERIA FOR RHEUMATOID ARTHRITIS

Criterion	Score
Target population (who should be tested?): Patients who have the following: 1. At least 1 joint with definite clinical synovitis (swelling)[a] 2. Synovitis that is not better explained by another disease[b]	
Classification criteria for RA (score-based algorithm: add score of categories A–D; a score greater than or equal to 6/10 is needed for classification of a patient as having definite RA)[c]	
A. Joint Involvement[d]	
1 large joint[e]	0
2–10 large joints	1
1–3 small joints (with or without involvement of large joints)[f]	2
4–10 small joints (with or without involvement of large joints)	3
>10 joints (at least 1 small joint)[g]	5
B. Serology (at least 1 test result is needed for classification)[h]	
Negative RF *and* negative ACPA	0
Low-positive RF *or* low-positive ACPA	2
High-positive RF *or* high-positive ACPA	3
C. Acute-Phase Reactants (at least 1 test result is needed for classification[i])	
Normal CRP *and* normal ESR	0
Abnormal CRP *or* abnormal ESR	1
D. Duration of Symptoms[j]	
Less than 6 weeks	0
At least 6 weeks	1

From: www.rheumatology.org/practice/clinical/classification/ra/ra_2010.asp

** American College of Rheumatology/European League Against Rheumatism*

a. The criteria are aimed at classification of newly presenting patients. In addition, patients with erosive disease typical of rheumatoid arthritis (RA) with a history compatible with prior fulfillment of the 2010 criteria should be classified as having RA. Patients with long-standing disease, including those whose disease is inactive (with or without treatment) and who, based on retrospectively available data, have previously fulfilled the 2010 criteria, should be classified as having RA.

b. Differential diagnoses vary among patients with different presentations but may include conditions such as systemic lupus erythematosus, psoriatic arthritis, and gout. If it is unclear about the relevant differential diagnoses to consider, an expert rheumatologist should be consulted.

c. Although patients with a score of less than 6/10 are not classifiable as having RA, their status can be reassessed and the criteria might be fulfilled cumulatively over time.

d. Joint involvement refers to any swollen *or* tender *joint on examination, which may be confirmed by imaging evidence of synovitis. Distal interphalangeal joints, first carpometacarpal joints, and first metatarsophalangeal joints are* excluded from assessment. *Categories of joint distribution are classified according to the location and number of involved joints, with placement into the highest category possible based on the pattern of joint involvement.*

e. Large joints *refer to shoulders, elbows, hips, knees, and ankles.*

f. Small joints *refer to the metacarpophalangeal joints, proximal interphalangeal joints, second through fifth metatarsophalangeal joints, thumb interphalangeal joints, and wrists.*

g. In this category, at least one of the involved joints must be a small joint; the other joints can include any combination of large and additional small joints, as well as other joints not specifically listed elsewhere (e.g., temporomandibular, acromioclavicular, sternoclavicular, etc.).

h. Negative *refers to IU values that are less than or equal to the upper limit of normal (ULN) for the laboratory and assay;* low-positive *refers to IU values that are higher than the ULN but are less than or equal to 3 times the ULN for the laboratory and assay;* high-positive *refers to IU values that are greater than 3 times the ULN for the laboratory and assay. Where rheumatoid factor (RF) information is only available as positive or negative, a positive result should be scored as low-positive for RF. ACPA = anti-citrullinated protein antibody.*

i. Normal/abnormal is determined by local laboratory standards. CRP = C-reactive protein; ESR = erythrocyte sedimentation rate.

j. Duration of symptoms *refers to patient self-report of the duration of signs or symptoms of synovitis (e.g., pain, swelling, tenderness) of joints that are clinically involved at the time of assessment, regardless of treatment status.*

Immune Basis for Rheumatoid Arthritis

The initiating factor in RA is unknown. However, it is apparent that the underlying basis of this disease consists of an autoimmune response in genetically susceptible individuals.[13] Some precipitating factor such as a virus or other infectious agent, or an environmental trigger such as cigarette/tobacco use, appears to initiate the formation of antibodies that are later recognized by the host as antigens.[14,15] Subsequent formation of new antibodies to these antigens then initiates a complex chain of events involving a variety of immune system components such as mononuclear phagocytes, T lymphocytes, and B lymphocytes (Fig. 16-1).[14,16] These cells interact with each other to produce several arthritogenic mediators, including cytokines (**interleukins, tumor necrosis factor**-alpha), eicosanoids (prostaglandins, leukotrienes), and destructive enzymes (proteases, collagenases).[16,17] These substances act either directly or through other cellular components of the immune system to induce synovial cell proliferation and destruction of articular cartilage and bone.[3,18] Thus, the joint destruction in RA is the culmination of a series of events resulting from an inherent defect in the patient's immune response.[14,16]

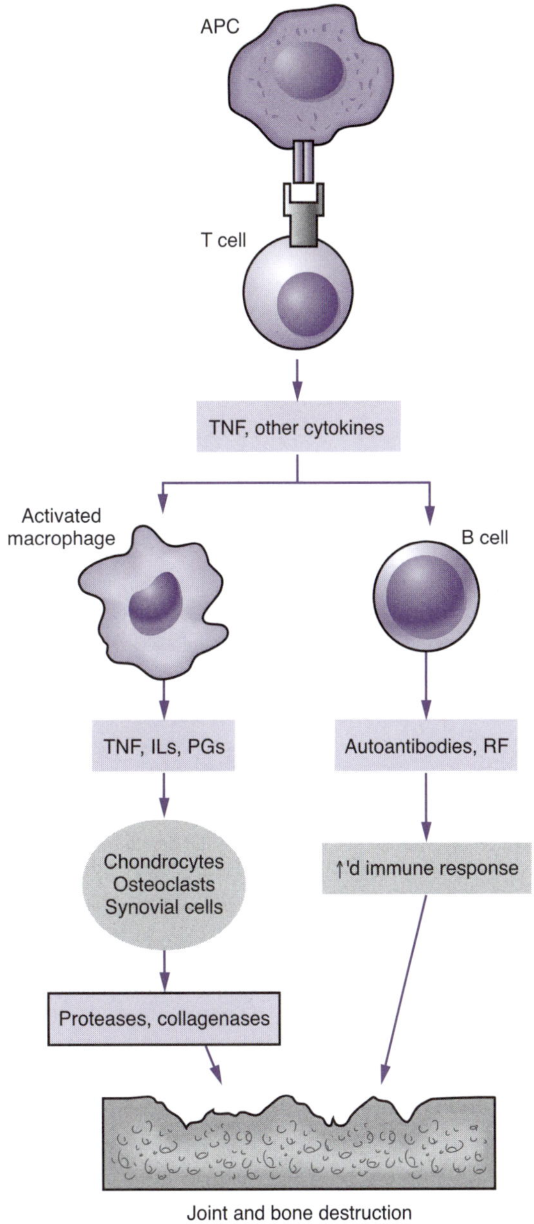

Figure ■ 16-1
Cellular and chemical responses in rheumatoid arthritis. An antigen-presenting cell (APC) initiates a complex autoimmune response that involves various other cells and chemical mediators such as tumor necrosis factor (TNF), interleukins (ILs), prostaglandins (PGs), rheumatoid factor (RF), and other components that ultimately lead to inflammation and damage to bone and joint tissues.

Overview of Drug Therapy in Rheumatoid Arthritis

The drug treatment of RA has two goals: to decrease joint inflammation and to arrest the progression of the disease. Three general categories of drugs are available to accomplish these goals:

- NSAIDs
- Glucocorticoids
- A diverse group of agents known as *disease-modifying antirheumatic drugs* (DMARDs; Table 16-2).[3,19]

NSAIDs and glucocorticoids are used primarily to decrease joint inflammation, but these agents do not necessarily halt the progression of RA. DMARDs, including the newer "biological" agents that attempt to modify the immune response in RA, have become increasingly popular as the primary form of drug therapy.[20] Each of these major drug categories, as well as specific disease-modifying drugs, is discussed in the following sections.

Table 16-2
DRUG CATEGORIES USED IN RHEUMATOID ARTHRITIS

I. Nonsteroidal Anti-Inflammatory Drugs	
Aspirin (many trade names)	Ketoprofen (Orudis, others)
Celecoxib (Celebrex)*	Meclofenamate (Meclomen)
Diclofenac (Voltaren)	Meloxicam (Mobic)
Diflunisal (Dolobid)	Nabumetone (Relafen)
Etodolac (Lodine)	Naproxen (Anaprox, Naprosyn, others)
Fenoprofen (Nalfon)	Oxaprozin (Daypro)
Flurbiprofen (Ansaid)	Piroxicam (Feldene)
Ibuprofen (many trade names)	Sulindac (Clinoril)
Indomethacin (Indocin)	Tolmetin (Tolectin)
II. Corticosteroids	
Betamethasone (Celestone)	Methylprednisolone (Medrol, others)
Cortisone (Cortone acetate)	Prednisolone (Prelone, others)
Dexamethasone (Decadron, others)	Prednisone (Deltasone, others)
Hydrocortisone (Cortef, others)	Triamcinolone (Aristocort, others)
III. Disease-Modifying Antirheumatic Drugs	
Abatacept (Orencia)	Gold sodium thiomalate (Myochrysine)
Adalimumab (Humira)	Golimumab (Simponi)
Anakinra (Kineret)	Hydroxychloroquine (Plaquenil)
Auranofin (Ridaura)	Infliximab (Remicade)
Azathioprine (Imuran)	Leflunomide (Arava)
Certolizumab (Cimzia)	Methotrexate (Rheumatrex, others)
Chloroquine (Aralen)	Penicillamine (Cuprimine, Depen)
Cyclophosphamide (Cytoxan)	Sulfasalazine (Azulfidine)
Cyclosporine (Neoral, Sandimmune)	Tocilizumab (Actemra)
Etanercept (Enbrel)	

**Subclassified as a cyclooxygenase type 2 (COX-2) inhibitor; see Chapter 15.*

NSAIDs

Aspirin and the other NSAIDs were once considered the first line of defense in treating RA. This idea has changed somewhat because early and aggressive use of DMARDs (discussed later in this chapter) can help deter the progression of RA and provide better long-term management. Nonetheless, NSAIDs remain an important short-term option for controlling pain and inflammation throughout the course of the disease. Although NSAIDs are not as powerful in reducing inflammation as glucocorticoids, they are associated with fewer side effects, and they offer the added advantage of analgesia. See Chapter 15 for a thorough discussion of aspirin and other NSAIDs, their mechanism of action, and adverse side effects.

NSAIDs that can be used for RA are listed in Table 16-2. Usually it is not advisable to use two different NSAIDs simultaneously, because there is an increased risk of side effects without any appreciable increase in therapeutic benefit. Some amount of trial and error may be involved in selecting the optimal NSAID. As discussed in Chapter 15, aspirin appears approximately equal to the newer, more expensive NSAIDs in terms of anti-inflammatory and analgesic effects, but some of the newer drugs may produce less gastrointestinal (GI) discomfort. In particular, the cyclooxygenase-2 (COX-2) selective drugs (see below) may be especially helpful in people with a history of peptic ulcers or other risk factors for GI problems.[21]

On the other hand, COX-2 inhibitors and traditional NSAIDs are associated with heart attack and stroke in some patients, and concern about these cardiovascular risks has raised questions about the long-term use of these drugs in people with RA. Hence, NSAIDs remain a potential tool for short-term treatment of exacerbation of pain and inflammation[3] related to RA, but the emergence of other drugs (DMARDs) and concerns about safety have relegated NSAIDs to a secondary role.[22]

Finally, acetaminophen (paracetamol) products may provide some temporary analgesic effects in people with RA, but these products are not optimal because they lack anti-inflammatory effects. As discussed in Chapter 15, acetaminophen can be used to treat mild-to-moderate pain, but the lack of anti-inflammatory effects means acetaminophen provides questionable benefits for patients with RA.[23] As a result, acetaminophen products are not typically used for the routine treatment of this disease.

Mechanism of Action

The pharmacology of the NSAIDs was discussed in Chapter 15. To review, aspirin and the other NSAIDs exert most or all of their anti-inflammatory and analgesic effects by inhibiting the synthesis of prostaglandins.[24,25] Certain prostaglandins (i.e., prostaglandin E_2

[PGE_2]) are believed to participate in the inflammatory response by increasing local blood flow and vascular permeability and by exerting a chemotactic effect on leukocytes.[26] Prostaglandins are also believed to sensitize pain receptors to the nociceptive effects of other pain mediators such as bradykinin.[27] Aspirin and other NSAIDs prevent the production of prostaglandins by inhibiting the COX enzyme that initiates prostaglandin synthesis. As discussed in Chapter 15, aspirin and most other NSAIDs inhibit all COX forms—that is, these drugs inhibit the COX-1 form of the enzyme that produces beneficial and protective prostaglandins in certain tissues while also inhibiting the COX-2 form that synthesizes prostaglandins in painful and inflamed tissues.[25]

However, newer NSAIDs are known as COX-2 inhibitors because these drugs inhibit the specific form of COX-2 that synthesizes prostaglandins during pain and inflammation. COX-2 drugs such as celecoxib (Celebrex) often spare the production of normal or protective prostaglandins produced by COX-1 in the stomach, kidneys, and platelets (see Chapter 15).[28] Hence, COX-2 selective drugs may be an option for certain patients with RA because they may be less toxic to the stomach and other tissues.[29]

Adverse Effects

The problems and adverse effects of aspirin and other NSAIDs are discussed in Chapter 15. To review, the most common problem with chronic use is stomach irritation, which can lead to gastric ulceration and hemorrhage. This can be resolved to some extent by taking aspirin in an enteric-coated form so that release is delayed until the drug reaches the small intestine. Other pharmacological interventions such as prostaglandin analogs (misoprostol) and proton pump inhibitors (e.g., omeprazole [Prilosec]) can also be used if gastropathy continues to be a limiting factor during NSAID use. Chronic NSAID use can also produce bleeding problems (because of platelet inhibition) and impaired renal function, especially in an older or debilitated patient.

As indicated earlier, COX-2 selective drugs may reduce the risk of toxicity to the stomach, kidneys, and other tissues because they may spare the production of normal or protective prostaglandins in these tissues.[28,29] These drugs may cause other problems such as diarrhea, heartburn, GI cramps, and an increased risk of upper respiratory tract infection. COX-2 drugs have also been associated with serious cardiovascular problems (e.g., heart attack, stroke). But this problem does not seem limited to just the COX-2 selective drugs, and an increased risk of heart attack and stroke may also occur with all NSAIDs. Hence, the role of traditional and newer (COX-2 selective) NSAIDs in the long-term treatment of RA has been questioned recently, and the routine use of these drugs has declined somewhat in favor of other drug strategies such as the DMARDs.

Glucocorticoids

Glucocorticoids such as prednisone are extremely effective anti-inflammatory agents. When used alone, glucocorticoids (known also as *corticosteroids*) can provide symptomatic relief by decreasing joint inflammation and the pain associated with RA. There is also evidence that early use of these drugs can decrease joint erosion and damage, thus potentially slowing the progression of RA.[30] In this regard, glucocorticoids can be said to have disease-modifying properties analogous to the DMARDs. However, relatively high glucocorticoid doses may be needed to achieve these modifying effects if glucocorticoids are used as the only drug treatment for RA. This treatment may ultimately be counterproductive because administration of high does for prolonged periods can cause serious musculoskeletal problems and other adverse effects (see below). Hence, these drugs are used cautiously to treat inflammatory symptoms.

Alternatively, glucocorticoids can supplement the effects of DMARDs throughout all phases of this disease.[31,32] Glucocorticoids, for example, can help control pain and inflammation during earlier stages of RA, especially when initiating DMARD treatments, which can take several weeks or months to exert therapeutic effects.[33] By controlling pain and inflammation in the early phases of RA, glucocorticoids provide a "bridge" between the debilitating symptoms and more long-term benefits that will occur after the DMARDs begin to take effect.[3] Glucocorticoids also seem to work synergistically with DMARDs, thus providing optimal control of disease progression and sustained joint health.[34] Hence, some patients may remain on relatively low "maintenance" doses of glucocorticoids used in combination with one or more DMARDs throughout the course of their disease.

Glucocorticoids can also facilitate remission during acute flare-ups and decrease disability by enabling the patient to remain more active during exacerbations of this disease.[31] If necessary, these drugs can be given systemically at high doses for short periods (a week or two) to provide anti-inflammatory effects. This "pulse treatment" may be especially helpful in managing acute exacerbations of RA without producing the severe side effects associated with long-term use.[3] The ultimate goal, of course, is to return to a lower maintenance dose as soon as possible for long-term management of RA.

Glucocorticoids can also be injected directly into the arthritic joint, a technique that can be invaluable in managing acute exacerbations. There is considerable controversy about whether intra-articular glucocorticoids will produce harmful catabolic effects in joints that are already weakened by arthritic changes. At the very least, the number of injections into an arthritic joint should be limited, and a common rule of thumb is to not exceed more than two to three injections in one joint within 1 year.[3]

Mechanism of Action

The details of the cellular effects of steroids are discussed in Chapter 29. Briefly, glucocorticoids exert their primary effects by binding to a receptor in the cytoplasm of certain cells (macrophages, leukocytes), thereby forming a glucocorticoid-receptor complex.[35,36] This complex then moves to the cell's nucleus, where it binds to specific genes that regulate the inflammatory process. By binding to these genes, the glucocorticoid-receptor complex inhibits the production of many proinflammatory substances while also increasing the production of several anti-inflammatory proteins.[35,37]

In particular, glucocorticoids exert many of their beneficial effects by inhibiting the production of transcription factors that initiate synthesis of proinflammatory cytokines (e.g., interleukin-1, tumor necrosis factor), enzymes (e.g., COX-2, nitric oxide synthase), and receptor proteins (e.g., natural killer receptors).[38,39] These inflammatory products are normally responsible for promoting the destructive changes in joint tissues, and reduced synthesis of these products can be invaluable in reducing joint pathology related to RA.

Glucocorticoids also increase the production of proteins called *annexins* (previously known as *lipocortins*).[40,41] Annexins inhibit the phospholipase A_2 enzyme that normally liberates fatty acid precursors at the start of prostaglandin and leukotriene biosynthesis. Therefore, glucocorticoid-induced production of annexins blocks the first step in the synthesis of proinflammatory prostaglandins and leukotrienes.[42] Glucocorticoids also increase the production of proteins such as interleukin-10, interleukin-1 receptor antagonist, and neutral endopeptidase.[43] These other proteins contribute to anti-inflammatory effects by inhibiting, destroying, or blocking various other inflammatory chemicals, peptides, and proteins.[43]

Finally, glucocorticoids may exert some of their effects via a membrane-bound receptor that regulates activity of macrophages, eosinophils, T lymphocytes, and several other types of cells involved in the inflammatory response.[37] Consequently, glucocorticoids affect many aspects of inflammation, and their powerful anti-inflammatory effects in RA result from their ability to blunt various cellular and chemical components of the inflammatory response.

Adverse Effects

The side effects of glucocorticoids are numerous (see Chapter 29). These drugs exert a general catabolic effect on all types of supportive tissue (i.e., muscle, tendon, bone). Osteoporosis is a particular problem in the patient with arthritis because many of these patients have significant bone loss before even beginning steroid therapy. Glucocorticoids can increase bone loss in patients with arthritis, especially when they are used at higher doses for prolonged periods.[44] Glucocorticoids may also cause muscle wasting and weakness, as well as hypertension, aggravation of diabetes mellitus, glaucoma, cataracts, and increased risk of infection.[3,45] These side effects emphasize the need to limit glucocorticoid therapy as much as possible in patients with arthritis.

Disease-Modifying Antirheumatic Drugs

Disease-modifying antirheumatic drugs (DMARDs) are defined as "medications that retard or halt the progression of [rheumatoid] disease."[46] These drugs comprise an eclectic group of agents that are now recognized as essential in the early treatment of RA—that is, early and aggressive use of DMARDs can slow the progression of this disease and promote remission before there is extensive damage to affected joints. When used in conjunction with glucocorticoids and NSAIDs, DMARDs can help improve the long-term outcomes of patients with RA and can contribute to substantial improvements in quality of life.[32]

Disease-modifying drugs are typically used to control synovitis and erosive changes during the active stages of rheumatoid joint disease.[47] However, there is still considerable concern over the safety and efficacy of

DMARDs. Older DMARDs, such as penicillamine and oral gold, were especially problematic, and many patients who started treatment on these drugs eventually discontinued drug therapy due to side effects or lack of therapeutic benefits.[48] Some of the newer DMARDs are substantially more effective, but they can still produce serious side effects such as hepatic toxicity and an increased risk of infection.[49,50] Despite these limitations, there has been a definite trend toward more frequent DMARD use and to use these drugs earlier in the course of RA before excessive joint destruction has occurred.[32,47]

Disease-modifying agents currently used in treating RA are listed in Table 16-3. As the name implies, DMARDs attempt to induce remission by modifying the pathological process inherent to RA. In general, DMARDs inhibit certain aspects of the immune response thought to underlie rheumatoid disease. For example, these drugs can inhibit the function of monocytes and T and B lymphocytes or affect specific inflammatory mediators (e.g., cytokines) that are responsible for perpetuating joint inflammation and destruction.[49] The pharmacology of specific DMARDs is discussed below.

Traditional (Nonbiological) DMARDs

Antimalarial Drugs

Originally used in the treatment of malaria, the drugs chloroquine (Aralen) and hydroxychloroquine

Table 16-3
DISEASE-MODIFYING ANTIRHEUMATIC DRUGS

Drug	Trade Name	Usual Adult Dosage for Rheumatoid Arthritis	Special Considerations
Traditional (Nonbiological) DMARDs			
Antimalarials			
Chloroquine	Aralen	Oral: 150 mg/d initially; reduce dosage after maximum response is achieved	Periodic ophthalmic exams recommended to check for retinal toxicity
Hydroxychloroquine	Plaquenil	Oral: 400–600 mg/d initially; reduce whenever possible to maintenance dose of 200–400 mg/d	Similar to chloroquine.
Azathioprine	Azasan, Imuran	Oral: 1 mg/kg body weight per day; can be increased after 6–8 wk up to maximum dose of 2.5 mg/kg body weight.	Relatively high toxicity; should be used cautiously in debilitated patients or patients with renal disease.
Cyclosporine	Neoral	Oral: 2.5 mg/kg body weight per day; can be increased after 8 wk by 0.5–0.75 mg/kg body weight per day; dose can be increased after another 4 wk to a maximum daily dose of 4 mg/kg body weight per day.	May cause nephrotoxicity and gastrointestinal problems.
Gold Compounds			
Auranofin	Ridaura	Oral: 6 mg/d; may increase to 3 mg tid if no improvement after 6 mo	May have a long latency (6–9 mo) before onset of benefits.
Gold sodium thiomalate	Aurolate	Intramuscular: 10 mg the 1st wk, 25 mg the 2nd and 3rd wk, then 25–50 mg each wk until improvement or toxicity occurs (up to a total dose of 1 g). Maintenance doses of 25–50 mg every 2–4 wk for up to 20 wk can follow.	Effects occur somewhat sooner than oral gold, but often still has long delay (4 mo).
Other Nonbiological DMARDs			
Leflunomide	Arava	Oral: 100 mg/d for the first 3 days; continue with a maintenance dosage of 20 mg/day thereafter.	May decrease joint erosion/destruction with relatively few serious side effects; effects of long-term use remains to be determined.
Methotrexate	Rheumatrex, others	Oral: 2.5 mg every 12 hr for a total of 3 doses, or a single dose up to 20 mg/wk. Dosage can be decreased somewhat when maximal response occurs.	Often the primary drug used initially when treating RA; other agents can be added if response to methotrexate monotherapy is inadequate.

Continued

Table 16-3
DISEASE-MODIFYING ANTIRHEUMATIC DRUGS—cont'd

Drug	Trade Name	Usual Adult Dosage for Rheumatoid Arthritis	Special Considerations
Penicillamine	Cuprimine, Depen	Oral: 125 or 250 mg/d; can be increased to a maximum of 1.5 g/day.	Relatively high incidence of toxicity with long-term use.
Sulfasalazine	Azulfidine	Oral: 0.5–1 g/day for the first week; dose can be increased by 500 mg each week up to a maximum daily dose of 2–3 g/day.	Relatively high toxicity; may produce serious hypersensitivity reactions and blood dyscrasias.
Biological DMARDs			
Tumor Necrosis Factor Inhibitors			
Adalimumab	Humira	Subcutaneous injection: 40 mg every week if used alone; 40 mg every other week if used in combination with other antiarthritic agents such as methotrexate.	Relatively low incidence of serious side effects compared to traditional DMARDs. Risk of infection increased if used with other immunosuppressants (glucocorticoids, methotrexate).
Certolizumab	Cimzia	Subcutaneous injection: 400 mg initially and at wk 2 and 4, followed by 200 mg every other wk. Typical maintenance dose is 400 mg once each mo.	Similar to adalimumab.
Etanercept	Enbrel	Subcutaneous injection: 50 mg once each week.	Similar to adalimumab.
Golimumab	Simponi	Subcutaneous injection: 50 mg once each month.	Similar to adalimumab.
Infliximab	Remicade	Slow IV infusion: 3 mg/kg body weight. Additional 3 mg/kg doses at 2 and 6 weeks after first infusion, then every 8 weeks thereafter.	Similar to adalimumab.
Other Biological DMARDs			
Abatacept	Orencia	IV infusion: one dose every 2 wk for 3 doses, then every 4 wk; Doses adjusted by body wt: less than 60 kg: 500 mg 60–100 kg: 750 mg more than 100 kg: 1,000 mg	Inhibits T cell activation; typically used when disease progression occurs despite other DMARD treatments.
Anakinra	Kineret	Subcutaneous injection: 100 mg/day	Blocks interleukin-1 receptors; can be used alone or with other antiarthritic agents, but should not be used with tumor necrosis factor inhibitors.
Tocilizumab	Actemra	IV infusion: 4 mg/kg body wt initially; increase up to 8 mg/kg based on response	Blocks interleukin-6 receptors; can be used alone but is often combined with methotrexate if other DMARDs are not effective.

(Plaquenil) can also be used to treat RA. In the past, physicians were reluctant to use these drugs because of the fear of retinal toxicity.[51] There is now evidence that these agents can be used safely, although they may not be as effective in treating RA compared to newer DMARDs. Antimalarials are therefore not usually the first choice, but they remain an option for patients who cannot tolerate other DMARDs, or they can be used in combination with another DMARD (e.g., methotrexate) for more comprehensive treatment. At present, only hydroxychloroquine is FDA approved for treating RA, but chloroquine may be prescribed off-label for selected patients with severe RA.

Mechanism of Action. Antimalarials exert several effects, although it is unclear exactly which of these contributes to halting the progression of RA.[52] The drugs affect immune cell responses by stabilizing lysosomes, increasing the pH of intracellular structures, inhibiting T cell function, and impairing DNA and RNA synthesis.[53] However, the significance of these cellular effects in their role as antiarthritics remains unclear.[54] More recently, it has been suggested that these drugs inhibit specific cellular receptors known as toll-like receptors (TLRs). The receptors play a role in allowing macrophages and dendritic cells to recognize foreign materials, and activation of TLRs initiates certain immune responses. Antimalarials may exert their antirheumatic effects by inhibiting TLRs, thus suppressing excessive or inappropriate immune responses that cause RA.[54,55] Additional research will be needed to clarify the effects of antimalarials on TLRs and other immune cell actions.

Adverse Effects. Chloroquine and hydroxychloroquine are relatively safe compared to other DMARDs.[3,56] The major concern is that high doses of these drugs can produce irreversible retinal damage. Retinal toxicity is rare, however, when daily dosages are maintained below 6 to 6.5 mg/kg per day for hydroxychloroquine and less than 3.5 to 4 mg/kg per day for chloroquine.[51] Doses that are effective in treating RA are typically well below these limits. Nonetheless, ocular examinations should be scheduled periodically during prolonged administration.[57] Other side effects such as headache and GI distress can occur, but these are relatively infrequent and usually transient.

Azathioprine

Azathioprine (Azasan, Imuran) is an immunosuppressant drug that is often used to prevent tissue rejection following organ transplants. Because of its immunosuppressant properties, physicians have been employing azathioprine to treat cases of severe, active RA that have not responded to other agents.

Mechanism of Action. Azathioprine's mechanism of action in RA is not fully understood. This drug has been shown to impair the synthesis of DNA and RNA precursors, but it is unclear exactly how (or if) this is related to its immunosuppressant effects. Azathioprine can also inhibit many aspects of B and T cell function, thereby impairing immune responses mediated by these cells.[53] These actions probably account for the immunosuppressant effects and explain how azathioprine can blunt the autoimmune responses that govern rheumatoid disease.

Adverse Effects. Azathioprine is relatively toxic, with more frequent and more severe side effects than other DMARDs.[58] The primary side effects include fever, chills, sore throat, fatigue, loss of appetite, and nausea or vomiting; these effects often limit the use of this drug.

Gold Therapy

Compounds containing elemental gold were among the first drugs identified as DMARDs. In the past, oral and parenteral gold therapy was often used to arrest further progression of rheumatoid joint disease. When used now, specific compounds such as aurothioglucose (Solganal) and gold sodium thiomalate (Myochrysine) are usually administered by intramuscular injection. An orally active gold compound, auranofin (Ridaura), offers the advantage of oral administration.[59] Although auranofin is easier to administer than parenteral gold compounds, concerns about long-term suppression of immune function has limited the use of this drug in recent years.[60] Because safer and more effective agents are available, gold compounds in general are reserved for patients who fail to respond to other DMARDs.[60]

Mechanism of Action. Although the exact mechanism is not fully understood, gold compounds probably induce remission in patients with RA by inhibiting enzymes that influence the growth and function of T cells and mononuclear phagocytes.[61] That is, gold compounds bind strongly to specific proteins (enzymes) in immune cells, thus suppressing the ability of these cells to mediate damaging autoimmune responses. Several additional cellular effects have been noted, including increased expression of anti-inflammatory proteins, decreased expression of COX-2 and other proinflammatory enzymes, and reduced synthesis of prostaglandin E_2 and other inflammatory mediators.[62,63] Clearly, gold compounds exert many complex effects on cellular immune responses, and the exact way that these drugs exert antirheumatoid effects remains to be determined.

Adverse Effects. Adverse effects are relatively common with gold therapy, and many patients are unable to continue treatment because of intolerable side effects,[64,65] primarily GI distress (diarrhea, indigestion), irritation of the oral mucosa, and rashes and itching of the skin.[3,66] Other side effects include proteinuria, conjunctivitis, and blood dyscrasias (e.g., thrombocytopenia, leukopenia). On the other hand, gold compounds may be less hepatotoxic than other DMARDs, including the newer biological agents (see "Biological DMARDs"). Hence, gold compounds may be a suitable alternative for patients with RA who have liver diseases (e.g., hepatitis B) or patients who cannot tolerate other DMARDs because of liver toxicity.[67,68]

Leflunomide

Leflunomide (Arava) is a relative newcomer to the antirheumatic drug arsenal. This drug helps decrease pain, inflammation, and joint effusion in rheumatoid joint disease and has been shown to slow the formation of bone erosions in arthritic joints.[69] Leflunomide is also fairly well tolerated by most patients and may produce beneficial effects fairly soon (i.e., 1 month) after beginning treatment.[70] This drug is therefore a potential alternative for people who fail to respond to, or cannot tolerate, other DMARDs such as methotrexate.[71,72] In certain patients, leflunomide can also be combined with methotrexate to provide greater effects than could be achieved using only one of these drugs.[73,74]

Mechanism of Action. Leflunomide acts primarily by inhibiting the synthesis of RNA precursors (pyrimidines) in lymphocytes.[75,76] When stimulated, lymphocytes must radically increase their RNA synthesis to proliferate and become activated during the inflammatory response. Leflunomide blocks a key enzyme responsible for RNA synthesis, so that these lymphocytes cannot progress to a more activated state and cannot cause as much joint inflammation.[77]

Adverse Effects. Leflunomide's primary side effects include GI distress, allergic reactions (skin rashes), and hair loss.[78] This drug can also affect the liver; liver function may need to be monitored periodically.[79] Finally, leflunomide has been associated with pneumonitis and interstitial lung disease and should probably be avoided in patients with a history of respiratory problems.[71,80]

Methotrexate

Methotrexate (Folex, Rheumatrex, others) is an antimetabolite used frequently in the treatment of cancer (see Chapter 36). It has also emerged as the drug of choice for treating RA in both adults and children.[19,81] For example, this drug has been shown to slow the effects of RA as evidenced by decreased synovitis, decreased bone erosion, and less narrowing of the joint space.[82,83] Its therapeutic effects appear to be superior to older DMARDs (gold compounds, azathioprine), and it may offer an advantage in terms of a rapid onset (within 2 to 3 weeks) in some patients.[3,46] Some patients can use methotrexate alone to manage RA, but this drug may be especially beneficial when combined with various other DMARDs[84] (see "DMARD Combinations Used in Rheumatoid Arthritis").

Mechanism of Action. The ability of methotrexate and similar anticancer drugs to impair DNA and RNA synthesis is well known (see Chapter 36). At the doses used to treat cancer, methotrexate inhibits the synthesis of folic acid, thus inhibiting the formation of nucleoproteins that serve as DNA precursors.[85] This action inhibits cellular replication by impairing the cell's ability to produce new genetic material, an effect that helps attenuate tumor cell replication in cancer. However, doses of methotrexate used to treat RA are considerably lower than those used in cancer, and it is not entirely clear how this drug exerts beneficial effects in RA.[86] Methotrexate could affect immune function by inhibiting folic acid metabolism, thereby limiting the proliferation of lymphocytes and other cells that cause the autoimmune responses in rheumatoid disease. However, methotrexate also exerts other effects, including inhibition of inflammatory cytokines and stimulation of adenosine release.[86] The effects on adenosine release may be especially important because increased amounts of endogenous adenosine can inhibit various components of inflammation and the immune response.[53,87]

Adverse Effects. Even at lower doses, methotrexate is still a relatively toxic drug, and several adverse side effects can occur.[88] The primary problems involve the GI tract and include loss of appetite, nausea, and other forms of GI distress (including intragastrointestinal hemorrhage).[88] Long-term methotrexate use in patients with RA has also been associated with pulmonary problems, hematological disorders, liver dysfunction, and hair loss.[88,89]

Administering folic acid along with methotrexate may reduce the incidence of GI problems, liver dysfunction, and perhaps other side effects.[90,91] This makes sense because methotrexate inhibits folic acid synthesis, and folic acid supplementation may help offset certain side effects.[92] Folic acid supplementation is somewhat controversial, however. Its use is based on the idea that methotrexate exerts at least part of its therapeutic effects by inhibiting folic acid synthesis, and providing exogenous folic acid will negate this drug's therapeutic effects in RA.[90] Nonetheless, methotrexate offers a favorable benefit-to-risk ratio in many patients with RA, and this drug has a relatively good safety record compared to many of the other commonly used DMARDs.[93]

Penicillamine

Penicillamine (Cuprimine), a derivative of penicillin, is officially classified as a chelating agent that is often used in the treatment of heavy metal intoxication (e.g., lead poisoning, copper accumulation in Wilson's disease).[94] However, penicillamine tends to be substantially more toxic than other DMARDs, and questions have been raised about whether this drug is really effective in slowing the progression of RA.[48] Therefore, penicillamine is no longer considered a primary treatment for people with RA and is reserved for selected patients who have not responded to other agents.

Mechanism of Action. The basis for the antiarthritic effects of penicillamine is unknown. It has been suggested that penicillamine can sequester harmful chemical products (reactive aldehydes), thus preventing the damage caused by these products in joint tissues.[95] This drug can also influence T cell activity and immune function, but evidence suggests this effect *increases* autoimmune responses in experimental animals rather than suppresses the autoimmune responses in RA.[96] Hence, the exact mechanisms of this drug in treating RA remain to be determined.

Adverse Effects. Penicillamine is considered to be fairly toxic when compared with other DMARDs.[97] It can produce serious renal toxicity and blood disorders such as aplastic anemia. Other common side effects include allergic reactions and autoimmune blistering of the skin and mucous membranes (pemphigus). This drug has also been associated with myasthenia gravis in certain patients, thus adding to its limitations in treating RA and other disorders.[98]

Biological DMARDs

Tumor Necrosis Factor Inhibitors

Several agents are now available that inhibit the action of tumor necrosis factor-alpha (TNF-α). TNF-α is a small protein (cytokine) that is released from cells involved in the inflammatory response. TNF-α seems to be a key chemical mediator that promotes inflammation and joint erosion in RA.[99] Drugs that inhibit this chemical will therefore help delay the progression of this disease by decreasing TNF-α's destructive effects.[100,101]

Drugs in this group include adalimumab (Humira), certolizumab (Cimzia), etanercept (Enbrel), golimumab (Simponi), and infliximab (Remicade). These drugs are also referred to as *biological DMARDs* because they affect the biological response to a specific cytokine (TNF-α).[20] Etanercept was the first biological DMARD—it was created by fusing human immunoglobulin (IgG) with an amino acid sequence that mimics the binding portion of the TNF receptor. TNF-α recognizes the binding portion on the drug and attaches to it; therefore, it cannot bind to the real TNF receptor on immune cells.

The newer TNF-α inhibitors (i.e., adalimumab, certolizumab, golimumab, infliximab) were developed using monoclonal antibody techniques. These techniques enable the drug to bind tightly to antigenic components on TNF-α, thereby forming a drug-cytokine molecule that is too large to bind to the real TNF receptor. These monoclonal antibody-derived drugs can also help destroy cells that express TNF-α, thus further reducing the destructive effects of this cytokine.[102]

There is substantial evidence that TNF-α inhibitors can retard the progression of inflammatory joint disease and promote improvements in symptoms and quality of life in people with RA.[103-105] These drugs can be used as the initial treatment but are often substituted for another DMARD or added to other agents (e.g., methotrexate), if patients do not have an adequate response to the other antirheumatoid drugs.[100,106] There is some concern about toxicity (see below), and these drugs must be given parenterally, usually by subcutaneous injection or by slow IV infusion (see Table 16-3). Nonetheless, TNF-α inhibitors represent an important breakthrough in the drug treatment of RA.

Mechanism of Action. As indicated, these agents bind selectively to TNF-α (Fig. 16-2).[99,107] This action prevents TNF-α from binding to surface receptors located on other inflammatory cells. TNF is therefore unable to activate other inflammatory cells that cause inflammation and joint destruction in RA.[107]

Adverse Effects. Patients taking TNF-α inhibitors may be prone to upper respiratory tract infections and other serious infections, including sepsis.[49,101] This increased risk of infection probably occurs because the drug inhibits a key component of the immune response—namely, TNF-α. These drugs are therefore contraindicated in people with infections, and administration should be discontinued if an infection develops.

Other potential adverse responses include malignancy (e.g., lymphoma), liver disease, heart failure, lupuslike disease, irritation around the injection site, and demyelinating disorders that mimic multiple sclerosis.[49,53] However, the incidence of these adverse effects seems to be fairly low and may, in some cases, be related more to the severity of the underlying rheumatoid disease rather than the drugs used to treat it.[108] For the most part, these drugs provide an acceptable risk-to-benefit ratio for most people with RA. Patients should be screened carefully for any risk factors before beginning drug therapy and should be monitored periodically for any potential adverse reactions to these drugs.

Abatacept

Abatacept (Orencia) is unique in treating RA because it specifically targets T cell activation. Normally, T lymphocytes play a critical role in mediating immune and inflammatory responses. By limiting the activation of these cells, abatacept can suppress abnormal autoimmune responses associated with RA. It is used primarily

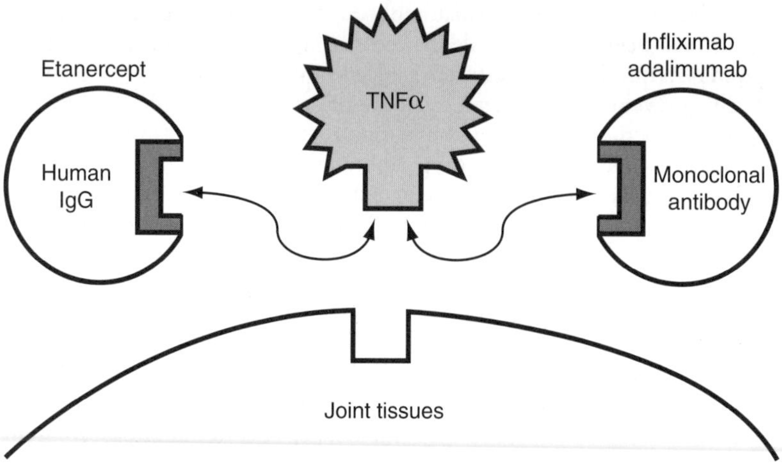

Figure ■ 16-2
Schematic diagram illustrating the effects of tumor necrosis factor-alpha (TNF-α) inhibitors. Drugs such as etanercept, infliximab, and adalimumab attach directly to TNF-α, thereby preventing this destructive cytokine from reaching joint tissues.

as a second-line drug for patients who fail to respond to one or more tumor necrosis factor inhibitors.[109]

Mechanism of Action. As indicated, abatacept suppresses T cell activation. T lymphocytes normally become activated when presented with antigens by B cells and other antigen-presenting cells.[110] This presentation initiates a complex interaction between the T cell and the antigen-presenting cell that ultimately enhances T cell proliferation and production of proinflammatory mediators. Abatacept interrupts the signals sent back and forth between the T cell and the antigen-presenting cell, thus inhibiting the ability of these signals to ultimately activate the T cell.[111,112]

Adverse Effects. Abatacept is similar to, or slightly better tolerated than, other DMARDs in terms of serious adverse reactions.[113] There is some concern about pulmonary infection,[50] and serious allergic reactions can occur in rare cases. Other minor, but common side effects, include headache and dizziness.

Anakinra

Anakinra (Kineret) blocks the effects of interleukin-1 on joint tissues. Like TNF-α, interleukin-1 is a cytokine that promotes inflammation and joint destruction in RA.[114] By blocking interleukin-1 receptors on joint tissues, anakinra prevents the destructive events mediated by this cytokine. This drug is generally well tolerated but is only moderately effective in limiting the progression of RA.[115,116] Anakinra is therefore not a primary option for most people with RA but can be used alone in selected patients or in combination with other DMARDs such as methotrexate.[117]

Mechanism of Action. As indicated, anakinra is an antagonist (blocker) that is specific for the interleukin-1 receptor found on joint tissues, other tissues, and organs.[118,119] By blocking this receptor, the drug prevents this cytokine from binding and exerting destructive effects on joint tissues.

Adverse Effects. Anakinra is administered via subcutaneous injection. Irritation at the injection site is fairly common but is usually not severe.[120] Patients receiving high doses of anakinra may be more susceptible to bacterial infections and other infectious agents.[121] More serious systemic allergic reactions may also occur in a small number of susceptible patients.[122]

Rituximab

Rituximab (Rituxan) is another DMARD that was developed using monoclonal antibody techniques. This drug acts primarily on specific B lymphocytes, and therefore offers a different strategy than other DMARDs such as the TNF-α inhibitors.[123] Studies suggest that rituximab can produce beneficial effects in selected patients with RA who have failed to respond to the TNF-α inhibitors.[109,124] Rituximab can be used as the primary drug but is often combined with methotrexate to provide optimal effects in suppressing the progression of RA.[125]

Mechanism of Action. Rituximab targets specific (CD20) B lymphocytes and depletes the number of these lymphocytes by several biochemical mechanisms that result in the death of these cells.[126] B lymphocytes are normally responsible for presenting antigens to T lymphocytes and for producing cytokines and other chemical signals that mediate an inflammatory response.[53] Rituximab decreases the contribution of key cells associated with the autoimmune response in RA. However, approximately 30 to 40 percent of patients do not respond to rituximab, even though this drug clearly decreases the number of functioning B cells in these patients.[127] This suggests that some of rituximab's beneficial effects in RA may be related to cellular responses other than just depletion of B lymphocytes. Future studies may clarify exactly how rituximab affects the cellular responses in patients with RA who respond positively to this drug.

Adverse Effects. Similar to other DMARDs, rituximab may increase the risk of infection.[128,129] Many patients also develop skin reactions (rashes, itching) when this drug is initially administered, but these reactions are often minor and do not necessarily require that the drug be discontinued. Other fairly minor side effects include headache, nausea, vomiting, and nasopharyngitis.[128] More serious allergic reactions (e.g.., anaphylaxis, angioedema) may occur, and rituximab may also cause blood dyscrasias (e.g., anemia, neutropenia, thrombocytopenia) in certain patients. This drug has also been associated with progressive multifocal leukoencephalopathy in susceptible patients,[130] and clinicians should look for signs such as headache, confusion, seizures, and loss of vision, which might indicate this serious adverse effect.

Tocilizumab

Tocilizumab (Actemra) is an antibody derived from human cells that blocks the interleukin-6 receptor located on various tissues. Interleukin-6 (IL-6) is a small protein (cytokine) produced by T and B lymphocytes, joint synovial tissues, and many other cells. This cytokine is involved in mediating many physiological responses (e.g., fever, stress reactions), but IL-6 seems especially important as a chemical signal in inflammation.[131] Tocilizumab blocks the receptor for IL-6, thus reducing inflammation normally mediated by this cytokine. Tocilizumab provides an alternative strategy to other DMARDs that affect TNF-α and other chemical signals in RA, including anakinra, which affects the interleukin-1 receptor (see earlier). Tocilizumab is therefore used primarily in patients who failed to respond to methotrexate or DMARDs such as the TNF-α inhibitors.[132] Preliminary reports also suggest that tocilizumab may be superior to methotrexate as the initial drug used in RA, and future clinical studies will be needed to confirm if tocilizumab should be used alone as the primary drug for certain patients.[106]

Mechanism of Action. As discussed above, tocilizumab works by blocking the IL-6 receptors and negating the proinflammatory effects of IL-6. Specifically, tocilizumab binds to the IL-6 receptor on cell membranes and to the soluble receptor in the bloodstream, thus reducing the adverse effects of this cytokine on autoimmune-mediated joint inflammation.

Adverse Effects. The safety profile and incidence of severe side effects with tocilizumab are similar to other DMARDs. However, this drug is also associated with an increased risk of serious infections in some patients (e.g., tuberculosis, disseminated fungal infections) and blood dyscrasias such as neutropenia, thrombocytopenia, and hyperlipidemia.[132] There is also concern that this drug may cause GI perforation, resulting in severe abdominal pain, nausea, vomiting, chills, and fever.[50]

Other DMARDs

Because of the autoimmune basis of RA, physicians can employ various other drugs that suppress the immune response to a certain extent. For instance, cyclosporine (Sandimmune) is an immunosuppressant agent normally used to prevent rejection of organ transplants (see Chapter 37).[133] Sulfasalazine (Azulfidine) is typically used to treat inflammatory bowel disease.[133,134] Cyclophosphamide (Cytoxan) is used primarily for cancer treatment.[53]

In general, these drugs are more toxic and are usually reserved for patients who have not responded to more traditional DMARDs such as methotrexate. Drugs with immunosuppressant activity may also be used in combination with more traditional DMARDs to provide optimal benefits in certain patients. Combination drug therapy in RA is addressed in the next section.

DMARD Combinations Used in Rheumatoid Arthritis

There has been a great deal of interest in using several DMARDs simultaneously to achieve remission in patients with RA. The strategy of combination therapy is to attack the underlying disease process from several pharmacological vantage points, much in the same way that combination therapies are used in other disorders such as hypertension (Chapter 21) and cancer (Chapter 36). Although the benefits of combining DMARDs have been questioned, most practitioners currently advocate a combination of two or more drugs so that optimal benefits can be achieved with a relatively low dose of each drug.[19,135] Researchers continue to investigate various combinations of new and old DMARDs for efficacy and toxicity.[84,136]

At present, methotrexate is typically the cornerstone of treatment, with other DMARDs added, depending on the needs of each patient.[19,84] In particular, a TNF-α inhibitor (e.g., etanercept, infliximab, adalimumab, golimumab, certolizumab) can be combined with methotrexate as the initial treatment for certain patients, or a TNF-α inhibitor can be added to methotrexate if the patient exhibits an inadequate response to methotrexate used alone.[137] Other biological or nonbiological DMARDs can be substituted for the TNF-α inhibitor as needed to achieve optimal effects in each patient.[32,136]

The drawback of combination therapy is the potential for increased toxicity and drug interactions when several DMARDs are used simultaneously.[138] This fact is understandable, considering that many DMARDs have a relatively high risk of toxicity when used alone, and combining these drugs might increase the risk of adverse drug reactions. However, there is evidence that the incidence of side effects is not necessarily greater with DMARD combinations, especially if methotrexate is combined with one of the newer biological agents such as a TNF-α inhibitor.[135] Hence, combination therapy continues to gain acceptance, and the use of two or more DMARDs early in the course of the disease may provide patients with the best hope for halting the progression of RA.[32] Continued research will hopefully lend additional insight to the best way that DMARDs can be combined to safely and effectively treat patients with RA.

Dietary Implications for Rheumatoid Arthritis

Investigators are searching for nonpharmacological interventions that can help arrest the progression of rheumatoid joint disease. There is some evidence, for example, that dietary manipulation can alleviate some of the symptoms of RA.[139] Diets that are high in fish oil and certain fatty acids (e.g., omega-3 fatty acids) have been advocated for patients.[140,141] These dietary fatty acids may supply the precursors for the biosynthesis of endogenous lipids that control several aspects of inflammation, including regulation of T cell function, inhibition of proinflammatory mediators, and other cellular responses that suppress inflammatory signals.[142,143] Foods that have antioxidant properties (e.g., fruits, vegetables) may also have beneficial effects in people with RA.[144,145] On the other hand, certain dietary factors and environmental influences may increase the risk of RA. It is thought, for example, that diets rich in meat and protein may exacerbate RA, but this has not been proven conclusively.[146] Cigarette smoking is now believed to substantially increase the risk of this disease in susceptible individuals (i.e., people with genetic predisposition for RA).[147] Hence, certain dietary and lifestyle changes used in combination with drug therapy may provide additional benefits for some people with RA.

OSTEOARTHRITIS

Osteoarthritis (OA) far exceeds RA as the most common form of joint disease, especially in older adults. Approximately 50 percent of people aged 65 years have OA to some extent, with the prevalence of this disease rising to 85 percent in people aged 75 or older.[148] Unlike rheumatoid joint disease, OA does not seem to be caused by an immune response but is likely due to an intrinsic defect in remodeling of the joint cartilage and underlying (subchondral) bone.[149] That is, trauma or excessive loads cause increased cartilage and bone turnover within the joint surfaces, but the joint surfaces are essentially being broken down faster than they can be successfully repaired. The result is a progressive deterioration of articular cartilage that is accompanied by degenerative bony changes, including thickening of the subchondral bone, creation of subchondral bone cysts, and formation of large bony protrusions (osteophytes) at the joint margins.[148] OA typically occurs in large weight-bearing joints such as the knees and hips, as well as the spine and some of the smaller joints in the hands and feet.[150] Patients are described as having primary OA when there is no apparent reason for the onset of joint destruction; in secondary OA, a factor such as previous joint trauma, infection, or metabolic disease is responsible for triggering articular changes.[148] Obesity, genetic susceptibility, and joint vulnerability (e.g., malalignment, weakness, etc.) have also been implicated as predisposing factors in OA.[150,151]

Clearly, OA is a different form of joint disease than RA. Hence, treatment of these conditions also differs somewhat. As discussed previously, RA is characterized by a severe inflammatory response that is perpetuated by a cellular immune reaction. Drug therapy in rheumatoid disease consists of agents that are focused on directly relieving these inflammatory symptoms (i.e., NSAIDs or glucocorticoids) or drugs that attempt to arrest the cellular immune response that causes this inflammation (DMARDs). Treatment of joint inflammation is not a major focus of drug therapy in OA. A mild inflammatory synovitis does occur in OA, but this is secondary to the articular damage inherent to this disease.[148,150] Also, drug therapy represents one of the primary interventions in RA, whereas treatment of OA should focus more on nonpharmacological measures such as physical therapy, weight loss, and joint replacement in the advanced stages of this disease.[152-154]

Consequently, drug therapy in OA is used primarily to help patients manage their pain and maintain an active lifestyle. When joint pain begins to be a problem, simple analgesics such as acetaminophen and NSAIDs have been the major form of drug therapy. Newer pharmacological strategies are also emerging that attempt to slow or reverse the pathological changes in OA. These newer strategies use disease-modifying osteoarthritic drugs (DMOADs) rather than drugs that treat only the symptoms of OA.[155] Two types of DMOADs will be addressed: drugs that attempt to directly improve the viscosity and function of synovial fluid (**viscosupplementation**) and agents that serve as precursors to the normal constituents of joint tissues (glucosamine and chondroitin sulfate).

Acetaminophen and NSAIDs

Acetaminophen is often the first drug used to treat OA.[148,156] As indicated in Chapter 15, acetaminophen is as effective as NSAIDs in controlling pain, but it does not have anti-inflammatory effects. This is of less concern when acetaminophen is used in OA because the inflammatory symptoms are milder. Because the drug does not cause gastric irritation, it provides a relatively safe and effective form of analgesia for patients with mild-to-moderate OA,[148,157] especially when it needs to be administered for long periods of time.[148,156,157]

NSAIDs are also used for the symptomatic treatment of pain in OA.[148,158] These drugs are used primarily for their analgesic properties, although the anti-inflammatory effects of NSAIDs can help control the mild synovitis that typically occurs in advanced OA secondary to joint destruction.[148] In addition, NSAIDs often provide better pain relief than acetaminophen, especially in patients with moderate to severe OA-related pain.[159] Traditional NSAIDs can cause more gastric irritation than acetaminophen, and this side effect is often a limiting factor in the long-term use of NSAIDs. The newer COX-2 selective NSAIDs (i.e., celecoxib; see Chapter 15) do not typically cause as much gastric irritation as traditional NSAIDs, and they may be a valuable alternative to acetaminophen and traditional NSAIDs in the long-term treatment of OA.[21,160] However, COX-2 drugs may increase the risk of serious cardiovascular problems (heart attack, stroke), and patients should be screened carefully for cardiovascular risk factors before beginning treatment with these drugs.[21]

Alternatively, certain NSAIDs can be administered topically to the skin over the osteoarthritic joint.[161,162] Some of the topically applied drug will be absorbed through the skin into the joint and periarticular tissues. This action may provide local pain relief without causing GI irritation or other adverse effects on the kidneys and cardiovascular system.[163,164] Diclofenac seems especially beneficial as a topical agent, and it is available in several topical forms (i.e., patch, gel, solution). Data suggest that topical administration of diclofenac is equivalent to orally administered NSAIDs in relieving the symptoms of osteoarthritic pain in the knees and hands.[164]

Regardless of the exact drug or administration techniques, there is no doubt that the analgesia produced by NSAIDs or acetaminophen plays a valuable role in the management of OA. These drugs allow the patient to maintain a more active lifestyle and to participate in various activities, including exercise programs and other forms of physical therapy and occupational therapy. However, these drugs do not alter the progressive course of joint destruction and osteoarthritic changes. In fact, there is preliminary evidence that some of the NSAIDs may actually impair bone healing following fractures or surgery, but their effects on cartilage formation and soft tissue repair remain unclear (see Chapter 15).[165] At the present time, however, acetaminophen and NSAIDs remain the cornerstone of the pharmacological treatment of joint pain in OA.

Viscosupplementation

Viscosupplementation is a clinical procedure increasingly in use for the treatment of OA. This technique uses a substance known as hyaluronan (hyaluronic acid) to restore the lubricating properties of synovial fluid in osteoarthritic joints.[166,167] Hyaluronan is a polysaccharide that can be injected into an arthritic joint to help restore the normal viscosity of the synovial fluid.[168] This treatment helps reduce joint stress, thus limiting the progression of articular destruction seen in OA.[169] Therefore, viscosupplementation has been shown to reduce pain and improve function in OA.[167,170]

When used to treat OA, viscosupplementation typically consists of three to five weekly injections of hyaluronan, depending on the brand used (e.g., Hyalgan, Synvisc, others). Patients often experience a decrease in pain within days after injection, and pain continues to diminish within the first weeks after treatment. Duration of relief is variable, but most patients who respond to viscosupplementation experience beneficial effects for 6 months to 1 year after a series of injections.[171] This intervention is also tolerated fairly well, although a pseudoseptic reaction that produces local pain and swelling may occur.[172]

Hence, viscosupplementation may temporarily attenuate the progressive changes in joint structure and function typically seen in OA. Although these benefits are relatively modest and transient, viscosupplementation can delay the need for more invasive surgical treatments such as joint replacement. Future clinical studies will be needed to determine how viscosupplementation can be used most effectively in the comprehensive treatment of people with OA.

Glucosamine and Chondroitin Sulfate

It has been suggested that dietary supplements such as glucosamine and chondroitin sulfate may help protect articular cartilage and halt or reverse joint degeneration in OA. These two compounds are key ingredients needed for the production of several components of articular cartilage and synovial fluid, including glycosaminoglycans, proteoglycans, and hyaluronic acid.[173,174] It seems reasonable that increased amounts of these ingredients should facilitate the repair of joint tissues, improve synovial fluid viscosity, and help restore joint function in conditions like OA.[175] It has also been suggested that glucosamine and chondroitin may stabilize cartilage turnover and suppress the production of cytokines that contribute to pain and destructive changes in osteoarthritic joints.[176,177] As a result, several products containing glucosamine, or glucosamine combined with chondroitin sulfate, are currently available as nonprescription dietary supplements. These supplements typically contain oral dosages of 1,500 mg/d glucosamine and 1,200 mg/d chondroitin sulfate.[148]

However, it is not clear if glucosamine and chondroitin are actually beneficial in people with OA. Although several studies suggest that these supplements can decrease pain and improve function in some patients with OA, these effects have not been proven conclusively in all clinical trials.[178-180] Discrepancies in the results from various studies may be due in part to differences in study design, sample size, patient characteristics, and other factors that affect the credibility of each study.[148] Based on the current evidence, it seems that glucosamine and chondroitin may not produce beneficial effects in all patients with OA. These supplements, however, might be helpful in a subgroup of patients with a high rate of cartilage turnover because they will provide the necessary substrates to sustain this turnover and maintain joint integrity.[181]

Consequently, it appears that glucosamine and chondroitin supplements are certainly worth a trial for many patients with OA. Some GI problems may occur, but these supplements are usually well tolerated. Although these supplements are available over the counter in the United States, people with OA should consult their physician and pharmacist before self-administration. Patients should be educated on the proper dosage and should be reminded that these products may need to be consumed for several weeks or months before beneficial effects become apparent. Long-term studies on the effects of these supplements are currently being conducted, and it remains to be determined how glucosamine and chondroitin might be used effectively with other pharmacological and nonpharmacological treatments for OA. Clinicians should try to stay abreast of any new information about the potential benefits of glucosamine and chondroitin.

Special Concerns for Rehabilitation Patients

Drugs used to treat RA and OA often play a vital role in permitting optimal rehabilitation of patients with joint disease. By decreasing pain and inflammation, these drugs help facilitate a more active and vigorous program of exercise and functional activity. Some drugs, such as the disease-modifying drugs used in RA and OA, appear to be able to impair or even halt the progression of joint destruction. This may enable the therapist to help restore muscle strength and joint function rather than simply employ a program of maintenance therapy during a steady downward progression in patients with arthritis.

The influence of antiarthritic drugs on the rehabilitative process depends primarily on the type of drugs used. Beginning with the NSAIDs, there is little concern for adverse effects on physical therapy procedures. These drugs are relatively safe and are not usually associated with the type of side effects that will directly influence the physical rehabilitation of people with RA or OA. If glucocorticoids are used, the therapist must be aware of adverse side effects; in particular, the catabolic effects of these agents on supporting tissues (muscle, tendon, bone, skin) must be considered. Range-of-motion and strengthening programs must be used judiciously to avoid fractures and soft-tissue injuries. Care must also be taken to prevent skin breakdown, especially when splints and other protective orthotic devices are employed.

The disease-modifying agents used in RA are associated with several side effects that could influence rehabilitation. Some of these drugs, such as methotrexate and the tumor necrosis factor-α inhibitors, may cause headache and nausea, which may be bothersome during the therapy session. Joint pain and swelling may also occur with drugs such as methotrexate and penicillamine, and these effects may also become a problem during rehabilitation. Most DMARDs are associated with an increased risk of infection, so clinicians should be careful about sterilizing equipment and should avoid exposing patients to other individuals who might be contagious. A variety of other side effects can occur, depending on the particular DMARD being used and the patient's sensitivity. Therapists should be aware of any changes in patient response when a new drug is being started and during the prolonged use of DMARDs.

Finally, the use of DMOADs (i.e., viscosupplementation, glucosamine, chondroitin) to restore joint function in OA may have a positive effect on the patient's ability to participate in physical rehabilitation. It remains to be seen how rehabilitation techniques (exercise, physical agents) can be used most effectively to capitalize on the beneficial effects of DMOADs. It is hoped that these pharmacological techniques will work synergistically with physical therapy to improve function in patients with osteoarthritic joints.

CASE STUDY

RHEUMATOID ARTHRITIS

Brief History. A.T., a 75-year-old woman, was diagnosed with rheumatoid joint disease several years ago. She is currently being seen three times each week in physical therapy as an outpatient for a program of paraffin and active exercise to her wrists and hands. Resting splints were also fabricated for both hands, and these are worn at night to prevent joint deformity. The patient was also instructed in a home exercise program to maintain joint mobility in both upper extremities. Pharmacological management

Continued on following page

CASE STUDY (Continued)

in this patient originally consisted of NSAIDs, beginning with aspirin and later switching to ibuprofen. As her condition worsened, she was also placed on prednisone, an anti-inflammatory steroid (glucocorticoid) that can decrease joint inflammation and perhaps also suppress the autoimmune response underlying RA. Prednisone was administered orally at a dosage of 20 mg each day.

Problem/Influence of Medication. The combination of an NSAID, a glucocorticoid, and the physical therapy program seemed to be quite effective in reducing the patient's pain and joint stiffness. However, while preparing the patient for her paraffin treatment, the therapist noticed the skin on A.T.'s hands and wrists was very thin and bruised very easily. Likewise, her skeletal muscles were weaker than would be expected even with her advanced age, and substantial skeletal muscle wasting was apparent throughout her trunk and extremities.

1. ***What is causing the skin changes and muscle wasting?***
2. ***What might be an alternative drug strategy to modify disease progression in RA?***
3. ***What can the therapist do to try to offset the general loss of muscle mass and strength?***

See Appendix C, "Answers to Case Study Questions."

SUMMARY

Rheumatoid arthritis and osteoarthritis represent two distinct forms of joint disease that can produce devastating effects on the structure and function of synovial joints. Fortunately, management of these conditions has improved substantially through advancements in drug therapy. RA can be treated pharmacologically with NSAIDs, glucocorticoids, and various DMARDs. NSAIDs, including aspirin, represent the primary form of drug therapy in the early stages of this disease, and they are often used in conjunction with other drugs as the arthritic condition increases in severity. Glucocorticoids are often effective in decreasing the joint inflammation typically found in RA, but long-term use of these agents is limited because of their toxic effects. Disease-modifying drugs can slow or halt the progressive nature of RA by suppressing the immune response inherent in this disease. Although there is some concern about the efficacy and safety of these drugs, DMARDs have been a welcome addition to the rather limited arsenal of drugs used to treat RA.

Drug treatment of OA differs somewhat from that of RA, with NSAIDs and acetaminophen constituting the major forms of drug therapy to manage pain. A technique known as *viscosupplementation* can help restore the lubricating properties of the synovial fluid in osteoarthritic joints. Dietary supplements containing glucosamine and chondroitin sulfate may also help provide constituents that protect joint structure and function, and some people with OA have benefited from their long-term use. In any event, drug therapy along with nonpharmacological measures such as physical therapy can provide an effective way of dealing with the potentially devastating effects of RA and OA.

REFERENCES

1. Ngian GS. Rheumatoid arthritis. *Aust Fam Physician.* 2010;39:626-628.
2. Schett G, Gravallese E. Bone erosion in rheumatoid arthritis: mechanisms, diagnosis and treatment. *Nat Rev Rheumatol.* 2012;8:656-664.
3. Schuna AA. Rheumatoid arthritis. In: DiPiro JT, et al, eds. *Pharmacotherapy: A Pathophysiologic Approach.* 8th ed. New York: McGraw-Hill; 2011.
4. Espinosa M, Gottlieb BS. Juvenile idiopathic arthritis. *Pediatr Rev.* 2012;33:303-313.
5. Restrepo R, Lee EY. Epidemiology, pathogenesis, and imaging of arthritis in children. *Orthop Clin North Am.* 2012;43:213-225.
6. Kahn P. Juvenile idiopathic arthritis—an update on pharmacotherapy. *Bull NYU Hosp Jt Dis.* 2011;69:264-276.
7. Carmona L, Cross M, Williams B, et al. Rheumatoid arthritis. *Best Pract Res Clin Rheumatol.* 2010;24:733-745.

8. Scott DL, Wolfe F, Huizinga TW. Rheumatoid arthritis. *Lancet.* 2010;376:1094-1108.
9. Kingsley G, Scott IC, Scott DL. Quality of life and the outcome of established rheumatoid arthritis. *Best Pract Res Clin Rheumatol.* 2011;25:585-606.
10. Charles-Schoeman C. Cardiovascular disease and rheumatoid arthritis: an update. *Curr Rheumatol Rep.* 2012;14:455-462.
11. Gullick NJ, Scott DL. Co-morbidities in established rheumatoid arthritis. *Best Pract Res Clin Rheumatol.* 2011;25:469-483.
12. Her M, Kavanaugh A. Critical analysis of economic tools and economic measurement applied to rheumatoid arthritis. *Clin Exp Rheumatol.* 2012;30(suppl 73):S107-111.
13. Ruyssen-Witrand A, Constantin A, Cambon-Thomsen A, Thomsen M. New insights into the genetics of immune responses in rheumatoid arthritis. *Tissue Antigens.* 2012;80:105-118.
14. Boissier MC, Semerano L, Challal S, et al. Rheumatoid arthritis: from autoimmunity to synovitis and joint destruction. *J Autoimmun.* 2012;39:222-228.
15. Javierre BM, Hernando H, Ballestar E. Environmental triggers and epigenetic deregulation in autoimmune disease. *Discov Med.* 2011;12:535-545.
16. Choy E. Understanding the dynamics: pathways involved in the pathogenesis of rheumatoid arthritis. *Rheumatology.* 2012;51(suppl 5):v3-11.
17. Astry B, Harberts E, Moudgil KD. A cytokine-centric view of the pathogenesis and treatment of autoimmune arthritis. *J Interferon Cytokine Res.* 2011;31:927-940.
18. Komatsu N, Takayanagi H. Autoimmune arthritis: the interface between the immune system and joints. *Adv Immunol.* 2012;115:45-71.
19. Upchurch KS, Kay J. Evolution of treatment for rheumatoid arthritis. *Rheumatology.* 2012;51(suppl 6):vi28-36.
20. Malaviya AP, Ostör AJ. Rheumatoid arthritis and the era of biologic therapy. *Inflammopharmacology.* 2012;20:59-69.
21. McCormack PL. Celecoxib: a review of its use for symptomatic relief in the treatment of osteoarthritis, rheumatoid arthritis and ankylosing spondylitis. *Drugs.* 2011;71:2457-2489.
22. Suresh E. Recent advances in rheumatoid arthritis. *Postgrad Med J.* 2010;86:243-250.
23. Hazlewood G, van der Heijde DM, Bombardier C. Paracetamol for the management of pain in inflammatory arthritis: a systematic literature review. *J Rheumatol Suppl.* 2012;90:11-16.
24. Botting RM. Vane's discovery of the mechanism of action of aspirin changed our understanding of its clinical pharmacology. *Pharmacol Rep.* 2010;62:518-525.
25. Grosser T, Smyth E, FitzGerald GA. Anti-inflammatory, antipyretic, and analgesic agents: pharmacotherapy of gout. In: Brunton LL, et al, eds. *The Pharmacological Basis of Therapeutics.* 12th ed. New York: McGraw Hill; 2011.
26. Khanapure SP, Garvey DS, Janero DR, Letts LG. Eicosanoids in inflammation: biosynthesis, pharmacology, and therapeutic frontiers. *Curr Top Med Chem.* 2007;7:311-340.
27. Ricciotti E, FitzGerald GA. Prostaglandins and inflammation. *Arterioscler Thromb Vasc Biol.* 2011;31:986-1000.
28. Shi S, Klotz U. Clinical use and pharmacological properties of selective COX-2 inhibitors. *Eur J Clin Pharmacol.* 2008;64:233-252.
29. Frampton JE, Keating GM. Celecoxib: a review of its use in the management of arthritis and acute pain. *Drugs.* 2007;67:2433-2472.
30. Bijlsma JW. Disease control with glucocorticoid therapy in rheumatoid arthritis. *Rheumatology.* 2012;51(suppl 4):iv9-13.
31. Jacobs JW. Optimal use of non-biologic therapy in the treatment of rheumatoid arthritis. *Rheumatology.* 2012;51(suppl 4): iv3-8.
32. Keystone EC, Smolen J, van Riel P. Developing an effective treatment algorithm for rheumatoid arthritis. *Rheumatology.* 2012;51(suppl 5):v48-54.
33. Malysheva O, Baerwald CG. Low-dose corticosteroids and disease modifying drugs in patients with rheumatoid arthritis. *Clin Exp Rheumatol.* 2011;29(suppl 68):S113-115.
34. Bakker MF, Jacobs JW, Welsing PM, et al. Low-dose prednisone inclusion in a methotrexate-based, tight control strategy for early rheumatoid arthritis: a randomized trial. *Ann Intern Med.* 2012;156:329-339.
35. Schimmer BP, Funder JW. ACTH, adrenal steroids, and pharmacology of the adrenal cortex. In: Brunton L, et al, eds. *The Pharmacological Basis of Therapeutics.* 12th ed. New York: McGraw-Hill; 2011.
36. Strehl C, Spies CM, Buttgereit F. Pharmacodynamics of glucocorticoids. *Clin Exp Rheumatol.* 2011;29(suppl 68):S13-18.
37. Stahn C, Buttgereit F. Genomic and nongenomic effects of glucocorticoids. *Nat Clin Pract Rheumatol.* 2008;4:525-533.
38. Barnes PJ. Corticosteroid effects on cell signalling. *Eur Respir J.* 2006;27:413-426.
39. Hayashi R, Wada H, Ito K, Adcock IM. Effects of glucocorticoids on gene transcription. *Eur J Pharmacol.* 2004;500:51-62.
40. D'Acquisto F, Perretti M, Flower RJ. Annexin-A1: a pivotal regulator of the innate and adaptive immune systems. *Br J Pharmacol.* 2008;155:152-169.
41. Perretti M, D'Acquisto F. Annexin A1 and glucocorticoids as effectors of the resolution of inflammation. *Nat Rev Immunol.* 2009;9:62-70.
42. Smyth E, Grosser T, FitzGerald GA. Lipid-derived autocoids: eicosanoids and platelet-activating factor. In: Brunton LL, et al, eds. *The Pharmacological Basis of Therapeutics.* 12th ed. New York: McGraw Hill; 2011.
43. Adcock IM, Ito K. Molecular mechanisms of corticosteroid actions. *Monaldi Arch Chest Dis.* 2000;55:256-266.
44. Weinstein RS. Glucocorticoid-induced osteoporosis and osteonecrosis. *Endocrinol Metab Clin North Am.* 2012;41:595-611.
45. da Cunha VR, Brenol CV, Brenol JC, et al. Metabolic syndrome prevalence is increased in rheumatoid arthritis patients and is associated with disease activity. *Scand J Rheumatol.* 2012;41:186-191.
46. O'Dell JR. Therapeutic strategies for rheumatoid arthritis. *N Engl J Med.* 2004;350:2591-2602.
47. Birch JT Jr, Bhattacharya S. Emerging trends in diagnosis and treatment of rheumatoid arthritis. *Prim Care.* 2010;37:779-792.
48. Gaujoux-Viala C, Smolen JS, Landewé R, et al. Current evidence for the management of rheumatoid arthritis with synthetic disease-modifying antirheumatic drugs: a systematic literature review informing the EULAR recommendations for the management of rheumatoid arthritis. *Ann Rheum Dis.* 2010;69:1004-1009.
49. Rubbert-Roth A. Assessing the safety of biologic agents in patients with rheumatoid arthritis. *Rheumatology.* 2012;51(suppl 5): v38-47.
50. Ruderman EM. Overview of safety of non-biologic and biologic DMARDs. *Rheumatology.* 2012;51(suppl 6):vi37-43.
51. Michaelides M, Stover NB, Francis PJ, Weleber RG. Retinal toxicity associated with hydroxychloroquine and chloroquine: risk factors, screening, and progression despite cessation of therapy. *Arch Ophthalmol.* 2011;129:30-39.

52. Ben-Zvi I, Kivity S, Langevitz P, Shoenfeld Y. Hydroxychloroquine: from malaria to autoimmunity. *Clin Rev Allergy Immunol.* 2012;42:145-153.
53. Furst DE, Ulrich RW, Prakash S. Nonsteroidal anti-inflammatory drugs, disease-modifying antirheumatic drugs, nonopioid analgesics, and drugs used in gout. In: Katzung BG, Masters SB, Trevor AJ, eds. *Basic and Clinical Pharmacology.* 12th ed. New York: Lange Medical Books/McGraw Hill; 2012.
54. Katz SJ, Russell AS. Re-evaluation of antimalarials in treating rheumatic diseases: re-appreciation and insights into new mechanisms of action. *Curr Opin Rheumatol.* 2011;23:278-281.
55. Kuznik A, Bencina M, Svajger U, Jeras M, Rozman B, Jerala R. Mechanism of endosomal TLR inhibition by antimalarial drugs and imidazoquinolines. *J Immunol.* 2011;186:4794-4804.
56. Abarientos C, Sperber K, Shapiro DL, et al. Hydroxychloroquine in systemic lupus erythematosus and rheumatoid arthritis and its safety in pregnancy. *Expert Opin Drug Saf.* 2011;10:705-714.
57. Stelton CR, Connors DB, Walia SS, Walia HS. Hydrochloroquine retinopathy: characteristic presentation with review of screening. *Clin Rheumatol.* 2013;32:895-898. 58. Sahasranaman S, Howard D, Roy S. Clinical pharmacology and pharmacogenetics of thiopurines. *Eur J Clin Pharmacol.* 2008;64:753-767.
59. Madeira JM, Gibson DL, Kean WF, Klegeris A. The biological activity of auranofin: implications for novel treatment of diseases. *Inflammopharmacology.* 2012;20:297-306.
60. Kean WF, Kean IR. Clinical pharmacology of gold. *Inflammopharmacology.* 2008;16:112-125.
61. Bhabak KP, Bhuyan BJ, Mugesh G. Bioinorganic and medicinal chemistry: aspects of gold(I)-protein complexes. *Dalton Trans.* 2011;40:2099-2111.
62. Nieminen R, Korhonen R, Moilanen T, et al. Aurothiomalate inhibits cyclooxygenase 2, matrix metalloproteinase 3, and interleukin-6 expression in chondrocytes by increasing MAPK phosphatase 1 expression and decreasing p38 phosphorylation: MAPK phosphatase 1 as a novel target for antirheumatic drugs. *Arthritis Rheum.* 2010;62:1650-1659.
63. Nieminen R, Vuolteenaho K, Riutta A, et al. Aurothiomalate inhibits COX-2 expression in chondrocytes and in human cartilage possibly through its effects on COX-2 mRNA stability. *Eur J Pharmacol.* 2008;587:309-316.
64. Maetzel A, Wong A, Strand V, et al. Meta-analysis of treatment termination rates among rheumatoid arthritis patients receiving disease-modifying anti-rheumatic drugs. *Rheumatology.* 2000;39:975-981.
65. van Jaarsveld CH, Jahangier ZN, Jacobs JW, et al. Toxicity of anti-rheumatic drugs in a randomized clinical trial of early rheumatoid arthritis. *Rheumatology.* 2000;39:1374-1382.
66. Eisler R. Chrysotherapy: a synoptic review. *Inflamm Res.* 2003;52:487-501.
67. Buckley WA, Stump AL, Monger RM, Lookabill SK. Gold sodium thiomalate for the treatment of rheumatoid arthritis in a patient with hepatitis B. *Ann Pharmacother.* 2011;45:e23.
68. Cheung JM, Scarsbrook D, Klinkhoff AV. Characterization of patients with arthritis referred for gold therapy in the era of biologics. *J Rheumatol.* 2012;39:716-719.
69. Cutolo M, Bolosiu H, Perdriset G; for the LEADER Study Group. Efficacy and safety of leflunomide in DMARD-naive patients with early rheumatoid arthritis: comparison of a loading and a fixed-dose regimen. *Rheumatology.* 2013;52:1132-1140.
70. Li EK, Tam LS, Tomlinson B. Leflunomide in the treatment of rheumatoid arthritis. *Clin Ther.* 2004;26:447-459.
71. Behrens F, Koehm M, Burkhardt H. Update 2011: leflunomide in rheumatoid arthritis—strengths and weaknesses. *Curr Opin Rheumatol.* 2011;23:282-287.
72. Golicki D, Newada M, Lis J, et al. Leflunomide in monotherapy of rheumatoid arthritis: meta-analysis of randomized trials. *Pol Arch Med Wewn.* 2012;122:22-32.
73. Bird P, Griffiths H, Tymms K, et al. The SMILE study—safety of methotrexate in combination with leflunomide in rheumatoid arthritis. *J Rheumatol.* 2013;40:228-235.
74. Singer O, Gibofsky A. Methotrexate versus leflunomide in rheumatoid arthritis: what is new in 2011? *Curr Opin Rheumatol.* 2011;23:288-292.
75. Leban J, Vitt D. Human dihydroorotate dehydrogenase inhibitors, a novel approach for the treatment of autoimmune and inflammatory diseases. *Arzneimittelforschung.* 2011;61:66-72.
76. Munier-Lehmann H, Vidalain PO, Tangy F, Janin YL. On dihydroorotate dehydrogenases and their inhibitors and uses. *J Med Chem.* 2013;56:3148-3167.
77. Fox RI, Herrmann ML, Frangou CG, et al. How does leflunomide modulate the immune response in rheumatoid arthritis? *BioDrugs.* 1999;12:301-315.
78. Wiacek R, Kolossa K, Jankowski T, et al. The efficacy and safety of leflunomide in patients with active rheumatoid arthritis. *Adv Clin Exp Med.* 2012;21:337-342.
79. Gupta R, Bhatia J, Gupta SK. Risk of hepatotoxicity with add-on leflunomide in rheumatoid arthritis patients. *Arzneimittelforschung.* 2011;61:312-316.
80. Chikura B, Lane S, Dawson JK. Clinical expression of leflunomide-induced pneumonitis. *Rheumatology.* 2009;48:1065-1068.
81. Gutiérrez-Suárez R, Burgos-Vargas R. The use of methotrexate in children with rheumatic diseases. *Clin Exp Rheumatol.* 2010;28(suppl 61):S122-127.
82. Gaujoux-Viala C, Paternotte S, Combe B, Dougados M. Evidence of the symptomatic and structural efficacy of methotrexate in daily practice as the first disease-modifying drug in rheumatoid arthritis despite its suboptimal use: results from the ESPOIR early synovitis cohort. *Rheumatology.* 2012;51:1648-1654.
83. Kosta PE, Voulgari PV, Zikou AK, et al. Effect of very early treatment in rheumatoid arthritis on bone oedema and synovitis, using magnetic resonance imaging. *Scand J Rheumatol.* 2012;41:339-344.
84. Rath T, Rubbert A. Drug combinations with methotrexate to treat rheumatoid arthritis. *Clin Exp Rheumatol.* 2010;28(suppl 61):S52-57.
85. Visentin M, Zhao R, Goldman ID. The antifolates. *Hematol Oncol Clin North Am.* 2012;26:629-648.
86. Cronstein B. How does methotrexate suppress inflammation? *Clin Exp Rheumatol.* 2010;28(suppl 61):S21-23.
87. Chan ES, Cronstein BN. Methotrexate—how does it really work? *Nat Rev Rheumatol.* 2010;6:175-178.
88. Albrecht K, Müller-Ladner U. Side effects and management of side effects of methotrexate in rheumatoid arthritis. *Clin Exp Rheumatol.* 2010;28(suppl 61):S95-101.
89. Gilani ST, Khan DA, Khan FA, Ahmed M. Adverse effects of low dose methotrexate in rheumatoid arthritis patients. *J Coll Physicians Surg Pak.* 2012;22:101-104.
90. Morgan SL, Baggott JE. Folate supplementation during methotrexate therapy for rheumatoid arthritis. *Clin Exp Rheumatol.* 2010;28(suppl 61):S102-109.

91. Prey S, Paul C. Effect of folic or folinic acid supplementation on methotrexate-associated safety and efficacy in inflammatory disease: a systematic review. *Br J Dermatol.* 2009;160:622-628.
92. Whittle SL, Hughes RA. Folate supplementation and methotrexate treatment in rheumatoid arthritis: a review. *Rheumatology.* 2004;43:267-271.
93. Yazici Y. Long-term safety of methotrexate in the treatment of rheumatoid arthritis. *Clin Exp Rheumatol.* 2010;28(suppl 61):S65-67.
94. Delangle P, Mintz E. Chelation therapy in Wilson's disease: from D-penicillamine to the design of selective bioinspired intracellular Cu(I) chelators. *Dalton Trans.* 2012;41:6359-6370.
95. Wood PL, Khan MA, Moskal JR. Mechanism of action of the disease-modifying anti-arthritic thiol agents D-penicillamine and sodium aurothiomalate: restoration of cellular free thiols and sequestration of reactive aldehydes. *Eur J Pharmacol.* 2008;580:48-54.
96. Zhu X, Li J, Liu F, Uetrecht JP. Involvement of T helper 17 cells in D-penicillamine-induced autoimmune disease in Brown Norway rats. *Toxicol Sci.* 2011;120:331-338.
97. Habib GS, Saliba W, Nashashibi M, Armali Z. Penicillamine and nephrotic syndrome. *Eur J Intern Med.* 2006;17:343-348.
98. Poulas K, Koutsouraki E, Kordas G, et al. Anti-MuSK- and anti-AChR-positive myasthenia gravis induced by d-penicillamine. *J Neuroimmunol.* 2012;250:94-98.
99. Taylor PC, Feldmann M. Anti-TNF biologic agents: still the therapy of choice for rheumatoid arthritis. *Nat Rev Rheumatol.* 2009;5:578-582.
100. Aaltonen KJ, Virkki LM, Malmivaara A, et al. Systematic review and meta-analysis of the efficacy and safety of existing TNF blocking agents in treatment of rheumatoid arthritis. *PLoS One.* 2012;7:e30275.
101. Thalayasingam N, Isaacs JD. Anti-TNF therapy. *Best Pract Res Clin Rheumatol.* 2011;25:549-567.
102. Makrygiannakis D, Catrina AI. Apoptosis as a mechanism of action of tumor necrosis factor antagonists in rheumatoid arthritis. *J Rheumatol.* 2012;39:679-685.
103. Curtis JR, Singh JA. Use of biologics in rheumatoid arthritis: current and emerging paradigms of care. *Clin Ther.* 2011;33: 679-707.
104. Furst DE. Development of TNF inhibitor therapies for the treatment of rheumatoid arthritis. *Clin Exp Rheumatol.* 2010;28(suppl 59):S5-12.
105. Smith HS, Smith AR, Seidner P. Painful rheumatoid arthritis. *Pain Physician.* 2011;14:E427-458.
106. Gómez-Reino J. Biologic monotherapy as initial treatment in patients with early rheumatoid arthritis. *Rheumatology.* 2012;51(suppl 5):v31-37.
107. Geiler J, Buch M, McDermott MF. Anti-TNF treatment in rheumatoid arthritis. *Curr Pharm Des.* 2011;17:3141-3154.
108. Rosenblum H, Amital H. Anti-TNF therapy: safety aspects of taking the risk. *Autoimmun Rev.* 2011;10:563-568.
109. Moots RJ, Naisbett-Groet B. The efficacy of biologic agents in patients with rheumatoid arthritis and an inadequate response to tumour necrosis factor inhibitors: a systematic review. *Rheumatology.* 2012;51:2252-2261.
110. Herrero-Beaumont G, Martínez Calatrava MJ, Castañeda S. Abatacept mechanism of action: concordance with its clinical profile. *Reumatol Clin.* 2012;8:78-83.
111. Iannone F, Lapadula G. The inhibitor of costimulation of T cells: abatacept. *J Rheumatol Suppl.* 2012;89:100-102.
112. Solomon GE. T-cell agents in the treatment of rheumatoid arthritis. *Bull NYU Hosp Jt Dis.* 2010;68:162-165.
113. Khraishi M, Russell A, Olszynski WP. Safety profile of abatacept in rheumatoid arthritis: a review. *Clin Ther.* 2010;32: 1855-1870.
114. Gabay C, Lamacchia C, Palmer G. IL-1 pathways in inflammation and human diseases. *Nat Rev Rheumatol.* 2010;6:232-241.
115. Mertens M, Singh JA. Anakinra for rheumatoid arthritis. *Cochrane Database Syst Rev.* 2009;1:CD005121.
116. Singh JA, Cameron DR. Summary of AHRQ's comparative effectiveness review of drug therapy for rheumatoid arthritis (RA) in adults—an update. *J Manag Care Pharm.* 2012; 18(suppl C):S1-18.
117. Clark W, Jobanputra P, Barton P, Burls A. The clinical and cost-effectiveness of anakinra for the treatment of rheumatoid arthritis in adults: a systematic review and economic analysis. *Health Technol Assess.* 2004;8:1-105.
118. Dinarello CA, Simon A, van der Meer JW. Treating inflammation by blocking interleukin-1 in a broad spectrum of diseases. *Nat Rev Drug Discov.* 2012;11:633-652.
119. Goldbach-Mansky R. Blocking interleukin-1 in rheumatic diseases. *Ann NY Acad Sci.* 2009;1182:111-123.
120. Kaiser C, Knight A, Nordström D, et al. Injection-site reactions upon Kineret (anakinra) administration: experiences and explanations. *Rheumatol Int.* 2012;32:295-299.
121. Salliot C, Dougados M, Gossec L. Risk of serious infections during rituximab, abatacept and anakinra treatments for rheumatoid arthritis: meta-analyses of randomised placebo-controlled trials. *Ann Rheum Dis.* 2009;68:25-32.
122. Desai D, Goldbach-Mansky R, Milner JD, et al. Anaphylactic reaction to anakinra in a rheumatoid arthritis patient intolerant to multiple nonbiologic and biologic disease-modifying antirheumatic drugs. *Ann Pharmacother.* 2009;43:967-972.
123. Korhonen R, Moilanen E. Anti-CD20 antibody rituximab in the treatment of rheumatoid arthritis. *Basic Clin Pharmacol Toxicol.* 2010;106:13-21.
124. Emery P. Optimizing outcomes in patients with rheumatoid arthritis and an inadequate response to anti-TNF treatment. *Rheumatology.* 2012;51(suppl 5):v22-30.
125. Lee YH, Bae SC, Song GG. The efficacy and safety of rituximab for the treatment of active rheumatoid arthritis: a systematic review and meta-analysis of randomized controlled trials. *Rheumatol Int.* 2011;31:1493-1499.
126. Goldblatt F, Isenberg DA. Anti-CD20 monoclonal antibody in rheumatoid arthritis and systemic lupus erythematosus. *Handb Exp Pharmacol.* 2008;181:163-181.
127. Verweij CL, Vosslamber S. New insight in the mechanism of action of rituximab: the interferon signature towards personalized medicine. *Discov Med.* 2011;12:229-236.
128. Haraoui B, Bokarewa M, Kallmeyer I, Bykerk VP; RESET Investigators. Safety and effectiveness of rituximab in patients with rheumatoid arthritis following an inadequate response to 1 prior tumor necrosis factor inhibitor: the RESET Trial. *J Rheumatol.* 2011;38:2548-2556.
129. Leandro MJ, Becerra-Fernandez E. B-cell therapies in established rheumatoid arthritis. *Best Pract Res Clin Rheumatol.* 2011;25:535-548.
130. Tavazzi E, Ferrante P, Khalili K. Progressive multifocal leukoencephalopathy: an unexpected complication of modern therapeutic monoclonal antibody therapies. *Clin Microbiol Infect.* 2011;17:1776-1780.

131. Tanaka T, Kishimoto T. Immunotherapeutic implication of IL-6 blockade. *Immunotherapy*. 2012;4:87-105.
132. Navarro-Millán I, Singh JA, Curtis JR. Systematic review of tocilizumab for rheumatoid arthritis: a new biologic agent targeting the interleukin-6 receptor. *Clin Ther.* 2012;34:788-802.
133. Soriano ER. The actual role of therapy with traditional disease-modifying antirheumatic drugs in psoriatic arthritis. *J Rheumatol Suppl.* 2012;89:67-70.
134. Plosker GL, Croom KF. Sulfasalazine: a review of its use in the management of rheumatoid arthritis. *Drugs*. 2005;65: 1825-1849.
135. Ma MH, Kingsley GH, Scott DL. A systematic comparison of combination DMARD therapy and tumour necrosis inhibitor therapy with methotrexate in patients with early rheumatoid arthritis. *Rheumatology*. 2010;49:91-98.
136. Pavelka K, Kavanaugh AF, Rubbert-Roth A, Ferraccioli G. Optimizing outcomes in rheumatoid arthritis patients with inadequate responses to disease-modifying anti-rheumatic drugs. *Rheumatology*. 2012;51(suppl 5):v12-21.
137. Demoruelle MK, Deane KD. Treatment strategies in early rheumatoid arthritis and prevention of rheumatoid arthritis. *Curr Rheumatol Rep*. 2012;14:472-480.
138. Katchamart W, Trudeau J, Phumethum V, Bombardier C. Efficacy and toxicity of methotrexate (MTX) monotherapy versus MTX combination therapy with non-biological disease-modifying antirheumatic drugs in rheumatoid arthritis: a systematic review and meta-analysis. *Ann Rheum Dis.* 2009;68: 1105-1112.
139. Li S, Micheletti R. Role of diet in rheumatic disease. *Rheum Dis Clin North Am.* 2011;37:119-133.
140. Calder PC. Omega-3 fatty acids and inflammatory processes. *Nutrients*. 2010;2:355-374.
141. Miles EA, Calder PC. Influence of marine n-3 polyunsaturated fatty acids on immune function and a systematic review of their effects on clinical outcomes in rheumatoid arthritis. *Br J Nutr.* 2012;107(suppl 2):S171-184.
142. Calder PC. Fatty acids and inflammation: the cutting edge between food and pharma. *Eur J Pharmacol.* 2011;668(suppl 1): S50-58.
143. Issazadeh-Navikas S, Teimer R, Bockermann R. Influence of dietary components on regulatory T cells. *Mol Med.* 2012;18:95-110.
144. Pattison DJ, Winyard PG. Dietary antioxidants in inflammatory arthritis: do they have any role in etiology or therapy? *Nat Clin Pract Rheumatol.* 2008;4:590-596.
145. Zadák Z, Hyspler R, Tichá A, et al. Antioxidants and vitamins in clinical conditions. *Physiol Res.* 2009;58(suppl 1):S13-17.
146. Liao KP, Alfredsson L, Karlson EW. Environmental influences on risk for rheumatoid arthritis. *Curr Opin Rheumatol.* 2009;21:279-283.
147. Hoovestol RA, Mikuls TR. Environmental exposures and rheumatoid arthritis risk. *Curr Rheumatol Rep.* 2011;13:431-439.
148. Buys LM, Elliott ME. Osteoarthritis. In: DiPiro JT, et al, eds. *Pharmacotherapy: A Pathophysiologic Approach.* 8th ed. New York: McGraw-Hill; 2011.
149. Burr DB, Gallant MA. Bone remodelling in osteoarthritis. *Nat Rev Rheumatol.* 2012;8:665-673.
150. Bian Q, Wang YJ, Liu SF, Li YP. Osteoarthritis: genetic factors, animal models, mechanisms, and therapies. *Front Biosci* (elite ed). 2012;4:74-100.
151. Zhang Y, Jordan JM. Epidemiology of osteoarthritis. *Clin Geriatr Med.* 2010;26:355-369.
152. Brakke R, Singh J, Sullivan W. Physical therapy in persons with osteoarthritis. *PM R.* 2012;4(suppl):S53-58.
153. Iversen MD. Rehabilitation interventions for pain and disability in osteoarthritis. *Am J Nurs.* 2012;112(suppl 1):S32-37.
154. Vincent HK, Heywood K, Connelly J, Hurley RW. Obesity and weight loss in the treatment and prevention of osteoarthritis. *PM R.* 2012;4(suppl):S59-67.
155. Le Graverand-Gastineau MP. Disease modifying osteoarthritis drugs: facing development challenges and choosing molecular targets. *Curr Drug Targets.* 2010;11:528-535.
156. Flood J. The role of acetaminophen in the treatment of osteoarthritis. *Am J Manag Care.* 2010;16(suppl management): S48-54.
157. Reid MC, Shengelia R, Parker SJ. Pharmacologic management of osteoarthritis-related pain in older adults. *Am J Nurs.* 2012;112(suppl 1):S38-43.
158. Sinusas K. Osteoarthritis: diagnosis and treatment. *Am Fam Physician.* 2012;85:49-56.
159. Towheed TE, Maxwell L, Judd MG, et al. Acetaminophen for osteoarthritis. *Cochrane Database Syst Rev.* 2006;1:CD004257.
160. Mallen SR, Essex MN, Zhang R. Gastrointestinal tolerability of NSAIDs in elderly patients: a pooled analysis of 21 randomized clinical trials with celecoxib and nonselective NSAIDs. *Curr Med Res Opin.* 2011;27:1359-1366.
161. Altman RD. New guidelines for topical NSAIDs in the osteoarthritis treatment paradigm. *Curr Med Res Opin.* 2010;26: 2871-2876.
162. Arnstein PM. Evolution of topical NSAIDs in the guidelines for treatment of osteoarthritis in elderly patients. *Drugs Aging.* 2012;29:523-531.
163. Argoff CE. Recent developments in the treatment of osteoarthritis with NSAIDs. *Curr Med Res Opin.* 2011;27:1315-1327.
164. Derry S, Moore RA, Rabbie R. Topical NSAIDs for chronic musculoskeletal pain in adults. *Cochrane Database Syst Rev.* 2012;9:CD007400.
165. Chen MR, Dragoo JL. The effect of nonsteroidal anti-inflammatory drugs on tissue healing. *Knee Surg Sports Traumatol Arthrosc.* 2013;21:540-549.
166. Axe JM, Snyder-Mackler L, Axe MJ. The role of viscosupplementation. *Sports Med Arthrosc.* 2013;21:18-22.
167. Clegg TE, Caborn D, Mauffrey C. Viscosupplementation with hyaluronic acid in the treatment for cartilage lesions: a review of current evidence and future directions. *Eur J Orthop Surg Traumatol.* 2013;23:119-124.
168. Gigante A, Callegari L. The role of intra-articular hyaluronan (Sinovial) in the treatment of osteoarthritis. *Rheumatol Int.* 2011;31:427-444.
169. Cianflocco AJ. Viscosupplementation in patients with osteoarthritis of the knee. *Postgrad Med.* 2013;125:97-105.
170. Bellamy N, Campbell J, Robinson V, et al. Viscosupplementation for the treatment of osteoarthritis of the knee. *Cochrane Database Syst Rev.* 2006;2:CD005321.
171. Abate M, Pulcini D, Di Iorio A, Schiavone C. Viscosupplementation with intra-articular hyaluronic acid for treatment of osteoarthritis in the elderly. *Curr Pharm Des.* 2010;16: 631-640.
172. Tahiri L, Benbouazza K, Amine B, Hajjaj-Hassouni N. Acute pseudoseptic arthritis after viscosupplementation of the knee: a case report. *Clin Rheumatol.* 2007;26:1977-1979.
173. Huskisson EC. Glucosamine and chondroitin for osteoarthritis. *J Int Med Res.* 2008;36:1161-1179.

174. Jerosch J. Effects of glucosamine and chondroitin sulfate on cartilage metabolism in OA: outlook on other nutrient partners especially omega-3 fatty acids. *Int J Rheumatol.* 2011;2011:969012.
175. Matsuno H, Nakamura H, Katayama K, et al. Effects of an oral administration of glucosamine-chondroitin-quercetin glucoside on the synovial fluid properties in patients with osteoarthritis and rheumatoid arthritis. *Biosci Biotechnol Biochem.* 2009;73:288-292.
176. Imagawa K, de Andrés MC, Hashimoto K, et al. The epigenetic effect of glucosamine and a nuclear factor-kappa B (NF-kB) inhibitor on primary human chondrocytes—implications for osteoarthritis. *Biochem Biophys Res Commun.* 2011;405:362-367.
177. Sherman AL, Ojeda-Correal G, Mena J. Use of glucosamine and chondroitin in persons with osteoarthritis. *PM R.* 2012;4(suppl):S110-116.
178. Black C, Clar C, Henderson R, et al. The clinical effectiveness of glucosamine and chondroitin supplements in slowing or arresting progression of osteoarthritis of the knee: a systematic review and economic evaluation. *Health Technol Assess.* 2009;13:1-148.
179. Miller KL, Clegg DO. Glucosamine and chondroitin sulfate. *Rheum Dis Clin North Am.* 2011;37:103-118.
180. Wandel S, Jüni P, Tendal B, et al. Effects of glucosamine, chondroitin, or placebo in patients with osteoarthritis of hip or knee: network meta-analysis. *BMJ.* 2010;341:c4675.
181. Clegg DO, Reda DJ, Harris CL, et al. Glucosamine, chondroitin sulfate, and the two in combination for painful knee osteoarthritis. *N Engl J Med.* 2006;354:795-808.

CHAPTER 17

Patient-Controlled Analgesia

Patient-controlled analgesia (PCA) was first introduced into clinical practice in the early 1980s as an alternative way to administer analgesic medications. The basic principle behind PCA is that the patient can self-administer small doses of the drug (usually an opioid) at relatively frequent intervals to provide optimal pain relief.[1] These small doses are typically delivered intravenously or into the spinal canal by some type of machine (i.e., pump) that is controlled by the patient. Patient-controlled analgesia has several advantages over more traditional dosing regimens. In particular, PCA systems allow the patient to better match his or her need for analgesic medication to the dose to treat a specific amount of pain at any given point in time—that is, as pain fluctuates, the patient can self-administer more or less drug to provide the appropriate level of anesthesia. PCA therefore provides equivalent or increased analgesic effects with better patient satisfaction compared to conventional analgesia.[2,3] This has generated increased use of PCA in a variety of clinical situations. For instance, PCA systems are used to help manage acute pain following surgery, and they are used to treat pain in patients with cancer and other conditions associated with chronic pain.[4,5]

Because PCA is used extensively to treat acute and chronic pain, rehabilitation specialists should be aware of some of the fundamental principles governing it. This chapter begins by discussing the basic concepts and strategies of PCA, followed by some of its practical aspects, including the types of analgesics used, the types of machines used to administer the drugs, and the possible routes of drug administration. An indication of why PCA is often clinically superior to more traditional methods of analgesia is then presented. Finally, potential problems associated with PCA and the specific ways that PCA can affect patients receiving physical therapy and occupational therapy are discussed. This review should provide you with a better understanding of why PCA systems are often a preferred method of managing pain in contemporary practice.

PHARMACOKINETIC BASIS FOR PCA

To provide optimal management of pain, analgesic drugs should be delivered into the bloodstream or other target tissues (epidural space, within joints, etc.) in a predictable and fairly constant manner. The goal is to maintain drug levels within a fairly well-defined therapeutic window.[5] Such a therapeutic window for systemic (IV) dosages is represented schematically by the shaded area in Figure 17-1. If drug levels are below this window, the analgesic is below the minimum analgesic concentration, and the patient is in pain. Drug levels above the window may produce adequate analgesia but may also produce side effects such as sedation. The traditional method of administering analgesics is to give relatively large doses with relatively large time intervals between each dosage. For instance, opioid analgesics are sometimes injected intramuscularly every 3 to 4 hours to manage severe pain, thus creating large fluctuations in the amount of drug

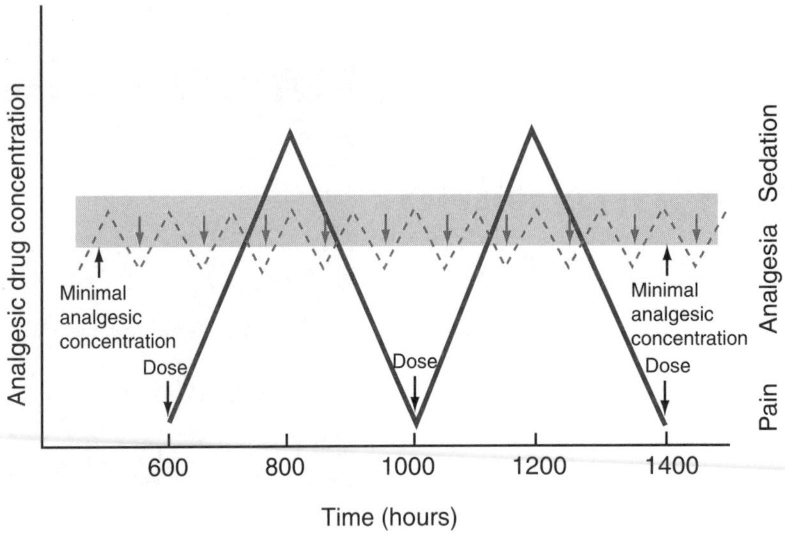

Figure ■ 17-1
Pharmacokinetic model for PCA using opioid drugs. Conventional intramuscular injection is indicated by the long solid lines, PCA is indicated by the short dashed lines, and the therapeutic window for analgesia is indicated by the shaded area. *(From Ferrante, et al. Anesth Analg. 1988;67: 457–461; with permission.)*

present in the body. The dark solid lines in Figure 17-1 illustrate these large fluctuations. This method of administration is associated with long periods of time when the drug concentration falls below the therapeutic window, allowing pain to occur, or above the therapeutic window, causing sedation.

Figure 17-1 also illustrates why PCA systems are better at maintaining drug levels within the therapeutic window. Systems using some form of PCA deliver small doses of the analgesic on a relatively frequent basis, as indicated by the dashed lines. Drug levels are maintained within the analgesic range; there are shorter periods of time when the drug concentration falls below the therapeutic window (i.e., below the shaded area), and there is virtually no time when side effects occur because the concentration has risen above the therapeutic window. Hence, analgesia can be achieved more effectively with a reduced incidence of side effects.

PCA DOSING STRATEGIES AND PARAMETERS

The fact that PCA enables the patient to self-deliver small doses of the analgesic at frequent intervals illustrates the need for specific dosing parameters that control the amount and frequency of analgesic administration. Several terms are used to describe these parameters and indicate each parameter's role in safeguarding against excessive drug delivery.[5,6] The basic terms that describe PCA dosing strategies are indicated here:

Loading dose. A single large dose is given initially to establish analgesia. This loading dose is used to bring levels of the analgesic to the therapeutic window, as illustrated by the shaded area in Figure 17-1.

Demand dose. The amount of drug that is self-administered by the patient each time he or she activates the PCA delivery mechanism is known as the *demand dose*. The magnitude of these doses for some commonly used opioid analgesics is listed in Table 17-1.

Lockout interval. The minimum amount of time allowed between each demand dose is called the *lockout interval*. After the patient self-administers a dose, the PCA delivery system will not deliver the next dose until the lockout interval has expired. Typical lockout intervals for commonly used opioids are listed in Table 17-1.

1- and 4-hour limits. Some PCA systems can be set to limit the total amount of drug given in a 1- or 4-hour period. The use of these parameters is somewhat questionable, however, because other parameters such as the demand dose and lockout interval automatically limit the total amount of drug that can be given in a specific period of time.

Background infusion rate. In some patients, a small amount of the analgesic is infused continuously to maintain a low background level of analgesia.

Table 17-1
PARAMETERS FOR INTRAVENOUS PCA USING OPIOID MEDICATIONS*

Drug (Concentration)	Demand Dose	Lockout Interval (min)
Alfentanil (0.1 mg/mL)	0.1–0.2 mg	5–8
Buprenorphine (0.03 mg/mL)	0.03–0.1 mg	8–20
Fentanyl (10 μg/mL)	10–20 μg	4–10
Hydromorphone (0.2 mg/mL)	0.05–0.25 mg	5–10
Meperidine (10 mg/mL)	5–25 mg	5–10
Methadone (1 mg/mL)	0.5–2.5 mg	8–20
Morphine (1 mg/mL)	0.5–2.5 mg	5–10
Nalbuphine (1 mg/mL)	1–5 mg	5–15
Oxymorphone (0.25 mg/mL)	0.2–0.4 mg	8–10
Pentazocine (10 mg/mL)	5–30 mg	5–15
Sufentanil (2 μg/mL)	2–5 μg	4–10

**Concentrations and demand doses are those typically administered to adults who are not tolerant to opioid medications.*

Source: Hurley RW, Wu CL. Acute postoperative pain. In: Miller RD, ed. Miller's Anesthesia. 7th ed. Philadelphia, PA: Churchill Livingstone/Elsevier; 2010:2762, with permission.

Demand doses are superimposed on the background infusion whenever the patient feels an increase in pain (e.g., the breakthrough pain that may occur when the patient coughs or changes position). The use of background infusion basically combines the technique of continuous infusion with PCA, which may provide optimal analgesia with less chance of analgesic levels falling well below the therapeutic window.[7] Background infusion, for example, can maintain adequate analgesia even when patients are asleep or otherwise unable to activate the pump manually.

However, routine use of background infusion has been questioned, especially when opioids are administered systemically (intravenously) by PCA. It appears that background infusions may not provide any additional analgesic benefits in most patients, but they can lead to an increased risk of side effects such as respiratory depression because patients ultimately receive a larger total amount of opioid (i.e., the background infusion plus the demand doses).[8-10] Hence, the use of background infusion rates with PCAs have been discouraged for most patients. Techniques are being explored that combine background infusions with mandatory programmed bolus doses or that use computerized systems that automatically adjust bolus doses based on the patient's previous demands for analgesia.[11,12] Future clinical studies will help clarify the role of these techniques.

Successful versus total demands. Successful demands occur when the patient activates the PCA delivery system and receives a demand dose. Demands made during the lockout interval are not considered successful but are added to the number of successful demands to indicate the total demands. A large number of unsuccessful demands may indicate that the PCA parameters are not effective in providing adequate analgesia. Therefore, most PCA systems record the number of total demands so that the demand dose can be adjusted if a large number of unsuccessful demands are being made.

TYPES OF ANALGESICS USED FOR PCA

Opioid analgesics (see Chapter 14) are the primary medications used during PCA.[3] Opioids such as morphine, meperidine, tramadol, fentanyl, and fentanyl derivatives (alfentanil, remifentanil, sufentanil) are powerful analgesics that act primarily on the spinal cord and brain to inhibit the transmission and perception of nociceptive impulses. Opioids must be used cautiously because these drugs can cause serious side effects and have the potential for patient overdose. As explained earlier, PCA often provides a safer and more effective way to administer these powerful drugs by preventing large fluctuations in plasma opioid levels.

Practitioners can combine non-opioid analgesics with opioids during systemic (IV) PCA to decrease the amount of opioid needed for adequate analgesia. This "opioid sparing" effect is achieved by combining morphine or other opioids with ketorolac (an NSAID; see Chapter 15), ketamine (an anesthetic agent; see Chapter 11), or droperidol (an antipsychotic; see Chapter 8) in specific clinical situations.[13-16] Alternatively, a very low dose of an opioid receptor antagonist (blocker) such as naloxone (see Chapter 14) is administered along with the opioid during PCA. Preliminary evidence suggests that a low dosage of the opioid antagonist may block certain opioid side effects (nausea, pruritus) while still allowing an adequate level of analgesia.[17,18]

PCAs can also deliver local anesthetics such as bupivacaine and ropivacaine (see Chapter 12). These drugs block transmission along afferent sensory neurons and thus decrease sensation at the spinal cord level when administered epidurally. Local anesthetics are often administered when an epidural PCA is used during labor and childbirth.[12] These drugs, mixed with opioids, can provide effective epidural PCA during labor or following surgery.[19,20] Local anesthetics can also be applied to a specific site, such as the subacromial space or around a particular peripheral nerve. This technique, known as *patient controlled regional anesthesia* (PCRA), is discussed later. Hence, local anesthetics serve as an alternative or adjunct to opioids during several types of PCA.

PCA PUMPS

The increase in popularity and use of PCA has largely been because of the development of infusion devices that can administer the analgesic in a safe and accurate manner. These devices, or *pumps*, vary in technological sophistication and cost, but they share common features (some are summarized in Table 17-2).[21,22] PCA pumps essentially allow the practitioner to set specific parameters of drug delivery (demand dose, lockout interval, etc.). The pump must then provide features to safeguard the patient against pump malfunction and to warn the patient or caregiver if drug delivery is interrupted. Likewise, contemporary pumps often have software that detects errors in the programmed dose and alerts practitioners that the dose may exceed preset limits for a specific drug and clinical indication. This type of safeguard, known commonly as a dose error reduction system (DERS), can be invaluable in preventing overdose.[21]

Pumps used for PCA fall into two basic categories: external and internal (implantable).[22,23] The most basic type of external pump is a simple syringe driver (Fig. 17-2). A syringe containing the medication is placed in a viselike machine that advances the syringe a small amount when the patient activates the pump. A second type of pump uses a peristaltic action that sequentially compresses a piece of tubing to milk the medication through the tubing toward the patient. A third pump, known as a *cassette system*, works by drawing the medication into a fluid container within the pump and expelling the selected amount of medication out of the chamber into tubing that leads to the patient. In most cases, these external pumps are activated when the patient pushes a button located on the end of a pendant that is connected to the pump (see Fig. 17-2).

Disposable models of external PCA pumps are also available, offering a simple and cost-effective alternative

Table 17-2
BASIC FEATURES OF SOME COMMON PCA PUMPS

Feature	CareFusion Alaris	Hospira LifeCare PCA	Smiths Medical CADD-Solaris	Moog Curlin 6000 CMS
Ambulatory use*	No	No	Yes	Yes
DERS**	Excellent	Excellent	Good	Good
Ease of use	Excellent	Good	Excellent	Good
Primary application(s)	IV-PCA	IV-PCA	IV-PCA Epidural Subcutaneous Peripheral nerve block	Multitherapy***
Other features	Integrated respiratory monitoring is available; can monitor pulse oximetry and capnography (end tidal CO_2 levels).	Has an integrated bar code reader to help ensure that correct drug and dose concentration are selected.	Small, lightweight pump; good choice when an ambulatory pump is needed for multiple pain applications.	Relatively small, ambulatory pump that can be used for pain control as well as other types of drug infusion.

**Ambulatory pumps are smaller and can be carried/worn by the patient; larger pumps are pole mounted and are typically used at bedside.*

***DERS: dose error reduction system; pump has software that checks the dosing variables for each drug and alerts the clinician if the programmed dose exceeds preset limits for that drug.*

****Multitherapy: can be used for pain control and other applications such as parenteral nutrition, antibiotic infusion, and chemotherapy.*

Source: Adapted from Patient-controlled analgesic infusion pumps. Health Devices. 2011;40:42-58; with permission.

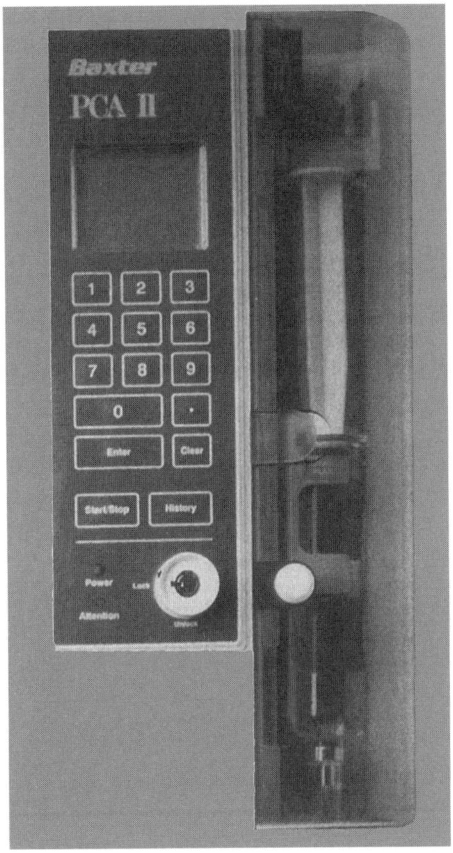

Figure ■ 17-2
An example of a commonly used syringe driver pump for a PCA.

for pain management.[24,25] The device is either controlled electronically or the patient can activate it manually by squeezing a small bulb containing a small dose (i.e., the demand dose) of medication. As with other PCA pumps, built-in safeguards limit how often these demand doses can be administered. Patients can use disposable PCA pumps in the hospital or after discharge following surgery.[24]

Internal, or implantable, pumps are placed surgically beneath the patient's skin and connected to a catheter leading to the patient's bloodstream or perispinal spaces (epidural or intrathecal). This basically creates a closed system within the patient's body. These pumps typically contain a reservoir filled with medication. The reservoir can be refilled by inserting a Huber needle through the skin and into the pump via a resealable septum located on the outside of the pump (Fig. 17-3). Some implantable pumps use a rotatory peristaltic mechanism to milk the medication

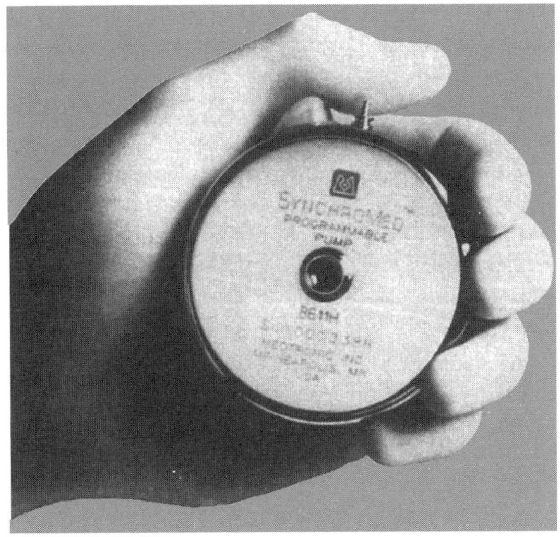

Figure ■ 17-3
An example of an implantable, electronically controlled PCA pump. This pump is implanted surgically in the patient's abdomen and is refilled periodically through a self-sealing septum.

out of the pump. Other pumps use a bellows system to compress a chamber within the pump, thus expelling a given quantity of the drug. Implantable pumps are often programmed through the skin with an electronic control device.

The type of pump that is selected depends primarily on which method (external or implantable) will best serve the patient's needs, as well as cost and availability of a given type of pump. Advances in pump technology will continue to improve the available devices, and future developments will undoubtedly provide devices that are even more efficient in providing PCA.

ADMINISTRATION ROUTES DURING PCA

IV PCA

Intravenous patient-controlled analgesia (IV-PCA) is perhaps the most common method of systemic PCA administration. IV-PCA is typically administered by inserting a needle into a peripheral vein and then connecting the needle to a catheter or IV line. The catheter is then connected to a PCA pump, and small intermittent doses of the analgesic are administered through the catheter and delivered directly into the systemic circulation. This technique is often effective in allowing the patient to regulate his or her level of analgesia for a short period of time (e.g., for the first few days after surgery).

When IV-PCA is needed for longer periods, a catheter can be implanted surgically in a large central vein, with the tip of the catheter advanced to the right atrium of the heart. The catheter is then tunneled through subcutaneous tissues and brought out through the patient's skin to allow administration of PCA. Alternatively, the catheter can be connected to a small container known as an *access port*, which is implanted subcutaneously in the upper chest, arm, or abdomen (Fig. 17-4). This type of catheter-port system, also known as a *central venous access device* (CVAD), provides a method of IV drug delivery that is located entirely within the patient's body. Injections can be made through the skin and into the port through a self-sealing silicone rubber septum located on the port. When these ports are used during PCA, the external PCA source is connected to the port via a special (Huber) needle that is inserted through the skin and into the port (see Fig. 17-4). The analgesic drug is then given from the PCA pump through a catheter into the port and ultimately into the systemic circulation. This provides an effective way of getting small, frequent doses of the drug into the bloodstream with less risk of infection or IV catheter displacement. The PCA-port delivery also enables the patient to be disconnected from the PCA delivery system for short periods of time by removing the needle from the port. This allows the patient to bathe or get dressed without risking damage to the indwelling port-IV system.[26]

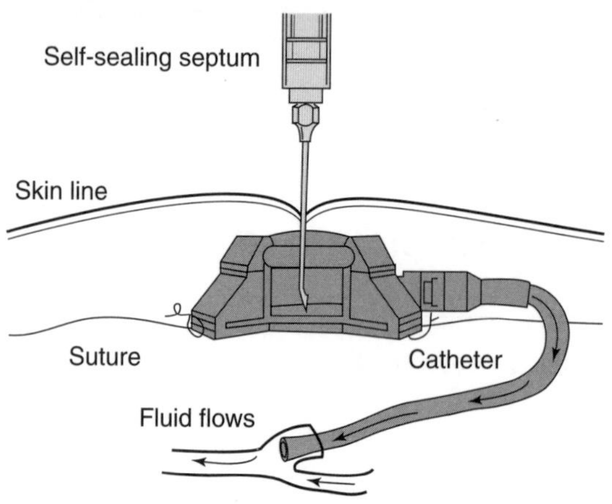

Figure ■ 17-4
Schematic representation of an implantable vascular access port for a PCA. The port is connected to a PCA pump via a percutaneous needle, and a catheter leads from the port to a large central vein. *(From Knox LS. Crit Care Nurse. 1987;7:71; with permission.)*

Epidural PCA

Patient-controlled epidural analgesia (PCEA) is achieved by administering drugs directly into the area outside of the membranes (meninges) surrounding the spinal cord.[11,27] This is typically done by inserting a small catheter so that its tip lies in the epidural space at a specific level of the spinal cord (Fig. 17-5). Alternatively, the tip of the catheter can be placed in the subarachnoid space—this type of delivery is known as *spinal* or *intrathecal administration*—that is, the drug is

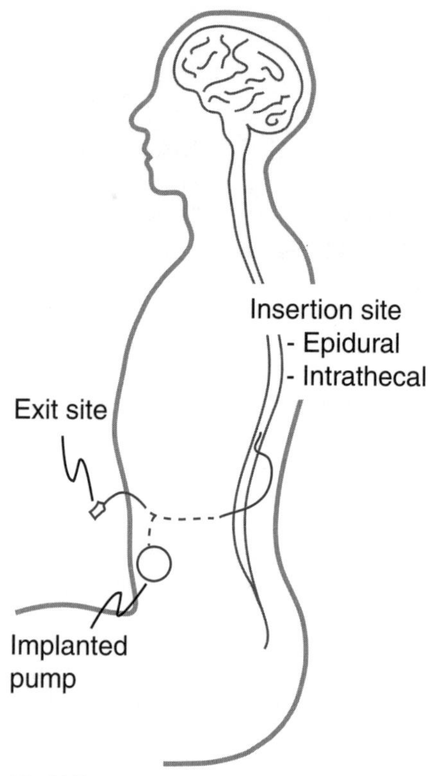

Figure ■ 17-5
Schematic illustration of PCA spinal delivery. The catheter delivers the analgesic into either the epidural or intrathecal (subarachnoid) space. Catheters for long-term use are tunneled under the skin (*dashed line*) and can either be connected directly to an implanted PCA pump or exit the anterior-lateral flank for connection to an external pump.

delivered into the space between the middle (arachnoid) layer of the meninges and the inner (pia mater) meningeal membrane (*intrathecal* means "within a sheath"; see Chapter 2). Although intrathecal administration can be used in certain situations, the epidural route seems to be the preferred method during PCA because it is safer and there is less risk of damaging the meninges.

If PCEA is intended for short-term use, the catheter can be externalized through the skin on the midline of the patient's back and held in place by surgical tape. For long-term use, the catheter is often tunneled through the subcutaneous tissues in the patient's abdominal wall, after which the catheter can either be brought out through the skin on the patient's side (see Fig. 17-5) or connected to an implanted access port or drug reservoir. In either case, PCEA is achieved by using a pump to deliver the drug through the catheter and into the area directly surrounding the spinal cord.

Administration of drugs into the epidural space is obviously more difficult than simple IV delivery using a peripheral vein. Epidural delivery does, however, offer advantages in terms of providing more effective analgesia with a smaller amount of drug. For instance, it is estimated that epidural morphine is 5 to 10 times more potent than IV morphine, indicating that less drug needs to be administered by the epidural route to achieve adequate analgesia.[26] This fact makes sense, considering that PCEA administers the drug closer and more directly to the spinal cord compared with IV-PCA, which must get the drug to the spinal cord via the systemic circulation. Likewise, there have been numerous studies that directly compared PCEA with other parenteral administration routes, including IV-PCA. Although these studies varied in the type of analgesic drugs used and the clinical indication (i.e., pain control following various types of surgery), they routinely found that PCEA provided superior pain control without a significant increase in side effects.[5,28-30] By improving pain control after surgery, PCEA can also facilitate early recovery and rehabilitation in situations such as total knee arthroplasty.[31]

Regional PCA

Patient-controlled regional analgesia (PCRA) occurs when the patient self-administers the medication directly into a specific anatomical site, such as a peripheral joint, near a peripheral nerve, or into a wound. This technique helps localize the drug to the site of administration, thereby providing adequate pain control with minimal effects on other tissues and organs. Although this technique has been used to administer analgesic medications such as morphine, PCRA typically uses some type of local anesthetic, such as bupivacaine or ropivacaine (see Chapter 12). Hence, this technique is really analogous to patient-controlled regional *anesthesia* rather than a strictly analgesic intervention. Regardless, PCRA is an excellent way to provide safe and effective pain control.

PCRA is typically accomplished by inserting a small catheter into the affected site and then attaching the catheter to some type of pump that enables the patient to self-administer small amounts of medication as needed. For example, a PCA system was developed to deliver local anesthetics such as bupivacaine and ropivacaine into the subacromial space following acromial decompression surgery.[32] Administration of a local anesthetic directly into the joint, however, can cause breakdown of articular surfaces (chondrolysis).[33,34] Hence, this technique is no longer recommended when articular cartilage remains in the joint.[35] Intra-articular administration of local anesthetics, however, might be useful after total joint arthroplasty because the joint surfaces have been removed and replaced by synthetic components.[36]

Instead of injecting the drug intra-articularly, it is now more feasible to deliver a local anesthetic continuously to the area around a peripheral nerve (femoral, popliteal, etc.). These perineural applications, known commonly as *continuous nerve blocks* (see Chapter 12), can provide excellent pain control following surgery and in other clinical situations.[37,38] As indicated, the local anesthetic is typically infused continuously and automatically rather than via a patient-controlled device. Hence, the future of patient-controlled regional analgesia and anesthesia seems uncertain at the present time. Additional studies will be needed to determine if PCRA can be used alone or incorporated into more traditional analgesic regimens as an effective way to control local pain in various clinical situations.

Transdermal PCA

Patient-controlled transdermal analgesia (PCTA) uses iontophoresis techniques to deliver a small dose of analgesic medication through the skin (transdermally) and into the systemic circulation. Specifically, a relatively short (10-minute) burst of electricity facilitates transdermal administration of the drug, thus eliminating the need for needles or catheters. The patient has the ability to activate this electrical burst, thus adding an aspect of patient control to this method of analgesia. PCTA typically uses a delivery system consisting of a patch that is approximately the size of a credit card.[39,40] This patch is adhered to the patient's skin, usually on the arm or upper chest. The patch is impregnated with an opioid such as fentanyl, and the patient can self-administer a small dose of the drug by pushing a button on the patch.

The first commercially available system was designed to deliver 40 μg of fentanyl over a 10-minute period each time the patient activated the patch.[39,41] Several studies have suggested that PCTA using this type of fentanyl device can provide pain control that is superior to placebo and comparable to standard postoperative analgesic techniques such as morphine IV-PCA.[42,43]

Questions were raised, however, about the accuracy of the fentanyl iontophoretic transdermal system—that is, the actual dose of fentanyl may not be adequate when the device is first applied to the patient.[3,39] Moreover, problems with safety and possible overdose due to electronic malfunction caused this device to be withdrawn from the market in 2008.[3] Hence, the future of PCTA using fentanyl or other analgesics remains uncertain at the present time. Perhaps improvements in these iontophoretic delivery systems will permit more extensive use of PCTA in the future.

Other Potential Administration Routes for PCA

Several other techniques allow patients to self-administer small analgesic doses as needed for pain but without the safety issues associated with IV lines, epidural catheters, or other invasive delivery methods.[3] Perhaps the simplest alternative PCA technique uses the oral route. In this situation, a bedside device provides a pill containing a small dose of opioid such as morphine, hydromorphone, or oxycodone. The device is programmed to provide the pill only upon activation by the patient via a wristband or similar electronic mechanism and after an appropriate lockout interval has ended. The patient must, of course, be able to swallow the pill without choking or vomiting, and patients with "nothing by mouth" (NPO) restrictions cannot use this technique. Nonetheless, this technique does allow the patient to self-administer small, frequent oral doses as needed for pain, without requiring the nurse or other health-care provider to intervene.

In addition, inhalation devices can administer a small dose of opioid (morphine, fentanyl) to the lungs for absorption into the systemic circulation. The device is equipped with technical features that control the demand dose and lockout interval, thus limiting the amount and frequency of drug administration, respectively. Similarly, devices are being considered that can deliver opioids intranasally, thus taking advantage of the highly vascularized absorptive surface of the nasal mucosa. Sublingual PCA may also be feasible, by placing a small (3-mm diameter) container beneath the tongue that releases opioids (e.g. sufentanil) upon activation by the patient via a handheld device.

Most of the newer PCA techniques described above are still in development or in clinical trials. Nonetheless, these techniques might eventually provide safe and effective alternatives to more traditional PCA administration using the IV and epidural routes. It will be interesting to see if these alternative techniques are eventually accepted into routine clinical practice.

COMPARISON OF PCA TO OTHER METHODS OF ANALGESIC ADMINISTRATION

Considering the vast array of analgesic drugs, dosing patterns, and administration techniques, direct comparisons between these techniques becomes a complex and extensive topic. Nonetheless, some key comparisons between PCA and other techniques may be helpful. In particular, it is apparent that giving small, frequent doses of analgesic through PCA is superior to administering large doses at infrequent intervals. Many clinical studies have attempted to verify this by comparing PCA using opioid drugs with traditional intramuscular (IM) opioid injection. Although some studies have not shown any clear advantages or disadvantages of IV-PCA,[44] most controlled trials indicate that PCA administered either intravenously or epidurally provides improved analgesia without a substantial increase in side effects.[2,45-48]

Many studies also reported that patients were more satisfied with the pain control provided by PCA versus traditional intermittent dosing, which seems to be related to the increased feeling of control over pain.[2,47,49-51] Some studies also suggested that patients receiving opioid PCA are generally able to ambulate sooner and tend to have shorter hospital stays than patients receiving opioids by the traditional IM route.[52,53] Other studies, however, failed to find a significant difference in factors such as length of stay[2,46,54] or in ability to ambulate sooner.[55] These discrepancies in the results from different studies are understandable, considering that they often differed in research design and patient populations (various types of surgical procedures, different analgesic drugs, etc.). Nonetheless, the preponderance of evidence suggests that PCA systems afford some obvious advantages in certain patients over more traditional methods such as periodic IM injection.

One must then consider how PCA-like administration would compare with continuous infusion of an analgesic drug. As discussed in Chapter 14, it is sometimes feasible to administer opioid analgesics by slow, continuous infusion into the bloodstream or into some other area such as the epidural or intrathecal space. Continuous infusion would obviously provide the best way of maintaining drug concentration within a given therapeutic range. Several studies suggest that continuous epidural infusion of an opioid, local anesthetic, or some combination of these agents provides better pain control than techniques that allow the patient to self-administer the drug via the IV or epidural route.[56,57] Hence, continuous epidural infusion is an option for patients who do not achieve adequate pain control using PCEA or some other PCA technique. Continuous infusion, however, tends to supply more total drug than patient-controlled techniques, and the additional drug quantities may pose unnecessary costs and expose patients to an increased risk of side effects.[58-60]

An advantage of PCA over intermittent IM injection or continuous epidural infusion is that PCA decreases the need for other health professionals (physicians, nurses, pharmacists) to be directly involved in administering analgesics or adjusting the rate of analgesic delivery. Intramuscular injection, for instance, requires that the nurse be available at the proper time to inject the proper amount of the correct drug into the correct patient. This clearly takes the locus of control out of the patient's hands and makes the patient feel more dependent on an outside person to provide pain relief. When PCA systems are used appropriately, pain control is literally in the patient's hands. Likewise, continuous infusion often requires frequent adjustments by a qualified person who must attempt to match the dose of analgesic to the patient's pain level. This is especially difficult if pain levels are changing, such as in the patient recovering from surgery. With PCA, the patient is able to automatically adjust the amount of analgesia according to his or her pain. Again, this underscores a key advantage of PCA: it is superior to more traditional methods of analgesia because the person most qualified to judge his or her pain is empowered to self-administer the analgesic according to his or her own needs.

COMPARISON OF PCA TO CONTINUOUS NERVE BLOCKS

As discussed earlier and in Chapter 12, continuous infusion of a local anesthetic near a peripheral nerve can provide anesthesia to a specific area of the body. These continuous nerve blocks have become very popular as a method of pain control following various surgical procedures. When compared to IV-PCA using opioids, continuous nerve blocks have typically been shown to provide better immediate postoperative pain control with fewer opioid-related side effects such as sedation, nausea, and pruritis.[61-63] This idea makes sense considering that the continuous nerve block provides a local *anesthetic* effect rather than an analgesic effect on the CNS. When compared with opioid PCEA, continuous nerve blocks seem to be fairly similar in providing postoperative pain control.[64,65] However, introducing a catheter into the epidural space may be associated with more serious safety concerns than placing a catheter near a peripheral nerve.

Pain control may be excellent with continuous local anesthetic administration because the patient literally cannot feel any sensation in the affected area. On the other hand, continuous nerve blocks are associated with certain problems such as loss of motor function in the affected area, infection, possible injury to the peripheral nerve, and the chance for serious toxicity if the local anesthetic reaches the systemic circulation.[66]

Clearly, continuous nerve blocks and PCA techniques are each associated with certain advantages and disadvantages when controlling postoperative pain or other acute and chronic pain syndromes. Ultimately, selection of a specific method for pain control depends on each patient, the type and location of surgery performed, and the experience of the practitioner. In fact, some patients may obtain optimal pain control by combining different techniques. Such "multimodal" techniques might include perineural application of a local anesthetic (either continuous infusion or a single shot of drug at the end of surgery) plus opioid IV-PCA to supplement the nerve block or serve as "rescue" therapy if the nerve block is inadequate.[63] Regardless of the exact techniques used, patients with acute or chronic pain must be treated effectively to allow physical rehabilitation and to achieve optimal functional outcomes. Researchers continue to clarify which techniques can be used alone or together to provide effective analgesia in specific clinical situations.

PROBLEMS AND ADVERSE EFFECTS OF PCA

Pharmacological Adverse Effects

When opioids are used for PCA, side effects typically include sedation, pruritus, and gastrointestinal problems (nausea, vomiting). However, the incidence of these side effects during PCA is normally similar to, or less than, the incidence associated with other administration techniques such as continuous infusion and intermittent IV or intramuscular dosing.[47,59,67] Respiratory depression is another common side effect of opioid use, but again, there is no increased incidence of this problem when appropriate amounts of opioids are given via PCA.[68,69] In fact, patients receiving IV-PCA may have a reduced risk of post-operative respiratory depression compared to other techniques such as a single dose of extended-release morphine that is administered epidurally.[70] Likewise, the risk of respiratory depression during IV-PCA can be minimized if a background infusion is not used (i.e., only on-demand doses are administered).[71-73] Furthermore, respiratory depression is believed to be negligible when patients receive opioids through spinal routes (epidural and intrathecal).[28,74] Therefore, when PCA techniques are used to administer opioids, there does not seem to be an increase in the side effects commonly associated with these drugs. In fact, the side effects may even be reduced during certain types of PCA application.

The incidence of side effects during PCA with local anesthetics is not well defined. Local anesthetics could conceivably cause sensory loss and motor weakness below the level of administration during PCEA. The possibility of these effects is directly dependent on the dose and type of local anesthetic. Practitioners usually try to use agents such as bupivacaine and ropivacaine because these drugs tend to produce sensory effects with minimal motor loss. Also, local anesthetic side effects can be minimized during PCEA by combining the local anesthetic with an opioid, thus reducing the total amount of each drug.[74] Some degree of sensory and motor loss will also occur when local anesthetics are administered into other peripheral sites, especially near specific peripheral nerves (i.e., single-shot perineural PCRA or continuous nerve blocks). Hence, transient sensory and motor loss must always be considered as a potential side effect when local anesthetics are used during PCA.

Problems With PCA Delivery

Other problems that can occur with PCA systems include operator errors (errors on the part of the nurse, physician, etc.), patient errors, and mechanical problems with the pump-delivery system.[75] These problems are summarized in Table 17-3. Operator errors

Table 17-3
SUMMARY OF PROBLEMS THAT CAN OCCUR DURING PCA THERAPY

Operator Errors	Patient Errors	Mechanical Problems
Misprogramming PCA device	Failure to understand PCA therapy	Failure to deliver on demand
Failure to clamp or unclamp tubing	Misunderstanding PCA pump device	Cracked drug vials or syringes
Improperly loading syringe or cartridge	Intentional analgesic abuse	Defective one-way valve at Y connector
Inability to respond to safety alarms		Faulty alarm system
Misplacing PCA pump key		Malfunctions (e.g., lock)

Source: White PF. Mishaps with patient-controlled analgesia. Anesthesiology. 1987;66:81-83; with permission.

typically occur because the pump is not programmed correctly or some other error occurs in loading the analgesic.[75,76] Fortunately, technological developments in PCA pumps have helped minimize operator errors by incorporating better safeguards for programming the pump properly (e.g., the DERS technologies discussed earlier) and for administering drugs correctly.[77] Likewise, implementing regular training programs and safety guidelines for health-care providers can help reduce the incidence of adverse effects associated with PCA.[76,78]

Patient errors can likewise compromise safety and effectiveness if the patient is not properly educated in PCA use or if he or she lacks adequate cognitive skills to use the PCA correctly.[22] Problems can likewise occur if the patient intentionally tries to administer more drug than necessary to adequately control pain—that is, the patient attempts to use the PCA as a form of drug abuse. Although the safeguards provided by the device (small demand dose, appropriate lockout interval) should prevent addiction, these PCA systems are not usually as successful in controlling pain in people with a history of opioid addiction. Finally, mechanical problems, including pump malfunction and clogging or displacement of the delivery tubing, may preclude delivery of the analgesic. Members of the health-care team should be alert for signs that the drug is being overdelivered during PCA, as evidenced by an increase in analgesic side effects, or that the analgesic is being underdelivered, as indicated by inadequate pain control.

Special Concerns for Rehabilitation Patients

When used appropriately, PCA offers several advantages to patients receiving physical therapy and occupational therapy. As discussed previously, PCA often provides analgesia with a lower chance of side effects such as sedation. Patients will be more alert and will have a clearer sensorium while still receiving optimal pain control. Likewise, PCA prevents large fluctuations in plasma analgesic concentration and helps maintain analgesic concentration within a more finite range (see Fig. 17-1). This decreases the need to schedule rehabilitation at a time when analgesic concentrations are at optimal levels because concentrations should always be within the appropriate range. Patients may also be more mobile using various PCA systems as compared with more traditional analgesic methods. The use of PCA may allow patients to begin ambulation sooner following surgery, and PCA systems can help decrease the need for the patient to be bed-bound for long periods because of severe pain or the side effects from high, intermittent doses of analgesics.[41,53,79] Rehabilitation specialists should therefore capitalize on the advantages of PCA whenever possible.

Rehabilitation specialists should also be aware of potential problems that can occur in patients receiving PCA. In particular, therapists should monitor the patient's signs and symptoms to help detect problems in PCA delivery. Therapists should use visual analog scales or some other valid measurement tool to routinely assess pain in patients receiving PCA. Patients exhibiting inadequate pain management or an unexplained increase in pain may be using a PCA system that is underdelivering the analgesic drug. The medical and nursing staff should be notified so that the delivery problem can be identified and rectified. Conversely, signs of respiratory depression or excessive sedation may indicate that the patient is being overdosed by the PCA system. This can obviously be a life-threatening situation that requires immediate attention. It is the responsibility of all health-care workers, including rehabilitation specialists, to look for signs of PCA malfunction every time they interact with the patient.

CASE STUDY

PATIENT-CONTROLLED ANALGESIA

Brief History. S.G., a 61-year-old man, was being treated for severe osteoarthritis in the right knee. Following an unsuccessful course of conservative therapy, S.G. was admitted to the hospital for a total knee replacement. The surgery was performed successfully, and PCA was instituted for postoperative pain management. PCA consisted of an external syringe pump connected to an IV catheter. The analgesic, meperidine (Demerol), was used at a concentration of 10 mg/mL. Parameters for PCA were set by the physician to allow a demand dose of 1 mL (10 mg) with a lockout interval of 10 minutes. An initial or loading dose of 10 mg was also provided at the conclusion of the surgery. Physical therapy was initiated at the patient's bedside on the afternoon following surgery. The therapist found the patient asleep and impossible to arouse. Family members who were present in the room said that he had been asleep since returning to his room.

Problem/Influence of Drug Therapy. The therapist was concerned because the patient was unresponsive to any commands. His breathing seemed labored and the color of his skin and mucous membranes had a slight, distinct bluish twinge indicative of cyanosis. The therapist noticed the pulse oximeter on his finger, which indicated hemoglobin saturation was 86 percent, well below normal values (i.e., 95 to 100 percent). The pulse oximeter normally has an alarm set for 90 percent, but this alarm had been shut off. The therapist immediately notified the nurses, who intervened and discontinued the PCA drug delivery. This device had been administering excessive amounts of opioid, resulting in unresponsiveness and decreased respiration.

1. *How can PCA cause respiratory problems?*
2. *What are some possible reasons for the apparent overdose observed in this case?*

See Appendix C, "Answers to Case Study Questions."

SUMMARY

PCA allows the patient to self-administer a small amount of analgesic medication on a relatively frequent basis. This technique has been used to administer drugs such as opioids and local anesthetics. PCA can often provide better pain control, especially with regard to increased patient satisfaction about their analgesic regimen. The patient is encouraged to self-administer a small dose of the drug by pressing a button that is connected to a pump. These PCA pumps vary in cost, level of sophistication, and location (external versus surgically implanted), but all pumps are capable of being programmed to prevent the patient from exceeding certain dosing parameters. PCA systems continue to be a mainstay in the management of patients with acute and chronic pain. Rehabilitation specialists should be aware that PCA can improve pain control and enhance the patient's recovery. Human error or mechanical malfunction during PCA, however, may cause excessive or inadequate drug delivery, so therapists should also be alert for any signs that patients are receiving too much or too little analgesic during PCA.

REFERENCES

1. Mann C, Ouro-Bang'na F, Eledjam JJ. Patient-controlled analgesia. *Curr Drug Targets.* 2005;6:815-819.
2. Hudcova J, McNicol E, Quah C, et al. Patient controlled opioid analgesia versus conventional opioid analgesia for postoperative pain. *Cochrane Database Syst Rev.* 2006;4:CD003348.
3. Palmer PP, Miller RD. Current and developing methods of patient-controlled analgesia. *Anesthesiol Clin.* 2010;28:587-599.
4. Brogan SE, Winter NB. Patient-controlled intrathecal analgesia for the management of breakthrough cancer pain: a retrospective review and commentary. *Pain Med.* 2011;12:1758-1768.

5. Momeni M, Crucitti M, De Kock M. Patient-controlled analgesia in the management of postoperative pain. *Drugs*. 2006;66:2321-2337.
6. Stratmann G, Gambling DR, Moeller-Bertram T, et al. A randomized comparison of a five-minute versus fifteen-minute lockout interval for PCEA during labor. *Int J Obstet Anesth*. 2005;14:200-207.
7. White I, Ghinea R, Avital S, et al. Morphine at "sub-analgesic" background infusion rate plus low-dose PCA bolus control pain better and is as safe as twice a bolus-only PCA regimen: a randomized, double blind study. *Pharmacol Res*. 2012;66:185-191.
8. Chen WH, Liu K, Tan PH, Chia YY. Effects of postoperative background PCA morphine infusion on pain management and related side effects in patients undergoing abdominal hysterectomy. *J Clin Anesth*. 2011;23:124-129.
9. George JA, Lin EE, Hanna MN, et al. The effect of intravenous opioid patient-controlled analgesia with and without background infusion on respiratory depression: a meta-analysis. *J Opioid Manag*. 2010;6:47-54.
10. Sam WJ, MacKey SC, Lötsch J, Drover DR. Morphine and its metabolites after patient-controlled analgesia: considerations for respiratory depression. *J Clin Anesth*. 2011;23:102-106.
11. Capogna G, Stirparo S. Techniques for the maintenance of epidural labor analgesia. *Curr Opin Anaesthesiol*. 2013;26:261-267.
12. Sia AT, Leo S, Ocampo CE. A randomised comparison of variable-frequency automated mandatory boluses with a basal infusion for patient-controlled epidural analgesia during labour and delivery. *Anaesthesia*. 2013;68:267-275.
13. Carstensen M, Møller AM. Adding ketamine to morphine for intravenous patient-controlled analgesia for acute postoperative pain: a qualitative review of randomized trials. *Br J Anaesth*. 2010;104:401-406.
14. Chen JY, Ko TL, Wen YR, et al. Opioid-sparing effects of ketorolac and its correlation with the recovery of postoperative bowel function in colorectal surgery patients: a prospective randomized double-blinded study. *Clin J Pain*. 2009;25:485-489.
15. Mathews TJ, Churchhouse AM, Housden T, Dunning J. Does adding ketamine to morphine patient-controlled analgesia safely improve post-thoracotomy pain? *Interact Cardiovasc Thorac Surg*. 2012;14:194-199.
16. McKeage K, Simpson D, Wagstaff AJ. Intravenous droperidol: a review of its use in the management of postoperative nausea and vomiting. *Drugs*. 2006;66:2123-2147.
17. Movafegh A, Shoeibi G, Ansari M, et al. Naloxone infusion and post-hysterectomy morphine consumption: a double-blind, placebo-controlled study. *Acta Anaesthesiol Scand*. 2012;56:1241-1249.
18. Murphy JD, Gelfand HJ, Bicket MC, et al. Analgesic efficacy of intravenous naloxone for the treatment of postoperative pruritus: a meta-analysis. *J Opioid Manag*. 2011;7:321-327
19. Bang EC, Lee HS, Kang YI, et al. Onset of labor epidural analgesia with ropivacaine and a varying dose of fentanyl: a randomized controlled trial. *Int J Obstet Anesth*. 2012;21:45-50.
20. Tveit TO, Seiler S, Halvorsen A, Rosland JH. Labour analgesia: a randomised, controlled trial comparing intravenous remifentanil and epidural analgesia with ropivacaine and fentanyl. *Eur J Anaesthesiol*. 2012;29:129-136.
21. [No authors listed]. Patient-controlled analgesic infusion pumps. Making a painless purchase. *Health Devices*. 2011;40:42-58.
22. Chumbley G, Mountford L. Patient-controlled analgesia infusion pumps for adults. *Nurs Stand*. 2010;25:35-40.
23. Ilias W, Todoroff B. Optimizing pain control through the use of implantable pumps. *Med Devices*. 2008;1:41-47.
24. Skryabina EA, Dunn TS. Disposable infusion pumps. *Am J Health Syst Pharm*. 2006;63:1260-1268.
25. Zimmermann M, Friedrich K, Kirchner R. Electronically monitored single-use patient-controlled analgesia pumps in postoperative pain control. *J Opioid Manag*. 2005;1:267-272.
26. Chrubasik J, Chrubasik S, Martin E. Patient-controlled spinal opiate analgesia in terminal cancer. Has its time really arrived? *Drugs*. 1992;43:799-804
27. Choi PT, Bhandari M, Scott J, Douketis J. Epidural analgesia for pain relief following hip or knee replacement. *Cochrane Database Syst Rev*. 2003;3:CD003071.
28. Behera BK, Puri GD, Ghai B. Patient-controlled epidural analgesia with fentanyl and bupivacaine provides better analgesia than intravenous morphine patient-controlled analgesia for early thoracotomy pain. *J Postgrad Med*. 2008;54:86-90.
29. Clarke H, Chandy T, Srinivas C, et al. Epidural analgesia provides better pain management after live liver donation: a retrospective study. *Liver Transpl*. 2011;17:315-323.
30. Mann C, Pouzeratte Y, Eledjam JJ. Postoperative patient-controlled analgesia in the elderly: risks and benefits of epidural versus intravenous administration. *Drugs Aging*. 2003;20:337-345.
31. Horlocker TT. Pain management in total joint arthroplasty: a historical review. *Orthopedics*. 2010;33(suppl):14-19.
32. Harvey GP, Chelly JE, AlSamsam T, Coupe K. Patient-controlled ropivacaine analgesia after arthroscopic subacromial decompression. *Arthroscopy*. 2004;20:451-455.
33. Anakwenze OA, Hosalkar H, Huffman GR. Case reports: two cases of glenohumeral chondrolysis after intraarticular pain pumps. *Clin Orthop Relat Res*. 2010;468:2545-2549.
34. Busfield BT, Romero DM. Pain pump use after shoulder arthroscopy as a cause of glenohumeral chondrolysis. *Arthroscopy*. 2009;25:647-652.
35. Fredrickson MJ, Krishnan S, Chen CY. Postoperative analgesia for shoulder surgery: a critical appraisal and review of current techniques. *Anaesthesia*. 2010;65:608-624.
36. Goyal N, McKenzie J, Sharkey PF, et al. The 2012 Chitranjan Ranawat award: intraarticular analgesia after TKA reduces pain: a randomized, double-blinded, placebo-controlled, prospective study. *Clin Orthop Relat Res*. 2013;471:64-75.
37. Chelly JE, Ghisi D, Fanelli A. Continuous peripheral nerve blocks in acute pain management. *Br J Anaesth*. 2010;105 (suppl 1):i86-96.
38. Ilfeld BM. Continuous peripheral nerve blocks: a review of the published evidence. *Anesth Analg*. 2011;113:904-925.
39. Herndon CM. Iontophoretic drug delivery system: focus on fentanyl. *Pharmacotherapy*. 2007;27:745-754.
40. Sathyan G, Phipps B, Gupta SK. Passive absorption of fentanyl from the fentanyl HCl iontophoretic transdermal system. *Curr Med Res Opin*. 2009;25:363-366.
41. Bourne MH, Chelly JE, Damaraju CV, Nelson WW, Schein JR, Hewitt DJ. Physical therapists' perceptions of ease of care in patients receiving 2 forms of analgesia after total hip arthroplasty. *Phys Ther*. 2010;90:707-713.
42. Mattia C, Coluzzi F, Sonnino D, Anker-Møller E. Efficacy and safety of fentanyl HCl iontophoretic transdermal system compared with morphine intravenous patient-controlled analgesia for postoperative pain management for patient subgroups. *Eur J Anaesthesiol*. 2010;27:433-440.

43. Minkowitz HS, Rathmell JP, Vallow S, et al. Efficacy and safety of the fentanyl iontophoretic transdermal system (ITS) and intravenous patient-controlled analgesia (IV PCA) with morphine for pain management following abdominal or pelvic surgery. *Pain Med.* 2007;8:657-668.
44. Macintyre PE. Intravenous patient-controlled analgesia: one size does not fit all. *Anesthesiol Clin North America.* 2005;23:109-123.
45. Bainbridge D, Martin JE, Cheng DC. Patient-controlled versus nurse-controlled analgesia after cardiac surgery—a meta-analysis. *Can J Anaesth.* 2006;53:492-499.
46. Crisp CC, Bandi S, Kleeman SD, et al. Patient-controlled versus scheduled, nurse-administered analgesia following vaginal reconstructive surgery: a randomized trial. *Am J Obstet Gynecol.* 2012;207:433.e1-6.
47. Ebneshahidi A, Akbari M, Heshmati B. Patient-controlled versus nurse-controlled post-operative analgesia after caesarean section. *Adv Biomed Res.* 2012;1:6.
48. Ng TK, Cheng BC, Chan WS, et al. A double-blind randomized comparison of intravenous patient-controlled remifentanil with intramuscular pethidine for labour analgesia. *Anaesthesia.* 2011;66:796-801.
49. Birnbaum A, Schechter C, Tufaro V, et al. Efficacy of patient-controlled analgesia for patients with acute abdominal pain in the emergency department: a randomized trial. *Acad Emerg Med.* 2012;19:370-377.
50. Rahman NH, DeSilva T. A randomized controlled trial of patient-controlled analgesia compared with boluses of analgesia for the control of acute traumatic pain in the emergency department. *J Emerg Med.* 2012;43:951-957.
51. Tveit TO, Halvorsen A, Seiler S, Rosland JH. Efficacy and side effects of intravenous remifentanil patient-controlled analgesia used in a stepwise approach for labour: an observational study. *Int J Obstet Anesth.* 2013;22:19-25.
52. Conner M, Deane D. Patterns of patient-controlled analgesia and intramuscular analgesia. *Appl Nurs Res.* 1995;8:67-72.
53. Saeki H, Ishimura H, Higashi H, et al. Postoperative management using intensive patient-controlled epidural analgesia and early rehabilitation after an esophagectomy. *Surg Today.* 2009;39:476-480.
54. Asha SE, Curtis KA, Taylor C, Kwok A. Patient-controlled analgesia compared with interval analgesic dosing for reducing complications in blunt thoracic trauma: a retrospective cohort study. *Emerg Med J.* 2013;30:1024-1028.
55. Choinière M, Rittenhouse BE, Perreault S, et al. Efficacy and costs of patient-controlled analgesia versus regularly administered intramuscular opioid therapy. *Anesthesiology.* 1998;89:1377-1388.
56. Ali M, Winter DC, Hanly AM, et al. Prospective, randomized, controlled trial of thoracic epidural or patient-controlled opiate analgesia on perioperative quality of life. *Br J Anaesth.* 2010;104:292-297.
57. Bartha E, Carlsson P, Kalman S. Evaluation of costs and effects of epidural analgesia and patient-controlled intravenous analgesia after major abdominal surgery. *Br J Anaesth.* 2006;96:111-117.
58. Haydon ML, Larson D, Reed E, et al. Obstetric outcomes and maternal satisfaction in nulliparous women using patient-controlled epidural analgesia. *Am J Obstet Gynecol.* 2011;205:271.e1-6.
59. Shen MK, Wu ZF, Zhu AB, et al. Remifentanil for labour analgesia: a double-blinded, randomised controlled trial of maternal and neonatal effects of patient-controlled analgesia versus continuous infusion. *Anaesthesia.* 2013;68:236-244.
60. Vallejo MC, Ramesh V, Phelps AL, Sah N. Epidural labor analgesia: continuous infusion versus patient-controlled epidural analgesia with background infusion versus without a background infusion. *J Pain.* 2007;8:970-975.
61. Baranović S, Maldini B, Milosević M, et al. Peripheral regional analgesia with femoral catheter versus intravenous patient controlled analgesia after total knee arthroplasty: a prospective randomized study. *Coll Antropol.* 2011;35:1209-1214.
62. Chan EY, Fransen M, Sathappan S, et al. Comparing the analgesia effects of single-injection and continuous femoral nerve blocks with patient controlled analgesia after total knee arthroplasty. *J Arthroplasty.* 2013;28:608-613.
63. Paul JE, Arya A, Hurlburt L, et al. Femoral nerve block improves analgesia outcomes after total knee arthroplasty: a meta-analysis of randomized controlled trials. *Anesthesiology.* 2010;113:1144-1162.
64. Fowler SJ, Symons J, Sabato S, Myles PS. Epidural analgesia compared with peripheral nerve blockade after major knee surgery: a systematic review and meta-analysis of randomized trials. *Br J Anaesth.* 2008;100:154-164.
65. Pöpping DM, Zahn PK, Van Aken HK, et al. Effectiveness and safety of postoperative pain management: a survey of 18 925 consecutive patients between 1998 and 2006 (2nd revision): a database analysis of prospectively raised data. *Br J Anaesth.* 2008;101:832-840.
66. Swenson JD. Use of catheters in the postoperative patient. *Orthopedics.* 2010;33(suppl):20-22.
67. Morad A, Winters B, Stevens R, et al. The efficacy of intravenous patient-controlled analgesia after intracranial surgery of the posterior fossa: a prospective, randomized controlled trial. *Anesth Analg.* 2012;114:416-423.
68. Lehmann KA. Recent developments in patient-controlled analgesia. *J Pain Symptom Manage.* 2005;29(suppl):S72-89.
69. Weber LM, Ghafoor VL, Phelps P. Implementation of standard order sets for patient-controlled analgesia. *Am J Health Syst Pharm.* 2008;65:1184-1191.
70. Sumida S, Lesley MR, Hanna MN, et al. Meta-analysis of the effect of extended-release epidural morphine versus intravenous patient-controlled analgesia on respiratory depression. *J Opioid Manag.* 2009;5:301-305.
71. George JA, Lin EE, Hanna MN, et al. The effect of intravenous opioid patient-controlled analgesia with and without background infusion on respiratory depression: a meta-analysis. *J Opioid Manag.* 2010;6:47-54.
72. Grissinger M. Beware of basal opioid infusions with patient-controlled analgesia. *P T.* 2012;37:605-619.
73. Sam WJ, MacKey SC, Lötsch J, Drover DR. Morphine and its metabolites after patient-controlled analgesia: considerations for respiratory depression. *J Clin Anesth.* 2011;23:102-106.
74. Liu SS, Bieltz M, Wukovits B, John RS. Prospective survey of patient-controlled epidural analgesia with bupivacaine and hydromorphone in 3736 postoperative orthopedic patients. *Reg Anesth Pain Med.* 2010;35:351-354.
75. Schein JR, Hicks RW, Nelson WW, et al. Patient-controlled analgesia-related medication errors in the postoperative period: causes and prevention. *Drug Saf.* 2009;32:549-559.

76. Paul JE, Bertram B, Antoni K, et al. Impact of a comprehensive safety initiative on patient-controlled analgesia errors. *Anesthesiology*. 2010;113:1427-1432.
77. Tran M, Ciarkowski S, Wagner D, Stevenson JG. A case study on the safety impact of implementing smart patient-controlled analgesic pumps at a tertiary care academic medical center. *Jt Comm J Qual Patient Saf.* 2012;38:112-119.
78. Ferguson R, Williams ML, Beard B. Combining quality improvement and staff development efforts to decrease patient-controlled analgesia pump errors. *J Nurses Staff Dev*. 2010; 26:E1-4.
79. Izumi Y, Amaya F, Hosokawa K, et al. Five-day pain management regimen using patient-controlled analgesia facilitates early ambulation after cardiac surgery. *J Anesth*. 2010;24:187-191.

SECTION

5

Autonomic and Cardiovascular Pharmacology

CHAPTER 18

Introduction to Autonomic Pharmacology

The human nervous system can be divided into two major functional areas: the somatic nervous system and the autonomic nervous system (ANS). The somatic division is concerned primarily with voluntary function—that is, control of the skeletal musculature. The ANS is responsible for controlling bodily functions that are largely involuntary, or automatic, in nature. For instance, the control of blood pressure (BP) and other aspects of cardiovascular function are under the influence of the ANS. This system also controls other involuntary, or vegetative, functions such as digestion, elimination, and thermoregulation.

Considering the potential problems that can occur in various systems, such as the cardiovascular and digestive systems, the use of therapeutic drugs to alter autonomic function is one of the major areas of pharmacology. Drugs affecting autonomic function are prescribed routinely to patients, including those seen for physical therapy and occupational therapy. The purpose of this chapter is to review some of the primary anatomical and physiological aspects of the ANS. This review is intended to provide you with a basis for understanding the pharmacological effects and clinical applications of the autonomic drugs, which are discussed in subsequent chapters.

ANATOMY OF THE AUTONOMIC NERVOUS SYSTEM: SYMPATHETIC AND PARASYMPATHETIC DIVISIONS

The ANS can be roughly divided into two primary areas: the sympathetic and parasympathetic nervous systems.[1,2] The *sympathetic*, or thoracolumbar, division arises primarily from neurons located in the thoracic and upper lumbar regions of the spinal cord. The *parasympathetic*, or craniosacral, division is composed of neurons originating in the midbrain, brainstem, and sacral region of the spinal cord. Some sources also consider the *enteric nervous system* to be a third ANS division. This system is comprised of an extensive network of neurons in the wall of the gastrointestinal (GI) tract that controls various aspects of GI function.[1,3] The enteric nervous system, however, contains both sympathetic and parasympathetic components and is therefore often considered part of the two primary ANS divisions. Hence, this chapter will focus on the sympathetic and parasympathetic systems, and the physiological and functional characteristics that differentiate these two primary ANS divisions. For a more detailed discussion of the anatomic and functional organization of the ANS, the references at the end of this chapter list several excellent sources.[1-4]

Preganglionic and Postganglionic Neurons

The somatic nervous system uses one neuron to reach from the central nervous system (CNS) to the periphery. In the somatic motor system, for instance, the alpha motor neuron begins in the spinal cord and extends all the way to the skeletal muscle—that is, it does not synapse until it reaches the muscle cell. In both the sympathetic and parasympathetic divisions, however, two neurons are used in sequence to reach from the CNS (i.e., brain or spinal cord) to the peripheral organ or tissue that is being supplied. The first neuron begins at a specific location in the CNS and extends a certain distance toward the periphery before synapsing with a second neuron, which completes the journey to the final destination. The synapse of these two neurons is usually in one of the autonomic ganglia (see the "Sympathetic Organization" and "Parasympathetic Organization" sections). Hence, the first neuron in sequence is termed the *preganglionic neuron*, and the second is referred to as the *postganglionic neuron*.

In both the sympathetic and parasympathetic divisions, preganglionic fibers are myelinated type B fibers, and postganglionic fibers are the small, unmyelinated type C fibers. In the sympathetic division, preganglionic neurons tend to be short, while the sympathetic postganglionic neurons are long. The opposite is true for the parasympathetic division—preganglionic neurons are long and postganglionic neurons are short. The location of preganglionic and postganglionic fibers in each autonomic division is presented here.

Sympathetic Organization

The cell bodies for the sympathetic preganglionic fibers arise from the intermediolateral gray columns of the thoracic and upper lumbar spinal cord. The preganglionic fibers leave the spinal cord via the ventral root of the spinal nerve and end in a sympathetic ganglion. The sympathetic ganglia are located in three areas:

- The paired paravertebral, or chain, ganglia, which lie bilaterally on either side of the vertebral column
- A group of unpaired prevertebral ganglia, which lie anterior to the aorta (e.g., the celiac plexus, the superior and inferior mesenteric ganglia)
- A small number of terminal ganglia, which lie directly in the tissue that is innervated (e.g., the bladder and rectum).

When the preganglionic fiber reaches one of the sympathetic ganglia, it synapses with a postganglionic fiber. Actually, one sympathetic preganglionic neuron may synapse with many postganglionic fibers. (The ratio of preganglionic to postganglionic fibers in the sympathetic chain ganglia is usually 1:15 to 1:20.)[2] The postganglionic fiber then leaves the ganglion to travel to the effector tissue that it supplies (i.e., the heart, peripheral arteriole, sweat gland, etc.).

Parasympathetic Organization

Parasympathetic preganglionic neurons originate in the midbrain and brainstem (cranial portion) or the sacral region of the spinal cord. Neurons comprising the cranial portion of the parasympathetics exit the CNS via cranial nerves III, VII, IX, and X. Cranial nerve X (vagus nerve) is particularly significant because it contains approximately 75 percent of the efferent component of the entire parasympathetic division. Neurons composing the preganglionic fibers of the sacral portion exit the spinal cord via the pelvic splanchnic nerves.

As in the sympathetic division, parasympathetic preganglionic neurons synapse in the periphery with a postganglionic fiber. This synapse usually takes place in a terminal ganglion that is located directly in the organ or tissue supplied by the postganglionic neuron. Consequently, the parasympathetic ganglia are usually embedded directly in the innervated organ or tissue.

Functional Aspects of the Sympathetic and Parasympathetic Divisions

Except for skeletal muscle, virtually all tissues in the body are innervated in some way by the ANS.[3] Table 18-1 summarizes the innervation and effects of the sympathetic and parasympathetic divisions on some of the major organs and tissues in the body. Some organs, such as the heart, are innervated by both sympathetic and parasympathetic neurons. Other tissues, however, may be supplied only by the sympathetic division. For instance, the sympathetic division innervates the peripheral arterioles, but these arterioles receive no parasympathetic innervation.

If an organ *is* innervated by both the sympathetic and parasympathetic divisions, a physiological antagonism typically exists between these divisions—that is, if both divisions innervate the tissue, one division usually increases function, whereas the other decreases

Table 18-1
RESPONSE OF EFFECTOR ORGANS TO AUTONOMIC STIMULATION

Organ	Sympathetic*	Parasympathetic†
Heart	Increased heart rate (beta-1, -2)	Decreased heart rate (M_2)
	Increased contractility (beta-1, -2)	Slight decrease in atrial contractility (M_2)
Arterioles	Vasoconstriction of skin and viscera (alpha-1, -2)	No parasympathetic innervation
	Vasodilation of skeletal muscle and liver (beta-2)	No parasympathetic innervation
Lung		
Airway smooth muscle	Bronchodilation (beta-2)	Bronchoconstriction (M_3)
Bronchial secretions	Increased secretion (beta-2); decreased secretion (alpha-1)	Increased secretion (M_2)
Eye		
Radial muscle of iris	Contraction (alpha-1)	No parasympathetic innervation
Circular muscle of iris	No sympathetic innervation	Contraction (M_3)
Ciliary muscle	Relaxation (beta-2)	Contraction (M_3)
GI function	Decreased motility and secretions (alpha-1, -2; beta-1, -2)	Increased motility and secretion (M_3)
Kidney	Increased renin secretion (beta-1)	No parasympathetic innervation
Urinary bladder		
Detrusor	Relaxation (beta-2)	Contraction (M_3)
Trigone and sphincter	Contraction (alpha-1)	Relaxation (M_3)
Sweat glands	Increased secretion (M‡)	No parasympathetic innervation
Liver	Glycogenolysis and gluconeogenesis (alpha-1, beta-2)	No parasympathetic innervation
Fat cells	Lipolysis (alpha-2, beta-1, -2, -3)	No parasympathetic innervation

**The primary receptor subtypes mediating each response are listed in parentheses (e.g., alpha-1, beta-2).*

†Organ responses to parasympathetic stimulation are mediated via muscarinic (M) receptors; the primary receptor subtype mediating each response is indicated by subscript numerals (M_2, M_3).

‡Represents response due to sympathetic postganglionic cholinergic fibers; the subtype of muscarinic receptor controlling human sweat glands has not been fully determined.

activity. For instance, the sympathetics increase heart rate and stimulate cardiac output, whereas the parasympathetics cause bradycardia. However, it is incorrect to state that the sympathetics are always excitatory in nature and that the parasympathetics are always inhibitory. In tissues such as the GI tract, the parasympathetics tend to increase intestinal motility and secretion, whereas the sympathetics slow down intestinal motility. The effect of each division on any tissue must be considered according to the particular organ or gland.

One generalization that can be made regarding sympathetic and parasympathetic function is that the sympathetic division tends to mobilize body energy, whereas the parasympathetic division tends to conserve and store it. Typically, sympathetic discharge is increased when the individual is faced with some stressful situation. This situation initiates the classic fight-or-flight scenario in which the body prepares for unusually strenuous exertion. Sympathetic discharge causes increased cardiac output, decreased visceral blood flow (thus leaving more blood available for skeletal muscle), increased cellular metabolism, and several other physiological changes that facilitate vigorous activity. In contrast, the parasympathetic division tends to have the opposite effect. Parasympathetic discharge slows down the heart and brings about changes that generally encourage inactivity. Parasympathetic discharge tends to increase intestinal digestion and absorption, an activity that stores energy for future needs.

Finally, activation of the sympathetic division tends to result in a more massive and diffuse reaction than does parasympathetic activation. Parasympathetic reactions, on the other hand, tend to be fairly discrete and affect only one organ or tissue. For instance, the parasympathetic fibers to the myocardium can be activated to slow down the heart without a concomitant emptying of the bowel through an excitatory effect on the lower GI tract. When the sympathetic division is activated, effects are commonly observed on many tissues throughout the body. The more diffuse sympathetic reactions routinely produce a simultaneous effect on the heart, total peripheral vasculature, general cellular metabolism, and so on.

FUNCTION OF THE ADRENAL MEDULLA

The adrenal medulla synthesizes and secretes norepinephrine and epinephrine directly into the bloodstream. Typically, the secretion from the adrenal medulla contains about 20 percent norepinephrine and 80 percent epinephrine.[5] These two hormones are fairly similar in action, except that epinephrine increases cardiac function and cellular metabolism to a greater extent because it has a higher affinity for certain receptors than norepinephrine (i.e., epinephrine binds more readily to the beta subtype of adrenergic receptors; see "Autonomic Receptors").[5]

The adrenal medulla is innervated by sympathetic neurons. During normal, resting conditions, the adrenal medulla secretes small amounts of epinephrine and norepinephrine. During periods of stress, however, a general increase in sympathetic discharge causes an increased release of epinephrine and norepinephrine from the adrenal medulla. Because these hormones are released directly into the bloodstream, they tend to circulate extensively throughout the body. Circulating epinephrine and norepinephrine can reach tissues that are not directly innervated by the sympathetic neurons, thus augmenting the general sympathetic effect. Also, the circulating epinephrine and norepinephrine are removed from the body more slowly than norepinephrine that is produced locally at the sympathetic postganglionic nerve terminals. As a result, adrenal release of epinephrine and norepinephrine tends to prolong the effect of the sympathetic reaction.

Consequently, the adrenal medulla serves to augment the sympathetic division of the ANS. In situations where a sudden increase in sympathetic function is required (i.e., the fight-or-flight scenario), the adrenal medulla works with the sympathetics to produce a more extensive and lasting response.

AUTONOMIC INTEGRATION AND CONTROL

Most of the autonomic control over various physiological functions is manifested through autonomic reflexes—that is, homeostatic control of BP, thermoregulation, and GI function depend on the automatic reflex adjustment in these systems through the sympathetic and/or parasympathetic divisions.[3,5] Autonomic reflexes are based on the following strategy: A peripheral sensor monitors a change in the particular system. This information is relayed to a certain level of the CNS, where it is integrated. An adjustment is made in the autonomic discharge to the specific organ or tissue, which will alter its activity to return physiological function back to the appropriate level.

A practical example of this type of autonomic reflex control is the baroreceptor reflex, which is important in the control of BP. In this example, pressure sensors (i.e., baroreceptors) located in the large arteries of the thorax and neck monitor changes in BP and heart rate. The baroreceptors sense a sudden drop in BP, and this information is relayed to the brainstem. In the brainstem, this information is integrated, and a compensatory increase occurs in sympathetic discharge to the heart and peripheral vasculature, and parasympathetic outflow to the heart is decreased. The result is an increase in cardiac output and an increase in peripheral vascular resistance, which effectively brings BP back to the appropriate level. The baroreceptor reflex also works in the opposite fashion—if BP were to suddenly increase, a decrease in sympathetic outflow and an increase in cardiac parasympathetic discharge would ultimately bring a return to normal pressure levels.

The baroreceptor response is just one example of the type of reflex activity the ANS employs. The control of other involuntary functions usually follows a similar pattern of peripheral monitoring, central integration, and altered autonomic discharge. Body temperature, for instance, is monitored by thermoreceptors located in the skin, viscera, and hypothalamus. When a change in body temperature is monitored by these sensors, this information is relayed to the hypothalamus and appropriate adjustments are made in autonomic discharge to maintain thermal homeostasis (e.g., sweating is increased or decreased and blood flow is redistributed). Many other autonomic reflexes that control visceral and involuntary functions operate in a similar manner.

Integration of autonomic responses is often fairly complex and may occur at several levels of the CNS. Some reflexes, such as emptying of the bowel and bladder, are integrated primarily at the level of the sacral spinal cord. Other reflexes, such as the baroreceptor reflex, are integrated at higher levels in the vasomotor center located in the brainstem. Also, the hypothalamus is important in regulating the ANS, and many functions—including body temperature, water balance, and energy metabolism—are controlled and integrated at the hypothalamus. To add to the complexity, higher levels of the brain, such as the cortex and limbic system, can also influence autonomic function through their interaction with the hypothalamus, brainstem, and spinal cord. This information is important pharmacologically because drugs that act on the CNS have the potential to alter autonomic function by influencing the central integration of autonomic responses. Drugs that affect the cortex, limbic system, and brainstem may indirectly alter the response of some of the autonomic reflexes by altering the relationship between afferent input and efferent sympathetic and parasympathetic outflow.

AUTONOMIC NEUROTRANSMITTERS

Acetylcholine and Norepinephrine

There are four sites of synaptic transmission in the efferent limb of the ANS:

- The synapse between the preganglionic and postganglionic neurons in the sympathetic division
- The analogous preganglionic-postganglionic synapse in the parasympathetic division
- The synapse between the sympathetic postganglionic neuron and the effector cell
- The parasympathetic postganglionic–effector cell synapse

Figure 18-1 summarizes the chemical neurotransmitter that is present at each synapse. The transmitter at the preganglionic-postganglionic synapse in both divisions is acetylcholine, as is the transmitter at the parasympathetic postganglionic–effector cell synapse. The transmitter at the sympathetic postganglionic–effector cell synapse is usually norepinephrine. A small number of sympathetic postganglionic fibers also use acetylcholine as their neurotransmitter.

Consequently, all preganglionic neurons and parasympathetic postganglionic neurons are said to be cholinergic in nature because of the presence of acetylcholine at their respective synapses. Most sympathetic postganglionic neurons use norepinephrine and are referred to as **adrenergic**. (Norepinephrine is sometimes referred to as *noradrenaline*, hence the term *adrenergic*.) An exception to this scheme is the presence of certain sympathetic postganglionic fibers that use acetylcholine as their neurotransmitter. These sympathetic cholinergic neurons innervate sweat glands and certain blood vessels in the face, neck, and lower extremities.

Other Autonomic Neurotransmitters

In recent years, it has become apparent that several nonadrenergic, noncholinergic neurotransmitters may also be present in the ANS. Purinergic substances such

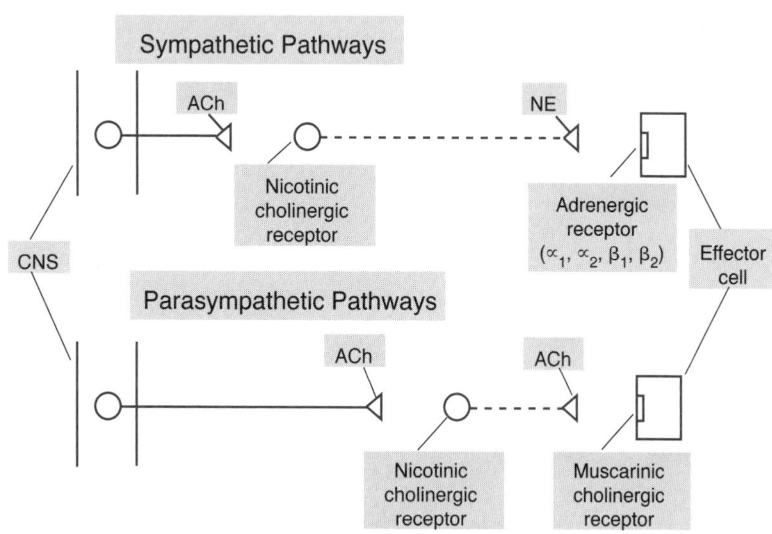

Figure ■ 18-1
Autonomic neurotransmitters and receptors. Preganglionic neurons (solid lines) release acetylcholine (ACh). Postganglionic neurons (dashed lines) release ACh in the parasympathetic pathways and norepinephrine (NE) in the sympathetic pathways.

as adenosine and adenosine triphosphate have been implicated as possible transmitters in the GI tract, cardiovascular system, and several other organs and systems influenced by autonomic nerves.[6-8] Researchers identified several peptides such as neuropeptide Y, vasoactive intestinal polypeptide, calcitonin gene-related peptide, orexin, cholecystokinin, and angiotensin II as possibly participating in the autonomic control of various organs and systems.[1,9-12] Nitric oxide may also help regulate various peripheral autonomic responses, and this substance may also control CNS autonomic activity.[8,13]

It is still uncertain whether all of these nonadrenergic, noncholinergic substances are true neurotransmitters. They may act as cotransmitters that are released from the synaptic terminal along with the classic autonomic transmitters (i.e., acetylcholine and norepinephrine). These other substances, however, may simply be produced locally and serve to modulate synaptic activity without actually being released from the presynaptic terminal. Nonetheless, future research will continue to clarify the role of these nonadrenergic, noncholinergic substances and identify how they affect normal physiological function as well as autonomic dysfunction in specific pathological conditions.[6,14]

AUTONOMIC RECEPTORS

Because there are two primary neurotransmitters involved in autonomic discharge, there are two primary classifications of postsynaptic receptors. Cholinergic receptors are located at acetylcholine synapses, and adrenergic receptors are located at norepinephrine synapses. As indicated in Figure 18-2, each type of receptor has several subclassifications. The location and functional significance of these classifications and subclassifications are presented here.

Cholinergic Receptors

Cholinergic receptors are subdivided into two categories: nicotinic and muscarinic. Although acetylcholine will bind to all cholinergic receptors, certain receptors bind preferentially with the drug nicotine. Other receptors have a specific affinity for muscarine, a naturally occurring compound found in certain poisonous mushrooms. Thus the terms *nicotinic* and *muscarinic* were derived.

Nicotinic cholinergic receptors are located at the junction between preganglionic and postganglionic neurons in both the sympathetic and parasympathetic pathways (see Fig. 18-1). This is significant pharmacologically because any drug that affects these nicotinic receptors will affect activity in both divisions of the ANS. The cholinergic nicotinic receptor located in the ANS is sometimes referred to as a type I (or N_N) nicotinic receptor to differentiate it from the type II (or N_M) nicotinic receptors, which are located at the skeletal neuromuscular junction.

Muscarinic cholinergic receptors are located at all of the synapses between cholinergic postganglionic neurons and the terminal effector cell, including all the parasympathetic terminal synapses and the sympathetic postganglionic cholinergic fibers that supply sweat glands and some specialized blood vessels. Current research suggests that there may be five subtypes of muscarinic receptors, classified as M_1, M_2, M_3, and so forth, based on their structural and chemical characteristics.[15] These receptors are found extensively throughout the body, with some tissues and organs

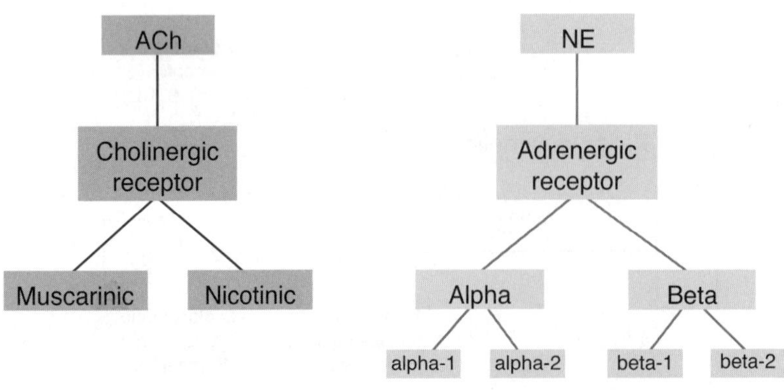

Figure ■ 18-2
Receptor classifications and subclassifications for acetylcholine (ACh) and norepinephrine (NE), the two primary neurotransmitters used in the autonomic nervous system.

containing more than one muscarinic receptor subtype. Specific muscarinic subtypes, however, may predominate at certain organ systems. For example, the M_1, M_4, and M_5 subtypes are abundant throughout the CNS,[4,16] whereas the M_2 receptor is predominant in the heart, and the M_3 subtype controls the bladder detrusor muscle and helps control pancreatic insulin release and other peripheral metabolic responses.[17,18] The exact role of these muscarinic receptor subtypes continues to be elucidated through ongoing research. Future studies will lend more insight to how each receptor subtype participates in normal function and whether drugs can be developed that affect specific muscarinic receptors in specific pathological conditions.

Thus, cholinergic muscarinic receptors ultimately mediate the effect on the tissue itself. Table 18-2 summarizes the primary physiological responses when muscarinic receptors are stimulated on various tissues in the body. Note that the specific response to stimulation of a muscarinic cholinergic receptor depends on the tissue in question. Stimulation of muscarinic receptors on the myocardium, for instance, causes a decrease in heart rate, whereas stimulation of muscarinic receptors in the intestinal wall leads to increases in smooth muscle contraction and glandular secretion.

Table 18-2
AUTONOMIC RECEPTOR LOCATIONS AND RESPONSES

Receptor	Primary Location(s)	Response*
Cholinergic		
Nicotinic	Autonomic ganglia	Mediate transmission to postganglionic neuron (N_N)
Muscarinic	CNS	Mediate effects of acetylcholine in various parts of brain (M_1–M_5)
	Visceral and bronchiole smooth muscle	Contraction (generally) (M_2, M_3)
	Cardiac muscle	Decreased heart rate (M_2)
	Exocrine glands (salivary, intestinal, lacrimal)	Increased secretion (M_1, M_3)
	Sweat glands	Increased secretion (M)†
Adrenergic		
Alpha-1	Vascular smooth muscle	Contraction
	Intestinal smooth muscle	Relaxation
	Radial muscle iris	Contraction (mydriasis)
	Ureters	Increased motility
	Urinary sphincter	Contraction
	Spleen capsule	Contraction
Alpha-2	CNS inhibitory synapses	Decreased sympathetic discharge from CNS
	Presynaptic terminal at peripheral adrenergic synapses	Decreased norepinephrine release
	GI tract	Decreased motility and secretion
	Pancreatic islet cells	Decreased insulin secretion
	Some arterioles (skeletal muscle, liver, kidneys)	Vasoconstriction
Beta-1	Cardiac muscle	Increased heart rate and contractility
	Kidney	Increased renin secretion
	Fat cells	Increased lipolysis

Continued

Table 18-2
AUTONOMIC RECEPTOR LOCATIONS AND RESPONSES—cont'd

Receptor	Primary Location(s)	Response*
Beta-2	Bronchiole smooth muscle	Relaxation (bronchodilation)
	Some arterioles (skeletal muscle, liver)	Vasodilation
	GI smooth muscle	Decreased motility
	Skeletal muscle and liver cells	Increased cellular metabolism
	Uterus	Relaxation
	Gallbladder	Relaxation
Beta-3	Fat cells	Increased lipolysis
	Bladder	Decreased contraction of detrusor muscle
	Heart	Decreased contractility

**Primary response that occurs when each receptor subtype is stimulated. Abbreviations: N_N: nicotinic receptor in autonomic ganglia; M: muscarinic receptor, with the subscript numeral indicating the primary receptor subtype(s) mediating each response (M_1, M_2, etc.).*

†Represents response due to sympathetic postganglionic cholinergic fibers; the subtype of muscarinic receptor controlling human sweat glands has not been fully determined.

Adrenergic Receptors

As shown in Figure 18-2, the adrenergic receptors are subdivided into two primary categories: alpha- and beta-adrenergic receptors. Alpha receptors are further subdivided into alpha-1 and alpha-2 receptors, and beta receptors are subdivided into beta-1, beta-2, and beta-3 receptors.[4] These divisions are based on the different sensitivities of each receptor subcategory to different endogenous and exogenous agents. Alpha-1 receptors, for instance, bind more readily with certain agonists and antagonists, whereas alpha-2 receptors bind preferentially with other agents. Specific agents that bind to each adrenergic receptor subcategory are identified in Chapter 20.

In the ANS, the various types of adrenergic receptors are found on the effector cell in the innervated tissue. In other words, these receptors are located at the terminal synapse between sympathetic postganglionic adrenergic neurons and the tissue they supply. The basic characteristics of each adrenergic receptor subtype are briefly outlined here.

Alpha-1 Receptors

A primary location of these receptors is the smooth muscle located in various tissues throughout the body. Alpha-1 receptors are located on the smooth muscle located in the peripheral vasculature, intestinal wall, radial muscle of the iris, ureters, urinary sphincter, and spleen capsule. The response of each tissue when the alpha-1 receptor is stimulated varies, depending on the tissue (see Table 18-2). Research also suggests that there might be three subtypes of alpha-1 receptors, identified as alpha-1A, alpha-1B, and alpha-1D receptors.[19] Much of this research, however, has focused on the characteristics of alpha-1 receptor subtypes in various animal models. Studies are currently under way to determine the exact location and functional significance of these alpha-1 receptor subtypes in humans.

Alpha-2 Receptors

The alpha-2 receptors were originally identified by their presence on the presynaptic terminal of certain adrenergic synapses.[20] These presynaptic alpha-2 receptors are sometimes called *autoreceptors* because they modulate the release of neurotransmitters from the presynaptic terminal. In other words, they decrease the release of norepinephrine and other chemicals, thus serving as a form of negative feedback that limits the amount of neurotransmitter released from the presynaptic terminal.[20] As discussed in Chapter 13, alpha-2 receptors are also on spinal interneurons, and stimulation of these alpha-2 receptors may cause decreased neurotransmitter release and diminished stimulation of the interneurons that influence the alpha motor neuron. Thus, alpha-2 stimulants (agonists), such as tizanidine, can decrease neuronal excitability in the spinal cord and thereby decrease muscle hyperexcitability in conditions such as spasticity. Also, alpha-2 receptors have been found postsynaptically on certain CNS adrenergic synapses involved in the control of sympathetic discharge.[21] Stimulation of these centrally located alpha-2 receptors is believed to inhibit sympathetic discharge from the brainstem. The importance of central alpha-2 receptors in controlling cardiovascular function and the possible use of alpha-2 agonists to control BP are discussed in Chapter 21.

Alpha-2 receptors are also located on CNS nonadrenergic neurons and seem to be important in regulating various other responses, including sedation and analgesia.[20] Stimulation of alpha-2 receptors located in the pancreas and GI tract causes decreased insulin secretion and decreased intestinal motility, respectively. Finally, alpha-2 receptors can be found in the vasculature of many tissues and organs such as the liver, kidneys, and skeletal muscle; stimulation of these receptors generally causes vasoconstriction in these tissues.

As is the case with alpha-1 receptors, we now believe that at least three subtypes of alpha-2 receptors may exist, namely alpha-2A, alpha-2B, and alpha-2C.[20] The functional and pharmacological significance of these different alpha-2 receptors remains to be fully determined.

Beta-1 Receptors

These receptors predominate in the heart and kidneys (see Table 18-2).[21] The cardiac beta-1 receptors have received a tremendous amount of attention with regard to pharmacological antagonism of their function through the use of beta blockers.

Beta-2 Receptors

Beta-2 receptors are found primarily on the smooth muscle of certain vasculatures, the bronchioles, the gallbladder, and the uterus.[1,21] Their presence in bronchiole smooth muscle is especially important in the pharmacological management of respiratory conditions such as asthma (see Chapter 26). These receptors are also responsible for mediating changes in the metabolism of skeletal muscle and liver cells. Beta-2 receptors are also located on the heart, although the predominant effects on cardiac tissue seem to be mediated through the beta-1 subtype.

Beta-3 Receptors

Although it was originally thought that only two subtypes of beta receptors existed, we now know that a third subtype, the beta-3 receptor, plays a functional role in certain tissues. In particular, beta-3 receptors are located on adipose tissue, and stimulation of beta-3 receptors increases lipolysis (see Table 18-2).[21] In addition, beta-3 receptors are found on the heart and bladder, and stimulation of these receptors generally inhibits muscular contraction in these tissues.[22-24]

PHARMACOLOGICAL SIGNIFICANCE OF AUTONOMIC RECEPTORS

Perhaps no area of research has contributed more to pharmacology than the identification, classification, and subclassification of autonomic receptors. The realization that various tissues have distinct subtypes of receptors has enabled the use of drugs affecting certain tissues and organs while causing minimal effects on other tissues. For instance, a beta-1 antagonist (i.e., a drug that specifically blocks the beta-1 adrenergic receptor) will slow down the heart rate and decrease myocardial contractility without causing any major changes in the physiological functions that are mediated by the other autonomic receptors.

However, there are several limitations of autonomic drugs to be considered. First, a drug that binds preferentially to one receptor subtype will bind to that receptor at all of its locations. For example, a muscarinic antagonist that decreases activity in the GI tract may also decrease bronchial secretions in the lungs and cause urinary retention because of relaxation of the detrusor muscle of the bladder. Also, no drug is entirely specific for only one receptor subtype. For instance, the beta-1–specific antagonists atenolol and metoprolol have a much greater affinity for beta-1 receptors than for beta-2 receptors.[25] At high enough concentrations, however, these drugs will affect beta-2 receptors as well. Finally, organs and tissues in the body do not contain only one subtype of receptor. For example, the predominant receptor in the bronchioles is the beta-2 subtype, but some beta-1 receptors are also present. Thus, a patient using a beta-1–specific drug such as metoprolol (Lopressor) may experience some respiratory effects as well.[25]

Consequently, the many side effects and beneficial effects of autonomic drugs can be attributed to the interaction of various agents with different receptors. The significance of autonomic receptor subtypes as well as the use of specific cholinergic and adrenergic drugs in treating various problems are covered in more detail in Chapters 19 and 20.

SUMMARY

The ANS is primarily responsible for controlling involuntary, or vegetative, functions in the body. The sympathetic and parasympathetic divisions of the ANS often function as physiological antagonists to maintain homeostasis of various activities, including BP control, thermoregulation, digestion, and elimination. The primary neurotransmitters used in synaptic transmission within the ANS are acetylcholine and norepinephrine. These chemicals are found at specific locations in each autonomic division, as are their respective cholinergic and adrenergic receptors. The two primary types of autonomic receptors (cholinergic and adrenergic) are classified according to differences in drug affinity. Cholinergic receptors are subclassified as muscarinic and nicotinic receptors, and adrenergic receptors are subclassified as alpha and beta receptors. Each subclass can be further categorized according to its location and affinity for certain substances. Receptor subtypes located on specific tissues are responsible for mediating a given tissue response when stimulated by an appropriate substance.

Autonomic drugs typically exert their therapeutic effects by either stimulating or blocking a specific subtype of cholinergic or adrenergic receptor. For example, drugs that block beta-1 adrenergic receptors on the heart will slow heart rate, while drugs that stimulate specific muscarinic cholinergic receptors in the GI tract will generally increase GI movement. The next several chapters will address other situations where autonomic drugs promote beneficial effects on specific tissues.

REFERENCES

1. Katzung BG. Introduction to autonomic pharmacology. In: Katzung BG, ed. *Basic and Clinical Pharmacology*. 12th ed. New York: Lange Medical Books/McGraw Hill; 2012.
2. Standring S, ed. *Gray's Anatomy*. 40th ed. New York: WB Saunders; 2008.
3. Kandel ER, Scwartz JH, Jessell TM, et al. The basal ganglia. In: *Principles of Neural Science*. 5th ed. New York: McGraw-Hill; 2013:982-998.
4. Westfall TC, Westfall DP. Neurotransmission: the autonomic and somatic motor nervous systems. In: Brunton L, et al, eds. *The Pharmacological Basis of Therapeutics*. 12th ed. New York: McGraw-Hill; 2011.
5. Hall JE, Guyton AC. *Textbook of Medical Physiology*. 12th ed. Philadelphia, PA: WB Saunders/Elsevier; 2011.
6. Burnstock G. Introduction to purinergic signalling in the brain. *Adv Exp Med Biol.* 2013;986:1-12.
7. Burnstock G. Introductory overview of purinergic signalling. *Front Biosci.* 2011;3:896-900.
8. Macarthur H, Wilken GH, Westfall TC, Kolo LL. Neuronal and non-neuronal modulation of sympathetic neurovascular transmission. *Acta Physiol.* 2011;203:37-45.
9. Bohlender J, Imboden H. Angiotensinergic neurotransmission in the peripheral autonomic nervous system. *Front Biosci.* 2012;17:2419-2432.
10. Harmar AJ, Fahrenkrug J, Gozes I, et al. Pharmacology and functions of receptors for vasoactive intestinal peptide and pituitary adenylate cyclase-activating polypeptide: IUPHAR review 1. *Br J Pharmacol.* 2012;166:4-17.
11. Kuwaki T. Orexin links emotional stress to autonomic functions. *Auton Neurosci.* 2011;161:20-27.
12. Nattie E, Li A. Respiration and autonomic regulation and orexin. *Prog Brain Res.* 2012;198:25-46. PMID: 22813968.
13. Hirooka Y, Kishi T, Sakai K, et al. Imbalance of central nitric oxide and reactive oxygen species in the regulation of sympathetic activity and neural mechanisms of hypertension. *Am J Physiol Regul Integr Comp Physiol.* 2011;300:R818-826.
14. Liu Y, Scherlag BJ, Fan Y, et al. Inducibility of atrial fibrillation after GP ablations and "autonomic blockade": evidence for the pathophysiological role of the nonadrenergic and noncholinergic neurotransmitters. *J Cardiovasc Electrophysiol.* 2013;24: 188-195.
15. Eglen RM. Overview of muscarinic receptor subtypes. *Handb Exp Pharmacol.* 2012;208:3-28.
16. Conn PJ, Jones CK, Lindsley CW. Subtype-selective allosteric modulators of muscarinic receptors for the treatment of CNS disorders. *Trends Pharmacol Sci.* 2009;30:148-155.
17. Gautam D, Jeon J, Li JH, et al. Metabolic roles of the M3 muscarinic acetylcholine receptor studied with M3 receptor mutant mice: a review. *J Recept Signal Transduct Res.* 2008;28:93-108.
18. Ruiz de Azua I, Gautam D, Jain S, et al. Critical metabolic roles of β-cell M3 muscarinic acetylcholine receptors. *Life Sci.* 2012;91:986-991.
19. Du L, Li M. Modeling the interactions between alpha(1)-adrenergic receptors and their antagonists. *Curr Comput Aided Drug Des.* 2010;6:165-178.
20. Gilsbach R, Hein L. Are the pharmacology and physiology of α_2 adrenoceptors determined by α_2-heteroreceptors and autoreceptors respectively? *Br J Pharmacol.* 2012;165:90-102.
21. Westfall TC, Westfall DP. Adrenergic agonists and antagonists. In: Brunton L, et al, eds. *The Pharmacological Basis of Therapeutics*. 12th ed. New York: McGraw-Hill; 2011.
22. Dessy C, Balligand JL. Beta3-adrenergic receptors in cardiac and vascular tissues emerging concepts and therapeutic perspectives. *Adv Pharmacol.* 2010;59:135-163.
23. Gauthier C, Rozec B, Manoury B, Balligand JL. Beta-3 adrenoceptors as new therapeutic targets for cardiovascular pathologies. *Curr Heart Fail Rep.* 2011;8:184-192.
24. Michel MC. β-Adrenergic receptor subtypes in the urinary tract. *Handb Exp Pharmacol.* 2011;202:307-318.
25. Robertson D, Biaggioni I. Adrenoceptor antagonist drugs. In: Katzung BG, ed. *Basic and Clinical Pharmacology*. 12th ed. New York: Lange Medical Books/McGraw Hill; 2012.

CHAPTER 19

Cholinergic Drugs

Cholinergic drugs affect the activity at cholinergic synapses—that is, synapses using acetylcholine as a neurotransmitter. Cholinergic synapses are important in several physiological systems. As discussed in Chapter 18, acetylcholine is one of the primary neurotransmitters in the autonomic nervous system (ANS), especially in the parasympathetic autonomic division. Consequently, physicians administer many of the drugs discussed in this chapter to alter the response of various tissues to autonomic parasympathetic control. Acetylcholine is also the neurotransmitter at the skeletal neuromuscular junction. Certain cholinergic stimulants are used to treat a specific problem at the skeletal neuromuscular junction (e.g., myasthenia gravis). The brain contains cholinergic synapses in specific areas, and some anticholinergic drugs decrease the symptoms of diverse problems such as parkinsonism and motion sickness. Cholinergic stimulants effectively increase activity at acetylcholine synapses, whereas anticholinergic drugs decrease synaptic activity. Cholinergic stimulants and anticholinergic agents can be further characterized according to functional or pharmacodynamic criteria, and these criteria will be discussed as well.

Considering the diverse clinical applications of cholinergic and anticholinergic agents, you will likely encounter patients taking these drugs. Knowledge of the pharmacodynamics of these medications will enable you to understand the therapeutic rationale behind drug administration as well as the patient's response to the drug.

CHOLINERGIC RECEPTORS

Many autonomic cholinergic drugs affect synaptic activity by interacting with the acetylcholine receptor located on the postsynaptic membrane. At each cholinergic synapse, postsynaptic receptors are responsible for recognizing the acetylcholine molecule and transducing the chemical signal into a postsynaptic response. As discussed in Chapter 18, cholinergic receptors can be subdivided into muscarinic and nicotinic receptors according to their affinity for certain drugs.[1]

Muscarinic cholinergic receptors are generally found on the peripheral tissues supplied by parasympathetic postganglionic neurons—that is, on effector organs such as the gastrointestinal (GI) tract, urinary bladder, heart, eye, and so on. Acetylcholine synapses found in specific areas of the central nervous system (CNS) also use the muscarinic subtype of cholinergic receptor. Nicotinic cholinergic receptors are located in the autonomic ganglia (i.e., the N_N nicotinic subtype) and at the skeletal neuromuscular junction (the N_M nicotinic subtype). Refer to Chapter 18 for a more detailed discussion of cholinergic receptor subclassification.

The existence of these different varieties of cholinergic receptors is important pharmacologically. Some drugs are relatively specific for a certain cholinergic receptor subtype, whereas others tend to bind rather indiscriminately to all cholinergic receptors. Obviously, specific drugs are preferable because they tend to produce a more precise response with fewer side effects. However, specificity is only a relative term, and drugs that bind preferentially to one receptor subtype may still produce a variety of responses.

CHOLINERGIC STIMULANTS

Cholinergic stimulants increase activity at acetylcholine synapses. Chemically, many agents are capable of potently and effectively stimulating cholinergic activity. However, only a few drugs exhibit sufficient safety and relative specificity for use in clinical situations. These clinically relevant drugs can be subdivided into two categories, depending on their mechanism of action. Direct-acting cholinergic stimulants exert their effects by binding directly with the cholinergic receptor (Fig. 19-1). Indirect-acting cholinergic stimulants increase synaptic activity by inhibiting the acetylcholinesterase enzyme located at the cholinergic synapse (see Fig. 19-1). Table 19-1 lists specific direct-acting and indirect-acting cholinergic stimulants. The direct-acting cholinergic stimulants and the rationale for their use are presented first.

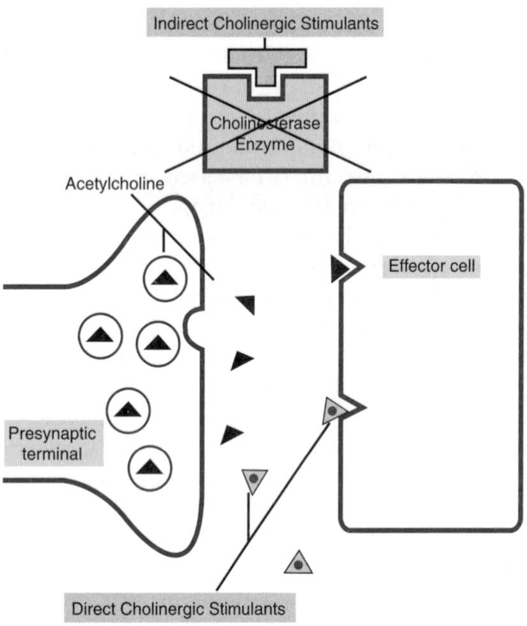

Figure ■ 19-1
Mechanism of action of cholinergic stimulants. Direct-acting stimulants bind directly to the postsynaptic cholinergic receptor. Indirect-acting stimulants inhibit the cholinesterase enzyme, thus allowing acetylcholine to remain in the synaptic cleft.

Direct-Acting Cholinergic Stimulants

Direct-acting stimulants bind directly to the cholinergic receptor to activate it, which in turn initiates a cellular response. These stimulants may be considered true cholinergic agonists, and they function in a manner similar to the acetylcholine molecule. By definition, acetylcholine is a direct-acting cholinergic stimulant. Exogenously administered acetylcholine is not used therapeutically, however, because it is degraded rapidly and extensively by the acetylcholinesterase enzyme, which is found ubiquitously throughout the body.

As mentioned previously, there are many pharmacological agents that can directly stimulate cholinergic receptors. A certain degree of drug specificity is desirable, though, when considering these agents for therapeutic purposes. For instance, drugs that have a greater specificity for the muscarinic cholinergic receptor are more beneficial. These muscarinic cholinergic stimulants will primarily affect the peripheral tissues while exerting a minimal effect on the cholinergic receptors located in the autonomic ganglia and the neuromuscular junction. (Recall that the cholinergic receptors found in the autonomic ganglia and at the skeletal neuromuscular junction are the N_N and N_M, respectively.)

Consequently, only a few agents are suitable for clinical use as direct-acting cholinergic stimulants. For systemic administration, bethanechol (Urecholine, others) is the primary direct-acting cholinergic stimulant (see Table 19-1). Bethanechol appears to preferentially stimulate muscarinic cholinergic receptors, especially those on GI and bladder tissues.[2,3] Hence, this drug is sometimes used to increase GI or bladder contractions, especially when motility in these tissues is reduced following abdominal surgery. Pilocarpine is another direct-acting cholinergic stimulant that can be administered orally to treat dry mouth associated with autoimmune diseases (Sjögren syndrome) or when damage has occurred to the salivary glands following radiation treatments for cancer. Other direct-acting cholinergic stimulants such as carbachol are typically limited to topical use in ophthalmologic conditions, especially glaucoma. These antiglaucoma drugs produce too many side effects if administered systemically but are relatively specific when administered directly to the eye. Likewise, methacholine is a direct-acting cholinergic stimulant that can

Table 19-1
CHOLINERGIC STIMULANTS

Generic Name	Trade Name(s)	Primary Clinical Use(s)*
Direct-Acting (Cholinergic Agonists)		
Bethanechol	Duvoid, Urecholine	Postoperative GI and urinary atony
Carbachol	Carboptic, Isopto Carbachol	Glaucoma
Methacholine	Provocholine	Diagnose asthma (used to test for airway hyper-responsiveness)
Pilocarpine	Pilocar, Isopto Carpine, many others	Glaucoma
Indirect-Acting (Cholinesterase Inhibitors)		
Ambenonium	Mytelase	Myasthenia gravis
Donepezil	Aricept	Alzheimer-type dementia
Echothiophate	Phospholine Iodide	Glaucoma
Edrophonium	Enlon, Reversol, Tensilon	Myasthenia gravis, reversal of neuromuscular blocking drugs
Galantamine	Razadyne, Reminyl	Alzheimer-type dementia
Isoflurophate	Diflupyl	Glaucoma
Neostigmine	Prostigmin	Postoperative GI and urinary atony, myasthenia gravis, reversal of neuromuscular blocking drugs
Physostigmine	Antilirium, Eserine Opht	Glaucoma, reversal of CNS toxicity caused by anticholinergic drugs
Pyridostigmine	Mestinon, Regonol	Myasthenia gravis, reversal of neuromuscular blocking drugs
Rivastigmine	Exelon	Dementia of the Alzheimer's type
Tacrine	Cognex	Alzheimer-type dementia

**Agents used to treat glaucoma and other visual disturbances are administered directly to the eye. Agents used for other problems are given systemically by oral administration or injection.*

be administered locally to the lungs via inhalation to test for airway hyper-responsiveness when diagnosing patients for asthma. Clinical applications of direct-acting cholinergic stimulants are summarized in Table 19-1.

Indirect-Acting Cholinergic Stimulants

Indirect-acting stimulants increase activity at cholinergic synapses by inhibiting the acetylcholinesterase enzyme.[4,5] This enzyme is normally responsible for destroying acetylcholine after this neurotransmitter is released from the presynaptic terminal. Indirect-acting stimulants inhibit the acetylcholinesterase, thus allowing more acetylcholine to remain at the synapse. The result is an increase in cholinergic synaptic transmission.

Because of their effect on the acetylcholinesterase enzyme, indirect-acting stimulants are also referred to as *cholinesterase inhibitors* or *anticholinesterase agents*. The exact way in which these drugs inhibit the acetylcholinesterase enzyme varies depending on the individual agent. The net effect is similar, however, in that the enzyme's ability to degrade acetylcholine is diminished by these drugs.

Unlike the systemic direct-acting cholinergic stimulants (e.g., bethanechol), cholinesterase inhibitors display a relative lack of specificity regarding which cholinergic synapses they stimulate. These drugs tend to inhibit the acetylcholinesterase found at many cholinergic synapses. Thus, they may exert a stimulatory effect on the peripheral muscarinic cholinergic synapses and on the cholinergic synapses found at the autonomic ganglia, at the skeletal neuromuscular junction, and within certain aspects of the CNS. In appropriate doses, certain agents exert some degree of specificity at peripheral versus CNS synapses. Indirect-acting stimulants such as neostigmine, for example, tend to predominantly affect the skeletal neuromuscular junction and peripheral tissues containing muscarinic receptors. In contrast, newer agents such as tacrine and donepezil show more specificity for cholinergic synapses in certain regions of the brain—hence, these newer drugs are being used to boost cholinergic function in conditions such as Alzheimer disease. Still, none of the indirect-acting cholinergic stimulants affect only one type of tissue, and some adverse side effects can be caused by their relatively nonspecific activity.

Indirect-acting cholinergic stimulants currently in use include neostigmine and pyridostigmine. Several other agents are also used therapeutically to treat systemic conditions such as myasthenia gravis, ophthalmologic disorders such as glaucoma, and diminished acetylcholine activity associated with degenerative brain syndromes such as Alzheimer disease (see Table 19-1).

Clinical Applications of Cholinergic Stimulants

Direct- and indirect-acting cholinergic stimulants are used to treat the decrease in smooth-muscle tone that sometimes occurs in the GI tract and urinary bladder following abdominal surgery or trauma. Indirect-acting stimulants are also used to treat glaucoma, myasthenia gravis, and in Alzheimer disease and to reverse the effects from an overdose of other drugs, such as neuromuscular blocking agents and anticholinergics. Each of these applications is briefly discussed here.

Alzheimer Disease

Alzheimer disease is a progressive neurodegenerative disorder that affects older adults. It is characterized by neuronal atrophy and other pathological changes in neuron structure and function throughout the brain (neurofibrillary tangles, formation of plaques, and so forth). Included in this neuronal degeneration are cholinergic neurons that are critical in memory, cognition, and other higher cortical functions.[6-8] Although there is no cure for this disease, indirect cholinergic stimulants such as tacrine (Cognex), donepezil (Aricept), galantamine (Reminyl), and rivastigmine (Exelon) (see Table 19-1) may help decrease some of the symptoms during the early stages of Alzheimer disease.[4,9,10] By inhibiting acetylcholine breakdown, these drugs prolong the effects of any acetylcholine released from neurons that are still functioning in the cerebral cortex.

Regrettably, these drugs do not alter the progression of Alzheimer disease, and they tend to lose effectiveness as the disease progresses into the advanced stages.[10,11] This loss of effectiveness makes sense because these drugs can only prolong the effects of endogenously released acetylcholine; they will have no effect when cortical neurons degenerate to the point where acetylcholine is no longer being synthesized and released within the brain. Nonetheless, drugs such as tacrine, donepezil, and other CNS cholinesterase inhibitors can help patients retain better cognitive function during the early stages of Alzheimer disease, which can help sustain a better quality of life for as long as possible.[9]

Gastrointestinal and Urinary Bladder Atony

After surgical manipulation or other trauma to the viscera, there is often a period of atony (i.e., lack of tone) in the smooth muscle of these organs. As a result, intestinal peristalsis is diminished or absent, and the urinary bladder becomes distended, leading to urinary retention. Under normal circumstances, acetylcholine released from parasympathetic postganglionic neurons would stimulate smooth-muscle contraction in these tissues. Consequently, medical practitioners administer cholinergic agonists (i.e., drugs that mimic or enhance the effects of acetylcholine) to treat atony. Bethanechol and neostigmine, a direct-acting and an indirect-acting cholinergic stimulant, respectively, are the drugs most frequently used for this condition until normal GI and urinary function is resumed.

Glaucoma

Glaucoma is an increase in intraocular pressure brought on by an accumulation of aqueous humor within the eye.[12] Normally, cholinergic stimulation via the parasympathetic supply to the eye increases the outflow of aqueous humor, thus preventing excessive accumulation that leads to impaired vision and blindness if left untreated.

To treat glaucoma, direct-acting and indirect-acting cholinergic drugs are usually applied topically to the eye by placing the drug directly within the conjunctival sac (see Table 19-1). This application concentrates the action of the drug, thus limiting the side effects that might occur if these agents were given systemically. These agents are not typically the first drugs used to treat glaucoma, but they can be used if other agents are not effective.[13-15]

Myasthenia Gravis

Myasthenia gravis affects the skeletal neuromuscular junction and is characterized by skeletal muscle weakness and profound fatigability.[16] As the disease progresses, fatigue increases in severity and in the number of muscles involved. In advanced stages, the patient requires respiratory support because of a virtual paralysis of the respiratory musculature. In myasthenia gravis, the number of functional cholinergic receptors located postsynaptically at the neuromuscular junction is diminished.[17,18] As a result, acetylcholine released from the presynaptic terminal cannot sufficiently excite the muscle cell to reach threshold. The decreased receptivity of the muscle cell accounts for the clinical symptoms of weakness and fatigue.

Myasthenia gravis appears to be caused by an autoimmune response whereby an antibody is produced that affects the neuromuscular cholinergic receptor and enzymes related to the skeletal neuromuscular junction (i.e., muscle-specific tyrosine kinase).[16,19] Although no cure is available, cholinesterase inhibitors such as ambenonium, neostigmine, and pyridostigmine may help reduce the muscular fatigue associated with this disease. These indirect-acting cholinergic agonists inhibit the acetylcholinesterase enzyme at the neuromuscular junction, allowing the endogenous acetylcholine released from the presynaptic terminal to remain at the myoneural junction for a longer period of time. The endogenously released acetylcholine is able to provide adequate excitation of the skeletal muscle cell and thus allow a more sustained muscular contraction.

Reversal of Neuromuscular Blockage

Anesthesia providers often use drugs that block transmission at the skeletal neuromuscular junction to maintain skeletal muscle paralysis during surgical procedures requiring general anesthesia (see Chapter 11). These skeletal muscle paralytic agents include curare-like drugs (e.g., tubocurarine, gallamine, pancuronium). Occasionally, the neuromuscular blockage caused by these drugs must be reversed. For instance, an accelerated recovery from the paralytic effects of these neuromuscular blockers may be desired at the end of the surgical procedure. Consequently, indirect-acting cholinergic stimulants are sometimes used to inhibit the acetylcholinesterase enzyme at the neuromuscular junction, thus allowing endogenously released acetylcholine to remain active at the synaptic site and effectively overcome the neuromuscular blockade until the curare-like agents have been metabolized.

Reversal of Anticholinergic-Induced CNS Toxicity

Indirect-acting cholinergic stimulants (e.g., physostigmine) are sometimes used to reverse the toxic effects of anticholinergic drugs on the CNS. An overdose of anticholinergic drugs may produce toxic CNS effects such as delirium, hallucinations, and coma. By inhibiting acetylcholine breakdown, indirect-acting stimulants enable endogenously released acetylcholine to overcome the anticholinergic drug effects.

Problems and Adverse Effects of Cholinergic Stimulants

Cholinergic stimulants are frequently associated with several adverse side effects caused by the relative nonspecificity of these drugs. Even bethanechol, which is relatively specific for muscarinic receptors, may stimulate muscarinic receptors on many different tissues. For example, administering bethanechol to increase GI motility may also result in bronchoconstriction if this drug reaches muscarinic receptors in the upper respiratory tract. Many indirect-acting stimulants (i.e., the cholinesterase inhibitors) show even less specificity and may increase synaptic activity at all synapses that they reach, including nicotinic cholinergic synapses.

The adverse effects associated with both the direct- and indirect-acting cholinergic stimulants mimic the effects that occur during exaggerated parasympathetic activity. This notion is logical considering that the parasympathetic autonomic division exerts its effects on peripheral tissues by releasing acetylcholine from postganglionic neurons. Consequently, the primary adverse effects of cholinergic stimulants include GI distress (e.g., nausea, vomiting, diarrhea, abdominal cramping), increased salivation, bronchoconstriction, bradycardia, and difficulty in visual accommodation. Increased sweating and vasodilation of facial cutaneous blood vessels (flushing) may also occur because of an effect on the respective tissues supplied by special sympathetic postganglionic neurons that release acetylcholine. The incidence of these side effects varies from patient to patient, but the onset and severity increases as higher drug doses are administered.

ANTICHOLINERGIC DRUGS

In contrast to drugs that stimulate cholinergic activity, anticholinergic drugs attempt to diminish the response of tissues to cholinergic stimulation. In general, these drugs are competitive antagonists of the postsynaptic cholinergic receptors—that is, they bind reversibly to the cholinergic receptor but do not activate it. This binding blocks the receptor from the effects of endogenously released acetylcholine, thus diminishing the cellular response to cholinergic stimulation. (See Chapter 4 for a more detailed description of the mechanism by which drugs function as competitive antagonists.)

Anticholinergic drugs can be classified as antimuscarinic or antinicotinic agents, depending on their specificity for the two primary subtypes of cholinergic receptors. Antinicotinic drugs, such as the N_N antagonists mecamylamine and trimethaphan, are relatively specific for the nicotinic receptor located in the autonomic ganglia (the N_N subtype). These antinicotinic drugs are sometimes used to treat extremely high blood pressure and hypertensive emergencies (see Chapter 21). As mentioned earlier, anesthesia providers may use antinicotinic drugs that block the skeletal neuromuscular junction (i.e., the N_M antagonists) to produce skeletal muscle paralysis during surgery. These neuromuscular blockers are discussed in Chapter 11. However, this section will focus on the antimuscarinic agents.

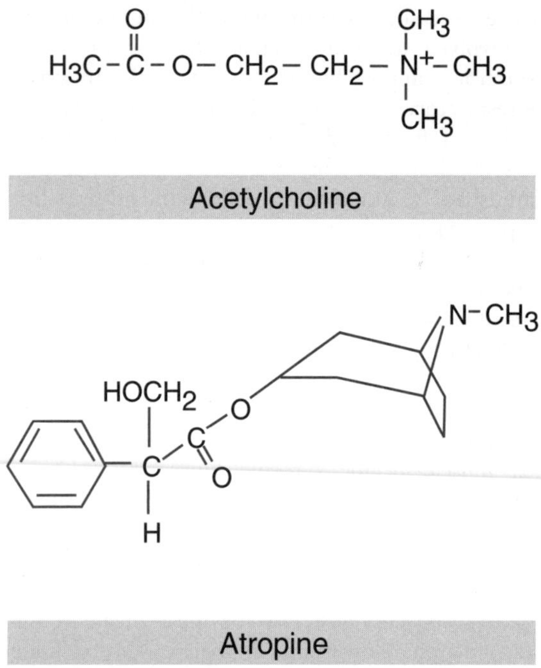

Figure ■ 19-2
Structures of acetylcholine and atropine. Atropine and similar agents antagonize the effects of acetylcholine by blocking muscarinic cholinergic receptors.

Source and Mechanism of Action of Antimuscarinic Anticholinergic Drugs

The prototypical antimuscarinic anticholinergic drug is atropine (Fig. 19-2). Atropine is a naturally occurring substance that can be obtained from the extract of plants such as belladonna and jimsonweed. Other natural, semisynthetic, and synthetic antimuscarinic anticholinergic agents are available that are similar in structure or function to atropine.

As mentioned previously, antimuscarinic anticholinergic drugs all share the same basic mechanism of action: They block the postsynaptic cholinergic muscarinic receptor. However, certain antimuscarinic agents seem to preferentially affect some tissues more than others. For instance, there are antimuscarinics that seem to preferentially antagonize GI muscarinic receptors, whereas other antimuscarinics have a predominant effect on CNS cholinergic synapses. This fact suggests some degree of specificity of these drugs, which may be because of differences in the muscarinic receptor at GI versus central synapses. As indicated in Chapter 18, there are at least five muscarinic receptor subtypes located throughout the body; these receptor subtypes are designated M_1, M_2, M_3, M_4, and M_5.[20] Some drugs may be more selective for a certain receptor subtype than for others. This drug-receptor specificity is far from complete, however, and virtually every antimuscarinic drug will antagonize cholinergic receptors on a number of tissues, which leads to various side effects (see "Problems and Adverse Effects of Anticholinergic Drugs"). Perhaps as more is learned about muscarinic receptor subtypes, more selective anticholinergic drugs may be developed.

Clinical Applications of Antimuscarinic Drugs

The primary clinical applications of antimuscarinic anticholinergic drugs include the treatment of particular GI disorders. These drugs may also be helpful in managing Parkinson disease and helping to treat various clinical disorders involving other physiological systems (Table 19-2).[21]

Gastrointestinal System

Stimulation of the GI tract via parasympathetic cholinergic neurons generally produces an increase in gastric

Table 19-2
COMMON ANTICHOLINERGIC DRUGS*

Generic Name	Trade Name(s)	Primary Clinical Use(s)*
Atropine	AtroPen	Peptic ulcer, IBS, neurogenic bladder, bronchospasm, preoperative antisecretory agent, cardiac arrhythmias (e.g., sinus bradycardia, postmyocardial infarction, asystole), reversal of neuromuscular blockade, antidote to cholinesterase inhibitor poisoning
Belladonna	Generic	Peptic ulcer, IBS, dysmenorrhea, nocturnal enuresis, antivertigo
Clidinium	Quarzan	Peptic ulcer, IBS
Cyclopentolate	Ocu-Pentolate, Cyclogyl, others	Induces mydriasis for ophthalmologic procedures
Darifenacin	Enablex	Overactive bladder
Dicyclomine	Bentyl, others	IBS
Fesoterodine	Toviaz	Overactive bladder
Glycopyrrolate	Cuvposa, Robinul	Peptic ulcer, preoperative antisecretory agent, reversal of neuromuscular blockade, prevent excessive drooling
Homatropine	Isopto Homapin	Induces mydriasis for ophthalmologic procedures
Hyoscyamine	Cystospaz, Levsin, others	Peptic ulcer, IBS, urinary bladder hypermotility, preoperative antisecretory agent
Ipratropium	Atrovent	Bronchodilator
Mepenzolate	Cantil	Peptic ulcer
Oxybutynin	Ditropan, Oxytrol	Neurogenic or overactive bladder
Methscopolamine	Pamine	Peptic ulcer
Propantheline	Pro-Banthine, Probanthel	Peptic ulcer, IBS, urinary incontinence
Scopolamine	Transderm-Scop, others	Motion sickness, preoperative antisecretory agent, postoperative nausea and vomiting, antivertigo
Solifenacin	Vesicare	Overactive bladder
Tiotropium	Spiriva	Bronchodilator
Tolterodine	Detrol	Overactive bladder
Trospium	Sanctura	Overactive bladder

**Clinical uses listed for a specific agent reflect that agent's approved indication(s). Actual clinical use, however, may be limited because anticholinergics have often been replaced by agents that are more effective and better tolerated. Anticholinergic drugs used specifically to treat Parkinson disease are listed in Table 10-1.*

secretions and an increase in GI motility. Certain antimuscarinic anticholinergics tend to reverse this stimulation by blocking the effects of endogenously released acetylcholine. Consequently, physicians administer these drugs as an adjunct in peptic ulcer treatment. The rationale is that they will limit secretion of gastric acid, thus reducing irritation of the stomach mucosa. Also, the Food and Drug Administration approved antimuscarinic anticholinergic drugs for treatment of irritable bowel syndrome (IBS). This condition is characterized by hyperactivity of GI smooth muscle and includes problems such as irritable colon and spastic colon. These antimuscarinic agents are sometimes referred to as *antispasmodics* because of their reported ability to decrease GI smooth-muscle tone or spasms.

Drugs used to treat peptic ulcer and IBS are listed in Table 19-2. Although the FDA approved the drugs to treat these GI disorders, considerable doubt exists as to how effective they are in actually resolving the conditions. Other agents such as the H_2 histamine receptor blockers and proton pump inhibitors have essentially replaced antimuscarinic agents in treating peptic ulcer (see Chapter 27). However, antimuscarinic anticholinergics may still be used if other drugs are ineffective or poorly tolerated.[21] These drugs will not cure peptic ulcer or prevent its recurrence when the medication is discontinued. In essence, they only treat a symptom of the problem (e.g., increased gastric secretion), without really addressing the cause of the increased secretion (e.g., emotional stress, poor eating habits, bacterial infection, etc.).

Finally, antimuscarinic anticholinergic drugs used to treat GI problems are often combined with other agents, such as antianxiety drugs. Librax, for instance, is the trade name for a combination of chlordiazepoxide and clidinium (an antianxiety agent and an anticholinergic agent, respectively). These combination products are supposedly better at relieving GI problems where emotional factors are also present.

Parkinson Disease

A detailed review of the pharmacological management of Parkinson disease is in Chapter 10. Consequently, this section will mention only briefly the use of anticholinergic drugs in this disorder. Parkinsonism is a movement disorder caused by a deficiency of the neurotransmitter dopamine in the basal ganglia. This deficiency leads to an overactivity of central cholinergic synapses. Hence, anticholinergic drugs should be beneficial in helping to resolve this increase in central cholinergic influence.[22]

Certain anticholinergic drugs such as benztropine, biperiden, and trihexyphenidyl are approved for use in treating Parkinson disease (see Table 10-1 for a more complete list). These drugs seem to preferentially block the central muscarinic cholinergic synapses involved in parkinsonism. This does not mean that the drugs do not affect other peripheral muscarinic receptors. Indeed, antiparkinsonian drugs are associated with several side effects, such as dry mouth, constipation, and urinary retention, which are caused by their antagonistic effect on muscarinic receptors located outside of the brain. Their primary effect, however, is to decrease the influence of central cholinergic synapses in parkinsonism.

Cardiovascular System

Atropine is sometimes used to block the effects of the vagus nerve (cranial nerve X) on the myocardium. Release of acetylcholine from vagal efferent fibers slows heart rate and the conduction of the cardiac action potential throughout the myocardium. Atropine reverses the effects of excessive vagal discharge and is used to treat the symptomatic bradycardia that may accompany myocardial infarction, intubation of critically ill children, and other situations involving increased vagal activity.[21,23] Atropine may also be useful in treating other cardiac arrhythmias such as atrioventricular nodal block and ventricular asystole.

Motion Sickness

Antimuscarinics (scopolamine in particular) are frequently used in the treatment of motion sickness.[24,25] Scopolamine appears to block cholinergic transmission from areas of the brain and brainstem that mediate motion-related nausea and vomiting (i.e., the vestibular system, reticular formation, and cortical locations).[24] These drugs are often administered transdermally via small patches that adhere to the skin.[26]

Preoperative Medication

Anesthesia providers occasionally administer atropine and related antimuscarinics preoperatively to decrease respiratory secretions during general anesthesia. This use of these agents has declined considerably, however, because the newer inhalation forms of general anesthesia do not stimulate bronchial secretions to the same extent as earlier general anesthetics (see Chapter 11).[27] Anticholinergic medications can sometimes be used pre- and perioperatively with other agents (sedatives, antianxiety agents, etc.) to help control postoperative nausea and vomiting.[28,29] Medical practitioners may also administer antimuscarinics to prevent bradycardia during surgery, especially in children.

Urinary Tract

Atropine and several synthetic antimuscarinics can alleviate urinary frequency and incontinence caused by hypertonicity of the urinary bladder.[30,31] Increased bladder tone results if the normal reflex control of bladder function is disrupted (i.e., neurogenic bladder syndrome) or if a urinary tract infection irritates the bladder. Some people might also exhibit increased urinary frequency and nocturia without any obvious pathological findings, a condition known as *overactive bladder*.[32-34] Regardless of the cause, antimuscarinics can help reduce bladder hypertonicity by inhibiting contraction of the bladder detrusor muscle, thus allowing the bladder to fill more normally, with a decrease in frequency of urination and a lesser chance of incontinence.

Respiratory Tract

Stimulation of the upper respiratory tract via the vagus causes bronchoconstriction. Anticholinergic drugs that block the effects of vagal-released acetylcholine will relax bronchial smooth muscle. Consequently, practitioners have been using atropine and some synthetic derivatives (ipratropium, tiotropium) to treat bronchospasms occurring in patients with asthma and chronic obstructive pulmonary disease (COPD).[35-37] Although anticholinergics are not usually the initial drugs chosen to treat bronchoconstriction, they can be used in combination with other drugs (e.g., beta-2 agonists) to provide optimal bronchodilation.[38] The use of anticholinergics in treating respiratory disorders is discussed in more detail in Chapter 26.

Eye

Atropine and similar antimuscarinics block the acetylcholine-mediated contraction of the pupillary sphincter muscle, thus causing dilation of the pupil (mydriasis).[1] During an ophthalmologic exam, these drugs may be applied topically to dilate the pupil, thus allowing a more detailed inspection of internal eye structures such as the retina.

Cholinergic Poisoning

Cholinergic poisoning can occur in several situations such as eating wild mushrooms, being exposed to certain pesticides, or being exposed to certain types of chemical warfare.[39,40] This type of poisoning often occurs because organophosphates and similar toxic compounds inhibit the acetylcholinesterase enzyme throughout the body, thereby causing severe overstimulation of nicotinic and muscarinic receptors in organs and physiological systems. These potentially life-threatening occurrences typically require emergency treatment with atropine or an analogous anticholinergic agent. In cases of severe poisoning, fairly high doses of these drugs must often be administered for several days.

Problems and Adverse Effects of Anticholinergic Drugs

Considering the diverse uses of the previously named anticholinergics, these drugs can obviously affect several different tissues. A systemically administered anticholinergic agent cannot be targeted for one specific organ without also achieving a response in other tissues as well. For instance, an antimuscarinic drug administered to decrease motility in the GI tract may also affect other tissues containing muscarinic receptors (e.g., the bladder, bronchial smooth muscle, eye, heart). As higher doses are administered for any given problem, the chance of additional effects in tissues other than the target organ is also increased.

Consequently, antimuscarinic anticholinergic drugs are associated with numerous side effects. Exactly which symptoms (if any) will be encountered depends on several factors, such as the specific anticholinergic agent, the dosage of the drug, and the individual response of each patient. The most common side effects include dry mouth, blurred vision, urinary retention, constipation, and tachycardia. Each of these side effects is caused by the blockade of muscarinic receptors on the tissue or organ related to the effect. Some patients also report symptoms such as confusion, dizziness, nervousness, and drowsiness, presumably because of an interaction of antimuscarinic drugs with CNS cholinergic receptors. These CNS-related symptoms occur more frequently with anticholinergic drugs that readily cross the blood-brain barrier.

SUMMARY

Drugs affecting acetylcholine-mediated responses are classified as cholinergic stimulants and anticholinergic drugs. Cholinergic stimulants increase cholinergic activity by binding to the acetylcholine receptor and activating the receptor (direct-acting stimulants) or by inhibiting the acetylcholinesterase enzyme, thus allowing more acetylcholine to remain active at the cholinergic synapse (indirect-acting stimulants). Anticholinergic drugs inhibit cholinergic activity by acting as competitive antagonists—that is, they bind to the cholinergic receptor but do not activate it.

Cholinergic stimulants and anticholinergic drugs affect many tissues in the body and are used to treat a variety of clinical problems. Cholinergic stimulants are often administered to increase GI and urinary bladder tone; to treat conditions such as glaucoma, myasthenia gravis, and Alzheimer disease; and to reverse the neuromuscular blockade produced by curare-like drugs. Anticholinergic drugs are used principally to treat overactive bladder, bronchoconstriction, and excessive GI motility and secretions and to decrease the symptoms of Parkinson disease, but they may also be used to treat problems in several other physiological systems. Because of the ability of cholinergic stimulants and anticholinergic drugs to affect different tissues, these drugs may be associated with several side effects. Considering the diverse clinical applications of cholinergic stimulants and anticholinergics, physical therapists and occupational therapists may frequently encounter patients taking these drugs. Rehabilitation specialists should be aware of the rationale for drug administration as well as possible side effects of cholinergic stimulants and anticholinergic agents.

REFERENCES

1. Westfall TC, Westfall DP. Neurotransmission: the autonomic and somatic motor nervous systems. In: Brunton L, et al, eds. *The Pharmacological Basis of Therapeutics*. 12th ed. New York: McGraw-Hill; 2011.
2. Braverman AS, Miller LS, Vegesna AK, et al. Quantitation of the contractile response mediated by two receptors: M2 and M3 muscarinic receptor-mediated contractions of human gastroesophageal smooth muscle. *J Pharmacol Exp Ther*. 2009;329: 218-224.
3. Manchana T, Prasartsakulchai C. Bethanechol chloride for the prevention of bladder dysfunction after radical hysterectomy in gynecologic cancer patients: a randomized controlled trial study. *Int J Gynecol Cancer*. 2011;21:730-736.
4. Pohanka M. Acetylcholinesterase inhibitors: a patent review (2008–present). *Expert Opin Ther Pat*. 2012;22:871-886.
5. Pappano AJ. Cholinoceptor-activating and cholinesterase-inhibiting drugs. In: Katzung BG, Masters SB, Trevor AJ, eds. *Basic and Clinical Pharmacology*. 12th ed. New York: Lange Medical Books/McGraw Hill; 2012:97-113.
6. Hirano S, Shinotoh H, Eidelberg D. Functional brain imaging of cognitive dysfunction in Parkinson's disease. *J Neurol Neurosurg Psychiatry*. 2012;83:963-969.
7. Pinto T, Lanctôt KL, Herrmann N. Revisiting the cholinergic hypothesis of behavioral and psychological symptoms in dementia of the Alzheimer's type. *Ageing Res Rev*. 2011;10:404-412.
8. Schliebs R, Arendt T. The cholinergic system in aging and neuronal degeneration. *Behav Brain Res*. 2011;221:555-563.
9. Atri A. Effective pharmacological management of Alzheimer's disease. *Am J Manag Care*. 2011;17(suppl 13):S346-355.
10. Sabbagh M, Cummings J. Progressive cholinergic decline in Alzheimer's disease: consideration for treatment with donepezil 23 mg in patients with moderate to severe symptomatology. *BMC Neurol*. 2011;11:21.
11. Massoud F, Léger GC. Pharmacological treatment of Alzheimer disease. *Can J Psychiatry*. 2011;56:579-588.
12. Casson RJ, Chidlow G, Wood JP, et al. Definition of glaucoma: clinical and experimental concepts. *Clin Experiment Ophthalmol*. 2012;40:341-349.
13. Costagliola C, dell'Omo R, Romano MR, et al. Pharmacotherapy of intraocular pressure: part I. Parasympathomimetic, sympathomimetic and sympatholytics. *Expert Opin Pharmacother*. 2009;10: 2663-2677.
14. Toris CB. Pharmacotherapies for glaucoma. *Curr Mol Med*. 2010;10:824-840.
15. Burr J, Azuara-Blanco A, Avenell A, Tuulonen A. Medical versus surgical interventions for open angle glaucoma. *Cochrane Database Syst Rev*. 2012;9:CD004399.
16. Silvestri NJ, Wolfe GI. Myasthenia gravis. *Semin Neurol*. 2012;32:215-226.
17. Gomez AM, Van Den Broeck J, Vrolix K, et al. Antibody effector mechanisms in myasthenia gravis-pathogenesis at the neuromuscular junction. *Autoimmunity*. 2010;433:353-370.
18. Serra A, Ruff RL, Leigh RJ. Neuromuscular transmission failure in myasthenia gravis: decrement of safety factor and susceptibility of extraocular muscles. *Ann NY Acad Sci*. 2012;1275: 129-135.
19. Meriggioli MN, Sanders DB. Autoimmune myasthenia gravis: emerging clinical and biological heterogeneity. *Lancet Neurol*. 2009;8:475-490.
20. Eglen RM. Overview of muscarinic receptor subtypes. *Handb Exp Pharmacol*. 2012;208:3-28.
21. Pappano AJ. Cholinoceptor-blocking drugs. In: Katzung BG, Masters SB, Trevor AJ, eds. *Basic and Clinical Pharmacology*. 12th ed. New York: Lange Medical Books/McGraw Hill; 2012: 115-127.
22. Yuan H, Zhang ZW, Liang LW, et al. Treatment strategies for Parkinson's disease. *Neurosci Bull*. 2010;26:66-76.
23. Jones P, Dauger S, Denjoy I, et al. The effect of atropine on rhythm and conduction disturbances during 322 critical care intubations. *Pediatr Crit Care Med*. 2013;14:289-297.
24. Schmäl F. Neuronal mechanisms and the treatment of motion sickness. *Pharmacology*. 2013;91:229-241.
25. Spinks A, Wasiak J. Scopolamine (hyoscine) for preventing and treating motion sickness. *Cochrane Database Syst Rev*. 2011;6:CD002851.
26. Nachum Z, Shupak A, Gordon CR. Transdermal scopolamine for prevention of motion sickness: clinical pharmacokinetics and therapeutic applications. *Clin Pharmacokinet*. 2006;45: 543-566.
27. White PF, Eng MR. Ambulatory (outpatient) anesthesia. In: Miller RD, et al, eds. *Miller's Anesthesia*. Vol 1. 7th ed. Philadelphia, PA: Churchill Livingstone Elsevier; 2010:667-718.
28. Apfel CC, Zhang K, George E, et al. Transdermal scopolamine for the prevention of postoperative nausea and vomiting: a systematic review and meta-analysis. *Clin Ther*. 2010;32: 1987-2002.
29. Baciarello M, Cornini A, Zasa M, et al. Intrathecal atropine to prevent postoperative nausea and vomiting after Cesarean section: a randomized, controlled trial. *Minerva Anestesiol*. 2011;77:781-788.
30. Elser DM. Stress urinary incontinence and overactive bladder syndrome: current options and new targets for management. *Postgrad Med*. 2012;124:42-49.
31. Madhuvrata P, Singh M, Hasafa Z, Abdel-Fattah M. Anticholinergic drugs for adult neurogenic detrusor overactivity: a systematic review and meta-analysis. *Eur Urol*. 2012;62: 816-830.
32. Geoffrion R. Treatments for overactive bladder: focus on pharmacotherapy. *J Obstet Gynaecol Can*. 2012;34:1092-1101.
33. Madhuvrata P, Cody JD, Ellis G, et al. Which anticholinergic drug for overactive bladder symptoms in adults. *Cochrane Database Syst Rev*. 2012;1:CD005429.

34. Rai BP, Cody JD, Alhasso A, Stewart L. Anticholinergic drugs versus non-drug active therapies for non-neurogenic overactive bladder syndrome in adults. *Cochrane Database Syst Rev.* 2012;12:CD003193.
35. Kanazawa H. Anticholinergic agents in asthma: chronic bronchodilator therapy, relief of acute severe asthma, reduction of chronic viral inflammation and prevention of airway remodeling. *Curr Opin Pulm Med.* 2006;12:60-67.
36. Novelli F, Malagrinò L, Dente FL, Paggiaro P. Efficacy of anticholinergic drugs in asthma. *Expert Rev Respir Med.* 2012;6:309-319.
37. Tashkin DP. Impact of tiotropium on the course of moderate-to-very severe chronic obstructive pulmonary disease: the UPLIFT trial. *Expert Rev Respir Med.* 2010;4:279-289.
38. Williams DM, Bourdet SV. Chronic obstructive pulmonary disease. In: DiPiro JT, et al, eds. *Pharmacotherapy: A Pathophysiologic Approach.* 8th ed. New York: McGraw-Hill; 2011:471-495.
39. Husain K, Ansari RA, Ferder L. Pharmacological agents in the prophylaxis/treatment of organophosphorous pesticide intoxication. *Indian J Exp Biol.* 2010;48:642-650.
40. Soukup O, Tobin G, Kumar UK, et al. Interaction of nerve agent antidotes with cholinergic systems. *Curr Med Chem.* 2010;17:1708-1718.

CHAPTER 20

Adrenergic Drugs

Adrenergic refers to physiological responses related to adrenaline and noradrenaline, two neurohormones that are also known commonly as *epinephrine* and *norepinephrine*, respectively. Adrenergic drugs either stimulate activity in tissues that respond to epinephrine and norepinephrine (adrenergic agonists) or inhibit epinephrine and norepinephrine influence (adrenergic antagonists). Epinephrine and norepinephrine are released from the adrenal gland and reach the heart, kidneys, and various other tissues and organs via the systemic circulation (see Chapter 18).

Norepinephrine is also the neurotransmitter typically found at the junction between sympathetic postganglionic neurons and peripheral tissues. Consequently, medical practitioners administer most of the adrenergic agonists to augment sympathetic responses, while they administer adrenergic antagonists to attenuate sympathetic-induced activity. In fact, adrenergic agonists are sometimes referred to as *sympathomimetic*, and antagonists are referred to as *sympatholytic* because of their ability to increase and decrease sympathetic activity, respectively.

This chapter focuses specifically on the adrenergic drugs that primarily influence activity in the sympathetic nervous system through their effect on adrenergic synapses. As a result, the drugs are categorized according to a common mode of action rather than according to common clinical applications. Most of the drugs introduced in this chapter will also appear elsewhere in the text when they are classified according to their use in treating specific problems. For instance, the beta-selective adrenergic antagonists, or beta blockers, are collectively introduced in the section "Beta Antagonists." Individual beta blockers are also discussed in subsequent chapters with regard to their use in specific problems such as hypertension (see Chapter 21), angina pectoris (see Chapter 22), cardiac arrhythmias (see Chapter 23), and congestive heart failure (see Chapter 24).

Adrenergic drugs are used to treat a variety of disorders, ranging from severe cardiovascular and respiratory problems to symptoms of the common cold. Therefore, many of the patients you will see in physical therapy and occupational therapy may be taking adrenergic agonists or antagonists. In this chapter, the discussion is limited to the basic pharmacodynamic mechanisms, clinical applications, and adverse effects of these drugs. The relevance of specific adrenergic drugs to physical rehabilitation is addressed in more detail in subsequent chapters, where their use is categorized according to certain disorders (hypertension, angina, asthma, etc.).

Many adrenergic agonists and antagonists exert their effects by binding directly to the appropriate postsynaptic receptor. Because a great deal of the specificity (or lack of specificity) of these drugs depends on the drug-receptor interaction, the first section is a brief review of the adrenergic receptor classes and subclasses.

ADRENERGIC RECEPTOR SUBCLASSIFICATIONS

Adrenergic receptors can be divided into two primary categories: alpha and beta receptors (see Chapter 18). Each category can then be subdivided, so that five receptor subtypes are commonly identified: alpha-1, alpha-2, beta-1, beta-2, and beta-3.[1] Alpha-1 receptors have been further categorized as alpha-1a, -1b, and -1d receptors, and alpha-2 receptors have been subdivided into alpha-2a, -2b, and -2c receptors. The functional significance of these subclassifications remains unclear, so for the purposes of this chapter, the categorization of drugs affecting alpha receptors is restricted to the primary alpha receptor that they affect (e.g., alpha-1 or alpha-2). Adrenergic receptor subtypes are located on specific tissues throughout the body, and the response mediated by each receptor depends on the interaction between that receptor and the respective tissue. Refer to Chapter 18 for a more detailed description of adrenergic receptor locations and responses.

Table 20-1 summarizes the primary uses of adrenergic agonists and antagonists according to their selectivity for individual receptor subtypes. In general, a specific agonist is used to mimic or increase the receptor-mediated response, whereas the antagonist is used to decrease the receptor-mediated response.

Clinically useful adrenergic agonists and antagonists display variable amounts of specificity for each receptor subtype. Some drugs are fairly specific and bind to only one receptor subtype. For example, a specific alpha-1 agonist like phenylephrine preferentially stimulates the alpha-1 subtype. Other drugs show a moderate amount of specificity, perhaps affecting one major receptor category. An example is the nonselective beta antagonist propranolol, which blocks beta-1 and beta-2 receptors but has little or no effect on alpha receptors. Finally, other drugs such as epinephrine are rather nonspecific and affect alpha and beta receptors equally. In some clinical situations, administering a selective drug may be desirable, whereas in others, a drug that interacts with more than one receptor subtype is beneficial. The use of selective versus nonselective adrenergic drugs is considered in the sections "Adrenergic Agonists" and "Adrenergic Antagonists."

However, *receptor selectivity* is a relative term. Even though an adrenergic drug is reported to be selective for only one receptor subtype, a certain affinity for other receptor subtypes may also occur to a lesser degree. A beta-1-specific drug, for instance, binds preferentially to beta-1 receptors but may also show

Table 20-1
SUMMARY OF ADRENERGIC AGONIST/ANTAGONIST USE ACCORDING TO RECEPTOR SPECIFICITY

Primary Receptor Location: Response When Stimulated	Agonist Use(s)*	Antagonist Use(s)*
Alpha-1 Receptor		
Vascular smooth muscle: vasoconstriction	Hypotension Nasal congestion Paroxysmal supraventricular tachycardia	Hypertension Benign prostatic hyperplasia
Alpha-2 Receptor		
CNS synapses (inhibitory)	Hypertension Spasticity	No significant clinical use
Beta-1 Receptor		
Heart: increased heart rate and force of contraction	Cardiac decompensation	Hypertension Arrhythmia Angina pectoris Heart failure Prevention of reinfarction
Beta-2 Receptor		
Bronchioles: bronchodilation	Prevent bronchospasm	No significant clinical use
Uterus: relaxation	Prevent premature labor	

**Primary clinical condition(s). See text for specific drugs in each category and a discussion of treatment rationale.*

some slight affinity for beta-2 receptors. Selectivity is also dose-related, with the relative degree of receptor selectivity decreasing as higher doses are administered. Consequently, some side effects of the selective drugs may be caused by stimulation of other receptor subtypes, especially at higher drug doses.

ADRENERGIC AGONISTS

This section presents drugs that stimulate the adrenergic receptors according to their relative specificity for each receptor subtype. The drugs that primarily activate alpha receptors are discussed first, followed by beta-selective drugs and drugs that have mixed alpha- and beta-agonist activity.

Alpha-1-Selective Agonists

Alpha-1 agonists bind directly to and activate the alpha-1 receptor located primarily on vascular smooth muscle, thus leading to smooth-muscle contraction and vasoconstriction.[1] Because of their vasoconstrictive properties, these drugs are able to increase blood pressure by increasing peripheral vascular resistance. Consequently, certain alpha-1 agonists are administered systemically to treat acute hypotension occurring in emergencies such as shock or during general anesthesia. A second common clinical application of these drugs is the treatment of nasal congestion (i.e., the runny nose and stuffy head associated with the common cold). In appropriate doses, alpha-1 agonists preferentially constrict the vasculature in the nasal and upper respiratory mucosa, thus decreasing the congestion and mucosal discharge. A third application of alpha-1 agonists is to decrease heart rate during attacks of paroxysmal supraventricular tachycardia. By increasing peripheral vascular resistance, these drugs bring about a decrease in heart rate through the cardiac baroreceptor reflex.

Specific Agents

Mephentermine (Wyamine). This alpha-1 stimulant is used primarily to maintain or restore blood pressure during hypotensive episodes that may occur during spinal anesthesia. It is typically administered by intravenous or intramuscular injection.

Methoxamine (Vasoxyl). This drug is used primarily to increase and maintain blood pressure in severe, acute hypotension, especially during general anesthesia and spinal anesthesia. It can also be used to treat paroxysmal supraventricular tachycardia by causing peripheral vasoconstriction and activation of the baroreceptor reflex. Methoxamine is usually administered by injection (intramuscularly or intravenously) to provide a rapid onset.

Midodrine (ProAmatine). Midodrine can be administered orally to treat resistant cases of orthostatic hypotension. This drug can also prevent hypotension in patients undergoing dialysis, and it can offset the hypotensive effects of certain psychotropic drugs (e.g., antipsychotic medications).

Oxymetazoline (Afrin, OcuClear, many others). This drug, administered in nose drops and nasal sprays, decreases nasal congestion through alpha-1-mediated vasoconstriction. Higher or systemic doses may also cause hypotension, presumably because central nervous system (CNS) alpha-2 receptors are stimulated in a manner similar to clonidine (see "Alpha-2-Selective Agonists"). Oxymetazoline can also be administered as eyedrops to decrease redness and minor eye irritation.

Phenylephrine (Neo-Synephrine, others). Like methoxamine, phenylephrine can be administered systemically to treat hypotension, and phenylephrine can also be used to terminate certain episodes of supraventricular tachycardia. In addition, phenylephrine is administered orally or via nasal spray to treat nasal congestion and can be applied topically as eyedrops to treat redness and minor eye irritation. Phenylephrine is found in many over-the-counter products and is often combined with other cough/cold medications (antitussives, antihistamines, mucolytics, expectorants).

Pseudoephedrine (Drixoral, Sudafed, many others). Pseudoephedrine is administered orally for its decongestant effects. It is found in many over-the-counter preparations and is commonly used to help relieve cold symptoms.

Xylometazoline (Otrivin, others). This drug is used primarily as a nasal spray to decrease congestion during colds and allergies.

Adverse Effects

The primary side effects associated with alpha-1-specific agonists are caused by excessive stimulation of alpha-adrenergic responses. Some of the more frequent side effects include increased blood pressure, headache, and an abnormally slow heart rate (because of reflex bradycardia). Some patients also report chest pain, difficulty breathing, and feelings of nervousness. These side effects are quite variable and are usually dose-related (i.e., they occur more frequently at higher doses).

Alpha-2-Selective Agonists

Alpha-2-selective drugs are used primarily in the treatment of hypertension and spasticity. When treating hypertension, these drugs stimulate alpha-2 receptors located in the brain and brainstem. When stimulated, these central alpha-2 receptors exert an *inhibitory* effect on sympathetic discharge from the vasomotor center in the brainstem.[2] Diminished sympathetic discharge results in decreased blood pressure. The use of alpha-2 agonists in lowering blood pressure is discussed in more detail in Chapter 21.

Alpha-2 receptors have also been identified on interneurons in the spinal cord. Stimulation of these receptors causes interneuron inhibition and a subsequent decrease in excitability of motor neurons supplied by the interneurons.[3] Alpha-2 agonists have therefore been used to normalize neuronal activity in conditions such as spasticity (see Chapter 13).

Alpha-2 agonists appear to exert their antihypertensive effects and antispasticity effects by preferentially stimulating alpha-2 receptors in the brain and spinal cord, respectively. In both situations, it is unclear whether alpha-2 agonists exert their primary effects on presynaptic or postsynaptic receptors. Stimulation of presynaptic alpha-2 receptors located at adrenergic synapses results in a decrease in norepinephrine release from the presynaptic terminal.[4] Similarly, alpha-2 receptors have also been identified postsynaptically at specific central synapses. These postsynaptic receptors are believed to directly inhibit neuronal excitation, and drugs that stimulate these postsynaptic alpha-2 receptors may be helpful in treating attention deficit-hyperactivity disorder.[5] Thus, alpha-2 agonists may exert their effects by stimulating either central presynaptic or postsynaptic receptors or by acting on inhibitory presynaptic and postsynaptic receptors simultaneously. Alpha-2 receptors may also exist on other tissues such as the eye, and the use of alpha-2 agonists continues to expand as more is learned about the location and function of these receptors.

Specific Agents

Brimonidine (Alphagan). This drug is administered locally to the eye to treat glaucoma. It stimulates ocular alpha-2 receptors, which decreases intraocular pressure by decreasing vitreous humor production and increasing drainage of vitreous humor from the eye.

Clonidine (Catapres, Duraclon). Clonidine is used as an antihypertensive as well as an analgesic. Clonidine's antihypertensive effects occur because the drug stimulates alpha-2 receptors in the vasomotor center of the brainstem and decreases sympathetic discharge to the heart and vasculature. Clonidine, however, is not usually successful when used alone in long-term treatment of essential hypertension. This drug is usually reserved for use in short-term management or in combination with other antihypertensive drugs, especially in patients who are unable to tolerate alpha-1 antagonists such as prazosin (Minipress) (see "Alpha Antagonists"). Clonidine also has sedative properties and medical practitioners have been prescribing it as an antianxiety drug, an adjunct in general anesthesia, and an analgesic. In particular, this drug can be combined with other analgesics (opioids) for treating severe pain in people with cancer. Clonidine's analgesic effects are probably mediated by stimulation of alpha-2 receptors located in the spinal cord. Because of its effects on alpha-2 receptors in the spinal cord, clonidine has antispasticity effects. Use of this drug in spasticity, however, is often limited because it also causes hypotension. Finally, clonidine affects specific postsynaptic alpha-2 receptors in the prefrontal cortex, and therefore practitioners have been prescribing it with other medications to treat attention deficit-hyperactivity disorder.[6]

Guanabenz (Wytensin). Guanabenz is used primarily to decrease blood pressure via its effect on alpha-2 receptors in the brainstem. This drug is similar to clonidine in efficacy and clinical use.

Guanfacine (Tenex). This drug is similar to guanabenz and is typically used to treat advanced or resistant cases of high blood pressure.

Methyldopa (Aldomet). Methyldopa has been used as an antihypertensive drug for some time, but its mechanism of action is poorly understood. Methyldopa is believed to exert its effects by converting to alpha-methylnorepinephrine in the body.[1] Alpha-methylnorepinephrine is a potent alpha-2 agonist that lowers blood pressure by stimulating inhibitory central adrenergic receptors in a manner similar to clonidine and guanabenz.

Tizanidine (Zanaflex). Tizanidine is used primarily for treating spasticity.[7,8] This drug is similar to clonidine but has fewer vasomotor effects and is therefore less likely to cause hypotension and other cardiovascular problems. As indicated earlier, tizanidine stimulates alpha-2 receptors in the spinal cord, which results in decreased excitatory input onto the alpha motor neuron. Decreased excitation of the alpha motor neuron results in decreased spasticity of the skeletal muscle supplied by that neuron.

Adverse Effects

Use of alpha-2-specific drugs may be associated with some relatively minor side effects such as dizziness, drowsiness, and dry mouth. More pronounced adverse effects such as difficulty breathing, an unusually slow heart rate, and persistent fainting may indicate a toxic accumulation or overdose of these drugs.

Beta-1-Selective Agonists

The beta-1 receptor is located primarily on the myocardium, and stimulation of the receptor results in increased heart rate and increased force of myocardial contraction (i.e., increased cardiac output). Consequently, beta-1 agonists are used primarily to increase cardiac output in emergency situations such as cardiovascular shock or if complications develop during cardiac surgery. Beta-1 agonists may also be used to increase cardiac function in the short-term treatment of certain types of heart disease, including heart failure.

Specific Agents

Dobutamine (Dobutrex). Dobutamine is used for short-term management of cardiac decompensation that sometimes occurs during exacerbations of heart disease or following cardiac surgery.[9] This drug increases the force of cardiac contraction (positive inotropic effect) by stimulating cardiac beta-1 receptors. Dobutamine is often administered via IV pump infusion to provide relatively stable plasma levels.

Dopamine (Intropin). In addition to its ability to stimulate dopamine receptors, this drug directly stimulates beta-1-adrenergic receptors. Depending on the dose, this drug also exerts complex effects on other dopaminergic and adrenergic receptors.[1] At low doses, for example, dopamine may cause peripheral vasodilation in the viscera and kidneys by stimulating dopamine receptors in the vasculature of these tissues. This effect may help sustain kidney function in people with heart failure because cardiac output is increased (beta-1 effect) as renal blood flow is also increased. At higher doses, however, dopamine may cause peripheral vasoconstriction by directly stimulating vascular alpha-1 receptors and increasing the release of norepinephrine from vascular sympathetic neurons. This effect can help sustain blood pressure in people with severe hypotension.

Clinically, dopamine is used to treat cardiac decompensation in a manner similar to dobutamine. In particular, dopamine is used to increase cardiac output in severe congestive heart failure and to treat other forms of acute or severe hypotension—that is, moderate to high doses of dopamine can stimulate the heart (beta-1 effect) while simultaneously increasing peripheral vascular resistance (alpha-1 effect). When used as a cardiac medication, dopamine is typically administered via IV drip to help maintain stable and consistent plasma levels.

Adverse Effects

Because of their cardiostimulatory effects, beta-1-selective drugs may induce side effects such as chest pain and cardiac arrhythmias in some patients. Shortness of breath and difficulty in breathing (i.e., feelings of chest constriction) have also been reported.

Beta-2-Selective Agonists

One important location of beta-2 receptors is on bronchiole smooth muscle. When stimulated, the receptor mediates relaxation of the bronchioles. Consequently, medical practitioners administer most beta-2 agonists to treat the bronchospasm associated with respiratory ailments such as asthma, bronchitis, and emphysema.[10] Because a nonselective beta agonist will also stimulate the myocardium (beta-1 effect), beta-2-selective agonists are often used preferentially in treating bronchoconstriction, especially if the patient has a cardiac abnormality such as arrhythmias or heart failure.[11,12]

Another clinically important location of beta-2 receptors is on uterine muscle. When stimulated, these receptors cause inhibition or relaxation of the uterus. As a result, the use of beta-2-selective drugs such as terbutaline will inhibit premature uterine contractions during pregnancy, thus preventing premature labor and delivery.[13,14] There is considerable controversy, however, about whether beta-selective agonists actually result in beneficial outcomes for the newborn child, and there is considerable evidence that these drugs may actually be harmful to the mother (see "Adverse Effects" below).[15] Hence, other drugs such as nifedipine (a calcium channel blocker) and atosiban (an oxytocin receptor blocker) have largely replaced beta-2 agonists to prevent preterm labor.

Specific Agents

Beta-2-Selective Bronchodilators. This group of drugs includes albuterol (Proventil, Ventolin, others), metaproterenol (Alupent, others), pirbuterol (Maxair), salmeterol (Serevent), and terbutaline (Brethaire, Bricanyl). These agents are similar pharmacologically and stimulate beta-2 receptors located on pulmonary smooth muscle, thus causing bronchodilation in patients with asthma and similar conditions. Isoproterenol (Isuprel) can also be included with this group, but it is somewhat less beta-2-selective and affects beta-1 receptors as well. Beta-2 bronchodilators are often administered by oral inhalation so that the drug is applied directly to bronchial membranes. The patient uses small aerosol inhalers to self-administer albuterol and similar agents at the onset of a bronchospastic attack. Chapter 26 addresses the use of these drugs to treat respiratory conditions in more detail.

Adverse Effects

The primary side effects associated with beta-2-specific drugs include nervousness, restlessness, and trembling. These adverse symptoms may be caused by stimulation of central beta-adrenergic receptors. There is also some suggestion that excessive use of beta-2 agonists may cause increased airway hyperresponsiveness in some patients, which could lead to severe and possibly fatal asthmatic attacks.[10,16] This fact has generated debate about the safe and effective use of these drugs in treating asthma (see Chapter 26). When used to prevent premature labor, drugs such as terbutaline have also been associated with increases in maternal heart rate and systolic blood pressure, as well as maternal pulmonary edema. These changes in maternal cardiopulmonary function can be quite severe and may be fatal to the mother.

Drugs With Mixed Alpha- and Beta-Agonist Activity

Several drugs are available that display a mixed agonistic activity with regard to adrenergic receptor subtypes. Some drugs, like epinephrine, appear to be able to stimulate all four adrenergic receptor subtypes. Other drugs, such as norepinephrine, bind to both types of alpha receptors and bind to beta-1 receptors to a lesser extent, and they show little or no affinity for beta-2 receptors. Another group of indirect adrenergic agonists (ephedrine, metaraminol) appear to act as nonselective agonists because they increase the release of norepinephrine from presynaptic storage sites. Because many of these multiple-receptor drugs can affect several adrenoceptor subtypes, their clinical uses are quite varied. Specific agents with mixed agonistic activity and their respective applications are presented below.

Specific Agents

Amphetamines. Drugs such as amphetamine (generic), dextroamphetamine (Dexedrine, others), and methamphetamine (Desoxyn) are known for their powerful sympathomimetic effects. These drugs appear to increase norepinephrine release while decreasing norepinephrine reuptake and breakdown at adrenergic synapses, thus increasing activity at synapses with norepinephrine-sensitive receptors (i.e., alpha-1, alpha-2, and beta-1 receptors). These drugs may also exert similar effects on certain dopaminergic synapses. Amphetamines are used on a limited basis to treat attention-deficit disorder in children and to increase mental alertness in adults with narcolepsy. The use of these drugs to suppress appetite or to combat normal sleepiness is discouraged because of their high potential for abuse. These drugs are classified in the United States as schedule II controlled substances (see Chapter 1 for a description of controlled substance classification).

Ephedrine (generic). Ephedrine appears to directly stimulate alpha-1, alpha-2, and beta-1 adrenoceptors and may also stimulate these receptors indirectly by increasing the release of norepinephrine at synapses that use these receptor subtypes. This drug is used primarily for its alpha-1 effects and can be used to treat severe, acute hypotension. When treating hypotension in emergency situations (e.g., shock), practitioners administer ephedrine systemically by injection (intravenously, intramuscularly, or subcutaneously). Ephedrine is also a nasal decongestant because of its ability to stimulate alpha-1 receptors in the nasal mucosa. As a decongestant, ephedrine is typically combined with other agents (antitussives, antihistamines) to form cough and cold products. Ephedrine is also sometimes administered as a bronchodilator (beta-2 agonist effect), but safer agents have generally replaced the use of this drug in asthma and related conditions (see Chapter 26). Finally, medical practitioners have been administering ephedrine to produce a general excitatory effect on central adrenergic receptors and to treat conditions associated with a decrease in CNS arousal (e.g., narcolepsy).

Epinephrine (Adrenalin, Bronkaid Mist, Primatene Mist, others). Epinephrine appears to directly stimulate all adrenergic receptor subtypes and is administered for a variety of reasons. Epinephrine is found in many antiasthmatic inhalation products because of its ability to stimulate beta-2 receptors on the bronchi. Because it stimulates vascular alpha-1 receptors, epinephrine may be applied topically to produce local vasoconstriction and control bleeding during minor surgical procedures (e.g., suturing superficial wounds). Likewise, epinephrine may be mixed with a local anesthetic when the anesthetic is injected during minor surgical and dental procedures. The vasoconstriction produced by epinephrine prevents the anesthetic from being washed away by the local blood flow, thus prolonging the anesthetic's effects. Because of a potent ability to stimulate the heart (beta-1 effect), epinephrine can reestablish normal cardiac rhythm during cardiac arrest. Finally, epinephrine is often the drug of choice in treating anaphylactic shock, which is a hypersensitive allergic reaction marked by cardiovascular collapse (decreased cardiac output, hypotension) and severe bronchoconstriction. Epinephrine is ideally suited to treat this problem because of its ability to stimulate the heart (beta-1 effect), vasoconstrict the periphery (alpha-1 effect), and dilate the bronchi (beta-2 effect).

Metaraminol (Aramine). Metaraminol appears to act like ephedrine—that is, it directly stimulates alpha-1, alpha-2, and beta-1 receptors and indirectly stimulates them by increasing the release of presynaptic norepinephrine. This drug is usually administered by injection (intramuscularly, intravenously, or subcutaneously) to treat severe hypotension occurring in shock or general anesthesia.

Norepinephrine (Levophed). Norepinephrine stimulates both types of alpha receptors as well as beta-1 receptors but displays very little agonistic activity toward beta-2 receptors. It is usually administered intravenously to treat hypotension during shock or general anesthesia.

Adverse Effects

Because of the general ability of many of the drugs previously described to produce CNS excitation, some of the primary side effects are nervousness, restlessness, and anxiety. These agents also tend to stimulate the cardiovascular system; therefore, prolonged or excessive use may lead to complications such as hypertension, arrhythmias, and even cardiac arrest. When used to treat bronchospasm, prolonged administration via inhalation may also cause some degree of bronchial irritation with some agents.

ADRENERGIC ANTAGONISTS

Adrenergic antagonists or blockers bind to adrenergic receptors but do not activate them. These agents are often referred to as *sympatholytic drugs* because of their ability to block the receptors that typically mediate sympathetic responses (i.e., alpha and beta receptors). Clinically useful adrenergic antagonists usually show a fairly high degree of specificity for one of the major receptor classifications. They tend to bind preferentially to either alpha- or beta-adrenergic receptors. Specific drugs may show an additional degree of specificity within the receptor class. For instance, a beta blocker may bind rather selectively to only beta-1 receptors, or it may bind equally to both beta-1 and beta-2 receptors. This section begins with the general clinical applications of alpha antagonists.

Alpha Antagonists

Alpha antagonists are administered primarily to reduce peripheral vascular tone by blocking the alpha-1 receptors located on vascular smooth muscle. When stimulated by endogenous catecholamines (norepinephrine, epinephrine), the alpha-1 receptor initiates vasoconstriction. Consequently, alpha antagonists are used in conditions where peripheral vasodilation would be beneficial. A principal application of these agents is in treating hypertension.[17,18]

These drugs seem to attenuate the peripheral vasoconstriction mediated by excessive adrenergic influence, thus decreasing blood pressure through a decrease in peripheral vascular resistance. These agents may also be used in patients with a pheochromocytoma, a tumor that produces large quantities of epinephrine and norepinephrine. Alpha antagonists are often administered prior to and during the removal of such a tumor, thus preventing the hypertensive crisis that may occur from excessive alpha-1 stimulation from catecholamines released from the tumor. Similarly, alpha antagonists can successfully prevent and treat the sudden increase in blood pressure occurring during an autonomic crisis. These drugs have been used to promote vasodilation in conditions of vascular insufficiency, including peripheral vascular disease and Raynaud phenomenon. However, the success of these drugs in treating vascular insufficiency has been somewhat limited.

Certain alpha-1 blockers, such as doxazosin, tamsulosin, and silodosin, are used extensively to treat benign prostatic hyperplasia (BPH).[19,20] Alpha-1 receptors located on smooth muscle in the prostate capsule, neck of the bladder, and urethra cause muscle constriction that restricts urine flow and the ability to empty the bladder. By blocking these receptors, alpha-1 antagonists relax these smooth muscles and allow men with BPH to void urine more easily and completely.[19,20]

A group of drugs known collectively as *ergot derivatives* display some alpha-blocking ability and other unique properties. Ergot alkaloids and ergoloid mesylates are used clinically for diverse problems, including the treatment of vascular headache and improvement of mental function in presenile dementia.

Because the primary uses of alpha antagonists involve their ability to decrease vascular tone, the clinically useful alpha antagonists tend to be somewhat alpha-1 selective. Alpha-2 receptors should not be selectively antagonized because this may ultimately lead to an *increase* in peripheral vascular tone through an increase in sympathetic discharge. Certain alpha-2 receptors are located in the brainstem, and stimulation of these receptors appears to decrease sympathetic outflow from the vasomotor center. Thus, blocking these centrally located alpha-2 receptors is counterproductive when a decrease in vascular tone is desired.

Specific Agents

Alfuzosin (Uroxatral). This drug is relatively selective for postsynaptic alpha-1 receptors on smooth muscle in the prostate gland and lower urinary tract. By blocking these receptors, alfuzosin inhibits smooth muscle contraction and is therefore used to treat urinary retention and other symptoms of BPH.

Doxazosin (Cardura, others). This drug shows a high degree of alpha-1 selectively and promotes relaxation of smooth muscle in the vasculature and other tissues. It was developed as an antihypertensive and can be taken orally to reduce blood pressure because it decreases peripheral vascular resistance.[17,21] In addition, doxazosin may have beneficial effects on the plasma lipid profile (decreased total cholesterol, decreased triglycerides) and may decrease insulin resistance in people with type 2 diabetes mellitus (see Chapter 32).[17,22,23] Hence, this drug is useful in treating high blood pressure in people with metabolic problems, including various hyperlipidemias and glucose intolerance. In addition, doxazosin can reduce urinary retention in men with BPH. As indicated above, this drug relaxes smooth muscle in the prostate and urethra, thereby allowing urine to flow more freely during micturition.

Ergot alkaloids. Ergotamine (Ergomar, others) and similar drugs, such as dihydroergotamine (Migranal, D. H. E. 45) and ergonovine (Ergometrine, Ergotrate), exert several pharmacological effects. At higher doses, these drugs act as competitive alpha antagonists, hence their inclusion here. However, these drugs appear to produce vasoconstriction in blood vessels that have low vascular tone and vasodilation in blood vessels that have high vascular tone. Exactly how they accomplish these rather contradictory effects is unclear, but these drugs essentially function as partial agonists because they display agonistic (stimulatory) activity in vessels with low tone and antagonistic (inhibitory) activity in vessels with high tone. These drugs, however, can also affect serotonin and dopamine receptors. Hence, they exert numerous complex effects throughout the body, and it is difficult to attribute their therapeutic effects to only one type of receptor. In the past, these drugs were used primarily for their ability to prevent or abort vascular headaches (migraine, cluster headaches) by vasoconstricting cerebral vessels.[24,25] Their antimigraine effects, however, may be due to their agonistic effect on vascular serotonin receptors rather than an effect on cerebral alpha-1 receptors. Hence, medical practitioners have replaced these drugs with serotonin-selective agonists, such as sumatriptan (Imitrex) and rizatriptan (Maxalt), to treat headaches in many patients. Alpha-1 blockers are also useful for preventing or treating postpartum hemorrhage. They stimulate the uterus to contract, thereby helping compress and occlude bleeding vessels in the uterine wall. Occasionally, these drugs can also be used to diagnosis angina pectoris because they cause transient constriction of the coronary arteries.

Ergoloid mesylate. These compounds, which appear under trade names such as Gerimal and Hydergine, exhibit some ability to produce peripheral vasodilation by blocking peripheral alpha-1 receptors. The primary clinical application of ergoloid mesylates is to increase mental acuity and alertness in geriatric patients with dementia related to Alzheimer disease.[26] These drugs supposedly increase mental function by increasing cerebral blood flow or by increasing oxygen utilization in the brain. These drugs' mechanism of action is probably a moot point, however, because there is little evidence that they produce any significant clinical benefits in treating Alzheimer dementia.[27] These drugs are usually administered orally or sublingually.

Phenoxybenzamine (Dibenzyline). Phenoxybenzamine is a noncompetitive alpha-1 blocker that binds irreversibly to the alpha-1 receptor. This drug tends to have a slow onset, but its effects last much longer than those of the competitive blockers (e.g., phentolamine and prazosin). Phenoxybenzamine is used primarily to control blood pressure prior to and during the removal of a pheochromocytoma. This drug is not typically used for the long-term management of hypertension, however, because it produces several side effects, including reflex tachycardia. Other indications for phenoxybenzamine include treatment of urinary retention in benign prostatic hypertrophy and treatment of vasospastic disease (Raynaud phenomenon). Phenoxybenzamine is usually administered orally.

Phentolamine (Regitine). Phentolamine is a competitive alpha antagonist used primarily to control blood pressure during management of pheochromocytoma. The drug is usually administered via IV or intramuscular injection. Phentolamine is not typically used to treat essential hypertension because with prolonged use, effectiveness tends to decrease and patients begin to develop adverse side effects.

Prazosin (Minipress). Prazosin is a competitive alpha-1 antagonist and one of the main alpha-1 selective agents. It tends to produce vasodilation in both arteries and veins, and its primary use is for the long-term management of essential hypertension.[17] Prazosin is also used to reduce alpha-1-receptor mediated activity in congestive heart failure, Raynaud phenomenon, pheochromocytoma, and BPH. In addition, this drug appears to be effective in reducing nightmares related to post-traumatic stress disorder, presumably by decreasing the excitatory effects of norepinephrine in the brain.[28] Prazosin is administered orally.

Silodosin (Rapaflo). This drug is similar to alfuzosin.

Tamsulosin (Flomax). This drug is similar to alfuzosin.

Terazosin (Hytrin). This drug is similar to doxazosin.

Adverse Effects

One of the primary adverse effects associated with alpha antagonists is reflex tachycardia. By blocking alpha-1 receptors, these drugs tend to decrease blood pressure by decreasing peripheral vascular resistance. As blood pressure falls, a compensatory increase in cardiac output is initiated via the baroreceptor reflex. The increased cardiac output is mediated in part by an increase in heart rate, hence the reflex tachycardia. A second major problem with these drugs is orthostatic hypotension. Dizziness and syncope following changes in posture are quite common due to the decrease in peripheral vascular tone. With alpha antagonists, orthostatic hypotension may be a particular problem just after drug therapy is initiated, in geriatric patients, or following exercise.

Beta Antagonists

Beta antagonists, or beta blockers, are generally administered for their effect on the beta-1 receptors located on the heart.[29] When stimulated, these receptors mediate an increase in cardiac contractility and rate of contraction. By blocking these receptors, beta antagonists reduce the rate and force of myocardial contractions. Consequently, medical practitioners frequently administer beta antagonists to decrease cardiac workload in conditions such as hypertension and certain types of angina pectoris. Beta blockers may also be used to normalize heart rate in certain forms of cardiac arrhythmias. Specific clinical applications of individual beta blockers are summarized in Table 20-2.

Another important function of beta blockers is their ability to limit the extent of myocardial damage following a heart attack and to reduce the risk of fatality following myocardial infarction.[30] Apparently, these drugs help reduce the workload of the damaged heart, thus allowing the heart to recover more completely following infarction. Substantial evidence shows that some beta blockers can help improve cardiac function in certain types of heart failure[31,32] (see Chapter 24).

Clinically useful beta antagonists are classified as beta-1-selective if they predominantly affect the beta-1 subtype; they are classified as beta-nonselective if they have a fairly equal affinity for beta-1 and beta-2 receptors (see Table 20-2). Beta-1-selective drugs are also referred to as *cardioselective* because of their preferential effect on the myocardium. Even if a beta antagonist is nonselective (i.e., blocks both beta-1 and beta-2 receptors), the beta-1 blockade is clinically beneficial. When stimulated, beta-2 receptors, which are found primarily on bronchial smooth muscle, cause bronchodilation. Blocking these beta-2 receptors may lead to smooth-muscle contraction and bronchoconstriction. Thus, drugs that selectively block beta-2 receptors have no real clinical significance because they promote bronchoconstriction.[10]

The selection of a specific beta blocker depends on factors such as cardioselectivity, duration of action (half-life), and several other ancillary properties of each drug.[29,33] Certain beta blockers, for instance, produce added effects such as mild peripheral vasodilation or stabilization of cardiac membranes that can be beneficial in treating certain cardiovascular

Table 20-2
SUMMARY OF COMMON BETA BLOCKERS

Generic Name	Trade Name(s)	Selectivity	Primary Indications*
Acebutolol	Sectral	Beta-1	Hypertension, arrhythmias
Atenolol	Tenormin	Beta-1	Angina pectoris, hypertension, prevent reinfarction
Betaxolol	Kerlone	Beta-1	Hypertension
Bisoprolol	Zebeta	Beta-1	Hypertension
Carteolol	Cartrol	Nonselective	Hypertension
Carvedilol	Coreg	Nonselective	Hypertension, congestive heart failure, prevent reinfarction
Esmolol	Brevibloc	Beta-1	Arrhythmias
Labetalol	Normodyne, Trandate	Nonselective	Hypertension
Metoprolol	Lopressor, Toprol-XL	Beta-1	Angina pectoris, hypertension, prevent reinfarction
Nadolol	Corgard	Nonselective	Hypertension, angina pectoris
Nebivolol	Bystolic	Beta-1	Hypertension
Penbutolol	Levatol	Nonselective	Hypertension
Pindolol	Visken	Nonselective	Hypertension
Propranolol	Inderal	Nonselective	Angina pectoris, arrhythmias, hypertension, prevent reinfarction, prevent vascular headache
Sotalol	Betapace	Nonselective	Arrhythmias
Timolol	Blocadren	Nonselective	Hypertension, prevent reinfarction, prevent vascular headache

**This table includes only indications listed in the United States product labeling. All drugs are fairly similar pharmacologically, and some may be used for appropriate cardiovascular conditions not specifically listed in product labeling.*

conditions.[34,35] Primary indications and relative selectivity of these drugs are summarized in Table 20-2. Chapters 21 through 24 cover clinical applications of specific beta blockers in more detail.

Specific Agents

Acebutolol (Sectral). Acebutolol is described as a relatively cardioselective beta blocker that tends to bind preferentially to beta-1 receptors at low doses but binds to both types of beta receptors as the dosage increases. This drug also exerts mild to moderate intrinsic sympathomimetic activity, which means that acebutolol blocks the beta receptor from the effects of endogenous catecholamines and stimulates the receptor to some extent (i.e., it acts as a partial beta agonist). This advantage protects the beta receptor from excessive endogenous stimulation while still preserving a low level of background sympathetic activity. Primary clinical applications are for treatment of hypertension and prevention and treatment of cardiac arrhythmias. The drug is usually administered orally.

Atenolol (Tenormin). Like acebutolol, atenolol is regarded as beta-1 selective but tends to be less beta-specific at higher doses. The drug is administered orally for the long-term treatment of hypertension and chronic, stable angina. Atenolol is also administered immediately following a myocardial infarction to prevent reinfarction and to promote recovery of the myocardium.

Betaxolol (Kerlone). This drug is a relatively beta-1-selective agent that is administered orally for treating hypertension.

Bisoprolol (Zebeta). This drug is similar to betaxolol.

Carteolol (Cartrol). Carteolol is a nonselective beta blocker that also has moderate intrinsic sympathomimetic activity. It is typically administered orally to treat hypertension.

Carvedilol (Coreg). Carvedilol is a nonselective beta blocker that can also cause systemic vasodilation by blocking alpha-1 receptors on the peripheral vasculature. The drug is administered orally to treat hypertension, congestive heart failure, and recovery from myocardial infarction.

Esmolol (Brevibloc). This drug is a selective beta blocker that is administered intravenously for the short-term treatment of specific arrhythmias.

Labetalol (Normodyne, Trandate). Labetalol is a nonselective beta blocker. It appears to also have some alpha-1-selective blocking effects. Labetalol is used primarily in the management of hypertension and, while usually given orally, may be injected intravenously in emergency hypertensive situations.

Metoprolol (Lopressor, Toprol-XL). Metoprolol is considered a cardioselective beta blocker and has been approved for treating hypertension, preventing angina pectoris, and preventing myocardial reinfarction. As an antihypertensive and antianginal, metoprolol is usually administered orally. In the prevention of reinfarction, metoprolol is initiated by IV injection and then followed up by oral administration.

Nadolol (Corgard). Nadolol is a nonselective beta blocker that is administered orally as an antihypertensive and antianginal agent. The drug has an advantage over other nonselective beta blockers (propranolol) in that nadolol often needs to be taken only once each day.

Nebivolol (Bystolic). This drug is a relatively beta-1-selective agent that is administered orally for treating hypertension.

Penbutolol (Levatol). This drug is similar to carteolol.

Pindolol (Visken). Pindolol is a nonselective beta blocker that exhibits the highest level of intrinsic sympathomimetic activity of all the beta blockers. Pindolol is used primarily in the long-term management of hypertension, but it may also be used to prevent certain types of angina pectoris.

Propranolol (Inderal, many others). Propranolol, the classic nonselective beta blocker, is approved for use in hypertension, angina pectoris, cardiac arrhythmias, and prevention of myocardial reinfarction. In addition, propranolol has been used in the prevention of vascular headache and as an adjunct to alpha blockers in treating pheochromocytoma. Propranolol is usually administered orally for the long-term management of the previously listed conditions, but it may be administered via IV injection for the immediate control of arrhythmias.

Sotalol (Betapace, Sorine). This drug is a nonselective beta blocker that is administered primarily to treat arrhythmias, although it is sometimes used as an antihypertensive or antianginal agent. It is administered orally.

Timolol (Blocadren, others). This nonselective beta blocker is administered orally for the treatment of hypertension and prevention of myocardial reinfarction. It may also be used to treat angina or prevent vascular headaches.

Adverse Effects

Some antagonism of beta-2 receptors occurs with the use of nonselective beta blockers.[29,36] The antagonism of beta-2 receptors on bronchiole smooth muscle often leads to a degree of bronchoconstriction and an increase in airway resistance. Although this event is usually not a problem in individuals with normal pulmonary function, patients with respiratory problems such as asthma, bronchitis, and emphysema may be adversely affected by nonselective beta antagonists. These patients should use one of the beta-1-selective drugs.

Selective and nonselective beta blockers are also associated with several other adverse effects. The most serious of these effects results from excessive depression of cardiac function.[37] By slowing down the heart too much, these agents can lead to cardiac failure, especially if there is some preexisting cardiac disease. Because of their antihypertensive properties, beta blockers may produce orthostatic hypotension, and dizziness and syncope may occur following abrupt changes in posture. Patients taking beta blockers for prolonged periods have also been reported to have an increase in centrally related side effects such as depression, lethargy, and sleep disorders.[38,39] These behavioral side effects may be due to the interaction of beta blockers with CNS beta receptors.

Various other relatively minor side effects have also been reported, including gastrointestinal (GI) disturbances (nausea, vomiting) and allergic responses (fever, rash). However, these are fairly uncommon and tend to be resolved by adjusting the dosage or specific medication type.

Other Drugs That Inhibit Adrenergic Neurons

Several agents inhibit activity at adrenergic synapses by interfering with the release of norepinephrine. Rather than directly blocking the postsynaptic receptor, these drugs typically inhibit or deplete the presynaptic terminal of stored norepinephrine. The drugs are used primarily to decrease peripheral adrenergic influence and to treat problems such as hypertension and cardiac arrhythmias.

Specific Agents

Bretylium (Bretylol). Bretylium appears to directly inhibit the release of norepinephrine from adrenergic nerve terminals. With prolonged use, this drug may also replace presynaptic norepinephrine in a manner similar to guanethidine (listed below). Bretylium is used primarily in the treatment of cardiac arrhythmias (see Chapter 23). In addition to its effect on norepinephrine release, bretylium also appears to have a direct stabilizing effect on cardiac muscle cells that contributes to its antiarrhythmic properties. While usually given orally for the long-term management of ventricular arrhythmias, bretylium is also injected intravenously for the emergency treatment of ventricular tachycardia and ventricular fibrillation.

Guanethidine (Ismelin). This drug acts on postganglionic sympathetic neurons, including the neurons that innervate the peripheral arterioles. Guanethidine is actively transported into the presynaptic terminal of these neurons, where it inhibits norepinephrine release and later replaces stored norepinephrine. Guanethidine therefore acts as a false neurotransmitter that is unable to stimulate alpha-1 receptors on the vasculature, which results in vasodilation. Guanethidine selectively affects postganglionic sympathetic adrenergic nerve terminals but does not affect release of norepinephrine from the adrenal medulla. Because of its vasodilating effects, guanethidine is usually administered orally for the management of moderate-to-severe hypertension.

Metyrosine (Demser). Metyrosine inhibits the enzyme initiating catecholamine synthesis (epinephrine, norepinephrine). Medical practitioners administer the drug to diminish catecholamine stores prior to removal of a catecholamine-producing tumor (pheochromocytoma) or to prevent hypertension in patients when removal of such a tumor is not possible.

Rauwolfia alkaloids. This chemical group includes reserpine (Reserfia, others), deserpidine (Harmonyl), and rauwolfia serpentina (Rauwolfemms, others). These drugs all inhibit the synthesis of catecholamines (norepinephrine, epinephrine) and 5-hydroxytryptamine (serotonin) in peripheral and CNS sympathetic nerve endings. This inhibition eventually causes a depletion of presynaptic neurotransmitter stores in several tissues, including in postganglionic nerve terminals, the adrenal medulla, and the brain. Unlike guanethidine, these agents do not appear to actually replace the presynaptic neurotransmitter but simply prevent more transmitter from being resynthesized. Reserpine and the other rauwolfia alkaloids are administered orally to treat mild-to-moderate hypertension. The antihypertensive effects of these drugs are caused, in part, by the inhibition of peripheral adrenergic nerve terminals, although some of their antihypertensive effects may also be because of the inhibition of CNS catecholamine activity.

Adverse Effects

Orthostatic hypotension is occasionally a problem with the aforementioned drugs, and dizziness and syncope sometimes occur after a sudden change in posture. Some patients also experience GI disturbances, including nausea, vomiting, and diarrhea. Peripheral edema as evidenced by swelling in the feet and legs has also been reported.

SUMMARY

A variety of drugs have stimulatory (agonistic) or inhibitory (antagonistic) effects on adrenergic function. In general, adrenergic agonists are administered according to their ability to evoke specific tissue responses via specific adrenergic receptors. Alpha-1-adrenergic agonists are used as antihypotensive agents because of their ability to increase peripheral vascular resistance; they may also be used as nasal decongestants because of their ability to vasoconstrict the nasal mucosa. Agonists selective for alpha-2 receptors are administered to treat hypertension and spasticity because of their ability to inhibit neuronal activity in the brainstem and spinal cord, respectively. Cardioselective beta-1 agonists are used primarily for their ability to stimulate the heart, and beta-2 agonists are used in the treatment of asthma and premature labor because of their ability to relax bronchiole and uterine smooth muscle, respectively.

Alpha-adrenergic antagonists are used primarily as antihypertensive drugs because of their ability to block vascular alpha-1 receptors. Beta-adrenergic antagonists (beta blockers) are administered primarily for their inhibitory effects on myocardial function and are used in the prevention and treatment of hypertension, angina pectoris, arrhythmias, and myocardial reinfarction. Many of the drugs introduced in this chapter are discussed further in chapters that deal with the specific clinical conditions (e.g., hypertension, asthma, and other disorders).

REFERENCES

1. Westfall TC, Westfall DP. Adrenergic agonists and antagonists. In: Brunton L, et al, eds. *The Pharmacological Basis of Therapeutics*. 12th ed. New York: McGraw-Hill; 2011.
2. Vongpatanasin W, Kario K, Atlas SA, Victor RG. Central sympatholytic drugs. *J Clin Hypertens*. 2011;13:658-661.
3. Rank MM, Murray KC, Stephens MJ, et al. Adrenergic receptors modulate motoneuron excitability, sensory synaptic transmission and muscle spasms after chronic spinal cord injury. *J Neurophysiol*. 2011;105:410-422.
4. Gilsbach R, Hein L. Are the pharmacology and physiology of α_2 adrenoceptors determined by α_2-heteroreceptors and autoreceptors respectively? *Br J Pharmacol*. 2012;165:90-102.
5. Arnsten AF. The use of alpha-2A adrenergic agonists for the treatment of attention-deficit/hyperactivity disorder. *Expert Rev Neurother*. 2010;10:1595-1605.
6. Childress AC, Sallee FR. Revisiting clonidine: an innovative add-on option for attention-deficit/hyperactivity disorder. *Drugs Today*. 2012;48:207-217.
7. Kamen L, Henney HR 3rd, Runyan JD. A practical overview of tizanidine use for spasticity secondary to multiple sclerosis, stroke, and spinal cord injury. *Curr Med Res Opin*. 2008;24:425-439.
8. Vakhapova V, Auriel E, Karni A. Nightly sublingual tizanidine HCl in multiple sclerosis: clinical efficacy and safety. *Clin Neuropharmacol*. 2010;33:151-154.
9. Parissis JT, Rafouli-Stergiou P, Stasinos V, et al. Inotropes in cardiac patients: update 2011. *Curr Opin Crit Care*. 2010;16:432-441.
10. Cazzola M, Page CP, Rogliani P, Matera MG. β2-agonist therapy in lung disease. *Am J Respir Crit Care Med*. 2013;187:690-696.
11. Matera MG, Martuscelli E, Cazzola M. Pharmacological modulation of beta-adrenoceptor function in patients with coexisting chronic obstructive pulmonary disease and chronic heart failure. *Pulm Pharmacol Ther*. 2010;23:1-8.
12. Warnier MJ, Rutten FH, Kors JA, et al. Cardiac arrhythmias in adult patients with asthma. *J Asthma*. 2012;49:942-946.
13. Haas DM, Caldwell DM, Kirkpatrick P, et al. Tocolytic therapy for preterm delivery: systematic review and network meta-analysis. *BMJ*. 2012;345:e6226.
14. Motazedian S, Ghaffarpasand F, Mojtahedi K, Asadi N. Terbutaline versus salbutamol for suppression of preterm labor: a randomized clinical trial. *Ann Saudi Med*. 2010;30:370-375.
15. Gaudet LM, Singh K, Weeks L, et al. Effectiveness of terbutaline pump for the prevention of preterm birth. A systematic review and meta-analysis. *PLoS One*. 2012;7:e31679.
16. Khianey R, Oppenheimer J. Controversies regarding long-acting β2-agonists. *Curr Opin Allergy Clin Immunol*. 2011;11:345-354.
17. Chapman N, Chen CY, Fujita T, et al. Time to re-appraise the role of alpha-1 adrenoceptor antagonists in the management of hypertension? *J Hypertens*. 2010;28:1796-1803.
18. Grimm RH Jr, Flack JM. Alpha 1 adrenoreceptor antagonists. *J Clin Hypertens*. 2011;13:654-657.
19. Lepor H, Kazzazi A, Djavan B. α-Blockers for benign prostatic hyperplasia: the new era. *Curr Opin Urol*. 2012;22:7-15.

20. Osman NI, Chapple CR, Cruz F, et al. Silodosin: a new subtype selective alpha-1 antagonist for the treatment of lower urinary tract symptoms in patients with benign prostatic hyperplasia. *Expert Opin Pharmacother.* 2012;13:2085-2096.
21. Wykretowicz A, Guzik P, Wysocki H. Doxazosin in the current treatment of hypertension. *Expert Opin Pharmacother.* 2008;9: 625-633.
22. Chapman N, Chang CL, Dahlöf B, et al. Effect of doxazosin gastrointestinal therapeutic system as third-line antihypertensive therapy on blood pressure and lipids in the Anglo-Scandinavian Cardiac Outcomes Trial. *Circulation.* 2008;118:42-48.
23. Shibasaki S, Eguchi K, Matsui Y, et al. Adrenergic blockade improved insulin resistance in patients with morning hypertension: the Japan Morning Surge-1 Study. *J Hypertens.* 2009;27:1252-1257.
24. Dahlöf C, Maassen Van Den Brink A. Dihydroergotamine, ergotamine, methysergide and sumatriptan—basic science in relation to migraine treatment. *Headache.* 2012;52:707-714.
25. Reddy DS. The pathophysiological and pharmacological basis of current drug treatment of migraine headache. *Expert Rev Clin Pharmacol.* 2013;6:271-288.
26. Olin J, Schneider L, Novit A, Luczak S. Hydergine for dementia. *Cochrane Database Syst Rev.* 2001;2:CD000359.
27. Howland RH. Alternative drug therapies for dementia. *J Psychosoc Nurs Ment Health Serv.* 2011;49:17-20.
28. Hudson SM, Whiteside TE, Lorenz RA, Wargo KA. Prazosin for the treatment of nightmares related to posttraumatic stress disorder: a review of the literature. *Prim Care Companion CNS Disord.* 2012;14:2.
29. Frishman WH, Saunders E. β-Adrenergic blockers. *J Clin Hypertens.* 2011;13:649-653.
30. Kezerashvili A, Marzo K, De Leon J. Beta blocker use after acute myocardial infarction in the patient with normal systolic function: when is it "ok" to discontinue? *Curr Cardiol Rev.* 2012;8:77-84.
31. Chatterjee S, Biondi-Zoccai G, Abbate A, et al. Benefits of β blockers in patients with heart failure and reduced ejection fraction: network meta-analysis. *BMJ.* 2013;346:f55.
32. Ong HT, Ong LM, Kow FP. Beta-blockers for heart failure: an evidence based review answering practical therapeutic questions. *Med J Malaysia.* 2012;67:7-11.
33. Gorre F, Vandekerckhove H. Beta-blockers: focus on mechanism of action. Which beta-blocker, when and why? *Acta Cardiol.* 2010;65:565-570.
34. Fares H, Lavie CJ, Ventura HO. Vasodilating versus first-generation β-blockers for cardiovascular protection. *Postgrad Med.* 2012;124:7-15.
35. Rath G, Balligand JL, Dessy C. Vasodilatory mechanisms of beta receptor blockade. *Curr Hypertens Rep.* 2012;14: 310-317.
36. Manrique C, Giles TD, Ferdinand KC, Sowers JR. Realities of newer beta-blockers for the management of hypertension. *J Clin Hypertens.* 2009;11:369-375.
37. Shepherd G. Treatment of poisoning caused by beta-adrenergic and calcium-channel blockers. *Am J Health Syst Pharm.* 2006;63:1828-1835.
38. Kountz DS. Are tolerability concerns a class effect of beta-blockers in treating patients with hypertension? *Postgrad Med.* 2009;121:14-24.
39. Verbeek DE, van Riezen J, de Boer RA, et al. A review on the putative association between beta-blockers and depression. *Heart Fail Clin.* 2011;7:89-99.

CHAPTER 21

Antihypertensive Drugs

Hypertension is a sustained, reproducible increase in blood pressure. It is one of the most common diseases affecting adults living in industrialized nations. In the United States, for example, hypertension occurs in approximately 30 percent of the general population aged 20 and over.[1,2] The prevalence of this disease can be even higher in certain subpopulations (e.g., 44 to 45 percent in African Americans), and the incidence of hypertension increases with age.[2,3] If left untreated, the sustained increase in blood pressure associated with hypertension can lead to cardiovascular problems (stroke, heart failure), renal disease, and blindness.[4,5] These and other medical problems ultimately lead to an increased mortality rate in hypertensive individuals.

Although there is a general consensus regarding the adverse effects of hypertension, some debate exists as to exactly how much of an increase in blood pressure constitutes hypertension. Generally, diastolic values greater than 90 mm Hg and/or systolic values greater than 140 mm Hg warrant a diagnosis of hypertension. Patients are classified as prehypertensive, stage 1, or stage 2, depending on the extent of their elevated blood pressure. A more detailed classification scheme is shown in Table 21-1.

Hypertension is often described as a silent killer because of the lack of symptoms throughout most of the disease course. Patients may feel fine into the advanced stages of hypertension. As might be expected, the incidence of morbidity and mortality increases as the hypertension becomes more severe. Hence, pharmacological and nonpharmacological methods are implemented to decrease blood pressure to an optimal diastolic value of 80 mm Hg or less and an optimal systolic value less than 120 mm Hg.

When you are dealing with hypertensive patients, you are usually treating a problem other than the increased blood pressure—that is, hypertension is not the reason the patient is referred to physical therapy and occupational therapy. Due to the prevalence of hypertension, however, many patients receiving therapy for other problems will also be taking antihypertensive drugs. These drugs can also affect heart rate and vascular responses to aerobic exercise, mobility training, physical agents, and various other rehabilitation interventions. Hence, it is essential that you have knowledge of the pharmacology of these agents.

The pharmacological management of hypertension has evolved to where blood pressure can be controlled for extended periods in most patients. Several major categories of antihypertensive agents are currently available, and new drugs are continually being added to the antihypertensive arsenal. Each group of antihypertensive drugs is discussed under the appropriate section in this chapter, as well as how several different drugs can be used together when treating hypertension. To help you better understand how these drugs work in decreasing blood pressure, the first section is a brief review of the normal control of blood pressure and the possible mechanisms that generate a hypertensive state.

Table 21-1
CLASSIFICATION OF BLOOD PRESSURE

Category	Systolic BP (mm Hg)	Diastolic BP (mm Hg)
Optimal	<120	<80
Prehypertension	120–139	80–89
Hypertension		
Stage 1	140–159	90–99
Stage 2	≥160	≥100

BP = blood pressure.

Source: From the Seventh Report of the Joint National Committee on Prevention, Detection, Evaluation, and Treatment of High Blood Pressure (JNC-VII). JAMA. 2003;289:2560-2571, with permission.

NORMAL CONTROL OF BLOOD PRESSURE

Blood pressure is normally maintained by the complex interaction of several physiological systems.[6] Rapid control of blood pressure is accomplished primarily by the baroreceptor reflex (see Chapter 18),[7] which monitors and corrects changes in blood pressure within a matter of seconds by altering cardiac output and peripheral vascular resistance. The long-term management of blood pressure is accomplished primarily by the kidneys through their control of fluid balance.[8] Changes in blood pressure through the renal handling of fluid and electrolytes usually take place over a period of several hours to several days. Humoral factors such as circulating catecholamines (from the adrenal gland), arginine-vasopressin (from the pituitary gland), and angiotensin II (from a reaction involving the kidneys) can also play a role in regulating blood pressure, especially if blood pressure decreases suddenly.[9] Other substances such as nitric oxide and endothelins are produced locally within the vascular system; these chemicals are also involved in regulating blood pressure through their effects on vascular tone and sodium homeostasis.[10] Hence, various systems interact to maintain blood pressure within a fairly narrow range.

Although the control of blood pressure is a fairly complex subject, the actual factors that determine blood pressure can be simplified. At any given time, blood pressure is the product of cardiac output and the total resistance in the peripheral vasculature. This relationship is illustrated by the following equation:

$$BP = (CO) \times (TPR)$$

where *BP* is blood pressure, *CO* is the cardiac output, and *TPR* is the total peripheral resistance in the systemic vasculature. As indicated by this equation, BP can be maintained at a relatively constant level by changes in either CO or TPR. A decrease in CO, for instance, can potentially be offset by an increase in TPR so that BP does not appreciably change. Conversely, a sudden fall in TPR will necessitate an increase in CO to maintain BP.

The relevance of this simple equation to antihypertensive therapy will become apparent as different drugs are discussed. Some antihypertensive drugs exert their effects by primarily acting on CO, others primarily affect TPR, and some agents decrease both factors.

PATHOGENESIS OF HYPERTENSION

Essential Versus Secondary Hypertension

Hypertension can be divided into two major categories: secondary hypertension and primary, or essential, hypertension. In secondary hypertension, the elevated blood pressure can be attributed to some specific abnormality such as chronic kidney disease, renal artery stenosis, certain drugs, catecholamine-producing tumors, endocrine disorders, or cerebral damage. The treatment of secondary hypertension is rather straightforward, with efforts focusing on correcting the underlying pathology (i.e., the cause of the problem can be dealt with directly by surgery, discontinuing specific drugs, etc.). Secondary hypertension, however, accounts for less than 10 percent of the patients diagnosed with hypertension.[2] The remaining 90 percent of hypertensive individuals are classified as having primary, or essential, hypertension. In essential hypertension, there is no clear, readily discernible cause of the elevated blood pressure.

Consequently, the exact cause of hypertension in the majority of patients is unknown. Many theories have been proposed to explain how blood pressure increases and eventually becomes sustained in essential hypertension. The literature dealing with potential causes and mechanisms of essential hypertension is voluminous and cannot be reviewed extensively in this chapter. Nonetheless, some of the major factors that may account for the increased blood pressure in essential hypertension are presented here.

Possible Mechanisms in Essential Hypertension

It appears there is a rather complex interaction of genetic and environmental factors that ultimately leads to adaptive changes in the cardiovascular system of patients with essential hypertension.[11-13] Diet, stress, and other external factors are associated with increased blood pressure. These factors seem to be more influential in certain patients, suggesting a possible genetic predisposition to hypertension. Other risk factors such as cigarette smoking and alcohol abuse clearly play a role in potentiating the onset and maintenance of hypertension. Obesity is also an important risk factor for hypertension and various other types of cardiovascular disease.[14,15] Thus, essential hypertension is probably not caused by a single factor but likely by a subtle, complex interaction of many factors. The exact way in which these factors interact probably varies from person to person, so the cause of this disease must be regarded individually rather than being based on one common etiology.

Although the exact cause of hypertension is unknown, studies in humans and in animal models that mimic essential hypertension have suggested that the sympathetic nervous system may be a final common pathway in mediating and perpetuating the hypertensive state—that is, the factors described earlier may interact in such a way as to cause a general increase in sympathetic activity, which then becomes the common denominator underlying the elevated blood pressure in essential hypertension.[16-18] Increased sympathetic activity should produce a hypertensive effect because of the excitatory effect of sympathetic neurons on the heart and peripheral vasculature. Increased sympathetic drive may initially increase blood pressure by increasing cardiac output. In later stages, cardiac output often returns to normal levels, with the increased blood pressure being due to an increase in vascular resistance. The reasons for the shift from elevated cardiac output to elevated peripheral vascular resistance are somewhat unclear, but a sustained increase in sympathetic activity may be the initiating factor that begins a sequence of events ultimately resulting in essential hypertension.

Once blood pressure becomes elevated, hypertension seems to become self-perpetuating to some extent. For example, mechanisms that control blood pressure (the baroreceptor reflex) may decrease in sensitivity, thus blunting the normal response to elevated pressure.[19,20] Increased sympathetic discharge to the kidneys and altered renal hemodynamics may also cause changes in renal function, contributing to the sustained increase in blood pressure.[16,21] Moreover, it is apparent that hypertension is often associated with metabolic abnormalities, including impaired glucose metabolism (due to insulin resistance), hyperinsulinemia, dyslipidemia, and abdominal obesity.[15,22,23] This cluster of problems, known commonly as **metabolic syndrome,** places the patient at risk for type 2 diabetes mellitus (see Chapter 32). Although the exact link between hypertension and metabolic syndrome is not clear, it is apparent that a chronic elevation in blood pressure is associated with metabolic impairments that further jeopardize the health of patients with this disease.[23-25]

Increased blood pressure may also invoke adaptive changes in the peripheral vasculature so that peripheral vessels become less compliant and vascular resistance increases.[26,27] That is, increased pressure on the vascular wall actually causes thickening of the wall, which further increases the resistance to blood flow through the thickened vessels. The peripheral vasculature may also become more reactive to pressor substances, such as norepinephrine and angiotensin II.[28,29] Hypertension is also associated with a defect in the production of vasoactive substances by the cells lining the peripheral vasculature—the vascular endothelium. These cells normally produce several vasoactive substances, including vasodilators (nitric oxide, bradykinin, prostaglandin I_2) and vasoconstrictors (angiotensin II, endothelin-I).[10,30] These endothelial-derived substances help maintain local control over vascular resistance.[30,31] In hypertension, however, there may be a defect in the production of these substances, especially a decreased production of nitric oxide.[32,33] A relative deficiency of this vasodilator would result in increased vascular resistance, which helps increase the hypertensive condition.

The possible factors involved in initiating and maintaining essential hypertension are summarized in Figure 21-1. Ultimately, certain environmental factors may turn on the sympathetic division of the autonomic nervous system in susceptible individuals. Increased sympathetic discharge then creates a vicious cycle whereby increased sympathetic effects—in conjunction with the increased blood pressure itself—help perpetuate hypertension. Exactly how various factors initiate the increased sympathetic discharge is not fully

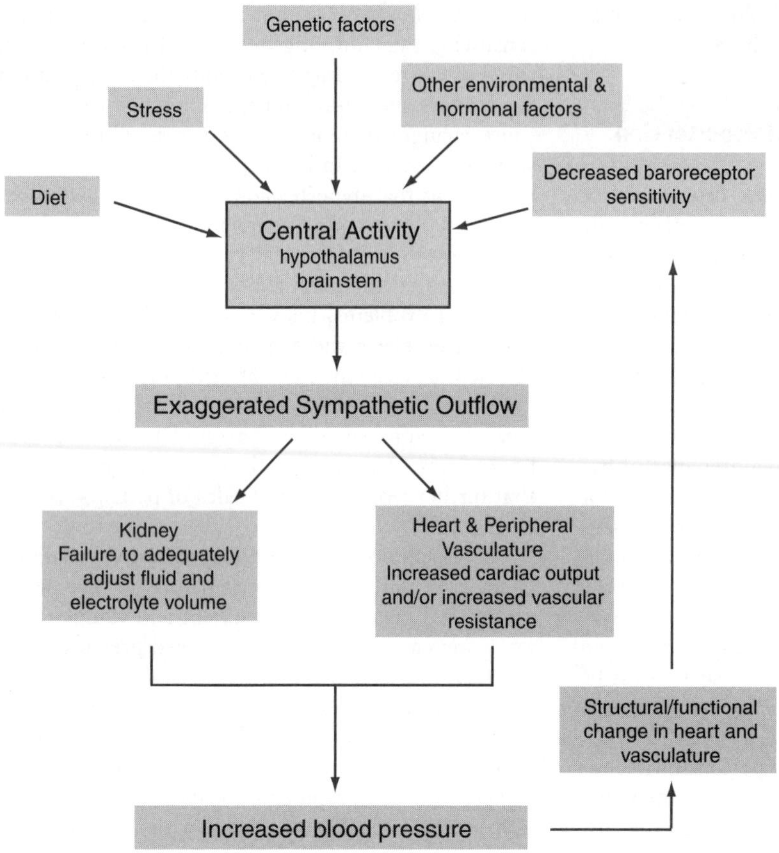

Figure ■ 21-1 Schematic diagram of the possible mechanisms in essential hypertension. Various factors interact to turn on sympathetic outflow to the kidneys, heart, and peripheral vasculature, resulting in elevated blood pressure. Hypertension also causes structural and functional changes in the vasculature that help maintain the elevated pressure.

understood and may in fact vary from patient to patient. Hopefully future studies will elaborate on the exact role of factors causing essential hypertension, and treatment can then be focused on preventing the changes that initially increase blood pressure.

DRUG THERAPY

Several major categories of drugs exist for the treatment of essential hypertension, including diuretics, sympatholytic drugs, vasodilators, drugs that inhibit the renin-angiotensin system, and calcium channel blockers. The primary sites of action and effects of each category are summarized in Table 21-2. This section surveys the mechanism of action, rationale for use, specific agents, and adverse effects of drugs in each category.

Diuretics

Diuretics increase the formation and excretion of urine. These drugs are used as antihypertensive agents because of their ability to increase the renal excretion of water and sodium, thus decreasing the volume of fluid within the vascular system. This is somewhat analogous to the decrease in pressure that occurs inside a balloon when some of the air inside leaks out. Consequently, diuretics appear to have a rather direct effect on blood pressure through their ability to simply decrease the amount of fluid in the vascular system.

Diuretics have been instrumental in treating hypertension for over 50 years.[34] They are relatively inexpensive and seem to work well in a large percentage of patients with mild-to-moderate hypertension.[35] Results from a large clinical trial suggested that thiazide diuretics might be superior to calcium channel blockers and angiotensin converting enzyme

Table 21-2
ANTIHYPERTENSIVE DRUG CATEGORIES

Category	Primary Site(s) of Action	Primary Antihypertensive Effect(s)
Diuretics	Kidneys	Decrease in plasma fluid volume
Sympatholytics	Various sites within the sympathetic division of the autonomic nervous system	Decrease sympathetic influence on the heart and/or peripheral vasculature
Vasodilators	Peripheral vasculature	Lower vascular resistance by directly vasodilating peripheral vessels
Inhibition of the renin-angiotensin system (ACE inhibitors, angiotensin II receptor blockers, direct renin inhibitors)	Peripheral vasculature and certain organs with a functional renin-angiotensin system (heart, kidneys, others)	ACE inhibitors: prevent the conversion of angiotensin I to angiotensin II. Angiotensin II receptor blockers: block the effects of angiotensin II on the vasculature and various other tissues. Direct renin inhibitors: block renin's ability to convert angiotensinogen to angiotensin I.
Calcium channel blockers	Limit calcium entry into vascular smooth muscle and cardiac muscle	Decrease vascular smooth-muscle contraction; decrease myocardial force and rate of contraction

ACE = angiotensin converting enzyme.

inhibitors in preventing major cardiac events such as myocardial infarction, stroke, and heart failure in people with hypertension.[36] Hence, diuretics remain one of the primary methods for treating this condition in a large number of people. These drugs can be used alone or combined with other antihypertensives as needed to control hypertension in specific clinical situations (see "Drug Selection for Specific Patients With Hypertension").

Although they differ chemically, all diuretics exert their beneficial effects by acting directly on the kidneys to increase water and sodium excretion.[37]

Classification of Diuretics

Diuretics can be classified according to their chemical structure or the manner in which they affect kidney function. The classifications include thiazide, loop, and potassium-sparing drugs (Table 21-3).

Thiazide Diuretics. Thiazide drugs share a common chemical nucleus and a common mode of action. These drugs act primarily on the early portion of the distal tubule of the nephron, where they inhibit sodium reabsorption. By inhibiting sodium reabsorption, more sodium is retained within the nephron, creating an osmotic force that also retains more water in the nephron. Because more sodium and water are passed through the nephron, where they will ultimately be excreted from the body, a diuretic effect is produced. Thiazides are the most frequently used type of diuretic for hypertension.

Loop Diuretics. These drugs act primarily on the ascending limb of the loop of Henle (hence the term *loop diuretic*). They exert their diuretic effect by inhibiting the reabsorption of sodium and chloride from the nephron, thereby preventing the reabsorption of the water that follows these electrolytes (see Table 21-3).

Potassium-Sparing Diuretics. The potassium-sparing diuretics are able to prevent the secretion of potassium into the distal tubule. Normally, a sodium-potassium exchange occurs in the distal tubule, where sodium is reabsorbed and potassium is secreted. Potassium-sparing agents interfere with this exchange in various ways (depending on the specific drug), and sodium remains in the tubule, where it is excreted. Although these agents do not produce a diuretic effect to the same extent as the loop and thiazide diuretics, potassium-sparing drugs have the advantage of reducing potassium loss and thus preventing hypokalemia (see Table 21-3).

Adverse Effects

The most serious side effects of diuretics are fluid depletion and electrolyte imbalance.[37,38] By the very nature of their action, diuretics decrease extracellular fluid volume and produce sodium depletion (hyponatremia) and potassium depletion (hypokalemia).

Table 21-3
DIURETIC DRUGS USED TO TREAT HYPERTENSION

Thiazide Diuretics	
Bendroflumethiazide (Naturetin)	Methyclothiazide (Aquatensen, Enduron)
Chlorothiazide (Diuril)	Metolazone (Mykrox, Zaroxolyn)
Chlorthalidone (Hygroton, Thalidone)	Polythiazide (Renese)
Hydrochlorothiazide (Aquazide, others)	Quinethazone (Hydromox)
Hydroflumethiazide (Diucardin, Saluron)	Trichlormethiazide (Metahydrin, Naqua, others)
Indapamide (Lozol)	
Loop Diuretics	
Bumetanide (Bumex)	Furosemide (Lasix, others)
Ethacrynic acid (Edecrin)	Torsemide (Demadex)
Potassium-Sparing Diuretics	
Amiloride (Midamor)	Triamterene (Dyrenium)
Spironolactone (Aldactone)	

Hypokalemia is a particular problem with the thiazide and loop diuretics but occurs less frequently when the potassium-sparing agents are used. Hypokalemia and other disturbances in fluid and electrolyte balance can produce serious metabolic and cardiac problems and may even prove fatal in some individuals. Consequently, patients must be monitored closely, and the drug dosage should be maintained at the lowest effective dose. Also, potassium supplements are used in some patients to prevent hypokalemia.

Fluid depletion may also be a serious problem during diuretic therapy. A decrease in blood volume may cause a reflex increase in cardiac output and peripheral vascular resistance because of activation of the baroreceptor reflex (see Chapter 18). This occurrence may produce an excessive demand on the myocardium, especially in patients with cardiac disease. Decreased blood volume may also activate the renin-angiotensin system, thereby causing further peripheral vasoconstriction and increased cardiac workload. Again, the effects of fluid depletion may be especially serious in patients with certain types of heart failure.

Loop and thiazide diuretics may also impair glucose and lipid metabolism.[39,40] This risk may be especially problematic in patients with concomitant metabolic disorders such as the metabolic syndrome described earlier in this chapter—that is, patients may have hypertension combined with insulin resistance and **hyperlipidemia**. Hence, diuretics should be used cautiously in patients who are prone to metabolic disorders, and concerns about metabolic side effects should be minimized by using the lowest possible dose.[40]

Other less serious, but bothersome, side effects of diuretic therapy include GI disturbances and weakness/fatigue. **Orthostatic hypotension** may occur because of the relative fluid depletion produced by these drugs. Changes in mood and confusion may also occur in some patients.

Sympatholytic Drugs

As discussed previously, the preponderance of evidence indicates that an increase in sympathetic activity may be an underlying factor in essential hypertension. Consequently, drugs that interfere with sympathetic discharge (i.e., sympatholytic agents) should be valuable as antihypertensive agents. These sympatholytic drugs can be classified according to where and how they interrupt sympathetic activity. Sympatholytic drugs used to treat hypertension include beta-adrenergic blockers, alpha-adrenergic blockers, presynaptic adrenergic neurotransmitter depletors, centrally acting drugs, and ganglionic blockers (Table 21-4).

Beta Blockers

Beta-adrenergic blockers have been used extensively to decrease blood pressure and are a mainstay of antihypertensive therapy in many patients.[41,42] Beta blockers exert their primary effect on the heart, where they decrease heart rate and myocardial contraction force. In hypertensive patients, these drugs lower blood pressure by slowing down the heart and reducing cardiac output. This is probably an oversimplification of how beta blockers produce an antihypertensive effect. In addition to their direct effect on the myocardium, beta blockers also produce a general decrease in sympathetic tone.[43,44] Although their exact effects on sympathetic activity remain to be determined, beta blockers may decrease sympathetic activity via the following: a central inhibitory effect on the brainstem, decreased renin release from the kidneys and within the central nervous system (CNS), impaired sympathetic activity in the ganglia or at the presynaptic adrenergic terminals, increased baroreceptor sensitivity, or via a combination of these and other factors.[43] Regardless of the

Table 21-4
SYMPATHOLYTIC DRUGS USED TO TREAT HYPERTENSION

Beta Blockers	
Acebutolol (Sectral)	Metoprolol (Lopressor, others)
Atenolol (Tenormin)	Nadolol (Corgard)
Betaxolol (Kerlone)	Nebivolol (Bystolic)
Bisoprolol (Zebeta)	Penbutolol (Levatol)
Esmolol (Brevibloc)	Pindolol (Visken)
Carteolol (Cartrol)	Propranolol (Inderal, others)
Carvedilol (Coreg)	Sotalol (Betapace, Sorine)
Labetalol (Normodyne, Trandate)	Timolol (Blocadren)
Alpha Blockers	
Doxazosin (Cardura, others)	Prazosin (Minipress)
Phenoxybenzamine (Dibenzyline)	Terazosin (Hytrin)
Presynaptic Adrenergic Inhibitors	
Reserpine (Novoreserpine, Reserfia)	
Centrally Acting Agents	
Clonidine (Catapres)	Guanfacine (Intuniv, Tenex)
Guanabenz (Wytensin)	Methyldopa (Aldomet)
Ganglionic Blockers	
Mecamylamine (Inversine, Vecamyl)	Trimethaphan (Arfonad)

exact mechanism of their action, beta blockers often complement the effects of other antihypertensives (diuretics, angiotensin converting enzyme [ACE] inhibitors, etc.) and are therefore included in the drug regimen of many patients with hypertension. The use of beta blockers in combination with these other agents is addressed in more detail in "Drug Selection for Specific Patients With Hypertension" later in this chapter.

Specific Agents. Beta-adrenergic blockers that are approved for use in hypertension are all effective in decreasing blood pressure (see Table 21-4), but certain beta blockers have additional properties that make them more suitable in specific patients.[45] As discussed in Chapter 20, some beta blockers are relatively selective for beta-1 receptors (cardioselective) and tend to affect the heart more than the lungs and other tissues (see Table 20-2). Beta blockers such as pindolol and acebutolol function as partial agonists and are said to have intrinsic sympathomimetic activity because they block the effects of excessive endogenous catecholamines while producing a normal background level of sympathetic stimulation to the heart.[42] Beta blockers such as labetalol and propranolol are able to normalize the excitability of the cardiac cell membrane; these drugs have membrane-stabilizing activity—other beta blockers may also exhibit this membrane-stabilizing effect at higher doses.[42] Finally, some of the newer "third-generation" beta blockers, such as carvedilol and nebivolol, produce peripheral vasodilation and a cardiac beta blockade, making these drugs especially useful in decreasing blood pressure.[46,47] Some of these newer agents like carvedilol may also have other beneficial effects, such as antioxidant properties and the ability to decrease lipid abnormalities and insulin resistance.[48-50] Hence, the selection of a specific beta blocker is based on these properties along with consideration for the individual needs of each patient.

Adverse Effects. Nonselective beta blockers (i.e., those with a fairly equal affinity for beta-1 and beta-2 receptors) may produce bronchoconstriction in patients with asthma and similar respiratory disorders. Cardiovascular side effects include excessive depression of heart rate and myocardial contractility as well as orthostatic hypotension. Some of the traditional beta blockers may impair glucose and lipid metabolism, but this effect can be reduced by using one of the newer vasodilating beta blockers such as carvedilol.[50] Other side effects include depression, fatigue, GI disturbances, and allergic reactions. However, beta blockers are generally well tolerated by most patients, and the incidence of side effects is relatively low.

Alpha Blockers

Drugs that block the alpha-1–adrenergic receptor on vascular smooth muscle will promote a decrease in vascular resistance.[51,52] Given that total peripheral vascular resistance often increases in essential hypertension, blocking vascular adrenergic receptors should be an effective course of action. In a sense, alpha blockers act directly on the tissues that ultimately mediate the increased blood pressure—that is, the peripheral vasculature. In the past, the use of alpha blockers in mild-to-moderate essential hypertension was somewhat limited because these drugs are sometimes too effective and tend to cause problems with hypotension and dizziness.[53]

It is now recognized that alpha-1 antagonists may offer specific advantages in treating hypertension, including an ability to improve blood lipid profiles (e.g., decreased triglycerides and total cholesterol, increased high-density lipoprotein–cholesterol ratio). They may produce a favorable effect on glucose metabolism and insulin resistance as well.[51] Newer agents such as doxazosin (Cardura) also appear to have less adverse cardiovascular side effects—such as reflex tachycardia—presumably because these agents act longer and do not cause a sudden fall in blood pressure.[54] A controlled-release formulation of this drug, known as *doxazosin gastrointestinal therapeutic system* (GITS), allows slower drug absorption into the bloodstream, thereby further reducing sudden adverse effects and improving tolerability.[55] Hence, alpha-1 blockers are gaining acceptance for use with certain patients with moderate hypertension and are being included in the antihypertensive regimen of patients having more severe cases of high blood pressure.

Alpha-1 blockers can also be used to treat the symptoms of benign prostatic hypertrophy because they decrease sympathetic-mediated contraction of smooth muscle located in the prostate gland.[52] Reduction of muscle tone in the prostate decreases constriction of the ureter, thereby improving urinary flow and the ability to empty the bladder.[56]

Specific Agents. The characteristics of individual alpha blockers were discussed in Chapter 20. Basically, these drugs can be differentiated according to their relative alpha-1 selectivity, their duration of action, and other pharmacokinetic properties. Prazosin (Minipress) has been the primary alpha blocker used in the past, but newer agents such as doxazosin and terazosin (Hytrin) are gaining acceptance in treating hypertension. Prazosin and other alpha blockers approved as antihypertensives are listed in Table 21-4.

Adverse Effects. One of the primary problems with alpha blockers is reflex tachycardia. When peripheral vascular resistance falls due to the effects of these drugs, the baroreceptor reflex often responds by generating a compensatory increase in heart rate. This tachycardia may be a significant problem, especially if there is a history of cardiac disease. To prevent reflex tachycardia, a beta blocker may be administered with the alpha blocker. The beta blocker will negate the increase in heart rate normally mediated through the sympathetic innervation to the heart. Alternatively, use of a longer-acting or controlled-release drug (doxazosin) may reduce the risk of reflex tachycardia because these agents produce a milder and more prolonged decrease in blood pressure following administration. Hence, reflex mechanisms controlling blood pressure (i.e., the baroreceptor reflex) are not suddenly activated as would be the case if blood pressure was reduced more rapidly with a shorter-acting drug.

Another major adverse effect with alpha blockers is orthostatic hypotension. Blockade of alpha-1 receptors in peripheral arteries and veins often promotes pooling of blood in the lower extremities when a patient stands up. Therapists should be alert for the symptoms of orthostatic hypotension (i.e., dizziness and syncope), especially for the first few days of alpha-blocker administration.

Finally, there is concern that alpha blockers may increase the risk of cardiac disease, including congestive heart failure.[52] By causing vasodilation, these drugs can increase plasma volume, thereby increasing the workload on the heart and predisposing certain patients to heart failure and other cardiac events (stroke, infarction). Hence, alpha blockers should probably be avoided in patients at risk for heart failure and related cardiovascular problems. Alpha blockers are usually not prescribed alone when treating hypertension but are used in advanced cases along with diuretics (to control fluid balance) or other antihypertensives such as beta blockers and ACE inhibitors. Likewise, alpha blockers may be a good choice for men with advanced hypertension and benign prostatic hypertrophy because these drugs may help resolve both problems simultaneously.[52]

Presynaptic Adrenergic Inhibitors

Drugs that inhibit the release of norepinephrine from the presynaptic terminals of peripheral adrenergic neurons may be used effectively in some individuals with hypertension. Some agents, such as reserpine, inhibit the presynaptic synthesis and storage of norepinephrine in peripheral and CNS adrenergic neurons.[57] Other agents, such as guanadrel, replace norepinephrine in peripheral sympathetic neurons, thus creating a false neurotransmitter.[43] In either case, depletion of norepinephrine from the presynaptic terminal decreases sympathetic-mediated excitation of the heart and peripheral vasculature, resulting in decreased blood pressure.

Specific Agents. Chapter 20 covers the drugs that inhibit the presynaptic synthesis and storage of norepinephrine. These agents have been available for several decades, but their use has declined over the years in favor of newer antihypertensives that are often better tolerated. Hence, reserpine is the only drug in this category that is still used commonly in the United States to treat hypertension (see Table 21-4). This drug is typically used in conjunction with other agents in resistant cases of hypertension (see "Drug Selection for Specific Patients With Hypertension").

Adverse Effects. A slow heart rate (bradycardia) and other arrhythmias are sometimes a problem with reserpine. Other bothersome side effects include drowsiness, depression, and GI disturbances such as nausea, vomiting, and diarrhea.

Centrally Acting Agents

Several antihypertensives work by inhibiting sympathetic discharge from the brainstem (see Table 21-4). Sympathetic discharge from the vasomotor center appears to be influenced by two types of neuronal receptors located in the brainstem: alpha-2 adrenergic receptors and imidazoline type I1 receptors. Stimulation of these receptors results in a *decrease* in sympathetic discharge to the heart and vasculature. Centrally acting sympatholytics are therefore characterized as agonists for either one or possibly both types of these receptors. Clonidine, for example, is considered to be primarily an alpha-2 agonist, although this drug also has some ability to stimulate imidazoline receptors.[58] Newer agents in this category (e.g., moxonidine, rilmenidine) may be more selective for imidazoline receptors, but these drugs are not currently available in the United States.[44,59] In either case, stimulation of these centrally located receptors results in a decrease in sympathetic outflow and a subsequent decrease in cardiovascular stimulation and blood pressure.[44] Consequently, centrally acting drugs offer a rather unique approach to hypertension because these drugs limit sympathetic activity at the source (i.e., the brainstem vasomotor center) rather than at the periphery (i.e., the cardiovascular neuroeffector junction).

Specific Agents. Of the primary drugs in this category, clonidine, guanabenz, and guanfacine act directly on the alpha-2 receptor, whereas methyldopa acts as an alpha-2 agonist after being converted in vivo to alpha-methylnorepinephrine. As indicated, moxonidine and rilmenidine act primarily on imidazoline receptors.

Adverse Effects. At therapeutic doses, these drugs are associated with some troublesome but relatively minor side effects, including dry mouth, dizziness, and sedation. The incidence of sedation seems to be related to these drugs' alpha-2 stimulatory effects. Hence, agents that are more selective for imidazoline receptors may seem better tolerated because patients are more alert and have less psychomotor slowing.[59]

Ganglionic Blockers

Drugs that block synaptic transmission at autonomic ganglia will dramatically and effectively reduce blood pressure by decreasing systemic sympathetic activity.[60] These agents are essentially nicotinic cholinergic antagonists (see Chapter 18), which block transmission at the junction between presynaptic and postsynaptic neurons in sympathetic and parasympathetic pathways. Because of the effect of these agents on both divisions of the autonomic nervous system, ganglionic blockers are used sparingly in treating hypertension. In the past, these drugs were used to reduce blood pressure in hypertensive emergencies.[60] Their routine use, however, has been largely replaced by vasodilators such as nitroprusside, calcium channel blockers, and other agents that are safer and produce fewer side effects.[61,62]

Specific Agents. Ganglionic blockers such as trimethaphan may be used to rapidly decrease blood pressure in certain emergencies, such as acute aortic dissection or autonomic crisis in people with spinal cord injury.[63] Lower doses of mecamylamine may help treat various CNS disorders (e.g., addiction, Tourette syndrome, schizophrenia, other cognitive and mood disorders) because of its ability to block cholinergic receptors in the brain.[63,64]

Adverse Effects. As might be expected, ganglionic blockers produce a multitude of side effects because of the inhibition of both sympathetic and parasympathetic responses. Some adverse effects include GI discomfort (e.g., nausea, constipation), urinary retention, visual disturbances, and orthostatic hypotension. At higher doses, they may even exhibit some neuromuscular blocking activity. These and other side effects may be quite severe in some patients. Fortunately, ganglionic blockers are usually not used for extended periods because the patient is placed on other antihypertensive drugs when the hypertensive crisis is resolved.

Vasodilators

Drugs that directly vasodilate the peripheral vasculature will produce an antihypertensive effect by decreasing peripheral vascular resistance.[65,66] Although other drugs such as the alpha blockers may ultimately produce vasodilation by interrupting adrenergic supply to the vasculature, the vasodilators exert an inhibitory effect directly on vascular smooth-muscle cells. Vasodilators are believed to inhibit smooth-muscle contraction by increasing the intracellular production of second messengers, such as cyclic guanosine monophosphate (cGMP; see Chapter 4). Increased amounts of cGMP inhibit the function of the contractile process in the vascular smooth-muscle cell, thus leading to vasodilation.

Specific Agents

The primary vasodilators used in hypertension are hydralazine (Apresoline) and minoxidil (Loniten) (Table 21-5). These drugs are not usually the first medications used in patients with hypertension but tend to be added to the drug regimen if other agents (e.g., diuretics, beta blockers) do not produce an adequate response.[65] Hydralazine is also used to lower blood pressure in emergency situations, such as severe preeclampsia or malignant hypertension.[65,67] Other vasodilators include diazoxide (Hyperstat), fenoldopam (Corlopam), and nitroprusside (Nipride, Nitropress), but these drugs are usually given only in emergency situations to treat a patient in hypertensive crisis.[43,62]

Nitric oxide also produces vasodilation in vascular smooth muscle. As indicated earlier, hypertension may be perpetuated by a defect in the production of nitric oxide by the vascular endothelium. It follows that providing nitric oxide directly or administering precursors for nitric oxide production may help reduce vascular resistance and decrease arterial pressure in specific hypertensive syndromes.[68] Practitioners are using inhaled nitric oxide to treat acute pulmonary hypertension associated with respiratory distress syndrome in newborns and adults.[69-71] Researchers are trying to determine if nitric oxide also could be used to treat systemic (essential) hypertension or if other drugs could be used to restore the production of endogenous nitric oxide in people with hypertension.[72] Additional studies are needed to determine if nitric oxide production in the peripheral vasculature can be manipulated to treat essential hypertension.

Table 21-5
ANTIHYPERTENSIVE VASODILATORS, ACE INHIBITORS, ANGIOTENSIN II RECEPTOR BLOCKERS, DIRECT RENIN INHIBITOR, AND CALCIUM CHANNEL BLOCKERS

Vasodilators	
Diazoxide (Hyperstat)	Minoxidil (Loniten)
Hydralazine (Apresoline)	Nitroprusside (Nitropress)
Fenoldopam (Corlopam)	
ACE* Inhibitors	
Benazepril (Lotensin)	Moexipril (Univasc)
Captopril (Capoten)	Perindopril (Aceon)
Enalapril (Vasotec)	Quinapril (Accupril)
Fosinopril (Monopril)	Ramipril (Altace)
Lisinopril (Prinivil, Zestril)	Trandolapril (Mavik)
Angiotensin II Receptor Blockers	
Azilsartan (Edarbi)	Olmesartan (Benicar)
Candesartan (Atacand)	Telmisartan (Micardis)
Irbesartan (Avapro)	Valsartan (Diovan)
Losartan (Cozaar)	
Direct Renin Inhibitor	
Aliskiren (Tekturna)	
Calcium Channel Blockers (dihydropyridine)	
Amlodipine (Norvasc)	Nicardipine (Cardene)
Clevidipine (Cleviprex)	Nifedipine (Adalat, Procardia, others)
Felodipine (Plendil)	Nisoldipine (Sular)
Isradipine (DynaCirc)	
Calcium Channel Blockers (Nondihydropyridine)	
Diltiazem (Cardizem, Dilacor, others)	Verapamil (Calan, Isoptin, others)

**ACE = angiotensin converting enzyme.*

Adverse Effects

Although vasodilators are effective in lowering blood pressure, these drugs are associated with several adverse effects. Reflex tachycardia often occurs because the baroreceptor reflex attempts to compensate for the fall in vascular resistance that these drugs produce. This side effect is analogous to the increased heart rate occurring when alpha blockers are used to decrease peripheral vascular resistance. Other common reactions include dizziness, orthostatic hypotension, weakness, nausea, fluid retention, and headache. Minoxidil also increases hair growth on the face, ears, forehead, and other hairy body surfaces. This increased hair growth is often a cause for the discontinuation of this drug in women. Some men, however, have applied minoxidil cutaneously to treat baldness, and a topical preparation of this drug (Rogaine) is marketed as a potential hair-growth stimulant.

Renin-Angiotensin System Inhibitors

The renin-angiotensin system involves several endogenous components that help regulate vascular tone and regulate sodium and water balance in the body.[9,73,74] In systemic circulation, the normally functioning renin-angiotensin system acts by a sequence of events summarized in Figure 21-2. Renin is an enzyme produced primarily in the kidneys. When blood pressure falls, renin is released from the kidneys into the systemic circulation. Angiotensinogen is a peptide that is produced by the liver and circulates continually in the bloodstream. When renin contacts angiotensinogen, angiotensinogen is transformed into angiotensin I. The circulating angiotensin I is then transformed by angiotensin-converting enzyme into angiotensin II. The converting enzyme is located in the vasculature of many tissues, especially the lungs.

Angiotensin II is an extremely potent vasoconstrictor. Consequently, the fall in blood pressure that activated the renin-angiotensin system is rectified by the increase in vascular resistance caused by angiotensin II. Angiotensin II, or possibly its by-product angiotensin III, also increases **aldosterone** secretion from the adrenal cortex. Aldosterone directly increases sodium reabsorption from the kidneys, which creates osmotic forces in the kidneys that encourage water reabsorption, thus helping maintain plasma volume. Hence, some sources consider aldosterone an integral part of renin-angiotensin function and often refer to the "renin-angiotensin-aldosterone system" to identify the more comprehensive aspects of this system.

Exactly what goes wrong with the renin-angiotensin system in patients with essential hypertension is not fully understood. Some patients display increased levels of circulating renin, hence their classification as having high-renin hypertension. Why plasma renin production is elevated in these patients is often unclear. In addition to problems in circulating levels of renin and angiotensin II, there may also be problems with the renin-angiotensin system in specific tissues or organs. For instance, a complete, functioning renin-angiotensin system has been identified within the brain, heart, vascular walls, kidneys, GI tract, liver, endocrine system, and hemopoietic system.[74,75-78] This suggests that some of the hypertensive effects of this system may be mediated through CNS mechanisms or by changes directly in the vascular tissues, kidneys, or other systems.

Nonetheless, activation of the renin-angiotensin system is extremely detrimental in people with high blood pressure. Excess production of angiotensin II causes vasoconstriction that perpetuates the hypertensive condition. More importantly, angiotensin II is a powerful stimulant of vascular tissue growth, and sustained production of angiotensin II results in the thickening and hypertrophy of the vascular wall.[79] The thickened vascular wall causes a decrease in the lumen of the vessel, thereby causing additional resistance to blood flow and increased hypertension. Excessive

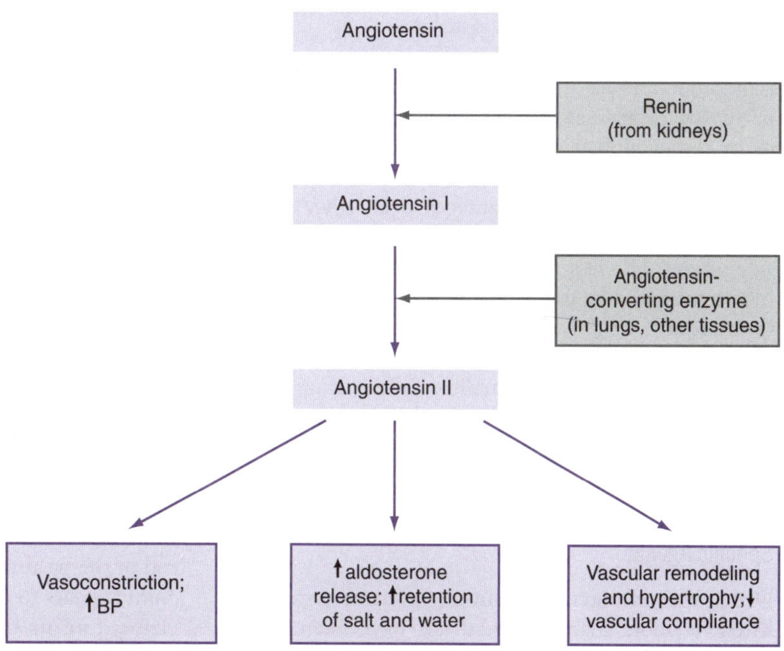

Figure ■ 21-2
The renin-angiotensin system and the effects of angiotensin II. Angiotensin converting enzyme inhibitors interrupt this system by blocking the conversion of angiotensin I to angiotensin II, and angiotensin II receptor blockers prevent angiotensin II from stimulating cardiovascular tissues. *(From: Ciccone. Medications. In: DeTurk WE, Cahalin LP, eds. Cardiovascular and Pulmonary Physical Therapy. New York: McGraw-Hill; 2004:193, with permission.)*

production of angiotensin II may have other detrimental effects on the vasculature, including inflammation of the vascular endothelium and increased lipid accumulation within the vascular wall.[80,81] These changes in the vascular wall can lead to hypertension and related cardiovascular events (i.e., stroke, myocardial infarction, heart failure).[82,83]

Fortunately, researchers have been developing three pharmacological strategies to inhibit the effects of abnormal renin-angiotensin system activation.[84,85] The first strategy involves drugs that inhibit the enzyme that converts angiotensin I to angiotensin II. These drugs are commonly referred to as angiotensin converting enzyme (ACE) inhibitors. ACE inhibitors decrease the hypertensive effects of angiotensin II by limiting the production of this compound. A second strategy uses drugs that block angiotensin II receptors on various tissues.[86,87] Angiotensin II stimulates vascular and other tissues by binding to a protein receptor (specifically, the AT1 angiotensin II receptor) on these tissues.[88] Hence, pharmacologists have been developing drugs known as *angiotensin II blockers* or *antagonists* to block these receptors, thereby negating the harmful effects of angiotensin II on vascular and other tissues. Finally, a third strategy uses drugs that directly inhibit renin[87,89] or, more precisely, inhibit renin's ability to convert angiotensinogen to angiotensin I (see Fig. 21-2). By reducing the formation of angiotensin I, direct renin inhibitors decrease the precursor substance for subsequent products in the renin-angiotensin pathway, namely angiotensin II and aldosterone.

ACE inhibitors, angiotensin II blockers, and direct renin inhibitors are an important addition to the antihypertensive drug arsenal. These drugs can be used alone or in conjunction with other drugs for the long-term control of high blood pressure.[84] In fact, these drugs appear to have several advantages over other antihypertensives, such as a lower incidence of cardiovascular side effects (i.e., less reflex tachycardia and orthostatic hypotension).[2] The drugs' ability to inhibit angiotensin II–induced vascular hypertrophy and remodeling is also recognized as an important benefit during the treatment of high blood pressure.[84] In addition, these drugs are extremely beneficial in decreasing morbidity and mortality associated with congestive heart failure, and their use in heart failure will be addressed in Chapter 24.

Specific Agents

Drugs that inhibit the renin-angiotensin system are listed in Table 21-5. These drugs have been shown to be effective in many cases of mild-to-moderate essential hypertension, and they may be used alone or in combination with beta blockers or diuretics. At present, the only direct-acting renin inhibitor is aliskiren (Tekturna).

Adverse Effects

ACE inhibitors are generally well tolerated in most patients. Some individuals may experience an allergic reaction as evidenced by skin rash. This reaction usually disappears when the dosage is reduced or when administration is discontinued. Patients may also experience a persistent, dry cough that is annoying but relatively harmless. Although the incidence is rare, hematological effects (neutropenia, agranulocytosis) and renal problems (glomerulonephritis, renal failure) may occur in susceptible patients; these drugs should be use cautiously in certain patients with preexisting blood or kidney diseases. ACE inhibitors have a slight chance of causing angioedema as indicated by rashes, raised patches of red or white skin (welts), burning/itching skin, swelling in the face, and difficulty breathing. Angioedema is an emergency situation that requires immediate medical attention.[90] Other problems (e.g., GI discomfort, dizziness, chest pain) may occur in some patients, but major adverse effects are relatively rare.

Angiotensin II blockers are likewise well tolerated; these drugs do not cause the cough associated with ACE inhibitors.[2] Hence, angiotensin II blockers may be an effective alternative in patients who experience side effects such as coughing.[91] The direct-acting renin inhibitor aliskiren (Tekturna) has side effects similar to ACE inhibitors, including dry cough, GI problems (e.g., diarrhea, stomach upset, abdominal pain), and rare cases of angioedema. The incidence of these side effects, however, may be lower than those occurring with ACE inhibitors, making this drug an attractive method of decreasing activity in the renin-angiotensin system.[92]

Calcium Channel Blockers

Drugs that selectively block calcium entry into vascular smooth-muscle cells were originally developed to treat certain forms of angina pectoris and cardiac arrhythmias (Chapters 22 and 23, respectively). Calcium channel blockers are now recognized as being beneficial in the treatment of essential hypertension.[93,94] Calcium appears to play a role in activating the contractile element in smooth muscle much in the same way that calcium initiates actin-myosin interaction in skeletal muscle cells. Certain calcium channel blockers, known as the *dihydropyridine agents* (nifedipine, amlodipine, and others; see Table 21-5), block calcium entry into vascular smooth muscle. This action will inhibit the contractile process, leading to vasodilation and decreased vascular resistance.[93] Other (nondihydropyridine) calcium channel blockers, such as diltiazem and verapamil, tend to have a greater effect on calcium influx into myocardial cells, and the primary effect of these drugs is to decrease heart rate and myocardial contraction force. These nonhydropyridine agents may be more useful in treating certain arrhythmias, although they can also treat high blood pressure because of their inhibitory effect on heart rate and myocardial contraction force.[94]

Calcium channel blockers generally have a relatively small incidence of metabolic side effects, such as impaired glucose or lipid metabolism,[95] and they may help overcome vascular endothelial dysfunction, which can be especially helpful in people with hypertension-related kidney disease.[96,97] Consequently, calcium channel blockers have gained popularity over the last several decades as one of the primary treatments for high blood pressure.[94]

However, the safety of these drugs in treating hypertension may be somewhat questionable. Several studies noted that use of certain calcium channel blockers (i.e., the short-acting form of nifedipine) was associated with an increased risk of myocardial infarction when these drugs were administered to certain hypertensive patients (i.e., patients who were older, had diabetes, or had unstable angina).[98] The risk of infarction, however, seems minimal if long-acting or sustained-release formulations are used, presumably because these formulations do not cause a sudden change in blood pressure as do their shorter-acting counterparts.[99] Other studies suggested that calcium channel blockers may increase the risk of cancer, presumably because these drugs interfere with the normal role that calcium plays in regulating cell growth and turnover.[100] Subsequent studies, however, have failed to establish a clear link between calcium channel blockers and cancer.[101]

Consequently, calcium channel blockers still play an important role in the antihypertensive arsenal, but practitioners are more cautious about using these drugs to lower blood pressure in certain patients.[94] As mentioned above, the longer-acting or sustained-release forms of these drugs are somewhat safer and should be used whenever possible.[93]

Specific Agents

The primary calcium channel blockers used to treat hypertension differ somewhat from one another, and they can be subclassified in categories according to their chemistry and how they block calcium channels (see Table 21-5).[2] Despite their chemical diversity, however, calcium channel blockers all act by limiting calcium entry into cardiovascular tissues.[94]

The selection of a specific agent is typically based on the side-effect profile of each drug and the individual needs of each patient. As mentioned earlier, several agents are also available in longer-acting (sustained-release) forms, and use of these agents may help reduce the risk of cardiovascular side effects (e.g., reflex tachycardia, orthostatic hypotension). Because calcium channel blockers are important in treating angina, the pharmacology of these drugs is discussed in more detail in Chapter 22.

Adverse Effects

These drugs may cause excessive vasodilation as evidenced by swelling in the feet and ankles, and some patients may also experience orthostatic hypotension. Abnormalities in heart rate (too fast, too slow, irregular) may also occur, and reflex tachycardia—caused by excessive peripheral vasodilation—has been noted with certain drugs, such as the short-acting form of nifedipine. Other bothersome side effects include dizziness, headache, and nausea.

DRUG SELECTION FOR SPECIFIC PATIENTS WITH HYPERTENSION

Choice of drugs for patients with hypertension should be tailored according to the amount that blood pressure is elevated in each patient and any other comorbidities or factors that could affect blood pressure in that patient. In patients with uncomplicated stage 1 hypertension (see Table 21-1), initial drug therapy often consists of a single "first-line" drug such as a thiazide-type diuretic, calcium channel blocker, or renin-angiotensin system inhibitor (i.e., an ACE inhibitor or angiotensin II receptor blocker).[2] Some experts, however, advocate that stage 1 hypertension can be treated more aggressively in many patients by combining two of the first-line drugs. For example, a calcium channel blocker can be combined with an angiotensin II receptor blocker. These two drugs can even be administered at a fixed dose in the same pill for effective treatment of stage 1 hypertension.[102,103] Usually, two first-line drugs are combined when the hypertension is relatively uncomplicated but has already reached stage 2—that is, a thiazide diuretic or a calcium channel blocker is combined with a renin-angiotensin system inhibitor. Clearly, there are many options for the initial treatment of uncomplicated hypertension, and the choice of a specific drug or drugs is ultimately left to the discretion of the prescribing physician.

Drug selection is also influenced by any comorbidities or "compelling indications" in each patient.[2] Recommended treatment in specific clinical situations is summarized in Table 21-6. As indicated, certain drug regimens are preferred if other factors are present that may also affect blood pressure and organ function. For example, patients with diabetes mellitus seem to respond best to standard treatment with an ACE inhibitor or angiotensin II receptor blocker, with additional drugs such as a diuretic, calcium channel blocker, and beta blocker being added to the regimen as needed. These recommendations still enable the prescribing physician to tailor drug therapy by selecting specific drugs from each category and adjusting dosages to provide optimal treatment. Recommendations for drug treatment will continue to be reevaluated as new drugs become available, and additional clinical trials help investigate the effects of various drug interventions.

NONPHARMACOLOGICAL TREATMENT OF HYPERTENSION

Although several effective and relatively safe drugs exist for treating hypertension, the use of nondrug methods in decreasing blood pressure should not be overlooked, especially in cases of prehypertension and stage 1 hypertension.[104,105] Dietary modifications such as the Dietary Approaches to Stop Hypertension (DASH) program advocate sodium restriction and diets that are rich in fruits, vegetables, and low-fat dairy products.[106] Decreasing the use of alcohol and tobacco may also help lower blood pressure, although modest alcohol consumption (i.e., 1 drink/day for women; 2 drinks/day for men) may actually have some beneficial effects on blood pressure and the risk of heart disease.[104] Generally, a decrease in body weight will produce an antihypertensive effect[107]; regular exercise may help decrease blood pressure by decreasing body weight or by mechanisms unrelated to weight loss.[108] Many forms of behavior modification and stress management techniques have also been suggested as nonpharmacological methods of blood pressure control.

Hence, changes in lifestyle and behavior can positively influence blood pressure, and these changes should be encouraged in all hypertensive patients, even if blood pressure is reduced pharmacologically. Ideally, successful implementation of these lifestyle changes can control blood pressure to the point where drug therapy is no longer necessary in some people.

Table 21-6
DRUG SELECTION FOR SPECIFIC PATIENTS WITH HYPERTENSION

Patient Indication/Comorbidity	Standard Pharmacotherapy	Add-on Pharmacotherapy
Left ventricular dysfunction	Diuretic with ACE inhibitor; then add beta blocker	Aldosterone antagonist or ARB
Post-myocardial infarction	Beta blocker; then add ACE inhibitor or ARB	None
Coronary artery disease	Beta blocker; then add ACE inhibitor or ARB	CCB, diuretic
Diabetes mellitus	ACE inhibitor or ARB	Diuretic; then add CCB, beta blocker
Chronic kidney disease	ACE inhibitor or ARB	None
Recurrent stroke prevention	Diuretic with ACE inhibitor	None

ACE = angiotensin converting enzyme; ARB = angiotensin receptor blocker; CCB = calcium channel blocker.

Adapted from: Saseen JJ, Maclaughlin EJ. Hypertension. In: DiPiro JT, et al, eds. Pharmacotherapy: A Pathophysiologic Approach. 8th ed. New York: McGraw-Hill; 2011:111.

Special Concerns for Rehabilitation Patients

Considering the prevalence of hypertension, therapists will undoubtedly work with many patients taking blood pressure medications. These drugs produce a diverse array of side effects that can influence the rehabilitation session. Primary among these are hypotension and orthostatic hypotension. Because the major action of these drugs is to lower blood pressure, physical therapists and occupational therapists should be cautious when their patients change posture suddenly or engage in other activities that may lower blood pressure.

Activities producing widespread vasodilation must be avoided or used very cautiously, especially if the patients are taking vasodilating drugs. For instance, systemically applied heat (whirlpool, Hubbard tank) may cause blood pressure to fall precipitously if the patients are taking alpha blockers, calcium channel blockers, or direct-acting vasodilators. Similarly, exercise may cause vasodilation in skeletal musculature, which may potentiate the peripheral vasodilation induced by antihypertensive drugs. Additionally, if the patients are taking beta blockers, cardiac responses to exercise (i.e., increased heart rate and cardiac output) may be somewhat blunted because the myocardial response to sympathetic stimulation will be diminished.

Aside from being aware of the side effects of antihypertensive drugs, therapists may also play an important role in encouraging patients to adhere to drug therapy when dealing with high blood pressure. Although drug therapy can control blood pressure, patients are often forgetful or hesitant about taking their medications, largely because hypertension is usually asymptomatic until the late stages of this disease. The patient will probably feel fine even when the drug is not taken, or the patient may actually avoid taking the drug because of some bothersome side effect (i.e., the patient may actually feel better without the drug). The idea that hypertension is a silent killer must be reinforced continually. Through their close contact with the patient, rehabilitation specialists are often in a good position to remind the patient of the consequences of nonadherence. In addition, therapists can help suggest and supervise nonpharmacological methods of lowering blood pressure (e.g., exercise programs, stress management, relaxation techniques). Physical therapists and occupational therapists can play a valuable role in helping patients realize the importance of long-term pharmacological and nonpharmacological management of hypertension.

CASE STUDY

HYPERTENSION

Brief History. H.C. is a 55-year-old man who works as an attorney for a large corporation. He is consistently faced with a demanding work schedule, often working 12- to 14-hour days, 6 days each week. In addition, he is 25 to 30 pounds overweight and is a habitual cigarette smoker. He has a long history of high blood pressure, which has been managed fairly successfully over the past 15 years through the use of different drugs. Currently, he is receiving a diuretic (furosemide [Lasix], 160 mg/d), a cardioselective beta blocker (metoprolol [Lopressor], 200 mg/d), and a vasodilator (hydralazine [Apresoline], 200 mg/d). He

Continued on following page

CASE STUDY (Continued)

also takes 81 mg of aspirin each day to prevent myocardial infarction, 20 mg of rosuvastatin (Crestor) to reduce plasma cholesterol, and 10 mg of zolpidem (Ambien) at bedtime when he has trouble falling asleep.

While rushing to a business luncheon, H.C. was hit by an automobile as he was crossing the street. He was admitted to the hospital, where radiological examination revealed a fracture of the right pelvis. Further examination did not reveal any other significant internal injuries. The pelvic fracture appeared stable at the time of admission, and internal fixation was not required. H.C. remained in the hospital and was placed on bed rest. Two days after admission, a physical therapist was called in to consult on the case. The physical therapist suggested a progressive ambulation program using the facility's therapeutic pool. The buoyancy provided by the pool would allow a gradual increase in weight bearing while protecting the fracture site.

Problem/Influence of Medication. To guard against patient hypothermia, the water temperature in the therapeutic pool was routinely maintained at 95°F. The therapist was concerned that immersing the patient in the pool would cause excessive peripheral vasodilation.

1. ***How would the combination of the drug regimen and the vasodilation caused by the therapeutic pool affect H.C.'s cardiovascular system?***
2. ***What precautions should the therapist take to avoid adverse cardiovascular changes during the pool interventions?***

See Appendix C, "Answers to Case Study Questions."

SUMMARY

Hypertension is a common disease marked by a sustained increase in blood pressure. If untreated, hypertension leads to serious problems such as stroke, renal failure, and problems in several other physiological systems. Although the cause of hypertension is discernible in a small percentage of patients, the majority of hypertensive individuals are classified as having essential hypertension, which means that the exact cause of their elevated blood pressure is unknown. Fortunately, several types of drugs are currently available to adequately control blood pressure in essential hypertension. Drugs such as diuretics, sympatholytics (alpha blockers, beta blockers, etc.), vasodilators, renin-angiotensin system inhibitors, and calcium channel blockers have all been used in treating hypertension. These agents are usually prescribed according to the degree of hypertension and any other comorbidities that also affect blood pressure and organ function. Rehabilitation specialists should be aware of the potential side effects of these drugs. Physical therapists and occupational therapists assume an important role in making patients aware of the sequelae of hypertension and should actively encourage patients to adhere to pharmacological and nonpharmacological methods of lowering blood pressure.

REFERENCES

1. Crim MT, Yoon SS, Ortiz E, et al. National surveillance definitions for hypertension prevalence and control among adults. *Circ Cardiovasc Qual Outcomes*. 2012;5:343-351.
2. Saseen JJ, Maclaughlin EJ. Hypertension. In: DiPiro JT, et al, eds. *Pharmacotherapy: A Pathophysiologic Approach*. 8th ed. New York: McGraw-Hill; 2011.
3. Pimenta E, Oparil S. Management of hypertension in the elderly. *Nat Rev Cardiol*. 2012;9:286-296.
4. Arima H, Barzi F, Chalmers J. Mortality patterns in hypertension. *J Hypertens*. 2011;29(suppl 1):S3-7.
5. Leone A, Landini L, Leone A. Epidemiology and costs of hypertension-related disorders. *Curr Pharm Des*. 2011;17:2955-2972.
6. Hall JE, Guyton AC. *Textbook of Medical Physiology*. 12th ed. Philadelphia: WB Saunders/Elsevier; 2011.
7. Fadel PJ. Arterial baroreflex control of the peripheral vasculature in humans: rest and exercise. *Med Sci Sports Exerc*. 2008;40:2055-2062.
8. Hamm LL, Hering-Smith KS. Pivotal role of the kidney in hypertension. *Am J Med Sci*. 2010;340:30-32.

9. Crowley SD, Coffman TM. Recent advances involving the renin-angiotensin system. *Exp Cell Res.* 2012;318:1049-1056.
10. Hyndman KA, Pollock JS. Nitric oxide and the A and B of endothelin of sodium homeostasis. *Curr Opin Nephrol Hypertens.* 2013;22:26-31.
11. Bochud M, Guessous I. Gene-environment interactions of selected pharmacogenes in arterial hypertension. *Expert Rev Clin Pharmacol.* 2012;5:677-686.
12. Landsbergis PA, Dobson M, Koutsouras G, Schnall P. Job strain and ambulatory blood pressure: a meta-analysis and systematic review. *Am J Public Health.* 2013;103:e61-71.
13. Simino J, Rao DC, Freedman BI. Novel findings and future directions on the genetics of hypertension. *Curr Opin Nephrol Hypertens.* 2012;21:500-507.
14. Aghamohammadzadeh R, Heagerty AM. Obesity-related hypertension: epidemiology, pathophysiology, treatments, and the contribution of perivascular adipose tissue. *Ann Med.* 2012;44(suppl 1): S74-84.
15. Nikolopoulou A, Kadoglou NP. Obesity and metabolic syndrome as related to cardiovascular disease. *Expert Rev Cardiovasc Ther.* 2012;10:933-939.
16. DiBona GF. Sympathetic nervous system and hypertension. *Hypertension.* 2013;61:556-560.
17. Grassi G, Bertoli S, Seravalle G. Sympathetic nervous system: role in hypertension and in chronic kidney disease. *Curr Opin Nephrol Hypertens.* 2012;21:46-51.
18. Parati G, Esler M. The human sympathetic nervous system: its relevance in hypertension and heart failure. *Eur Heart J.* 2012;33:1058-1066.
19. Fardin NM, Oyama LM, Campos RR. Changes in baroreflex control of renal sympathetic nerve activity in high-fat-fed rats as a predictor of hypertension. *Obesity.* 2012;20:1591-1597.
20. Okada Y, Galbreath MM, Shibata S, et al. Relationship between sympathetic baroreflex sensitivity and arterial stiffness in elderly men and women. *Hypertension.* 2012;59:98-104.
21. Masuo K, Lambert GW, Esler MD, et al. The role of sympathetic nervous activity in renal injury and end-stage renal disease. *Hypertens Res.* 2010;33:521-528.
22. McCullough AJ. Epidemiology of the metabolic syndrome in the USA. *J Dig Dis.* 2011;12:333-340.
23. Swislocki AL, Siegel D, Jialal I. Pharmacotherapy for the metabolic syndrome. *Curr Vasc Pharmacol.* 2012;10:187-205.
24. Goldberg RB, Mather K. Targeting the consequences of the metabolic syndrome in the Diabetes Prevention Program. *Arterioscler Thromb Vasc Biol.* 2012;32:2077-2090.
25. Rask-Madsen C, Kahn CR. Tissue-specific insulin signaling, metabolic syndrome, and cardiovascular disease. *Arterioscler Thromb Vasc Biol.* 2012;32:2052-2059.
26. Koumaras C, Tzimou M, Stavrinou E, et al. Role of antihypertensive drugs in arterial "de-stiffening" and central pulsatile hemodynamics. *Am J Cardiovasc Drugs.* 2012;12:143-156.
27. Palatini P, Casiglia E, G_sowski J, et al. Arterial stiffness, central hemodynamics, and cardiovascular risk in hypertension. *Vasc Health Risk Manag.* 2011;7:725-739.
28. Hassellund SS, Flaa A, Sandvik L, et al. Long-term stability of cardiovascular and catecholamine responses to stress tests: an 18-year follow-up study. *Hypertension.* 2010;55:131-136.
29. Turoni CJ, Marañón RO, Proto V, et al. Nitric oxide modulates reactivity to angiotensin II in internal mammary arterial grafts in hypertensive patients without associated risk factors. *Clin Exp Hypertens.* 2011;33:27-33.
30. Bauer V, Sotníková R. Nitric oxide—the endothelium-derived relaxing factor and its role in endothelial functions. *Gen Physiol Biophys.* 2010;29:319-340.
31. Lamas S, Rodríguez-Puyol D. Endothelial control of vasomotor tone: the kidney perspective. *Semin Nephrol.* 2012;32: 156-166.
32. Ghiadoni L, Taddei S, Virdis A. Hypertension and endothelial dysfunction: therapeutic approach. *Curr Vasc Pharmacol.* 2012;10:42-60.
33. Giles TD, Sander GE, Nossaman BD, Kadowitz PJ. Impaired vasodilation in the pathogenesis of hypertension: focus on nitric oxide, endothelial-derived hyperpolarizing factors, and prostaglandins. *J Clin Hypertens* (Greenwich). 2012;14:198-205.
34. Wright JM, Musini VM. First-line drugs for hypertension. *Cochrane Database Syst Rev.* 2009;3:CD001841.
35. Sica DA, Carter B, Cushman W, Hamm L. Thiazide and loop diuretics. *J Clin Hypertens.* 2011;13:639-643.
36. Einhorn PT, Davis BR, Wright JT Jr, et al. ALLHAT: still providing correct answers after 7 years. *Curr Opin Cardiol.* 2010;25: 355-365.
37. Wile D. Diuretics: a review. *Ann Clin Biochem.* 2012;49(Pt 5): 419-431.
38. Sarafidis PA, Georgianos PI, Lasaridis AN. Diuretics in clinical practice. Part II: electrolyte and acid-base disorders complicating diuretic therapy. *Expert Opin Drug Saf.* 2010;9:259-273.
39. Duarte JD, Cooper-DeHoff RM. Mechanisms for blood pressure lowering and metabolic effects of thiazide and thiazide-like diuretics. *Expert Rev Cardiovasc Ther.* 2010;8:793-802.
40. Palmer BF. Metabolic complications associated with use of diuretics. *Semin Nephrol.* 2011;31:542-552.
41. Chrysant SG, Chrysant GS. Current status of β-blockers for the treatment of hypertension: an update. *Drugs Today.* 2012;48: 353-366.
42. Frishman WH, Saunders E. β-Adrenergic blockers. *J Clin Hypertens.* 2011;13:649-653.
43. Michel T, Hoffman BB. Treatment of myocardial ischemia and hypertension. In: Brunton L, et al, eds. *The Pharmacological Basis of Therapeutics.* 12th ed. New York: McGraw-Hill; 2011.
44. Parati G, Esler M. The human sympathetic nervous system: its relevance in hypertension and heart failure. *Eur Heart J.* 2012;33:1058-1066.
45. Gorre F, Vandekerckhove H. Beta-blockers: focus on mechanism of action. Which beta-blocker, when and why? *Acta Cardiol.* 2010;65:565-570.
46. DiNicolantonio JJ, Hackam DG. Carvedilol: a third-generation β-blocker should be a first-choice β-blocker. *Expert Rev Cardiovasc Ther.* 2012;10:13-25.
47. Toblli JE, DiGennaro F, Giani JF, Dominici FP. Nebivolol: impact on cardiac and endothelial function and clinical utility. *Vasc Health Risk Manag.* 2012;8:151-160.
48. Chen-Scarabelli C, Saravolatz L Jr, Murad Y, et al. A critical review of the use of carvedilol in ischemic heart disease. *Am J Cardiovasc Drugs.* 2012;12:391-401.
49. DiNicolantonio JJ, Lavie CJ, Fares H, et al. Meta-analysis of carvedilol versus beta 1 selective beta-blockers (atenolol, bisoprolol, metoprolol, and nebivolol). *Am J Cardiol.* 2013;111:765-769.
50. Leonetti G, Egan CG. Use of carvedilol in hypertension: an update. *Vasc Health Risk Manag.* 2012;8:307-322.
51. Chapman N, Chen CY, Fujita T, et al. Time to re-appraise the role of alpha-1 adrenoceptor antagonists in the management of hypertension? *J Hypertens.* 2010;28:1796-1803.

52. Grimm RH Jr, Flack JM. Alpha 1 adrenoreceptor antagonists. *J Clin Hypertens*. 2011;13:654-67.
53. Santillo VM, Lowe FC. Treatment of benign prostatic hyperplasia in patients with cardiovascular disease. *Drugs Aging*. 2006;23:795-805.
54. Wykretowicz A, Guzik P, Wysocki H. Doxazosin in the current treatment of hypertension. *Expert Opin Pharmacother.* 2008;9: 625-633.
55. Chapman N, Chang CL, Dahlöf B, et al. Effect of doxazosin gastrointestinal therapeutic system as third-line antihypertensive therapy on blood pressure and lipids in the Anglo-Scandinavian Cardiac Outcomes Trial. *Circulation*. 2008;118:42-48.
56. Lepor H, Kazzazi A, Djavan B. α-Blockers for benign prostatic hyperplasia: the new era. *Curr Opin Urol*. 2012;22:7-15.
57. Slim HB, Black HR, Thompson PD. Older blood pressure medications-do they still have a place? *Am J Cardiol*. 2011;108: 308-316.
58. Nikolic K, Agbaba D. Imidazoline antihypertensive drugs: selective i(1)-imidazoline receptors activation. *Cardiovasc Ther*. 2012;30:209-216.
59. Edwards LP, Brown-Bryan TA, McLean L, Ernsberger P. Pharmacological properties of the central antihypertensive agent, moxonidine. *Cardiovasc Ther*. 2012;30:199-208.
60. Pappano AJ. Cholinoceptor blocking drugs. In: Katzung BG, ed. *Basic and Clinical Pharmacology.* 12th ed. New York: Lange Medical Books/McGraw Hill; 2012.
61. Rodriguez MA, Kumar SK, De Caro M. Hypertensive crisis. *Cardiol Rev*. 2010;18:102-107.
62. Sarafidis PA, Georgianos PI, Malindretos P, Liakopoulos V. Pharmacological management of hypertensive emergencies and urgencies: focus on newer agents. *Expert Opin Investig Drugs*. 2012;21:1089-1106.
63. Nickell JR, Grinevich VP, Siripurapu KB, et al. Potential therapeutic uses of mecamylamine and its stereoisomers. *Pharmacol Biochem Behav.* 2013;108:28-43.
64. Bacher I, Wu B, Shytle DR, George TP. Mecamylamine—a nicotinic acetylcholine receptor antagonist with potential for the treatment of neuropsychiatric disorders. *Expert Opin Pharmacother.* 2009;10:2709-2721.
65. Cohn JN, McInnes GT, Shepherd AM. Direct-acting vasodilators. *J Clin Hypertens*. 2011;13:690-692.
66. Kandler MR, Mah GT, Tejani AM, et al. Hydralazine for essential hypertension. *Cochrane Database Syst Rev.* 2011;11:CD004934.
67. McCoy S, Baldwin K. Pharmacotherapeutic options for the treatment of preeclampsia. *Am J Health Syst Pharm*. 2009;66:337-344.
68. Tousoulis D, Kampoli AM, Tentolouris C, et al. The role of nitric oxide on endothelial function. *Curr Vasc Pharmacol.* 2012;10:4-18.
69. Hagan G, Pepke-Zaba J. Pulmonary hypertension, nitric oxide and nitric oxide-releasing compounds. *Expert Rev Respir Med.* 2011;5:163-171.
70. Love LE, Bradshaw WT. Efficacy of inhaled nitric oxide in preterm neonates. *Adv Neonatal Care*. 2012;12:15-20.
71. Porta NF, Steinhorn RH. Pulmonary vasodilator therapy in the NICU: inhaled nitric oxide, sildenafil, and other pulmonary vasodilating agents. *Clin Perinatol.* 2012;39:149-164.
72. Roe ND, Ren J. Nitric oxide synthase uncoupling: a therapeutic target in cardiovascular diseases. *Vascul Pharmacol.* 2012;57: 168-172.
73. Iwanami J, Mogi M, Iwai M, Horiuchi M. Inhibition of the renin-angiotensin system and target organ protection. *Hypertens Res.* 2009;32:229-237.
74. Nguyen Dinh Cat A, Touyz RM. A new look at the renin-angiotensin system—focusing on the vascular system. *Peptides.* 2011;32:2141-2150.
75. Durik M, Sevá Pessôa B, Roks AJ. The renin-angiotensin system, bone marrow and progenitor cells. *Clin Sci.* 2012;123: 205-223.
76. Fändriks L. The renin-angiotensin system and the gastrointestinal mucosa. *Acta Physiol.* 2011;201:157-167.
77. Thatcher S, Yiannikouris F, Gupte M, Cassis L. The adipose renin-angiotensin system: role in cardiovascular disease. *Mol Cell Endocrinol.* 2009;302:111-117.
78. Wright JW, Harding JW. Brain renin-angiotensin—a new look at an old system. *Prog Neurobiol.* 2011;95:49-67.
79. Patel BM, Mehta AA. Aldosterone and angiotensin: role in diabetes and cardiovascular diseases. *Eur J Pharmacol.* 2012;697:1-12.
80. Marchesi C, Paradis P, Schiffrin EL. Role of the renin-angiotensin system in vascular inflammation. *Trends Pharmacol Sci.* 2008;29:367-374.
81. Silva PM. From endothelial dysfunction to vascular occlusion: role of the renin-angiotensin system. *Rev Port Cardiol.* 2010;29:801-824.
82. de la Sierra A. Renin-angiotensin system blockade and reduction of cardiovascular risk: future perspectives. *Expert Rev Cardiovasc Ther.* 2011;9:1585-1591.
83. van Vark LC, Bertrand M, Akkerhuis KM, et al. Angiotensin-converting enzyme inhibitors reduce mortality in hypertension: a meta-analysis of randomized clinical trials of renin-angiotensin-aldosterone system inhibitors involving 158,998 patients. *Eur Heart J.* 2012;33:2088-2097.
84. Epstein BJ, Leonard PT, Shah NK. The evolving landscape of RAAS inhibition: from ACE inhibitors to ARBs, to DRIs and beyond. *Expert Rev Cardiovasc Ther*. 2012;10:713-725.
85. Powers B, Greene L, Balfe LM. Updates on the treatment of essential hypertension: a summary of AHRQ's comparative effectiveness review of angiotensin-converting enzyme inhibitors, angiotensin II receptor blockers, and direct renin inhibitors. *J Manag Care Pharm*. 2011;17(suppl):S1-14.
86. Abramov D, Carson PE. The role of angiotensin receptor blockers in reducing the risk of cardiovascular disease. *J Renin Angiotensin Aldosterone Syst.* 2012;13:317-327.
87. Volpe M, Pontremoli R, Borghi C. Direct renin inhibition: from pharmacological innovation to novel therapeutic opportunities. *High Blood Press Cardiovasc Prev.* 2011;18:93-105.
88. Naik P, Murumkar P, Giridhar R, Yadav MR. Angiotensin II receptor type 1 (AT1) selective nonpeptidic antagonists—a perspective. *Bioorg Med Chem*. 2010;18:8418-8456.
89. Brunetti ND, De Gennaro L, Pellegrino PL, et al. Direct renin inhibition: update on clinical investigations with aliskiren. *Eur J Cardiovasc Prev Rehabil.* 2011;18:424-437.
90. Kloth N, Lane AS. ACE inhibitor-induced angioedema: a case report and review of current management. *Crit Care Resusc.* 2011;13:33-37.
91. Caldeira D, David C, Sampaio C. Tolerability of angiotensin-receptor blockers in patients with intolerance to angiotensin-converting enzyme inhibitors: a systematic review and meta-analysis. *Am J Cardiovasc Drugs.* 2012;12:263-277.
92. Fisher ND, Meagher EA. Renin inhibitors. *J Clin Hypertens.* 2011;13:662-666.
93. Coca A, Mazón P, Aranda P, et al. Role of dihydropyridinic calcium channel blockers in the management of hypertension. *Expert Rev Cardiovasc Ther*. 2013;11:91-105.

94. Elliott WJ, Ram CV. Calcium channel blockers. *J Clin Hypertens.* 2011;13:687-689.
95. Karagiannis A, Tziomalos K, Anagnostis P, et al. The effect of antihypertensive agents on insulin sensitivity, lipids and haemostasis. *Curr Vasc Pharmacol.* 2010;8:792-803.
96. Ishizawa K, Yamaguchi K, Horinouchi Y, et al. Drug discovery for overcoming chronic kidney disease (CKD): development of drugs on endothelial cell protection for overcoming CKD. *J Pharmacol Sci.* 2009;109:14-19.
97. Preston Mason R. Pleiotropic effects of calcium channel blockers. *Curr Hypertens Rep.* 2012;14:293-303.
98. Lundy A, Lutfi N, Beckey C. Review of nifedipine GITS in the treatment of high risk patients with coronary artery disease and hypertension. *Vasc Health Risk Manag.* 2009;5:429-440.
99. Eisenberg MJ, Brox A, Bestawros AN. Calcium channel blockers: an update. *Am J Med.* 2004;116:35-43.
100. Shapovalov G, Skryma R, Prevarskaya N. Calcium channels and prostate cancer. *Recent Pat Anticancer Drug Discov.* 2013;8:18-26.
101. Epstein BJ, Vogel K, Palmer BF. Dihydropyridine calcium channel antagonists in the management of hypertension. *Drugs.* 2007;67:1309-1327.
102. Kjeldsen SE, Messerli FH, Chiang CE, et al. Are fixed-dose combination antihypertensives suitable as first-line therapy? *Curr Med Res Opin.* 2012;28:1685-1697.
103. Suárez C. Single-pill telmisartan and amlodipine: a rational combination for the treatment of hypertension. *Drugs.* 2011;71: 2295-2305.
104. Frisoli TM, Schmieder RE, Grodzicki T, Messerli FH. Beyond salt: lifestyle modifications and blood pressure. *Eur Heart J.* 2011;32:3081-3087.
105. Woolf KJ, Bisognano JD. Nondrug interventions for treatment of hypertension. *J Clin Hypertens.* 2011;13:829-835.
106. Tyson CC, Nwankwo C, Lin PH, Svetkey LP. The Dietary Approaches to Stop Hypertension (DASH) eating pattern in special populations. *Curr Hypertens Rep.* 2012;14:388-396.
107. Landsberg L, Aronne LJ, Beilin LJ, et al. Obesity-related hypertension: pathogenesis, cardiovascular risk, and treatment: a position paper of the Obesity Society and the American Society of Hypertension. *J Clin Hypertens.* 2013;15:14-33.
108. Fagard RH. Exercise therapy in hypertensive cardiovascular disease. *Prog Cardiovasc Dis.* 2011;53:404-411.

CHAPTER 22

Treatment of Angina Pectoris

Angina pectoris is pain that occurs in the chest region during ischemic heart disease. Attacks of angina pectoris begin suddenly and are often described as a sensation of intense compression and tightness in the retrosternal region, with pain sometimes radiating to the jaw or left arm. In many patients, episodes of angina pectoris are precipitated by physical exertion. Some forms of angina may occur spontaneously even when the patient is at rest or asleep.

The basic problem in angina pectoris is that the supply of oxygen to the heart is insufficient to meet myocardial demands at a given point in time, which results in an imbalance between myocardial oxygen supply and demand (Fig. 22-1).[1,2] This imbalance leads to myocardial ischemia, which results in several metabolic, electrophysiological, and contractile changes in the heart. The painful symptoms inherent to angina pectoris seem to result from the accumulation of metabolic by-products such as lactic acid. Presumably, these metabolic by-products act as nociceptive substances and trigger the painful compressive sensations characteristic of angina pectoris.

Although angina pectoris is believed to be caused by the buildup of lactic acid and other metabolites, the exact mechanisms responsible for mediating anginal pain remain unknown. Also, the patient's emotional state and other factors that influence central pain perception play an obvious role in angina pectoris.[3] In fact, the majority of anginal attacks may be silent in many patients, and myocardial ischemia may frequently occur without producing any symptoms.[3,4] Certain patients may also exhibit symptoms of angina even though their coronary arteries appear to be normal and there is no obvious obstruction to coronary blood flow.[2] Clearly, there is much information regarding the nature of angina pectoris still remaining to be clarified.

Considering the prevalence of ischemic heart disease in the United States, many patients receiving physical therapy and occupational therapy may suffer from angina pectoris. These patients may be undergoing rehabilitation for a variety of clinical disorders, including (but not limited to) coronary artery disease. This chapter describes the primary drug groups used to treat angina pectoris, as well as the pharmacological management of specific forms of angina. You should be aware of the manner in which these drugs work and the ways in which antianginal drugs can influence patient performance in rehabilitation sessions.

DRUGS USED TO TREAT ANGINA PECTORIS

Three drug groups are typically used to treat the symptoms of angina pectoris: organic nitrates, beta blockers, and calcium channel blockers. These drugs exert various effects that help restore or maintain the balance between myocardial oxygen supply and myocardial oxygen demand.

Organic Nitrates

Organic nitrates consist of drugs such as nitroglycerin, isosorbide dinitrate, and isosorbide mononitrate

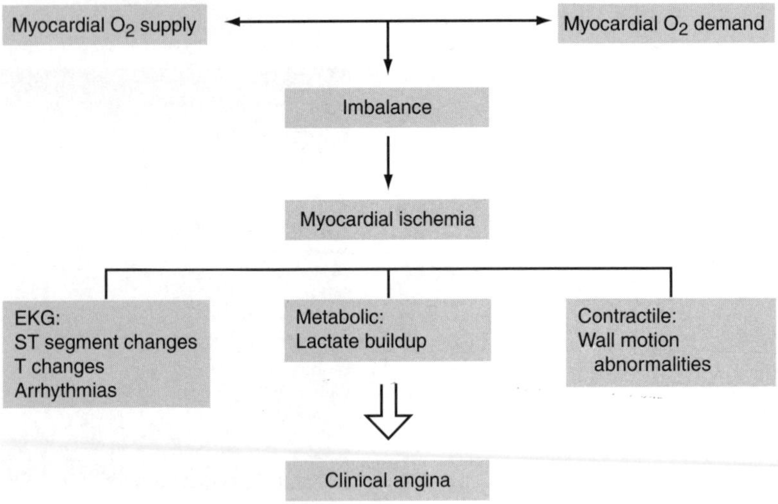

Figure ■ 22-1
Myocardial ischemia equation. *(Adapted from: Miller AB. Mixed ischemic subsets. Comparison of the mechanism of silent ischemia and mixed angina. Am J Med. 1985;79 [suppl 3a]:25, with permission.)*

(Table 22-1). The ability of these agents to dilate vascular smooth muscle is well established. Nitrates are actually drug precursors (prodrugs) that become activated when they are converted to nitric oxide within vascular smooth muscle.[5,6] Nitric oxide causes vasodilation by increasing the production of cyclic guanosine monophosphate (cGMP) within the muscle cell. Cyclic GMP acts as a second messenger that inhibits smooth-muscle contraction, probably by initiating the phosphorylation of specific contractile proteins.[7]

For years, nitrates were believed to relieve angina attacks by dilating the coronary arteries—that is, they supposedly increased blood flow to the myocardium, thereby increasing myocardial oxygen supply. We now know, however, that these drugs exert their primary antianginal effects by producing a general vasodilation in the vasculature throughout the body, not just in the coronary vessels.[8] By producing dilation in the systemic venous system, nitrates decrease the amount of blood returning to the heart (cardiac preload). By dilating systemic peripheral arterioles, these drugs decrease the pressure against which the heart must pump (cardiac afterload). A decrease in cardiac preload and afterload decreases the amount of work the heart must perform; hence, myocardial oxygen demand decreases.

Consequently, nitroglycerin and other organic nitrates seem to primarily decrease myocardial oxygen demand rather than directly increase oxygen supply. Nitrates can also dilate the coronary arteries to some extent; these drugs are documented to cause an increase in coronary artery flow.[9] The *primary* way that these drugs relieve angina pectoris, however, is through their ability to decrease cardiac work, thus decreasing myocardial oxygen demand.

Table 22-1
ORGANIC NITRATES

Dosage Form	Onset of Action	Duration of Action
Nitroglycerin		
IV	Immediate	Several minutes
Oral (extended release)	40–60 min	8–12 hr
Sublingual/lingual	1–3 min	30–60 min
Transdermal ointment	20–60 min	4–8 hr
Transdermal patches	40–60 min	8–24 hr
Isosorbide Dinitrate		
Oral	20–40 min	4–6 hr
Oral (extended release)	30 min	12 hr
Chewable	2–5 min	1–2 hr
Sublingual	2–5 min	1–2 hr
Isosorbide Mononitrate		
Oral	30–60 min	6–8 hr
Amyl nitrite		
Inhaled	30 sec	5–10 min

Specific Agents

Nitroglycerin (Nitro-Bid, Nitrostat, Nitro-Dur, many others). In addition to being used as a powerful explosive, nitroglycerin is perhaps the most well-known antianginal drug. The explosive nature of this agent is rendered inactive by diluting it with lactose, alcohol, or propylene glycol. Nitroglycerin is administered for both the prevention and treatment of anginal attacks and can be administered by oral, buccal, sublingual, translingual, transdermal, and intravenous routes (see Table 22-1).

Sublingual administration of nitroglycerin is perhaps the best method to treat an acute attack of angina. Placed under the tongue, the drug is rapidly absorbed through the oral mucosa into the systemic circulation. Therapeutic effects usually begin within 2 minutes when nitroglycerin is administered sublingually. Sublingual administration also spares the nitroglycerin from the first-pass effect because the drug can reach the systemic circulation before first passing through the liver, where it is inactivated (see Chapter 2).

Nitroglycerin can also be delivered via an aerosol form that is sprayed on or under the tongue (translingual spray). Oral preparations are available but this method of administration is limited because—as previously mentioned—nitroglycerin undergoes extensive first-pass degradation in the liver when absorbed directly from the intestines.

For prophylaxis of angina, nitroglycerin can also be administered transdermally via ointment or medicated patches placed on the skin (see Table 22-1). Nitroglycerin-impregnated patches or disks are applied cutaneously like a small bandage, with the drug slowly and continuously absorbed through the skin and into the systemic circulation[10] (Fig. 22-2). Patients are favorable toward nitroglycerin patches because of their ease and convenience. By providing fairly continuous and sustained administration, nitroglycerin patches can also help prevent the onset of an anginal episode in many patients.

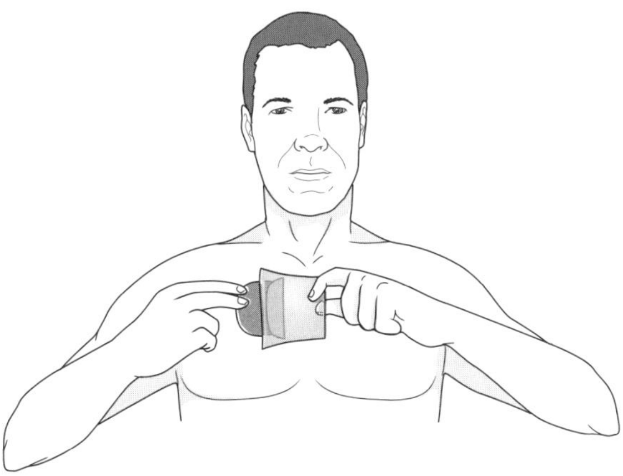

Figure ■ 22-2
Placement of a nitroglycerin patch. Patches adhere to the skin on the upper body or upper arms and are typically worn for 12 to 14 hours each day.

One drawback to the use of patches is that some patients develop drug tolerance when nitroglycerin is delivered continuously. This effect will reduce the antianginal effectiveness of this medication and may cause other harmful changes in the vascular endothelium.[11,12] The exact reasons for nitrate tolerance are not fully understood and may involve a decrease in the ability to convert nitroglycerin to nitric oxide, local production of reactive oxygen species (oxygen free radicals), neurohumoral responses that cause vasoconstriction, or a combination of these and other factors.[12,13] Tolerance to nitrate drugs is rather short-lived, however, and normal responses to nitrate drugs can be restored within only a few hours after withdrawing these agents.[14]

Consequently, patients may benefit from a daily regimen of wearing the patch for 12 to 16 hours followed by an 8- to 12-hour nitrate-free interval.[14] This method of intermittent nitroglycerin administration may result in less chance of developing drug tolerance.[11] The drawback, of course, is that the patient will be more susceptible to angina attacks during the nitrate-free interval. Hence, intermittent nitrate use must be monitored carefully in each patient to make sure that the patch provides adequate protection during the part of day or night when angina is likely to occur, without leaving the patient especially vulnerable during the nondrug interval.

Nitroglycerin ointment is another way to provide continuous transdermal administration.[14] These nitroglycerin ointments are somewhat messy and inconvenient, however, and use of nitroglycerin ointments for treating angina has been largely replaced by other methods such as the transdermal patch. On the other hand, nitroglycerin ointments, or ointments containing glyceryl trinitrate (a similar compound), may be helpful in treating wounds and tendon injuries—that is, local nitroglycerin application can cause vasodilation and other beneficial effects that might enhance tissue growth and promote wound healing. Hence, these ointments may be useful in promoting tendon healing in various tendiopathies[15] and promoting wound healing in chronic anal fissures, diabetic foot ulcers, and other types of wounds.[16,17]

Isosorbide Dinitrate. Like nitroglycerin, isosorbide dinitrate is used for the treatment of acute episodes of angina and for the prevention of anginal attacks. The antianginal and hemodynamic effects last longer with isosorbide dinitrate, so this drug is often classified as a long-acting nitrate. The longer duration of action, however, may occur after this drug is converted to active metabolites such as isosorbide mononitrate (see below).[14] For acute attacks, isosorbide dinitrate is administered sublingually, buccally, or by chewable tablets (see Table 22-1). For prevention of angina, oral tablets are usually given.

Isosorbide Mononitrate. This drug is another long-acting nitrate that is similar in structure and function to isosorbide dinitrate. It is typically given orally for prevention of anginal attacks.

Amyl Nitrite. This drug is supplied in small ampules that can be broken open to inhale during acute anginal attacks. Absorption of the drug through the nasal membranes causes peripheral vasodilation and decreased cardiac preload and afterload. Clinical use of inhaled amyl nitrite is very limited, however, and safer and more convenient methods of nitrate administration (e.g., nitroglycerin patches) generally have replaced this type of antianginal treatment.

Adverse Effects

The primary adverse effects associated with organic nitrates are headache, dizziness, and orthostatic hypotension.[18,19] These effects are related to the drugs' ability to dilate peripheral blood vessels and decrease peripheral resistance. Nausea may also be a problem in some patients. As indicated earlier, tolerance to the beneficial effects of nitrates can occur during continuous administration, but providing daily nitrate-free intervals should prevent this problem.

Beta-Adrenergic Blockers

By antagonizing beta-1 receptors on the myocardium, beta blockers tend to decrease heart rate and the force of myocardial contractions.[20] The effect is an obvious decrease in the work that the heart must perform and a decrease in myocardial oxygen demand. Beta blockers help certain patients with angina maintain an appropriate balance between myocardial oxygen supply and demand by preventing an increase in myocardial oxygen demand.[21,22] The prophylactic administration prevents the onset of an anginal attack. The use of beta blockers in specific forms of angina is reviewed later in this chapter.

Specific Agents

Individual beta blockers were discussed in Chapter 20; beta blockers effective in treating angina pectoris are listed in Table 22-2. Various beta blockers seem to display a fairly equal ability to decrease episodes of stable angina pectoris.[14] However, certain beta-blockers may be more favorable in some patients because the side effects are more tolerable or because the dosing schedule is more convenient (i.e., the drug needs to be given only once each day rather than in several doses). Likewise, some beta blockers may have other properties that might provide additional benefits. Agents such as carvedilol (Coreg), for example, produce peripheral vasodilation that can be advantageous in patients with angina who also have hypertension.[23] Certain beta blockers are also helpful in preventing sudden death after myocardial infarction, so these agents may be especially useful in treating angina in a patient recovering from a heart attack.[23,24] Therefore, the choice of a specific beta blocker depends on the pharmacological profile of each drug in conjunction with the particular needs of each patient.[20]

Adverse Effects

Beta blockers that bind to both beta-1 and beta-2 receptors (nonselective agents) may induce bronchoconstriction in patients with asthma or similar respiratory

Table 22-2
BETA BLOCKERS USED TO TREAT ANGINA PECTORIS

Generic Name	Common Trade Name(s)	Usual Oral Dose*
Acebutolol	Monitan, Sectral	200–600 mg, 2 times a day
Atenolol	Tenormin	50–200 mg, once a day
Carteolol	Cartrol	2.5–10 mg, once a day
Carvedilol	Coreg	6.25–25 mg, 2 times a day
Labetalol	Trandate	200–400 mg, 2 times a day
Metoprolol	Lopressor, others	50–200 mg, 2 times a day
Nadolol	Corgard	40–240 mg, once a day
Penbutolol	Levatol	20 mg, once a day
Pindolol	Visken	5–30 mg, 2 times a day
Propranolol	Inderal, others	40–80 mg, 2–4 times a day
Sotalol	Betapace, others	80–120 mg, 2 times a day
Timolol	Blocadren, others	10–30 mg, 2 times a day

**Indicates typical dosage range used to treat chronic, stable angina. Initial doses may be lower and increased gradually to reach this range.*

problems. These patients should be given one of the more cardioselective beta antagonists, such as atenolol (Tenormin) or metoprolol (Lopressor, others). Beta blockers may also produce excessive cardiac depression in individuals with certain types of cardiac disease. These drugs are generally well tolerated in most patients, however, and major problems are infrequent.

Calcium Channel Blockers

These drugs block the entry of calcium into vascular smooth muscle,[25] where calcium ions facilitate contraction by initiating actin-myosin interaction. Calcium channel blockers decrease the entry of calcium into vascular smooth-muscle cells, thus causing relaxation and vasodilation. By blocking calcium entry into coronary artery smooth muscle, these drugs mediate coronary vasodilation, with a subsequent increase in the supply of oxygen to the myocardium. Consequently, a primary role of calcium channel blockers in angina pectoris is to directly increase coronary blood flow, thus increasing myocardial oxygen supply.[9,26]

Calcium channel blockers also cause some degree of systemic vasodilation, and some of their antianginal effects may be related to a decrease in myocardial oxygen demand caused by a decrease in cardiac preload and afterload—that is, they may exert some of their beneficial effects in a manner similar to that of organic nitrates.[25] Also, calcium channel blockers limit the entry of calcium into cardiac striated cells, thus decreasing myocardial contractility and oxygen demand. The *primary* beneficial effects of these drugs in angina pectoris, however, are related to their ability to dilate the coronary arteries and peripheral vasculature. Certain calcium channel blockers can also affect myocardial excitability by altering the conduction of electrical activity throughout the myocardium.[27] This effect seems to be more important when these drugs are used to treat cardiac arrhythmias (see Chapter 23).

The calcium channel blockers currently used to treat angina pectoris are listed in Table 22-3. Although the chemistry and exact mechanism of action of each drug are somewhat distinct, all of these agents exert their effects by limiting calcium entry into specific cardiovascular tissues. Certain calcium channel blockers known as the *dihydropyridine agents* (e.g., nifedipine, other *-ipine* drugs; see below) affect vascular smooth muscle more than myocardial tissues. Other nondihydropyridine calcium channel blockers such as

Table 22-3
CALCIUM CHANNEL BLOCKERS

Generic Name	Trade Name(s)	Usual Oral Antianginal Dose*
Amlodipine	Norvasc	5–10 mg, once a day
Diltiazem	Cardizem, Dilacor, others	30–120 mg, 3–4 times a day
Felodipine	Plendil, Renedil	5–10 mg, once a day
Isradipine	DynaCirc	2.5–10 mg, 2 times a day
Nicardipine	Cardene	20–40 mg, 3 times a day
Nifedipine	Adalat, Procardia, others	10–30 mg, 3 times a day
Verapamil	Calan, Isoptin, Verelan, others	80–120 mg, 3 times a day

**Indicates typical dosage range for standard preparations. Extended and sustained release dosages may be somewhat different.*

diltiazem and verapamil primarily affect the heart and inhibit calcium entry into cardiac muscle cells. Individual agents are discussed below.

Specific Agents

Diltiazem (Cardizem, Dilacor). Like the other calcium channel blockers, diltiazem is able to vasodilate the coronary arteries and the peripheral vasculature. Diltiazem also produces some depression of electrical conduction in the sinoatrial and atrioventricular nodes, an effect that may cause slight bradycardia. This bradycardia can be worsened by beta blockers or in patients with myocardial conduction problems, and diltiazem should probably be avoided in these individuals.[28]

Nifedipine (Adalat, Procardia) and Other Dihydropyridines. Nifedipine and similar drugs are members of the dihydropyridine class of calcium channel blockers. This class is distinguished by drugs with an *-ipine* suffix, including felodipine (Plendil), isradipine (DynaCirc), and nicardipine (Cardene). These drugs are relatively selective for vascular smooth muscle as compared to cardiac striated muscle, and they vasodilate the coronary arteries and peripheral vasculature without exerting any direct effects on cardiac excitability or contractility.[14] These drugs are therefore advantageous when treating patients with angina who also have certain types of cardiac arrhythmias or problems with cardiac excitation and conduction—that is, they may reduce angina without directly aggravating cardiac arrhythmias.[25] However, nifedipine and similar drugs may produce reflex tachycardia, which is a compensatory increase in heart rate occurring when peripheral vascular resistance decreases because of the drug-induced vasodilation. Other nondihydropyridine drugs (diltiazem, verapamil) also lower vascular resistance but do not produce reflex tachycardia because these drugs also have an inhibitory effect on heart rate (negative chronotropic effect). If reflex tachycardia does occur with nifedipine, this problem can be controlled by using sustained-release or long-acting forms of these drugs (see "Adverse Effects").

Verapamil (Calan, Isoptin, others). Verapamil can be used to treat angina because of its ability to vasodilate the coronary vessels. However, it seems to be moderately effective compared to the other antianginal drugs, and it depresses myocardial excitability and decreases heart rate.[25] Because of its negative effects on cardiac excitation, verapamil is probably more useful in controlling certain cardiac arrhythmias (see Chapter 23).

Adverse Effects

The primary problems associated with the calcium channel blockers are related to the peripheral vasodilation produced by these agents. Headache, flushing or feelings of warmth, and dizziness may occur in some patients. Peripheral edema, as evidenced by swelling in the feet and legs, may also occur, and nausea is fairly common. Certain calcium channel blockers that primarily affect the myocardium (e.g., diltiazem, verapamil) can cause disturbances in cardiac rhythm. As indicated, reflex tachycardia can also be a problem, especially with nifedipine and other dihydropyridine calcium channel blockers (i.e., the *-ipine* drugs) that selectively decrease vascular resistance without simultaneously inhibiting heart rate.

Researchers have raised some concern about the safety of the calcium channel blockers. In particular, reports indicated that certain calcium channel blockers, such as the short-acting form of nifedipine, may be associated with an increased risk of myocardial infarction in certain patients (i.e., older patients with hypertension and patients with unstable angina).[29,30] The short-acting or immediate-release form of nifedipine and other *-ipine* calcium channel blockers can be problematic because they may cause a fairly rapid decrease in peripheral vascular resistance and blood pressure.[14] This can precipitate reflex hemodynamic changes (increased heart rate, decreased myocardial perfusion), which leads to ischemia and infarction in susceptible patients. Sustained-release or longer-acting forms of nifedipine and similar agents may be somewhat safer because they do not cause as rapid a change in vascular resistance as the short-acting drugs.[31]

As indicated in Chapter 21, preliminary studies also suggested that calcium channel blockers may increase the risk of cancer.[29] Intracellular calcium levels are important in regulating cell division. By modifying calcium influx, calcium channel blockers could conceivably accelerate cell proliferation and lead to cancerous growths. Fortunately for the large number of patients that must take the drugs, the carcinogenic potential of these drugs has not been proven conclusively by subsequent studies.[29] Hence, calcium channel blockers are used cautiously but effectively.

OTHER DRUGS AFFECTING MYOCARDIAL OXYGEN BALANCE IN ANGINA PECTORIS

Ranolazine (Ranexa) decreases calcium concentration in heart muscle cells. The drug inhibits specific sodium channels that allow sodium to enter heart cells during cardiac excitation and depolarization.[32,33] This effect ultimately decreases calcium concentration in heart cells via a mechanism involving the sodium-calcium exchanger, which is a transport protein located on the surface of the heart cell. As sodium enters via this exchanger, calcium is extruded from the heart cell. By inhibiting sodium channels during depolarization, the gradient for sodium to enter via the sodium-calcium exchanger is increased—that is, if less sodium enters through activated sodium channels, the amount of sodium inside the cell is reduced and there is a greater tendency for sodium to enter the cell via the sodium-calcium exchanger. As more sodium enters the cell via the exchanger, calcium efflux from the cell is increased, thus decreasing the amount of calcium in the myocardial tissues. Decreased calcium concentration leads to a reduced contraction force, thereby reducing cardiac workload, oxygen demand, and symptoms of angina.

Hence, ranolazine is distinct from other drugs that decrease calcium concentration in heart cells (i.e., the channel blockers). This drug may also be advantageous in certain patients because it does not promote arrhythmias or reduce blood pressure. Ranolazine is not usually the first drug used to treat angina but is typically reserved for patients who have not responded adequately to more conventional agents, such as nitrates, beta blockers, or dihydropyridine calcium channel blockers (e.g., amlodipine).[34]

USE OF ANTICOAGULANTS IN ANGINA PECTORIS

Angina pectoris is typically associated with some degree of coronary artery occlusion. Practitioners may administer certain anticoagulant drugs so that a partially occluded artery does not become completely blocked and cause myocardial infarction.[35,36] This strategy seems especially important in patients with unstable angina and other acute coronary syndromes that predispose the patient to coronary occlusion and infarction. Agents commonly used in this situation include the platelet inhibitors such as aspirin and other agents that inhibit specific aspects of blood coagulation.[35] The pharmacology and anticoagulant effects of these drugs are discussed in detail in Chapter 25, and their use in angina is addressed briefly here.

Aspirin and other drugs that reduce platelet activity are essential in preventing platelet-induced clotting in the coronary arteries and other vascular tissues.[37] As discussed in Chapter 15, aspirin inhibits the biosynthesis of prostaglandins, and certain prostaglandins are responsible for activating platelets during the clotting process. In angina pectoris, aspirin administration can prevent platelets from becoming activated in partially occluded coronary vessels and therefore helps maintain blood flow through these vessels.[38]

People with angina often take aspirin orally for the long-term management of platelet-induced clotting. Aspirin, however, only produces a moderate amount of platelet inhibition, and stronger antiplatelet drugs are available. Drugs such as clopidogrel (Plavix) and prasugrel (Effient), for example, block a specific receptor known as the P2Y12 receptor located on the platelet. This receptor is normally stimulated by adenosine diphosphate (ADP); hence these P2Y12 blockers reduce the ability of ADP to bind to this receptor and activate the platelet.[35,37] These stronger antiplatelet drugs can be used alone or added to aspirin therapy in patients who are at high risk for infarction.[39]

Heparin is often used during the initial or acute phase of unstable angina to prevent clot formation at atherosclerotic plaques that may have ruptured in the coronary arteries.[40,41] Heparin is a fast-acting anticoagulant that leads to the inhibition of thrombin, a key component of the clotting mechanism. With regard to their use in angina, low molecular weight heparins (LMWH) such as enoxaparin (Lovenox) seem to be especially advantageous because they produce a more predictable anticoagulant response and are tolerated better than more traditional (unfractionated) heparin.[41,42] However, heparin must be administered parenterally, and LMWHs are usually given via subcutaneous injection.

Pharmacologists have been developing several newer anticoagulant strategies to prevent adverse outcomes in unstable angina and acute coronary syndromes. These strategies include direct thrombin inhibitors (hirudin, bivalirudin), clotting factor Xa inhibitors (fondaparinux, rivaroxaban), and platelet glycoprotein IIb–IIIa receptor inhibitors (abciximab, tirofiban, eptifibatide).[43] These newer drugs all inhibit a specific aspect of the clotting process (see Chapter 25), and their effects in preventing adverse effects in patients with angina continue to be investigated.

Antiplatelet drugs, heparin, and various other anticoagulant strategies are therefore used in various forms of angina to help prevent infarction. When administered with the traditional antianginal medications, these anticoagulants can help decrease morbidity and mortality in people with ischemic heart disease. For more details on the effects of anticoagulant medications, please refer to Chapter 25.

TREATMENT OF SPECIFIC TYPES OF ANGINA PECTORIS

All forms of angina pectoris are not the same. Traditionally, angina has been subclassified according to factors that precipitate the angina and the pathophysiological mechanisms responsible for producing myocardial ischemia.[44] The major forms of angina and the primary drugs used to treat each type are discussed here and summarized in Table 22-4.

Stable Angina

Stable angina is the most common form of ischemic heart disease.[2] The primary problem in stable angina is that myocardial oxygen demand greatly exceeds oxygen supply. Stable angina is also frequently referred to as *effort*, or *exertional*, *angina*, because a certain level of

Table 22-4
TYPES OF ANGINA PECTORIS

Classification	Cause	Drug Therapy
Stable angina	Myocardial oxygen demand exceeds oxygen supply Usually brought on by physical exertion	Sublingual/lingual nitroglycerin is typically used at the onset of an acute episode A beta blocker or a long-acting nitrate is often used to prevent attacks
Variant angina	Myocardial oxygen supply decreases due to coronary vasospasm May occur while patient is at rest	A calcium channel blocker primarily
Unstable angina	Myocardial oxygen supply decreases at the same time oxygen demand increases Can occur at any time secondary to atherosclerotic plaque rupture within the coronary artery	May require a combination of drugs (e.g., a calcium channel blocker plus a beta blocker). Anticoagulant drugs are also helpful in preventing thrombogenesis and coronary occlusion.

physical exertion usually precipitates attacks. If the patient exercises beyond the level of his or her capacity, the coronary arteries are unable to deliver the oxygen needed to sustain that level of myocardial function, and an anginal episode occurs. The inability of the coronary arteries to adequately deliver oxygen in stable angina is usually caused by some degree of permanent coronary artery occlusion (e.g., coronary artery atherosclerosis or stenosis).

Because stable angina is caused primarily by an increase in myocardial oxygen demand, treatment of this form of angina has mainly consisted of beta blockers, calcium channel blockers, and organic nitrates.[45] Beta blockers are often the first drugs used in the long-term management of stable angina because they decrease the workload of the heart, thus limiting myocardial oxygen requirements. Hence, beta blockers are often taken orally on a daily basis to prevent the onset of an angina episode.

The primary drug strategy for managing an acute attack consists of an organic nitrate in the form of nitroglycerin.[46,47] Nitroglycerin is often applied via sublingual tablets or lingual sprays at the onset of an attack or just before exercise or other activities that routinely precipitate an attack. As previously mentioned, the sublingual route allows rapid drug effects while avoiding the first pass effect. Nitrates can also be given as a preventive measure to blunt myocardial oxygen needs, and nitroglycerin can be administered transdermally through patches or ointments, or a long-acting nitrate (isosorbide dinitrate, isosorbide mononitrate) can be administered orally. As discussed earlier, however, long-term use of nitrates can cause tolerance, and an intermittent dosing procedure (i.e., daily nitrate-free intervals) should be instituted when these drugs are taken regularly to prevent angina.[14]

Calcium channel blockers can also be given to treat stable angina, especially if beta blockers are not tolerated or are contraindicated in specific patients.[45] These drugs decrease cardiac workload directly by limiting calcium entry into myocardial cells and indirectly by producing peripheral vasodilation, thus decreasing cardiac preload and afterload.[25] Hence, calcium channel blockers are administered in stable angina primarily for their effect on the myocardium and peripheral vasculature rather than for their ability to dilate the coronary arteries. Nonetheless, these drugs also produce some degree of coronary vasodilation, and this action may produce additional beneficial effects in certain patients with stable angina.[25]

Ranolazine is another option for treating chronic stable angina.[33] As indicated earlier, this drug decreases calcium concentration in heart cells by a complex mechanism involving the exchange of sodium and calcium ions across the cell membrane. Reduced intracellular calcium concentration leads to less actin-myosin interaction with a subsequent decrease in myocardial contraction force and cardiac workload. Ranolazine is usually not the first choice for treating chronic angina but may be prescribed if the response to other antianginal drugs is inadequate.[34]

The drugs discussed above can be used separately, but a combination of these antianginal drugs is also used in many patients with stable angina.[2] For example, a beta blocker and long-acting nitrate may be administered together, especially when either drug by itself is not completely successful in managing anginal episodes. Likewise, a beta blocker and calcium channel blocker may be used in combination,[46] but care must be taken to avoid excessive negative chronotropic and negative ionotropic effects on the heart (i.e., nondihydropyridine calcium channel blockers can decrease heart rate and contraction force, which can add to the inhibitory effects of beta blockers on the heart).[45] Hence, beta blockers are typically combined with nifedipine or another dihydropyridine agent (*-ipine* drugs) when these two types of antianginal agents are used together.[25]

Finally, other drugs can be included to improve the general health and outcome in patients with stable angina. In particular, low-dose aspirin therapy or other antiplatelet strategies are important in decreasing the risk of thrombus formation and coronary infarction.[48] Drugs that decrease plasma lipids (e.g., statin drugs; see Chapter 25) and certain antihypertensives (e.g., angiotensin converting enzyme inhibitors; see Chapter 21) also play a prominent role in decreasing mortality in people with stable angina.[48,49] Any medication regimen should be comprehensive and optimally tailored to meet the individual needs of each patient.

Variant Angina (Prinzmetal Ischemia)

In variant angina, the primary problem is that oxygen supply to the myocardium *decreases* because of coronary artery vasospasm.[9,26] Vasospasm causes oxygen supply to decrease even though oxygen demand has not changed, and this phenomenon can occur even when the patient is at rest. In some patients with variant angina, the coronary arteries appear to be supersensitive to endogenous vasoconstrictive agents, and a variety of emotional or environmental stimuli may trigger coronary vasospasm.[45] In many patients, however, the reason for this spontaneous coronary vasoconstriction is unknown.

Calcium channel blockers are especially effective in treating variant angina and are usually the drugs of choice. Most patients with this form of angina respond well to these agents. These drugs limit the entry of calcium into the coronary vessels, thus attenuating or preventing the vasospasm underlying variant angina.[25] If patients do not respond to a single calcium channel blocker, long-acting nitrates may be added for management of severe variant angina.[45] If necessary, short-acting nitrates can be applied sublingually or translingually during an acute attack of variant angina, presumably because these drugs can dilate the coronary arteries. If calcium channel blockers are not tolerated, long-acting nitrates may be used instead.

Unstable Angina

The more severe form of angina is often classified as "unstable" angina. This type of angina is often initiated by sudden rupture of atherosclerotic plaques within the coronary arteries, which precipitates coronary vasoconstriction and thrombus formation.[50,51] Plaque rupture can be brought on by exertion, or it may occur spontaneously when the patient is at rest. Therefore, the primary defect in unstable angina is a decrease in myocardial oxygen supply, although myocardial oxygen demand may be increasing simultaneously if the patient is exercising. Because unstable angina is also associated with thrombosis and increased platelet aggregation in the affected coronary arteries, this type of angina is often a precursor to acute myocardial infarction.[51] Together, unstable angina and myocardial infarction comprise the category of acute coronary syndromes.[52] Unstable angina is therefore regarded as the most serious and potentially dangerous form of angina.[50]

Various traditional antianginal drugs have been used alone or in combination to treat the ischemic symptoms of unstable angina and acute coronary syndrome.[52,53] Beta blockers, for example, are among the primary drugs because they decrease cardiac workload and thereby prevent subsequent damage to the ischemic myocardium.[54] Beta blockers can be combined with the two other types of traditional antianginal medications (nitrates and calcium channel blockers), depending on the specific needs and responses of each patient.[53] Most important is the recognition that unstable angina is often associated with coronary artery thrombosis and that anticoagulant and antiplatelet therapy is critical in preventing this type of angina from progressing to myocardial infarction.[35,36,55] Hence, anticoagulant drugs are often administered in the early stages of unstable angina, with antiplatelet drugs (aspirin, clopidogrel) being continued indefinitely to help prevent coronary occlusion.[45] Likewise, other drugs such as the ACE inhibitors (see Chapter 21) can help protect the heart and vasculature in acute coronary syndromes,[56] and lipid-lowering drugs such as the statins (see Chapter 25) can provide immediate and long-term beneficial effects in preventing coronary occlusion in patients with unstable angina.[50,57]

NONPHARMACOLOGICAL MANAGEMENT OF ANGINA PECTORIS

The primary drugs used to treat angina (i.e., nitrates, beta blockers, calcium channel blockers) are effective and relatively safe for long-term use. These agents, however, really only treat a symptom of heart disease—namely, the pain associated with myocardial ischemia. Traditional antianginal drugs do not cure any cardiac conditions, nor do they exert any beneficial long-term effects on cardiac function. Consequently, practitioners encourage many patients with angina to make efforts to resolve the underlying disorder responsible for causing an imbalance in myocardial oxygen supply and demand.

Nonpharmacological treatment usually begins by identifying any potentiating factors that might initiate or exacerbate anginal attacks. For instance, hypertension, congestive heart failure, anemia, and thyrotoxicosis may all contribute to the onset of angina. In some cases, treatment of one of these potentiating factors may effectively resolve the angina, thus making subsequent drug therapy unnecessary. Lifestyle changes, including exercise, weight control, smoking cessation, and stress management, may also be helpful in decreasing or even eliminating the need for antianginal drugs. Finally, several surgical techniques that increase coronary blood flow may be attempted. Revascularization procedures such as coronary artery bypass and coronary artery angioplasty may be successful in increasing myocardial oxygen supply, thus attenuating anginal attacks in some patients. Regardless of what strategy is pursued, the medical team, including rehabilitation therapists, should explore a permanent solution to the factors that precipitate myocardial ischemia in all patients with angina pectoris.

Special Concerns for Rehabilitation Patients

Physical therapists and occupational therapists must be aware of patients who are taking medications for angina pectoris and whether the medications are taken prophylactically or during an attack. For the patient with stable angina taking nitroglycerin at the onset of an anginal episode, therapists must make sure the drug is always nearby during therapy sessions. Because many activities in rehabilitation (exercise, functional training, etc.) increase myocardial oxygen demand, anginal attacks may occur during the therapy session. If the nitroglycerin tablets are in the patient's hospital room (inpatients) or were left at home (outpatients), the anginal attack will be prolonged and possibly quite severe. A little precaution in making sure patients bring their nitroglycerin to therapy can prevent some tense moments while waiting to see if an anginal attack will subside.

For patients taking antianginal drugs prophylactically (i.e., at regular intervals), having the drug actually present during the rehabilitation session is not as crucial, providing that the patient has been taking the medication as prescribed. Therapists must still be aware, however, that many rehabilitation activities may disturb the balance between myocardial oxygen supply and demand, particularly by increasing oxygen demand beyond the ability of the coronary arteries to increase oxygen supply to the heart. Consequently, therapists must be aware of the cardiac limitations in their patients with angina and use caution in not overtaxing the heart to the extent that the antianginal drugs are ineffective.

Another important consideration in rehabilitation is the effect of antianginal drugs on the response to an exercise bout. Some patients taking nitrates, for example, may experience an *increase* in exercise tolerance because the patient is not as limited by symptoms of angina.[58] Certain drugs, however, may blunt the ability of the heart to respond to an acute exercise bout. Beta blockers and certain calcium channel blockers, for instance, slow down heart rate and decrease myocardial contractility during

Special Concerns for Rehabilitation Patients (Continued)

exercise.[59,60] At any absolute exercise workload, the myocardial response (e.g., heart rate) of the patient taking these drugs will be lower than if the drug was not taken. Consequently, the heart may not be able to handle some workloads. This blunted exercise response must be taken into account when patients engage in cardiac conditioning activities, and exercise workloads should be adjusted accordingly.

Finally, therapists should be aware of how the side effects of the antianginal drugs may affect the therapy session. The nitrates and calcium channel blockers both produce peripheral vasodilation and can lead to hypotension. This decrease in blood pressure may be exaggerated when the patient suddenly sits or stands up (orthostatic hypotension). Also, conditions that produce peripheral vasodilation, such as heat or exercise, may produce an additive effect on the drug-induced hypotension, thus leading to dizziness and syncope. Therapists should be aware that patients taking nitrates and calcium channel blockers may experience hypotension when systemic heat is applied or when patients perform exercises that use large muscle groups.

CASE STUDY

ANTIANGINAL DRUGS

Brief History. T.M. is a 73-year-old man who is retired from his job as an accountant. He has a long history of type 2 diabetes mellitus, which has progressively worsened over the past decade despite oral antidiabetic medication and insulin treatment. He also has a history of stable (classic) angina that has been managed by nitroglycerin. The patient self-administers a nitroglycerin tablet (0.4 mg) sublingually at the onset of an anginal attack. Recently, the patient was admitted to the hospital for treatment of a gangrenous lesion on his left foot. When this lesion failed to respond to conservative treatment, a left below-knee amputation was performed. Following the amputation, the patient was referred to physical therapy for strengthening and a preprosthetic evaluation.

Problem/Influence of Medication. The therapist initiated a program of general conditioning and strengthening at the patient's bedside the day following surgery. On the third day, the therapist decided to bring the patient to the physical therapy department for a more intensive program, including standing activities with the parallel bars. The patient arrived in the department via wheelchair and began complaining immediately of chest pains. The patient had not brought his nitroglycerin tablets with him to the therapy session.

1. ***What immediate action should the therapist take to help this patient during an angina attack?***
2. ***Why did T.M. experience angina before even beginning any exercises or other rehabilitation regimens?***
3. ***What can be done to prevent similar situations in the future?***

See Appendix C, "Answers to Case Study Questions."

SUMMARY

Pain in the chest region, or angina pectoris, is a common symptom of ischemic heart disease. Anginal pain usually occurs because of an imbalance between myocardial oxygen supply and myocardial oxygen demand. Organic nitrates, beta blockers, and calcium channel blockers are the primary drugs used to treat angina pectoris. Organic nitrates and beta blockers primarily exert their effects by decreasing myocardial oxygen demand, whereas calcium channel blockers primarily increase myocardial oxygen supply. The forms of angina pectoris include stable, variant, and unstable. Specific types of antianginal drugs are used alone or in combination with each other to treat or prevent the various forms of angina.

Rehabilitation specialists must be aware of any patients who have angina pectoris and the possibility of patients having an anginal attack during a therapy session. Therapists should also be mindful of what drugs the patients are taking, as well as any side effects that may influence certain rehabilitation procedures.

REFERENCES

1. Arrebola-Moreno A, Dungu J, Kaski JC. Treatment strategies for chronic stable angina. *Expert Opin Pharmacother.* 2011;12:2833-2844.
2. Tarkin JM, Kaski JC. Pharmacological treatment of chronic stable angina pectoris. *Clin Med.* 2013;13:63-70.
3. Rosen SD. From heart to brain: the genesis and processing of cardiac pain. *Can J Cardiol.* 2012;28(suppl):S7-19.
4. Gutterman DD. Silent myocardial ischemia. *Circ J.* 2009;73:785-797.
5. Iachini Bellisarii F, Radico F, Muscente F, et al. Nitrates and other nitric oxide donors in cardiology: current positioning and perspectives. *Cardiovasc Drugs Ther.* 2012;26:55-69.
6. Katsumi H, Nishikawa M, Hashida M. Development of nitric oxide donors for the treatment of cardiovascular diseases. *Cardiovasc Hematol Agents Med Chem.* 2007;5:204-208.
7. Kots AY, Bian K, Murad F. Nitric oxide and cyclic GMP signaling pathway as a focus for drug development. *Curr Med Chem.* 2011;18:3299-3305.
8. Nossaman VE, Nossaman BD, Kadowitz PJ. Nitrates and nitrites in the treatment of ischemic cardiac disease. *Cardiol Rev.* 2010;18:190-197.
9. Looi KL, Grace A, Agarwal S. Coronary artery spasm and ventricular arrhythmias. *Postgrad Med J.* 2012;88:465-471.
10. Uxa A, Thomas GR, Gori T, Parker JD. Standard versus low-dose transdermal nitroglycerin: differential effects on the development of tolerance and abnormalities of endothelial function. *J Cardiovasc Pharmacol.* 2010;56:354-359.
11. Daiber A, Münzel T, Gori T. Organic nitrates and nitrate tolerance—state of the art and future developments. *Adv Pharmacol.* 2010;60:177-227.
12. Münzel T, Gori T. Nitrate therapy and nitrate tolerance in patients with coronary artery disease. *Curr Opin Pharmacol.* 2013;13:251-259.
13. Daiber A, Wenzel P, Oelze M, Münzel T. New insights into bioactivation of organic nitrates, nitrate tolerance and cross-tolerance. *Clin Res Cardiol.* 2008;97:12-20.
14. Michel T, Hoffman BB. Treatment of myocardial ischemia and hypertension. In: Brunton L, et al, eds. *The Pharmacological Basis of Therapeutics.* 12th ed. New York: McGraw-Hill; 2011.
15. Gambito ED, Gonzalez-Suarez CB, Oquiñena TI, Agbayani RB. Evidence on the effectiveness of topical nitroglycerin in the treatment of tendinopathies: a systematic review and meta-analysis. *Arch Phys Med Rehabil.* 2010;91:1291-1305.
16. Gagliardi G, Pascariello A, Altomare DF, et al. Optimal treatment duration of glyceryl trinitrate for chronic anal fissure: results of a prospective randomized multicenter trial. *Tech Coloproctol.* 2010;14:241-248.
17. Hotkar MS, Avachat AM, Bhosale SS, Oswal YM. Preliminary investigation of topical nitroglycerin formulations containing natural wound healing agent in diabetes-induced foot ulcer. *Int Wound J.* 2013 [Epub ahead of print].
18. Bagdy G, Riba P, Kecskeméti V, et al. Headache-type adverse effects of NO donors: vasodilation and beyond. *Br J Pharmacol.* 2010;160:20-35.
19. Scatena R, Bottoni P, Pontoglio A, Giardina B. Pharmacological modulation of nitric oxide release: new pharmacological perspectives, potential benefits and risks. *Curr Med Chem.* 2010;17:61-73.
20. Frishman WH, Saunders E. β-Adrenergic blockers. *J Clin Hypertens.* 2011;13:649-653.
21. Guha S, Ray S. Beta blockers in coronary artery disease with and without hypertension. *Indian Heart J.* 2010;62:126-131.
22. Shu de F, Dong BR, Lin XF, et al. Long-term beta blockers for stable angina: systematic review and meta-analysis. *Eur J Prev Cardiol.* 2012;19:330-341.
23. Chen-Scarabelli C, Saravolatz L Jr, Murad Y, et al. A critical review of the use of carvedilol in ischemic heart disease. *Am J Cardiovasc Drugs.* 2012;12:391-401.
24. Fares H, Lavie CJ, Ventura HO. Vasodilating versus first-generation β-blockers for cardiovascular protection. *Postgrad Med.* 2012;124:7-15.
25. Elliott WJ, Ram CV. Calcium channel blockers. *J Clin Hypertens.* 2011;13:687-689.
26. Kusama Y, Kodani E, Nakagomi A, et al. Variant angina and coronary artery spasm: the clinical spectrum, pathophysiology, and management. *J Nippon Med Sch.* 2011;78:4-12.
27. Frommeyer G, Eckardt L, Milberg P. Calcium handling and ventricular tachyarrhythmias. *Wien Med Wochenschr.* 2012;162:283-286.
28. Mills TA, Kawji MM, Cataldo VD, et al. Profound sinus bradycardia due to diltiazem, verapamil, and/or beta-adrenergic blocking drugs. *J La State Med Soc.* 2004;156:327-331.
29. Epstein BJ, Vogel K, Palmer BF. Dihydropyridine calcium channel antagonists in the management of hypertension. *Drugs.* 2007;67:1309-1327.
30. Lundy A, Lutfi N, Beckey C. Review of nifedipine GITS in the treatment of high risk patients with coronary artery disease and hypertension. *Vasc Health Risk Manag.* 2009;5:429-440.

31. Eisenberg MJ, Brox A, Bestawros AN. Calcium channel blockers: an update. *Am J Med.* 2004;116:35-43.
32. Maier LS. A novel mechanism for the treatment of angina, arrhythmias, and diastolic dysfunction: inhibition of late I(Na) using ranolazine. *J Cardiovasc Pharmacol.* 2009;54:279-286.
33. Sossalla S, Maier LS. Role of ranolazine in angina, heart failure, arrhythmias, and diabetes. *Pharmacol Ther.* 2012;133:311-323.
34. Di Monaco A, Sestito A. The patient with chronic ischemic heart disease. Roleof ranolazine in the management of stable angina. *Eur Rev Med Pharmacol Sci.* 2012;16:1611-1636.
35. Angiolillo DJ, Ferreiro JL. Antiplatelet and anticoagulant therapy for atherothrombotic disease: the role of current and emerging agents. *Am J Cardiovasc Drugs.* 2013;13:233-250.
36. Verheugt FW. Low-dose anticoagulation for secondary prevention in acute coronary syndrome. *Am J Cardiol.* 2013;111: 618-626.
37. Pankert M, Quilici J, Cuisset T. Role of antiplatelet therapy in secondary prevention of acute coronary syndrome. *J Cardiovasc Transl Res.* 2012;5:41-51.
38. Bailey AL, Campbell CL. Oral antiplatelet therapy for acute coronary syndromes: aspirin, P2Y12 inhibition and thrombin receptor antagonists. *Curr Drug Targets.* 2011;12:1805-1812.
39. Sadanandan S, Singh IM. Clopidogrel: the data, the experience, and the controversies. *Am J Cardiovasc Drugs.* 2012;12:361-374.
40. Gresele P, Busti C, Paganelli G. Heparin in the prophylaxis and treatment of venous thromboembolism and other thrombotic diseases. *Handb Exp Pharmacol.* 2012;207:179-209.
41. Nicolau JC, Cohen M, Montalescot G. Differences among low-molecular-weight heparins: evidence in patients with acute coronary syndromes. *J Cardiovasc Pharmacol.* 2009;53:440-445.
42. Iqbal Z, Cohen M. Enoxaparin: a pharmacologic and clinical review. *Expert Opin Pharmacother.* 2011;12:1157-1170.
43. Showkathali R, Natarajan A. Antiplatelet and antithrombin strategies in acute coronary syndrome: state-of-the-art review. *Curr Cardiol Rev.* 2012;8:239-249.
44. Cassady SL, Cahalin LP. Cardiovascular pathophysiology. In: DeTurk WE, Cahalin LP, eds. *Cardiovascular and Pulmonary Physical Therapy.* 2nd ed. New York: McGraw-Hill; 2011.
45. Talbert RL. Ischemic heart disease. In: DiPiro JT, et al, eds. *Pharmacotherapy: A Pathophysiologic Approach.* 8th ed. New York: McGraw-Hill; 2011.
46. Taggart D. Tailor treatment to the patient in stable angina. *Practitioner.* 2011;255:25-28.
47. Zimmerman FH, Fass AE, Katz DR, et al. Nitroglycerin prescription and potency in patients participating in exercise-based cardiac rehabilitation. *J Cardiopulm Rehabil Prev.* 2009;29: 376-379.
48. Palaniswamy C, Aronow WS. Treatment of stable angina pectoris. *Am J Ther.* 2011;18:e138-152.
49. Siama K, Tousoulis D, Papageorgiou N, et al. Stable angina pectoris: current medical treatment. *Curr Pharm Des.* 2013;19: 1569-1580.
50. Braunwald E. Unstable angina and non-ST elevation myocardial infarction. *Am J Respir Crit Care Med.* 2012;185:924-932.
51. Welch TD, Yang EH, Reeder GS, Gersh BJ. Modern management of acute myocardial infarction. *Curr Probl Cardiol.* 2012;37:237-310.
52. Mistry NF, Vesely MR. Acute coronary syndromes: from the emergency department to the cardiac care unit. *Cardiol Clin.* 2012;30:617-627.
53. Kireyev D, Yun EC, Page BJ, Boden WE. Medical therapy in acute coronary syndromes: which medicines and at what doses? *Curr Cardiol Rep.* 2009;11:267-275.
54. de Peuter OR, Lussana F, Peters RJ, et al. A systematic review of selective and non-selective beta blockers for prevention of vascular events in patients with acute coronary syndrome or heart failure. *Neth J Med.* 2009;67:284-294.
55. Kar S, Bhatt DL. Anticoagulants for the treatment of acute coronary syndrome in the era of new oral agents. *Coron Artery Dis.* 2012;23:380-390.
56. Ferrari R, Guardigli G, Ceconi C. Secondary prevention of CAD with ACE inhibitors: a struggle between life and death of the endothelium. *Cardiovasc Drugs Ther.* 2010;24:331-339.
57. Angeli F, Reboldi G, Mazzotta G, et al. Statins in acute coronary syndrome: very early initiation and benefits. *Ther Adv Cardiovasc Dis.* 2012;6:163-174.
58. Boden WE, Finn AV, Patel D, et al. Nitrates as an integral part of optimal medical therapy and cardiac rehabilitation for stable angina: review of current concepts and therapeutics. *Clin Cardiol.* 2012;35:263-271.
59. Dorian P, Connors SP. Pharmacological and nonpharmacological methods for rate control. *Can J Cardiol.* 2005;21(suppl B): 26B-30B.
60. Goss FL, Robertson RJ, Haile L, et al. Use of ratings of perceived exertion to anticipate treadmill test termination in patients taking beta-blockers. *Percept Mot Skills.* 2011;112:310-318.

CHAPTER 23

Treatment of Cardiac Arrhythmias

An **arrhythmia** can be broadly defined as any significant deviation from normal cardiac rhythm.[1] Various problems in the origination and conduction of electrical activity in the heart can lead to distinct types of arrhythmias. If untreated, disturbances in normal cardiac rhythm result in impaired cardiac pumping ability, and certain arrhythmias are associated with cerebrovascular accidents, cardiac failure, and other sequelae that can be fatal.[2,3] Fortunately, a variety of drugs are available to help establish and maintain normal cardiac rhythm.

This chapter presents the primary antiarrhythmic drugs and therapeutic rationale for their use. As indicated throughout this chapter, antiarrhythmic drugs are associated with many side effects, including an increased chance of arrhythmias (pro-arrhythmic effect). Hence, the overall use of these drugs has declined somewhat in recent years, due largely to the development of nonpharmacological interventions such as implantable defibrillator devices and surgical interventions that offer a more permanent solution to rhythm disturbances.[4] Nonetheless, antiarrhythmic drugs remain a primary option for many patients with arrhythmias or as an adjunct to maintain normal rhythm after cardiac surgery.

You will often work directly with cardiac patients in cardiac rehabilitation and fitness programs. Many of these patients may be taking antiarrhythmics to help control and prevent the onset of arrhythmias. The cardiac patients taking antiarrhythmic drugs also may be in rehabilitation for any number of other neuromuscular or musculoskeletal disorders. These drugs can have a positive effect on physical rehabilitation by stabilizing heart rate and allowing the patient to engage in more strenuous exercise and functional activities. On the other hand, these drugs can produce abnormal heart rate and blood pressure responses in certain patients, and you may be in an ideal position to identify these untoward responses before they produce severe adverse reactions. Consequently, you should have some knowledge of the clinical use of these drugs.

To understand how antiarrhythmic drugs exert their effects, the chapter begins with a review on the origin and spread of electrical activity throughout the heart (cardiac electrophysiology). This is followed by a presentation of the basic mechanisms responsible for producing disturbances in cardiac rhythm and the common types of arrhythmias seen clinically. Finally, antiarrhythmic drugs are presented according to their mechanism of action and clinical use.

CARDIAC ELECTROPHYSIOLOGY

Cardiac Action Potentials

The action potential recorded from a cardiac Purkinje fiber is shown in Figure 23-1. At rest, the interior of the cell is negative relative to the cell's exterior. As in other excitable tissues (neurons, skeletal muscle), an action potential occurs when the cell interior suddenly

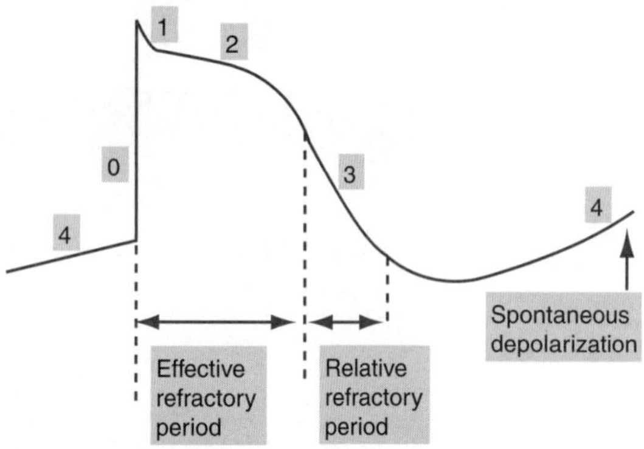

Figure ■ 23-1
The cardiac action potential recorded from a Purkinje cell. The effective refractory period is the time during which the cell cannot be depolarized, and the relative refractory period is the time in which a supranormal stimulus is required to depolarize the cell. *(From: Keefe DLD, Kates RE, Harrison DC. New antiarrhythmic drugs: their place in therapy. Drugs.1981;22:363; with permission.)*

becomes positive (*depolarizes*), primarily because of sodium ion influx. The cell interior then returns to a negative potential (*repolarizes*), primarily because of the efflux of potassium ions. The cardiac action potential has several features that distinguish it from action potentials recorded in other nerves and muscles.[5,6] The cardiac action potential is typically divided into several phases. The ionic movement that occurs in each phase is outlined here.

Phase 0. Rapid depolarization occurs because of the sudden influx of sodium ions into the cell. At some threshold level, the cell membrane suddenly becomes permeable to sodium ions because of the opening of sodium channels or gates, similar to the spike seen in skeletal muscle depolarization.

Phase 1. An early, brief period of repolarization occurs because specific potassium channels in the cell membrane open to allow potassium to leave the cell.

Phase 2. The action potential undergoes a plateau phase, primarily because the calcium channels open, and there is a slow, prolonged influx of calcium ions into the cell. There is no net change in the charge within the cell because the efflux of positively charged potassium ions that occurred in phase 1 is balanced by the influx of positively charged calcium ions. Thus, the cell's potential remains relatively constant for a brief period, which creates the distinctive plateau that can be seen in Figure 23-1. The phase 2 plateau is important in cardiac cells because it prolongs the cell's effective refractory period (i.e., the time interval between successive action potentials). The plateau basically enables the heart to enter a period of rest (*diastole*) so that the cardiac chambers can fill with blood before the next contraction (*systole*).

Phase 3. At the end of the plateau, repolarization is complete. This is primarily because of the closing (*inactivation*) of the calcium channels, which terminates the entry of calcium into the cell. Repolarization is completed by the unopposed exit of potassium ions.

Phase 4. Phase 4 consists of a slow, spontaneous depolarization in certain cardiac pacemaker cells (such as the one shown in Fig. 23-1). This spontaneous depolarization occurs because membrane ion channels allow the continuous leak of sodium ions into the cell along with a gradual decrease in potassium exit from the cell. Intracellular release of calcium from the myocardial sarcoplasmic reticulum also helps regulate the automatic depolarization that initiates each heartbeat. Hence, the coordinated action of membrane ion movements and intracellular calcium release causes a progressive accumulation of positive charge within the cell, which causes the cell to become more and more positive until it reaches threshold and phase 0 is initiated again.[7]

Action potentials recorded from various cardiac cells may vary somewhat from the action potential described previously. Some cells, for instance, totally lack phase 1 and have a slower phase 0. Such cells are said to have a slow response as opposed to the fast response just described. Also, action potentials from the nodal cells (see the next section, "Normal Cardiac Rhythm") differ somewhat from the fast response cells. Nonetheless, the fundamental ionic fluxes occurring during cardiac action potentials are similar in all cardiac cells. This ionic activity is pharmacologically significant because various antiarrhythmic drugs will affect the movement of sodium and other ions in an attempt to establish and maintain normal cardiac rhythm.

Normal Cardiac Rhythm

Certain cardiac cells are able to initiate and maintain a spontaneous automatic rhythm. Even in the absence of any neural or hormonal input, these cells will automatically generate an action potential. They are usually referred to as *pacemaker cells* in the myocardium. As described previously, pacemaker cells have the ability to depolarize spontaneously because of a rising phase 4 in the cardiac action potential (see Fig. 23-1).

Pacemaker cells are found primarily in the sinoatrial (SA) node and the atrioventricular (AV) node. Although many other cardiac cells also have the ability to generate an automatic rhythm, the pacemaker cells in the SA node usually dominate and control cardiac rhythm in the normal heart.

Normal Conduction of the Cardiac Action Potential

The cardiac action potential is normally conducted throughout the heart in a coordinated and predictable pattern (Fig. 23-2).[6] The action potential originates in the SA node and is conducted throughout both atria via the atrial muscle cells. While spreading through the atria, the action potential reaches the AV node. From the AV node, the action potential is passed on to the ventricles via a specialized conducting system known as the *bundle of His*. The bundle of His is composed primarily of specialized conducting cells known as *Purkinje fibers*. As the bundle leaves the AV node, it divides into left and right branches, which supply the respective ventricles. The action potential is distributed to all parts of the ventricles via the bundle branches and Purkinje fibers.

MECHANISMS OF CARDIAC ARRHYTHMIAS

The origin of the cardiac action potential and system of action potential propagation represents normal cardiac excitation and conduction. Any number of factors can disrupt the normal cardiac excitation process, thus resulting in arrhythmic contractions. Such factors include metabolic and electrolyte imbalances, abnormal autonomic influence on the heart, toxicity to other drugs (e.g., cancer chemotherapy), psychological distress, and other cardiac diseases (e.g., myocardial ischemia, infarction, heart failure, hypertension).[8-12] In addition, it is now recognized that genetic factors can predispose individuals to certain arrhythmias.[3,13,14] Specifically, mutations in certain genes can cause altered expression and function of channel proteins that control movements of sodium, potassium, or calcium ions across the cardiac cell membrane.[15-17] Thus, inherited alterations in ion channel function can cause serious and fatal arrhythmias, even if the heart appears structurally intact and has not been damaged by infarction or other factors that stress the heart.[18,19]

Regardless of what the initiating factor is in producing arrhythmias, the mechanism underlying a disturbance in cardiac rhythm can be attributed to one of the three basic abnormalities listed below.[5]

Abnormal impulse generation. The normal automatic rhythm of the cardiac pacemaker cells has been disrupted. Injury and disease may directly render the SA and AV cells incapable of

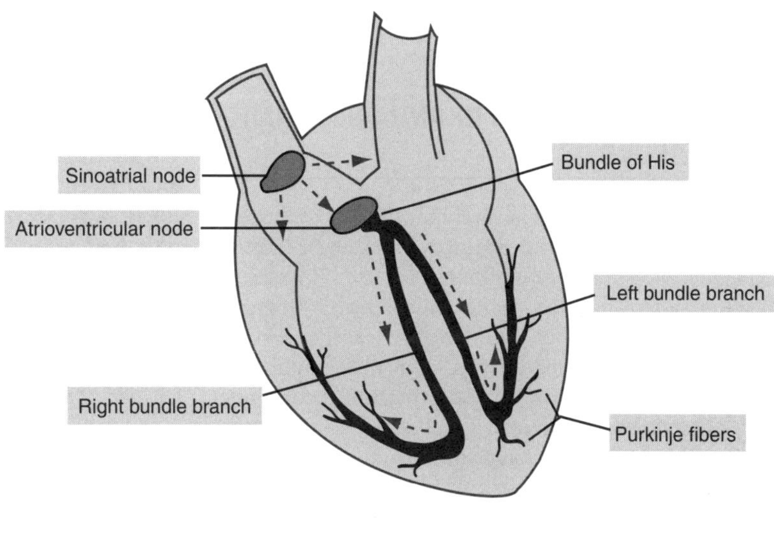

Figure ■ 23-2
Schematic representation of the conduction system of the heart. Conduction normally follows the pathways indicated by the dashed lines. Impulses originate in the sinoatrial node and are transmitted to the atrioventricular node. Impulses are then conducted from the atrioventricular node to the ventricles by the bundle of His and bundle branches.

maintaining normal rhythm. Also, cells that do not normally control cardiac rhythm may begin to compete with pacemaker cells, thus creating multiple areas of automaticity.

Abnormal impulse conduction. The conduction of impulses throughout the myocardium has been interrupted. Various diseases and local damage may result in the delay or failure of an action potential to reach certain areas. These conduction impairments or heart blocks can prevent a smooth and synchronous transmission of electrical activity thus creating an abnormal rhythm.

Simultaneous abnormalities of impulse generation and conduction. A combination of both previously listed factors may cause cardiac arrhythmias.

TYPES OF ARRHYTHMIAS

Cardiac arrhythmias are described by many different terms according to their site of origin, nature of disturbed heartbeat, or impairment in cardiac conduction.[20] This text cannot fully describe all of the various forms of the clinically occurring arrhythmias. To understand when various antiarrhythmic drugs are used, however, some basic terms describing cardiac arrhythmias must be defined. Specific arrhythmias, for example, are often defined by a heart rate that is too slow (bradycardia), too fast (tachycardia), or simply variable. Some of the more commonly occurring arrhythmias and the heart rates that identify bradycardia and tachycardia are listed in Table 23-1. For a more detailed description of the electrophysiological nature and diagnosis of these arrhythmias, the references at the end of this chapter include additional sources.[1,6,20]

Table 23-1
COMMON FORMS OF ARRHYTHMIAS

Classification	Characteristic Rhythm
Sinus Arrhythmias	
Sinus tachycardia	>100 beats/min
Sinus bradycardia	<60 beats/min
Sick sinus syndrome	Severe bradycardia (<50 beats/min); periods of sinus arrest
Supraventricular Arrhythmias	
Atrial fibrillation and flutter	Atrial rate >300 beats/min
Atrial tachycardia	Atrial rate >140–200 beats/min
Premature atrial contractions	Variable
Atrioventricular Junctional Arrhythmias	
Junctional rhythm	40–55 beats/min
Junctional tachycardia	100–200 beats/min
Conduction Disturbances	
Atrioventricular block	Variable
Bundle branch block	Variable
Fascicular block	Variable
Ventricular Arrhythmias	
Premature ventricular contractions	Variable
Ventricular tachycardia	140–200 beats/min
Ventricular fibrillation	Irregular; totally uncoordinated rhythm

CLASSIFICATION OF ANTIARRHYTHMIC DRUGS

Drugs used to treat cardiac arrhythmias are traditionally placed in one of four distinct classes according to their mechanism of action (Table 23-2).[5,21] The classification system has been criticized somewhat because it has several limitations, including the fact that certain drugs may have characteristics from more than one class, and certain drugs with antiarrhythmic properties (e.g., digitalis) do not fit into this system. Nonetheless, this method of categorizing antiarrhythmic drugs is still commonly used.[4,5]

Class I: Sodium Channel Blockers

Class I antiarrhythmic drugs are essentially sodium channel blockers.[5] These drugs bind to membrane sodium channels in various excitable tissues, including myocardial cells. In cardiac tissues, class I drugs normalize the rate of sodium entry into cardiac tissues and thereby help control cardiac excitation and conduction.[16,22] Certain class I agents (e.g., lidocaine) are also used as local anesthetics; the way that these drugs bind to sodium channels is discussed in more detail in Chapter 12.

Because sodium influx plays an important role during action potential generation in phase 0 of the cardiac action potential, inhibition of sodium channels tends to decrease membrane excitability. Thus, class I drugs help stabilize the cardiac cell membrane and normalize the rate of cardiac cell firing. Although

Table 23-2
CLASSIFICATION OF ANTIARRHYTHMIC DRUGS

Generic Names	Trade Names
Class I: Sodium Channel Blockers	
Subclass A	
Disopyramide	Norpace, Rythmodan
Procainamide	Pronestyl
Quinidine	Apo-Quin, Apo-Quinidine
Subclass B	
Lidocaine	Xylocaine, others
Mexiletine	Mexitil
Tocainide	Tonocard
Subclass C	
Flecainide	Tambocor
Propafenone	Rythmol
Class II: Beta Blockers	
Acebutolol	Monitan, Sectral
Atenolol	Tenormin
Esmolol	Brevibloc
Metoprolol	Lopressor, others
Nadolol	Corgard
Propranolol	Inderal, others
Sotalol*	Betapace, Sorine, Sotacor
Timolol	Blocadren
Class III: Drugs That Prolong Repolarization	
Amiodarone†	Cordarone, Pacerone
Dofetilide	Tikosyn
Dronedarone†	Multaq
Ibutilide	Corvert
Class IV: Calcium Channel Blockers	
Diltiazem	Cardizem, Dilacor, others
Verapamil	Calan, Isoptin, Verelan, others

**Also has some class III properties*
†Also has some class I, II, and IV properties.

all class I drugs exert their antiarrhythmic effects by inhibiting sodium channel function, various agents affect myocardial excitation and conduction in slightly different ways. Class I drugs are typically subclassified according to how they influence cardiac electrophysiology (see Table 23-2).[4,5]

Specific Agents

Class IA. Drugs in this group are similar in that they produce a moderate slowing of phase 0 depolarization and a moderate slowing of action potential propagation throughout the myocardium. These drugs also prolong repolarization of the cardiac cell, thus lengthening the interval before a second action potential can occur (i.e., they increase the effective refractory period). Class IA agents include quinidine, procainamide, and disopyramide; these drugs are used to treat a variety of arrhythmias originating in the ventricles or atria.

Class IB. These drugs display a minimal ability to slow phase 0 depolarization and produce a minimal slowing of cardiac conduction. In contrast to IA drugs, class IB drugs usually shorten cardiac repolarization—that is, the effective refractory period is decreased. Class IB drugs include lidocaine and mexiletine and are primarily used to treat ventricular arrhythmias such as ventricular tachycardia and premature ventricular contractions (PVCs). However, Class IB drugs are typically reserved for people with more severe types of ventricular arrhythmias, and their use in relatively minor or asymptomatic arrhythmias has been replaced by safer drugs or nonpharmacological management (see "Nonpharmacological Treatment of Arrhythmias" later in this chapter).

Class IC. These drugs produce both a marked decrease in the rate of phase 0 depolarization and a marked slowing of cardiac conduction. They have little effect on repolarization. Class IC drugs include flecainide and propafenone and appear to be best suited to treat ventricular arrhythmias such as ventricular tachycardia and PVCs.

Adverse Effects

Despite their use in treating arrhythmias, the most common side effect of all antiarrhythmic drugs is their tendency to increase rhythm disturbances (proarrhythmic effects). While attempting to control one type of arrhythmia, these agents can aggravate or initiate other cardiac rhythm abnormalities.[23,24] This fact seems especially true with all class I agents.[25,26] Because these drugs affect sodium channel function and cardiac excitability, they may produce some serious proarrhythmic effects in certain patients. For example, patients with heart failure, myocardial ischemia, and structural heart disease (including previous infarction) seem to be especially prone to class I–induced arrhythmias, and these drugs should be avoided in these patients.[1,5] Likewise, people with inherited sodium channel mutations that decrease sodium entry may be susceptible to proarrhythmic effects of class I agents.[27] Class I drugs are also associated with a variety of side effects such as dizziness, visual disturbances, gastrointestinal problems (nausea, vomiting, diarrhea), and other untoward effects, depending on the specific drug.[5] These symptoms are often important because they may indicate the presence of arrhythmias even when the pulse or electrocardiogram (ECG) is not being directly monitored. Class I drugs are still important in treating certain arrhythmias, but they are used less and with more caution than in the past.[1]

Class II: Beta Blockers

Drugs that block beta-1 receptors on the myocardium are one of the mainstays in arrhythmia treatment. Beta blockers are effective because they decrease the excitatory effects of the sympathetic nervous system and related catecholamines (norepinephrine and epinephrine) on the heart.[28] This effect typically decreases cardiac automaticity and prolongs the effective refractory period, thus slowing heart rate.[1] Beta blockers also slow down conduction through the myocardium and are especially useful in controlling function of the atrioventricular node.[29] Hence, these drugs are often effective in treating atrial tachycardias such as atrial fibrillation.[29,30] Beta blockers can also be used to treat ventricular arrhythmias and can reduce mortality in serious rhythm disturbances such as ventricular tachycardia.[31]

Specific Agents

Beta blockers that are effective in treating arrhythmias include acebutolol, atenolol, esmolol, metoprolol, nadolol, propranolol, sotalol, and timolol (see Table 23-2). The individual beta blockers are presented in Chapter 20. Choice of a specific beta blocker depends to a large extent on the exact type of arrhythmia present and the individual patient's response to the drug.

Adverse Effects

Nonselective beta blockers affect beta-2 receptors on the lungs and beta-1 receptors on the heart, and these nonselective agents can increase bronchoconstriction in patients with asthma and chronic obstructive pulmonary disease. Hence, a drug that is more specific for beta-1 receptors is preferred in these patients. Beta blockers can also produce excessive slowing of cardiac conduction in some patients, resulting in an increase in arrhythmias. Severe adverse reactions are rare, however, and beta blockers are well tolerated by most patients when used appropriately to treat arrhythmias.

Class III: Drugs That Prolong Repolarization

Class III agents delay repolarization of cardiac cells, which prolongs the effective refractory period of the cardiac action potential.[4,5] This delay lengthens the time interval before a subsequent action potential can be initiated, thus slowing and stabilizing the heart rate. The effects of class III drugs are complex, but their ability to lengthen the cardiac action potential is most likely mediated by inhibition of potassium efflux during repolarization.[4,32] That is, these drugs limit the ability of potassium to leave the cell during phases 2 and 3 of the action potential, which prolongs repolarization and prevents the cell from firing another action potential too rapidly. Class III drugs are used to treat ventricular arrhythmias such as ventricular tachycardia and ventricular fibrillation, and supraventricular arrhythmias such as postoperative atrial fibrillation.[4,33] Interest in using these drugs and developing new class III agents has increased recently because they affect both atrial and ventricular problems and are relatively safe compared to other agents such as the class I drugs.[34]

Specific Agents

Class III drugs currently in use include amiodarone, dofetilide, dronedarone, and ibutilide (see Table 23-2). These drugs all exert their primary effects by prolonging repolarization in cardiac cells. Amiodarone, however, has emerged as the most widely used antiarrhythmic drug.[35] In addition to prolonging repolarization, amiodarone also appears to have some properties similar to drugs in other classes and may help control arrhythmias by inhibiting sodium channel function (class I effect), by blocking beta-1 receptors (class II effect), or even by blocking calcium channels (class IV effect).[4] Hence, this drug seems rather versatile and is able to control a variety of rhythm disturbances.

Adverse Effects

An initial increase in cardiac arrhythmias (proarrhythmic effect) may occur when class III drugs are instituted. The most important proarrhythmia is known as *torsades de pointes*, which is a form of ventricular tachycardia that can be fatal in susceptible patients.[36,37]

Specific class III agents are associated with various other side effects. Amiodarone, for example, is associated with pulmonary toxicity, thyroid problems, and liver damage.[35] Newer class III drugs such as dronedarone (a derivative of amiodarone) may have a more favorable side-effect profile but may not be as effective in controlling arrhythmias.[38-40] Side effects of other class III drugs vary from agent to agent, and any untoward effects should be monitored carefully.

Class IV: Calcium Channel Blockers

Class IV drugs have a selective ability to block calcium entry into myocardial and vascular smooth-muscle cells. These drugs inhibit calcium influx by binding to specific channels in the cell membrane.[41] As discussed previously, calcium entry plays an important role in the generation of the cardiac action potential, especially during phase 2. By inhibiting calcium influx into myocardial cells, calcium channel blockers can alter the excitability and conduction of cardiac tissues.

Calcium channel blockers decrease the rate of discharge of the SA node and inhibit conduction velocity through the AV node.[4,5] These drugs are most successful in treating arrhythmias caused by atrial dysfunction, such as supraventricular tachycardia and atrial fibrillation.[42,43]

Specific Agents

Of the calcium channel blockers currently in use, verapamil and diltiazem are currently approved for treating arrhythmias (see Table 23-2). Although these drugs differ chemically, both normalize heart rate by reducing calcium effects on SA and AV nodal tissues. Preliminary studies suggest that verapamil might be more effective than diltiazem, but their antiarrhythmic effects seem to be fairly similar when administered orally at therapeutic doses.[5,44] Other calcium channel blockers, however, such as nifedipine and similar dihydropyridines (see Chapter 22), do not have any substantial effects on cardiac rhythm. These other calcium channel blockers are more effective in dilating vascular smooth muscle and are used more frequently to treat hypertension and angina pectoris (see Chapters 21 and 22).

Adverse Effects

Because drugs like verapamil slow down the heart rate by inhibiting calcium entry into cardiac muscle cells, excessive bradycardia (less than 50 beats per minute) may occur in some patients receiving these drugs. Calcium channel blockers also limit calcium entry into vascular smooth muscle, which may cause peripheral vasodilation and lead to dizziness and headaches in some patients.

OTHER DRUGS USED TO TREAT ARRHYTHMIAS

Several other drug strategies can be used to treat certain arrhythmias, even though these drugs are not classified according to the traditional categories described above.[5] Digitalis glycosides, for example, are typically used to treat congestive heart failure (see Chapter 24), but these drugs can also be used to prevent or treat certain arrhythmias, including severe atrial fibrillation and paroxysmal AV nodal reentrant tachycardia. Large doses of magnesium (1 to 2 gm) can be infused intravenously to treat severe ventricular arrhythmias such as torsades de pointes. Magnesium is thought to control these arrhythmias by normalizing cardiac ion channel function, but the exact mechanism of magnesium's effects is not fully understood. Adenosine, a substance found naturally in the body, can also be administered intravenously to terminate severe arrhythmias such as reentrant supraventricular tachycardia. This substance binds to specific adenosine receptors on the heart, and it affects heart rate by decreasing calcium entry into myocardial tissues. Finally, the antianginal drug ranolazine (Ranexa) has complex effects on sodium and calcium movement across myocardial cell membranes (see Chapter 22). This drug may help control atrial and ventricular arrhythmias with minimal proarrhythmic effects.[45] Researchers continue to investigate the use of ranolazine and other nontraditional antiarrhythmic drugs that are effective in treating specific rhythm problems with fewer side effects compared to the typical antiarrhythmic agents.

NONPHARMACOLOGICAL TREATMENT OF ARRHYTHMIAS

Although drug therapy remains a common treatment for people with arrhythmias, many patients may also use a nonpharmacological approach to help provide a more long-term solution for certain rhythm disturbances. Antiarrhythmic drugs do not usually cure cardiac arrhythmias because they do not typically resolve the source of the arrhythmia. As indicated earlier, many antiarrhythmic drugs are also associated with potentially serious side effects, including the risk of increased arrhythmias.[23] As a result, the overall use of antiarrhythmic drugs has declined somewhat in recent years, due largely to the development of better implantable devices (pacemakers, cardioverter defibrillators) and surgical interventions (electrode catheter ablation).[46-49] Research also indicates that these nonpharmacological techniques may also decrease mortality and improve quality of life compared to traditional antiarrhythmic drug treatment.[46,50]

Special Concerns for Rehabilitation Patients

The primary problems associated with antiarrhythmic drugs in rehabilitation patients are related to the side effects of these agents. Therapists should be aware of the potential for increased arrhythmias or changes in the nature of arrhythmias. This concern may be especially important in patients involved in exercise and cardiac rehabilitation programs. Therapists who supervise such patients can often detect the presence of arrhythmias by monitoring ECG recordings. If an ECG recording is not available, palpation of pulses for rate and regularity may detect rhythm disturbances. Also, the presence of other side effects such as faintness or dizziness may signal the presence of cardiotoxic drug effects and increased arrhythmias. Consequently, therapists treating patients for both cardiac and noncardiac disorders may help detect the cardiotoxic effects of antiarrhythmic drugs by staying alert for any side effects. By playing a role in the early detection of increased arrhythmias, therapists can alert the physician to a problem and avert any potentially serious or even fatal consequences.

Other concerns related to side effects are fairly minor. Hypotension may occur with some agents, especially with beta blockers (class II) and calcium channel blockers (class IV). Therapists should be aware that patients may become faint or dizzy, especially if blood pressure drops after sudden changes in posture (orthostatic hypotension). Likewise, therapists should monitor blood pressure and pulse to help differentiate whether the faintness and dizziness is caused by orthostatic hypotension, or if these responses might be due to abnormal heart rate caused by the proarrhythmic effects of drug therapy.

CASE STUDY

ANTIARRHYTHMIC DRUGS

Brief History. M.R. is a 48-year-old man with a history of coronary artery disease and cardiac rhythm disturbances. Specifically, he has experienced episodes of paroxysmal supraventricular tachycardia, with his heart rate often exceeding 180 beats per minute. He has been treated for several years with the beta blocker propranolol (Inderal). Taking this drug orally at a dose of 60 mg/d has successfully diminished his episodes of tachycardia. M.R. had also been a cigarette smoker but quit recently to improve his health and reduce the risk of cigarette-related diseases. In an effort to improve his myocardial function and overall cardiovascular fitness, M.R. underwent a graded exercise test and

CASE STUDY (Continued)

was subsequently enrolled as an outpatient in a cardiac rehabilitation program. Under the supervision of a physical therapist, he attended cardiac training sessions three times each week. A typical session consisted of warm-up calisthenics, bicycle ergometry, and cool-down stretching activities. Each session lasted approximately 45 minutes.

Problem/Influence of Medication. During the initial rehabilitation sessions, the therapist noticed that M.R. seemed to be having some trouble breathing during the bicycle exercises. The therapist placed a stethoscope over M.R.'s chest and heard distinct wheezing sounds indicative of bronchoconstrictive disease. M.R. apparently had some residual effects of cigarette smoking, most likely in the form of mild to moderate emphysema.

1. ***Could M.R.'s current drug regimen be contributing to the bronchoconstrictive symptoms?***
2. ***What potential change in drug therapy may reduce the risk of bronchoconstriction?***

See Appendix C, "Answers to Case Study Questions."

SUMMARY

Cardiac arrhythmias may arise due to disturbances in the origination and conduction of electrical activity in the heart. These changes in cardiac rhythm can be controlled to a large extent by several groups of drugs, including sodium channel blockers, beta blockers, calcium channel blockers, and drugs that prolong the cardiac action potential. These agents work by different cellular mechanisms to stabilize heart rate and improve the conduction of electrical impulses throughout the myocardium. Although these drugs are often successful in preventing or resolving arrhythmias, rehabilitation specialists should be aware of patients who are taking these agents. Therapists should also be alert for any changes in cardiac function or other side effects that may signal toxicity of these drugs.

REFERENCES

1. Sampson KJ, Kass RS. Anti-arrhythmic drugs. In: Brunton L, et al, eds. *The Pharmacological Basis of Therapeutics*. 12th ed. New York: McGraw-Hill; 2011.
2. Marcus GM, Keung E, Scheinman MM. The year in review of clinical cardiac electrophysiology. *J Am Coll Cardiol*. 2013;61: 772-782.
3. Merghani A, Sharma S. Identifying patients at risk of sudden arrhythmic death. *Practitioner*. 2012;256:15-18.
4. Sanoski CA, Bauman JL. The arrhythmias. In: DiPiro JT, et al, eds. *Pharmacotherapy: A Pathophysiologic Approach*. 8th ed. New York: McGraw-Hill; 2011.
5. Hume JR, Grant AO. Agents used in cardiac arrhythmias. In: Katzung BG, ed. *Basic and Clinical Pharmacology*. 12th ed. New York: Lange Medical Books/McGraw Hill; 2012.
6. Rubart M, Zipes DP. Genesis of cardiac arrhythmias: electrophysiological considerations. In: Bonow RO, et al, eds. *Braunwald's Heart Disease*. 9th ed. Philadelphia, PA: Elsevier Saunders; 2012.
7. Lakatta EG, Maltsev VA, Vinogradova TM. A coupled SYSTEM of intracellular Ca2+ clocks and surface membrane voltage clocks controls the timekeeping mechanism of the heart's pacemaker. *Circ Res*. 2010;106:659-673.
8. Bonita R, Pradhan R. Cardiovascular toxicities of cancer chemotherapy. *Semin Oncol*. 2013;40:156-167.
9. El-Sherif N, Turitto G. Electrolyte disorders and arrhythmogenesis. *Cardiol J*. 2011;18:233-245.
10. Mischke K, Knackstedt C, Marx N, Vollmann D. Insights into atrial fibrillation. *Minerva Med*. 2013;104:119-130.
11. Peacock J, Whang W. Psychological distress and arrhythmia: risk prediction and potential modifiers. *Prog Cardiovasc Dis*. 2013;55:582-589.
12. Shen MJ, Choi EK, Tan AY, et al. Neural mechanisms of atrial arrhythmias. *Nat Rev Cardiol*. 2011;9:30-39.
13. George AL Jr. Molecular and genetic basis of sudden cardiac death. *J Clin Invest*. 2013;123:75-83.
14. Giudicessi JR, Ackerman MJ. Genetic testing in heritable cardiac arrhythmia syndromes: differentiating pathogenic mutations from background genetic noise. *Curr Opin Cardiol*. 2013;28:63-71.
15. Giudicessi JR, Ackerman MJ. Potassium-channel mutations and cardiac arrhythmias—diagnosis and therapy. *Nat Rev Cardiol*. 2012;9:319-332.
16. Remme CA, Bezzina CR. Sodium channel (dys)function and cardiac arrhythmias. *Cardiovasc Ther*. 201;28:287-294.

17. Venetucci L, Denegri M, Napolitano C, Priori SG. Inherited calcium channelopathies in the pathophysiology of arrhythmias. *Nat Rev Cardiol.* 2012;9:561-575.
18. Hofman N, van Lochem LT, Wilde AA. Genetic basis of malignant channelopathies and ventricular fibrillation in the structurally normal heart. *Future Cardiol.* 2010;6:395-408.
19. Roberts JD, Gollob MH. The genetic and clinical features of cardiac channelopathies. *Future Cardiol.* 2010;6:491-506.
20. Olgin J, Zipes DP. Specific arrhythmias: diagnosis and treatment. In: Bonow RO, et al, eds. *Braunwald's Heart Disease.* 9th ed. Philadelphia, PA: Elsevier Saunders: 2012.
21. Miller JM, Zipes DP. Therapy for cardiac arrhythmias. In: Bonow RO, et al, eds. *Braunwald's Heart Disease.* 9th ed. Philadelphia, PA: Elsevier Saunders; 2012.
22. Burashnikov A, Antzelevitch C. Role of late sodium channel current block in the management of atrial fibrillation. *Cardiovasc Drugs Ther.* 2013;27:79-89.
23. Camm J. Antiarrhythmic drugs for the maintenance of sinus rhythm: risks and benefits. *Int J Cardiol.* 2012;155:362-371.
24. Gramley F, Himmrich E, Mollnau H, et al. Recent advances in the pharmacological treatment of cardiac arrhythmias. *Drugs Today.* 2009;45:807-824.
25. Coronel R, Wilms-Schopman FJ, Janse MJ. Anti- or profibrillatory effects of Na(+) channel blockade depend on the site of application relative to gradients in repolarization. *Front Physiol.* 2010;1:10.
26. Darbar D. Standard anti-arrhythmic drugs. In: Zipes DP, Jaliffe J, eds. *Cardiac Electrophysiology. From Cell to Bedside.* 5th ed. Philadelphia, PA: Elsevier Saunders: 2009.
27. Kaufman ES. Mechanisms and clinical management of inherited channelopathies: long QT syndrome, Brugada syndrome, catecholaminergic polymorphic ventricular tachycardia, and short QT syndrome. *Heart Rhythm.* 2009;6(suppl):S51-55.
28. Frishman WH, Saunders E. β-Adrenergic blockers. *J Clin Hypertens.* 2011;13:649-653.
29. Workman AJ. Cardiac adrenergic control and atrial fibrillation. *Naunyn Schmiedebergs Arch Pharmacol.* 2010;381:235-249.
30. Gillis AM, Verma A, Talajic M, et al. Canadian Cardiovascular Society atrial fibrillation guidelines 2010: rate and rhythm management. *Can J Cardiol.* 2011;27:47-59.
31. Aronow WS. Management of ventricular arrhythmias. *Minerva Cardioangiol.* 2010;58:657-676.
32. Islam MA. Pharmacological modulations of cardiac ultra-rapid and slowly activating delayed rectifier currents: potential antiarrhythmic approaches. *Recent Pat Cardiovasc Drug Discov.* 2010;5:33-46.
33. Omae T, Kanmura Y. Management of postoperative atrial fibrillation. *J Anesth.* 2012;26:429-437.
34. Singla S, Karam P, Deshmukh AJ, et al. Review of contemporary antiarrhythmic drug therapy for maintenance of sinus rhythm in atrial fibrillation. *J Cardiovasc Pharmacol Ther.* 2012;17:12-20.
35. Santangeli P, Di Biase L, Burkhardt JD, et al. Examining the safety of amiodarone. *Expert Opin Drug Saf.* 2012;11:191-214.
36. Camm AJ. Safety considerations in the pharmacological management of atrial fibrillation. *Int J Cardiol.* 2008;127:299-306.
37. Taira CA, Opezzo JA, Mayer MA, Höcht C. Cardiovascular drugs inducing QT prolongation: facts and evidence. *Curr Drug Saf.* 2010;5:65-72.
38. Cohen M, Boiangiu C. The management of patients with atrial fibrillation and dronedarone's place in therapy. *Adv Ther.* 2011;28:1059-1077.
39. Kozlowski D, Budrejko S, Lip GY, et al. Dronedarone: an overview. *Ann Med.* 2012;44:60-72.
40. Oyetayo OO, Rogers CE, Hofmann PO. Dronedarone: a new antiarrhythmic agent. *Pharmacotherapy.* 2010;30:904-915.
41. Elliott WJ, Ram CV. Calcium channel blockers. *J Clin Hypertens.* 2011;13:687-689.
42. Colucci RA, Silver MJ, Shubrook J. Common types of supraventricular tachycardia: diagnosis and management. *Am Fam Physician.* 2010;82:942-952.
43. Scheuermeyer FX, Grafstein E, Stenstrom R, et al. Safety and efficiency of calcium channel blockers versus beta-blockers for rate control in patients with atrial fibrillation and no acute underlying medical illness. *Acad Emerg Med.* 2013;20:222-230.
44. Medi C, Kalman JM, Freedman SB. Supraventricular tachycardia. *Med J Aust.* 2009;190:255-260.
45. Tzeis S, Andrikopoulos G. Antiarrhythmic properties of ranolazine—from bench to bedside. *Expert Opin Investig Drugs.* 2012;21:1733-1741.
46. Corcoran SJ, Davis LM. Cardiac implantable electronic device therapy for bradyarrhythmias and tachyarrhythmias. *Heart Lung Circ.* 2012;21:328-337.
47. Kircher S, Hindricks G, Sommer P. Long-term success and follow-up after atrial fibrillation ablation. *Curr Cardiol Rev.* 2012;8:354-361.
48. Lee G, Sanders P, Kalman JM. Catheter ablation of atrial arrhythmias: state of the art. *Lancet.* 2012;380:1509-1519.
49. Olshansky B, Sullivan RM. Sudden death risk in syncope: the role of the implantable cardioverter defibrillator. *Prog Cardiovasc Dis.* 2013;55:443-453.
50. John RM, Tedrow UB, Koplan BA, et al. Ventricular arrhythmias and sudden cardiac death. *Lancet.* 2012;380:1520-1529.

CHAPTER 24

Treatment of Congestive Heart Failure

Congestive heart failure is a chronic condition in which the heart is unable to pump a sufficient quantity of blood to meet the needs of peripheral tissues.[1,2] Essentially, the heart's pumping ability has been compromised by some form of myocardial disease or dysfunction. The congestive aspect of heart failure arises from the tendency for fluid to accumulate in the lungs and peripheral tissues because the heart is unable to maintain proper circulation.

The primary symptoms associated with congestive heart failure are peripheral edema and a decreased tolerance for physical activity.[3,4] Dyspnea and shortness of breath are also common, especially if the left heart is failing and pulmonary congestion is present. In severe cases, cyanosis develops because the heart cannot deliver oxygen to peripheral tissues.

Congestive heart failure is one of the major illnesses present in industrialized nations.[2,5] In the United States, approximately 5 million people have been diagnosed with this disease,[3] and the incidence of heart failure (number of new cases each year) approaches 700,000.[2] The prevalence of heart failure also increases in the elderly, and the number of people with heart failure will undoubtedly increase as a larger percentage of our population reaches advanced age.[6] This disease is also associated with serious consequences, and the prognosis for congestive heart failure is often poor.[2,4] Despite recent advances in medical treatment, approximately 50 percent of patients die within 5 years after they are diagnosed with heart failure.[3]

Consequently, effective treatment of congestive heart failure is a critical and challenging task. Pharmacotherapy represents one of the primary methods of treating congestive heart failure, and the drugs discussed in this chapter play a vital role in the optimal management of this disease. As with other cardiac problems, the prevalence of congestive heart failure necessitates that members of the health-care community be aware of the pharmacological management of this disease. You will often treat patients with heart failure, and you should be aware of the drugs used to manage this problem. These drugs can, for example, increase myocardial pumping ability, thus allowing the patient to participate more actively in cardiac rehabilitation and other therapeutic interventions.

Drug therapy can likewise have a positive influence on exercise therapy, and vice versa. If drug therapy helps improve myocardial function, that patient will be able to exercise more effectively, which can further strengthen cardiac function, and so forth. Certain heart failure drugs, however, can cause potentially severe side effects that adversely affect the patient's well-being, and you must be alert for these, especially during exercise sessions. This chapter begins with a brief overview of the pathophysiological changes and characteristics of heart failure. The remainder of the chapter then explores the primary drug strategies used to improve cardiac pumping ability or decrease workload in patients with heart failure.

PATHOPHYSIOLOGY OF CONGESTIVE HEART FAILURE

The mechanisms underlying chronic heart failure are complex and may include biochemical disturbances in the cardiac cell, altered genetic expression of myocardial proteins, and systemic changes in hemodynamic and neurohormonal factors.[7,8] Heart failure also tends to be self-perpetuating because an aberration in cardiac function often initiates a vicious cycle that leads to further decrements in cardiac function.[3,9]

The Vicious Cycle of Heart Failure

Figure 24-1 illustrates the way in which a vicious cycle might be generated by the interaction of cardiac and neurohormonal factors. The sequence of events depicted in Figure 24-1 is as follows:

1. *Decreased cardiac performance.* Any number of factors that affect cardiac pumping ability may be responsible for initiating a change in myocardial performance. Factors such as ischemic heart disease, myocardial infarction, valve dysfunction, and hypertension may all compromise the heart's pumping ability.[3,5,10] Also, cardiomyopathy may result from other diseases and infections.[11]
2. *Neurohormonal compensations.* The body responds to the decreased cardiac pumping ability in several ways. In the early stages of failure, cardiac output decreases, and the delivery of oxygen and nutrients to tissues and organs is diminished. To compensate for this initial decrease, several neural and neurochemical changes occur that increase cardiac contractility and help maintain blood pressure. In particular, the sympathetic nervous system and renin-angiotensin system are activated, and secretion of aldosterone and antidiuretic hormone increases.[7,12] Although these compensations are initially helpful in maintaining cardiac function, they actually place more stress on the failing heart.[3] This increased stress initiates the cycle because it causes more damage to the myocardium, which further compromises cardiac pumping ability, causing more neurohormonal activation, more stress to the heart, and so on.
3. *Increased cardiac workload.* The neurohormonal changes previously described contribute to peripheral vasoconstriction as well as a general increase in sodium and water retention.[13] These effects place additional strain on the heart by increasing cardiac preload (i.e., the volume of blood returning to the heart) and cardiac afterload (i.e., the pressure that the heart must pump against).[14]
4. *Changes in myocardial cell function.* The increased workload on the heart can lead to, or cause, exaggerated alterations in cell function and further structural damage to the already compromised myocardial cell.[9,10] Also, studies on the molecular basis of heart failure have suggested that alterations in calcium transport, contractile protein function, energy production and utilization, free-radical production, and beta-receptor density may occur.[15-17] Continued stress on the heart may exacerbate these changes, leading to more cellular dysfunction and inappropriate adaptive changes in myocardial cell structure and function, which ultimately leads to abnormal changes in the size, shape, and function of the heart (cardiac remodeling).[10,18,19] The pathological remodeling results in a further decrease in cardiac performance, thus completing the cycle.

This sequence of events represents a simplification of the interaction of central and peripheral factors in congestive heart failure. The description does, however, illustrate the primary problems that occur in this disease, as well as the manner in which heart failure tends to self-perpetuate.

Heart failure is not always associated with systolic dysfunction and an obvious decline in cardiac pumping ability. In approximately half the cases of symptomatic heart failure, systolic function and cardiac output may appear normal when the patient is at rest.[4,20] In this type of heart failure, cardiac function is impaired because the left ventricle is stiff and unable to relax during the filling phase, resulting in increased pressures at the end of diastole.[21] This condition is often described as "diastolic" heart failure, but it is also identified by other names such as *heart failure with preserved left ventricular function* and *heart failure with normal ejection fraction*.[20] The increased stress on the myocardium leads to progressive changes in cellular function and cardiac remodeling that are detrimental to cardiac function.

Diastolic heart failure is more common in older adults, especially older women.[22,23] The pathophysiology of this type of heart failure may also differ from heart failure associated with left ventricular or systolic

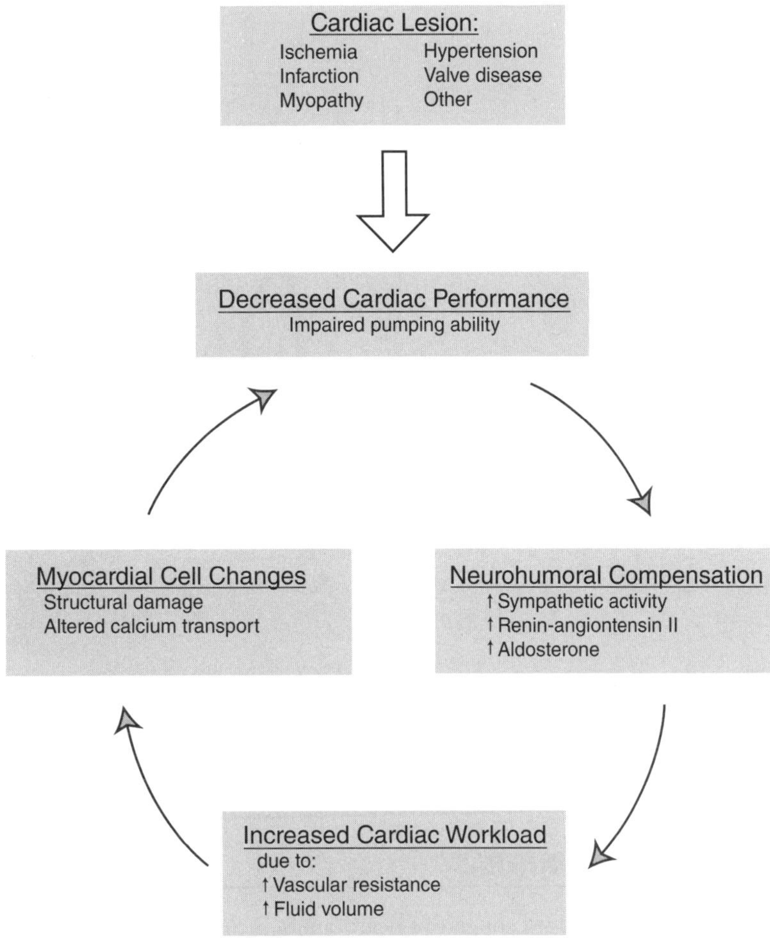

Figure ■ 24-1 The vicious cycle of congestive heart failure. An initial cardiac lesion begins a self-perpetuating decrease in myocardial performance.

dysfunction, with hypertension being relatively more important in the cause of diastolic heart failure.[24] Drug therapy for diastolic heart failure therefore focuses on lowering blood pressure and reducing other factors that increase the risk of developing heart failure.[24,25] The drugs discussed in this chapter are generally more effective in patients with systolic heart failure—that is, patients with reduced ejection fraction.[26]

Congestion in Left and Right Heart Failure

The primary problem in advanced heart failure is that the heart is unable to push blood forward through the circulatory system, thus causing pressure to build up in the veins returning blood to the heart. In effect, blood begins to back up in the venous system, increasing the pressure gradient for fluid to move out of the capillary beds. The net movement of fluid out of the capillaries causes the edema or congestion typically found in advanced stages of heart failure.

Although heart disease commonly affects the entire myocardium, congestive heart failure is sometimes divided into left and right heart failure (Fig. 24-2). In *left heart failure*, the left atrium and ventricle are unable to adequately handle the blood returning from the lungs. This causes pressure to build up in the pulmonary veins, and fluid accumulates in the lungs. Consequently, left heart failure is associated with pulmonary edema.

In *right heart failure*, the right atrium and ventricle are unable to handle blood returning from the systemic circulation. This causes fluid to accumulate in the peripheral tissues, and ankle edema and organ congestion

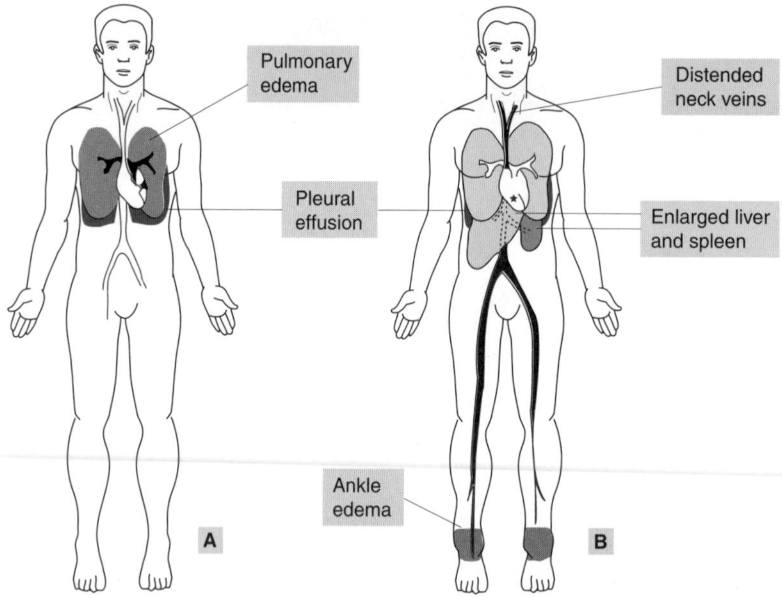

Figure ■ 24-2
Effects of congestive heart failure. (*A*) Left-sided heart failure results primarily in pulmonary edema. (*B*) Right-sided heart failure results in peripheral edema (swollen ankles, enlarged organs). *(Adapted from: Kent TH, Hart MN. Introduction to Human Disease. 2nd ed. Norwalk, CT: Appleton-Century-Crofts; 1987:141, with permission.)*

(liver, spleen) are typical manifestations. If both left and right heart failure occur simultaneously, congestion is found in the lungs as well as the periphery.

PHARMACOTHERAPY

One of the basic goals in congestive heart failure is to improve the heart's pumping ability. Drug administration should selectively increase cardiac contractile performance and produce what is referred to as a *positive inotropic effect.* **Inotropic** refers to the force of muscular contraction. The primary drugs used to exert a positive inotropic effect are the cardiac glycosides such as digoxin. Drugs are also recognized as beneficial for congestive heart failure if they decrease cardiac workload by affecting the heart or peripheral vasculature or by controlling fluid volume. Angiotensin-converting enzyme inhibitors, beta blockers, diuretics, and vasodilators are included in this group.

The primary drug groups used to treat congestive heart failure are listed in Table 24-1. The drugs in this table and in this chapter, are grouped according to their primary goal in treating heart failure—that is, drugs that improve myocardial contraction force (positive inotropic agents) and agents that decrease cardiac workload.

DRUGS THAT INCREASE MYOCARDIAL CONTRACTION FORCE (POSITIVE INOTROPIC AGENTS)

Digitalis

The digitalis glycosides are digoxin and digitoxin. At the time of this writing, only digoxin is available in the United States, whereas digitoxin may be available in other countries. For simplicity, the term *digitalis* is used to represent these drugs. Although the widespread use of digitalis has been questioned, it continues to be one of the primary drugs used to treat congestive heart failure.[27,28] There is little doubt that digitalis improves cardiac pumping ability and therefore improves the primary symptoms of congestive heart failure.[29] Digitalis typically increases cardiac output at rest and during exercise, and exercise tolerance often increases because the heart is able to pump blood more effectively.[30] There is questionable evidence, however, whether digitalis prolongs life expectancy in people with heart failure.[31] Also, the use of digitalis is limited to some extent by its toxic effects (see "Adverse Effects").

Nonetheless, the consensus is that digitalis is a useful drug because it can decrease the symptoms of heart failure and the number of hospitalizations and

Table 24-1
PRIMARY DRUGS USED IN CONGESTIVE HEART FAILURE

Drug Group	Primary Effect
Agents That Increase Myocardial Contraction Force (Positive Inotropic Agents)	
Digoxin (Digitek, Lanoxin)	Increases myocardial contractility by elevating intracellular calcium levels and facilitating actin-myosin interaction in cardiac cells; may also help normalize autonomic effects on the heart
Inamrinone (Inocor) Milrinone (Primacor)	Enhance myocardial contractility by prolonging effects of cyclic adenosine monophosphate (cAMP), which increases intracellular calcium levels and promotes stronger actin-myosin interaction in cardiac cells
Dopamine (Intropin, Revimine) Dobutamine (Dobutrex)	Stimulate cardiac beta-1 adrenergic receptors, which selectively increases myocardial contraction force
Agents That Decrease Cardiac Workload	
Angiotensin-converting enzyme inhibitors* • Captopril (Capoten) • Enalapril (Vasotec) • Fosinopril (Monopril) • Lisinopril (Prinivil, Zestril) • Quinapril (Accupril) • Ramipril (Altace) • Trandolapril (Mavik)	Reduce peripheral vascular resistance by preventing angiotensin II–induced vasoconstriction and vascular hypertrophy/remodeling; also help prevent sodium and water retention by limiting aldosterone secretion, and promote vasodilation by prolonging the effects of bradykinin
Angiotensin II receptor blockers** • Candesartan (Atacand) • Eprosartan (Teveten) • Irbesartan (Avapro) • Losartan (Cozaar) • Telmisartan (Micardis) • Valsartan (Diovan)	Reduce angiotensin II–induced peripheral vascular resistance and cardiovascular hypertrophy/remodeling by blocking angiotensin II receptors on the heart and vasculature
Direct renin inhibitor • Aliskiren (Tekturna)	Inhibits renin's ability to convert angiotensinogen to angiotensin I, thus decreasing the production of the precursor for angiotensin II
Beta adrenergic blockers*** • Acebutolol (Monitan, Sectral) • Atenolol (Tenormin) • Bisoprolol (Monocor, Zebeta) • Carteolol (Cartrol) • Carvedilol (Coreg) • Labetalol (Normodyne, Trandate) • Metoprolol (Lopressor)	Prevent sympathetic-induced overload on the heart by blocking the effects of epinephrine and norepinephrine on the myocardium; some agents (e.g., carvedilol) may also produce peripheral vasodilation
Diuretics****	Decrease the volume of fluid the heart must pump by promoting the excretion of excess sodium and water; also reduce fluid accumulation (congestion) in the lungs and other tissues
Vasodilators • Hydralazine (Apresoline) • Nesiritide (Natrecor) • Nitrates (isosorbide dinitrate, others) • Prazosin (Minipress) • Sildenafil (Viagra, Revatio)	Promote dilation in the peripheral vasculature, which decreases the amount of blood returning to the heart (cardiac preload) and decreases the pressure the heart must pump against (cardiac afterload)

Only the ACE inhibitors currently approved for treating heart failure are listed here. See Table 21-5 for a more complete list of ACE inhibitors.

***Only candesartan and valsartan are FDA approved to treat heart failure; other angiotensin II–receptor blockers may be prescribed for heart failure in specific situations.*

**** Only carvedilol and metoprolol are FDA approved to treat heart failure; other beta blockers may be prescribed for heart failure in specific situations.*

*****Loop diuretics are often preferred when treating heart failure, but various thiazide and potassium-sparing diuretics can also be used depending on the needs of each patient; see Table 21-3 for specific diuretic agents.*

other aspects of morbidity associated with this disease.[32,33] Digitalis must be used cautiously and specifically in certain cases of congestive heart failure, rather than as a panacea for all forms of this disease.[28] Specifically, digitalis seems most effective in patients with systolic heart failure and atrial fibrillation—that is, this drug can help improve left ventricular function and normalize heart rate in patients with reduced ejection fraction.[31,34] Likewise, digitalis is often added to the pharmacological regimen in patients with systolic heart failure who remain symptomatic despite treatment with other agents such as diuretics, angiotensin-converting enzyme (ACE) inhibitors, and beta blockers (see the respective headings later in this chapter).[35,36] Hence, the role of digitalis as a primary treatment for heart failure has declined in favor of other agents that decrease cardiac workload, and digitalis is now used as a secondary agent in specific patients who might benefit from the positive inotropic effects of this drug.[28]

Effects and Mechanism of Action

Mechanical Effects. Digitalis and the other cardiac glycosides increase the heart's mechanical pumping ability by bringing about an increase in intracellular calcium concentration. Increased intracellular calcium enhances contractility by facilitating the interaction between thick (myosin) and thin (actin) filaments in the myocardial cell.[34] Digitalis probably increases intracellular calcium concentration by a complex mechanism, which is illustrated in Figure 24-3. Details of this mechanism are also briefly outlined below.

1. Digitalis exerts its primary effect by inhibiting the sodium-potassium pump on the myocardial cell membrane.[37,38] The sodium-potassium pump is an active transport system that normally transports sodium out of the cell and transports potassium into it. Sodium enters the cardiac cell during the depolarization phase of each action potential, and the sodium-potassium pump is responsible for removing this sodium from the cell (see Chapter 23 for a description of ion movements during cardiac excitation). Inhibition of the sodium-potassium pump therefore causes sodium to accumulate within the cell.
2. An increase in intracellular sodium concentration leads to an increase in intracellular calcium.[34] During cardiac excitation, calcium ions normally enter the myocardial cell through specific calcium channels during each action potential (see Chapter 23). An enzyme known as the *sodium-calcium exchange protein* removes some of the calcium that enters. This enzyme uses the ionic gradient for sodium entry to help remove calcium from the cell, thus exchanging sodium entry for calcium exit from the cell. Because intracellular sodium concentration has increased, there is a smaller driving force (electrochemical gradient) for sodium to enter the cell. If less sodium enters, there is a reduction in the ability of the sodium-calcium exchange protein to remove calcium. Hence, intracellular calcium concentration increases.
3. The increased availability of calcium within the cardiac cell enables it to store more calcium in the sarcoplasmic reticulum.[38] As in any type of muscle cell, calcium is normally stored within the sarcoplasmic reticulum and released during each action potential to facilitate actin-myosin interaction and initiate muscle contraction. Because more calcium is stored in the cardiac cell, the sarcoplasmic reticulum releases more calcium during each action potential, thereby initiating greater actin-myosin interaction and a stronger cardiac contraction.

Autonomic and Electrophysiological Effects. In addition to its effects on cardiac contractility, digitalis has a direct inhibitory effect on sympathetic nervous system activity.[38] This effect is beneficial because it decreases stress on the failing heart by decreasing excessive sympathetic stimulation of the heart and peripheral vasculature.[39] Therapeutic levels of digitalis also stabilize the heart rate and slow impulse conduction through the myocardium. In fact, digitalis is used to prevent and treat certain arrhythmias, such as atrial tachycardia and atrial fibrillation (see Chapter 23).[40] Some of these electrical properties may be caused by the direct effect of digitalis on the sodium-potassium pump and can be attributed to alterations in sodium, potassium, and calcium fluxes. As indicated, digitalis also decreases excessive sympathetic stimulation of the heart, which helps normalize cardiac excitation and conduction. Digitalis also causes reflex stimulation of the vagus nerve, thus further slowing heart rate and conduction.[41] The autonomic and electrical properties of digitalis therefore improve cardiac excitation and function, and these effects generally complement the mechanical effects of this drug in treating congestive heart failure.

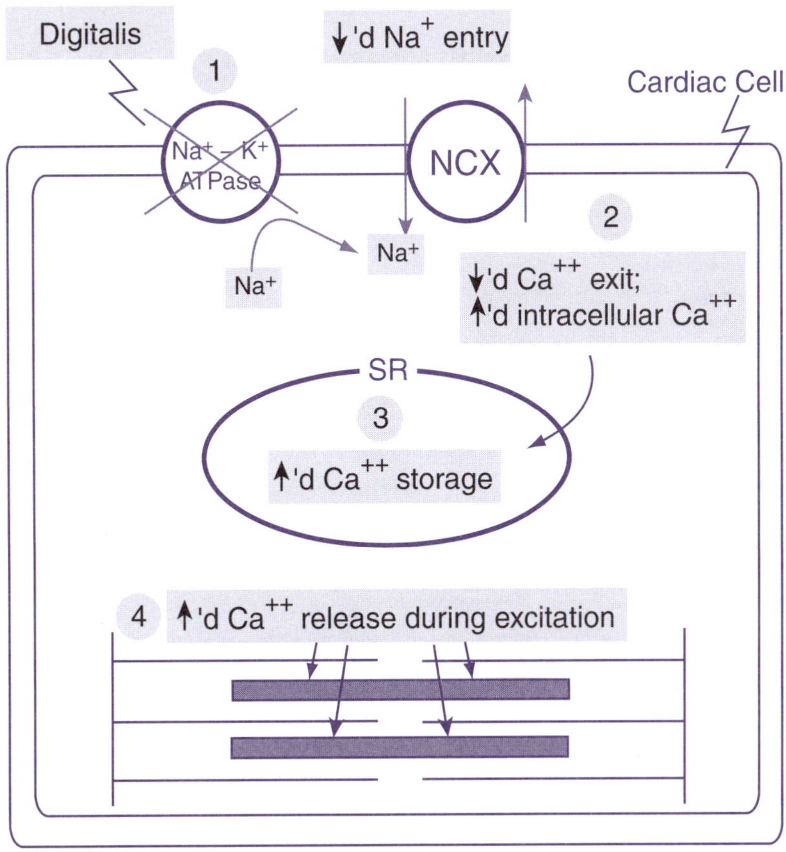

Figure ■ 24-3
Proposed mechanism of digitalis action on the sarcomere located within the myocardial cell. Digitalis inhibits the Na^+, K^+-ATPase (*1*) resulting in increased intracellular sodium (Na^+). Increased intracellular sodium alters the Na^+, Ca^{++} exchange (NCX) mechanism so that intracellular Ca^{++} also increases (*2*). As intracellular calcium increases, more calcium is available for storage in the sarcoplasmic reticulum (SR) (*3*). During cardiac excitation, more calcium is released from storage sites in the sarcoplasmic reticulum, which facilitates contractile protein binding, resulting in increased myocardial contractility (*4*).

Adverse Effects

Digitalis toxicity is a fairly common and potentially fatal adverse reaction to high blood levels of this drug.[42,43] Common signs of toxicity include gastrointestinal (GI) distress (nausea, vomiting, diarrhea) and central nervous system (CNS) disturbances (drowsiness, fatigue, confusion, visual disturbances; Table 24-2). Because digitalis alters the electrophysiological properties of the heart, abnormalities in cardiac function are also common during digitalis toxicity. Common adverse cardiac effects include arrhythmias such as premature atrial and ventricular contractions, paroxysmal atrial tachycardia, ventricular tachycardia, and high degrees of atrioventricular block. As toxicity increases, severe arrhythmias such as ventricular fibrillation can occur and may result in death.

To prevent digitalis toxicity, a low drug dosage should be maintained if possible. Plasma levels of digitalis should be monitored in suspected cases of toxicity to determine an appropriate decrease in dosage.[42] Health-care personnel should be warned to look for early signs of toxicity so that digitalis can be discontinued before the effects become life-threatening. Serious or life-threatening digitalis toxicity can be treated by IV administration of digoxin immune Fab (Digibind, DigiFab), which consists of antibody fragments that attach to digitalis glycosides and sequester the drug and terminate its toxic effects on the heart and other organs.[27]

Phosphodiesterase Inhibitors

Phosphodiesterase inhibitors include drugs such as inamrinone (known formally as *amrinone*) and milrinone. Inamrinone and milrinone exert their effects by inhibiting the phosphodiesterase enzyme that breaks down cyclic adenosine monophosphate (cAMP) in cardiac cells. Cyclic-AMP is a common second messenger in many cells (see Chapter 4), and drugs that inhibit the

Table 24-2
SIGNS AND SYMPTOMS OF DIGITALIS TOXICITY[a]

GI Symptoms	Visual Disturbances
Anorexia	Halos
Nausea	Photophobia
Vomiting	Problems with color perception
Abdominal pain	Scotomata
CNS Effects	**Cardiac Effects[b]**
Fatigue	Ventricular arrhythmias
Weakness	Premature ventricular depolarizations, bigeminy, trigeminy, ventricular tachycardia, ventricular fibrillation
Dizziness	Atrioventricular (A-V) block
Headache	First-degree, second-degree (Mobitz type 1), third-degree block
Neuralgia	A-V junctional escape rhythms, junctional tachycardia
Confusion	Atrial rhythms with slowed a-v conduction or A-V block
Delirium	Particularly paroxysmal atrial tachycardia with A-V block
Psychosis	Sinus bradycardia

[a]*Some adverse effects may be difficult to distinguish from the signs/symptoms of heart failure.*

[b]*Digitalis toxicity has been associated with almost every rhythm abnormality; only the more common manifestations are listed.*

Adapted from: *Parker RB, Cavallari LH. Heart failure. In: DiPiro JT, et al, eds.* Pharmacotherapy: A Pathophysiologic Approach. *8th ed. New York: McGraw-Hill; 2011, with permission.*

phosphodiesterase type III enzyme allow cAMP concentrations to increase in the cardiac cells.[38,44] In these cells, cAMP then acts on membrane calcium channels to allow more calcium to enter the cell.[45] Thus, inamrinone and milrinone cause a cAMP-mediated increase in intracellular calcium, which subsequently increases the force of contraction within the myocardial cell. These drugs also have some vasodilating properties, and some of their beneficial effects in congestive heart failure may be due to their ability to decrease cardiac preload and afterload in some patients.[46] On the other hand, vasodilation can lead to decreased arterial pressure and decreased perfusion of the heart and other organs in patients with low cardiac output, so vasodilation may be counterproductive in these patients.[38,45]

Phosphodiesterase inhibitors are classified as positive inotropic agents because they increase myocardial contractility in a relatively selective manner.[46] Inamrinone and milrinone, however, must be administered parenterally by IV infusion; hence, they are usually limited to short-term treatment of patients with severe congestive heart failure.[29,44] There is also little evidence that these drugs are more effective than digitalis in producing positive inotropic effects, and there is concern that these agents may actually result in more serious side effects, including an increase in patient mortality compared with other drug treatments.[44,47] Therefore, inamrinone and milrinone have limited use in treating heart failure and are usually administered in severe or acute cases of heart failure or in patients with severe heart failure who are awaiting a heart transplant.[38,48]

Dopamine and Dobutamine

Dopamine and dobutamine are sometimes used to stimulate the heart in cases of acute or severe heart failure (see Chapter 20). Dopamine and dobutamine exert a fairly specific positive inotropic effect, primarily through their ability to stimulate beta-1 receptors on the myocardium.[38,46] Other beta-1 agonists such as epinephrine will also increase myocardial contractility, but most of these other beta-1 agonists will also increase heart rate or have other side effects that prevent their use in congestive heart failure. Dopamine and dobutamine are usually reserved for certain patients with severe or advanced cases of congestive heart failure who do not respond to other positive inotropic drugs (e.g., digitalis).[46,49] Like the phosphodiesterase inhibitors, there is concern that these drugs do not improve the outcome for patients with heart failure and may actually be associated with increased mortality in some patients.[50] Hence, dobutamine and dopamine are not typically used to control chronic heart failure but are used more as a last resort to sustain cardiac output in specific cases of advanced heart failure.

AGENTS THAT DECREASE CARDIAC WORKLOAD

Drugs Affecting the Renin-Angiotensin System

As discussed previously in this chapter, the renin-angiotensin system is often activated in congestive heart failure; this results in increased production of a powerful vasoconstrictor known as *angiotensin II* (see Chapter 21 for details of the renin-angiotensin system). Excess production of angiotensin II is extremely detrimental to the cardiovascular system because it increases workload on the heart and causes abnormal structural changes (remodeling) of the heart and vasculature. Activation of the renin-angiotensin system also leads to increased production of aldosterone, which further stresses the cardiovascular system by increasing salt and water retention.

Fortunately, there are several drug strategies to deal with abnormal activation of the renin-angiotensin system. These strategies include the ACE inhibitors, angiotensin II receptor blockers, and direct renin inhibitors.

ACE Inhibitors

ACE inhibitors have been used successfully to treat hypertension (see Chapter 21) and are now recognized as critical in treating congestive heart failure with reduced left ventricular function (i.e., systolic heart failure).[2,51] ACE inhibitors interrupt the renin-angiotensin system and help decrease morbidity and mortality in patients with congestive heart failure by improving the patient's neurohormonal and hemodynamic function.[52,53] The ACE inhibitors commonly used in congestive heart failure include captopril (Capoten), enalapril (Vasotec), and several similar drugs listed in Table 24-1. In severe congestive heart failure, these drugs are often given in combination with diuretics and digitalis.

ACE inhibitors are one of the mainstays of treatment in many patients with congestive heart failure. They were the first agents shown to prolong the life span of people with this disease.[38] Although digitalis, diuretics, and other drugs commonly used to treat heart failure may all produce symptomatic improvements, the use of ACE inhibitors alone or in combination with these drugs actually results in decreased mortality.[52,53]

The use of ACE inhibitors in treating systolic heart failure has therefore increased dramatically over the last several years.[51] There is evidence that these drugs should be used even more extensively and in higher doses, especially in the early stages of this disease.[54,55] By reducing the detrimental effects of angiotensin II on the vascular system, early use of ACE inhibitors may prevent or delay the progression of the disease.

Effects and Mechanism of Action. As discussed in Chapter 21, ACE inhibitors suppress the enzyme that converts angiotensin I to angiotensin II in the bloodstream. Angiotensin II is a potent vasoconstrictor. By inhibiting the formation of angiotensin II, ACE inhibitors limit peripheral vasoconstriction. This effect decreases cardiac workload primarily by decreasing the pressure against which the heart must pump (cardiac afterload).[56] Decreased cardiac afterload eases the strain on the failing heart, resulting in improved cardiac performance and increased exercise tolerance.[2]

Angiotensin II also promotes abnormal growth and remodeling of the heart, and this substance is thought to be responsible for many of the pathological changes in left ventricular function in heart failure.[57,58] Angiotensin II also stimulates growth and hypertrophy of vascular tissues, which results in the thickening of peripheral blood vessels' walls.[59,60] This thickening reduces the size of the vessel lumen, which further increases cardiac afterload because the heart must force blood into these narrowed vessels. ACE inhibitors therefore prevent angiotensin II–induced cardiovascular remodeling, which helps reduce the workload on the heart and prevents the progression of heart failure.[57]

By directly inhibiting angiotensin II formation, ACE inhibitors also inhibit aldosterone secretion.[2] Angiotensin II promotes aldosterone secretion from the adrenal cortex (it is probably a by-product of angiotensin II—that is, angiotensin III, which directly stimulates aldosterone secretion). Aldosterone increases renal sodium reabsorption, with a subsequent increase in water reabsorption (i.e., the exact opposite effect produced by a diuretic). Inhibition of aldosterone secretion is beneficial in congestive heart failure because vascular fluid volume does not increase and overtax the failing heart. Consequently, ACE inhibitors may help decrease cardiac workload by both hemodynamic mechanisms (prevention of vasoconstriction by angiotensin II) and fluid-electrolyte mechanisms (inhibition of aldosterone secretion).

Finally, ACE inhibitors exert some of their beneficial effects by increasing bradykinin levels in the bloodstream.[61,62] Bradykinin is a vasodilator, and increased levels of this compound decrease cardiac workload. Normally, ACE is responsible for the enzymatic destruction of bradykinin in the bloodstream. ACE inhibitors reduce the breakdown of bradykinin, thereby prolonging the vasodilating effects of this substance.[61,63]

In summary, ACE inhibitors reduce the detrimental effects of excess angiotensin II and aldosterone and prolong the beneficial effects of bradykinin. These effects work in combination to sustain cardiovascular health in people with heart failure.

Angiotensin II Receptor Blockers

Angiotensin II receptor blockers (ARBs) represent a second strategy for treating disorders associated with the renin-angiotensin system.[51] These drugs include candesartan, losartan, and valsartan. As indicated in Chapter 21, these agents prevent angiotensin II from binding to receptors on vascular tissues, thus inhibiting angiotensin II–induced damage of the cardiovascular system. It appears that ARBs are as effective as ACE inhibitors in treating heart failure and preventing mortality.[64] It has also been suggested that combining an ARB with an ACE inhibitor might provide more benefits than using either drug alone.[64] This idea remains controversial, however, because some studies observed an increase in adverse effects without an increase in benefits when an ARB was added to an ACE inhibitor in the treatment of patients with heart failure.[65,66]

Consequently, ARBs are used primarily as an alternative for people who are unable to tolerate traditional ACE inhibitors.[2,64] Future studies comparing ACE inhibitors with angiotensin II receptor blockers should help clarify which type of drug—or perhaps a combination of specific renin-angiotensin system inhibitors—provides optimal treatment in heart failure.[67]

Direct Renin Inhibitors

Finally, direct renin inhibitors represent a third way to decrease activity in the renin-angiotensin system (see Chapter 21).[38] These drugs directly inhibit renin's ability to convert angiotensinogen to angiotensin I, thus decreasing the production of the precursor substance that is needed to produce angiotensin II. At present, the only direct-acting renin inhibitor is aliskiren (Tekturna), and the use of this drug in treating congestive heart failure continues to be investigated.[51] Additional research is needed to determine whether direct renin inhibitors such as aliskiren can be used alone or with other drugs in the treatment of specific types of heart failure.

Adverse Effects of Drugs Affecting the Renin-Angiotensin System

Adverse effects with ACE inhibitors are relatively rare. In fact, one of the primary advantages of these drugs over more toxic compounds such as digitalis is the low incidence of serious effects. ACE inhibitors are occasionally associated with bothersome side effects such as skin rashes, GI discomfort, and dizziness; these effects are often transient or can be resolved with an adjustment in dosage. Some patients taking ACE inhibitors develop a persistent dry cough, which is often the reason for discontinuing the drug or seeking an alternative treatment. As indicated above, the newer angiotensin II receptor blockers or direct renin inhibitors may be a suitable alternative to ACE inhibitors if patients are not able to tolerate a dry cough or other ACE inhibitor–induced side effects.

Beta Blockers

In the past, beta blockers were considered detrimental in patients with heart failure.[68] As indicated in Chapter 20, these drugs decrease heart rate and myocardial contraction force by blocking the effects of epinephrine and norepinephrine on the heart. Common sense dictated that a decrease in myocardial contractility would be counterproductive in heart failure, and beta blockers were therefore contraindicated in heart failure.[68,69] It is now recognized that beta blockers are actually beneficial in people with heart failure because they attenuate the excessive sympathetic activity associated with this disease.[70] As indicated earlier, increased sympathetic activity and other neurohormonal changes often contribute to the vicious cycle associated with heart failure, and excessive sympathetic stimulation can accelerate the pathological changes in the failing heart.[70,71] Beta blockers reduce the harmful effects of excessive sympathetic stimulation, and use of these drugs has been shown to reduce the morbidity and mortality associated with heart failure.[68,72] Hence, beta blockers are now considered one of the principal treatments of this disease, and use of these drugs along with ACE inhibitors and traditional agents (digitalis, diuretics, etc.) is advocated as state-of-the-art therapy for providing optimal treatment in heart failure.[2,73]

Effects and Mechanism of Action

Beta blockers bind to beta-1 receptors on the myocardium and block the effects of norepinephrine and epinephrine (see Chapter 20). These drugs therefore normalize sympathetic stimulation of the heart and help reduce heart rate (negative chronotropic effect) and myocardial contraction force (negative inotropic effect). Beta blockers may also prevent angina by reducing cardiac workload, and they may prevent certain arrhythmias by stabilizing heart rate.[74] These additional properties can be useful to patients with heart failure who also have other cardiac symptoms.

Finally, it has been suggested that some of the newer "third-generation" beta blockers, such as carvedilol (Coreg) and nebivolol (Bystolic), may be especially useful in heart failure because they block beta-1 receptors on the heart while also blocking alpha-1 receptors on the vasculature, thus causing peripheral vasodilation.[75,76] Vasodilation of peripheral vessels could further reduce myocardial stress by decreasing the pressure that the heart must work against in the peripheral vessels (cardiac afterload).

Adverse Effects

The primary problem associated with beta blockers is that they may cause excessive inhibition of the heart, resulting in an abnormally slow heart rate and reduced contraction force. This effect is especially problematic in heart failure because the heart is already losing its ability to pump blood. Nonetheless, the risk of this and other side effects is acceptable in most people with heart failure, and this risk is minimized by adjusting the dosage so that sympathetic activity is normalized rather than reduced to unacceptably low levels. The side effects and problems associated with beta blockers were addressed in Chapter 20.

Diuretics

Diuretics increase the excretion of sodium and water. These agents are useful in congestive heart failure primarily because of their ability to reduce congestion in the lungs and peripheral tissues by excreting excess fluid retained in these tissues.[77,78] Diuretics also decrease the amount of fluid the heart must pump (cardiac preload), thereby reducing the failing heart's workload.[79] Diuretics help improve the symptoms of heart failure, and they are often used with other agents (e.g., ACE inhibitors, beta blockers, digitalis) to provide optimal treatment of this disease.[80,81] Diuretic drugs, which are also used to treat hypertension, are discussed in more detail in Chapter 21. Diuretics that can be used in the treatment of congestive heart failure and hypertension are listed in Table 21-3.

Effects and Mechanism of Action

Diuretics work by inhibiting the reabsorption of sodium from the nephron, which, in turn, decreases the amount of water that is normally reabsorbed with sodium, thus increasing water excretion. This effect reduces congestion caused by fluids retained in the body and decreases cardiac preload by excreting excess fluid in the vascular system. In particular, diuretics that primarily affect the loop of Henle (i.e., loop diuretics) are used commonly to reduce fluid overload in people with congestive heart failure.[77,82] Chapter 21 provides a more detailed discussion on the mechanism of action of loop diuretics and other diuretic drugs.

It has also been suggested that certain diuretics, such as spironolactone (Aldactone) and eplerenone (Inspra), might be especially helpful in heart failure.[83,84] These drugs block aldosterone receptors in the kidneys and other tissues, thereby producing a diuretic effect and preventing adverse cardiovascular changes associated with excess aldosterone production. Hence, these drugs can also be categorized as aldosterone blockers or mineralocorticoid receptor antagonists.[84] Mineralocorticoid receptor antagonists have therefore gained acceptance as an important strategy in treating heart failure, and clinical studies continue to clarify the role of these drugs as part of the comprehensive treatment of congestive heart failure.[51,85]

Adverse Effects

By the very nature of their action, diuretics are often associated with disturbances in fluid and electrolyte balance. Volume depletion, hyponatremia, hypokalemia, and altered pH balance are among the most frequent problems.[81,86] These electrolyte and pH changes can produce serious consequences by affecting cardiac excitability and precipitating arrhythmias. Patients on diuretics should be monitored closely for symptoms such as fatigue, confusion, and nausea, which may indicate the presence of drug-induced disturbances in fluid-electrolyte balance. Some patients may also become resistant to diuretic drugs; the effectiveness of the diuretic is diminished primarily because the kidneys adapt to the drug-induced sodium excretion.[87,88] Resistance can often be prevented by altering the dose and type of diuretic or by adding a second diuretic.[87,88]

Vasodilators

Various drugs that vasodilate peripheral vessels have been successful in treating patients with cases of severe congestive heart failure.[89,90] By reducing peripheral vascular resistance, these agents decrease the amount of blood returning to the heart (cardiac preload) and reduce the pressure that the heart must pump against (cardiac afterload). Reduced cardiac preload and afterload helps alleviate some of the stress on the failing heart, thus slowing the disease progression. Vasodilators commonly used in heart failure include prazosin, hydralazine, and organic nitrates (e.g., nitroglycerin, isosorbide dinitrate, sodium nitroprusside; see Table 24-1). In particular, a combination of hydralazine and isosorbide dinitrate has been found to be helpful in reducing symptoms and improving survival, especially in African American patients with advanced heart failure.[91]

In addition to these traditional vasodilators, researchers developed nesiritide (Natrecor) as a newer method for producing arterial and venous dilation in people with heart failure.[92] They derived nesiritide from human B-type natriuretic peptide (BNP) using recombinant DNA techniques. BNP is a naturally occurring substance that is released from the ventricles when the heart is subjected to increased blood volume and pressure.[92] This substance dilates peripheral arteries and veins, thus reducing cardiac afterload and preload, respectively. Hence, nesiritide can be administered intravenously to reduce cardiac workload in certain patients with severe or acute heart failure.[93] Several other natriuretic peptides are produced endogenously, and researchers continue to investigate whether these compounds can be developed to treat congestive heart failure.[94]

Finally, other drugs such as sildenafil (Revatio, Viagra) can produce vasodilation by selectively inhibiting for the type-5 phosphodiesterase enzyme (PDE5). This PDE5 enzyme normally inactivates cyclic guanosine monophosphate (cGMP), which acts as a second messenger within endothelial cells to cause relaxation and vasodilation. By inhibiting PDE5, sildenafil prolongs the action of cGMP, thereby enhancing vasodilation.[95] Sildenafil and similar drugs are used commonly for treating erectile dysfunction, but they may also be useful as vasodilators in other cardiovascular conditions, such as pulmonary hypertension.[96] Hence, there is considerable interest in seeing whether sildenafil and other PDE5 inhibitors may enhance systemic vasodilation and thus reduce cardiac workload in certain patients with heart failure.[95,97] Future studies will clarify whether these drugs can provide a safe and effective method for treating heart failure compared to existing drugs.

Effects and Mechanism of Action

Prazosin produces vasodilation by blocking alpha-1 receptors on vascular smooth muscle (see Chapter 20); hydralazine, organic nitrates, and BNP produce vasodilation by a direct inhibitory effect on the vascular smooth-muscle cells (see Chapters 21 and 22). As indicated above, PDE5 inhibitors prolong the effects of cGMP, which promotes relaxation and vasodilation in vascular endothelial cells. Although these vasodilators work by different mechanisms, they all can decrease cardiac workload by decreasing peripheral vascular resistance. These drugs may be combined with other agents (e.g., digoxin, ACE inhibitors, beta blockers) to provide optimal benefits in patients with varying degrees of congestive heart failure.[38]

Adverse Effects

The primary side effects associated with vasodilators include headache, dizziness, hypotension, and orthostatic hypotension. These effects are all related to the tendency of these drugs to increase peripheral blood flow and decrease peripheral vascular resistance. Vasodilators may also cause reflex tachycardia in certain patients if the baroreceptor reflex increases heart rate in an attempt to maintain adequate blood pressure.

Special Concerns for Rehabilitation Patients

Therapists should be aware of the potential for drugs used to treat congestive heart failure to affect the patient's welfare and response to rehabilitation. Acute congestive heart failure may occur in patients with myocardial disease because of a lack of therapeutic drug effects or because of the toxic effects of some cardiac drugs. Therapists should remain alert for signs of acute congestive heart failure such as increased cough, difficulty in breathing (dyspnea), abnormal respiratory sounds (rales), and frothy sputum. Therapists should also remain alert for signs of digitalis toxicity such as dizziness, confusion, nausea, and arrhythmias. Early recognition by the therapist may prevent serious or even fatal consequences. Likewise, patients taking diuretics sometimes exhibit excessive fatigue and weakness—these may be the early signs of fluid and electrolyte depletion. Therapists may help detect serious metabolic and electrolyte imbalances that result from problems with diuretic drugs. Finally, use of vasodilators often causes hypotension and postural hypotension. Therapists must use caution when patients suddenly sit up or stand up. Also, therapeutic techniques that produce systemic vasodilation (whirlpool, exercise) may produce profound hypotension in patients taking vasodilators, and these modalities should therefore be used cautiously.

CASE STUDY

CONGESTIVE HEART FAILURE

Brief History. D.S. is a 67-year-old woman with a long history of congestive heart failure caused by myocarditis. She has been treated successfully with digitalis glycosides (digoxin [Lanoxin], 0.5 mg/d) for several years. Despite some swelling in her ankles and feet and a tendency to become winded, she has maintained a fairly active lifestyle and enjoys gardening and other hobbies. Recently, she developed some weakness and incoordination that primarily affected her right side. Subsequent testing revealed that she had suffered a cerebral vascular accident (stroke). She was not admitted to the hospital but remained living at home with her husband. Physical therapy was provided in the home to facilitate optimal recovery from her stroke. The therapist began seeing her three times each week for a program of therapeutic exercise and functional training.

Problem/Influence of Medication. The therapist initially found D.S. to be alert, coherent, and eager to begin therapy. Although there was some residual weakness and decreased motor skills, the prognosis for a full recovery appeared good. The therapist was impressed by the patient's enthusiasm and pleasant nature during the first two sessions. By the end of the first week, however, the therapist noted a distinct change in the patient's demeanor. She was confused and quite lethargic. Her husband confirmed that she also felt nauseous and had lost her appetite. The therapist initially suspected that she might have had another stroke. However, physical examination did not reveal any dramatic decrease in strength or coordination.

1. ***Could D.S.'s drug regimen be contributing to her current symptoms?***
2. ***Why did the symptoms probably begin to emerge at this point in time?***
3. ***What should the therapist do?***

See Appendix C, "Answers to Case Study Questions."

SUMMARY

Congestive heart failure is a serious cardiac condition in which the ability of the heart to pump blood becomes progressively worse. Decreased myocardial performance leads to a number of deleterious changes, including peripheral edema (i.e., congestion) and increased fatigue during physical activity. Moreover, heart failure is often perpetuated by a vicious cycle where the initial damage to cardiac cells causes neurohormonal changes that cause additional myocardial damage, which increases the neurohormonal reactions, and so on.

The pharmacological treatment of heart failure has undergone substantial changes over the past few decades. Digitalis, once the cornerstone of treatment, is associated with several serious side effects, and there is considerable doubt as to whether digitalis actually increases the rate of survival of patients with congestive heart failure.[2] Treatment is now centered on using drugs such as ACE inhibitors and beta blockers that decrease the counterproductive neurohormonal changes that increase cardiac workload in heart failure.[25] These drugs help resolve the symptoms of heart failure and can slow the progression of this disease and help prolong life expectancy. Other drugs such as digitalis, diuretics, and vasodilators can be added to the ACE inhibitor/beta blocker regimen as needed to help resolve symptoms or as heart failure becomes more pronounced.

In addition to using appropriate drugs, there is consensus that reduction of predisposing risk factors (e.g., coronary artery disease, hypertension, diabetes mellitus) and early intervention in the treatment of congestive heart failure is crucial in providing the best outcome.[38] Even with optimal treatment, however, the prognosis for patients with congestive heart failure is often poor. Therapists should be aware of the drugs used to manage this disorder and that certain side effects may adversely affect rehabilitation or signal a problem with drug treatment.

REFERENCES

1. Cassady SL, Cahalin LP. Cardiovascular pathophysiology. In: DeTurk WE, Cahalin LP, eds. *Cardiovascular and Pulmonary Physical Therapy.* 2nd ed. New York: McGraw-Hill; 2011.
2. Parker RB, Cavallari LH. Systolic heart failure. In: DiPiro JT, et al, eds. *Pharmacotherapy: A Pathophysiologic Approach*. 8th ed. New York: McGraw-Hill; 2011.
3. King M, Kingery J, Casey B. Diagnosis and evaluation of heart failure. *Am Fam Physician. 2012*;85:1161-1168.
4. Kemp CD, Conte JV. The pathophysiology of heart failure. *Cardiovasc Pathol.* 2012;21:365-371.
5. Rathi S, Deedwania PC. The epidemiology and pathophysiology of heart failure. *Med Clin North Am.* 2012;96:881-890.
6. Vigen R, Maddox TM, Allen LA. Aging of the United States population: impact on heart failure. *Curr Heart Fail Rep*. 2012;9: 369-374.
7. Chatterjee K. Pathophysiology of systolic and diastolic heart failure. *Med Clin North Am.* 2012;96:891-899.
8. Louridas GE, Lourida KG. Systems biology and biomechanical model of heart failure. *Curr Cardiol Rev.* 2012;8:220-230.
9. Kohlhaas M, Maack C. Interplay of defective excitation-contraction coupling, energy starvation, and oxidative stress in heart failure. *Trends Cardiovasc Med*. 2011;21:69-73.
10. Dhalla NS, Rangi S, Babick AP, et al. Cardiac remodeling and subcellular defects in heart failure due to myocardial infarction and aging. *Heart Fail Rev.* 2012;17:671-681.
11. Mocchegiani R, Nataloni M. Complications of infective endocarditis. *Cardiovasc Hematol Disord Drug Targets*. 2009;9: 240-248.
12. Messaoudi S, Azibani F, Delcayre C, Jaisser F. Aldosterone, mineralocorticoid receptor, and heart failure. *Mol Cell Endocrinol.* 2012;350:266-272.
13. Michael Felker G. Diuretic management in heart failure. *Congest Heart Fail.* 2010;16(suppl 1):S68-72.
14. Chaney E, Shaw A. Pathophysiology of fluid retention in heart failure. *Contrib Nephrol.* 2010;164:46-53.
15. Chen L, Knowlton AA. Mitochondrial dynamics in heart failure. *Congest Heart Fail.* 2011;17:257-261.
16. Marks AR. Calcium cycling proteins and heart failure: mechanisms and therapeutics. *J Clin Invest.* 2013;123:46-52.
17. Palazzuoli A, Nuti R. Heart failure: pathophysiology and clinical picture. *Contrib Nephrol.* 2010;164:1-10.
18. MacIver DH, Dayer MJ, Harrison AJ. A general theory of acute and chronic heart failure. *Int J Cardiol.* 2013;165:25-34.
19. Müller AL, Dhalla NS. Role of various proteases in cardiac remodeling and progression of heart failure. *Heart Fail Rev.* 2012;17:395-409.
20. Alagiakrishnan K, Banach M, Jones LG, et al. Update on diastolic heart failure or heart failure with preserved ejection fraction in the older adults. *Ann Med.* 2013;45:37-50.
21. Sohn DW. Heart failure due to abnormal filling function of the heart. *J Cardiol.* 2011;57:148-159.
22. Kaila K, Haykowsky MJ, Thompson RB, Paterson DI. Heart failure with preserved ejection fraction in the elderly: scope of the problem. *Heart Fail Rev*. 2012;17:555-562.
23. Scantlebury DC, Borlaug BA. Why are women more likely than men to develop heart failure with preserved ejection fraction? *Curr Opin Cardiol.* 2011;26:562-568.
24. Gradman AH, Wilson JT. Hypertension and diastolic heart failure. *Curr Cardiol Rep.* 2009;11:422-429.
25. Ginelli P, Bella JN. Treatment of diastolic dysfunction in hypertension. *Nutr Metab Cardiovasc Dis.* 2012;22:613-618.
26. Morrissey RP, Czer L, Shah PK. Chronic heart failure: current evidence, challenges to therapy, and future directions. *Am J Cardiovasc Drugs.* 2011;11(3):153-171.
27. Ehle M, Patel C, Giugliano RP. Digoxin: clinical highlights: a review of digoxin and its use in contemporary medicine. *Crit Pathw Cardiol.* 2011;10:93-98.

28. Mittal MK, Chockalingam P, Chockalingam A. Contemporary indications and therapeutic implications for digoxin use. *Am J Ther*. 2011;18:280-287.
29. Teerlink JR, Metra M, Zacà V, et al. Agents with inotropic properties for the management of acute heart failure syndromes. Traditional agents and beyond. *Heart Fail Rev.* 2009;14:243-253.
30. Dec GW. Digoxin remains useful in the management of chronic heart failure. *Med Clin North Am*. 2003;87:317-337.
31. Caccamo MA, Eckman PM. Pharmacologic therapy for New York Heart Association class IV heart failure. *Congest Heart Fail.* 2011;17:213-219.
32. Bourge RC, Fleg JL, Fonarow GC, et al. Digoxin reduces 30-day all-cause hospital admission in older patients with chronic systolic heart failure. *Am J Med*. 2013;126:701-708.
33. Cheng JW, Rybak I. Use of digoxin for heart failure and atrial fibrillation in elderly patients. *Am J Geriatr Pharmacother*. 2010;8:419-427.
34. Katzung BG. Drugs used in heart failure. In: Katzung BG, ed. *Basic and Clinical Pharmacology.* 12th ed. New York: Lange Medical Books/McGraw Hill; 2012.
35. Mörike K, Sindermann JR. Drug treatment for chronic systolic heart failure. *Thorac Cardiovasc Surg*. 2010;58(suppl 2):S170-172.
36. Sindone A, Naoum C. Chronic heart failure—improving life with modern therapies. *Aust Fam Physician*. 2010;39:898-901.
37. Katz A, Lifshitz Y, Bab-Dinitz E, et al. Selectivity of digitalis glycosides for isoforms of human Na,K-ATPase. *J Biol Chem*. 2010;285:19582-19592.
38. Maron BA, Rocco TP. Pharmacotherapy of congestive heart failure. In: Brunton L, et al, eds. *The Pharmacological Basis of Therapeutics.* 12th ed. New York: McGraw-Hill; 2011.
39. Kishi T. Heart failure as an autonomic nervous system dysfunction. *J Cardiol.* 2012;59:117-122.
40. Lane DA, Apostolakis S, Boos CJ, Lip GY. Atrial fibrillation (chronic). *Clin Evid (Online)*. 2011;2011.
41. Desai MY, Watanabe MA, Laddu AA, Hauptman PJ. Pharmacologic modulation of parasympathetic activity in heart failure. *Heart Fail Rev*. 2011;16:179-193.
42. Kanji S, MacLean RD. Cardiac glycoside toxicity: more than 200 years and counting. *Crit Care Clin*. 2012;28:527-535.
43. Yang EH, Shah S, Criley JM. Digitalis toxicity: a fading but crucial complication to recognize. *Am J Med.* 2012;125:337-343.
44. Movsesian MA, Kukreja RC. Phosphodiesterase inhibition in heart failure. *Handb Exp Pharmacol.* 2011;204:237-249.
45. Metra M, Bettari L, Carubelli V, Cas LD. Old and new intravenous inotropic agents in the treatment of advanced heart failure. *Prog Cardiovasc Dis*. 2011;54:97-106.
46. Rodgers JE, Lee CR. Acute decompensated heart failure. In: DiPiro JT, et al, eds. *Pharmacotherapy: A Pathophysiologic Approach*. 8th ed. New York: McGraw-Hill; 2011.
47. Metra M, Bettari L, Carubelli V, et al. Use of inotropic agents in patients with advanced heart failure: lessons from recent trials and hopes for new agents. *Drugs*. 2011;71:515-525.
48. Joseph SM, Cedars AM, Ewald GA, et al. Acute decompensated heart failure: contemporary medical management. *Tex Heart Inst J*. 2009;36:510-520.
49. Parissis JT, Rafouli-Stergiou P, Stasinos V, et al. Inotropes in cardiac patients: update 2011. *Curr Opin Crit Care*. 2010;16:432-441.
50. Tacon CL, McCaffrey J, Delaney A. Dobutamine for patients with severe heart failure: a systematic review and meta-analysis of randomised controlled trials. *Intensive Care Med*. 2012;38:359-367.
51. Lang CC, Struthers AD. Targeting the renin-angiotensin-aldosterone system in heart failure. *Nat Rev Cardiol.* 2013;10:125-134.
52. Hanif K, Bid HK, Konwar R. Reinventing the ACE inhibitors: some old and new implications of ACE inhibition. *Hypertens Res*. 2010;33:11-21.
53. Hoogwerf BJ. Renin-angiotensin system blockade and cardiovascular and renal protection. *Am J Cardiol.* 2010;105(suppl):30A-35A.
54. Thomas S, Geltman E. What is the optimal angiotensin-converting enzyme inhibitor dose in heart failure? *Congest Heart Fail.* 2006;12:213-218.
55. Volpe M. Should all patients at high cardiovascular risk receive renin-angiotensin system blockers? *QJM*. 2012;105:11-27.
56. Francis GS. Neurohormonal control of heart failure. *Cleve Clin J Med*. 2011;78(suppl 1):S75-79.
57. Katragadda S, Arora RR. Role of angiotensin-converting enzyme inhibitors in vascular modulation: beyond the hypertensive effects. *Am J Ther.* 2010;17:e11-23.
58. Kirkpatrick JN, St John Sutton M. Assessment of ventricular remodeling in heart failure clinical trials. *Curr Heart Fail Rep*. 2012;9:328-336.
59. Briet M, Schiffrin EL. Treatment of arterial remodeling in essential hypertension. *Curr Hypertens Rep*. 2013;15:3-9.
60. Tieu BC, Ju X, Lee C, et al. Aortic adventitial fibroblasts participate in angiotensin-induced vascular wall inflammation and remodeling. *J Vasc Res*. 2011;48:261-272.
61. Alhenc-Gelas F, Bouby N, Richer C, et al. Kinins as therapeutic agents in cardiovascular and renal diseases. *Curr Pharm Des*. 2011;17:2654-2662.
62. Regoli D, Plante GE, Gobeil F Jr. Impact of kinins in the treatment of cardiovascular diseases. *Pharmacol Ther*. 2012;135:94-111.
63. Izzo JL Jr, Weir MR. Angiotensin-converting enzyme inhibitors. *J Clin Hypertens.* 2011;13:667-675.
64. Werner C, Pöss J, Böhm M. Optimal antagonism of the renin-angiotensin-aldosterone system: do we need dual or triple therapy? *Drugs*. 2010;70:1215-1230.
65. Heran BS, Musini VM, Bassett K, et al. Angiotensin receptor blockers for heart failure. *Cochrane Database Syst Rev.* 2012;4:CD003040.
66. Makani H, Bangalore S, Desouza KA, et al. Efficacy and safety of dual blockade of the renin-angiotensin system: meta-analysis of randomized trials. *BMJ*. 2013;346:f360.
67. Volpe M, Danser AH, Menard J, et al. Inhibition of the renin-angiotensin-aldosterone system: is there room for dual blockade in the cardiorenal continuum? *J Hypertens.* 2012;30:647-654.
68. Kubon C, Mistry NB, Grundvold I, et al. The role of beta-blockers in the treatment of chronic heart failure. *Trends Pharmacol Sci*. 2011;32:206-212.
69. Sorrentino MJ. Beta-blockers for congestive heart failure. *Compr Ther.* 2003;29:210-214.
70. Hamdani N, Linke WA. Alteration of the beta-adrenergic signaling pathway in human heart failure. *Curr Pharm Biotechnol.* 2012;13:2522-2531.
71. Triposkiadis F, Karayannis G, Giamouzis G, et al. The sympathetic nervous system in heart failure physiology, pathophysiology, and clinical implications. *J Am Coll Cardiol.* 2009;54:1747-1762.
72. Chatterjee S, Biondi-Zoccai G, Abbate A, et al. Benefits of β blockers in patients with heart failure and reduced ejection fraction: network meta-analysis. *BMJ*. 2013;346:f55.

73. Nair AP, Timoh T, Fuster V. Contemporary medical management of systolic heart failure. *Circ J.* 2012;76:268-277.
74. Ramineni R, Bheemarasetti MK, Baranchuk A, et al. Management of arrhythmias in heart failure. What a practicing physician should know in the current times. *Cardiol J.* 2012;19:567-577.
75. DiNicolantonio JJ, Hackam DG. Carvedilol: a third-generation β-blocker should be a first-choice β-blocker. *Expert Rev Cardiovasc Ther.* 2012;10:13-25.
76. Fares H, Lavie CJ, Ventura HO. Vasodilating versus first-generation β-blockers for cardiovascular protection. *Postgrad Med.* 2012;124:7-15.
77. Basraon J, Deedwani PC. Diuretics in heart failure: practical considerations. *Med Clin North Am.* 2012;96:933-942.
78. Clark AL, Cleland JG. Causes and treatment of oedema in patients with heart failure. *Nat Rev Cardiol.* 2013;10:156-170.
79. Ives HE. Diuretic agents. In: Katzung BG, ed. *Basic and Clinical Pharmacology.* 12th ed. New York: Lange Medical Books/McGraw Hill; 2012.
80. Ito H, Ishii K, Kihara H, et al. Effect of ARB/Diuretics on Diastolic Function in Patients with Hypertension (EDEN) trial investigators. Adding thiazide to a renin-angiotensin blocker improves left ventricular relaxation and improves heart failure in patients with hypertension. *Hypertens Res.* 2012;35:93-99.
81. Sica DA, Carter B, Cushman W, Hamm L. Thiazide and loop diuretics. *J Clin Hypertens.* 2011;13:639-643.
82. Felker GM. Loop diuretics in heart failure. *Heart Fail Rev.* 2012;17:305-311.
83. Nagarajan V, Chamsi-Pasha M, Tang WH. The role of aldosterone receptor antagonists in the management of heart failure: an update. *Cleve Clin J Med.* 2012;79:631-639.
84. Seawell MR, Al Darazi F, Farah V, et al. Mineralocorticoid receptor antagonism confers cardioprotection in heart failure. *Curr Heart Fail Rep.* 2013;10:36-45.
85. Talatinian A, Chow SL, Heywood JT. Expanding role of mineralocorticoid receptor antagonists in the treatment of heart failure. *Pharmacotherapy.* 2012;32:827-837.
86. Wile D. Diuretics: a review. *Ann Clin Biochem.* 2012;49(Pt 5): 419-431.
87. Asare K. Management of loop diuretic resistance in the intensive care unit. *Am J Health Syst Pharm.* 2009;66:1635-1640.
88. De Bruyne LK. Mechanisms and management of diuretic resistance in congestive heart failure. *Postgrad Med J.* 2003;79:268-271.
89. Coons JC, McGraw M, Murali S. Pharmacotherapy for acute heart failure syndromes. *Am J Health Syst Pharm.* 2011;68:21-35.
90. Zamani P, Greenberg BH. Novel vasodilators in heart failure. *Curr Heart Fail Rep.* 2013;10:1-11.
91. Taylor AL, Sabolinski ML, Tam SW, et al. Effect of fixed-dose combined isosorbide dinitrate/hydralazine in elderly patients in the African-American heart failure trial. *J Card Fail.* 2012;18:600-606.
92. Gassanov N, Biesenbach E, Caglayan E, et al. Natriuretic peptides in therapy for decompensated heart failure. *Eur J Clin Pharmacol.* 2012;68:223-230.
93. Vogel MW, Chen HH. Novel natriuretic peptides: new compounds and new approaches. *Curr Heart Fail Rep.* 2011;8:22-27.
94. Reilly RF, Jackson EK. Regulation of renal function and vascular volume. In: Brunton L, et al, eds. *The Pharmacological Basis of Therapeutics.* 12th ed. New York: McGraw-Hill; 2011.
95. Kanwar M, Agarwal R, Barnes M, et al. Role of phosphodiesterase-5 inhibitors in heart failure: emerging data and concepts. *Curr Heart Fail Rep.* 2013;10:26-35.
96. Murray F, Maclean MR, Insel PA. Role of phosphodiesterases in adult-onset pulmonary arterial hypertension. *Handb Exp Pharmacol.* 2011;204:279-305.
97. Schwartz BG, Jackson G, Stecher VJ, et al. Phosphodiesterase type 5 inhibitors improve endothelial function and may benefit cardiovascular conditions. *Am J Med.* 2013;126:192-199.

CHAPTER 25

Treatment of Coagulation Disorders and Hyperlipidemia

Blood coagulation, or **hemostasis**, is necessary to prevent excessive hemorrhage from damaged blood vessels. Under normal conditions, clotting factors in the bloodstream spontaneously interact with damaged vessels to create a blood clot that plugs the leaking vessel. Obviously, inadequate blood clotting is harmful in that even minor vessel damage can lead to excessive blood loss. Overactive clotting is also detrimental because it will lead to *thrombogenesis* (i.e., the abnormal formation of blood clots, or thrombi).[1] **Thrombus** formation may lead directly to vessel occlusion and tissue infarction. Also, a piece of a thrombus may dislodge, creating an embolism that causes infarction elsewhere in the body, such as in the lungs or brain.

Consequently, normal hemostasis can be regarded as a balance between too much and too little blood coagulation.[2,3] This balance is often disrupted by several factors. Insufficient levels of blood-clotting factors typically cause inadequate clotting, as in patients with hemophilia. Excessive clotting often occurs during prolonged bed rest or when blood flow through vessels is partially obstructed, as in coronary atherosclerosis.

Restoration of normal hemostasis is accomplished through pharmacological methods. Excessive clotting and thrombus formation are rectified by drugs that prevent clot formation (anticoagulants, antiplatelet drugs) or facilitate the removal of previously formed clots (fibrinolytics). Inadequate clotting is resolved by replacing the missing clotting factors or facilitating the synthesis of specific clotting factors.

Hemostasis can also be influenced by **hyperlipidemia**, which is a chronic and excessive increase in plasma lipids. With hyperlipidemia, cholesterol and other lipids are progressively deposited onto arterial walls, forming plaquelike lesions indicative of atherosclerosis. These atherosclerotic lesions progressively occlude the arterial lumen, and atherosclerotic plaques can suddenly rupture, thus leading to thrombosis and infarction. Atherosclerotic heart disease is one of the leading causes of morbidity and mortality in the United States. Pharmacological methods to lower plasma lipids are often used in conjunction with dietary and lifestyle modifications to treat hyperlipidemia and prevent atherosclerosis.

Drugs that can normalize blood clotting or reduce hyperlipidemia are among the most common medications used clinically, and you will deal with many patients taking these agents. Many patients, in fact, will be treated in therapy for problems relating directly to thrombus formation (e.g., ischemic stroke, myocardial infarction, pulmonary embolism). You will also routinely see individuals with inadequate clotting, such as patients with hemophilia, who are in rehabilitation because of the intrajoint hemorrhaging and other problems associated with this disease. Consequently, the purpose of this chapter is to acquaint you with several common and important groups of drugs used to treat coagulation disorders and hyperlipidemia.

NORMAL MECHANISM OF BLOOD COAGULATION

To understand how various drugs affect hemostasis, it is necessary to review the normal way in which blood clots are formed. The physiological mechanisms involved in hemostasis are outlined in Figure 25-1, with clot formation and breakdown illustrated in the upper and lower parts of the figure, respectively.

Clot Formation

Clot formation involves the complex interaction of various cellular and chemical components.[4,5] Basically, specific clotting factors circulating in the bloodstream are responsible for initiating clot formation. These clotting factors are proteolytic enzymes synthesized in the liver that remain inactive until there is some injury to a blood vessel. Blood vessel damage begins a cascade effect, whereby one of the clotting factors is activated, which leads to the next factor's activation, and so forth.[4,6] As shown in Figure 25-1, clot formation occurs through two pathways: an intrinsic and an extrinsic pathway. In the intrinsic pathway (known also as the *plasma contact system*), direct contact of platelets and the first clotting factor (factor XII) with the damaged vessel wall initiates the cascade. In the extrinsic pathway, a substance known as *tissue factor* is released from the damaged vascular cell and other circulating cells. Tissue factor forms a complex with

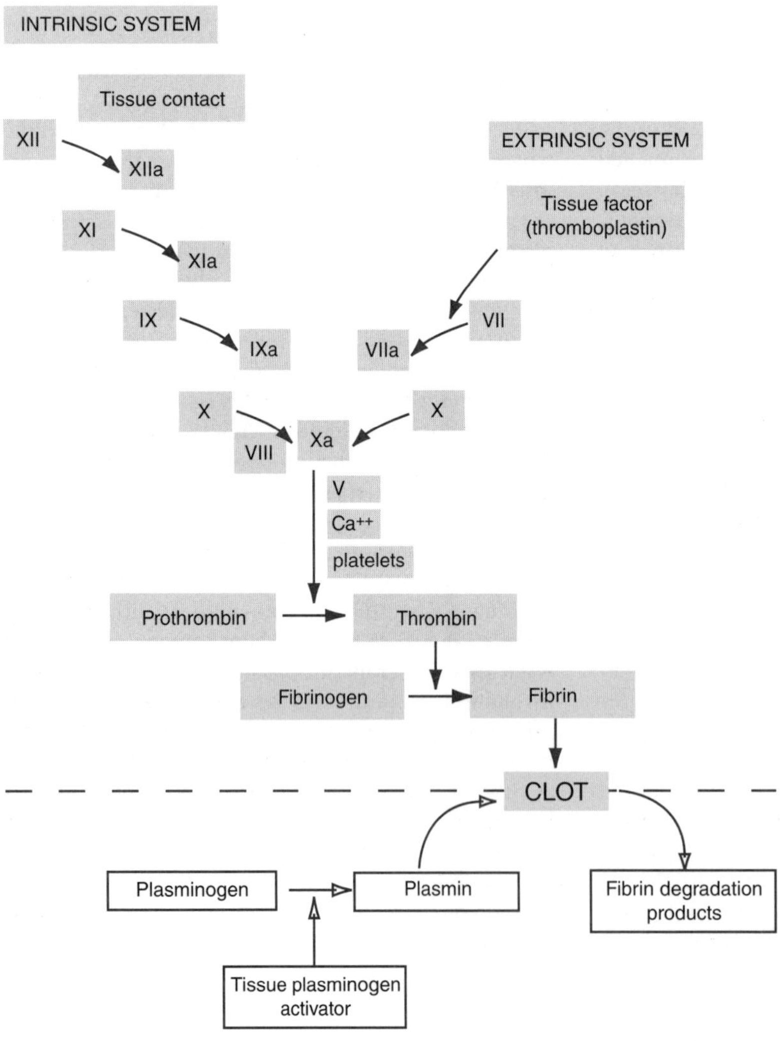

Figure ■ 25-1
Mechanism of blood coagulation. Factors involved in clot formation are shown above the dashed line; factors involved in clot breakdown are shown below the dashed line.

clotting factor VII, and this complex then activates subsequent factors in the clotting mechanism. Both the intrinsic and extrinsic pathways typically participate in normal blood clotting.

The ultimate goal of the intrinsic and extrinsic pathways is to convert prothrombin to thrombin.[5] *Thrombin* is an enzyme that quickly converts the inactive fibrinogen molecule to *fibrin*. Individual strands of fibrin bind together to form a meshlike structure, which forms the framework for the blood clot. Other cellular components, especially platelets, help reinforce the clot by sticking to the fibrin mesh.

Clot Breakdown

The breakdown of blood clots is illustrated in the lower part of Figure 25-1. *Tissue plasminogen activator (t-PA)* converts plasminogen to plasmin. *Plasmin*, also known as *fibrinolysin*, is an enzyme that directly breaks down the fibrin mesh, thus destroying the clot.

The balance between clot formation and breakdown is crucial in maintaining normal hemostasis. Obviously, clots should not be broken down as quickly as they are formed because then no coagulation will occur. Likewise, a lack of breakdown would enable clots to proliferate at an excessive rate, leading to thrombus formation.

The complex interaction of the factors described above, and a number of endogenous anticoagulant proteins such as protein C, protein S, and antithrombin III, normally control the balance between clot formation and clot breakdown.[7] Disease or inactivity, however, can alter this balance, leading to exaggerated clotting and venous or arterial thrombosis. Drugs used to treat overactive clotting are addressed in the next section.

DRUGS USED TO TREAT OVERACTIVE CLOTTING

Drugs used to treat excessive clot formation can be grouped into three primary categories: anticoagulant, antiplatelet, and fibrinolytic agents (Table 25-1). Anticoagulants exert their effect by controlling the function and synthesis of certain clotting factors; these drugs are used primarily to prevent clot formation in the venous system—that is, venous thrombosis. Antiplatelet drugs act primarily by inhibiting abnormal platelet activity and preventing thrombus formation in arteries that lead to myocardial infarction and ischemic stroke. Fibrinolytic drugs facilitate the destruction of blood clots and are used to reestablish blood flow through vessels that have been occluded by thrombi.

Anticoagulants

The primary anticoagulants are heparin, coumarin derivatives such as warfarin (Coumadin), direct thrombin inhibitors, and factor Xa inhibitors. These drugs are used primarily in the treatment of abnormal clot formation in the venous system. Venous clots typically form in the deep veins of the legs because of the relatively sluggish blood flow through those vessels. Hence, deep vein thrombosis is a primary indication for anticoagulant therapy.[8] When a piece of the clot breaks off and travels through the circulation to lodge elsewhere in the vascular system, deep vein thrombosis results in thromboembolism. Emboli originating in the venous system typically follow the venous flow back to the right side of the heart, where they are then pumped to the lungs. They finally lodge in the smaller vessels within the lungs, thus creating a pulmonary embolism.[9]

Anticoagulant drugs are administered for the acute treatment of venous thrombosis and thromboembolism; they may also be given prophylactically to individuals who are at high risk to develop venous thrombosis. For instance, physicians often administer these drugs after surgical procedures (joint replacement, mechanical heart valve replacement, etc.), following certain cardiovascular incidents (e.g., myocardial infarction, ischemic stroke, atrial fibrillation), and during medical conditions when patients will be relatively inactive for extended periods of time.[10-13]

Heparin

Heparin is often the primary drug used in the initial treatment of venous thrombosis.[14,15] The anticoagulant effects of heparin are seen almost instantly after administration. Heparin works by potentiating the activity of a circulating protein known as *antithrombin*.[16] Antithrombin binds to several of the active clotting factors (thrombin, IXa, Xa) and renders the clotting factors inactive. Heparin accelerates the antithrombin-induced inactivation of these clotting factors, thus reducing the tendency for clotting and thrombogenesis.

Heparin is a large, sugarlike molecule that is poorly absorbed from the gastrointestinal (GI) tract. Consequently, heparin must be administered parenterally. This agent was traditionally administered through IV infusion or repeated IV injection through a rubber-capped indwelling needle called a *heparin lock*. In the

Table 25-1
DRUGS USED TO TREAT OVERACTIVE CLOTTING

Drug Category	Primary Effect and Indication
Heparins	
Unfractionated heparin (Calciparin, Liquaemin, others) Low molecular weight heparins: Dalteparin (Fragmin) Enoxaparin (Lovenox) Tinzaparin (Innohep)	Inhibit synthesis and function of clotting factors (thrombin, IXa, Xa) Used primarily to prevent and treat acute venous thromboembolism
Coumarin Derivatives	
Warfarin (Coumadin)	Inhibits synthesis of specific clotting factors by impairing vitamin K function in the liver Often the primary drug used in the long-term prevention of venous thrombosis
Direct Thrombin Inhibitors	
Argatroban (Argatroban) Dabigatran (Pradaxa) Bivalirudin (Angiomax) Desirudin (Iprivask) Lepirudin (Refludan)	Bind directly to thrombin and impair thrombin's ability to activate fibrin Provide an alternative to more traditional agents in preventing and treating venous thrombosis
Factor Xa Inhibitors	
Apixaban (Eliquis) Fondaparinux (Arixtra) Rivaroxaban (Xarelto)	Directly inhibit the active form of clotting factor X Provide an alternative to heparin for preventing and treating acute venous thrombosis
Platelet Inhibitors	
Aspirin ADP receptor inhibitors • Clopidogrel (Plavix) • Prasugrel (Effient) • Ticlopidine (Ticlid) Glycoprotein IIb-IIIa receptor inhibitors: • Abciximab (ReoPro) • Eptifibatide (Integrilin) • Tirofiban (Aggrastat) Others • Cilostazol (Pletal) • Dipyridamole (Persantine, others) • Pentoxifylline (Trental)	Inhibit platelet aggregation and platelet-induced clotting Used primarily to prevent arterial thrombus formation and to prevent reocclusion after surgical procedures such as angioplasty or graft/shunt implantation
Fibrinolytics	
Alteplase, recombinant (Activase) Reteplase (Retavase) Tenecteplase (TNKase) Urokinase (Abbokinase)	Facilitate clot dissolution Used to reopen occluded vessels in arterial and venous thrombosis

past, heparin preparations were also somewhat heterogeneous and contained various forms of compounds with heparin-like activity. In recent years, pharmacologists made efforts to chemically extract certain types of heparin from the more general (unfractionated) forms of this compound.[17] These efforts led to the extraction and clinical use of specific forms of heparin known as *low-molecular-weight heparins* (LMWHs). These agents are enoxaparin (Lovenox), dalteparin (Fragmin), tinzaparin (Innohep), and other drugs identified by the *-parin* suffix.

The LMWHs appear to be as effective as unfractionated (mixed) heparins, but they offer certain advantages. For example, LMWHs can be administered by subcutaneous injection into fat tissues, thereby decreasing the need for repeated IV administration. Subcutaneous administration offers an easier and more convenient route, especially for people who are being treated at home or as outpatients.[17] Dosing schedules of LMWHs are typically easier (usually once per day), compared to two or more daily injections of unfractioned heparin.[18]

In addition, the LMWHs preferentially inhibit factor Xa (the active form of clotting factor X) rather than thrombin or factor IXa.[16] As a result, the anticoagulant effects of LMWHs are also more predictable, and these agents tend to normalize clotting with less risk of adverse effects such as hemorrhage and heparin-induced thrombocytopenia (see "Adverse Effects of Anticoagulant Drugs" later in this chapter).[18,19] The more predictable response to LMWHs also decreases or eliminates the need for repeated laboratory monitoring of clotting time in most patients—that is, traditional laboratory tests such as partial thromboplastin time and international normalized ratio (INR) are not typically used to monitor clotting activity in patients treated with LMWHs because these tests measure thrombin activity, and LMWHs affect factor Xa rather than thrombin. If necessary, clotting factor X activity can be measured using alternative tests in patients who are at high risk for bleeding while receiving LMWHs.[20]

The use of traditional (unfractionated) heparin has therefore essentially been replaced by LMWHs in most patients requiring heparin treatment.[21] LMWHs are clearly safer and more convenient than their unfractionated counterparts, and these drugs have become a primary method of treating acute venous thrombosis.[14,15] LMWHs are now used routinely to prevent or treat deep vein thrombosis (DVT) following various types of surgery or medical conditions (e.g., ischemic stroke, cancer).[19,22] LMWHs may produce optimal effects if they are administered for more than a few days, and some patients who are at high risk for thrombosis may receive LMWHs via subcutaneous injection for several weeks following discharge from the hospital.[23,24] Future research will help determine the best way to use LMWHs to prevent or treat venous thrombosis in specific clinical situations.

Warfarin

Warfarin (Coumadin) is the primary drug used in the long-term prevention of venous thrombosis. The drug is a member of the coumarin derivatives group; however, warfarin is the only drug in this group still used commonly in the United States. Warfarin exerts its anticoagulant effects by interfering with vitamin K metabolism in the liver and thus impairing the hepatic synthesis of several clotting factors.[16] The role of vitamin K in clotting factor biosynthesis, and the way that warfarin and other coumarin drugs affect vitamin K metabolism, are illustrated in Figure 25-2.

In the liver, vitamin K acts as a catalyst in the final step of the synthesis of clotting factors II, VII, IX, and X. In the process, vitamin K is oxidized to an altered form known as *vitamin K epoxide*. For the process to continue, vitamin K epoxide must be reduced to its original form.[16] As shown in Figure 25-2, warfarin blocks the conversion of vitamin K epoxide to vitamin K, thus impairing the synthesis of several clotting factors. With time, a decrease in the level of circulating clotting factors results in a decrease in blood coagulation and in thrombogenesis.

Unlike heparin, the primary advantage of warfarin and other coumarin drugs is that they are administered orally.[25] However, because of the nature of their action, there is often a lag time of several days before the decreased production of clotting factors is sufficient to interrupt the clotting cascade and an anticoagulant effect is appreciated.[26] Consequently, anticoagulant

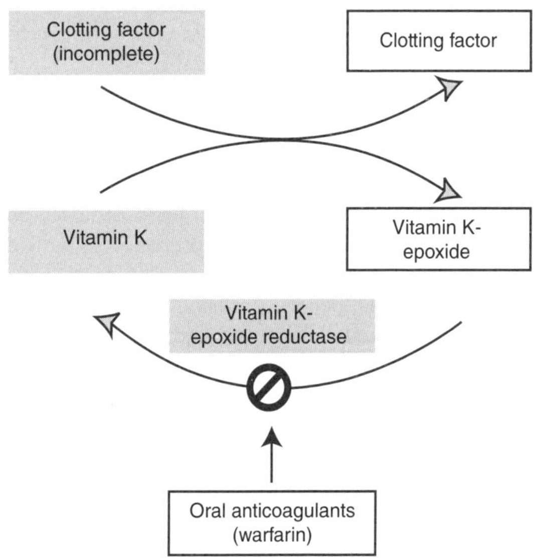

Figure ■ 25-2
Role of vitamin K in the synthesis of vitamin K–dependent clotting factors (II, VII, IX, and X). Vitamin K catalyzes the reaction necessary for completion of clotting factor synthesis, but it is oxidized in the process to vitamin K epoxide. Regeneration of vitamin K occurs via vitamin K epoxide reductase. Oral anticoagulants such as warfarin (Coumadin) block the regeneration of the vitamin K, thus halting further synthesis of the vitamin K–dependent factors.

therapy often begins with parenteral administration of heparin to achieve an immediate effect, followed by oral administration of warfarin.[27] Warfarin is then initiated, and heparin is discontinued after warfarin has had time to exert its anticoagulant effect. Oral administration of warfarin may then be continued for several weeks to 3 months or longer following an incident of thrombosis or pulmonary embolism.[8] However, patients on long-term warfarin therapy must typically be monitored periodically using standardized tests, such as prothrombin time and INR, to make sure clotting ability is in an acceptable range (e.g., an INR between 2 and 3).

Direct Thrombin Inhibitors

Certain drugs inhibit specific components in the clotting mechanism. For example, these drugs bind directly to the active site on thrombin and inhibit thrombin's ability to convert fibrinogen to fibrin.[28] The direct thrombin inhibitors include lepirudin (Refludan), dabigatran (Pradaxa), and several similar agents listed in Table 25-1. Although most of these agents must be administered parenterally (IV or subcutaneous injection), dabigatran is administered orally. Dabigatran is currently approved for preventing stroke and systemic embolism in patients with atrial fibrillation, but it may also be helpful in preventing other coagulation disorders, including DVT.[29,30]

Direct thrombin inhibitors offer an alternative to heparin, warfarin, and other traditional anticoagulant drugs. Preliminary evidence suggests that these drugs may be more effective than traditional drugs and may have an improved safety profile in terms of fewer side effects, less chance of drug-drug interactions, reduced risk of hemorrhagic stroke, and fewer adverse drug reactions such as heparin-induced thrombocytopenia.[26,31] As indicated, dabigatran is administered orally, thus adding to the convenience compared to heparins, which must be administered parenterally. Direct thrombin inhibitors have gained popularity as a primary method for treatment for thromboembolic disease, and future research will continue to clarify how these drugs can be used most effectively in preventing and treating clotting disorders.

Factor Xa Inhibitors

Factor Xa inhibitors directly affect the active form of this critical factor in the clotting cascade. Fondaparinux (Arixtra) was the first drug in this category. It can be administered by subcutaneous injection to prevent DVT following hip fractures, orthopedic procedures (e.g., hip, knee replacement), and other surgeries.[32,33] Fondaparinux first binds to antithrombin, which enhances the ability of antithrombin to selectively inactivate factor Xa. Studies suggest that fondaparinux may be more effective in preventing DVT than heparin (including LMWHs).[34] In addition, fondaparinux may be safer because it has a lower risk of causing heparin-induced thrombocytopenia.[35,36]

Oral factor Xa inhibitors, such as apixaban (Eliquis) and rivaroxaban (Xarelto), are available. These drugs appear to be a relatively safe, convenient, and effective way to treat venous thrombosis and other hypercoagulation disorders.[30] Hence, factor Xa inhibitors have gained acceptance as a primary way to prevent and treat DVT and other clotting problems, and their role as anticoagulants continues to expand in many clinical settings.

Adverse Effects of Anticoagulant Drugs

Predictably, hemorrhage is the primary and most serious problem with drugs used to decrease blood clotting.[26,37] Increased bleeding may occur with heparin and warfarin, and this bleeding may be quite severe in some patients. The risk of hemorrhage may be somewhat lower with the newer drugs such as the direct thrombin inhibitors and factor Xa inhibitors, but the possibility of increased bleeding cannot be ignored, especially in cases of overdose or if the metabolism of these drugs is reduced and their effects are prolonged (e.g., patients with renal disease).[38]

Consequently, any unusual bleeding, such as blood in the urine or stools; bleeding gums; unexplained nosebleeds; or an unusually heavy menstrual flow may indicate a problem. Also, back pain or joint pain may be an indication of abdominal or intrajoint hemorrhage, respectively. To prevent excessive bleeding, laboratory tests that measure hemostasis are sometimes used to monitor the patients. As indicated earlier, patients on long-term warfarin treatment are monitored routinely. Routine testing is not usually required for the newer drugs such as the LMWHs, direct thrombin inhibitors, and factor Xa inhibitors. However, specific tests may be performed on patients taking these newer drugs if bleeding or other problems occur, and adjustments in drug dosage are based on whether coagulation time falls within an acceptable range.[38]

Heparin may also produce a decrease in platelets (thrombocytopenia) in some patients.[39] This condition, known commonly as *heparin-induced thrombocytopenia* (HIT), is less common with LMWHs versus unfractionated heparin, but HIT can occur with any type of heparin treatment.[40] Heparin-induced thrombocytopenia can be asymptomatic and resolve spontaneously (type I HIT), or it can be severe (type II HIT). Type II HIT is mediated by an immune reaction, which can lead to serious complications, including *increased* thrombosis in vascular tissues throughout the body.[41,42] Development of type II HIT is therefore an emergency situation typically resolved by discontinuing heparin and substituting a nonheparin anticoagulant (e.g., a direct thrombin inhibitor).[42] Finally, oral anticoagulants may produce some GI distress (nausea, stomach cramps, diarrhea), and skin reactions, including dermal necrosis, may occur in rare cases.

Antiplateiet Drugs

Whereas anticoagulants affect the synthesis and function of specific clotting factors, antiplatelet drugs prevent excessive clotting caused by increased platelet activity.[43,44] In the bloodstream, platelets normally respond to vascular injury by changing their shape and adhering to one another (aggregation) at the site of clot formation. However, platelets may sometimes aggregate inappropriately, thus forming a thrombus and occluding certain blood vessels. In particular, arterial thrombi are often formed by abnormal platelet aggregation, especially in arteries with atherosclerotic plaques that rupture suddenly and initiate platelet clotting at the rupture site.[45] Hence, antiplatelet drugs are primarily used to prevent the formation of arterial clots, such as those that cause coronary artery occlusion or cerebral infarction. Specific antiplatelet drugs include aspirin, adenosine diphosphate (ADP) receptor blockers, and glycoprotein IIb-IIIa receptor blockers.

Aspirin

Aspirin suppresses platelet aggregation by inhibiting the synthesis of prostaglandins and thromboxanes.[46,47] As discussed in Chapter 15, aspirin exerts virtually all of its effects by inhibiting the cyclooxygenase enzyme that initiates the synthesis of lipidlike hormones known as *prostaglandins* and *thromboxanes*. Certain prostaglandins and thromboxanes, especially thromboxane A2, have a potent ability to induce platelet aggregation. By inhibiting the synthesis of these proaggregation substances, aspirin prevents platelet-induced thrombus formation.

Although the exact dose may vary in specific clinical situations, patients typically experience a meaningful antiplatelet and antithrombotic effect at very low aspirin doses. For example, many antithrombotic regimens suggest a daily dosage between 75 and 325 mg/d.[16,48] Considering that an adult aspirin tablet typically contains 325 mg of drug, these antithrombotic dosages represent taking the equivalent of one tablet or less each day. A pediatric (baby) aspirin tablet typically contains 81 mg of drug, and many patients achieve adequate antithrombotic effects with one baby aspirin tablet each day. Antithrombotic effects can be achieved at these remarkably low doses because aspirin inhibits platelet function irreversibly.[46] That is, when aspirin reaches a given platelet, that platelet is inhibited for the remainder of its life span (about 7 to 8 days).

Because of its antiplatelet effects, aspirin has received a great deal of attention regarding its use in treating and preventing myocardial infarction. During the acute phase of an infarction, aspirin is critical in helping to limit the progression of platelet-induced occlusion, thereby reducing the extent of damage to the myocardium.[49,50] Following the acute phase, aspirin is often administered for prolonged periods to maintain coronary artery patency and prevent reinfarction.[49] Also, low doses of aspirin may decrease the incidence of an initial infarction in susceptible individuals—that is, people who have not yet sustained an infarction but have one or more risk factors for coronary artery disease.[48,50]

These rather remarkable findings have prompted a great deal of debate about the chronic use of aspirin and possible side effects such as increased hemorrhage. In particular, the incidence of intracranial hemorrhage (hemorrhagic stroke) may be increased when aspirin is administered to decrease thrombosis.[51] Nonetheless, aspirin is considered standard therapy during the acute phase of myocardial infarction, and prolonged use of aspirin is one of the primary pharmacological methods used to prevent reinfarction.

Although aspirin increases the risk of hemorrhagic stroke, the drug may help prevent the type of stroke caused by cerebral ischemia and infarction.[52,53] The rationale is that aspirin will prevent infarction in cerebral vessels in the same manner that it prevents coronary infarction in heart attacks. Clearly, the use of aspirin must be limited to the types of stroke that result from insufficient blood flow, as opposed to hemorrhagic stroke.[50] Even so, the antithrombotic benefits of aspirin in some cerebral vessels must be weighed against the possible side effects such as increased bleeding in other vessels. Hence, aspirin therapy is probably beneficial to a certain percentage of stroke patients but should be used selectively.[54]

Consequently, there seems to be little doubt that aspirin can be a very cost-effective method for decreasing the morbidity and mortality associated with myocardial and cerebral infarction. Nonetheless, the long-term effects of aspirin on other organs such as the liver, kidneys, and GI tract must be considered. In addition, the therapeutic effects of low-dose aspirin therapy vary substantially from person to person, and some people may appear resistant to aspirin's antithrombotic effects.[55] Although the reasons are not clear, the antithrombotic effects of low-dose aspirin therapy may also differ between men and women—men experience greater protection against heart attack and women experience greater protection against ischemic stroke.[56] The emergence of newer antiplatelet drugs (discussed below) and the use of newer anticoagulants addressed earlier in this chapter have called into question whether aspirin is the most effective way to treat certain types of platelet-induced clots.[57] Hence, continued analysis of this topic promises to be an exciting and productive area of pharmacological research.

Finally, aspirin has also been used to prevent thrombus formation in peripheral veins (DVT), and aspirin is sometimes used as an adjunct or alternative to anticoagulants (heparin, warfarin) that are routinely used to treat DVT.[58] In addition, aspirin can be administered alone or with other antiplatelet drugs to prevent thromboembolism following surgical procedures such as coronary artery bypass, arterial grafts, endarterectomy, and valve replacement.[59,60] By preventing platelet-induced thrombogenesis, aspirin helps maintain patency and prevent reocclusion of vessels following these procedures.

It follows that aspirin is a primary antithrombotic agent with several important indications involving platelet-induced clots. This drug, however, is only a relatively weak inhibitor of platelet activity.[46] As indicated, aspirin may also increase the risk of intracranial hemorrhage and may be poorly tolerated in some patients due to gastric irritation, an allergic response, and so forth.[51,61] Researchers have therefore made progress in developing antiplatelet drugs that are stronger and safer than aspirin, and these drugs are addressed next.

ADP Receptor Blockers

Drugs that inhibit the adenosine diphosphate (ADP) receptor on the platelet membrane have proven to be an effective antiplatelet intervention.[46,62] ADP is a chemical signal that increases platelet activity, and platelet-induced clotting is reduced by drugs that inhibit the receptor for this compound.[62] Such drugs include clopidogrel (Plavix), prasugrel (Effient), and ticlopidine (Ticlid). These drugs are used primarily to prevent thrombosis in patients at risk for myocardial infarction or ischemic stroke, including patients with unstable angina, acute coronary syndrome, atrial fibrillation, and similar conditions (see Table 25-1). These drugs are also used to prevent infarction following percutaneous coronary angioplasty, placement of a coronary artery stent, and other surgical procedures.

ADP inhibitors produce moderate inhibition of platelet activity, making them somewhat more effective than aspirin but not as strong as the GP IIb-IIIa inhibitors (discussed below).[46] ADP inhibitors such as clopidogrel (Plavix) can also be added to low-dose aspirin therapy, and this "dual antiplatelet" strategy has been advocated for treatment after certain cardiac surgeries such as stent implantation and in other cases where aspirin alone does not provide adequate antithrombotic effects.[63,64] Combining aspirin with clopidogrel, however, has also raised concerns about an increased risk of bleeding, and researchers continue to study whether dual antiplatelet therapy can be used safely and effectively in specific clinical situations.[64]

ADP receptor inhibitors seem to be well tolerated, although the individual response to these drugs may vary considerably from patient to patient. In particular, up to 30 percent of patients may not respond adequately to clopidogrel, and one of the other ADP inhibitors (i.e., prasugrel or ticlopidine) may be preferred in these patients.[65]

Glycoprotein IIb-IIIa Receptor Blockers

Another antiplatelet strategy that has shown considerable promise is the use of drugs that inhibit the ability of fibrinogen and other chemical mediators to activate platelets.[46,66] These drugs are known as *glycoprotein (GP) IIb-IIIa inhibitors* because they block (antagonize) the GP receptor on the platelet membrane that is stimulated by fibrinogen and other chemical mediators.[66] Fibrinogen is unable to bind to the platelet, thereby decreasing platelet activation and reducing platelet-induced clotting.[67] Agents that are currently available include abciximab (ReoPro), eptifibatide (Integrilin), and tirofiban (Aggrastat) (see Table 25-1).[68]

GP IIb-IIIa inhibitors are the most powerful inhibitors of platelet activity,[67] and they are used primarily to prevent thrombosis in patients undergoing balloon angioplasty and other percutaneous coronary interventions that help reestablish coronary artery blood flow in patients with acute coronary syndromes.[69,70] GP IIb-IIIa inhibitors are administered intravenously before and during such procedures to help maintain coronary flow and decrease mortality, especially in people at high risk for reinfarction.[71] These drugs are often combined with other antithrombotics (e.g., heparin, aspirin, bivalirudin) during the procedure. The GP IIb-IIIa inhibitors are usually discontinued soon after the procedure, and the other antithrombotics are used to maintain coronary blood flow and prevent reinfarction.[72]

Other Antiplatelet Drugs

Dipyridamole (Persantine, other names) is another antiplatelet drug that is typically used in combination with aspirin to decrease platelet-induced clotting.[73] This drug may affect platelet function by impairing adenosine metabolism or by increasing the concentration of cyclic adenosine monophosphate within the platelet.[16] The exact mechanism of dipyridamole, however, is poorly understood, and the beneficial effects of this drug may actually be related to its ability to scavenge free radicals and decrease inflammation in vascular tissues.[74] Although it is not used as commonly as other antiplatelet drugs, dipyridamole has shown benefits in preventing ischemic stroke and myocardial infarction.[73,75] When combined with aspirin, dipyridamole provides greater benefits compared to using either drug alone.[73] Hence, dipyridamole is a potential alternative or adjunct to other antiplatelet agents (e.g., aspirin, ADP receptor inhibitors) in treating arterial thrombosis.

Finally, practitioners use cilostazol (Pletal) and pentoxifylline (Trental) primarily to reduce the symptoms of intermittent claudication in patients with peripheral arterial disease.[76] These drugs both decrease the breakdown of cAMP in platelets, thereby increasing intracellular cAMP levels. Increased cAMP in the platelet decreases platelet activity and aggregation, and this effect helps maintain blood flow through peripheral vessels. These drugs may also produce beneficial effects that are not related to platelet activity, such as increased erythrocyte flexibility and decreased blood viscosity.[77] Use of these drugs has therefore been reported to decrease leg pain and increase walking distance in people with intermittent claudication.[76] Ideally, these drugs should be combined with a supervised program of walking exercises to produce optimal improvements in patients with intermittent claudication.[78]

Adverse Effects of Antiplatelet Drugs

The primary concern with aspirin and other antiplatelet drugs is an increased risk of bleeding. Patients taking these agents should be especially alert for any unexplained or heavy bleeding or any other symptoms that might indicate hemorrhage (sudden increases in joint or back pain, severe headaches, etc.). Aspirin can also cause gastric irritation, and high doses of it may be toxic to the liver and kidneys (see Chapter 15). However, the likelihood of severe gastric disturbances and liver or renal toxicity is relatively low at the doses needed to create an antithrombotic effect. Other potential side effects of nonaspirin antiplatelet drugs include hypotension for the GP IIb-IIIa inhibitors (abciximab, eptifibatide, tirofiban), GI distress for clopidogrel and dipyridamole, and blood dyscrasias (neutropenia, agranulocytosis, thrombocytopenia) for ticlopidine.

Fibrinolytics

Fibrinolytic drugs facilitate the breakdown and dissolution of clots that have already formed. These drugs work by converting plasminogen (profibrinolysin) to plasmin (fibrinolysin).[79] As shown in Figure 25-1, plasmin is the active form of an endogenous enzyme that breaks down fibrin, the primary component of a clot. Fibrinolytics activate this enzyme by various mechanisms, thus helping to break down the fibrin. This effect helps dissolve clots that have already formed, thus reopening occluded blood vessels.

Fibrinolytic drugs are extremely valuable in treating acute myocardial infarction.[80,81] When administered at infarction onset, these drugs can reestablish blood flow through occluded coronary vessels, often preventing or reversing myocardial damage, which decreases the morbidity and mortality normally associated with a heart attack.[80] The drugs can help reopen occluded coronary vessels when administered up to 12 hours after symptom onset.[82] Fibrinolytics seem to produce the best results when they are administered much sooner after the symptom onset. For example, administration within 1 hour after symptom onset can result in a 50 percent reduction in mortality in patients with acute myocardial infarction.[83]

Hence, considerable efforts have been made to minimize the time between diagnosis of an infarction and administration of a fibrinolytic drug. This so-called door-to-needle time represents the shortest possible delay between when the patient arrives at the hospital and is correctly administered a fibrinolytic agent.[84] In fact, it might be possible in some situations to administer the fibrinolytic drug while the patient is in route to the hospital—that is, emergency medical technicians might be directed to begin drug administration when they first encounter the patient or in the ambulance to further save time and restore perfusion in a timely manner.[85] This idea has obvious benefits in rural geographic areas where it takes considerable time to transport the patient to the hospital. Consequently, fibrinolytic agents are typically administered as soon as possible after an acute myocardial infarction to achieve optimal results.

It was originally believed that these drugs had to be administered directly into the coronary arteries to reopen occluded coronary vessels.[86] However, it is now realized that these drugs will produce beneficial effects when injected intravenously into the systemic circulation; the drug can be injected into any accessible vein and eventually reach the coronary clot through the general circulation.[16] The IV route is a much more practical method of administration because it is easier, faster, and safer than the intracoronary route.

Intracranial hemorrhage and other bleeding problems are the primary drawbacks to fibrinolytic treatment because these drugs can also stimulate clot breakdown in other vessels, including the cerebral vasculature.[87] Fibrinolytics are therefore contraindicated in certain situations, including patients with a history of hemorrhagic stroke, intracranial neoplasm, active internal bleeding, possible aortic dissection, and several other factors representing the increased risk of hemorrhage.[80] Also, fibrinolytic therapy may not be curative, and reocclusion occurs in certain patients.

Fibrinolytic agents may also be used to treat specific cases of ischemic stroke.[88,89] Although the risk of intracranial hemorrhage remains a concern, fibrinolytic treatment can be used carefully in selected patients to dissolve clots within cerebral vessels and allow reperfusion of the brain, thus limiting the amount of damage from the infarction.[90] The window of opportunity for administration, however, is smaller when treating ischemic stroke compared to myocardial infarction, and fibrinolytic agents must typically be administered within 3 hours after cerebral infarction.[91] Also, certain fibrinolytics, such as recombinant tissue plasminogen activator (see below), may be better than other fibrinolytics when treating ischemic stroke.[89] Nonetheless, fibrinolytic treatment is regarded as an important option for patients who are experiencing an ischemic stroke and who have minimal risk factors for intracranial or systemic hemorrhage.

Fibrinolytic drugs are sometimes used to treat other types of arterial and venous occlusion. For example, fibrinolytic therapy can help dissolve clots in peripheral arteries (femoral, popliteal, etc.)[92] and can help resolve thrombus formation in the large veins (DVT).[93] This treatment is especially helpful during severe, limb-threatening occlusion or when surgical removal of the thrombus is not possible.[93] To minimize the risk of side effects, fibrinolytic drugs can be administered directly to the site of the clot through an intravascular catheter.[93,94]

Fibrinolytics may also play a role in treating acute, massive pulmonary embolism (PE).[95] Use of these drugs in PE is typically reserved for life-threatening situations, especially when the PE is so severe that function of the right ventricle is compromised.[96] Bypass grafts and shunts that have become occluded because of clot formation may also be cleaned out with fibrinolytic drug use.[97]

The most common fibrinolytic agents are listed below. Although these drugs differ chemically, they all ultimately activate fibrinolysis in some way. There has been considerable debate about which agent provides optimal long-term benefits following myocardial infarction. With regard to myocardial infarction, these agents are fairly similar in terms of efficacy and safety profile.[80] Making sure that the agent is used in a timely fashion is probably more important than the actual type of fibrinolytic agent.[98] Some of the newer agents can be administered by rapid (bolus) infusion and may therefore help decrease the time between when a patient is recognized as having an infarction and when meaningful amounts of the drug are able to reach the clot.[99] The relative benefits and unique aspects of each agent are presented here.

Streptokinase and Urokinase

Streptokinase was the first fibrinolytic agent and was developed originally from a protein produced by streptococcal bacteria. Urokinase is an enzyme produced by the human kidneys. Both of these agents activate plasmin but use somewhat different methods to bring about this activation. Streptokinase indirectly activates plasmin (fibrinolysin) by binding to the precursor molecule plasminogen (profibrinolysin) and facilitating activation by endogenous mechanisms. Urokinase directly converts plasminogen to plasmin by enzymatically cleaving a peptide bond within the plasminogen molecule. Both agents have been used successfully to resolve acute clot formation in coronary arteries and peripheral vessels. Streptokinase, however, has been largely replaced by newer agents (discussed below) and is therefore no longer marketed in the United States.

Likewise, a fibrinolytic product containing streptokinase combined with human plasminogen (anistreplase) is also no longer available in the United States.

Tissue Plasminogen Activator

In the endogenous control of hemostasis, plasminogen is activated by an intrinsic substance known as tissue plasminogen activator (t-PA) (see Fig. 25-1). Intravenous administration of t-PA rapidly and effectively initiates clot breakdown by directly activating plasmin (fibrinolysin). Extraction of t-PA from human blood is costly and impractical, but synthesis of t-PA is possible through the use of recombinant DNA techniques. Consequently, recombinant t-PA (rt-PA; also known by the generic name *alteplase*) is now available in commercial forms (Activase), and this agent has emerged as one of the primary fibrinolytic agents.

Tissue plasminogen activator has been used successfully to treat acute myocardial infarction, and the benefits of this treatment are well documented.[80,100] This drug, however, does not seem to be superior to other fibrinolytics when treating coronary artery thrombosis, and other drugs may be more cost-effective in treating myocardial infarction. Alternatively, rt-PA may be more effective than other fibrinolytics in its ability to initially reopen cerebral vessels; this drug is often used preferentially during ischemic stroke.[101,102]

Reteplase and Tenecteplase

Reteplase (Retavase) and tenecteplase (TNKase) are newer fibrinolytics. These agents are derived from human tissue plasminogen activator and therefore have actions similar to t-PA (alteplase).[80] Each drug, however, has an amino acid sequence that differs slightly from alteplase, hence they have certain pharmacological advantages over alteplase. In particular, these drugs can be given by more rapid (bolus) infusion; tenecteplase is typically administered by a single bolus injection, and reteplase is given by two bolus injections 30 minutes apart. Consequently, these drugs can be administered faster and more easily than other fibrinolytics that need to be infused slowly over several hours.[16] These newer agents, however, have generally not shown to be superior to alteplase or more traditional agents (streptokinase, urokinase) in terms of fibrinolytic efficacy.[71,80] On the other hand, tenecteplase may be somewhat superior to alteplase and reteplase in terms of having more prolonged effects due to its longer half-life, and it may also be more specific for activating plasminogen that is bound to clots rather than plasminogen that is circulating throughout the systemic vasculature.[99] As a result, tenecteplase may be associated with a lower risk of major bleeds and intracranial hemorrhage, and it has emerged as a preferred fibrinolytic option in many clinical situations.

Adverse Effects of Fibrinolytics

Hemorrhage is the major adverse effect associated with fibrinolytic agents. As indicated, intracranial hemorrhage may occur following fibrinolytic therapy, especially in patients who have predisposing risk factors such as advanced age, severe or untreated hypertension, or a history of hemorrhagic stroke.[103] GI bleeds can also occur, and patients may also experience bleeding gums, nosebleeds, and unusual or excessive bruising. Excessive bleeding may also occur during dressing changes, wound care, and other invasive procedures following fibrinolytic treatment. Fibrinolytic drugs may cause other side effects such as itching, nausea, and headache, and they can produce allergic reactions, including anaphylaxis, in susceptible individuals.

TREATMENT OF CLOTTING DEFICIENCIES

Hemophilia

Hemophilia is a hereditary disease in which an individual is unable to synthesize adequate amounts of a specific clotting factor. The two most common forms of hemophilia are hemophilia A, which is caused by deficiency of clotting factor VIII, and hemophilia B, which is a deficit in clotting factor IX.[104] In either form of this disease, patients are missing adequate amounts of a key clotting factor and have problems maintaining normal hemostasis. Even trivial injuries can produce serious or fatal hemorrhage. Also, patients with hemophilia often develop joint problems because of intra-articular hemorrhage (hemarthrosis).

Treatment of hemophilia consists of replacing the missing clotting factor. Depending on the severity of the disease, clotting factors can be administered on a regular basis (prophylaxis) or during an acute hemorrhagic episode.[105,106] Although this treatment seems relatively straightforward, obtaining sufficient amounts of the missing factor is a very costly procedure. At present, the primary source of clotting factors

VIII and IX is human blood extract. Obtaining an adequate supply can cost $40,000 to $50,000 per patient per year.

A more serious problem is the potential for clotting factor extract to contain viruses such as HIV or hepatitis B. The lack of proper blood screening has resulted in tragic consequences; for example, clotting factors extracted from patients infected with HIV have served as a vehicle for viral transmission to patients with hemophilia. More stringent screening procedures and other techniques such as heat treatment of clotting factor extracts have decreased the risk of transmission, but patients with hemophilia receiving exogenous factors remain at risk for viral infection.

New methods of drug production, such as genetic engineering and recombinant DNA techniques, are currently being used to manufacture specific clotting factors such as factors VIII and IX.[105,107,108] These techniques now offer a safer and more reliable source of missing clotting factors for patients with hemophilia and other disorders related to clotting factor deficiencies. However, certain patients receiving manufactured clotting factors can develop inhibitory antibodies (alloantibodies) that neutralize the clotting factor and render it ineffective.[109,110] Fortunately, alloantibody inhibitors such as rituximab have also been developed that can be administered to patients producing these antibodies, thus restoring the clotting factor activity.[110,111] Researchers continue to identify how clotting factor replacement can be used most effectively in patients with hemophilia and how production of alloantibodies can be avoided or managed in susceptible patients.

Deficiencies of Vitamin K-Dependent Clotting Factors

As indicated earlier in this chapter, the liver needs adequate amounts of vitamin K to synthesize clotting factors II, VII, IX, and X. As shown in Figure 25-2, vitamin K catalyzes the final steps in the synthesis of these factors. Normally, vitamin K is supplied through the diet or synthesized by intestinal bacteria and subsequently absorbed from the GI tract into the body. However, any defect in vitamin K ingestion, synthesis, or absorption may result in vitamin K deficiency. Insufficient vitamin K in the body results in an inadequate hepatic synthesis of the clotting factors listed previously, thus resulting in poor hemostasis and excessive bleeding.

Deficiencies in vitamin K and the related synthesis of the vitamin K–dependent clotting factors are treated by administering exogenous vitamin K.[16] Various commercial forms of this vitamin are available for oral or parenteral (intramuscular or subcutaneous) administration. Specifically, individuals with a poor diet, intestinal disease, or impaired intestinal absorption may require vitamin K to maintain proper hemostasis.

Vitamin K is routinely administered to newborn infants to prevent hemorrhage[112,113] and facilitate clotting factor synthesis. For the first 5 to 8 days following birth, newborns lack the intestinal bacteria necessary to help synthesize vitamin K. Finally, vitamin K can be administered to accelerate clotting factor production when clotting time is excessively long (e.g., INR between 4.5 and 10).[114] Specifically, patients with delayed blood clotting due to excess warfarin levels can be administered vitamin K either orally or by parenteral routes to help reestablish normal clotting time.[115]

Antifibrinolytics

The excessive bleeding that sometimes occurs following surgery, trauma, or advanced cancer may be caused by an overactive fibrinolytic system, or *hyperfibrinolysis*.[116,117] Hyperfibrinolysis results in excessive clot destruction and ineffective hemostasis. Patients with hemophilia who undergo surgery, including dental procedures (tooth extractions, restorations, etc.), will benefit if clot breakdown is inhibited because hemorrhage and the need for additional clotting factors are reduced. Antifibrinolytic agents, such as aminocaproic acid (Amicar) and tranexamic acid (Cyklokapron), are often used in these situations.[118-120] These drugs appear to inhibit activation of plasminogen (profibrinolysin) to plasmin (fibrinolysin). Plasmin is the enzyme responsible for breaking down fibrin clots (see Fig. 25-1). Antifibrinolytics prevent the activation of this enzyme, thus preserving clot formation.

Aminocaproic acid and tranexamic acid are administered either orally or intravenously for the acute treatment of hyperfibrinolysis or to prevent clot breakdown in patients with hemophilia who are undergoing surgery. Some adverse effects such as nausea, diarrhea, dizziness, and headache may occur when these drugs are administered, but these problems are relatively minor and usually disappear when the drug is discontinued.

AGENTS USED TO TREAT HYPERLIPIDEMIA

Hyperlipidemia, an abnormally high concentration of lipids in the bloodstream, is one of the primary causes of cardiovascular disease in industrialized nations. This condition typically causes deposition of fatty plaquelike lesions on the walls of large and medium-sized arteries (*atherosclerosis*), which can lead to thrombosis and infarction. Hence, elevated plasma lipids are related to some of the events discussed previously in this chapter because atherosclerosis can precipitate increased clotting and thromboembolic disease.

Hyperlipidemia is often caused by poor diet and lifestyle and by several genetic and metabolic conditions that cause disorders in lipid metabolism.[121-123] It is not possible to review the endogenous control of lipid metabolism or the various pathological processes involved in hyperlipidemia here—these topics are addressed in other sources.[124-126] It should be realized, however, that lipids such as cholesterol are transported in the bloodstream as part of a lipid-protein complex known as a *lipoprotein*. Certain lipoproteins are considered beneficial because they may decrease the formation of atherosclerotic plaques by removing cholesterol from the arterial wall. These beneficial complexes are known as high-density lipoproteins (HDLs) because of the relatively large amount of protein in the complex. Other lipoproteins are considered harmful because they transport and deposit cholesterol on the arterial wall. These atherogenic lipoproteins include intermediate-density lipoproteins (IDLs), low-density lipoproteins (LDLs), and very-low-density lipoproteins (VLDLs). Pharmacological and nonpharmacological strategies to reduce hyperlipidemia typically focus on reducing these atherogenic lipoproteins and increasing the beneficial HDLs.

Drugs used to treat hyperlipidemia are summarized in Table 25-2 and are discussed briefly below. Practitioners typically administer these agents when plasma lipid levels are unsuccessfully controlled by nonpharmacological methods such as low-fat diets, weight reduction, regular exercise, and smoking cessation.[127-129] However, these drugs can be used in conjunction with nonpharmacological methods, and optimal results are often realized through a combination of drug therapy and various dietary and lifestyle modifications.[130]

HMG-CoA Reductase Inhibitors (Statins)

This category includes atorvastatin (Lipitor), rosuvastatin (Crestor), and similar drugs listed in Table 25-2.These drugs, known commonly as **statins**, are characterized by their ability to inhibit 3-hydroxy-3-methylglutaryl coenzyme A (HMG-CoA) reductase.[131] This enzyme catalyzes one of the early steps of cholesterol synthesis, and drugs that inhibit HMG-CoA reductase decrease cholesterol production, especially in liver cells. Decreased hepatic cholesterol biosynthesis also causes more surface receptors for LDL cholesterol to be synthesized; this increase in surface receptors triggers an increase in the breakdown of LDL cholesterol and a decrease in the synthesis of VLDL, which serves as a precursor for LDL synthesis.[132] HMG-CoA reductase inhibitors can also decrease triglyceride levels to some extent[131] and can produce a modest increase in HDL levels.[133] However, the exact reasons for the beneficial effects on triglycerides and HDL levels are not entirely clear.

Furthermore, HMG-CoA reductase inhibitors may produce several favorable effects that are independent of their ability to affect plasma lipid levels.[131] It appears that certain by-products of cholesterol metabolism act directly on the vasculature or influence the production of other chemical signals that adversely affect cellular function in various tissues.[134] Increased production of these by-products could therefore influence a variety of pathological conditions. By controlling the production of these by-products, statins may produce a range of beneficial effects beyond their ability to improve plasma lipids.

Statins, for example, may increase the production and vasodilating effects of nitric oxide, which can directly benefit the vascular endothelium, and they may help stabilize atherosclerotic plaques on the arterial wall.[135,136] These drugs may also have anti-inflammatory and antioxidant effects that contribute to their ability to improve the vascular wall's function.[137,138] Statins' ability to reduce the risk of cardiovascular disease is probably the result of a combination of their favorable effects on plasma lipids combined with their ability to improve the function of the vascular endothelium.

Statins are helpful in decreasing morbidity and mortality in people with high cholesterol, as well as individuals who have normal cholesterol but other risk factors for cardiovascular disease.[139,140] It is estimated that these drugs decrease the risk of a major cardiac event by up to 50 percent, with the magnitude of these beneficial effects depending on the extent that cholesterol is reduced and the influence of other risk factors.[141,142] Hence, statins are now regarded as a mainstay

Table 25-2
DRUGS USED TO TREAT HYPERLIPIDEMIA

Generic Name	Trade Name(s)	Dosage*	Primary Effect
Statins			
Atorvastatin	Lipitor	10–80 mg once each day	Statins generally decrease total cholesterol and plasma LDL-C. Specific drugs may also increase HDL-C and decrease triglycerides.
Fluvastatin	Lescol	20–40 mg once each day in the evening	
Lovastatin	Mevacor, others	20–80 mg each day as a single dose or in divided doses with meals	
Pitavastatin	Livalo	2–4 mg once each day	
Pravastatin	Pravachol	10–40 mg once each day at bedtime	
Rosuvastatin	Crestor	5–40 mg once each day	
Simvastatin	Zocor	5–40 mg once each day in the evening	
Fibric Acids			
Fenofibrate	Fibricor, Tricor, others	45–200 mg once each day**	Fibrates typically decrease triglyceride levels and VLDL-C Some increase in HDL-C may also occur
Gemfibrozil	Lopid	1.2 g each day in 2 divided doses, 30 min before morning and evening meal	
Bile Acid Binding Drugs			
Cholestyramine	Questran, others	4 g 2–6 times each day before meals and at bedtime	These drugs decrease total cholesterol and LDL-C
Colestipol	Colestid	Granules: 5–30 mg per day in 1 or 2 doses Tablets: 2–16 mg per day in 1 or 2 doses	
Colesevelam	Welchol	3.75 g per day in 1 or 2 doses	
Others			
Niacin	Niacor, Niaspan, others	1–2 g 3 times each day (up to 8 g per day)	Lowers total cholesterol, triglycerides, LDL-C, and VLDL-C Increases HDL-C
Ezetimibe	Ezetrol, Zetia	10 mg once each day	Lowers total cholesterol, LDL-C, and triglycerides Increases HDL-C levels

**Doses represent typical adult oral maintenance dose.*
***Doses vary according to specific derivatives of fenofibric acid.*
HDL-C = high-density lipoprotein cholesterol; LDL-C = low-density lipoprotein cholesterol; VLDL-C = very low-density lipoprotein cholesterol.

in treating cardiovascular disease, and research is ongoing to determine the optimal dose of these drugs and how they can be used with other pharmacological and nonpharmacological interventions in cardiovascular disease.[130,139] Statins may even have anticancer effects, and investigators continue to explore their potential in preventing and treating certain malignancies.[143,144]

Fibric Acids

Fibric acids or "fibrates" include fenofibrate and gemfibrozil (see Table 25-2). These drugs primarily decrease triglyceride levels and are therefore most helpful in hyperlipidemias that are characterized by increased triglycerides.[145,146] Fibrates also produce beneficial increases in HDL production and can help lower LDL levels.[147,148] Fibrates are therefore helpful in treating a combination of lipid abnormalities (i.e., mixed hyperlipidemias) that include increased triglycerides and LDL levels along with low HDL levels.[147,149]

The exact mechanism of these drugs is unclear, but they probably work by binding to a specific nuclear receptor known as the *peroxisome proliferator activated receptor*.[146] This receptor, found primarily in the liver and adipose tissues, affects the transcription of genes that affect lipid metabolism.[150] By activating a specific type of this receptor (the alpha subtype), fibrates mediate several changes at the nuclear level that ultimately cause a decrease in triglycerides and other beneficial changes in plasma lipid metabolism.[151] In a manner similar to the statins, fibrates may also exert anti-inflammatory, antioxidant, and other beneficial effects in addition to their positive effects on plasma lipids.[146,152]

Although it is not exactly clear how much these agents can reduce the risk of a major cardiac event (e.g., infarction, stroke), these drugs will probably remain the first choice for people with certain hyperlipidemias (e.g., increased triglycerides). These drugs are also advocated for mixed hyperlipidemias that are common in metabolic disorders, such as type 2 diabetes mellitus (see Chapter 32).[148] Certain fibrates can be used with other drugs, such as statins or niacin, to provide more comprehensive pharmacological control of certain lipid disorders.[153,154] Such combinations, however, should be used carefully to prevent an increased risk of adverse neuromuscular effects such as myositis and rhabdomyolysis (see "Adverse Effects of Antihyperlipidemia Agents").

Other Lipid-Lowering Agents

Several other agents have beneficial effects on plasma lipid profiles occurring through various cellular mechanisms (see Table 25-2).[126] For example, several drugs are now available that attach to bile acids within the GI lumen and increase the fecal excretion of these acids. This action leads to decreased plasma cholesterol concentrations because cholesterol breakdown is accelerated to replace the bile acids that are lost in the feces. These bile-acid binding drugs include cholestyramine (Questran), colesevelam (Welchol), and colestipol (Colestid). Although these agents are not used routinely, they may be helpful in lowering LDL levels in certain patients.[155] These drugs may also have some ability to regulate glucose metabolism, although the reasons for this are not clear.[156] Hence, they may also be considered as part of the treatment for certain patients with type 2 diabetes mellitus (see Chapter 32).

Niacin (nicotinic acid, vitamin B3, Niaspan, other names) has received considerable attention as a "broad spectrum" antilipidemic because this drug produces beneficial effects on virtually all aspects of the lipid profile.[157,158] That is, high doses of niacin (several grams each day) help decrease LDL and triglyceride levels while raising HDL levels.[158,159] This drug apparently binds to a specific nicotinic acid receptor (i.e., the GPR109A receptor) in fat cells and initiates several metabolic effects, including decreased lipolysis and reduced entry of fatty acids into the bloodstream.[160] Niacin also may be used in combination with statins to produce optimal benefits in certain patients without increasing the risk of statin-induced myopathy.[161]

Finally, ezetimibe (Zetia) inhibits cholesterol absorption from the GI tract.[162,163] This action primarily results in decreased LDL-cholesterol levels, although a modest increase in HDL may also occur.[162] Ezetimibe seems especially useful in complementing the effects of the statin drugs, and it can be combined safely with a statin to produce optimal benefits in many patients.[164,165] Additional drugs limiting cholesterol absorption may ultimately be developed as part of the treatment against hyperlipidemia.

Adverse Effects of Antihyperlipidemic Agents

Most of the drugs used to treat hyperlipidemia are well tolerated. Some GI distress (nausea, diarrhea) is common with most of the drugs, but these problems are usually minor and do not require the discontinuation of drug therapy.

Other bothersome side effects are related to specific agents. Niacin, for instance, is often associated with cutaneous vasodilation and a sensation of warmth when doses are administered, but administering an extended-release form of this drug or administering niacin with a drug that blocks flushing (laropiprant) can reduce these sensations.[166,167] Some fairly serious problems, including liver dysfunction, gallstones, and pancreatitis, can occur with many antihyperlipidemic drugs, but the incidence of these side effects is rare. Cardiovascular problems such as arrhythmias, blood dyscrasias, and angioneurotic syndrome may also occur with fibric acids.

Neuromuscular problems have been noted with certain agents. In particular, myopathy (muscular pain, inflammation, weakness) is a potentially serious side effect of statin drugs.[168,169] It is estimated, for example, that 5 to 10 percent of patients taking statins will develop some degree of myopathy.[170] The reasons for these myotoxic effects are unclear, but statin-induced myopathy is associated with several risk factors such as high statin doses, advanced age, genetic factors, multiple diseases, frail stature, and immunosuppressant drugs.[171,172] Combining a statin with certain fibric acids (gemfibrozil) may also increase the risk of myopathy. Although statin-induced myopathy is usually reversible, this syndrome should be recognized early before it can progress to more severe forms of muscle disease and muscle damage (rhabdomyolysis).[169,173] Treatment typically consists of discontinuing the statin and allowing an adequate period of rest and recovery—4 to 6 weeks in most cases. Preliminary studies suggested that statins may also cause peripheral neuropathy, but more recent evidence suggested that these drugs may actually be somewhat neuroprotective in CNS disorders such as Alzheimer disease and Parkinson disease.[174,175] Future studies are needed to clarify the effects of these drugs on nervous tissue and to lend more insight to the prevention and treatment of statin-induced neuromuscular toxicity.

Special Concerns for Rehabilitation Patients

Therapists will frequently encounter patients taking drugs to alter hemostasis. Many patients on prolonged bed rest have a tendency for increased thrombus formation and are particularly susceptible to deep vein thrombosis. These patients will often be given anticoagulant drugs. Heparin followed by warfarin may be administered prophylactically or in response to the symptoms of thrombophlebitis in patients who have undergone hip surgery, heart valve replacement, and other surgical procedures. Therapists should be aware that the primary problem associated with anticoagulant drugs is an increased tendency for bleeding. Any rehabilitation procedures that deal with open wounds (dressing changes, debridement, etc.) should be carefully administered. Rigorous manual techniques, such as deep tissue massage or chest percussion, must also be used with caution since these procedures may directly traumatize tissues and induce bleeding in patients taking anticoagulants. Certain manual techniques such as upper cervical manipulation should be avoided or used very cautiously because of increased risk of damage to the vertebral artery in patients taking anticlotting drugs.

Anticoagulants and antithrombotic drugs may also be given to rehabilitation patients to prevent the recurrence of myocardial infarction, and these drugs are frequently employed in specific cases of cerebrovascular accidents (strokes) that are due to recurrent cerebral embolism and occlusion. Again, therapists should be cognizant of the possibility of increased bleeding with these agents. However, the long-term use of these agents, especially low-dose aspirin, usually does not create any significant problems in the course of rehabilitation.

Fibrinolytic drugs (t-PA, tenecteplase, others) usually do not have a direct impact on physical therapy or occupational therapy. Fibrinolytics are typically given in acute situations, immediately following myocardial infarction or ischemic stroke. Therapists may, however, benefit indirectly from the effects of these drugs because patients may recover faster and more completely from heart attacks and strokes. Fibrinolytics may also help reopen occluded peripheral vessels, thus improving tissue perfusion and wound healing in rehabilitation patients.

Therapists will often work with individuals who have chronic clotting deficiencies, such as patients with hemophilia. Intrajoint hemorrhage (*hemarthrosis*) with subsequent arthropathy is one of the primary problems associated with hemophilia.[176,177] The joints most often affected are the knees, ankles, elbows, hips, and shoulders.[178] Hemarthrosis is usually treated by replacing the missing clotting factor and by rehabilitating the affected joints. Therapists often work in conjunction with pharmacological management to employ a judicious program of exercise, joint support, and pain management to help improve joint function following hemarthrosis and other hemophilia-related joint disorders.[179]

Finally, therapists can encourage patients to comply with pharmacological and nonpharmacological methods used to lower plasma lipids. Hyperlipidemia drugs are typically used in conjunction with diet, exercise, and other lifestyle changes that reduce fat intake and improve plasma lipid profiles. Therapists can help design and implement exercise programs that enable patients to lose weight and increase plasma levels of antiatherogenic components such as HDL, thus maximizing the effects of drug therapy.

CASE STUDY

CLOTTING DISORDERS

Brief History. C.W. is an obese 47-year-old woman who sustained a compression fracture of the L-1 and L-2 vertebrae during a fall from a second-story window. (There was some suggestion that she may have been pushed during an argument with her husband, but the details remain unclear.) She was admitted to the hospital, where her medical condition was stabilized, and surgical procedures were performed to treat her vertebral fracture. Her injuries ultimately resulted in a partial transection of the spinal cord, with diminished motor and sensory function in both lower extremities. She began an extensive rehabilitation program, including physical therapy and occupational therapy. She was progressing well until she developed shortness of breath and an acute pain in her right thorax. Her systolic blood pressure also decreased and remained below 90 mm Hg. A pulmonary angiogram was administered to provide a definitive diagnosis of massive pulmonary embolism. Evidently, C.W. had developed deep vein thrombosis in both lower extremities, and a large embolism from the venous clots had lodged in her lungs, producing a pulmonary infarction.

Drug Treatment. Because of the extensive nature of the pulmonary infarction and her persistent hypotension, a fibrinolytic agent was used to attempt to resolve the clot. Alteplase (Activase) was administered intravenously, with 100 mg of the drug infused slowly over 2 hours. To prevent further thromboembolism, alteplase infusion was followed by heparin. A low-molecular weight heparin (enoxaparin [Lovenox], 1.5 mg/kg body weight) was administered subcutaneously once each day. Clotting time was monitored by periodic blood tests during the heparin treatment. After 7 days of heparin therapy, C.W. was switched to warfarin (Coumadin). Warfarin was administered orally, and the dosage was adjusted until she was receiving 5 mg/d. Oral warfarin was continued throughout the remainder of the patient's hospital stay, as well as after discharge.

1. ***What effect would the drugs administered to resolve the thromboembolic episode have on this patient's physical rehabilitation?***
2. ***What precautions should be considered when this patient is administered thrombolytic and anticoagulant drugs?***

See Appendix C, "Answers to Case Study Questions."

SUMMARY

Normal hemostasis is a balance between excessive and inadequate blood clotting. Overactive blood clotting is harmful because of the tendency for thrombus formation and occlusion of arteries and veins. Vessels may become directly blocked by the thrombus, or a portion of the thrombus may break off and create an embolism that lodges elsewhere in the vascular system. The tendency for excessive thrombus formation in the venous system is usually treated with anticoagulant drugs such as heparin and warfarin. Platelet inhibitors such as aspirin help prevent arterial thrombogenesis. Fibrinolytic drugs (t-PA, tenecteplase) that facilitate the dissolution of harmful clots may successfully reopen vessels that have suddenly become occluded because of acute thrombus formation.

The inadequate blood clotting and excessive bleeding that occur in patients with hemophilia are treated by replacing the missing clotting factor. Other conditions associated with inadequate coagulation may be treated by administering either vitamin K, which helps improve the synthesis of certain clotting factors, or antifibrinolytic agents (aminocaproic acid, tranexamic acid), which inhibit clot breakdown.

Hyperlipidemia can lead to atherosclerosis and subsequent cardiovascular incidents such as thrombosis and infarction. This condition is often treated by a combination of drug therapy and diet and lifestyle modifications. Pharmacological interventions are typically targeted toward decreasing the synthesis of harmful (atherogenic) plasma components, including certain lipoproteins (IDL, LDL, VLDL) that are associated with atherosclerotic plaque formation.

REFERENCES

1. Xu Z, Kim O, Kamocka M, et al. Multiscale models of thrombogenesis. *Wiley Interdiscip Rev Syst Biol Med.* 2012;4:237-246.
2. Kluft C, Burggraaf J. Introduction to haemostasis from a pharmacodynamics perspective. *Br J Clin Pharmacol.* 2011;72:538-546.
3. Reitsma PH, Versteeg HH, Middeldorp S. Mechanistic view of risk factors for venous thromboembolism. *Arterioscler Thromb Vasc Biol.* 2012;32:563-568.
4. Maas C, Renné T. Regulatory mechanisms of the plasma contact system. *Thromb Res.* 2012;129(suppl 2):S73-76.
5. Versteeg HH, Heemskerk JW, Levi M, Reitsma PH. New fundamentals in hemostasis. *Physiol Rev.* 2013;93:327-358.
6. Persson E, Olsen OH. Current status on tissue factor activation of factor VIIa. *Thromb Res.* 2010;125(suppl 1):S11-12.
7. Kubier A, O'Brien M. Endogenous anticoagulants. *Top Companion Anim Med.* 2012;27:81-87.
8. Andras A, Sala Tenna A, Crawford F. Vitamin K antagonists or low-molecular-weight heparin for the long term treatment of symptomatic venous thromboembolism. *Cochrane Database Syst Rev.* 2012;10:CD002001.
9. Prandoni P. Anticoagulant treatment of pulmonary embolism: impact and implications of the EINSTEIN PE study. *Eur J Haematol.* 2012;89:281-287.
10. Dobromirski M, Cohen AT. How I manage venous thromboembolism risk in hospitalized medical patients. *Blood.* 2012;120:1562-1569.
11. Falck-Ytter Y, Francis CW, Johanson NA, et al. Prevention of VTE in orthopedic surgery patients: *Antithrombotic Therapy and Prevention of Thrombosis*, 9th ed: American College of Chest Physicians Evidence-Based Clinical Practice Guidelines. *Chest.* 2012;141(suppl):e278S-325S.
12. Mischke K, Knackstedt C, Marx N, Vollmann D. Insights into atrial fibrillation. *Minerva Med.* 2013;104:119-130.
13. Toth PP. Practical management of anticoagulants in family medicine after orthopedic surgery. *Postgrad Med.* 2012;124:206-214.
14. Imberti D, Ageno W, Manfredini R, et al. Interventional treatment of venous thromboembolism: a review. *Thromb Res.* 2012;129:418-425.
15. Pendleton RC, Rodgers GM, Hull RD. Established venous thromboembolism therapies: heparin, low molecular weight heparins, and vitamin K antagonists, with a discussion of heparin-induced thrombocytopenia. *Clin Chest Med.* 2010;31:691-706.
16. Zehnder JL. Drugs used in disorders of coagulation. In: Katzung BG, ed. *Basic and Clinical Pharmacology.* 12th ed. New York: Lange Medical Books/McGraw Hill; 2012.
17. Guerrini M, Bisio A. Low-molecular-weight heparins: differential characterization/physical characterization. *Handb Exp Pharmacol.* 2012;207:127-157.
18. Abad Rico JI, Llau Pitarch JV, Páramo Fernández JA. Topical issues in venous thromboembolism. *Drugs.* 2010;70(suppl 2):11-18.
19. Sobieraj DM, Coleman CI, Tongbram V, et al. Comparative effectiveness of low-molecular-weight heparins versus other anticoagulants in major orthopedic surgery: a systematic review and meta-analysis. *Pharmacotherapy.* 2012;32:799-808.
20. Hammerstingl C. Monitoring therapeutic anticoagulation with low molecular weight heparins: is it useful or misleading? *Cardiovasc Hematol Agents Med Chem.* 2008;6:282-286.
21. Iqbal Z, Cohen M. Emerging antithrombotic agents: what does the intensivist need to know? *Curr Opin Crit Care.* 2010;16:419-425.
22. Piatek C, O'Connell CL, Liebman HA. Treating venous thromboembolism in patients with cancer. *Expert Rev Hematol.* 2012;5:201-209.
23. Huo MH, Muntz J. Extended thromboprophylaxis with low-molecular-weight heparins after hospital discharge in high-risk surgical and medical patients: a review. *Clin Ther.* 2009;31:1129-1141.
24. Rasmussen MS, Jørgensen LN, Wille-Jørgensen P. Prolonged thromboprophylaxis with low molecular weight heparin for abdominal or pelvic surgery. *Cochrane Database Syst Rev.* 2009;1:CD004318.
25. Sinauridze EI, Panteleev MA, Ataullakhanov FI. Anticoagulant therapy: basic principles, classic approaches and recent developments. *Blood Coagul Fibrinolysis.* 2012;23:482-493.
26. Scaglione F. New oral anticoagulants: comparative pharmacology with vitamin K antagonists. *Clin Pharmacokinet.* 2013;52:69-82.
27. Witt DM, Nutescu EA, Haines ST. Venous thromboembolism. In: DiPiro JT, et al, eds. *Pharmacotherapy: A Pathophysiologic Approach.* 8th ed. New York: McGraw-Hill; 2011.
28. Prandoni P, Dalla Valle F, Piovella C, et al. New anticoagulants for the treatment of venous thromboembolism. *Minerva Med.* 2013;104:131-139.
29. Eerenberg ES, van Es J, Sijpkens MK, et al. New anticoagulants: moving on from scientific results to clinical implementation. *Ann Med.* 2011;43:606-616.
30. King CS, Holley AB, Moores LK. Moving toward a more ideal anticoagulant: the oral direct thrombin and factor Xa inhibitors. *Chest.* 2013;143:1106-1116.
31. Dogliotti A, Paolasso E, Giugliano RP. Novel oral anticoagulants in atrial fibrillation: a meta-analysis of large, randomized, controlled trials vs warfarin. *Clin Cardiol.* 2013;36:61-67.
32. Marsland D, Mears SC, Kates SL. Venous thromboembolic prophylaxis for hip fractures. *Osteoporos Int.* 2010;21(suppl 4):S593-604.
33. Sharma T, Mehta P, Gajra A. Update on fondaparinux: role in management of thromboembolic and acute coronary events. *Cardiovasc Hematol Agents Med Chem.* 2010;8:96-103.
34. Nagler M, Haslauer M, Wuillemin WA. Fondaparinux—data on efficacy and safety in special situations. *Thromb Res.* 2012;129:407-417.
35. Badger NO. Fondaparinux (Arixtra(R)), a safe alternative for the treatment of patients with heparin-induced thrombocytopenia? *J Pharm Pract.* 2010;23:235-238.
36. Warkentin TE. Fondaparinux: does it cause HIT? Can it treat HIT? *Expert Rev Hematol.* 2010;3:567-581.
37. Jacobson A. Is there a role for warfarin anymore? *Hematology Am Soc Hematol Educ Program.* 2012;2012:541-546.
38. Tripodi A. The laboratory and the new oral anticoagulants. *Clin Chem.* 2013;59:353-362.
39. Lanzarotti S, Weigelt JA. Heparin-induced thrombocytopenia. *Surg Clin North Am.* 2012;92:1559-1572.

40. Alban S. Adverse effects of heparin. *Handb Exp Pharmacol.* 2012;207:211-263.
41. Cuker A. Recent advances in heparin-induced thrombocytopenia. *Curr Opin Hematol.* 2011;18:315-322.
42. Hess CN, Becker RC, Alexander JH, Lopes RD. Antithrombotic therapy in heparin-induced thrombocytopenia: guidelines translated for the clinician. *J Thromb Thrombolysis.* 2012;34:552-561.
43. Power RF, Hynes BG, Moran D, et al. Modern antiplatelet agents in coronary artery disease. *Expert Rev Cardiovasc Ther.* 2012;10:1261-1272.
44. Scharf RE. Drugs that affect platelet function. *Semin Thromb Hemost.* 2012;38:865-883.
45. Buch MH, Prendergast BD, Storey RF. Antiplatelet therapy and vascular disease: an update. *Ther Adv Cardiovasc Dis.* 2010;4:249-275.
46. Angiolillo DJ. The evolution of antiplatelet therapy in the treatment of acute coronary syndromes: from aspirin to the present day. *Drugs.* 2012;72:2087-2116.
47. De Caterina R, Renda G. Clinical use of aspirin in ischemic heart disease: past, present and future. *Curr Pharm Des.* 2012;18:5215-5223.
48. Meade T. Primary prevention of ischaemic cardiovascular disorders with antiplatelet agents. *Handb Exp Pharmacol.* 2012;210:565-605.
49. Hennekens CH, Dalen JE. Aspirin in the treatment and prevention of cardiovascular disease: past and current perspectives and future directions. *Am J Med.* 2013;126:373-378.
50. Tanguay JF. Antiplatelet therapy in acute coronary syndrome and atrial fibrillation: aspirin. *Adv Cardiol.* 2012;47:20-30.
51. Raju NC, Eikelboom JW. The aspirin controversy in primary prevention. *Curr Opin Cardiol.* 2012;27:499-507.
52. Apostolakis S, Marín F, Lip GY. Antiplatelet therapy in stroke prevention. *Adv Cardiol.* 2012;47:141-154.
53. Field TS, Benavente OR. Current status of antiplatelet agents to prevent stroke. *Curr Neurol Neurosci Rep.* 2011;11:6-14.
54. Albers GW, Amarenco P, Easton JD, et al. Antithrombotic and thrombolytic therapy for ischemic stroke: American College of Chest Physicians Evidence-Based Clinical Practice Guidelines (8th Edition). *Chest.* 2008;133(suppl):630S-669S.
55. Divani AA, Zantek ND, Borhani-Haghighi A, Rao GH. Antiplatelet therapy: aspirin resistance and all that jazz! *Clin Appl Thromb Hemost.* 2013;19:5-18.
56. Adelman EE, Lisabeth L, Brown DL. Gender differences in the primary prevention of stroke with aspirin. *Womens Health (Lond Engl).* 2011;7:341-352.
57. Kar S, Bhatt DL. Anticoagulants for the treatment of acute coronary syndrome in the era of new oral agents. *Coron Artery Dis.* 2012;23:380-390.
58. Stewart DW, Freshour JE. Aspirin for the prophylaxis of venous thromboembolic events in orthopedic surgery patients: a comparison of the AAOS and ACCP guidelines with review of the evidence. *Ann Pharmacother.* 2013;47:63-74.
59. Davis EM, Friedman SK, Baker TM. A review of antithrombotic therapy for transcatheter aortic valve replacement. *Postgrad Med.* 2013;125:59-72.
60. Kim FY, Marhefka G, Ruggiero NJ, et al. Saphenous vein graft disease: review of pathophysiology, prevention, and treatment. *Cardiol Rev.* 2013;21:101-109.
61. Patrono C, Rocca B. Aspirin and other COX-1 inhibitors. *Handb Exp Pharmacol.* 2012;210:137-164.
62. Bernlochner I, Sibbing D. Thienopyridines and other ADP-receptor antagonists. *Handb Exp Pharmacol.* 2012;210:165-198.
63. Mathur AP, Waller AH, Dhruvakumar S, et al. Dual antiplatelet therapy for primary and secondary prevention. *Minerva Cardioangiol.* 2012;60:611-628.
64. Shin DH, Hong MK. Optimal duration of dual antiplatelet therapy after drug-eluting stent implantation. *Expert Rev Cardiovasc Ther.* 2012;10:1273-1285.
65. Huber K. Clopidogrel in coronary artery disease: update 2012. *Adv Cardiol.* 2012;47:31-38.
66. Armstrong PC, Peter K. GPIIb/IIIa inhibitors: from bench to bedside and back to bench again. *Thromb Haemost.* 2012;107:808-814.
67. Starnes HB, Patel AA, Stouffer GA. Optimal use of platelet glycoprotein IIb/IIIa receptor antagonists in patients undergoing percutaneous coronary interventions. *Drugs.* 2011;71:2009-2030.
68. Hagemeyer CE, Peter K. Targeting the platelet integrin GPIIb/IIIa. *Curr Pharm Des.* 2010;16:4119-4133.
69. Aragam KG, Bhatt DL. Antiplatelet therapy in acute coronary syndromes. *J Cardiovasc Pharmacol Ther.* 2011;16:24-42.
70. Showkathali R, Natarajan A. Antiplatelet and antithrombin strategies in acute coronary syndrome: state-of-the-art review. *Curr Cardiol Rev.* 2012;8:239-249.
71. Weitz JI. Blood coagulation, and anticoagulant, fibrinolytic, and antiplatelet drugs. In: Brunton L, et al, eds. *The Pharmacological Basis of Therapeutics.* 12th ed. New York: McGraw-Hill; 2011.
72. Schneider DJ. Anti-platelet therapy: glycoprotein IIb-IIIa antagonists. *Br J Clin Pharmacol.* 2011;72:672-682.
73. Weber R, Brenck J, Diener HC. Antiplatelet therapy in cerebrovascular disorders. *Handb Exp Pharmacol.* 2012;210:519-546.
74. Eisert WG. Dipyridamole in antithrombotic treatment. *Adv Cardiol.* 2012;47:78-86.
75. Yip S, Benavente O. Antiplatelet agents for stroke prevention. *Neurotherapeutics.* 2011;8:475-487.
76. Stevens JW, Simpson E, Harnan S, et al. Systematic review of the efficacy of cilostazol, naftidrofuryl oxalate and pentoxifylline for the treatment of intermittent claudication. *Br J Surg.* 2012;99:1630-1638.
77. Salhiyyah K, Senanayake E, Abdel-Hadi M, et al. Pentoxifylline for intermittent claudication. *Cochrane Database Syst Rev.* 2012;1:CD005262.
78. Vodnala D, Rajagopalan S, Brook RD. Medical management of the patient with intermittent claudication. *Cardiol Clin.* 2011;29:363-379.
79. Murray V, Norrving B, Sandercock PA, et al. The molecular basis of thrombolysis and its clinical application in stroke. *J Intern Med.* 2010;267:191-208.
80. Kunadian V, Gibson CM. Thrombolytics and myocardial infarction. *Cardiovasc Ther.* 2012;30:e81-88.
81. Morse MA, Todd JW, Stouffer GA. Optimizing the use of thrombolytics in ST-segment elevation myocardial infarction. *Drugs.* 2009;69:1945-1966.
82. Menon V, Harrington RA, Hochman JS, et al. Thrombolysis and adjunctive therapy in acute myocardial infarction: the Seventh ACCP Conference on Antithrombotic and Thrombolytic Therapy. *Chest.* 2004;126(suppl):549S-575S.
83. Nee PA. Thrombolysis after acute myocardial infarction. *J Accid Emerg Med.* 1997;14:2-9.
84. Boden WE, Gupta V. Reperfusion strategies in acute ST-segment elevation myocardial infarction. *Curr Opin Cardiol.* 2008;23:613-619.

85. Crowder JS, Hubble MW, Gandhi S, et al. Prehospital administration of tenecteplase for ST-segment elevation myocardial infarction in a rural EMS system. *Prehosp Emerg Care*. 2011;15:499-505.
86. Goa KL, Henwood JM, Stolz JF, et al. Intravenous streptokinase. A reappraisal of its therapeutic use in acute myocardial infarction. *Drugs*. 1990;39:693-719.
87. Marder VJ, Stewart D. Towards safer thrombolytic therapy. *Semin Hematol*. 2002;39:206-216.
88. Kirmani JF, Alkawi A, Panezai S, Gizzi M. Advances in thrombolytics for treatment of acute ischemic stroke. *Neurology*. 2012;79(suppl 1):S119-125.
89. Kurz MW, Kurz KD, Farbu E. Acute ischemic stroke—from symptom recognition to thrombolysis. *Acta Neurol Scand Suppl*. 2013;196:57-64.
90. Hametner C, Ringleb PA, Hacke W, Kellert L. Selection of possible responders to thrombolytic therapy in acute ischemic stroke. *Ann NY Acad Sci*. 2012;1268:120-126.
91. Grotta J. Timing of thrombolysis for acute ischemic stroke: "timing is everything" or "everyone is different." *Ann NY Acad Sci*. 2012;1268:141-144.
92. Robertson I, Kessel DO, Berridge DC. Fibrinolytic agents for peripheral arterial occlusion. *Cochrane Database Syst Rev*. 2010;3:CD001099.
93. Fahrni J, Engelberger RP, Kucher N, et al. Catheter-based treatment of ilio-femoral deep vein thrombosis—an update on current evidence. *Vasa*. 2013;42:161-167.
94. Liu F, Lü P, Jin B. Catheter-directed thrombolysis for acute iliofemoral deep venous thrombosis. *Ann Vasc Surg*. 2011;25:707-715.
95. Tapson VF. Thrombolytic therapy for acute pulmonary embolism. *Semin Thromb Hemost*. 2013;39:452-458.
96. Lankeit M, Konstantinides S. Thrombolytic therapy for submassive pulmonary embolism. *Best Pract Res Clin Haematol*. 2012;25:379-389.
97. Tseke P, Kalyveza E, Politis E, et al. Thrombolysis with alteplase: a non-invasive treatment for occluded arteriovenous fistulas and grafts. *Artif Organs*. 2011;35:58-62.
98. Kunadian V, Gibson CM. Recombinant tissue-type plasminogen activators: "time matters." *Drugs Today*. 2011;47:559-570.
99. Melandri G, Vagnarelli F, Calabrese D, et al. Review of tenecteplase (TNKase) in the treatment of acute myocardial infarction. *Vasc Health Risk Manag*. 2009;5:249-256.
100. Van de Werf FJ, Topol EJ, Sobel BE. The impact of fibrinolytic therapy for ST-segment-elevation acute myocardial infarction. *J Thromb Haemost*. 2009;7:14-20.
101. Abou-Chebl A. Management of acute ischemic stroke. *Curr Cardiol Rep*. 2013;15:348.
102. DeMers G, Meurer WJ, Shih R, et al. Tissue plasminogen activator and stroke: review of the literature for the clinician. *J Emerg Med*. 2012;43:1149-1154.
103. Mokin M, Kan P, Kass-Hout T, et al. Intracerebral hemorrhage secondary to intravenous and endovascular intraarterial revascularization therapies in acute ischemic stroke: an update on risk factors, predictors, and management. *Neurosurg Focus*. 2012;32:E2.
104. Goodeve AC, Perry DJ, Cumming T, et al. Genetics of haemostasis. *Haemophilia*. 2012;18(suppl 4):73-80.
105. Franchini M, Frattini F, Crestani S, et al. Treatment of hemophilia B: focus on recombinant factor IX. *Biologics*. 2013;7:33-38.
106. Franchini M, Mannucci PM. Past, present and future of hemophilia: a narrative review. *Orphanet J Rare Dis*. 2012;7:24.
107. Mannucci PM, Mancuso ME, Santagostino E. How we choose factor VIII to treat hemophilia. *Blood*. 2012;119:4108-4114.
108. Schulte S. Pioneering designs for recombinant coagulation factors. *Thromb Res*. 2011;128(suppl 1):S9-12.
109. Kruse-Jarres R. Inhibitors: our greatest challenge. Can we minimize the incidence? *Haemophilia*. 2013;19(suppl 1):2-7.
110. Kruse-Jarres R. Current controversies in the formation and treatment of alloantibodies to factor VIII in congenital hemophilia A. *Hematology Am Soc Hematol Educ Program*. 2011;2011:407-412.
111. Astermark J. Immune tolerance induction in patients with hemophilia A. *Thromb Res*. 2011;127(suppl 1):S6-9.
112. Ipema HJ. Use of oral vitamin K for prevention of late vitamin k deficiency bleeding in neonates when injectable vitamin K is not available. *Ann Pharmacother*. 2012;46:879-883.
113. Lauer B, Spector N. Vitamins. *Pediatr Rev*. 2012;33:339-351.
114. Wilson SE, Watson HG, Crowther MA. Low-dose oral vitamin K therapy for the management of asymptomatic patients with elevated international normalized ratios: a brief review. *CMAJ*. 2004;170:821-824.
115. Hanslik T, Prinseau J. The use of vitamin K in patients on anticoagulant therapy: a practical guide. *Am J Cardiovasc Drugs*. 2004;4:43-55.
116. Breen KA, Grimwade D, Hunt BJ. The pathogenesis and management of the coagulopathy of acute promyelocytic leukaemia. *Br J Haematol*. 2012;156:24-36.
117. Ganter MT, Pittet JF. New insights into acute coagulopathy in trauma patients. *Best Pract Res Clin Anaesthesiol*. 2010;24:15-25.
118. Eubanks JD. Antifibrinolytics in major orthopaedic surgery. *J Am Acad Orthop Surg*. 2010;18:132-138.
119. McCormack PL. Tranexamic acid: a review of its use in the treatment of hyperfibrinolysis. *Drugs*. 2012;72:585-617.
120. Roberts I, Shakur H, Ker K, et al. Antifibrinolytic drugs for acute traumatic injury. *Cochrane Database Syst Rev*. 2012;12:CD004896.
121. Brouwers MC, van Greevenbroek MM, Stehouwer CD, et al. The genetics of familial combined hyperlipidaemia. *Nat Rev Endocrinol*. 2012;8:352-362.
122. Klop B, Elte JW, Cabezas MC. Dyslipidemia in obesity: mechanisms and potential targets. *Nutrients*. 2013;5:1218-1240.
123. Matikainen N, Taskinen MR. Management of dyslipidemias in the presence of the metabolic syndrome or type 2 diabetes. *Curr Cardiol Rep*. 2012;14:721-731.
124. Hassing HC, Surendran RP, Mooij HL, et al. Pathophysiology of hypertriglyceridemia. *Biochim Biophys Acta*. 2012;1821:826-832.
125. Lupattelli G, De Vuono S, Mannarino E. Patterns of cholesterol metabolism: pathophysiological and therapeutic implications for dyslipidemias and the metabolic syndrome. *Nutr Metab Cardiovasc Dis*. 2011;21:620-627.
126. Malloy MJ, Kane JP. Agents used in dyslipidemia. In: Katzung BG, ed. *Basic and Clinical Pharmacology*. 12th ed. New York: Lange Medical Books/McGraw Hill; 2012.
127. Ho M, Garnett SP, Baur L, et al. Effectiveness of lifestyle interventions in child obesity: systematic review with meta-analysis. *Pediatrics*. 2012;130:e1647-1671.
128. Manfredini F, D'Addato S, Laghi L, et al. Influence of lifestyle measures on hypertriglyceridaemia. *Curr Drug Targets*. 2009;10:344-355.

129. Tonstad S, Després JP. Treatment of lipid disorders in obesity. *Expert Rev Cardiovasc Ther.* 2011;1069-1080.
130. Ito MK. Dyslipidemia: management using optimal lipid-lowering therapy. *Ann Pharmacother.* 2012;46:1368-1381.
131. Koch CG. Statin therapy. *Curr Pharm Des.* 2012;18:6284-6290.
132. Goldstein JL, Brown MS. The LDL receptor. *Arterioscler Thromb Vasc Biol.* 2009;29:431-438.
133. Yamashita S, Tsubakio-Yamamoto K, Ohama T, et al. Molecular mechanisms of HDL-cholesterol elevation by statins and its effects on HDL functions. *J Atheroscler Thromb.* 2010;17:436-451.
134. Arnaud C, Veillard NR, Mach F. Cholesterol-independent effects of statins in inflammation, immunomodulation and atherosclerosis. *Curr Drug Targets Cardiovasc Haematol Disord.* 2005;5:127-134.
135. Antoniades C, Bakogiannis C, Leeson P, et al. Rapid, direct effects of statin treatment on arterial redox state and nitric oxide bioavailability in human atherosclerosis via tetrahydrobiopterin-mediated endothelial nitric oxide synthase coupling. *Circulation.* 2011;124:335-345.
136. Ylä-Herttuala S, Bentzon JF, Daemen M, et al. Stabilisation of atherosclerotic plaques. Position paper of the European Society of Cardiology (ESC) Working Group on Atherosclerosis and Vascular Biology. *Thromb Haemost.* 2011;106:1-19.
137. Antonopoulos AS, Margaritis M, Shirodaria C, Antoniades C. Translating the effects of statins: from redox regulation to suppression of vascular wall inflammation. *Thromb Haemost.* 2012;108:840-848.
138. Lahera V, Goicoechea M, de Vinuesa SG, et al. Endothelial dysfunction, oxidative stress and inflammation in atherosclerosis: beneficial effects of statins. *Curr Med Chem.* 2007;14:243-248.
139. Lewis SJ. Lipid-lowering therapy: who can benefit? *Vasc Health Risk Manag.* 2011;7:525-534.
140. Taylor F, Huffman MD, Macedo AF, et al. Statins for the primary prevention of cardiovascular disease. *Cochrane Database Syst Rev.* 2013;1:CD004816.
141. Baigent C, Keech A, Kearney PM, et al. Efficacy and safety of cholesterol-lowering treatment: prospective meta-analysis of data from 90,056 participants in 14 randomised trials of statins. *Lancet.* 2005;366:1267-1278.
142. Cholesterol Treatment Trialists' (CTT) Collaboration; Baigent C, Blackwell L, et al. Efficacy and safety of more intensive lowering of LDL cholesterol: a meta-analysis of data from 170,000 participants in 26 randomised trials. *Lancet.* 2010;376:1670-1681.
143. Lochhead P, Chan AT. Statins and colorectal cancer. *Clin Gastroenterol Hepatol.* 2013;11:109-118.
144. Lonardo A, Loria P. Potential for statins in the chemoprevention and management of hepatocellular carcinoma. *J Gastroenterol Hepatol.* 2012;27:1654-1664.
145. Maki KC, Bays HE, Dicklin MR. Treatment options for the management of hypertriglyceridemia: strategies based on the best-available evidence. *J Clin Lipidol.* 2012;6:413-426.
146. McKeage K, Keating GM. Fenofibrate: a review of its use in dyslipidaemia. *Drugs.* 2011;71:1917-1946.
147. McCullough PA, Ahmed AB, Zughaib MT, et al. Treatment of hypertriglyceridemia with fibric acid derivatives: impact on lipid subfractions and translation into a reduction in cardiovascular events. *Rev Cardiovasc Med.* 2011;12:173-185.
148. Tenenbaum A, Fisman EZ. Fibrates are an essential part of modern anti-dyslipidemic arsenal: spotlight on atherogenic dyslipidemia and residual risk reduction. *Cardiovasc Diabetol.* 2012;11:125.
149. Rubenfire M, Brook RD, Rosenson RS. Treating mixed hyperlipidemia and the atherogenic lipid phenotype for prevention of cardiovascular events. *Am J Med.* 2010;123:892-898.
150. Soskić SS, Dobutović BD, Sudar EM, et al. Peroxisome proliferator-activated receptors and atherosclerosis. *Angiology.* 2011;62:523-534.
151. Shah A, Rader DJ, Millar JS. The effect of PPAR-alpha agonism on apolipoprotein metabolism in humans. *Atherosclerosis.* 2010;210:35-40.
152. Balakumar P, Rohilla A, Mahadevan N. Pleiotropic actions of fenofibrate on the heart. *Pharmacol Res.* 2011;63:8-12.
153. Guo J, Meng F, Ma N, et al. Meta-analysis of safety of the coadministration of statin with fenofibrate in patients with combined hyperlipidemia. *Am J Cardiol.* 2012;110:1296-1301.
154. Jacobson TA. Myopathy with statin-fibrate combination therapy: clinical considerations. *Nat Rev Endocrinol.* 2009;5:507-518.
155. Shanes JG. A review of the rationale for additional therapeutic interventions to attain lower LDL-C when statin therapy is not enough. *Curr Atheroscler Rep.* 2012;14:33-40.
156. Out C, Groen AK, Brufau G. Bile acid sequestrants: more than simple resins. *Curr Opin Lipidol.* 2012;23:43-55.
157. Hochholzer W, Berg DD, Giugliano RP. The facts behind niacin. *Ther Adv Cardiovasc Dis.* 2011;5:227-240.
158. MacKay D, Hathcock J, Guarneri E. Niacin: chemical forms, bioavailability, and health effects. *Nutr Rev.* 2012;70:357-366.
159. Creider JC, Hegele RA, Joy TR. Niacin: another look at an underutilized lipid-lowering medication. *Nat Rev Endocrinol.* 2012;8:517-528.
160. Wanders D, Judd RL. Future of GPR109A agonists in the treatment of dyslipidaemia. *Diabetes Obes Metab.* 2011;13:685-691.
161. Al-Mohaissen MA, Pun SC, Frohlich JJ. Niacin: from mechanisms of action to therapeutic uses. *Mini Rev Med Chem.* 2010;10:204-217.
162. Phan BA, Dayspring TD, Toth PP. Ezetimibe therapy: mechanism of action and clinical update. *Vasc Health Risk Manag.* 2012;8:415-427.
163. Suchy D, Łabuzek K, Stadnicki A, Okopień B. Ezetimibe—a new approach in hypercholesterolemia management. *Pharmacol Rep.* 2011;63:1335-1348.
164. Ijioma N, Robinson JG. Lipid-lowering effects of ezetimibe and simvastatin in combination. *Expert Rev Cardiovasc Ther.* 2011;9:131-145.
165. Lyseng-Williamson KA. Ezetimibe/simvastatin: a guide to its clinical use in hypercholesterolemia. *Am J Cardiovasc Drugs.* 2012;12:49-56.
166. Kei A, Elisaf MS. Nicotinic acid: clinical considerations. *Expert Opin Drug Saf.* 2012;11:551-564.
167. Yadav R, France M, Younis N, et al. Extended-release niacin with laropiprant: a review on efficacy, clinical effectiveness and safety. *Expert Opin Pharmacother.* 2012;13:1345-1362.
168. Di Stasi SL, MacLeod TD, Winters JD, Binder-Macleod SA. Effects of statins on skeletal muscle: a perspective for physical therapists. *Phys Ther.* 2010;90:1530-1542.
169. Sathasivam S. Statin induced myotoxicity. *Eur J Intern Med.* 2012;23:317-324.

170. Rallidis LS, Fountoulaki K, Anastasiou-Nana M. Managing the underestimated risk of statin-associated myopathy. *Int J Cardiol.* 2012;159:169-176.
171. Abd TT, Jacobson TA. Statin-induced myopathy: a review and update. *Expert Opin Drug Saf.* 2011;10:373-387.
172. Chatzizisis YS, Koskinas KC, Misirli G, et al. Risk factors and drug interactions predisposing to statin-induced myopathy: implications for risk assessment, prevention and treatment. *Drug Saf.* 2010;33:171-187.
173. Hohenegger M. Drug induced rhabdomyolysis. *Curr Opin Pharmacol.* 2012;12:335-339.
174. Bełtowski J, Wójcicka G, Jamroz-Wiśniewska A. Adverse effects of statins—mechanisms and consequences. *Curr Drug Saf.* 2009;4:209-228.
175. Wang Q, Yan J, Chen X, et al. Statins: multiple neuroprotective mechanisms in neurodegenerative diseases. *Exp Neurol.* 2011;230:27-34.
176. Sherry DD. Avoiding the impact of musculoskeletal pain on quality of life in children with hemophilia. *Orthop Nurs.* 2008;27:103-108.
177. Simpson ML, Valentino LA. Management of joint bleeding in hemophilia. *Expert Rev Hematol.* 2012;5:459-468.
178. Luck JV Jr, Silva M, Rodriguez-Merchan EC, et al. Hemophilic arthropathy. *J Am Acad Orthop Surg.* 2004;12:234-245.
179. De la Corte-Rodriguez H, Rodriguez-Merchan EC. The role of physical medicine and rehabilitation in haemophiliac patients. *Blood Coagul Fibrinolysis.* 2013;24:1-9.

SECTION

6

Respiratory and Gastrointestinal Pharmacology

CHAPTER 26

Respiratory Drugs

The respiratory system is responsible for mediating gas exchange between the external environment and the bloodstream. The upper respiratory tract conducts air to the lower respiratory passages and ultimately to the lungs. It also humidifies and conditions inspired air and serves to protect the lungs from harmful substances. In the lungs, gas exchange takes place between the alveoli and the pulmonary circulation.

The drugs discussed in this chapter are directed primarily at maintaining proper airflow through the respiratory passages. Agents that treat specific problems in the lungs are not discussed here but are covered in other areas of this text. For instance, Section 8 (Chapters 33 to 35) includes drugs used to treat infectious diseases of the lower respiratory tract and lungs.

The respiratory agents presented here are divided into two primary categories. The first group includes drugs that treat acute and relatively minor problems, such as nasal congestion, coughing, or a seasonal **allergy**. The second category includes drugs that treat more chronic and serious airway obstructions, such as bronchial asthma, chronic bronchitis, and emphysema.

You will frequently treat patients with both acute and chronic respiratory conditions. Drug therapy can be critical in helping these patients breathe more easily and become more actively engaged in respiratory muscle training and various forms of aerobic and strengthening exercises. Patients will also be calmer and more engaged in rehabilitation activities if these medications improve difficult and labored breathing and reduce the anxiety and panicky sensation that occurs when patients feel they "cannot get enough air." Consequently, the overview of the drugs presented in this chapter is of interest.

DRUGS USED TO TREAT RESPIRATORY TRACT IRRITATION AND CONTROL RESPIRATORY SECRETIONS

The drugs presented below are used to treat symptomatic coughing and irritation resulting from problems such as the common cold, seasonal allergies, and upper respiratory tract infections. Many of these drugs are found in over-the-counter preparations. Often, several different agents are combined in the same commercial preparation; for example, a decongestant, an antitussive, and an expectorant may be combined and identified by a specific trade name. Also, agents within a specific category may have properties that overlap into other drug categories. Certain antihistamines, for instance, may also have antitussive properties.

Antitussives

Antitussive drugs suppress coughing associated with the common cold and other minor throat irritations. When used to treat cold and flu symptoms, these drugs are often combined with aspirin or acetaminophen and other respiratory tract agents.[1,2] Antitussives are typically recommended for short-term use in relieving symptomatic coughing.[3] Nonetheless, the extensive use of antitussives has been questioned in our society. Coughing is a type of defense mechanism that can help expel mucus and foreign material from the upper respiratory tract.[4] By inhibiting this mechanism, antitussives may reduce the ability of coughing to raise secretions. Hence, these agents may be helpful in treating an annoying dry cough, but their use to treat an active and productive cough may not be justified.[5]

The likelihood that many antitussives are not really effective in treating cough is also a concern. In particular, many over-the-counter products may not contain an adequate amount of the active medication, and it appears that these products may be no more effective than placebo in treating cough.[6] This fact seems especially true for children, where over-the-counter cough and cold products do not produce any beneficial effects but still contain chemicals that can harm the child.[7,8] Toxic effects may occur commonly in infants and very young children because of inappropriate dosing and overdose.[9,10] Many experts recommend that these products should not be used in infants and children younger than 4 to 6 years old.[7,11] Doses that contain sufficient active ingredients to be effective in treating cough may also produce serious side effects.[6] Hence, researchers continue to study the mechanisms underlying the cough reflex so that safer and more effective antitussives can be developed.[5]

Some of the commonly used antitussives are listed in Table 26-1. Codeine and similar opioid derivatives are the classic antitussive agents. Opioids exert at least some of their antitussive effects by suppressing the cough reflex center in the brainstem, and these drugs may also decrease the sensitivity of afferent (sensory) pathways that initiate the cough reflex.[12,13] Nonopioid antitussives work by inhibiting the irritant effects of histamine on the respiratory mucosa or by a local anesthetic action on the respiratory epithelium. The primary adverse effect associated with most antitussives is sedation. Dizziness and gastrointestinal (GI) upset may also occur. Chronic or excessive use of opioids may also lead to tolerance and dependence.

Table 26-1
COMMON ANTITUSSIVE AGENTS

Generic Name	Trade Name(s)*	Method of Action
Benzonatate	Tessalon	Local anesthetic effect on respiratory mucosa
Codeine	Many trade names	Inhibits cough reflex by direct effect on brainstem cough center May also inhibit peripheral afferent neurons that initiate coughing
Dextromethorphan	Many trade names	Inhibits cough reflex (similar to codeine) but is non-narcotic
Diphenhydramine	Benadryl (others)	Antihistamine
Hydrocodone	Hycodan, Tussigon, others	Similar to codeine
Hydromorphone	Dilaudid Cough	Similar to codeine

**Trade names often reflect combination of the antitussive with other agents (i.e., expectorants, decongestants).*

Decongestants

Congestion within and mucous discharge from the upper respiratory tract are familiar symptoms of many conditions. Allergies, the common cold, and various respiratory infections often produce a runny nose and a stuffy head sensation. Decongestants used to treat these symptoms are usually alpha-1–adrenergic agonists (see Chapter 20).[14] These agents bind to alpha-1 receptors located on the blood vessels of the nasal mucosa and stimulate vasoconstriction, thus effectively drying up the mucosal vasculature and decreasing local congestion in the nasal passages.[15]

Alpha-1 agonists used as decongestants are listed in Table 26-2. Depending on the preparation, these agents may be taken systemically or applied locally to the nasal mucosa via aerosol sprays. It appears that occasional use of these drugs can help the symptoms related to nasal congestion.[15,16] The drugs, however, can mimic the effects of increased sympathetic nervous system activity and can cause serious cardiovascular and central nervous system (CNS) excitation. Patients should avoid excessive use or abuse.

The primary adverse effects associated with decongestants are headache, dizziness, nervousness, nausea, and cardiovascular irregularities (e.g., increased blood pressure, palpitations). As indicated, these effects become more apparent at higher doses and during prolonged or excessive drug use.[17] Another problem associated with decongestants was the illicit manufacture of methamphetamine from ephedrine and pseudoephedrine derivatives found in nonprescription cold medications.[18] This fact led to the removal of these decongestants from many products and to the

Table 26-2
COMMON NASAL DECONGESTANTS

Generic Name	Trade Name(s)*	Dosage Forms
Ephedrine	Bronkaid, others	Oral
Oxymetazoline	Afrin, Dristan 12-Hr Nasal Spray, many others	Nasal spray
Phenylephrine	Sudafed PE, others	Nasal spray
Pseudoephedrine	Chlor Trimeton Nasal Decongestant, Sudafed, many others	Oral
Xylometazoline	Otrivin, Triaminic Decongestant	Nasal spray

**Trade names often reflect combination of the decongestant with other ingredients.*

restriction of the sale of over-the-counter products that still contain these medications.[19]

Antihistamines

Antihistamines are used for reasons ranging from sedation to the treatment of parkinsonism. However, two of the most common applications of antihistamines are the treatment of respiratory symptoms caused by viral infections such as the common cold and the respiratory allergic response to seasonal allergies (e.g., hay fever) and other allergens.[20,21]

Histamine is an endogenous chemical that is involved in the normal regulation of certain physiological functions (e.g., gastric secretion, CNS neural modulation) and various hypersensitivity (allergic) reactions.[22-24] Histamine exerts its effects on various cells through four primary receptor subtypes: the H_1, H_2, H_3, and H_4 receptors.[24] During allergic reactions, respiratory infections, and so forth, the effects of histamine are mediated primarily through the H_1 receptor located on vascular, respiratory, and other tissues.[20]

H_2 receptors are involved primarily in the regulation of gastric acid secretion. Drugs that selectively block the H_2 receptor (referred to simply as *H_2 antagonists*) may help control gastric secretion in conditions such as peptic ulcer (see Chapter 27). The H_3 receptor seems to be important in the control of several functions such as sleep-wake cycles, learning, cognition, and pain modulation.[25] Likewise, an H_4 receptor, found in various locations throughout the body, seems to be important in mediating inflammation in conditions such as asthma, allergic rhinitis, and other types of inflammation.[26] Researchers are investigating the clinical and pharmacological significance of H_3 and H_4 receptors.[27]

By definition, antihistamines are drugs that specifically block the H_1 subtype of histamine receptors. By blocking the effects of histamine on the upper respiratory tissues, these drugs help decrease nasal congestion, mucosal irritation and discharge (rhinitis, sinusitis), and conjunctivitis that are caused by inhaled allergens.[20,28] Similarly, antihistamines may decrease the coughing and sneezing associated with the common cold. Although these drugs do not reverse bronchospasm associated with asthma, antihistamines may be used as an adjunct in patients with asthma to help control rhinitis and sinusitis (see "Treatment of Bronchial Asthma").[29] Antihistamines used in the symptomatic treatment of hay fever and similar allergies are listed in Table 26-3.

The primary adverse effects associated with antihistamines are sedation, fatigue, dizziness, blurred vision, and incoordination. GI distress (nausea, vomiting) is also quite common. Certain side effects are related directly to each drug's ability to cross the blood-brain barrier (see Chapter 5 for a description of the blood-brain barrier). The original, or "first-generation," antihistamines readily cross the blood-brain barrier and enter the brain, thus causing CNS-related side effects such as sedation and psychomotor slowing.[20] Newer "second-generation" antihistamines do not easily cross the blood-brain barrier, and the risk of sedation and other CNS side effects is reduced substantially.[29,30] These newer agents, also known as *nonsedating antihistamines*, include cetirizine (Zyrtec), loratadine (Claritin), desloratadine (Clarinex), and fexofenadine (Allegra) (see Table 26-3). Newer antihistamines also seem to be more selective for the H_1 receptor subtype and produce fewer side effects related to other histamine receptors and receptors for other neurotransmitters (e.g., acetylcholine, serotonin, and norepinephrine).[20]

The newer drugs therefore represent a substantial improvement over original antihistamines. Likewise, certain first-generation antihistamines such as terfenadine and astemizole are no longer available in the United States because of an unacceptable risk of serious cardiovascular side effects. Nonetheless, the beneficial effects of the newer agents vary according to the drug and the patient, and practitioners should make efforts to find the drug and dose that produces antihistamine effects with the fewest side effects for each patient.[31] Several newer nonsedating agents are

Table 26-3
ANTIHISTAMINES

Generic Name	Trade Name(s)*	Dosage†	Sedation Potential§
Azatadine	Optimine	1–2 mg every 8–12 hr	Low
Azelastine	Astelin	2 sprays per nostril twice daily‡	Very low
Brompheniramine	Bromfenac, Dimetapp Allergy, others	4 mg every 4–6 hr	Low
Carbinoxamine	Arbinoxa, Pediatex, others	4–8 mg every 6–8 hr	Low to moderate
Cetirizine	Zyrtec	5–10 mg/d	Very low
Chlorpheniramine	Chlor-Trimeton, Telachlor, others	4 mg every 4–6 hr	Low
Clemastine	Dayhist, Tavist	1.34 mg twice daily; up to 2.68 mg 1–3 times daily	Low
Cyproheptadine	Periactin	4 mg every 8 hr	Moderate
Desloratadine	Clarinex	5 mg once a day	Very low
Dexchlorpheniramine	Polaramine	2 mg every 4–6 hr	Low
Dimenhydrinate	Dramamine, others	50–100 mg every 4–6 hr	High
Diphenhydramine	Benadryl, many others	25–50 mg every 4–6 hr	High
Doxylamine	Aldex AN, Unisom, Nytol Maximum Strength	10 mg every 4–6 hr	High
Fexofenadine	Allegra	60 mg twice daily or 180 mg/d	Very low
Hydroxyzine	Atarax, Vistaril, others	25–100 mg 3–4 times a day	Moderate
Levocetirizine	Xyzal	5 mg once a day in the evening	Low
Loratadine	Claritin, others	10 mg once a day	Very low
Olopatadine	Patanase	2 sprays per nostril twice daily‡	Very low
Phenindamine	Nolahist	25 mg every 4–6 hr	Low
Pyrilamine	Pyrlex	12–24 mg every 12 hr	Moderate
Tripelennamine	PBZ	25–50 mg every 4–6 hr	Moderate
Triprolidine	Actifed, others	2.5 mg every 4–6 hr	Low

**Some trade names reflect the combination of the antihistamine with other agents (decongestants, antitussives, etc.).*

†Normal adult dosage of standard release preparations when taken orally for antihistamine effects. Doses and dosing interval may vary for extended release preparations.

‡Administered by nasal spray.

§Sedation potential is based on comparison to other antihistamines and may vary considerably from person to person.

currently available, and these have become the agents of choice for many people because they decrease histamine-related symptoms without producing excessive sedation and other neuropsychiatric effects.

Mucolytics and Expectorants

Mucolytic drugs attempt to decrease the viscosity of respiratory secretions. Expectorant drugs facilitate the production and ejection of mucus. The intent of these drugs is to prevent the accumulation of thick, viscous secretions that can clog respiratory passages and lead to pulmonary problems. Expectorants and mucolytics can relieve acute disorders ranging from the common cold to pneumonia, as well as chronic disorders such as emphysema and chronic bronchitis.[3,32] These drugs are often taken in combination with other agents (e.g., antitussives, decongestants, bronchodilators). Although mucolytics and expectorants are widely used, there is some question about whether they actually produce beneficial effects in various types of respiratory disease.[33,34] Some studies have documented that these drugs can improve the ability to expel mucus and increase pulmonary function, but the extent of these benefits may vary widely according to the specific patient and type of respiratory illness.[34,35]

The primary mucolytic drug currently in use is acetylcysteine (Mucomyst, Mucosil).[36] This drug is thought to work by splitting the disulfide bonds of respiratory mucoproteins, thus forming a less viscous secretion. There is, however, some evidence that this drug also has antioxidant effects, and some of acetylcysteine's benefits may be due to its ability to decrease free-radical damage in the respiratory tissues.[36,37] Acetylcysteine can likewise be helpful in nonrespiratory conditions and is the primary drug used to prevent liver damage following acetaminophen overdose (see Chapter 15).[38] When used as a mucolytic, acetylcysteine is usually administered directly to the respiratory mucosa by inhalation or intratracheal instillation (through a tracheostomy). The primary adverse effects associated with this drug include nausea, vomiting, inflammation of the oral mucosa (stomatitis), and rhinorrhea. However, serious adverse effects are relatively rare.

Guaifenesin is the only expectorant currently acknowledged by the Food and Drug Administration (FDA) to have evidence of therapeutic effects.[35,39] This drug is administered to increase the production of respiratory secretions, thus encouraging ejection of phlegm and sputum. Exactly how guaifenesin exerts this effect is not fully understood. It is usually administered orally in some form of syrup or elixir and often combined with other agents in over-the-counter preparations, which are known by many different trade names. The primary adverse effect associated with guaifenesin is GI upset, which is exacerbated if excessive doses are taken or if this drug is taken on an empty stomach.

DRUGS USED TO MAINTAIN AIRWAY PATENCY IN OBSTRUCTIVE PULMONARY DISEASE

Airway obstruction is a major problem in respiratory disorders such as bronchial asthma, chronic bronchitis, and emphysema. The latter two disorders are usually grouped under the heading of *chronic obstructive pulmonary disease* (COPD).[40] Asthma and COPD are characterized by bronchospasm, airway inflammation, and mucous plugging of the airways.[40,41] One of the primary goals of drug treatment is to prevent or reverse the bronchial constriction and subsequent obstruction of the airways in these disorders by using bronchodilators (beta-adrenergic agonists, xanthine derivatives, anticholinergics) and anti-inflammatory agents (glucocorticoids, others).

Beta-Adrenergic Agonists

Respiratory smooth-muscle cells contain the beta-2 subtype of adrenergic receptors.[42] (See Chapter 18 for a discussion of adrenergic receptor classifications.) Stimulation of these beta-2 receptors results in *relaxation* of bronchiole smooth muscle. Hence, drugs that stimulate these beta-2 adrenergic receptors (i.e., beta-adrenergic agonists) produce bronchodilation and can be used to prevent or inhibit airway obstruction in bronchospastic diseases.[43]

Mechanisms of Action

Beta-adrenergic agonists are believed to induce smooth-muscle relaxation by the mechanism illustrated in Figure 26-1. Stimulation of the beta-2 receptor increases activity of the adenyl cyclase enzyme. This enzyme increases the production of intracellular cyclic adenosine monophosphate (cAMP). The cAMP acts as an intracellular second messenger, which then increases the activity of other enzymes such as protein kinase. The increased protein kinase activity ultimately inhibits smooth-muscle contraction, probably by adding a phosphate group to specific contractile proteins.

Specific Agents and Method of Administration

Beta-adrenergic agonists used to induce bronchodilation are listed in Table 26-4. Some of these drugs are nonselective and stimulate alpha and beta receptors fairly equally. Other agonists are more selective and preferentially stimulate the beta-adrenergic receptors. The beta-2–specific agents are the most selective and tend to bind preferentially to beta-2 receptors. Beta-2–selective agonists offer an advantage when administered systemically because there is less chance of side effects caused by stimulation of other adrenergic receptors located on other tissues (e.g., beta-1 receptors on the myocardium).[44] Likewise, administration of beta-2 selective drugs by some type of inhaler helps

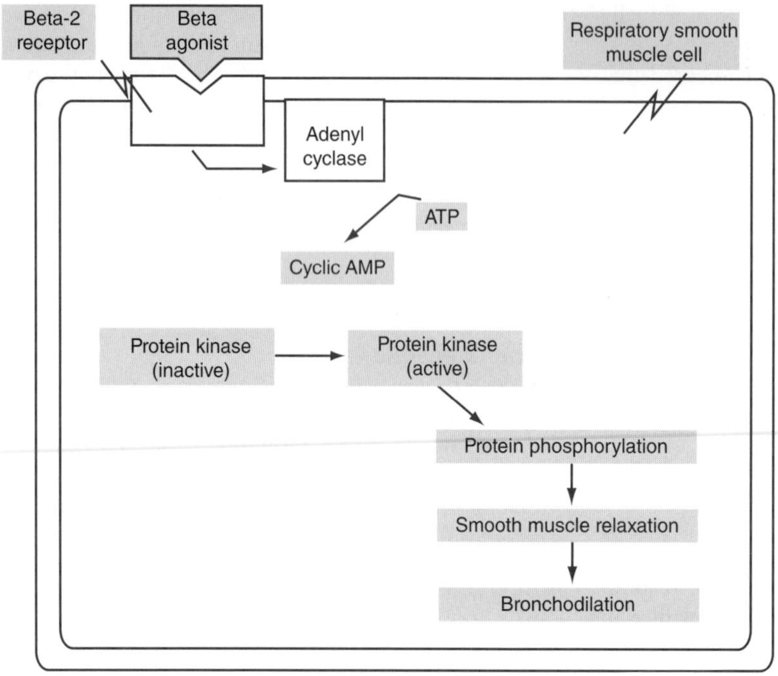

Figure ■ 26-1
Mechanism of action of beta agonists on respiratory smooth muscle. Beta agonists facilitate bronchodilation by stimulating adenyl cyclase activity, which in turn increases intracellular cyclic AMP production. Cyclic AMP activates protein kinase, which appears to add an inhibitory phosphate group to contractile proteins, thus causing muscle relaxation and bronchodilation.

apply the drug directly to the respiratory tissues, thus further reducing the chance of stimulating beta receptors on other tissues.[45] These agents also have different durations of action. Some drugs, such as formoterol and salmeterol, are considered to be long-acting beta-adrenergic agonists and are typically administered twice each day to prevent bronchoconstrictive attacks.[46] Newer beta-2 drugs such as indacaterol are classified as ultra-long acting and offer the advantage of once daily administration.[47,48] These long- and ultra-long-acting agents may provide more stable and sustained bronchodilation in conditions such as asthma and COPD.[46]

Beta-adrenergic drugs can be administered orally, subcutaneously, or by inhalation. Inhalation is often the preferred method. As indicated above, inhalation minimizes systemic side effects.[45] The onset of action is also more rapid with inhalation.

Oral or subcutaneous administration is usually associated with more side effects. However, when administered orally or subcutaneously, beta agonists may reach the more distal branches of the airway to a greater extent. The bronchioles are usually constricted during an asthmatic attack, and inhalation may not deliver the drug to the distal respiratory passages.

Several beta agonists are available in metered-dose inhalers (MDIs) for inhalation administration. MDIs contain the drug in a small aerosol canister, and a specific amount is dispensed each time the patient depresses the canister.[49] Although MDIs are convenient because of their small size and portability, there is a certain amount of coordination required on the patient's part to ensure adequate delivery of the drug. Some patients (e.g., young children) may have trouble timing the inhaled dose with a proper inspiratory effort.[50] In these patients, drug delivery can be facilitated by using a spacer or reservoir-like attachment that sequesters the drug between the MDI and the patient's mouth.[51] The patient can first dispense the drug into the reservoir and then take a deep breath, thus improving delivery to the respiratory tissues.

Another method of inhaling beta agonists is through a *nebulizer*.[52,53] These devices mix the drug with air to form a fine mist that is inhaled through a mask, thus reaching the lungs over a more prolonged period (10 minutes). Nebulizers originally were restricted to use in the home because they were large and required an electrical outlet. Newer devices, however, are portable and use batteries. It was thought that nebulizers would provide a more effective treatment than MDIs or dry powder inhalers because the nebulizer provides a fine mist over a longer time, which would enable better delivery of the drug to the more distal bronchioles. But this has not been proven conclusively,

Table 26-4
BETA-ADRENERGIC BRONCHODILATORS

Drug*	Primary Receptor	Route of Administration	Onset of Action (min)	Time to Peak Effect (hr)	Duration of Action (hr)
Albuterol (Proventil, Ventolin, others	Beta-2	Inhalation	5–15	1–1.5	3–6
		Oral	15–30	2–3	4–6 or more
Arformoterol (Brovana)	Beta-2	Inhalation	—	0.5	12
Epinephrine (Primatene, others)	Alpha, beta-1,2	Inhalation	1	—	1–3
		Intramuscular	6–12	—	<1–4
		Subcutaneous	5–10	0.3	<1–4
Formoterol (Foradil, Perforomist)	Beta-2	Inhalation	15	1–3	12
Indacaterol (Arcapta Neohaler)	Beta-2	Inhalation	5	1–4	24
Isoproterenol (Isuprel, Medihaler-Iso)	Beta-1,2	Inhalation	2–5	—	0.5–2
		Intravenous	Immediate	—	<1
Levalbuterol (Xopenex)	Beta-2	Inhalation	10–17	1.5	5-6
Metaproterenol (Alupent)	Beta-2	Inhalation (aerosol)	Within 1	1	1–5
		Oral	30	1	1–5
Pirbuterol (Maxair)	Beta-2	Inhalation	Within 5	1.5	6–8
Salmeterol (Serevent)	Beta-2	Inhalation	10–25	3–4	12
Terbutaline (Brethaire, Bricanyl)	Beta-2	Inhalation	15–30 Within 15	1–2 Within 0.5–1	3–6 1.5–4
		Oral	Within 60–120	Within 2–3	4–8
		Subcutaneous	Within 15	Within 0.5–1	1.5–4

**Common trade names are shown in parentheses.*

and the therapeutic benefits from nebulizers and other inhalers seem to be equivalent if the patient uses either device appropriately.[54,55] Still, nebulizers may be a useful alternative for people who cannot master the technique needed for MDI delivery.

Finally, beta-2 drugs can be delivered via a dry-powder inhaler (DPI).[56] This method offers the portability and convenience similar to an MDI. Again, the therapeutic effects of delivering a beta-2 drug via a DPI are not superior to other methods of inhalation (MDI, nebulizer), but DPIs may be easier for certain patients who lack the coordination and timing needed to use an MDI.[56,57]

Adverse Effects

With prolonged or excessive use, inhaled adrenergic agonists may actually increase bronchial responses to allergens and other irritants.[58,59] Although the exact reasons are not clear, excessive use of beta-2 drugs may promote airway irritation, thus increasing the incidence and severity of bronchospastic attacks.[60] Prolonged use of beta-2 drugs may also cause tolerance; the dose must be increased to achieve therapeutic effects when this occurs.[43,61] Hence, the regular and repeated use of adrenergic agonists has been questioned somewhat in recent years. These drugs are not typically used as the only method for treating asthma or COPD but may be helpful when combined with other anti-bronchospastic medications (see "Treatment of Bronchial Asthma").

Other side effects depend on the relative selectivity and route of administration of specific agents.[43] Adrenergic agonists that also stimulate beta-1 receptors may cause cardiac irregularities if they reach the myocardium through the systemic circulation. Similarly, stimulation of CNS adrenergic receptors may produce symptoms of nervousness, restlessness, and tremor. Adverse effects are relatively infrequent, however, when beta-adrenergic agonists are used as directed and administered locally via inhalation.

Xanthine Derivatives

Xanthine derivatives are a group of chemically similar compounds that exert a variety of pharmacological effects. Common xanthine derivatives include theophylline, caffeine, and theobromine (Fig. 26-2); these compounds are frequently found in various foods and beverages (e.g., tea, coffee, soft drinks). Theophylline and several theophylline derivatives are also administered therapeutically to produce bronchodilation in asthma and other forms of airway obstruction (e.g., bronchitis, emphysema).[62] Theophylline and caffeine are also potent CNS stimulants, and some of the more common side effects of these drugs are related to this CNS excitation (see "Adverse Effects").

Mechanisms of Action

Although the ability of xanthine derivatives to produce bronchodilation has been recognized for some time, the exact mechanism of action of theophylline and similar agents has been the subject of much debate. These drugs may enhance bronchodilation by inhibiting the phosphodiesterase (PDE) enzyme located in bronchial smooth-muscle cells.[62,63] PDE breaks down cAMP; inhibiting this enzyme results in higher intracellular cAMP concentrations. As discussed in the "Beta-Adrenergic Agonists" section, cAMP is the second messenger that brings about respiratory smooth-muscle relaxation and subsequent bronchodilation. By inhibiting PDE, theophylline can prolong the effects of this second messenger and increase bronchodilation. More important, PDE inhibition may decrease the function of inflammatory cells and inhibit the production of inflammatory mediators, thus accounting for theophylline's anti-inflammatory properties.[64] There is considerable evidence that much of theophylline's beneficial effects are related to this drug's anti-inflammatory properties rather than to a direct bronchodilating effect.[65,66] The importance of controlling airway inflammation is addressed in more detail later in this chapter.

Theophylline may also act as an adenosine antagonist.[64] Adenosine is thought to bind to specific receptors on the smooth-muscle cells and to stimulate contraction. By blocking this effect, theophylline would facilitate smooth-muscle relaxation. It may likewise help produce bronchodilation by other mechanisms, such as inhibition of intracellular calcium release, stimulation of catecholamine release, and activation of enzymes that promote the anti-inflammatory effects of glucocorticoids.[67,68] In reality, theophylline and similar drugs may induce bronchodilation and help protect the airways through a combination of several mechanisms, but the relative importance of each cellular effect remains to be determined.

Specific Agents and Method of Administration

Xanthine derivatives, when used in the treatment of bronchospastic disease, are administered orally, although certain drugs may be given rectally or by injection if the oral route is not tolerated (Table 26-5). When the oral route is used, sustained-release preparations of theophylline are available. These preparations enable the patient to take the drug just once or twice each day, thus improving patient adherence to the drug regimen.

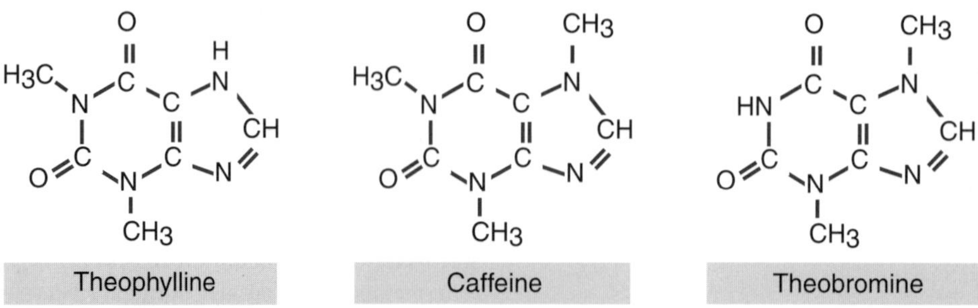

Figure ■ 26-2
Common xanthine derivatives. Theophylline is often administered therapeutically to reduce bronchoconstriction.

Table 26-5
XANTHINE DERIVATIVE BRONCHODILATORS

Generic Name	Trade Name(s)	Dosage Forms
Aminophylline	Phyllocontin, Truphylline	Oral; extended-release oral; rectal; IV injection
Dyphylline	Dilor, Lufyllin, others	Oral
Theophylline	Elixophyllin, Pulmophyllin, others	Oral; extended-release oral; IV injection

Adverse Effects

The most serious limitation in the use of xanthine bronchodilators is the possibility of toxicity.[69,70] Toxicity may appear when plasma levels are between 15 and 20 μg/mL. Because the recommended levels are between 10 and 20 μg/mL, signs of toxicity may occur in some patients even when blood levels are in the therapeutic range. Early signs of toxicity include nausea, confusion, irritability, and restlessness. When blood levels exceed 20 μg/mL, serious toxic effects such as cardiac arrhythmias and seizures may occur. In some patients, the serious toxic effects may be the first indication that there is a problem, because these effects are not always preceded by the more innocuous signs of toxicity. Theophylline-induced seizures are a life-threatening phenomenon, especially in patients who have been ingesting high levels of theophylline for prolonged periods.[69]

Consequently, during long-term use, care should be taken to avoid a toxic accumulation of theophylline. Patients in whom the metabolism of this drug is altered are especially prone to toxicity. In particular, factors such as liver disease, congestive heart failure, patient age (older than 55), infections such as pneumonia, and concomitant use of other drugs (e.g., cimetidine, ciprofloxacin, others) decrease theophylline clearance and therefore increase the likelihood of accumulation and toxicity.[67] To prevent toxicity, the dosage should be individualized for each patient, using the lowest possible dose (see "Treatment of Bronchial Asthma").

Anticholinergic Drugs

The lungs receive extensive parasympathetic innervation via the vagus nerve.[71] The efferent fibers of the vagus nerve release acetylcholine onto respiratory smooth-muscle cells, which contain muscarinic cholinergic receptors. When stimulated, these receptors mediate bronchoconstriction. Likewise, acetylcholine can be released from non-neuronal cells such as respiratory epithelial cells and local inflammatory cells, thus adding to acetylcholine's bronchoconstrictive effects in the lungs.[72]

Mechanisms of Action

Anticholinergic drugs block muscarinic cholinergic receptors and prevent acetylcholine-induced bronchoconstriction, thus improving airflow in certain types of bronchospastic disease. In particular, anticholinergics are often the drugs of choice in treating COPD.[73]

The primary factors that mediate bronchoconstriction in emphysema and chronic bronchitis appear to be increased vagal tone and acetylcholine release from neuronal (vagus nerve) and non-neuronal sources.[72,74] Moreover, excessive acetylcholine influence seems to contribute to other pathophysiological changes in COPD, including inflammation, increased mucus production, chronic cough, and cell proliferation (remodeling) of the airway.[72,75] Remodeling of the airway seems especially harmful because it causes irreversible bronchoconstriction, and thus a more permanent restriction of airflow in patients with COPD.[75]

Hence, drugs that reduce the effects of acetylcholine in the airways are the cornerstone of controlling bronchoconstriction in COPD. Anticholinergics are not typically the first-line treatment of asthma because the airway inflammation underlying asthma seems to be related to changes other than the direct effects of acetylcholine.[71,76] Nonetheless, these drugs can also be used to supplement anti-inflammatory drugs and other medications in treating acute episodes of moderate to severe asthma.[77,78]

Specific Agents and Route of Administration

The anticholinergic bronchodilators include ipratropium and tiotropium, which are muscarinic receptor blockers that are similar in structure and function to atropine. Although atropine is the prototypical muscarinic antagonist, its use in respiratory conditions is usually limited because it is readily absorbed into the systemic circulation and tends to produce many side effects even when administered by inhalation. Alternatively, ipratropium (Atrovent) is poorly absorbed into the systemic circulation and can be administered by an aerosol inhaler with substantially fewer systemic side effects.[79]

Tiotropium (Spiriva) is similar to ipratropium, but with longer-lasting effects.[80,81] Tiotropium only needs to be inhaled once each day, whereas ipratropium is often inhaled three or four times each day.[40,81] It appears that tiotropium may also be superior to ipratropium in improving pulmonary function and reducing the frequency and severity of exacerbations in people with COPD.[81] Future studies will continue to clarify how tiotropium can be used alone or with beta agonists and other bronchodilators to provide optimal treatment of COPD.[82]

Adverse Effects

Systemic side effects associated with atropine include dry mouth, constipation, urinary retention, tachycardia, blurred vision, and confusion. As stated previously, these effects appear to occur much less often with inhaled anticholinergics like ipratropium and tiotropium, which are not absorbed as readily into the systemic circulation.

Glucocorticoids

Inflammation appears to be a key underlying factor in the exaggerated responsiveness of the respiratory passages in asthma and other obstructive pulmonary disorders.[83,84] Because of their powerful anti-inflammatory effects, glucocorticoids are used to control inflammation-mediated bronchospasm and are undoubtedly the most effective agents for controlling asthma.[65,85]

Mechanisms of Action

Glucocorticoids (also known as *corticosteroids*) inhibit the inflammatory response in several important ways. These drugs directly affect the genes and transcription factors that produce inflammatory components.[86,87] As a result, the drugs inhibit the production of proinflammatory products (cytokines, prostaglandins, leukotrienes, etc.) while increasing the production of anti-inflammatory proteins. Glucocorticoids also exert some of their effects via a membrane-bound receptor that regulates activity of inflammatory cells (i.e., macrophages, eosinophils, T lymphocytes) and several other types of cells involved in the inflammatory response.[86] The mechanism of action of glucocorticoids and cellular responses mediated by the glucocorticoids is discussed in more detail in Chapter 29.

Specific Agents and Routes of Administration

Glucocorticoids used to treat asthma are listed in Table 26-6. During severe, acute episodes of bronchoconstriction (e.g., status asthmaticus), glucocorticoids are usually administered intravenously. For more prolonged use, glucocorticoids are given orally or by inhalation. As with the beta agonists, the inhaled route is preferable because of the decreased chance of systemic side effects.[88,89] Glucocorticoids that are currently available via inhalation include beclomethasone, budesonide, flunisolide, and triamcinolone. Inhalation of a glucocorticoid allows the drug to be applied directly to the respiratory mucosa, and any glucocorticoid that is absorbed into the systemic circulation is rapidly metabolized. When these drugs are administered appropriately by the inhalation route, the chance of adverse effects is greatly reduced, compared with the possible effects associated with systemic administration (see "Adverse Effects").[89] Patients should also be advised to rinse their mouths with water after using

Table 26-6
CORTICOSTEROIDS USED IN OBSTRUCTIVE PULMONARY DISEASE

Generic Name	Trade Name(s)	Dosage Forms*
Beclomethasone	Qvar	Inhalation
Betamethasone	Betaject, Celestone	Oral; IV or intramuscular injection
Budesonide	Pulmicort	Inhalation
Cortisone	Cortone	Oral; intramuscular injection
Dexamethasone	DexPak, others	Oral; IV or intramuscular injection
Flunisolide	AeroBid	Inhalation
Hydrocortisone	Cortef, others	Oral; IV or intramuscular injection
Methylprednisolone	Medrol, others	Oral; IV or intramuscular injection
Prednisolone	Prelone, others	Oral; IV or intramuscular injection
Prednisone	Sterapred	Oral
Triamcinolone	Azmacort, others	Inhalation; oral, intramuscular injection

**Dosage forms that use the inhalation route are often preferred in asthma and other obstructive pulmonary diseases. Systemic administration by the oral route or by injection is typically reserved for acute or severe bronchoconstrictive disease.*

oral glucocorticoid inhalers to prevent local irritation of the oral mucosa.

Adverse Effects

The major limitation of the glucocorticoids in any disease is the risk of serious adverse effects. Because of the general catabolic effect of these drugs on supporting tissues, problems with osteoporosis, skin breakdown, and muscle wasting can occur during prolonged systemic administration.[90,91] Other possible systemic effects include retardation of growth in children, cataracts, glaucoma, hyperglycemia, aggravation of diabetes mellitus, and hypertension.[92,93] Patients may also become resistant to anti-inflammatory effects during repeated exposure to these drugs, especially when they are used to treat COPD.[94] Prolonged or excessive use can have a negative feedback effect on the adrenal gland, resulting in loss of adrenal function (adrenal suppression) while these drugs are being administered.[95]

Fortunately, the risk of these adverse effects is minimal when these drugs are administered by inhalation. Inhalation provides a more direct and topical application of the glucocorticoid to the respiratory tissues, with fairly limited absorption of the drug into the systemic circulation. The risk of adverse effects is also minimized when the total dose of the glucocorticoid is kept below certain levels.[88,95] Consequently, patients should avoid prolonged systemic use of glucocorticoids and should use the lowest effective dose by inhalation. It is also prudent to periodically examine patients for bone mineral loss and other side effects when these drugs are used for prolonged periods.[96] Although these drugs are extremely effective in treating various types of bronchoconstriction, they should be used judiciously whenever possible.[89]

Cromones

Cromones such as cromolyn sodium (Intal, Nasalcrom) can help prevent bronchospasm in people with asthma. These drugs are not bronchodilators and will not reverse bronchoconstriction during an asthmatic attack. Hence, these agents must be taken prior to the onset of bronchoconstriction, and they must typically be administered prophylactically to prevent asthma attacks that are initiated by specific, well-defined activities (e.g., exercise, exposure to a friend's pet, pollen).[16,97,98] Likewise, the regular use of these drugs several times each day for several months may decrease airway hyperresponsiveness so that the incidence of asthmatic attacks decreases.[99]

Mechanism of Action

Cromolyn sodium and other cromones are believed to prevent bronchoconstriction by inhibiting the release of inflammatory mediators, such as histamine and leukotrienes from pulmonary mast cells.[100] That is, cromones are generally regarded as mast cell stabilizers because they desensitize these cells to allergens and other substances if the drug is administered before the mast cell is exposed to the precipitating factor. Cromolyn sodium is currently the only agent in this category that is available in the United States. This drug can be administered by inhalation using an MDI or a nebulizer. It is also available in a nonprescription nasal spray (Nasalcrom) that can be helpful in preventing allergic rhinitis associated with seasonal allergies, such as hay fever.[101]

Adverse Effects

Some irritation of the nasal and upper respiratory passages may occur following inhalation, but these drugs are remarkably free of serious adverse reactions. Hence, cromolyn sodium is often used to treat seasonal allergies and may be especially helpful in treating mild persistent asthma in children or people who are unable to tolerate the side effects of other antiasthma drugs.[98,101]

Leukotriene Inhibitors

Leukotrienes are inflammatory compounds that are especially important in mediating the airway inflammation that underlies bronchoconstrictive disease.[102,103] As indicated in Chapter 15, leukotrienes are 20-carbon fatty acids (eicosanoids) that are similar in structure and function to prostaglandins. Leukotrienes are actually derived from the same precursor as prostaglandins (arachidonic acid), but leukotrienes are synthesized by the lipoxygenase enzyme rather than by the cyclooxygenase enzyme (see Fig. 15-2). Pharmacologists developed leukotriene inhibitors to selectively decrease the effects or synthesis of leukotrienes.

Mechanism of Action

Zileuton (Zyflo) inhibits the lipoxygenase enzyme, thereby reducing the production of leukotrienes.[104] Other drugs such as montelukast (Singulair) and zafirlukast (Accolate) block the receptor for leukotrienes on respiratory tissues.[105,106] These drugs offer a fairly selective method for controlling a specific aspect of inflammation in bronchoconstrictive disease.[105]

Evidence also suggests that leukotriene inhibitors can be combined with other drugs (glucocorticoids, beta agonists) to provide optimal management in specific patients with asthma and COPD.[107,108] In particular, it appears that these drugs may enhance the anti-inflammatory effects of glucocorticoids and may therefore provide therapeutic effects at a relatively lower dose of glucocorticoid (glucocorticoid sparing effect).[109,110] Hence, the combination of a glucocorticoid and antileukotriene drug is a treatment option, especially for patients with severe or resistant bronchoconstrictive disease.[110,111]

Adverse Effects

Leukotriene inhibitors are safer than other anti-inflammatory agents, such as the glucocorticoids. Some hepatic impairment has been reported with these drugs, but cases of severe toxicity are relatively rare.

TREATMENT OF BRONCHIAL ASTHMA

Pathophysiology of Bronchial Asthma

Asthma is a disease of the respiratory system characterized by bronchial smooth-muscle spasm, airway inflammation, and mucous plugging of the airways.[112,113] Patients with asthma have an exaggerated bronchoconstrictor response of the airways to various stimuli.[113,114] In many patients, the stimuli that trigger an asthmatic attack are well defined (e.g., allergens like dust, pollen, chemicals, or certain drugs). Exercise, cold, psychological stress, and viral infections may trigger an asthmatic attack in some individuals. In other patients, the initiating factor may be unknown. Asthma is also associated with structural changes in the airway (remodeling) that contributes to the bronchoconstrictive nature of this disease.[113,115]

Although the exact cause of asthma remains to be determined, the basis for the increased airway reactivity has been elucidated somewhat. Airway inflammation is the critical factor in initiating the exaggerated bronchial reactions associated with this disease.[112,116] In asthmatic airways, there seems to be a complex interaction between several different cells, including macrophages, neutrophils, eosinophils, platelets, and the airway epithelial cells themselves.[117] These cells release proinflammatory chemical mediators such as prostaglandins, leukotrienes, bradykinin, histamine, and platelet activating factor.[112,117] The chemicals irritate the respiratory epithelium and stimulate the contraction of bronchiole smooth muscle. Thus, the localized inflammation appears to sensitize airway structures to asthmatic triggers, and the bronchoconstriction and other features of asthma seem to be related directly to the inflammatory response underlying this disease.

Long-Term Management of Asthma

The primary focus of treating asthma has undergone a shift within the last few years. In the past, treatment consisted primarily of bronchodilators such as the beta-adrenergic agonists and the xanthine derivatives, with systemic anti-inflammatory steroids (glucocorticoids) added only in more advanced and severe cases. Glucocorticoids, however, are now used as first-line agents in most patients, including cases of newly detected, mild asthma.[85,118] The increased use of glucocorticoids is largely due to the fact that certain types of glucocorticoids can now be administered by inhalation.

As indicated previously, inhaled glucocorticoids are not absorbed readily into the systemic circulation, and the risk of systemic side effects is therefore substantially reduced. Another reason for the shift toward increased glucocorticoid use is the recognition that these drugs directly reduce the inflammation that underlies asthmatic disease, whereas bronchodilators merely treat the secondary manifestations of this disease.[43] Put more simply, glucocorticoids directly affect the underlying disease process by decreasing the inflammation causing airway hyper-responsiveness.

Glucocorticoids can also be combined with a long-acting beta-2 agonist to provide optimal results.[119] That is, the glucocorticoid can help decrease the inflammatory response that causes airway hyper-responsiveness, while the beta-2 drug maintains bronchodilation in people with asthma. The addition of a beta-2 drug to an inhaled glucocorticoid seems especially helpful in patients who do not respond adequately to the use of only the inhaled glucocorticoid.[119,120] Combining a long-acting beta-2 drug with an inhaled glucocorticoid can also help provide anti-asthmatic effects at relatively lower and safer doses of the inhaled glucocorticoid. Effective use of combined treatment also helps reduce the need to administer the glucocorticoid orally, thus preventing the rather severe problems that can occur if glucocorticoids must be administered systemically to treat asthma.[121] The combination of a glucocorticoid and beta-2 drug can be found in several popular prescription medications listed in Table 26-7.

On the other hand, a short-acting beta-2 agonist can be used as the primary method for *symptomatically* treating asthma attacks. Many patients, for example, inhale short-acting beta-2 agonists through MDIs as "rescue" therapy at the onset of a bronchospastic attack; this technique is a mainstay in managing acute episodes of asthma.[122,123] However, excessive use of beta-2 drugs may be problematic, and patients who need repeated "rescue" therapy for acute attacks should be referred back to their physician for further evaluation and possible alternative drug treatments.

As indicated earlier, leukotrienes play a key role in mediating airway inflammation, and drugs that block leukotriene receptors (montelukast, zafirlukast), or inhibit the formation of leukotrienes (zileuton) can be helpful in the long-term control of asthma.[124] In particular, these drugs may be effective in certain situations, such as exercise-induced asthma.[125] Leukotriene inhibitors are also nonsteroidal and may therefore provide an alternative method for controlling airway inflammation in patients who do not respond adequately to inhaled glucocorticoids.[124,125] Likewise, leukotriene inhibitors may be helpful when combined with an anti-inflammatory steroid (glucocorticoid). The combination can provide optimal anti-inflammatory effects using lower doses of the glucocorticoid, thus preventing the systemic adverse effects associated with higher doses of steroids.[122,123] Hence, leukotriene inhibitors provide another way to control airway inflammation in asthma, and use of these drugs alone or in combination with other medications should be considered in certain patients.

Theophylline, once considered the foundation for asthma drug therapy, is now used sparingly compared to glucocorticoids and other antiasthmatic drugs (beta-2 agonists, leukotriene inhibitors). Theophylline is a powerful bronchodilator, but problems with toxicity often limit its use in the long-term management of asthma.[65,70] Currently, low doses of theophylline are sometimes added to the drug regimen of patients who are resistant to treatment using glucocorticoids and beta agonists.[123,126] The combination of theophylline with a glucocorticoid may provide optimal effects at lower doses of both drugs.[123] It is also recognized that theophylline may have anti-inflammatory effects, and some of the renewed interest in using low-dose theophylline therapy is based on this drug's ability to control airway inflammation rather than actually produce bronchodilation.[64] Hence, theophylline remains an important adjunct in treating certain patients with asthma, and practitioners may administer this drug more extensively as more is learned about the synergistic effects of theophylline and glucocorticoids.

In summary, inhaled glucocorticoids are often the cornerstone of drug therapy for patients with asthma. Leukotriene inhibitors, beta agonists, and theophylline can be used to supplement glucocorticoids as needed, with the specific drug regimen determined on a patient-by-patient basis. In addition, other drugs such as cromolyn sodium and antihistamines can be used to prevent the release or block the irritant effects of histamine in people with asthma.[29,98] Efforts should be made to find the optimal combination of agents for each patient, and the drug regimen must be reviewed constantly and adjusted in response to the patient's needs and the clinical course of the asthmatic disease.

Table 26-7

COMMERCIAL PRODUCTS CONTAINING AN ANTI-INFLAMMATORY STEROID COMBINED WITH A LONG-ACTING BETA-2 BRONCHODILATOR

Trade Name	Anti-inflammatory Steroid	Long-Acting Beta-2 Bronchodilator	Formulation and Dosing Frequency*
Advair HFA	Fluticasone	Salmeterol	Aerosol MDI; 1 inhalation twice each day
Advair Diskus	Fluticasone	Salmeterol	Dry powder inhaler; 1 inhalation twice each day
Dulera	Budesonide	Formoterol	Aerosol MDI; 1 inhalation twice each day
Symbicort	Mometasone	Formoterol	Aerosol MDI; 2 inhalations twice each day

**Recommended dosing frequencies administered by oral inhalation; MDI = metered dose inhaler.*

Along with drug therapy, several nonpharmacological interventions can be employed. If the initiating factors of an asthmatic attack are identified, patients can learn how to avoid these factors whenever possible. Also, considerable evidence shows that aerobic conditioning can improve the overall health and well-being of people with asthma.[127,128] Of course, exercise itself may be an asthmatic trigger in some individuals.[129] However, people with stable asthma that is well controlled by medications can usually exercise safely without an increased risk of bronchospastic attacks.[130]

TREATMENT OF REVERSIBLE BRONCHOSPASM IN COPD

As indicated previously, bronchospasm is often present in COPD—that is, in chronic bronchitis and emphysema.[40] *Chronic bronchitis* is a clinical diagnosis applied to a long-standing inflammation and remodeling of the bronchial tree. *Emphysema* is a pathological condition marked by the destruction of alveolar walls and enlargement of the terminal air spaces.

Drug therapy for COPD is directed primarily toward maintaining airway patency and preventing airflow restriction.[40,131] Thus, anticholinergics (e.g., ipratropium, tiotropium) are often the first drugs used, although long-acting beta-2 agonists can also be used initially to promote bronchodilation.[46,82] Likewise, a long-acting beta agonist can be combined with an anticholinergic such as tiotropium to provide optimal bronchodilation in some patients.[132] Theophylline can also be used as a bronchodilator in COPD and can be combined with other drugs or used as an alternative treatment for patients who fail to respond adequately to other bronchodilators.[131] It has been suggested that at relatively low doses, theophylline may also produce beneficial effects in COPD because of its anti-inflammatory effects rather than its bronchodilating properties.[66] Hence, there has been renewed interest in using theophylline as a part of COPD treatment.[40]

Glucocorticoids have also been used to treat airway inflammation in COPD, but their use in this situation remains somewhat controversial. Some research suggests that addition of glucocorticoids to bronchodilator drugs such as the long-acting beta-2 agonists may reduce exacerbations and improve lung function in certain situations, such as in patients with more severe airflow restriction or frequent exacerbations of COPD-related bronchospasm.[131,133] The commercial products that contain a long-acting beta-2 agonist and a glucocorticoid provide a convenient way to administer both drugs simultaneously to patients with COPD (see Table 26-7). However, the addition of glucocorticoids to bronchodilator therapy has not always produced clear therapeutic benefits in the long-term treatment of COPD.[134] Researchers therefore continue to investigate the role of glucocorticoids in COPD, and future studies may help clarify whether there is an ideal combination of specific glucocorticoids and bronchodilators that might be helpful in the long-term management of patients with COPD.

TREATMENT OF RESPIRATORY PROBLEMS IN CYSTIC FIBROSIS

Cystic fibrosis is one of the most common hereditary diseases in Caucasian populations—the autosomal-recessive trait is found in approximately 1 out of 2,000 to 4,000 Caucasian births.[135] Cystic fibrosis essentially affects all the major exocrine glands, resulting in very thick, viscous secretions. These thickened secretions often form mucous plugs, which obstruct major ducts in various glands and organs.[136] For instance, the pancreatic and bile ducts are often obstructed, resulting in problems with nutrient digestion and absorption. Mucous plugging of the bronchioles occurs quite frequently, leading to pulmonary problems such as pneumonia, bronchiectasis, pulmonary fibrosis, and various pulmonary infections (especially *Staphylococcus and Pseudomonas*). These respiratory problems are often the primary health threat to individuals with cystic fibrosis.[137]

Pharmacological management of respiratory problems in cystic fibrosis is focused on maintaining airway patency as much as possible. Bronchodilators and mucolytic and/or expectorant drugs may help limit the formation of mucous plugs. Systemic glucocorticoids (e.g., prednisone) may also be beneficial in some patients in limiting airway inflammation and improving pulmonary function.[138] The side effects and risks of long-term systemic glucocorticoids, however, may outweigh any benefits, especially in children.[139,140] Inhaled glucocorticoids could reduce the likelihood of severe adverse effects, but their beneficial effects are limited because inhaled forms of these drugs cannot penetrate through the thick mucus secretions in the airways of people with cystic fibrosis.[140] Other nonsteroidal anti-inflammatory interventions, including high doses of NSAIDs (e.g., ibuprofen), might also help control inflammation and possibly slow the progression of lung disease in children with cystic fibrosis.[141]

Anti-infectious agents also play a key role in the treatment of cystic fibrosis, and respiratory infections are treated with appropriate antibiotic agents.[135] In particular, azithromycin has shown considerable promise because it is an antibacterial drug with anti-inflammatory and immunomodulating properties.[142,143]

In addition to drug therapy, daily maintenance of respiratory hygiene (postural drainage, breathing exercises, etc.) is a key component in the management of cystic fibrosis. Evidence for the beneficial effects of chest physical therapy has been questioned somewhat, but there seems little doubt that a regular exercise program can help improve cardiovascular health and musculoskeletal function in people with cystic fibrosis.[144,145] Likewise, good nutrition and maintenance of healthy body weight may also help promote optimal health.[146] With recent advances in medical treatment, many people with cystic fibrosis are living into their third or fourth decade, and an exercise program seems especially important in helping maintain quality of life for these individuals.[147]

Although there is still no cure for cystic fibrosis, researchers have developed several pharmacological techniques that may help decrease the viscosity of respiratory secretions in patients with this disease. One technique uses aerosol preparations that contain enzymes known as *deoxyribonucleases*. These enzymes can be inhaled to break down the large quantities of DNA that are present in respiratory secretions of patients with cystic fibrosis.[148,149] Respiratory secretions in these patients often contain large amounts of DNA because the genetic material contained in airway inflammatory cells is deposited into the airway lumen when these cells are destroyed. DNA increases the viscosity and thickness of the respiratory secretions.

Preparations that contain recombinant human deoxyribonuclease (rhDNase; dornase alfa, Pulmozyme) can lyse this DNA, thus decreasing the viscosity of these secretions and improving pulmonary function and reducing the chance of lung collapse (atelectasis) and infection.[149,150] This treatment is typically administered by inhalation via a nebulizer, with the dose and frequency adjusted according to the needs of each patient. Researchers continue to investigate the optimal and most cost-effective way to incorporate deoxyribonuclease therapy into a drug for people with cystic fibrosis.[148]

Finally, considerable progress has been made to develop strategies to correct the defective gene causing cystic fibrosis.[151] This gene therapy may someday provide an effective long-term treatment by replacing the defective gene with a functionally correct gene.[152,153] These strategies and other new techniques are still experimental at present, but there is hope that these interventions may someday provide a means to alleviate the primary respiratory complications that often lead to illness and death in patients with cystic fibrosis.

Special Concerns for Rehabilitation Patients

Proper respiratory hygiene is crucial in preventing the serious adverse effects of respiratory infection and obstructive pulmonary disease. The accumulation of bronchial secretions can lead to decreased gas exchange, atelectasis, and additional infection. Rehabilitation specialists often play a critical role in preventing pulmonary mucus accumulation.[154,155] Therapists can facilitate the pharmacotherapeutic effects of mucolytic and expectorant drugs by performing postural drainage and breathing exercises. Even if patients are not being treated directly with chest physical therapy and respiratory hygiene, rehabilitation specialists should always encourage patients to cough and raise secretions for expectoration. Physical therapists and occupational therapists should also coordinate their treatments with respiratory therapy. Often, mucolytic and expectorant drugs are administered by the respiratory therapist through a nebulizer or positive-pressure ventilator. A program of chest physical therapy may

Continued on following page

Special Concerns for Rehabilitation Patients (Continued)

be most effective when administered 30 minutes to 1 hour after these agents are administered (i.e., after the drugs have had some time to exert an effect on respiratory secretions).

Therapists must be aware of which patients are prone to bronchospastic attacks. If patients use some sort of portable aerosol bronchodilator, they should always bring their medication to therapy. Rehabilitation procedures involving exercise may trigger a bronchospastic attack in some individuals, so it is important to have the medication close at hand.

Therapists must also be aware of the potential side effects of bronchodilator drugs. In particular, the cardiac side effects of the beta-adrenergic agonists and xanthine derivatives (theophylline, others) need to be considered. Therapists may notice cardiac arrhythmias while monitoring the electrocardiogram (ECG) or while taking the patient's pulse; these cardiac abnormalities may indicate a problem with the bronchodilator medications. Noncardiac symptoms such as nervousness, confusion, and tremors may also indicate bronchodilator toxicity and should be brought to the physician's attention. Early recognition of toxicity may be lifesaving, especially when the patient is using xanthine derivatives such as theophylline. Finally, patients receiving systemic glucocorticoid treatment may be prone to the well-known catabolic effects of these drugs. Therapists should be especially alert for skin breakdown and should take care not to overstress the bones and musculotendinous structures that may be weakened by the prolonged use of glucocorticoids.

CASE STUDY

RESPIRATORY DRUGS

Brief History. V.C., a 63-year-old man, has a long history of COPD and hypertension. Twelve years ago, he was diagnosed with emphysema. During the past 5 years, his symptoms of shortness of breath, wheezing, and bronchospasm have become progressively worse. He is also a chronic cigarette smoker and has had a cough for many years, which produces large amounts of sputum daily. Although his physician advised him repeatedly to quit smoking, the patient was unable to kick the habit. To control his bronchospasm, the patient self-administers an inhaled anticholinergic agent, tiotropium (Spiriva), via a dry powder inhaler (18 mcg/inhalation) once each day. To help resolve acute bronchospasm, he uses an inhaled beta-2 agonist, albuterol (Ventolin), via two inhalations from a metered dose inhaler (90 mcg/inhalation) at the onset of an attack. He is also taking a diuretic and an angiotensin-converting enzyme (ACE) inhibitor to control his hypertension. Two days ago, he was admitted to the hospital with weakness and incoordination in his left arm and leg. Subsequent medical tests indicated that he had suffered a cerebral vascular accident. Physical therapy was ordered to begin at the patient's bedside to facilitate optimal recovery from the stroke. The physical therapist began treating the patient with passive and active exercises to encourage motor return. The patient was also under the care of a respiratory therapist. The respiratory therapy treatments included administration of the mucolytic drug acetylcysteine (Mucomyst) via a nebulizer at a dose of 5 ml of 20 percent solution three times daily. The patient continued to self-administer the beta-2 agonist at the onset of bronchospasms.

Problem/Influence of Medication. Despite the program of respiratory therapy, bronchial secretions

CASE STUDY (Continued)

began to accumulate in the patient's airways. The patient had been instructed in deep-breathing and coughing exercises, and he was told by the respiratory therapist to perform these exercises periodically throughout the day. However, no postural drainage was being performed to encourage ejection of sputum.

1. ***What additional physical interventions can be used to complement the drug therapy?***
2. ***When should these physical interventions be administered to take optimal advantage of the effects of the pulmonary drugs?***

See Appendix C, "Answers to Case Study Questions."

SUMMARY

The drugs discussed in this chapter are used to control irritation and maintain airflow through the respiratory passages. Drugs such as the antitussives, decongestants, antihistamines, mucolytics, and expectorants are used primarily for the temporary relief of cold, flu, and seasonal allergy symptoms. These agents are frequently found in over-the-counter preparations, and several different agents are often combined in the same commercial product. Airway obstruction in chronic disorders such as bronchial asthma, chronic bronchitis, and emphysema is treated primarily with bronchodilator agents (beta-adrenergic agonists, xanthine derivatives, anticholinergics) and anti-inflammatory drugs (glucocorticoids, cromones, leukotriene inhibitors).

Rehabilitation specialists should be cognizant of which patients suffer from bronchospastic disorders (e.g., asthma) and of what medications are being used to control airway obstruction. Therapists can help facilitate the pharmacotherapeutic goals in patients with obstructive pulmonary disease by encouraging proper respiratory hygiene and breathing exercises and by helping improve overall cardiorespiratory endurance whenever possible.

REFERENCES

1. De Sutter AI, van Driel ML, Kumar AA, et al. Oral antihistamine-decongestant-analgesic combinations for the common cold. *Cochrane Database Syst Rev*. 2012;2:CD004976.
2. Jackson Allen P, Simenson S. Management of common cold symptoms with over-the-counter medications: clearing the confusion. *Postgrad Med*. 2013;125:73-81.
3. Smith SM, Schroeder K, Fahey T. Over-the-counter (OTC) medications for acute cough in children and adults in ambulatory settings. *Cochrane Database Syst Rev*. 2012;8:CD001831.
4. Rubin BK. The role of mucus in cough research. *Lung*. 2010; 188(suppl 1):S69-72.
5. Carr MJ. Antitussives: the pharmacological pipeline. *Pulm Pharmacol Ther*. 2009;22:152-154.
6. Chung KF. Clinical cough VI: the need for new therapies for cough: disease-specific and symptom-related antitussives. *Handb Exp Pharmacol*. 2009;187:343-368.
7. Fashner J, Ericson K, Werner S. Treatment of the common cold in children and adults. *Am Fam Physician*. 2012;86: 153-159.
8. Vassilev ZP, Kabadi S, Villa R. Safety and efficacy of over-the-counter cough and cold medicines for use in children. *Expert Opin Drug Saf*. 2010;9:233-242.
9. Isbister GK, Prior F, Kilham HA. Restricting cough and cold medicines in children. *J Paediatr Child Health*. 2012;48: 91-98.
10. Ryan T, Brewer M, Small L. Over-the-counter cough and cold medication use in young children. *Pediatr Nurs*. 2008;34: 174-180, 184.
11. Shefrin AE, Goldman RD. Use of over-the-counter cough and cold medications in children. *Can Fam Physician*. 2009;55: 1081-1083.
12. Gibson PG, Ryan NM. Cough pharmacotherapy: current and future status. *Expert Opin Pharmacother*. 2011;12:1745-1755.
13. Yaksh TL, Wallace MS. Opioids, analgesia, and pain management. In: Brunton L, et al, eds. *The Pharmacological Basis of Therapeutics*. 12th ed. New York: McGraw-Hill; 2011.
14. Westfall TC, Westfall DP. Adrenergic agonists and antagonists. In: Brunton L, et al, eds. *The Pharmacological Basis of Therapeutics*. 12th ed. New York: McGraw-Hill; 2011.
15. Mortuaire G, de Gabory L, François M. Rebound congestion and rhinitis medicamentosa: nasal decongestants in clinical practice. Critical review of the literature by a medical panel. *Eur Ann Otorhinolaryngol Head Neck Dis*. 2013;130:137-144.
16. Kushnir NM. The role of decongestants, cromolyn, guafenesin, saline washes, capsaicin, leukotriene antagonists, and other treatments on rhinitis. *Immunol Allergy Clin North Am*. 2011;31: 601-617.
17. Shah R, McGrath KG. Chapter 6: nonallergic rhinitis. *Allergy Asthma Proc*. 2012;33(suppl 1):S19-21.

18. Cunningham JK, Callaghan RC, Tong D, et al. Changing over-the-counter ephedrine and pseudoephedrine products to prescription only: impacts on methamphetamine clandestine laboratory seizures. *Drug Alcohol Depend.* 2012;126:55-64.
19. McKetin R, Sutherland R, Bright DA, Norberg MM. A systematic review of methamphetamine precursor regulations. *Addiction.* 2011;106:1911-1924.
20. Kalpaklioglu F, Baccioglu A. Efficacy and safety of H1-antihistamines: an update. *Antiinflamm Antiallergy Agents Med Chem.* 2012;11:230-237.
21. Simons FE, Simons KJ. Histamine and H1-antihistamines: celebrating a century of progress. *J Allergy Clin Immunol.* 2011;128:1139-1150.
22. Jutel M, Akdis M, Akdis CA. Histamine, histamine receptors and their role in immune pathology. *Clin Exp Allergy.* 2009;39: 1786-1800.
23. Tiligada E, Kyriakidis K, Chazot PL, Passani MB. Histamine pharmacology and new CNS drug targets. *CNS Neurosci Ther.* 2011;17:620-628.
24. Walter M, Stark H. Histamine receptor subtypes: a century of rational drug design. *Front Biosci.* 2012;4:461-488.
25. Schwartz JC. The histamine H3 receptor: from discovery to clinical trials with pitolisant. *Br J Pharmacol.* 2011;163: 713-721.
26. Kiss R, Keserű GM. Histamine H4 receptor ligands and their potential therapeutic applications: an update. *Expert Opin Ther Pat.* 2012;22:205-221.
27. Tiligada E, Zampeli E, Sander K, Stark H. Histamine H3 and H4 receptors as novel drug targets. *Expert Opin Investig Drugs.* 2009;18:1519-1531.
28. Cobanoğlu B, Toskala E, Ural A, Cingi C. Role of leukotriene antagonists and antihistamines in the treatment of allergic rhinitis. *Curr Allergy Asthma Rep.* 2013;13:203-208.
29. Bachert C, Maspero J. Efficacy of second-generation antihistamines in patients with allergic rhinitis and comorbid asthma. *J Asthma.* 2011;48:965-973.
30. Church DS, Church MK. Pharmacology of antihistamines. *World Allergy Organ J.* 2011;4(suppl):S22-27.
31. Church MK, Maurer M. H(1)-antihistamines and urticaria: how can we predict the best drug for our patient? *Clin Exp Allergy.* 2012;42:1423-1429.
32. Poole P, Black PN, Cates CJ. Mucolytic agents for chronic bronchitis or chronic obstructive pulmonary disease. *Cochrane Database Syst Rev.* 2012;8:CD001287.
33. Bolser DC. Pharmacologic management of cough. *Otolaryngol Clin North Am.* 2010;43:147-155.
34. Chang CC, Cheng AC, Chang AB. Over-the-counter (OTC) medications to reduce cough as an adjunct to antibiotics for acute pneumonia in children and adults. *Cochrane Database Syst Rev.* 2012;2:CD006088.
35. Storms W, Farrar JR. Guaifenesin in rhinitis. *Curr Allergy Asthma Rep.* 2009;9:101-106.
36. Sadowska AM. N-Acetylcysteine mucolysis in the management of chronic obstructive pulmonary disease. *Ther Adv Respir Dis.* 2012;6:127-135.
37. Nair GB, Ilowite JS. Pharmacologic agents for mucus clearance in bronchiectasis. *Clin Chest Med.* 2012;33:363-370.
38. Heard K, Green J. Acetylcysteine therapy for acetaminophen poisoning. *Curr Pharm Biotechnol.* 2012;13:1917-1923.
39. Paul IM. Therapeutic options for acute cough due to upper respiratory infections in children. *Lung.* 2012;190:41-44.
40. Williams DM, Bourdet SV. Chronic obstructive pulmonary disease. In: DiPiro JT, et al, eds. *Pharmacotherapy: A Pathophysiologic Approach.* 8th ed. New York: McGraw-Hill; 2011.
41. Athanazio R. Airway disease: similarities and differences between asthma, COPD and bronchiectasis. *Clinics (Sao Paulo).* 2012;67:1335-1343.
42. Hizawa N. Beta-2 adrenergic receptor genetic polymorphisms and asthma. *J Clin Pharm Ther.* 2009;34:631-643.
43. Cazzola M, Page CP, Rogliani P, Matera MG. β2-agonist therapy in lung disease. *Am J Respir Crit Care Med.* 2013;187:690-696.
44. Matera MG, Martuscelli E, Cazzola M. Pharmacological modulation of beta-adrenoceptor function in patients with coexisting chronic obstructive pulmonary disease and chronic heart failure. *Pulm Pharmacol Ther.* 2010;23:1-8.
45. Capstick TG, Clifton IJ. Inhaler technique and training in people with chronic obstructive pulmonary disease and asthma. *Expert Rev Respir Med.* 2012;6:91-101.
46. Decramer ML, Hanania NA, Lötvall JO, Yawn BP. The safety of long-acting β2-agonists in the treatment of stable chronic obstructive pulmonary disease. *Int J Chron Obstruct Pulmon Dis.* 2013;8:53-64.
47. Kerwin EM, Williams J. Indacaterol 75 μg once daily for the treatment of patients with chronic obstructive pulmonary disease: a North American perspective. *Ther Adv Respir Dis.* 2013;7: 25-37.
48. Ray SM, McMillen JC, Treadway SA, et al. Indacaterol: a novel long-acting β(2)-agonist. *Pharmacotherapy.* 2012;32:456-474.
49. Ehtezazi T. Recent patents in pressurised metered dose inhalers. *Recent Pat Drug Deliv Formul.* 2012;6:31-44.
50. Inhaler Error Steering Committee, Price D, Bosnic-Anticevich S, et al. Inhaler competence in asthma: common errors, barriers to use and recommended solutions. *Respir Med.* 2013;107:37-46.
51. Lavorini F, Fontana GA. Targeting drugs to the airways: the role of spacer devices. *Expert Opin Drug Deliv.* 2009;6:91-102.
52. Dhand R, Dolovich M, Chipps B, et al. The role of nebulized therapy in the management of COPD: evidence and recommendations. *COPD.* 2012;9:58-72.
53. Smith C, Goldman RD. Nebulizers versus pressurized metered-dose inhalers in preschool children with wheezing. *Can Fam Physician.* 2012;58:528-530.
54. Raissy HH, Kelly HW. MDI versus nebulizers for acute asthma. *J Pediatr Pharmacol Ther.* 2004;9:226-234.
55. Ramlal SK, Visser FJ, Hop WC, et al. The effect of bronchodilators administered via aerochamber or a nebulizer on inspiratory lung function parameters. *Respir Med.* 2013;107:1393-1399.
56. Selroos O, Borgström L, Ingelf J. Use of dry powder inhalers in acute exacerbations of asthma and COPD. *Ther Adv Respir Dis.* 2009;3:81-91.
57. Barrons R, Pegram A, Borries A. Inhaler device selection: special considerations in elderly patients with chronic obstructive pulmonary disease. *Am J Health Syst Pharm.* 2011;68: 1221-1232.
58. Salpeter SR. An update on the safety of long-acting beta-agonists in asthma patients using inhaled corticosteroids. *Expert Opin Drug Saf.* 2010;9:407-419.
59. Wijesinghe M, Weatherall M, Perrin K, et al. Risk of mortality associated with formoterol: a systematic review and meta-analysis. *Eur Respir J.* 2009;34:803-811.
60. Wraight JM, Smith AD, Cowan JO, et al. Adverse effects of short-acting beta-agonists: potential impact when anti-inflammatory therapy is inadequate. *Respirology.* 2004;9:215-221.

61. Yim RP, Koumbourlis AC. Tolerance & resistance to β2-agonist bronchodilators. *Paediatr Respir Rev.* 2013;14:195-198.
62. Tilley SL. Methylxanthines in asthma. *Handb Exp Pharmacol.* 2011;200:439-456.
63. Schudt C, Hatzelmann A, Beume R, Tenor H. Phosphodiesterase inhibitors: history of pharmacology. *Handb Exp Pharmacol.* 2011;204:1-46.
64. Haskó G, Cronstein B. Methylxanthines and inflammatory cells. *Handb Exp Pharmacol.* 2011;200:457-468.
65. Rottier BL, Duiverman EJ. Anti-inflammatory drug therapy in asthma. *Paediatr Respir Rev.* 2009;10:214-219.
66. Zhang WH, Zhang Y, Cui YY, et al. Can β2-adrenoceptor agonists, anticholinergic drugs, and theophylline contribute to the control of pulmonary inflammation and emphysema in COPD? *Fundam Clin Pharmacol.* 2012;26:118-134.
67. Barnes PJ. Pulmonary pharmacology. In: Brunton L, et al, eds. *The Pharmacological Basis of Therapeutics.* 12th ed. New York: McGraw-Hill; 2011.
68. Guerreiro S, Marien M, Michel PP. Methylxanthines and ryanodine receptor channels. *Handb Exp Pharmacol.* 2011;200: 135-150.
69. Boison D. Methylxanthines, seizures, and excitotoxicity. *Handb Exp Pharmacol.* 2011;200:251-266.
70. Boushey HA. Drugs used in asthma. In: Katzung BG, ed. *Basic and Clinical Pharmacology.* 12th ed. New York: Lange Medical Books/McGraw Hill; 2012.
71. Buels KS, Fryer AD. Muscarinic receptor antagonists: effects on pulmonary function. *Handb Exp Pharmacol.* 2012;208:317-341.
72. Pieper MP. The non-neuronal cholinergic system as novel drug target in the airways. *Life Sci.* 2012;91:1113-1138.
73. Joos GF. Potential for long-acting muscarinic antagonists in chronic obstructive pulmonary disease. *Expert Opin Investig Drugs.* 2010;19:257-264.
74. Meurs H, Dekkers BG, Maarsingh H, et al. Muscarinic receptors on airway mesenchymal cells: novel findings for an ancient target. *Pulm Pharmacol Ther.* 2013;26:145-155.
75. Karakiulakis G, Roth M. Muscarinic receptors and their antagonists in COPD: anti-inflammatory and antiremodeling effects. *Mediators Inflamm.* 2012;2012:409580.
76. Teoh L, Cates CJ, Hurwitz M, et al. Anticholinergic therapy for acute asthma in children. *Cochrane Database Syst Rev.* 2012;4:CD003797.
77. Kerstjens HA, Engel M, Dahl R, et al. Tiotropium in asthma poorly controlled with standard combination therapy. *N Engl J Med.* 2012;367:1198-1207.
78. O'Byrne PM, Naji N, Gauvreau GM. Severe asthma: future treatments. *Clin Exp Allergy.* 2012;42:706-711.
79. Scullion JE. The development of anticholinergics in the management of COPD. *Int J Chron Obstruct Pulmon Dis.* 2007;2:33-40.
80. Karner C, Chong J, Poole P. Tiotropium versus placebo for chronic obstructive pulmonary disease. *Cochrane Database Syst Rev.* 2012;7:CD009285.
81. Keating GM. Tiotropium bromide inhalation powder: a review of its use in the management of chronic obstructive pulmonary disease. *Drugs.* 2012;72:273-300.
82. Yohannes AM, Connolly MJ, Hanania NA. Ten years of tiotropium: clinical impact and patient perspectives. *Int J Chron Obstruct Pulmon Dis.* 2013;8:117-125.
83. Killeen K, Skora E. Pathophysiology, diagnosis, and clinical assessment of asthma in the adult. *Nurs Clin North Am.* 2013; 48:11-23.
84. Malmström K, Pelkonen AS, Mäkelä MJ. Remodeling, inflammation and airway responsiveness in early childhood asthma. *Curr Opin Allergy Clin Immunol.* 2013;13:203-210.
85. Kandeel M, Balaha M, Inagaki N, Kitade Y. Current and future asthma therapies. *Drugs Today.* 2013;49:325-339.
86. Stahn C, Buttgereit F. Genomic and nongenomic effects of glucocorticoids. *Nat Clin Pract Rheumatol.* 2008;4:525-533.
87. Strehl C, Spies CM, Buttgereit F. Pharmacodynamics of glucocorticoids. *Clin Exp Rheumatol.* 2011;29(suppl 68): S13-18.
88. Castro-Rodriguez JA, Pedersen S. The role of inhaled corticosteroids in management of asthma in infants and preschoolers. *Curr Opin Pulm Med.* 2013;19:54-59.
89. Ernst P, Suissa S. Systemic effects of inhaled corticosteroids. *Curr Opin Pulm Med.* 2012;18:85-89.
90. Pereira RM, Freire de Carvalho J. Glucocorticoid-induced myopathy. *Joint Bone Spine.* 2011;78:41-44.
91. Weinstein RS. Glucocorticoid-induced osteoporosis and osteonecrosis. *Endocrinol Metab Clin North Am.* 2012;41:595-611.
92. Coutinho AE, Chapman KE. The anti-inflammatory and immunosuppressive effects of glucocorticoids, recent developments and mechanistic insights. *Mol Cell Endocrinol.* 2011; 335:2-13.
93. Lui JC, Baron J. Effects of glucocorticoids on the growth plate. *Endocr Dev.* 2011;20:187-193.
94. Barnes PJ. Corticosteroid resistance in patients with asthma and chronic obstructive pulmonary disease. *J Allergy Clin Immunol.* 2013;131:636-645.
95. Schwartz RH, Neacsu O, Ascher DP, Alpan O. Moderate dose inhaled corticosteroid-induced symptomatic adrenal suppression: case report and review of the literature. *Clin Pediatr.* 2012;51:1184-1190.
96. Bolster MB. Osteoporosis and bone health in patients with lung disease. *Clin Chest Med.* 2010;31:555-563.
97. Melvin TA, Patel AA. Pharmacotherapy for allergic rhinitis. *Otolaryngol Clin North Am.* 2011;44:727-739.
98. Netzer NC, Küpper T, Voss HW, Eliasson AH. The actual role of sodium cromoglycate in the treatment of asthma—a critical review. *Sleep Breath.* 2012;16:1027-1032.
99. van der Wouden JC, Uijen JH, Bernsen RM, et al. Inhaled sodium cromoglycate for asthma in children. *Cochrane Database Syst Rev.* 2008;4:CD002173.
100. Amin K. The role of mast cells in allergic inflammation. *Respir Med.* 2012;106:9-14.
101. Ratner PH, Ehrlich PM, Fineman SM, et al. Use of intranasal cromolyn sodium for allergic rhinitis. *Mayo Clin Proc.* 2002;77: 350-354.
102. Di Gennaro A, Haeggström JZ. The leukotrienes: immune-modulating lipid mediators of disease. *Adv Immunol.* 2012;116: 51-92.
103. Okunishi K, Peters-Golden M. Leukotrienes and airway inflammation. *Biochim Biophys Acta.* 2011;1810:1096-1102.
104. Aparoy P, Reddy KK, Reddanna P. Structure and ligand based drug design strategies in the development of novel 5- LOX inhibitors. *Curr Med Chem.* 2012;19:3763-3778.
105. Amlani S, Nadarajah T, McIvor RA. Montelukast for the treatment of asthma in the adult population. *Expert Opin Pharmacother.* 2011;12:2119-2128.
106. Singh RK, Tandon R, Dastidar SG, Ray A. A review on leukotrienes and their receptors with reference to asthma. *J Asthma.* 2013;50:922-931.

107. Amlani S, McIvor RA. Montelukast in childhood asthma: what is the evidence for its use? *Expert Rev Respir Med.* 2011;5:17-25.
108. Bousquet J, Demoly P, Humbert M. Montelukast in guidelines and beyond. *Adv Ther.* 2009;26:575-587.
109. del Giudice MM, Pezzulo A, Capristo C, et al. Leukotriene modifiers in the treatment of asthma in children. *Ther Adv Respir Dis.* 2009;3:245-251.
110. Montuschi P, Peters-Golden ML. Leukotriene modifiers for asthma treatment. *Clin Exp Allergy.* 2010;40:1732-1741.
111. Bozek A, Warkocka-Szoltysek B, Filipowska-Gronska A, Jarzab J. Montelukast as an add-on therapy to inhaled corticosteroids in the treatment of severe asthma in elderly patients. *J Asthma.* 2012;49:530-534.
112. Kelly HW, Sorkness CA. Asthma. In: DiPiro JT, et al, eds. *Pharmacotherapy: A Pathophysiologic Approach.* 8th ed. New York: McGraw-Hill; 2011.
113. Killeen K, Skora E. Pathophysiology, diagnosis, and clinical assessment of asthma in the adult. *Nurs Clin North Am.* 2013;48:11-23.
114. Lommatzsch M. Airway hyperresponsiveness: new insights into the pathogenesis. *Semin Respir Crit Care Med.* 2012;33: 579-587.
115. Bergeron C, Tulic MK, Hamid Q. Airway remodelling in asthma: from benchside to clinical practice. *Can Respir J.* 2010;17: e85-93.
116. Myers TR, Tomasio L. Asthma: 2015 and beyond. *Respir Care.* 2011;56:1389-1410.
117. Naik SR, Wala SM. Inflammation, allergy and asthma, complex immune origin diseases: mechanisms and therapeutic agents. *Recent Pat Inflamm Allergy Drug Discov.* 2013;7: 62-95.
118. Kramer S, Rottier BL, Scholten RJ, Boluyt N. Ciclesonide versus other inhaled corticosteroids for chronic asthma in children. *Cochrane Database Syst Rev.* 2013;2:CD010352.
119. Tamm M, Richards DH, Beghé B, Fabbri L. Inhaled corticosteroid and long-acting β2-agonist pharmacological profiles: effective asthma therapy in practice. *Respir Med.* 2012;106 (suppl 1):S9-19.
120. Ducharme FM, Ni Chroinin M, Greenstone I, Lasserson TJ. Addition of long-acting beta2-agonists to inhaled corticosteroids versus same dose inhaled corticosteroids for chronic asthma in adults and children. *Cochrane Database Syst Rev.* 2010;5: CD005535.
121. Newton R, Leigh R, Giembycz MA. Pharmacological strategies for improving the efficacy and therapeutic ratio of glucocorticoids in inflammatory lung diseases. *Pharmacol Ther.* 2010;125:286-327.
122. FitzGerald JM, Shahidi N. Achieving asthma control in patients with moderate disease. *J Allergy Clin Immunol.* 2010;125: 307-311.
123. Weir NA, Levine SJ. Achieving symptom control in patients with moderate asthma. *Clin Med Insights Circ Respir Pulm Med.* 2012;6:1-11.
124. Sabin BR, Avila PC, Grammer LC, Greenberger PA. Chapter 15: lessons learned from clinical trials of asthma. *Allergy Asthma Proc.* 2012;33(suppl 1):S51-54.
125. Dumitru C, Chan SM, Turcanu V. Role of leukotriene receptor antagonists in the management of pediatric asthma: an update. *Paediatr Drugs.* 2012;14:317-330.
126. Dennis RJ, Solarte I, Rodrigo G. Asthma in adults. *Clin Evid (Online).* 2011;2011.
127. Avallone KM, McLeish AC. Asthma and aerobic exercise: a review of the empirical literature. *J Asthma.* 2013;50:109-116.
128. Eijkemans M, Mommers M, Draaisma JM, et al. Physical activity and asthma: a systematic review and meta-analysis. *PLoS One.* 2012;7:e50775.
129. Pongdee T, Li JT. Exercise-induced bronchoconstriction. *Ann Allergy Asthma Immunol.* 2013;110:311-315.
130. Chandratilleke MG, Carson KV, Picot J, et al. Physical training for asthma. *Cochrane Database Syst Rev.* 2012;5:CD001116.
131. Ohar JA, Donohue JF. Mono- and combination therapy of long-acting bronchodilators and inhaled corticosteroids in advanced COPD. *Semin Respir Crit Care Med.* 2010;31:321-333.
132. Gordon J, Panos RJ. Inhaled albuterol/salbutamol and ipratropium bromide and their combination in the treatment of chronic obstructive pulmonary disease. *Expert Opin Drug Metab Toxicol.* 2010;6:381-392.
133. Zervas E, Samitas K, Gaga M, Beghe B, Fabbri LM. Inhaled corticosteroids in COPD: pros and cons. *Curr Drug Targets.* 2013;14:192-224.
134. Nannini LJ, Lasserson TJ, Poole P. Combined corticosteroid and long-acting beta(2)-agonist in one inhaler versus long-acting beta(2)-agonists for chronic obstructive pulmonary disease. *Cochrane Database Syst Rev.* 2012;9:CD006829.
135. Wright CC, Vera YY. Cystic fibrosis. In: DiPiro JT, et al, eds. *Pharmacotherapy: A Pathophysiologic Approach.* 8th ed. New York: McGraw-Hill; 2011.
136. Sears EH, Gartman EJ, Casserly BP. Treatment options for cystic fibrosis: state of the art and future perspectives. *Rev Recent Clin Trials.* 2011;6:94-107.
137. de Vrankrijker AM, Wolfs TF, van der Ent CK. Challenging and emerging pathogens in cystic fibrosis. *Paediatr Respir Rev.* 2010;11:246-254.
138. Rebeyrol C, Saint-Criq V, Guillot L, et al. Glucocorticoids reduce inflammation in cystic fibrosis bronchial epithelial cells. *Cell Signal.* 2012;24:1093-1099.
139. Cheng K, Ashby D, Smyth RL. Oral steroids for long-term use in cystic fibrosis. *Cochrane Database Syst Rev.* 2011;10:CD000407.
140. Dinwiddie R. Anti-inflammatory therapy in cystic fibrosis. *J Cyst Fibros.* 2005;4(suppl 2):45-48.
141. Lands LC, Stanojevic S. Oral non-steroidal anti-inflammatory drug therapy for lung disease in cystic fibrosis. *Cochrane Database Syst Rev.* 2013;6:CD001505.
142. Yousef AA, Jaffe A. The role of azithromycin in patients with cysticfibrosis. *Paediatr Respir Rev.* 2010;11:108-114.
143. Zarogoulidis P, Papanas N, Kioumis I, et al. Macrolides: from in vitro anti-inflammatory and immunomodulatory properties to clinical practice in respiratory diseases. *Eur J Clin Pharmacol.* 2012;68:479-503.
144. Rand S, Prasad SA. Exercise as part of a cystic fibrosis therapeutic routine. *Expert Rev Respir Med.* 2012;6:341-351.
145. Wheatley CM, Wilkins BW, Snyder EM. Exercise is medicine in cystic fibrosis. *Exerc Sport Sci Rev.* 2011;39:155-160.
146. Gaskin KJ. Nutritional care in children with cystic fibrosis: are our patients becoming better? *Eur J Clin Nutr.* 2013;67: 558-564.
147. Dwyer TJ, Elkins MR, Bye PT. The role of exercise in maintaining health in cystic fibrosis. *Curr Opin Pulm Med.* 2011;17:455-460.
148. Konstan MW, Ratjen F. Effect of dornase alfa on inflammation and lung function: potential role in the early treatment of cystic fibrosis. *J Cyst Fibros.* 2012;11:78-83.

149. Wagener JS, Kupfer O. Dornase alfa (Pulmozyme). *Curr Opin Pulm Med.* 2012;18:609-614.
150. Jones AP, Wallis C. Dornase alfa for cystic fibrosis. *Cochrane Database Syst Rev.* 2010;3:CD001127.
151. Prickett M, Jain M. Gene therapy in cystic fibrosis. *Transl Res.* 2013;161:255-264.
152. Griesenbach U, Alton EW. Progress in gene and cell therapy for cystic fibrosis lung disease. *Curr Pharm Des.* 2012;18:642-662.
153. Oakland M, Sinn PL, McCray PB Jr. Advances in cell and gene-based therapies for cystic fibrosis lung disease. *Mol Ther.* 2012;20:1108-1115.
154. Flude LJ, Agent P, Bilton D. Chest physiotherapy techniques in bronchiectasis. *Clin Chest Med.* 2012;33:351-361.
155. Mejia-Downs A, Bishop KL. Physical therapy associated with airway clearance dysfunction. In: DeTurk WE, Cahalin LP, eds. *Cardiovascular and Pulmonary Physical Therapy*. 2nd ed. New York: McGraw-Hill; 2011.

CHAPTER 27

Gastrointestinal Drugs

The gastrointestinal (GI) tract is responsible for food digestion and the absorption of nutrients and water. Dietary constituents undergo a series of digestive processes as they progress through the GI system. Under normal conditions, the transit time of food and water is adequate to allow the processes of digestion and absorption to take place. Indigestible and nonabsorbable products are eliminated by defecation.

This chapter discusses drugs that are used to treat specific problems in the GI system. The primary disorders that occur in the GI tract are related to damage from gastric acid secretion and abnormal food movement through the GI tract. Problems may develop if digestive secretions in the stomach begin to damage the upper GI mucosa and cause a peptic ulcer. Certain drugs attempt to prevent or heal peptic ulcers by controlling gastric acid secretion and protecting the mucosal lining. Problems with GI motility may also respond to pharmacological management. Excessive motility (*diarrhea*) and inadequate bowel evacuation (*constipation*) are treated with various agents that normalize peristalsis and facilitate normal bowel movements. Drugs are also available to treat other problems with digestion and vomiting (*emesis*).

The GI system is susceptible to various infectious and parasitic invasions. The drugs used to treat these disorders are presented in Chapters 33 through 35, which deal with the chemotherapy of infectious diseases.

As a rehabilitation specialist, you will often treat patients taking some form of GI agent. The general public commonly uses these medications, as do hospitalized individuals and outpatients receiving physical therapy and occupational therapy. Although the direct impact of most GI drugs on physical rehabilitation is relatively small, an understanding of how these drugs are used will help you recognize their role in the patient's pharmacotherapeutic regimen.

DRUGS USED TO CONTROL GASTRIC ACIDITY AND SECRETION

The acidic nature of the gastric juices is essential for activating digestive protease activity and controlling intestinal bacteria. The gastric acids can cause severe ulceration and hemorrhage of the stomach lining if excessive amounts of it are produced or if the normal protection of the stomach mucosa is disturbed by irritants, drugs, or bacterial infection.[1] Consequently, several different types of drugs are available that attempt to control or prevent the detrimental effects of gastric acid. These agents are used to treat *peptic ulcers*—that is, ulcerations of the mucosal lining of the esophagus, stomach, and duodenum.[1,2] These drugs may also be helpful in treating general problems related to indigestion and epigastric pain (dyspepsia) and to heartburn sensations caused by the leakage of gastric acid into the distal esophagus, called *gastroesophageal reflux*.[3] Agents used to control gastric acidity and secretion are presented below.

Antacids

Antacids attempt to chemically neutralize stomach acids. These drugs typically contain a base such as carbonate or hydroxide combined with aluminum, magnesium, sodium, or calcium.[4] The base combines with excess hydrogen ions (H^+) in the stomach to increase intragastric pH. The basic strategy of this chemical neutralization is illustrated in Figure 27-1. There is some evidence that antacids containing aluminium may provide additional protection of the gastric mucosa by inhibiting *Helicobacter pylori* infection and by enhancing the production of prostaglandins, proteins, and growth factors that defend the stomach lining from gastric acids.[5]

One concern regarding antacids is that they may be abused because the public has come to regard antacids as a panacea for poor eating habits. In the past, antacids were often used to treat more serious and chronic conditions of peptic ulcer and chronic gastroesophageal reflux. However, the use of antacids in these more serious conditions has been replaced to a large extent by other drugs such as H_2 receptor blockers and proton pump inhibitors (see later).[3,4] Consequently, antacids are used primarily to treat fairly minor and transient dyspepsia occurring from overeating, eating spicy foods, and so forth.[6]

Basic Strategy:

antacid + hydrochloric acid → salt + water

Examples:

aluminum hydroxide
$$Al(OH)_3 + 3\,HCl \rightarrow AlCl_3 + 3\,H_2O$$

magnesium hydroxide
$$Mg(OH)_2 + 2\,HCl \rightarrow MgCl_2 + 2\,H_2O$$

calcium carbonate
$$CaCO_3 + 2\,HCl \rightarrow CaCl_2 + H_2O + CO_2$$

sodium bicarbonate
$$NaHCO_3 + HCl \rightarrow NaCl + H_2O + CO_2$$

Figure ■ 27-1
Neutralization of hydrochloric acid (HCl) by the primary forms of antacids. In each reaction, the antacid combines with HCl to form a salt and water. Carbon dioxide (CO_2) is also produced by calcium carbonate and sodium bicarbonate antacids.

Specific Agents

Antacids are identified by many trade names and frequently appear in over-the-counter products. There is such a plethora of antacids on the market that even a partial listing of commercial preparations is difficult. The primary antacids can be classified as:

- Aluminum-containing
- Magnesium-containing
- Calcium carbonate–containing
- Sodium bicarbonate–containing
- A combination of any of these classifications

These drugs are typically taken orally, either as tablets or as a liquid oral suspension.

Adverse Effects

Constipation is the most common side effect associated with the aluminum-containing antacids, whereas diarrhea often occurs with magnesium-containing preparations. Hence, many antacid products combine aluminum with magnesium to provide a more balanced effect on GI function, with the hope that the increased GI motility produced by magnesium will be offset by the decreased motility associated with aluminum.[7]

It was originally believed that gastric acid production might increase if antacids were suddenly discontinued after prolonged use. This idea, known as the *acid-rebound phenomenon*, has been largely disproven with antacid use but may still be a problem with other acid-reducing strategies, such as the proton-pump inhibitors (see "Proton Pump Inhibitors" later in this chapter).[8]

Electrolyte imbalances and altered pharmacokinetics can occur if antacids are used in high doses for prolonged periods.[6] Because antacids alter gastric pH, these drugs can affect the metabolism and solubility of medications that rely on gastric acidity to help dissolve the medication or activate the drug.[9] Hence, it is generally recommended that antacids should not be taken within 2 hours of other orally administered drugs such as warfarin, digoxin, iron supplements, and certain antibiotics (e.g., tetracyclines, fluoroquinolones, ketoconazole).[10] Likewise, excessive use of antacids can alter the absorption of electrolytes (especially phosphate) and other drugs from the GI tract and can cause an increase in urinary pH that affects drug elimination.

H_2 Receptor Blockers

The regulation of gastric acid secretion involves the complex interaction of many endogenous chemicals, including histamine.[11] Histamine stimulates specific receptors on stomach parietal cells to increase gastric acid secretion. These histamine receptors are classified as H_2 receptors in order to differentiate them from the H_1 receptors located on vascular, respiratory, and GI smooth muscle.[12] H_2 antagonists, or blockers, selectively bind to H_2 receptors without activating these receptors. These drugs prevent the histamine-activated release of gastric acid under basal conditions and during stimulation by food, and they can help decrease damage from gastric acid caused by NSAIDs and other factors that increase acid secretion.[13,14]

The H_2 blockers are therefore used for both acute and long-term management of peptic ulcer and other problems such as dyspepsia and gastroesophageal reflux disease (GERD).[13,15] These drugs have a good safety profile, and many of the H_2 blockers originally introduced as prescription agents are now available as over-the-counter preparations. H_2 blockers remain an option for treating mild or occasional gastric irritation, but the routine use of these drugs in serious gastric disease has diminished somewhat because of the superior effects achieved with proton pump inhibitors (see "Proton Pump Inhibitors" below).[16,17]

Specific Agents

The primary H_2 blockers used to control gastric secretions are listed in Table 27-1. Cimetidine was the first H_2 blocker to be widely used as an antiulcer agent. Newer drugs such as famotidine, nizatidine, and ranitidine appear to be at least as effective as cimetidine; they differ from one another primarily in their pharmacokinetics (absorption, metabolism, etc.) and their potential for interacting with other drugs.[7] Hence, all H_2 blockers seem to be essentially similar when used at moderate doses to control excess gastric acid secretion.

Adverse Effects

These drugs are generally well tolerated in most patients, and adverse effects are rare during short-term or periodic use. Problems that may occur include headache and dizziness. Mild, transient GI problems (nausea, diarrhea, constipation) may also occur with the H_2 blockers, and arthralgia and myalgia have been reported with cimetidine use. Following long-term use, sudden withdrawal of an H_2 blocker may result in increased acid secretion (acid rebound). This effect, however, is usually mild and may not be clinically important in most patients.[18] On the other hand, tolerance may occur during continuous (daily) use, so administering these drugs every other day may provide better long-term effects.[18]

Table 27-1
H_2 RECEPTOR BLOCKERS

Generic Name	Trade Name	Adult Oral Dosage*
Cimetidine	Tagamet, others	300 mg 4 times each day with meals and at bedtime, 400 or 600 mg in the morning and at bedtime, or 800 mg at bedtime
Famotidine	Pepcid, many others	40 mg once daily at bedtime or 20 mg bid
Nizatidine	Axid	300 mg once daily at bedtime or 150 mg bid
Ranitidine	Zantac	150 mg twice daily or 300 mg at bedtime

**Represents typical dose for short-term treatment of active gastric or duodenal ulcers. Doses for preventing ulcer recurrence or treating gastroesophageal reflux disease (heartburn) may be somewhat lower.*

Proton Pump Inhibitors

Proton pump inhibitors inhibit the H^+, K^+-ATPase enzyme that is ultimately responsible for secreting acid from gastric parietal cells into the lumen of the stomach[19] (Fig. 27-2). This enzyme is also known as the *proton pump*; hence these drugs are often referred to as proton pump inhibitors (PPIs). PPIs are extremely effective at inhibiting the proton pump, and therapeutic doses can reduce gastric acid secretion by 80 to 95 percent.[7]

There is some evidence that PPIs also have antibacterial effects against *H. pylori* infection and that they may have some anti-inflammatory properties that help decrease gastric irritation.[20,21] Evidence indicates that PPIs are more effective than H_2 blockers and antacids in controlling acid secretion and promoting the healing of ulcers in various conditions that

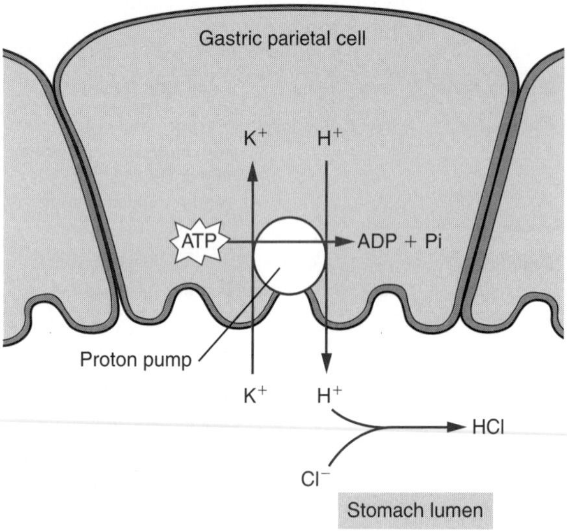

Figure ■ 27-2
Action of the gastric H^+, K^+-ATPase (proton pump). This enzyme actively transports hydrogen (H^+) ions into the stomach while reabsorbing potassium (K^+) ions into the gastric parietal cell. H^+ ions combine with chloride (Cl^-) ions in the stomach to form hydrochloric acid (HCl). Drugs classified as proton pump inhibitors (PPIs) suppress this enzyme, thus decreasing the transport of H^+ ions and subsequent formation of gastric acid.

cause increased gastric acid production.[22-24] PPIs have therefore gained prominence in treating gastric problems and are now the drug of choice in the long-term treatment of patients with gastric and duodenal ulcers and GERD.[16,25]

Specific Agents

Omeprazole (Prilosec) was the original PPI; this drug is now joined by esomeprazole (Nexium), lansoprazole (Prevacid), dexlansoprazole (Kapidex), pantoprazole (Protonix), and rabeprazole (AcipHex) (Table 27-2). All of these drugs are similar, with selection often depending on cost, availability, and the drug interaction potential of each agent.[7] Nonprescription forms of certain PPIs are now available, and these forms offer a convenient, effective, and remarkably safe option for patients who need to suppress gastric irritation and treat GERD.[26]

Adverse Effects

PPIs are usually well tolerated. However, increased secretion of gastric acid (acid rebound) can occur when PPIs are discontinued after prolonged use.[8,27] Research has also suggested that long-term use is associated with gastric polyps that might predispose patients to GI tumors.[28] Likewise, there is some evidence that prolonged inhibition of the proton pump can adversely affect calcium metabolism, thereby leading to decreased bone mineralization and an increased risk of hip and vertebral fractures.[29,30] Other potential problems include an increased risk of certain infections (*Clostridium difficile*, pneumonia), decreased absorption of certain nutrients (vitamin B, magnesium, iron), and kidney problems such as interstitial nephritis.[31-33]

On the other hand, there is substantial evidence that PPIs can decrease the morbidity associated with increased gastric acid secretion, and PPIs can decrease

Table 27-2
PROTON PUMP INHIBITORS: TYPICAL DAILY DOSE *

		Gastroesophageal Reflux Disease		*Gastric or Duodenal Ulcer*	
Generic Name	**Trade Name**	**Treatment: Healing**	**Maintenance: Prevent Recurrence**	**Treatment: Healing**	**Maintenance: Prevent Recurrence**
Dexlansoprazole	Kapidex	30 mg	30 mg	30–60 mg	30 mg
Esomeprazole	Nexium	20–40 mg	20 mg	40 mg	20–40 mg
Lansoprazole	Prevacid	15–30 mg	15 mg	15–30 mg	15 mg
Omeprazole	Prilosec, others	20–40 mg	20 mg	20–40 mg	20–40 mg
Pantoprazole	Pantoloc, Protonix	40 mg	20–40 mg	40 mg	40 mg
Rabeprazole	AcipHex, Pariet	20 mg	20 mg	20 mg	20 mg

**Doses are usually administered once each day, although exact doses and dosing schedule can be adjusted for specific patients. Time of administration (morning, bedtime, etc.) is also often determined according to each patient's symptoms and disease characteristics.*

the risk of esophageal damage and carcinoma associated with GERD.[25] The benefits of these drugs seem to outweigh the risks, but possible adverse effects should be monitored periodically in patients using these drugs for the long-term treatment of peptic ulcer and GI reflux disease.[28,33]

Treatment of *Helicobacter Pylori* Infection in Gastric Ulcer Disease

H. pylori is a gram-negative bacterium that is often present in the upper GI tract in people with gastric ulcer disease.[34] Research suggests that this bacterium may cause or potentiate gastroduodenal ulcers and that the treatment of an *H. pylori* infection is essential to treat these types of ulcers.[35] Use of various antibiotic regimens results in an increased healing rate and a decreased recurrence of gastric ulcers in many people who test positive for *H. pylori* infection.[36,37] The fact that *H. pylori* is present in certain patients should not eliminate the possibility that other factors (stress, diet, etc.) may also be contributing to gastric ulcer disease.[38] Likewise, there are patients who are infected with *H. pylori* who do *not* develop gastric ulcers.[34] Hence, the exact role of this bacterium as a causative factor in gastric ulcers remains uncertain. Nonetheless, *H. pylori* may contribute to the development of gastric ulcers in susceptible individuals, and antibacterial drugs should be considered in patients with ulcers who are infected with this bacterium.

Treatment of *H. pylori* infection typically consists of a combination therapy, using several drugs simultaneously or in a specific sequence.[39] For example, one common form of "triple therapy" consists of two antibacterials (amoxicillin and clarithromycin, or metronidazole and clarithromycin) and one of the PPIs described earlier.[10] Alternatively, various "quadruple therapies" combine bismuth compound (see "Antidiarrheal Agents" below) with a PPI and two antibacterials (e.g., tetracycline and metronidazole).[10] Because of concerns about antibacterial resistance, some clinicians may employ other antibacterial drugs or administer the antibacterial drugs in a specific sequence.[40] For example, a PPI might be administered for a 10-day period, but amoxicillin is administered for only the first 5 days of treatment, and metronidazole and clarithromycin are then administered for the last 5 days of treatment.[10]

Regardless of the exact drug regimen, drugs used to eradicate *H. pylori* are typically administered for 10 to 14 days. Antibacterial drugs are discontinued after this period, but some patients may need to remain on maintenance doses of the PPI or other antiulcer drugs to facilitate ulcer healing and prevent recurrence.[41]

Consequently, treatment of *H. pylori* infection may improve the prognosis of people with gastric ulcers and other forms of upper GI distress (dyspepsia, gastroesophageal reflux disease). Patients with clinical signs of ulcers who also test positive for this infection should receive a treatment regimen attempting to eradicate the infection. Successful treatment of an *H. pylori* infection may reduce or eliminate the need for subsequent antiulcer medications in patients with gastric ulcer disease.[10]

Other Agents Used to Control and Treat Gastric Ulcers

Several other agents besides the antacids, H_2 blockers, and PPIs have proved successful in preventing or treating problems associated with gastric acidity and mucosal breakdown. Some of the more frequently used agents are discussed below.

Anticholinergics

The role of muscarinic cholinergic antagonists in treating peptic ulcers was discussed in Chapter 19. Cholinergic stimulation of the gut via vagal efferent fibers produces a general increase in GI motility and secretion. Drugs that block the effects of acetylcholine on stomach parietal cells will decrease the release of gastric acid. Hence, atropine and similar anticholinergics (pirenzepine, telenzepine) can be used to control gastric acid secretion, but these drugs cause many side effects, such as dry mouth, constipation, urinary retention, and confusion.[7] Anticholinergics such as pirenzepine may still be used occasionally in countries outside the United States, but these drugs have been essentially replaced by safer and more effective H_2 receptor blockers and PPIs.

Metoclopramide (Reglan)

Metoclopramide is officially classified as a dopamine receptor antagonist but also appears to enhance the peripheral effects of acetylcholine. Primarily because of this latter effect, metoclopramide stimulates motility in the upper GI tract (prokinetic effect), which may be useful in moving the stomach contents toward the small intestine, thus decreasing the risk of gastric acid moving backward into the esophagus. Metoclopramide may therefore be helpful in treating gastroesophageal reflux disease in specific situations, such as certain children and neonates with GERD.[42] The primary side effects associated with metoclopramide are related to its antagonistic effects on central nervous system (CNS) dopamine receptors. Restlessness, drowsiness, and fatigue are fairly common. Some extrapyramidal symptoms (i.e., Parkinson-like tremor and rigidity) may also occur because of the central antidopamine effects.

Prostaglandins

There is little doubt that certain prostaglandins such as PGE_2 and PGI_2 inhibit gastric secretion and help protect the stomach mucosa by stimulating gastric mucus secretion.[43] The problem has been determining exactly how the prostaglandins are involved and whether exogenous prostaglandin analogs can be used to help treat peptic ulcer. Currently, misoprostol (Cytotec) is the only prostaglandin analog available for clinical use. Although this drug appears to be successful in treating ulcers, it does not seem to offer any advantages over more traditional antiulcer drugs such as PPIs.[44] Also, prostaglandin analogs may be effective only at doses that cause other GI effects, such as diarrhea.[10] Consequently, prostaglandin analogs have not gained overwhelming acceptance as antiulcer drugs, but they may be used in limited situations such as treatment of gastric damage caused by aspirin and similar NSAIDs.[45,46] Chapter 15 covers the use of misoprostol to reduce or prevent NSAID-induced gastropathy in more detail.

Sucralfate (Carafate, Sulcrate)

Sucralfate is a disaccharide that exerts a cytoprotective effect on the stomach mucosa.[7] Although the exact mechanism is unclear, sucralfate may form a protective gel within the stomach that adheres to ulcers and shields them from the contents of the stomach. The protective barrier formed by the drug prevents further erosion and permits healing of duodenal and gastric ulcers. Sucralfate is well tolerated, although constipation may occur in some patients.

ANTIDIARRHEAL AGENTS

Normal propulsion of food through the GI tract is crucial for proper absorption of nutrients and water. If transit time is too fast, diarrhea occurs, resulting in poor food absorption and dehydration. Diarrhea is often a temporary symptom of many relatively minor GI disorders, but it may also occur with more serious conditions such as dysentery, ulcerative colitis, and cholera. If diarrhea is sustained for even a few days, the resulting dehydration can be a serious problem, especially in infants or debilitated patients. Consequently, efforts should be made to control diarrhea as soon as possible. Antidiarrheal agents are listed in Table 27-3, and their pharmacology is discussed in the following sections.

Opioid Derivatives

The constipating effects of morphine and certain other opioid derivatives have been recognized for some time.

Table 27-3
COMMON ANTIDIARRHEAL AGENTS

Generic Name	Trade Names	Dosage
Bismuth salicylate	Pepto-Bismol, Kaopectate, many others	525 mg every half hour to 1 hour or 1,050 mg every hour if needed; total dose should not exceed 4,200 mg in any 24-hr period
Opioid Derivatives		
Diphenoxylate	Lomotil, others*	5 mg, 3 or 4 times daily
Loperamide	Imodium, others	4 mg initially, 2 mg after each loose stool; total dose should not exceed 16 mg in any 24-hr period
Opium tincture	—	0.6 mL (6 mg opium), 4 times daily
Paregoric	—	5–10 mL (2–4 mg opium), 1–4 times daily

**Commercial products often combine diphenoxylate (an opioid) with atropine (an anticholinergic).*

These drugs produce a general decrease in GI motility, and they may also reduce fluid loss by increasing the absorption of salt and water or by decreasing fluid and electrolyte excretion from the GI tract.[4] The exact manner in which opioids exert these effects is not known. As indicated in Chapter 14, opioids bind to CNS receptors and mediate analgesic effects, which may help decrease symptoms of cramping and abdominal discomfort. The primary effects of opioids on GI motility (antiperistalsis) seem to occur because opioids bind to neuronal receptors on the enteric nerve plexus within the gut wall or by a direct effect of opioids on GI epithelial and smooth muscle cells.[47] In particular, the mu and delta subtype of the opioid receptor seem to be important in mediating the GI effects of opioid drugs; stimulation of these receptors is the primary method for reducing GI motility and treating diarrhea.[48]

Specific Agents

Opioid derivatives used to treat diarrhea are listed in Table 27-3. Opium tincture (laudanum) and camphorated opium tincture (paregoric) are naturally occurring opiates that are very potent inhibitors of peristalsis. These natural agents are still available for treating diarrhea, but they have essentially been replaced by newer opioids such as diphenoxylate and loperamide. The newer opioids are somewhat less potent but may produce fewer side effects.

Adverse Effects

The primary side effects with opioid derivatives are nausea, abdominal discomfort, constipation, and other GI disturbances. Drowsiness, fatigue, and dizziness have also been reported. Although addiction is a potential problem when opioids are administered, the risk of tolerance and physical dependence is fairly small when these drugs are used in recommended dosages for the short-term treatment of diarrhea.

Bismuth Salicylate

Bismuth salicylate has several properties contributing to its antidiarrheal effects. This drug may stimulate water and electrolyte absorption from the lower GI tract, thus decreasing fecal fluid loss. In addition, the bismuth component of the compound may have antibacterial effects, and the salicylate component may inhibit the production of prostaglandins that irritate the intestinal lining. The combination of these properties makes this drug fairly effective in treating mild-to-moderate diarrhea.[4] Bismuth salicylate also decreases gastric acid secretion and exerts antacid effects, hence its use in stomach upset and minor gastric irritation. Individuals often use products containing bismuth salicylate to prevent and treat traveler's diarrhea (i.e., diarrhea caused by pathogens in food and water found in developing countries).[49] Bismuth salicylate is the active ingredient in Pepto-Bismol and Kaopectate, fairly inexpensive and readily available over-the-counter commercial products. As indicated earlier, bismuth compounds are also part of the antibacterial regimen in *H. pylori* infection.

Adverse Effects

This drug is relatively free from serious side effects. Problems with salicylate intoxication may occur during overdose or in people who are sensitive to aspirin and other salicylates.

Miscellaneous Agents Used to Treat Diarrhea

Various other drug strategies can be used in specific cases of diarrhea or in situations where conventional drug therapy is unsuccessful. For example, clonidine (Catapres) is a CNS alpha-2 receptor agonist that is normally used to treat hypertension (see Chapters 20 and 21). This drug, however, can also stimulate alpha-2 receptors in the GI tract, thereby decreasing secretion, increasing absorption, and normalizing GI movement.[50] Clonidine can therefore be used to control diarrhea in specific situations such as people with fecal incontinence and patients with autonomic neuropathy.[50,51] Octreotide (Sandostatin) is a complex drug that mimics the effects of endogenously produced somatostatin. It inhibits the secretion of serotonin and other peptides that stimulate GI function, and it is especially useful in treating diarrhea caused by tumors that secrete these substances into the GI tract.[52]

Cholestyramine (Questran), colestipol (Colestid), and colesevelam (Welchol) are drugs that sequester and bind bile acids within the GI tract (see Chapter 25). Bile-sequestering agents can be useful in treating diarrhea caused by excess bile acid secretion.[53]

Various other strategies to control diarrhea have been discontinued because of a lack of evidence for effectiveness. In particular, adsorbents such as kaolin, pectin, and attapulgite were once commonly used in over-the-counter antidiarrheals. Theoretically, these adsorbents could take up and hold bacteria and toxins in the intestinal lumen that cause diarrhea. However, there was considerable doubt as to whether they really helped improve stool production and decrease water loss. Hence, these adsorbents are no longer commonly available in the United States but may be found in various products in other countries.

LAXATIVES AND CATHARTICS

Laxatives promote evacuation of the bowel and defecation when normal bowel movements are impaired but no obstruction exists in the GI system. Cathartics, or purgatives, are also used to promote lower GI evacuation, but in a somewhat more rapid fashion than with typical laxatives. For this discussion, the term *laxative* includes both relatively slow-acting and fast-acting agents.

Laxatives may benefit patients on prolonged bed rest, patients with infrequent or painful bowel movements, patients with spinal cord injuries, or patients who should avoid straining during defecation (e.g., postpartum patients and those recovering from surgical procedures). Laxatives are also indicated for bowel evacuation prior to surgical or diagnostic procedures.

The problem with laxatives is that they are frequently abused. The long-term, chronic use of laxatives is usually unnecessary and often unhealthy. These agents are self-administered by individuals who are obsessed with maintaining daily bowel movements. The individuals may have the misconception that daily bowel evacuation is needed to maintain normal GI function. Also, laxatives are often relied on instead of other factors that promote normal bowel evacuation, such as a high-fiber diet, adequate hydration, and physical activity.[54] People with eating disorders (anorexia, bulimia) or athletes trying to lose weight to meet specific weight limits can also abuse laxatives.[54] Consequently, laxatives serve an important but finite role in GI function, but their use in helping maintain daily evacuation or promote weight loss should be discouraged.

Specific Agents and Mechanism of Action

The many available types of laxatives are usually classified by their apparent mode of action.[48,55] Often, two different laxatives, either from the same class or from two different classes, are combined in the same commercial preparation. Some of the more common laxatives, listed by their apparent mechanisms of action, are listed in Table 27-4. The major laxative classes and rationales for their use are outlined in the next few sections.

Bulk-Forming Laxatives

These agents absorb water and swell within the lower GI tract. The increased size of the water-laden laxative stretches the bowel, thus stimulating intestinal movement (peristalsis). Bulk laxatives commonly contain natural and semisynthetic dietary fiber such as bran, psyllium, and methylcellulose.

Stimulant Laxatives

The precise mechanism of stimulant laxatives is not known. They may activate peristalsis by a direct irritant effect on the intestinal mucosa or by stimulating the nerve plexus within the gut wall. Some evidence suggests that they may work by increasing

Table 27-4
LAXATIVES*

Bulk-Forming	**Trade Names**
Methylcellulose	Citrucel
Polycarbophil	Fiber Lax, Fiberall, others
Psyllium	Metamucil, many others
Stimulants	
Bisacodyl	Correctol, Dulcolax, Feen-A-Mint
Castor oil	—
Senna	Senokot; Ex-Lax; many others
Hyperosmotic	
Glycerin	Sani-Supp; Fleet Glycerin Laxative
Lactulose	Cholac; Constilac; Constulose, others
Magnesium hydroxide	Phillips' Milk of Magnesia, others
Magnesium sulfate	Epsom salts
Polyethylene glycol	MiraLax
Sodium phosphate	Fleet Phospho-Soda
Lubricants and Stool Softeners	
Docusate	Colace, many others
Mineral oil	Fleet Mineral Oil, Nujol

**Some of the more common agents are listed as examples in each laxative category. Common trade names are listed in the right-hand column. Many other preparations are available that combine two or more laxatives in the same commercial product.*

fluid accumulation within the small intestine. Common stimulant laxatives are castor oil, bisacodyl, and plant extracts such as senna and cascara.

Hyperosmotic Laxatives

Administration of osmotically active substances produces a gradient that draws water into the bowel and small intestine. This gradient increases stool fluid content and stimulates peristalsis. A variety of hyperosmotic substances—including magnesium salts, sodium salts, potassium salts, lactulose, polyethylene glycol, and glycerin—achieve this effect.

Lubricants and Stool Softeners

Agents like mineral oil and docusate facilitate the entry of water into the fecal mass, thus softening the stool and permitting easier defecation. These agents may also exert a laxative effect because of the increased pressure in the bowel secondary to the increased stool size.

Adverse Effects

Disturbances in the GI system, such as nausea and cramps, may occur with laxative use. With prolonged use, serious lower GI irritation, including spastic colitis, may occur. Fluid and electrolyte abnormalities are also a potential problem. Excessive loss of water and the concomitant loss of electrolytes may transpire, resulting in dehydration and possible acid-base imbalances.[54] These fluid and electrolyte abnormalities are especially significant in older or debilitated patients and can become life-threatening if renal and cardiovascular function is compromised. Finally, chronic administration may result in laxative dependence when bowel evacuation has become so subservient to laxative use that the normal mechanisms governing evacuation and defecation are impaired.

MISCELLANEOUS GASTROINTESTINAL DRUGS

Patients may take several other types of drugs for specific purposes in controlling GI function. These other drugs are introduced here only to alert you to their existence. For a more detailed description of the use of any of these agents, consult one of the drug indexes, such as *Davis's Drug Guide for Rehabilitation Professionals* or the *Physician's Desk Reference (PDR)*.

Digestants

Digestants aid the digestion of food. The primary digestant preparations contain pancreatic enzymes or bile salts. Pancreatic enzymes such as amylase, trypsin, and lipase are responsible for digestion of carbohydrates, proteins, and lipids, respectively. These enzymes are normally synthesized in the pancreas and secreted into the duodenum via the pancreatic duct. Bile salts are synthesized in the liver, stored in the gallbladder, and released into the duodenum via the common bile duct. Bile salts serve to emulsify lipids in the intestinal tract and are important in lipid digestion and absorption.

Digestant preparations can replace digestive constituents in the stomach and upper small intestine whenever the endogenous production of these constituents is impaired. In particular, individuals with cystic fibrosis often use digestants.[56] As discussed in Chapter 26, cystic fibrosis is a hereditary disease that affects all the major exocrine glands, resulting in thick, viscous secretions. These thickened secretions may form mucous plugs that obstruct certain ducts, such as the pancreatic and bile ducts. This condition leads to a chronic deficiency of pancreatic enzymes and bile salts; as a result, patients cannot digest and absorb nutrients from the GI tract. Oral preparations containing these digestants replace the missing compounds, thus improving digestion and nutrient absorption.

Emetics

Emetics induce vomiting. They are frequently administered to help empty the stomach of poisons or ingested toxins. The two primary emetics are apomorphine and ipecac. Both agents seem to work by stimulating the medullary emetic center, and ipecac also exerts a direct emetic effect on the stomach.

Antiemetics

Antiemetics decrease the nausea and vomiting associated with motion sickness, recovery from surgery, or other medical treatments, such as cancer chemotherapy and radiation treatment.[57-59] Antiemetic agents include antihistamines (dimenhydrinate, meclizine, others), anticholinergics (scopolamine), drugs that block specific CNS dopamine (D_2) and serotonin (5-HT_3) receptors, cannabinoids, and several other drugs that act at various sites in the CNS to suppress nausea and vomiting.[48] Other antiemetic drugs, such as antacids and adsorbents, act locally to soothe the gastric mucosa and decrease the irritation that may cause vomiting.

Cholelitholytic Agents

Drugs like ursodeoxycholic acid (ursodiol) and chenodeoxycholic acid (chenodiol) can dissolve certain types of gallstones.[60] These drugs decrease the cholesterol content of bile and may help dissolve gallstones that are supersaturated with cholesterol; however, the drugs do not appear effective in the treatment of calcified gallstones.[60]

Special Concerns for Rehabilitation Patients

Drugs affecting the GI system are important in rehabilitation patients by virtue of their frequent use. Critically ill patients will suffer some degree of stress-related damage to the stomach mucosa, especially if they are managed in the intensive care unit.[22,61] This stress ulceration syndrome appears to be especially prevalent in patients with burns, multiple traumas, renal failure, and CNS trauma. Drugs such as the PPIs (omeprazole, others) and H_2 receptor blockers (cimetidine, ranitidine, others) are often helpful in controlling gastric acid secretions, thus preventing damage to the mucosal lining.[22]

Patients seen in rehabilitation are often relatively inactive and suffer from many adverse effects of prolonged bed rest, including constipation. Constipation and fecal impaction may also be a recurrent and serious problem in patients with spinal cord injuries. Laxatives are used routinely in these patients to facilitate adequate bowel evacuation. Patients receiving cancer chemotherapy often have problems with nausea and vomiting, and antiemetic drugs may be helpful to these individuals. Various other GI disorders, including diarrhea and chronic indigestion, occur frequently in many rehabilitation patients and are often treated effectively with the appropriate agents.

Despite their frequent use, most GI drugs do not produce any significant side effects that will impair rehabilitation. Some dizziness and fatigue may occur with agents such as the opiates used to treat diarrhea or the antiulcer H_2 blockers, but these effects are fairly mild. Other problems with GI drugs are generally related to transient GI disturbances. In general, GI drugs are well tolerated and safe in most patients. In effect, these drugs indirectly facilitate physical rehabilitation by resolving annoying and uncomfortable GI symptoms, thus allowing the patient to participate more readily in the program.

CASE STUDY

GASTROINTESTINAL DRUGS

Brief History. M.B. is a 48-year-old insurance sales representative with a long history of back pain. He has had recurrent episodes of sciatica because of a herniated disk at the L5-S1 interspace. He frequently takes a nonprescription form of ibuprofen at 400 mg/dose to help alleviate his back pain. M.B. has a rather sedentary lifestyle and often eats poorly by consuming a high-fat, low-fiber diet. He frequently suffers from acid indigestion and often takes a nonprescription antacid preparation

CASE STUDY (Continued)

(Mylanta suspension) that contains magnesium hydroxide, aluminum hydroxide, and simethicone. Currently, he is being seen as an outpatient in a private physical therapy practice. Despite several treatments, his back pain has not improved. In fact, his pain was recently exacerbated when he was straining to pass a stool during a period of constipation. Evidently, the straining occurred often during defecation, and the patient's back problems were increased by the bowel-related problems that caused the straining.

1. *How is M.B.'s current behavior contributing to his constipation?*
2. *What advice should the therapist provide to reduce the chance of constipation and exacerbation of back pain?*

See Appendix C, "Answers to Case Study Questions."

SUMMARY

A variety of pharmacological agents are used to maintain proper function in the GI system. Drugs such as antacids, H_2 receptor antagonists, and PPIs help control gastric acid secretion and protect the stomach mucosa. These agents are widely used to prevent and treat peptic ulcer. Specific drugs are used to control GI motility. Drugs that inhibit excessive peristalsis (i.e., diarrhea) include the opiate derivatives, adsorbents, and bismuth salicylate. Decreased motility (constipation) is usually treated with various laxatives. Other GI agents attempt to treat specific problems such as poor digestion, emesis, or gallstones. GI drugs are used frequently in rehabilitation patients and, it is hoped, will produce beneficial effects that will allow the patient to participate more actively in the rehabilitation program.

REFERENCES

1. Yeomans ND. The ulcer sleuths: the search for the cause of peptic ulcers. *J Gastroenterol Hepatol.* 2011;26(suppl 1):35-41.
2. Banić M, Malfertheiner P, Babić Z, et al. Historical impact to drive research in peptic ulcer disease. *Dig Dis.* 2011;29:444-453.
3. Bredenoord AJ, Pandolfino JE, Smout AJ. Gastro-oesophageal reflux disease. *Lancet.* 2013;381:1933-1942.
4. McQuaid KR. Drugs used in the treatment of gastrointestinal diseases. In: Katzung BG, ed. *Basic and Clinical Pharmacology.* 12th ed. New York: Lange Medical Books/McGraw Hill; 2012.
5. Tarnawski A, Ahluwalia A, Jones MK. Gastric cytoprotection beyond prostaglandins: cellular and molecular mechanisms of gastroprotective and ulcer healing actions of antacids. *Curr Pharm Des.* 2013;19:126-132.
6. Maton PN, Burton ME. Antacids revisited: a review of their clinical pharmacology and recommended therapeutic use. *Drugs.* 1999;57:855-870.
7. Wallace JL, Sharkey KA. Pharmacotherapy of gastric acidity, peptic ulcers, and gastroesophageal reflux disease. In: Brunton L, et al, eds. *The Pharmacological Basis of Therapeutics.* 12th ed. New York: McGraw-Hill; 2011.
8. Lerotić I, Baršić N, Stojsavljević S, Duvnjak M. Acid inhibition and the acid rebound effect. *Dig Dis.* 2011;29:482-486.
9. Ogawa R, Echizen H. Clinically significant drug interactions with antacids: an update. *Drugs.* 2011;71:1839-1864.
10. Berardi RR, Fugit RV. Peptic ulcer disease. In: DiPiro JT, et al, eds. *Pharmacotherapy: A Pathophysiologic Approach.* 8th ed. New York: McGraw-Hill; 2011.
11. Chu S, Schubert ML. Gastric secretion. *Curr Opin Gastroenterol.* 2012;28:587-593.
12. Walter M, Stark H. Histamine receptor subtypes: a century of rational drug design. *Front Biosci.* 2012;4:461-488.
13. Loyd RA, McClellan DA. Update on the evaluation and management of functional dyspepsia. *Am Fam Physician.* 2011;83:547-552.
14. Tricco AC, Alateeq A, Tashkandi M, et al. Histamine H2 receptor antagonists for decreasing gastrointestinal harms in adults using acetylsalicylic acid: systematic review and meta-analysis. *Open Med.* 2012;6:e109-117.
15. Al Talalwah N, Woodward S. Gastro-oesophageal reflux. Part 2: medical treatment. *Br J Nurs.* 2013;22:277-284.
16. Sakaguchi M, Takao M, Ohyama Y, et al. Comparison of PPIs and H2-receptor antagonists plus prokinetics for dysmotility-like dyspepsia. *World J Gastroenterol.* 2012;18:1517-1524.
17. Sigterman KE, van Pinxteren B, Bonis PA, et al. Short-term treatment with proton pump inhibitors, H2-receptor antagonists and prokinetics for gastro-oesophageal reflux disease-like symptoms and endoscopy negative reflux disease. *Cochrane Database Syst Rev.* 2013;5:CD002095.

18. Takahashi M, Katayama Y. Reversal of the tolerance phenomenon by the intermittent administration of a histamine H2-receptor antagonist. *J Gastroenterol Hepatol.* 2010;25:1493-1497.
19. Schubert ML. Gastric secretion. *Curr Opin Gastroenterol.* 2011;27:536-542.
20. Bytzer P, Dahlerup JF, Eriksen JR, et al. Danish Society for Gastroenterology. Diagnosis and treatment of *Helicobacter pylori* infection. *Dan Med Bull.* 2011;58:C4271.
21. Kedika RR, Souza RF, Spechler SJ. Potential anti-inflammatory effects of proton pump inhibitors: a review and discussion of the clinical implications. *Dig Dis Sci.* 2009;54:2312-2317.
22. Alhazzani W, Alenezi F, Jaeschke RZ, et al. Proton pump inhibitors versus histamine 2 receptor antagonists for stress ulcer prophylaxis in critically ill patients: a systematic review and meta-analysis. *Crit Care Med.* 2013;41:693-705.
23. Barkun AN, Bardou M, Pham CQ, Martel M. Proton pump inhibitors vs. histamine 2 receptor antagonists for stress-related mucosal bleeding prophylaxis in critically ill patients: a meta-analysis. *Am J Gastroenterol.* 2012;107:507-520.
24. Nagahara A, Asaoka D, Hojo M, et al. Observational comparative trial of the efficacy of proton pump inhibitors versus histamine-2 receptor antagonists for uninvestigated dyspepsia. *J Gastroenterol Hepatol.* 2010;25(suppl 1):S122-128.
25. Williams DB, Schade RR. Gastroesophageal reflux disease. In: DiPiro JT, et al, eds. *Pharmacotherapy: A Pathophysiologic Approach.* 8th ed. New York: McGraw-Hill; 2011.
26. Holtmann G, Bigard MA, Malfertheiner P, Pounder R. Guidance on the use of over-the-counter proton pump inhibitors for the treatment of GERD. *Int J Clin Pharm.* 2011;33:493-500.
27. Waldum HL, Qvigstad G, Fossmark R, et al. Rebound acid hypersecretion from a physiological, pathophysiological and clinical viewpoint. *Scand J Gastroenterol.* 2010;45:389-394.
28. Lodato F, Azzaroli F, Turco L, et al. Adverse effects of proton pump inhibitors. *Best Pract Res Clin Gastroenterol.* 2010;24:193-201.
29. Lau YT, Ahmed NN. Fracture risk and bone mineral density reduction associated with proton pump inhibitors. *Pharmacotherapy.* 2012;32:67-79.
30. Yang YX. Chronic proton pump inhibitor therapy and calcium metabolism. *Curr Gastroenterol Rep.* 2012;14:473-479.
31. Abraham NS. Proton pump inhibitors: potential adverse effects. *Curr Opin Gastroenterol.* 2012;28:615-620.
32. Sheen E, Triadafilopoulos G. Adverse effects of long-term proton pump inhibitor therapy. *Dig Dis Sci.* 2011;56:931-950.
33. Vakil N. Prescribing proton pump inhibitors: is it time to pause and rethink? *Drugs.* 2012;72:437-445.
34. Salama NR, Hartung ML, Müller A. Life in the human stomach: persistence strategies of the bacterial pathogen *Helicobacter pylori. Nat Rev Microbiol.* 2013;11:385-399.
35. Shmuely H, Katicic M, Filipec Kanizaj T, Niv Y. *Helicobacter pylori* and nonmalignant diseases. *Helicobacter.* 2012;17(suppl 1):22-25.
36. Tepes B, O'Connor A, Gisbert JP, O'Morain C. Treatment of *Helicobacter pylori* infection 2012. *Helicobacter.* 2012;17(suppl 1):36-42.
37. Zullo A, De Francesco V, Hassan C, et al. Modified sequential therapy regimens for *Helicobacter pylori* eradication: a systematic review. *Dig Liver Dis.* 2013;45:18-22.
38. Overmier JB, Murison R. Restoring psychology's role in peptic ulcer. *Appl Psychol Health Well Being.* 2013;5:5-27.
39. Georgopoulos SD, Papastergiou V, Karatapanis S. Current options for the treatment of *Helicobacter pylori. Expert Opin Pharmacother.* 2013;14:211-223.
40. Iwańczak F, Iwańczak B. Treatment of *Helicobacter pylori* infection in the aspect of increasing antibiotic resistance. *Adv Clin Exp Med.* 2012;21:671-680.
41. Tang RS, Chan FK. Therapeutic management of recurrent peptic ulcer disease. *Drugs.* 2012;72:1605-1616.
42. Tighe MP, Afzal NA, Bevan A, Beattie RM. Current pharmacological management of gastro-esophageal reflux in children: an evidence-based systematic review. *Paediatr Drugs.* 2009;11:185-202.
43. Brzozowski T, Konturek PC, Konturek SJ, et al. Role of prostaglandins in gastroprotection and gastric adaptation. *J Physiol Pharmacol.* 2005;56(suppl 5):33-55.
44. Lazzaroni M, Porro GB. Management of NSAID-induced gastrointestinal toxicity: focus on proton pump inhibitors. *Drugs.* 2009;69:51-69.
45. Lee KN, Lee OY, Choi MG, et al. Prevention of NSAID-associated gastroduodenal injury in healthy volunteers-a randomized, double-blind, multicenter study comparing DA-9601 with misoprostol. *J Korean Med Sci.* 2011;26:1074-1080.
46. Satoh H, Takeuchi K. Management of NSAID/aspirin-induced small intestinal damage by GI-sparing NSAIDs, anti-ulcer drugs and food constituents. *Curr Med Chem.* 2012;19:82-89.
47. Holzer P. Opioid receptors in the gastrointestinal tract. *Regul Pept.* 2009;155:11-17.
48. Sharkey KA, Wallace JL. Treatment of disorders of bowel motility and water flux; anti-emetics; agents used in biliary and pancreatic disease. In: Brunton L, et al, eds. *The Pharmacological Basis of Therapeutics.* 12th ed. New York: McGraw-Hill; 2011.
49. Shlim DR. Update in traveler's diarrhea. *Infect Dis Clin North Am.* 2005;19:137-149.
50. Westfall TC, Westfall DP. Neurotransmission: the autonomic and somatic motor nervous systems. In: Brunton L, et al, eds. *The Pharmacological Basis of Therapeutics.* 12th ed. New York: McGraw-Hill; 2011.
51. Bharucha AE, Fletcher JG, Camilleri M, et al. Effects of clonidine in women with fecal incontinence. *Clin Gastroenterol Hepatol.* 2014;12:843-851.
52. Peeters M, Van den Brande J, Francque S. Diarrhea and the rationale to use Sandostatin. *Acta Gastroenterol Belg.* 2010;73:25-36.
53. Scaldaferri F, Pizzoferrato M, Ponziani FR, et al. Use and indications of cholestyramine and bile acid sequestrants. *Intern Emerg Med.* 2013;8:205-210.
54. Roerig JL, Steffen KJ, Mitchell JE, Zunker C. Laxative abuse: epidemiology, diagnosis and management. *Drugs.* 2010;70:1487-1503.
55. Emmanuel AV, Tack J, Quigley EM, Talley NJ. Pharmacological management of constipation. *Neurogastroenterol Motil.* 2009;21(suppl 2):41-54.
56. Kalnins D, Wilschanski M. Maintenance of nutritional status in patients with cystic fibrosis: new and emerging therapies. *Drug Des Devel Ther.* 2012;6:151-161.
57. Janelsins MC, Tejani MA, Kamen C, et al. Current pharmacotherapy for chemotherapy-induced nausea and vomiting in cancer patients. *Expert Opin Pharmacother.* 2013;14:757-766.
58. Kovac AL. Update on the management of postoperative nausea and vomiting. *Drugs.* 2013;73:1525-1547.
59. Spinks A, Wasiak J. Scopolamine (hyoscine) for preventing and treating motion sickness. *Cochrane Database Syst Rev.* 2011;6:CD002851.
60. Portincasa P, Di Ciaula A, Wang HH, et al. Medicinal treatments of cholesterol gallstones: old, current and new perspectives. *Curr Med Chem.* 2009;16:1531-1542.
61. Quenot JP, Thiery N, Barbar S. When should stress ulcer prophylaxis be used in the ICU? *Curr Opin Crit Care.* 2009;15:139-143.

SECTION

7

Endocrine Pharmacology

CHAPTER 28

Introduction to Endocrine Pharmacology

The endocrine system helps to maintain internal homeostasis through the use of endogenous chemicals known as *hormones*. A hormone is typically regarded as a chemical messenger that is released into the bloodstream to exert an effect on target cells located some distance from the hormonal release site.[1,2] Various endocrine glands manufacture and release specific hormones that help regulate physiological processes such as reproduction, growth and development, energy metabolism, fluid and electrolyte balance, and response to stress and injury.[1,3]

The use of drugs to help regulate and control endocrine function is an important area of pharmacology. In one sense, hormones can be considered drugs that are manufactured by the patient's body. This situation presents an obvious opportunity to use exogenous chemicals to either mimic or attenuate the effects of specific hormones during endocrine dysfunction.

Patients can take drugs as replacement therapy during hormonal deficiency—for example, insulin administration in diabetes mellitus. Likewise, exogenous hormone analogs can accentuate the effects of their endogenous counterparts, such as using glucocorticoids to help treat inflammation. Conversely, drugs can treat endocrine hyperactivity—for example, the use of antithyroid drugs in treating hyperthyroidism. Finally, drugs can regulate normal endocrine function to achieve a desired effect, as is done through the inhibition of ovulation by oral contraceptives.

The purpose of this chapter is to review the basic aspects of endocrine function, including the primary hormones and their effects. The factors regulating hormonal release and the cellular mechanisms of hormone action are also briefly discussed. Finally, the basic ways in which drugs can be used to alter endocrine function are presented. This overview is intended to provide you with a general review of endocrine and hormone activity. Chapters 29 through 32 deal with the physiology and pharmacology of the hormones of specific endocrine systems in more detail along with the specific endocrine drugs, and the problems the drugs treat.

PRIMARY ENDOCRINE GLANDS AND THEIR HORMONES

The primary endocrine glands include the hypothalamus, pituitary, thyroid, parathyroid, pancreas, adrenal, and gonads (Fig. 28-1). These glands and the physiological effects of their hormones are also summarized in Tables 28-1 and 28-2. For the purpose of this chapter, only the primary endocrine glands and their respective hormones are discussed. Substances such as prostaglandins and kinins, which are produced locally by a variety of different cells, are not discussed here but are referred to elsewhere in this text (e.g., see Chapter 15). Also, chemicals such as norepinephrine, which serve a dual purpose as hormones and neurotransmitters, are discussed in this chapter only with regard to their endocrine function.

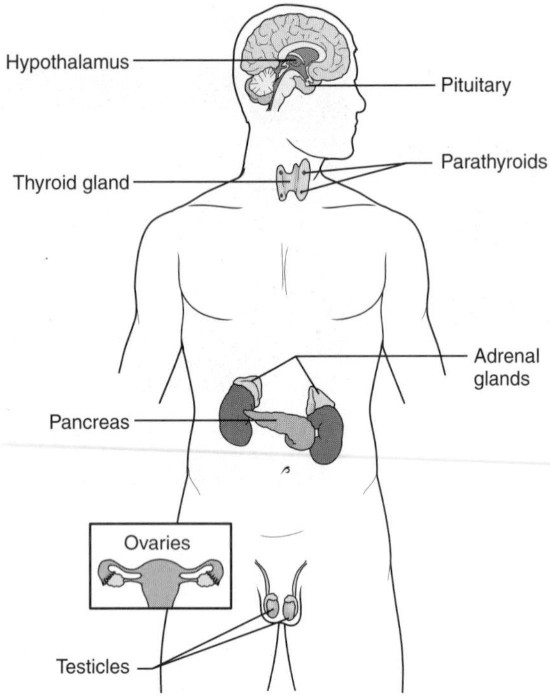

Figure ■ 28-1
The primary endocrine glands.

Table 28-1
HYPOTHALAMIC AND PITUITARY HORMONES

Hypothalamic Hormones and Releasing Factors	Effect
Growth hormone–releasing hormone (GHRH)	↑ GH release
Growth hormone–inhibitory hormone (GHIH)	↓ GH release
Gonadotropin-releasing hormone (GnRH)	↑ LH and FSH release
Thyrotropin-releasing hormone (TRH)	↑ TSH release
Corticotropin-releasing hormone (CRH)	↑ ACTH release
Prolactin-inhibitory factor (PIF)	↓ Pr release
Pituitary Hormones	**Principal Effects**
Anterior Lobe	
Growth hormone (GH)	↑ tissue growth and development
Luteinizing hormone (LH)	Female: ↑ ovulation; ↑ estrogen and progesterone synthesis from corpus luteum Male: ↑ testosterone synthesis
Follicle-stimulating hormone (FSH)	Female: ↑ follicular development and estrogen synthesis Male: enhance spermatogenesis
Thyroid-stimulating hormone (TSH)	↑ synthesis of thyroid hormones (T_3, T_4)
Adrenocorticotropic hormone (ACTH)	↑ adrenal steroid synthesis (e.g., cortisol)
Prolactin (Pr)	Initiates lactation
Posterior Lobe	
Antidiuretic hormone (ADH)	↑ renal reabsorption of water
Oxytocin	↑ uterine contraction; ↑ milk ejection during lactation

Hypothalamus and Pituitary Gland

The pituitary gland is a small, pea-shaped structure located within the sella turcica at the base of the brain. It lies inferior to the hypothalamus and is attached to the hypothalamus by a thin stalk of tissue known as the *infundibulum*. The structural and functional relationships between the hypothalamus and pituitary gland are briefly discussed later in this section. A more detailed presentation of the anatomic and physiological functions of the hypothalamus and pituitary gland can be found in several sources listed in the references.[4-7] Basically, the pituitary can be subdivided into an anterior, an intermediate, and a posterior lobe. These subdivisions and their respective hormones are listed in Table 28-1 and briefly discussed below.

Anterior Lobe

The anterior pituitary, or adenohypophysis, secretes six important peptide hormones. The anterior pituitary releases growth hormone (GH), luteinizing hormone (LH), follicle-stimulating hormone (FSH), thyroid-stimulating hormone (TSH), adrenocorticotropic hormone (ACTH), and prolactin (Pr). The physiological effects of these hormones are listed in Table 28-1.

Hormonal release from the anterior pituitary is controlled by specific hormones or releasing factors from the hypothalamus.[6] Basically, a releasing factor is sent from the hypothalamus to the anterior pituitary via local vascular structures known as the *hypothalamic-hypophysial portal vessels*. For example, to increase the secretion of growth hormone, the hypothalamus

Table 28-2
OTHER PRIMARY ENDOCRINE GLANDS

Gland	Hormone(s)	Principal Effects
Thyroid	Thyroxine (T_4), triiodothyronine (T_3)	Increase cellular metabolism; facilitate normal growth and development
Parathyroids	Parathormone (PTH)	Increase blood calcium
Pancreas	Glucagon	Increase blood glucose
	Insulin	Decrease blood glucose; increase carbohydrate, protein, and fat storage
Adrenal cortex	Glucocorticoids	Regulate glucose metabolism; enhance response to stress
	Mineralocorticoids	Regulate fluid and electrolyte levels
Adrenal medulla	Epinephrine, norepinephrine	Vascular and metabolic effects that facilitate increased physical activity
Testes	Testosterone	Spermatogenesis; male sexual characteristics
Ovaries	Estrogens, progesterone	Female reproductive cycle and sexual characteristics

first secretes growth hormone–releasing hormone (GHRH) into the portal vessels. The GHRH travels a short distance to the anterior pituitary via the hypothalamic-hypophysial portal system. Upon arriving at the pituitary, the GHRH causes the anterior pituitary to release growth hormone into the systemic circulation, where it can then travel to various target tissues in the periphery. Other hypothalamic-releasing factors that have been identified are listed in Table 28-1. Researchers are still investigating specific releasing factors, and the identification of additional factors (including those that inhibit anterior pituitary hormone release) will undoubtedly be forthcoming.

Intermediate Lobe

In mammals, there is a small intermediate lobe of the pituitary (pars intermedia) that may secrete melanocyte-stimulating hormone (MSH). Although it can influence skin pigmentation in lower vertebrates, the intermediate lobe does not produce MSH in meaningful amounts in humans. Humans can, however, produce MSH from a precursor protein (proopiomelacortin) that is synthesized in central tissues (anterior pituitary, hypothalamus) and the periphery (skin, lymphoid tissues).[8] MSH may play a role in controlling several diverse functions such as appetite, energy homeostasis, and inflammation.[9-11] MSH and similar hormones such as ACTH are key components of a neuroendocrine arrangement known as the *melanocortin system*; investigators continue to determine if this system can be manipulated pharmacologically to help control various physiological systems.

Posterior Lobe

The posterior pituitary, or neurohypophysis, secretes two hormones: antidiuretic hormone (ADH) and oxytocin.[12,13] ADH exerts its effect primarily on the kidneys, where it increases the reabsorption of water from the distal renal tubules. Oxytocin is important in parturition and stimulates the uterus to contract. It also promotes lactation by stimulating the ejection of milk from the mammary glands.

The hypothalamic control of the posterior pituitary is quite different than that of the anterior and intermediate lobes. Specific neurons have their cell bodies in certain hypothalamic nuclei. Cell bodies in the paraventricular nuclei manufacture oxytocin, whereas the supraoptic nuclei contain cell bodies that synthesize ADH. The axons from these cells extend downward through the infundibulum to terminate in the posterior pituitary. Hormones synthesized in the hypothalamic cell bodies are transported down the axon to be stored in neurosecretory granules in their respective nerve terminals (located in the posterior pituitary). When an appropriate stimulus is present, these neurons fire an action potential, which causes the hormones to release from their pituitary nerve terminals. The hormones are ultimately picked up by the systemic circulation and transported to their target tissues.

Thyroid Gland

The thyroid gland is located in the anterior neck region, approximately at the level of the fifth cervical to first thoracic vertebrae.[14] This gland consists of bilateral lobes that lie on either side of the trachea and are connected by a thin piece of the gland known as the *isthmus*. The thyroid synthesizes and secretes two hormones: thyroxine (T_4) and triiodothyronine (T_3). The synthesis of these hormones is controlled by the hypothalamic-pituitary system via thyroid-releasing hormone from the hypothalamus, which causes thyroid-stimulating hormone release from the anterior pituitary. Thyroid-stimulating hormone increases T_3 and T_4 synthesis and release from the thyroid gland.

The primary effect of the thyroid hormones is to increase cellular metabolism in most body tissues.[15,16] These hormones stimulate virtually all aspects of cellular function, including protein, fat, and carbohydrate metabolism. By exerting a stimulatory effect on the cellular level, thyroid hormones play a crucial role in helping maintain and regulate body heat (*thermogenesis*) in the whole organism. T_3 and T_4 also play an important role in growth and development, especially in the growth and maturation of normal bone. Finally, thyroid hormones play a permissive role in allowing other hormones, such as steroids, to exert their effects (see Chapter 31).

Parathyroid Gland

Parathyroid glands are small, egg-shaped structures embedded in the posterior surface of the thyroid gland. There are usually four parathyroid glands, with two glands located on each half of the thyroid gland. The parathyroids synthesize and release parathyroid hormone (PTH). PTH is essential in maintaining normal calcium homeostasis in the body; the primary effect of PTH is to increase the concentration of calcium in the bloodstream.[17] PTH increases circulating calcium levels primarily by mobilizing calcium from storage sites in bone.

The primary factor regulating PTH release is the level of calcium in the bloodstream.[18,19] The parathyroid glands contain a calcium-sensing receptor that monitors circulating calcium levels. As circulating calcium levels fall below a certain point, PTH secretion is increased. Conversely, elevated plasma calcium titers inhibit PTH secretion (see the "Parathyroid Hormone" section in Chapter 31).

Pancreas

The pancreas is located behind the stomach in the lower left area of the abdomen. This gland is unique in that it serves both endocrine and exocrine functions.[20,21] The exocrine aspect of this gland involves digestive enzymes that are excreted into the duodenum via the pancreatic duct. As an endocrine gland, the pancreas secretes several hormones into the systemic circulation. These hormones are synthesized and secreted by cells located in specialized clusters known as the Islets of Langerhans (see Chapter 32). The two primary pancreatic endocrines are insulin and glucagon. In the Islets of Langerhans, glucagon and insulin are synthesized by alpha and beta cells, respectively.

Insulin and glucagon are involved in the regulation of blood glucose, and the glucose concentration in the blood serves as the primary stimulus for the release of these hormones. For example, following a fast, glucagon is released from pancreatic alpha cells as blood glucose levels fall. Glucagon mobilizes the release of glucose from storage sites in the liver, thus bringing blood glucose levels back to normal. An increase in blood glucose after eating a meal stimulates insulin release from the beta cells. Insulin facilitates the storage of glucose in the liver and muscle, thus removing glucose from the bloodstream and returning blood glucose to normal levels. Insulin also exerts a number of other effects on protein and lipid metabolism. The effects of insulin and its pharmacological replacement in diabetes mellitus are discussed in more detail in Chapter 32.

Adrenal Gland

Adrenal glands are located at the superior poles of each kidney. Each adrenal gland is composed of an outer cortex and an inner medulla. The hormones associated with the adrenal cortex and adrenal medulla are described in the following sections.

Hormones of the Adrenal Cortex

The adrenal cortex synthesizes and secretes two primary groups of steroidal hormones: the glucocorticoids and the mineralocorticoids.[22,23] Small amounts of sex steroids (estrogens, androgens, progesterone) are also produced, but these amounts are essentially insignificant during normal adrenal function.

Glucocorticoids such as cortisol have several physiological effects.[24] Glucocorticoids are involved in the regulation of glucose metabolism and are important in enhancing the body's ability to handle stress. They also have significant anti-inflammatory and immunosuppressive properties and are often used therapeutically to control inflammation or suppress the immune response in various clinical situations (see Chapter 29). Glucocorticoid synthesis is controlled by the hypothalamic-pituitary system. Corticotropin-releasing hormone (CRH) from the hypothalamus stimulates ACTH release from the anterior pituitary, which in turn stimulates the synthesis of glucocorticoids.

Mineralocorticoids are involved in controlling electrolyte and fluid levels.[22,25] The primary mineralocorticoid produced by the adrenal cortex is aldosterone, which increases the reabsorption of sodium from the renal tubules (see Chapter 29). By increasing sodium reabsorption, aldosterone facilitates the reabsorption of water. It also inhibits the renal reabsorption of potassium, thus increasing potassium excretion. Mineralocorticoid release is regulated by fluid and electrolyte levels in the body and by other hormones, such as the renin-angiotensin system.

Hormones of the Adrenal Medulla

The adrenal medulla synthesizes and secretes epinephrine and norepinephrine.[22] These hormones have several physiological effects (see Chapters 18 and 20). Small amounts of epinephrine and norepinephrine are released under resting, basal conditions, but the primary significance of these hormones seems to be in helping to prepare the body for sudden physical activity. As discussed in Chapter 18, the sympathetic nervous system stimulates the adrenal gland to release epinephrine and norepinephrine into the bloodstream in certain situations. These substances cause many effects, including increased cardiac output, decreased visceral blood flow (thus leaving more blood available for skeletal muscle), increased cellular metabolism, and several other physiological changes that facilitate vigorous activity. The function of the adrenal medulla is therefore often characterized by the fight-or-flight reaction, in which a stressful challenge is presented to the individual and interpreted as requiring either a defense or a need to flee.

The release of epinephrine and norepinephrine from the adrenal medulla is controlled by the sympathetic division of the autonomic nervous system. Sympathetic cholinergic preganglionic neurons directly innervate this gland (see Chapter 18). An increase in sympathetic activity causes increased firing in these neurons, which in turn stimulates the release of epinephrine and norepinephrine from the adrenal medulla.

Gonads

Reproductive organs are the primary source of the steroid hormones that influence sexual and reproductive functions (see Chapter 30). In men, the testes produce *testosterone* and similar androgens that are responsible for spermatogenesis and the secondary sexual characteristics of adult males.[26,27] In women, sexual maturation and reproductive function are governed by the production of estrogens and progestins from the ovaries.[28,29] The release of male and female sex steroids is controlled by hormones from the hypothalamus and anterior pituitary.[26,30]

ENDOCRINE PHYSIOLOGY AND PHARMACOLOGY

Hormone Chemistry

Hormones can be divided into several primary categories according to their basic chemical structure. *Steroid hormones* share a common chemical framework that is derived from lipids, such as cholesterol.[31] Examples of steroids include the sex hormones (androgens, estrogens, progesterone), the glucocorticoids, and the mineralocorticoids. *Peptide hormones* consist of amino acids linked together in a specific sequence. These peptide chains can range in length from 3 to 180 amino acids. Primary examples of peptide hormones are the hypothalamic releasing factors and the pituitary hormones. Finally, several hormones are modified from a single amino acid. For instance, the thyroid hormones (T_3 and T_4) are manufactured from the amino acid tyrosine. In addition, hormones from the adrenal medulla (epinephrine, norepinephrine) are synthesized from either phenylalanine or tyrosine.

The basic chemical structure of various hormones is significant in determining how the hormone will exert its effects on target tissues (see "Hormone Effects on the Target Cell"). Different hormones that are fairly similar in structure can often have similar physiological and pharmacological effects (see Chapters 29 through 32). This is especially true for the steroids, in which one category of steroidal agents may have some of the same properties of a different category.[32] For instance, the endogenous glucocorticoids (e.g., cortisol) also exert some mineralocorticoid effects, presumably because of their similar chemical structure. The overlapping effects and their consequences are discussed in more detail in Chapters 29 through 32, which deal with specific endocrine systems.

Synthesis and Release of Hormones

Hormones are typically synthesized within the cells of their respective endocrine glands. Within the gland, most hormones are synthesized and packaged in storage granules. When the gland is stimulated, the storage granule fuses with the cell membrane, and the hormone is released by exocytosis. Notable exceptions to this are the steroid hormones, which are not stored to any great extent but are synthesized on demand when an appropriate stimulus is present.[33]

Extrinsic and intrinsic factors can initiate hormone synthesis and release.[34] Extrinsic factors include various environmental stimuli such as pain, temperature, light, and smell. Intrinsic stimuli include various humoral and neural factors. For instance, release of a hormone can be initiated by other hormones. These occurrences are particularly typical of the anterior pituitary hormones, which are controlled by releasing hormones from the hypothalamus. Hormonal release can be influenced by neural input; a primary example is the sympathetic neural control of epinephrine and norepinephrine release from the adrenal medulla. Other intrinsic factors that affect hormone release are the levels of ions and metabolites within the body. For instance, parathyroid hormone release is governed directly by the calcium concentration in the bloodstream, and the release of glucagon from pancreatic alpha cells is dependent on blood glucose levels.

Feedback Control Mechanisms in Endocrine Function

As mentioned previously, the endocrine system is concerned with maintaining homeostasis in the body. When a disturbance in physiological function occurs, hormones are released to rectify the disturbance. As function returns to normal, hormone release is attenuated and homeostasis is resumed. For example, an increase in the blood glucose level initiates the release of insulin from pancreatic beta cells. Insulin increases the incorporation into and storage of glucose in liver, skeletal muscle, and other tissues. Blood glucose levels then return to normal, and insulin release is terminated.

Hormonal release is also frequently regulated by some form of negative feedback system.[34,35] In these feedback systems, an increase in the release of a specific hormone ultimately serves to inhibit its own release, thus preventing the amount of the released hormone from becoming excessive. An example of a negative feedback system involving the hypothalamic-pituitary axis is illustrated in Figure 28-2. The endocrine hormone ultimately inhibits its own release by inhibiting the secretion of specific hypothalamic releasing factors and pituitary hormones. Numerous examples of such negative feedback loops are present in various endocrine pathways.

There are also a few examples of positive feedback mechanisms in the endocrine system.[35] In a positive feedback loop, rising concentrations of one hormone cause an increase in other hormones. The primary example of this type of feedback occurs in the menstrual cycle, where increasing levels of estrogen from the

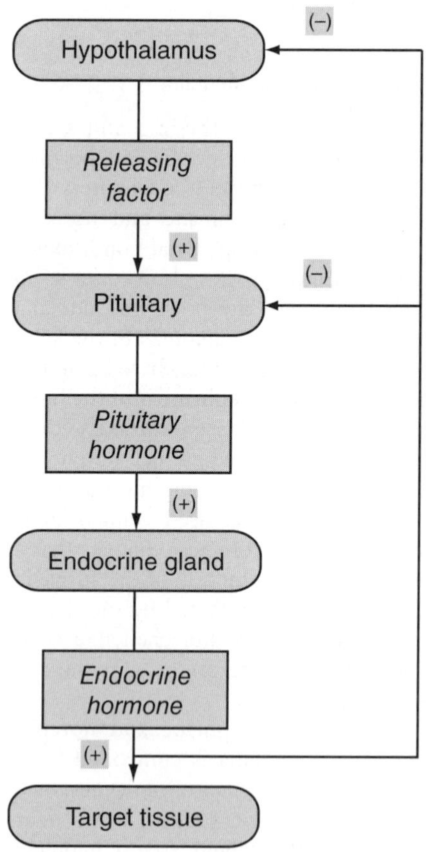

Figure ■ 28-2
Negative feedback control in the hypothalamic-pituitary endocrine pathways. Excitatory and inhibitory effects are indicated by (+) and (–), respectively. Negative feedback loops occur owing to inhibition of the endocrine hormone on the pituitary and hypothalamus.

developing follicle stimulate the release of hormones from the hypothalamus and pituitary. Specifically, a rise in estrogen above a critical point for an appropriate amount of time (36 hours) signals the hypothalamus to release gonadotropin-releasing hormone, which in turn causes a sudden increase in LH release (and, to a lesser extent, FSH production) from the anterior pituitary.[36] The sudden, sharp rise in LH from the anterior pituitary (i.e., the LH surge) triggers the release of the oocyte from the developing follicle. Thus, positive feedback of estrogen on the hypothalamic-pituitary axis facilitates the release of hormones that cause ovulation. Positive feedback mechanisms, however, are relatively rare in the endocrine system compared with negative feedback control of hormonal release.

The presence of feedback systems in endocrine function is important from a pharmacological perspective. Drugs can act through the intrinsic feedback loops to control endogenous hormone production. A primary example is the use of oral contraceptives, when women take exogenous estrogen and progesterone in controlled amounts to inhibit ovulation (see Chapter 30).

Therapeutic administration of hormonal agents may create problems, however, because of the negative feedback effects. For instance, glucocorticoid administration for various conditions (rheumatoid arthritis, asthma, certain cancers) may act as negative feedback to suppress the normal endogenous production of adrenal steroids.[37,38] If the body is unable to produce its own supply of adrenal steroids, abrupt withdrawal of the exogenous compounds can result in severe or even fatal consequences. Adrenocortical suppression is discussed in more detail in Chapter 29.

Hormone Transport

Hormones are usually carried from their site of origin to the target cell via the systemic circulation.[2,39] During transport in the bloodstream, certain hormones such as steroids are bound to specific plasma proteins such as corticosteroid binding globulin and sex hormone binding globulin. These protein carriers appear to help prolong the half-life of the hormone and prevent premature degradation. Other protein carriers may be important in the local effects of hormone function. For instance, the testes produce androgen-binding protein, which helps transport and concentrate testosterone within the seminiferous tubules of the testes (see Chapter 30). On the other hand, defects in the production or function of hormonal protein carriers may impair the delivery of hormones to their target sites, thus altering the effects of specific endocrines within the body.[40,41]

Hormone Effects on the Target Cell

Most hormones affect their target cell by interacting with a specific receptor. Hormone receptors are located at three locations: the surface of the plasma membrane, within the cytosol, and on the chromatin within the cell nucleus (Fig. 28-3). These primary

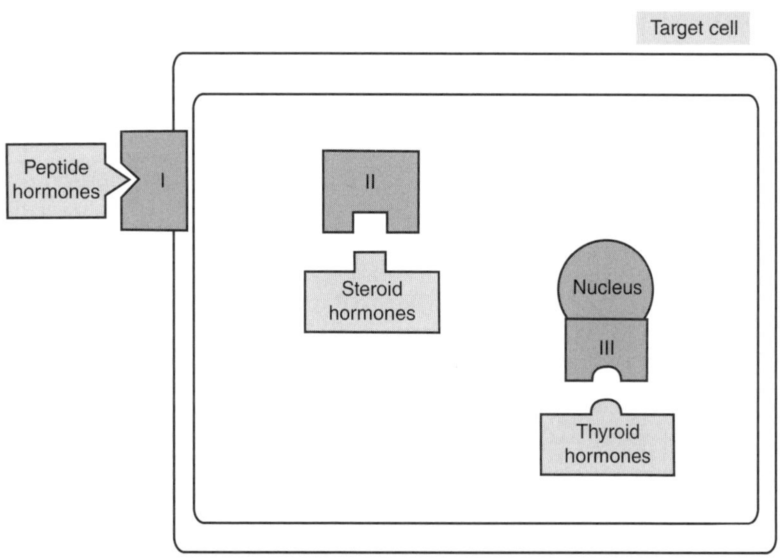

Figure ■ 28-3
Primary cellular locations of hormone receptors. Peptide hormones tend to bind to surface membrane receptors (site I), steroid hormones bind to cytosolic receptors (site II), and thyroid hormones bind to receptors in the cell nucleus (site III).

locations are on the cell's surface membrane, within the cytosol of the cell, or within the cell's nucleus.[1] Receptors at each location tend to be specific for different types of hormones and also tend to affect cell function in a specific manner. Each type of receptor is briefly discussed below.

Surface Membrane Receptors

These receptors are located on the outer surface of the plasma membrane (see Fig. 28-3).[42] Surface receptors tend to recognize the peptide hormones and some amino acid derivatives (e.g., pituitary hormones, catecholamines). They are typically linked to specific intracellular enzymes. When stimulated by a peptidelike hormone, the receptor initiates some change in the enzymatic machinery located within the cell. This event usually results in a change in the production of some intracellular chemical second messenger such as cyclic adenosine monophosphate (cAMP).[42]

An example of a hormone that exerts its effects through a surface receptor–second messenger system is ACTH,[4,43] which is a polypeptide that binds to a surface receptor on adrenal cortex cells. The surface receptor then stimulates the adenylate cyclase enzyme to increase production of cAMP, which acts as a second messenger (the hormone was the first messenger) and increases the activity of other enzymes within the cell to synthesize adrenal steroids such as cortisol. See Chapter 4 for a more detailed description of surface receptor–second messenger systems.

Cytosolic Hormone Receptors

Steroid hormones typically bind to protein receptors, some of which are located directly within the cytosol (see Fig. 28-3).[1,44] Of course, this means that the hormone must first enter the cell, which is easily accomplished by the steroid hormones because they are highly lipid soluble. After entering the cell, the hormone initiates a series of events that are depicted in Figure 28-4.

Basically, the hormone and receptor form a large activated steroid-receptor complex.[45] This complex travels to the cell's nucleus, where it binds to specific genes located within the DNA sequence.[1,46] This process initiates gene expression and transcription

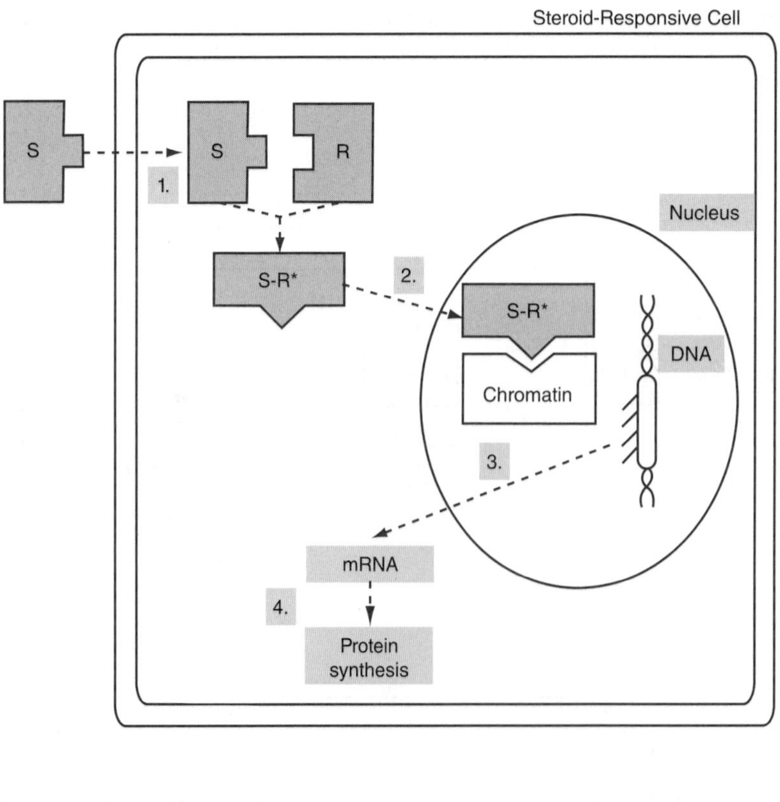

Figure ■ 28-4
Sequence of events of steroid hormone action. (1) Steroid hormone enters the cell, binds to a cytosolic receptor, and creates an activated steroid-receptor complex (S-R). (2) S-R complex travels to the cell's nucleus, where it binds to specific gene segments on nuclear chromatin. (3) DNA undergoes transcription into messenger RNA (mRNA) units. (4) mRNA undergoes translation in the cytosol into specific proteins that alter cell function.

of messenger RNA units, which go back to the cytosol and are translated into specific proteins by the endoplasmic reticulum.[1] These newly manufactured proteins are usually enzymes or structural proteins that change cell function in a specific manner. For instance, anabolic steroids increase muscle size by facilitating the production of more contractile proteins. Thus, steroids tend to exert their effects on target cells by directly affecting the cell's nucleus and subsequently altering the production of certain cellular proteins.

Hence, steroids exert their primary effects by acting on receptors located within the cytosol of the cell. As we discussed in Chapter 4, it is apparent that these substances also exert some of their effects by binding to a second set of receptors located on the cell surface.[45] Researchers continue to define the exact role of steroidal surface receptors and their contribution to the effects of each type of steroid.

Nuclear Hormone Receptors

Certain hormones interact directly with hormonal receptors that are located on the chromatin within the cell nucleus (see Fig. 28-3).[47] Thyroid hormones (T_3 and T_4) are a primary example of hormones that bind directly to nuclear receptors (see Chapter 31).[1,15] After binding, thyroid hormones invoke a series of changes similar to those caused by the steroid–cytosolic receptor complex—the nucleus begins to transcribe messenger RNA, which is ultimately translated into specific proteins. In the case of the thyroid hormones, these new proteins usually alter the cell's metabolism.

Hormone receptors have some obvious and important pharmacological distinctions. Drugs that can bind to and activate specific hormonal receptors (agonists) will mimic the effects of the endogenous compounds. Drugs that block the receptors (antagonists) will attenuate any unwanted hormonal effects. In fact, drugs can be produced that are even more specific for hormonal receptors than their endogenous counterparts. For instance, synthetic glucocorticoids, such as dexamethasone, exert anti-inflammatory effects in a manner similar to that of endogenous glucocorticoids, but with diminished mineralocorticoid-like side effects such as water and sodium retention. This increased specificity is presumably brought about by a more precise action of the synthetic compound on the glucocorticoid receptors rather than the mineralocorticoid receptors.

CLINICAL USE OF ENDOCRINE DRUGS

Physicians can administer pharmacological agents for replacement therapy, to treat excessive endocrine function, or to alter normal endocrine function. Furthermore, medical practitioners can also diagnose endocrine disorders with endocrine drugs. The following sections are brief overviews of these uses.

Replacement Therapy

If the endogenous production of a hormone is deficient or absent, therapeutic administration of the hormone can be used to restore normal endocrine function.[48-51] The exogenous hormone can be obtained from natural sources, such as extracts from animal tissues, or from chemical synthesis. In addition, researchers are using new recombinant DNA techniques to produce hormones from cell cultures, and these techniques have shown great promise in being able to generate hormones like human insulin.

Hormone substitution is sometimes referred to as *simple replacement therapy*. However, the use of exogenous hormones to replace normal endocrine function can be a complicated task. Problems such as regulation of optimal dosage, the interaction of the exogenous drug with other endogenous hormone systems, and drug-induced side effects are frequently encountered. Specific examples of hormone replacement therapy, and potential benefits and risks of these treatments, will be addressed in Chapters 29 through 32.

Diagnosis of Endocrine Disorders

Physicians may administer hormones or their antagonists to determine the presence of excess endocrine function or endocrine hypofunction. For example, hormones or their synthetic analogs can either increase or decrease pituitary secretion to determine if pituitary function is normal. Likewise, antagonists to specific hormones can help physicians see if symptoms are caused by excessive hormone production.

Treatment of Excessive Endocrine Function

Hyperactive or inappropriate endocrine function is often treated pharmacologically. Inhibition of hormone function can occur at several levels. For instance, patients take drugs that directly inhibit the synthesis of the hormone or inhibit its release through various negative feedback mechanisms (see earlier section, "Feedback Control Mechanisms in Endocrine Function"). Also, patients may use hormone antagonists (drugs that block hormone receptors) for prolonged periods to attenuate the effects of excessive hormone production.

Exploitation of Beneficial Hormone Effects

Hormones and their synthetic analogs are often administered to exaggerate the beneficial effects of their endogenous counterparts. The classic example is the use of glucocorticoids to treat inflammation. Doses of glucocorticoids that are much higher than the physiological levels produced by the body can be very effective in decreasing inflammation in a variety of clinical conditions (e.g., rheumatoid arthritis, allergic reactions). Of course, the use of high doses of hormones to accentuate beneficial effects may also cause some side effects and impair various aspects of endocrine function. However, short-term use of hormones in this capacity is often a useful therapeutic intervention.

Use of Hormones to Alter Normal Endocrine Function

Because of the intrinsic control mechanisms in the endocrine system, administration of exogenous hormones can often affect the normal release of hormones. This fact can be exploited in certain situations to cause a desired change in normal endocrine function. For instance, oral contraceptives containing estrogen and progesterone inhibit ovulation by inhibiting the release of LH and FSH from the anterior pituitary.

Use of Hormones in Nonendocrine Disease

There are many examples of how various hormones and hormone-related drugs can be used to treat conditions that are not directly related to the endocrine system. For example, certain forms of cancer respond to treatment with glucocorticoids (see Chapter 36). Drugs that block the cardiac beta-1 receptors may help control angina and hypertension by preventing excessive stimulation from adrenal medulla hormones (epinephrine, norepinephrine; see Chapters 21 and 22).

SUMMARY

The endocrine glands regulate a variety of physiological processes through the release of specific hormones. Hormones are the equivalent of endogenously produced drugs that usually travel through the bloodstream to exert an effect on specific target tissues. Hormones typically alter cell function by binding to receptors located at specific sites on or within the target cell. Pharmacological agents can be administered to mimic or exaggerate hormonal effects, inhibit excessive hormonal activity, and produce other desirable changes in endocrine activity.

REFERENCES

1. Barrett EJ. Organization of endocrine control. In: Boron WF, Boulpaep EL, eds. *Medical Physiology: A Cellular and Molecular Approach*. 2nd ed. New York: Elsevier/Saunders; 2012.
2. Kroneneberg HM, Melmed S, Larsen PR, Polonsky KS. Principles of endocrinology. In: Melmed S, et al, eds. *Williams Textbook of Endocrinology*. 12th ed. Philadelphia: Elsevier/Saunders; 2011.
3. White BA. Introduction to the endocrine system. In: Koeppen BM, Stanton BA, eds. *Berne and Levy Physiology*. 6th ed. Philadelphia: Mosby/Elsevier; 2010.
4. Melmed S, Kleinberg D. Pituitary physiology and diagnostic evaluation. In: Melmed S, et al, eds. *Williams Textbook of Endocrinology*. 12th ed. Philadelphia: Elsevier/Saunders; 2011.
5. Perez-Castro C, Renner U, Haedo MR, et al. Cellular and molecular specificity of pituitary gland physiology. *Physiol Rev*. 2012;92:1-38.
6. Sam S, Frohman LA. Normal physiology of hypothalamic pituitary regulation. *Endocrinol Metab Clin North Am*. 2008;37:1-22.
7. White BA. The hypothalamus and pituitary gland. In: Koeppen BM, Stanton BA, eds. *Berne and Levy Physiology*. 6th ed. Philadelphia: Mosby/Elsevier; 2010.
8. D'Agostino G, Diano S. Alpha-melanocyte stimulating hormone: production and degradation. *J Mol Med (Berl)*. 2010;88:1195-1201.
9. Brzoska T, Böhm M, Lügering A, et al. Terminal signal: anti-inflammatory effects of α-melanocyte-stimulating hormone related peptides beyond the pharmacophore. *Adv Exp Med Biol*. 2010;681:107-116.
10. Corander MP, Coll AP. Melanocortins and body weight regulation: glucocorticoids, Agouti-related protein and beyond. *Eur J Pharmacol*. 2011;660:111-118.
11. Parker JA, Bloom SR. Hypothalamic neuropeptides and the regulation of appetite. *Neuropharmacology*. 2012;63:18-30.

12. Calabrò RS, Italiano D, Ferrara D, et al. The hypothalamic-neurohypophyseal system: current and future treatment of vasopressin and oxytocyn related disorders. *Recent Pat Endocr Metab Immune Drug Discov*. 2012;6:235-250.
13. Robinson AG, Verbalis JG. Posterior pituitary. In: Melmed S, et al, eds. *Williams Textbook of Endocrinology.* 12th ed. Philadelphia: Elsevier/Saunders; 2011.
14. Barrett EJ. The thyroid gland. In: Boron WF, Boulpaep EL, eds. *Medical Physiology: A Cellular and Molecular Approach.* 2nd ed. New York: Elsevier/Saunders; 2012.
15. Boelen A, Kwakkel J, Fliers E. Thyroid hormone receptors in health and disease. *Minerva Endocrinol.* 2012;37:291-304.
16. Song Y, Yao X, Ying H. Thyroid hormone action in metabolic regulation. *Protein Cell.* 2011;2:358-368.
17. Silva BC, Costa AG, Cusano NE, et al. Catabolic and anabolic actions of parathyroid hormone on the skeleton. *J Endocrinol Invest.* 2011;34:801-810.
18. Kumar R, Thompson JR. The regulation of parathyroid hormone secretion and synthesis. *J Am Soc Nephrol.* 2011;22:216-224.
19. Ward DT, Riccardi D. New concepts in calcium-sensing receptor pharmacology and signalling. *Br J Pharmacol.* 2012;165:35-48.
20. Chen N, Unnikrishnan IR, Anjana RM, et al. The complex exocrine-endocrine relationship and secondary diabetes in exocrine pancreatic disorders. *J Clin Gastroenterol.* 2011;45:850-861.
21. Czakó L, Hegyi P, Rakonczay Z Jr, et al. Interactions between the endocrine and exocrine pancreas and their clinical relevance. *Pancreatology*. 2009;9:351-359.
22. Gorman LS. The adrenal gland: common disease states and suspected new applications. *Clin Lab Sci*. 2013;26:118-125.
23. Vinson GP. The adrenal cortex and life. *Mol Cell Endocrinol.* 2009;300:2-6.
24. Zanchi NE, Filho MA, Felitti V, et al. Glucocorticoids: extensive physiological actions modulated through multiple mechanisms of gene regulation. *J Cell Physiol.* 2010;224:311-315.
25. Fourkiotis VG, Hanslik G, Hanusch F, et al. Aldosterone and the kidney. *Horm Metab Res.* 2012;44:194-201.
26. Kicman AT. Biochemical and physiological aspects of endogenous androgens. *Handb Exp Pharmacol.* 2010;195:25-64.
27. Marchetti PM, Barth JH. Clinical biochemistry of dihydrotestosterone. *Ann Clin Biochem.* 2013;50:95-107.
28. Edson MA, Nagaraja AK, Matzuk MM. The mammalian ovary from genesis to revelation. *Endocr Rev.* 2009;30:624-712.
29. Farage MA, Neill S, MacLean AB. Physiological changes associated with the menstrual cycle: a review. *Obstet Gynecol Surv.* 2009;64:58-72.
30. Christensen A, Bentley GE, Cabrera R, et al. Hormonal regulation of female reproduction. *Horm Metab Res.* 2012;44:587-591.
31. Issop L, Rone MB, Papadopoulos V. Organelle plasticity and interactions in cholesterol transport and steroid biosynthesis. *Mol Cell Endocrinol.* 2013;371:34-46.
32. Schimmer BP, Funder JW. ACTH, adrenal steroids, and pharmacology of the adrenal cortex. In: Brunton L, et al, eds. *The Pharmacological Basis of Therapeutics.* 12th ed. New York: McGraw-Hill; 2011.
33. Poderoso C, Duarte A, Cooke M, et al. The spatial and temporal regulation of the hormonal signal. Role of mitochondria in the formation of a protein complex required for the activation of cholesterol transport and steroids synthesis. *Mol Cell Endocrinol.* 2013;371:26-33.
34. Parker KL, Schimmer BP. Introduction to endocrinology: the hypothalamic-pituitary axis. In: Brunton L, et al, eds. *The Pharmacological Basis of Therapeutics.* 12th ed. New York: McGraw-Hill; 2011.
35. Berga S, Naftolin F. Neuroendocrine control of ovulation. *Gynecol Endocrinol.* 2012;28(suppl 1):9-13.
36. Clarkson J, Herbison AE. Oestrogen, kisspeptin, GPR54 and the pre-ovulatory luteinising hormone surge. *J Neuroendocrinol.* 2009;21:305-311.
37. Gordijn MS, Gemke RJ, van Dalen EC, et al. Hypothalamic-pituitary-adrenal (HPA) axis suppression after treatment with glucocorticoid therapy for childhood acute lymphoblastic leukaemia. *Cochrane Database Syst Rev*. 2012;5:CD008727.
38. Smith A, Doan ML, Roy D, Pinsker JE. Adrenal insufficiency and growth failure secondary to inhaled corticosteroids: a paradoxical complication. *Clin Pediatr.* 2012;51:1194-1196.
39. Lin HY, Muller YA, Hammond GL. Molecular and structural basis of steroid hormone binding and release from corticosteroid-binding globulin. *Mol Cell Endocrinol.* 2010;316:3-12.
40. Hoppé E, Bouvard B, Royer M, et al. Sex hormone-binding globulin in osteoporosis. *Joint Bone Spine*. 2010;77:306-312.
41. Gagliardi L, Ho JT, Torpy DJ. Corticosteroid-binding globulin: the clinical significance of altered levels and heritable mutations. *Mol Cell Endocrinol.* 2010;316:24-34.
42. Spiegel AM, Carter-Su C, Taylor SI, Kulkarni RN. Mechanism of action of hormones that act at the cell surface. In: Melmed S, et al, eds. *Williams Textbook of Endocrinology.* 12th ed. Philadelphia: Elsevier/Saunders; 2011.
43. Gorrigan RJ, Guasti L, King P, et al. Localisation of the melanocortin-2-receptor and its accessory proteins in the developing and adult adrenal gland. *J Mol Endocrinol.* 2011;46:227-232.
44. Chrousos GP. Adrenocorticosteroids and adrenocortical antagonists. In: Katzung BG, ed. *Basic and Clinical Pharmacology.* 12th ed. New York: Lange Medical Books/McGraw Hill; 2012.
45. Strehl C, Spies CM, Buttgereit F. Pharmacodynamics of glucocorticoids. *Clin Exp Rheumatol.* 2011;29(suppl 68): S13-18.
46. Vandevyver S, Dejager L, Tuckermann J, Libert C. New insights into the anti-inflammatory mechanisms of glucocorticoids: an emerging role for glucocorticoid-receptor-mediated transactivation. *Endocrinology*. 2013;154:993-1007.
47. Burris TP, Solt LA, Wang Y, et al. Nuclear receptors and their selective pharmacologic modulators. *Pharmacol Rev.* 2013;65:710-778.
48. Appelman-Dijkstra NM, Claessen KM, Roelfsema F, et al. Long-term effects of recombinant human GH replacement in adults with GH deficiency: a systematic review. *Eur J Endocrinol.* 2013;169:R1-14.
49. Baer JT. Testosterone replacement therapy to improve health in older males. *Nurse Pract*. 2012;37:39-44.
50. Biondi B, Wartofsky L. Combination treatment with T4 and T3: toward personalized replacement therapy in hypothyroidism? *J Clin Endocrinol Metab.* 2012;97:2256-2271.
51. Rozenberg S, Vandromme J, Antoine C. Postmenopausal hormone therapy: risks and benefits. *Nat Rev Endocrinol.* 2013;9:216-227.

CHAPTER 29

Adrenocorticosteroids

The adrenal cortex produces two primary types of adrenal steroids: the glucocorticoids and mineralocorticoids. Small amounts of other steroids, such as the sex hormones (androgens, estrogens, and progestins), are also produced by the adrenal cortex (see Chapter 30). The adrenocorticosteroids have several important physiological and pharmacological functions. The **glucocorticoids** (cortisol, corticosterone) are primarily involved in the control of glucose metabolism and the body's ability to deal with stress. Glucocorticoids have other attributes, such as their ability to decrease inflammation and suppress the immune system. **Mineralocorticoids,** such as aldosterone, are involved in maintaining fluid and electrolyte balance in the body.

Physicians can administer adrenal steroids and their synthetic analogs to mimic the effects of their deficient endogenous counterparts. The quantity administered during this hormonal replacement therapy is roughly equivalent to the normal endogenous production and is often referred to as a **physiological dose.** The use of adrenal steroids in higher doses can capitalize on a particular beneficial effect, such as using glucocorticoids as anti-inflammatory agents. This larger dose is typically referred to as a **pharmacological dose** in order to differentiate them from the amount used to maintain normal endocrine function.

As a physical therapist or occupational therapist, you will encounter many patients who are receiving adrenal steroids for hormone replacement or for various other therapeutic reasons. Therefore, you should understand the pharmacotherapeutic and toxic characteristics of these compounds. This chapter discusses the biosynthesis of the adrenal steroids in an effort to show some of the structural and functional similarities between various steroid groups. The basic physiological and pharmacological properties of the glucocorticoids are then addressed, followed by a description of mineralocorticoid function.

STEROID SYNTHESIS

Adrenal steroids are manufactured by enzymes located in specific cellular organelles, such as the mitochondria and smooth endoplasmic reticulum. As shown in Figure 29-1, there are three primary pathways involved in steroid biosynthesis, each leading to one of the major types of steroid hormone.[1,2] The mineralocorticoid pathway synthesizes aldosterone, the glucocorticoid pathway synthesizes cortisol, and the androgen/estrogen pathway leads to the synthesis of sex hormones. Although all three pathways are present in the adrenal cortex, the mineralocorticoid and glucocorticoid pathways predominate. The appropriate enzymes for sex hormone biosynthesis are also present in the gonads, where hormones are synthesized in the testes (men) or ovaries (women).

Steroid hormones bear a remarkable structural similarity to one another (see Fig. 29-1). The precursor for steroid biosynthesis is cholesterol. Consequently, all of the steroid hormones share the same basic

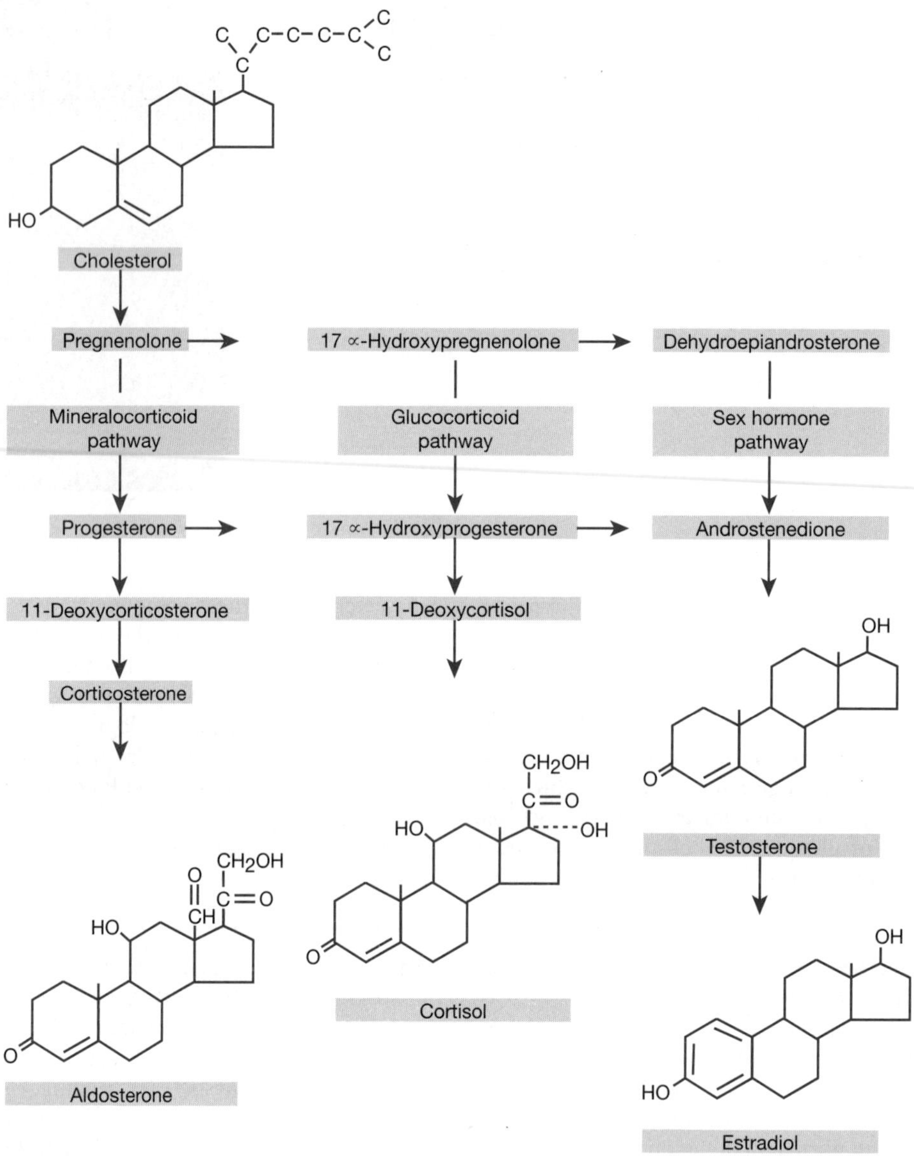

Figure ■ 29-1
Pathways of adrenal steroid biosynthesis. Cholesterol is the precursor for the three steroid hormone pathways. Note the similarity between the structures of the primary mineralocorticoid (aldosterone), the primary glucocorticoid (cortisol), and the sex hormones (testosterone, estradiol).

chemical configuration as their parent compound. This fact has several important physiological and pharmacological implications. First, even relatively minor changes in the side chains of the parent compound create steroids with dramatically different physiological effects. For instance, the addition of only one hydrogen atom in the sex steroid pathway changes testosterone (the primary male hormone) to estradiol (one of the primary female hormones). Second, the structural similarity between different types of steroids helps explain why there is often some crossover in the physiological effects of each major category. You can readily understand how aldosterone has some glucocorticoid-like activity and cortisol has some mineralocorticoid-like effects when you consider the similarity in their organic configuration.

Corticosterone (a glucocorticoid) is even the precursor to aldosterone (a mineralocorticoid).

Pharmacologists are manipulating the chemical side groups of these steroids to develop more effective and less toxic synthetic compounds. An example is the synthetic glucocorticoid dexamethasone, which is 25 times more potent than cortisol in reducing inflammation but has a smaller tendency to cause sodium retention than the naturally occurring glucocorticoid.[1] Also, excessive steroid production can be rectified in certain situations by using drugs that inhibit the enzymes that catalyze specific reactions during steroid biosynthesis.

GLUCOCORTICOIDS

The primary glucocorticoid released in humans is cortisol (also known as *hydrocortisone*). Cortisol synthesis and secretion are under the control of specific hypothalamic and pituitary hormones.[3,4] Corticotropin-releasing hormone (CRH) from the hypothalamus stimulates the release of adrenocorticotropic hormone (ACTH) from the anterior pituitary. ACTH travels in the systemic circulation to reach the adrenal cortex, where it stimulates cortisol synthesis. Cortisol then travels in the bloodstream to various target tissues to exert a number of physiological effects (see "Physiological Effects of Glucocorticoids").

Cortisol also helps control the release of CRH and ACTH from the hypothalamus and pituitary, respectively. As illustrated in Figure 29-2, the relationship between plasma cortisol and CRH and ACTH release is a classic example of a negative feedback control system. Increased plasma cortisol levels serve to inhibit subsequent release of CRH and ACTH, thus helping to maintain homeostasis by moderating glucocorticoid activity.

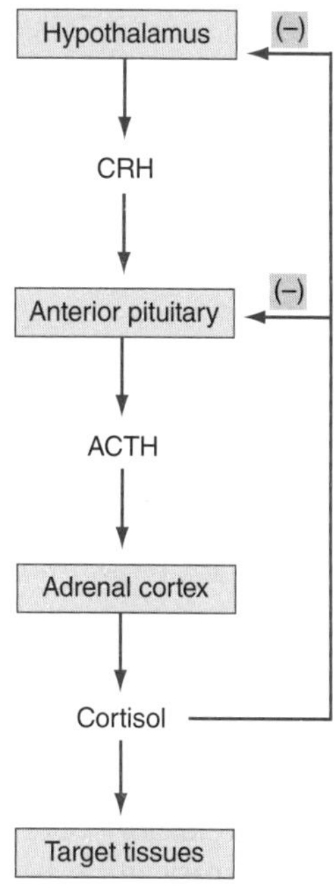

Figure ■ 29-2
Negative feedback control of glucocorticoid synthesis. Cortisol limits its own synthesis by inhibiting the release of corticotropin-releasing hormone (CRH) from the hypothalamus and adrenocorticotropic hormone (ACTH) from the anterior pituitary.

Role of Glucocorticoids in Normal Function

Under normal conditions, cortisol release occurs on a cyclic basis (Fig. 29-3). In an unstressed human, plasma cortisol levels rise slowly throughout the early morning hours and peak at approximately 8:00 a.m.[5] This type of physiological event is often referred to as a *circadian rhythm*, indicating that the cycle is repeated over a 24-hour period. The fact that plasma cortisol levels progressively increase as the individual is preparing to arise suggests that cortisol helps prepare the

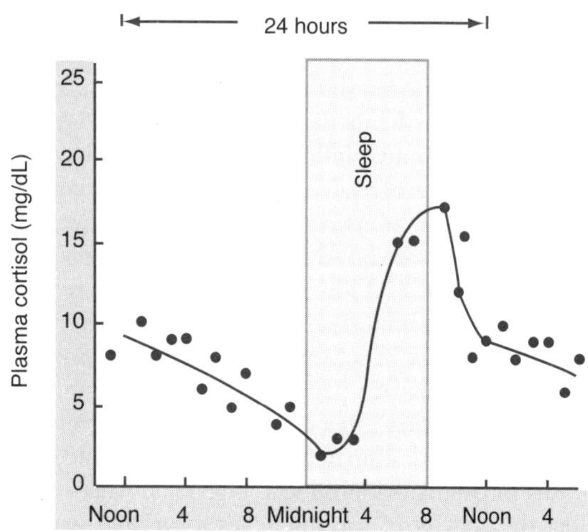

Figure ■ 29-3
Circadian rhythm of cortisol production in humans. Peak plasma cortisol levels normally occur approximately at the time an individual awakens (6:00 to 8:00 a.m.). *(From: Katzung BG. Basic and Clinical Pharmacology. 2nd ed. New York: Lange Medical Publications; 1984:454; after Liddle, 1966. Adapted with permission of the McGraw-Hill Companies.)*

organism for increased activity. Indeed, this belief is supported by the observation that in a rat, plasma glucocorticoid levels peak at around midnight, which corresponds to the time when nocturnal animals become active.

In addition to their normal circadian release, glucocorticoids are also released in response to virtually any stressful stimulus. For instance, trauma, infection, hemorrhage, temperature extremes, food and water deprivation, and any perceived psychological stress can increase cortisol release.[6-10] Various stressful events generate afferent input to the hypothalamus, thus evoking CRH and ACTH release from the hypothalamus and anterior pituitary, respectively.

Mechanism of Action of Glucocorticoids

Glucocorticoids affect various cells in a manner that is characteristic of steroid hormones (see Fig. 28-3). Steroids exert their primary effects by altering protein synthesis in responsive cells through a direct effect on the cell's nucleus. These hormones affect the transcription of specific DNA genes, which results in subsequent changes in RNA synthesis and the translation of RNA into cellular proteins.[11,12]

For example, glucocorticoids exert their primary anti-inflammatory effects by first entering the target cell and binding to a receptor located in the cytosol.[11,13] Binding the glucocorticoid to the receptor creates an activated hormone-receptor complex. This activated complex then travels (translocates) to the nucleus of the cell, where it binds directly to specific DNA gene segments that control inflammation and other cellular processes.[12,14] The activated hormone-receptor complex basically acts as a "transcription factor" because it modulates the transcription of DNA into messenger RNA (mRNA) units.[12,15] The activated hormone-receptor complex can also inhibit other transcription factors (nuclear factor-kappa B, activator protein-1) that normally activate inflammatory genes.[9,16,17] By inhibiting these transcription factors, glucocorticoids turn off proinflammatory genes and ultimately suppress the production of various inflammatory products. Hence, glucocorticoids affect the activity of specific genes associated with the inflammatory response, thereby altering mRNA transcription for products related to inflammation.[12]

Changes in mRNA transcription ultimately lead to a change in protein synthesis in the cell.[1] For example, glucocorticoids exert their anti-inflammatory effects by increasing the transcription of proteins that decrease inflammation while decreasing the transcription of inflammatory cytokines, enzymes, and other inflammatory proteins (see "Anti-Inflammatory Effects").[18-20] Other physiological and therapeutic effects of glucocorticoids are likewise mediated by altering the expression of proteins acting as cellular enzymes, membrane carriers, receptors, structural proteins, and so on. Fundamentally, glucocorticoids induce their primary effects by binding to specific genes that ultimately alter protein synthesis and lead to a change in the physiological status of the cell.

The genomic effect often takes several hours or days to occur because of the time required to alter protein synthesis and to create new proteins that reach meaningful concentrations in the cell. However, glucocorticoids may also have a more immediate effect on cell function that is independent of the hormonal action at the cell's nucleus.[21,22] This more rapid nongenomic effect is probably mediated through a different set of glucocorticoid receptors that are located on the cell membrane.[13,21] By binding to these surface receptors, glucocorticoids could induce rapid changes in cell function by altering membrane permeability, enzyme activity, and other factors.[22] Hence, glucocorticoids may actually affect cell function through at least two mechanisms: a rapid effect that is mediated by surface receptors and a delayed but more prolonged effect that is mediated by intracellular receptors affecting transcription at the genomic level.[21]

Finally, glucocorticoids may exert some of their effects through other mechanisms, including directly affecting the cell membrane (i.e., effects that are not mediated by the surface glucocorticoid receptor) and the activated cytosolic receptor outside of the nucleus (i.e., nongenomic effects of the activated intracellular receptor).[13] Future research will continue to provide insight into how glucocorticoids exert their effects on various tissues based on their interaction with specific receptors and other cellular components.

Physiological Effects of Glucocorticoids

Glucocorticoids exert several diverse physiological effects. The glucocorticoids are anti-inflammatory agents and are capable of immunosuppression. They also have an unusual and important effect on metabolism.

Effects on Glucose, Protein, and Lipid Metabolism

Cortisol and other glucocorticoids increase blood glucose and liver glycogen.[2,23] This fact is something of a metabolic paradox because circulating levels of glucose are increased at the same time that glucose storage is enhanced. This situation is analogous to being able to draw money out of a savings account while increasing the amount of money in the savings account. The withdrawn money is available to spend (i.e., the increased blood glucose is readily available as an energy source) while the savings account accrues additional funds (i.e., liver glycogen is increased).

Glucocorticoids accomplish this paradox by affecting the metabolism of glucose, fat, and protein (Fig. 29-4). Cortisol facilitates the breakdown of muscle into amino acids and lipids into free fatty acids, which can be transported to the liver to form glucose (gluconeogenesis). Glucose that is synthesized in the liver can either be stored as glycogen or released back into the bloodstream to increase blood glucose levels. Cortisol also inhibits the uptake of glucose into muscle and fat cells, thus allowing more glucose to remain available in the bloodstream.

Consequently, one of the primary effects of glucocorticoids is to maintain blood glucose and liver glycogen levels to enable a supply of this energy substrate to be readily available for increased activity. This effect occurs during the daily basal release of cortisol and to an even greater extent when high levels of cortisol are released in response to stress. However, the beneficial effects on glucose titers occur largely at the expense of muscle breakdown. This muscle catabolism is one of the primary problems that occur when patients take glucocorticoids for long periods as a therapeutic agent (see "Adverse Effects of Glucocorticoids").

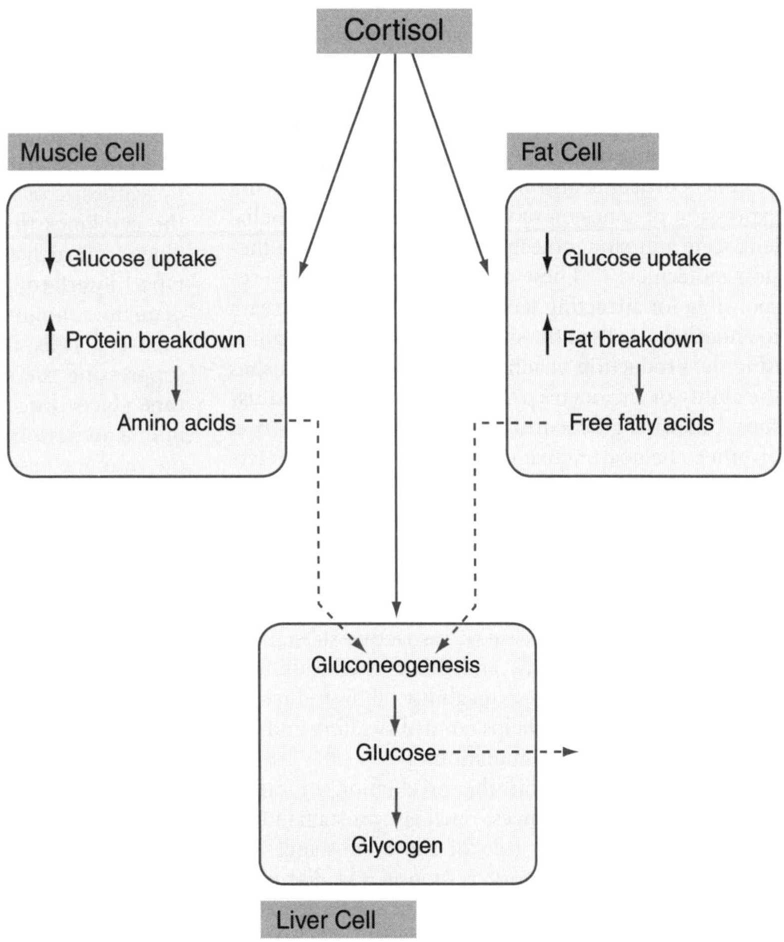

Figure ■ 29-4
Effects of cortisol on muscle, fat, and liver cells. Cortisol causes the breakdown of muscle and fat into amino acids and free fatty acids, which can be used by the liver to produce glucose.

Anti-Inflammatory Effects

Glucocorticoids are effective and potent anti-inflammatory agents. Regardless of the cause of the inflammation, glucocorticoids attenuate the heat, erythema, swelling, and tenderness of the affected area. The exact way that these agents intervene in the inflammatory process is complex and not completely understood. Some of the primary anti-inflammatory mechanisms are addressed here.

As indicated earlier, glucocorticoids inhibit the chemical signals and the concentration of cells that comprise the inflammatory response, thus reducing the ability of these cells to promote inflammation. For example, glucocorticoids act on macrophages, lymphocytes, and endothelial cells to inhibit the expression of inflammatory proteins (cytokines) such as interleukin-1, interleukin-6, tissue necrosis factor alpha, interferon gamma, and similar inflammatory cytokines.[2,19] These cytokines are the primary chemical signal for activating various inflammatory cells such as T lymphocytes, fibroblasts, and natural killer cells.[24] Glucocorticoids also reduce the number of circulating lymphocytes, eosinophils, and other cells that can promote inflammation.[1]

Glucocorticoids also inhibit the transcription and expression of adhesion molecules, such as endothelial leukocyte adhesion molecule-1 and intracellular adhesion molecule-1.[25] These adhesion molecules are responsible for attracting leukocytes in the bloodstream to endothelial cells at the site of inflammation.[26] Inhibiting the production of adhesion molecules diminishes the ability of leukocytes to find and enter inflamed tissues. Likewise, glucocorticoids inhibit the production of other chemoattractive chemicals, such as platelet-activating factor and interleukin-1.[2] By limiting the production of factors attracting leukocytes to the site of inflammation, glucocorticoids inhibit a critical step in the initiation of the inflammatory process.[27]

Glucocorticoids reduce vascular permeability by suppressing the local release of vasoactive substances such as histamine, kinins, and other chemicals that cause increased capillary permeability.[1] This reduction in vascular permeability helps control swelling and erythema at the site of inflammation.

Glucocorticoids inhibit the production of other proinflammatory substances, such as prostaglandins and leukotrienes.[28] The role of these substances in mediating the inflammatory response was discussed in Chapter 15. Glucocorticoids activate specific genes that promote the synthesis of a family of proteins known as *annexins*.[29,30] Annexins (known previously as *lipocortins*) exert many anti-inflammatory effects, including inhibition of the phospholipase A_2 enzyme. This enzyme is responsible for liberating phospholipids from cell membranes so that they can be transformed into prostaglandins and leukotrienes (see Fig. 15-1). By promoting annexin synthesis, glucocorticoids inhibit the formation of the precursor for prostaglandin and leukotriene biosynthesis, thus preventing the production of these proinflammatory substances.

Immunosuppression

Glucocorticoids have long been recognized for their ability to inhibit hypersensitivity reactions, especially delayed or cell-mediated allergic reactions. The exact way in which this immunosuppression occurs is unclear, but many immunosuppressive effects are mediated by the same actions that explain the anti-inflammatory effects of these drugs. As indicated previously, glucocorticoids inhibit the transcription of various factors that signal and direct other cells in the inflammatory and immune responses. Loss of these key signals results in decreased migration of leukocytes and macrophages to the location of a foreign tissue or antigen.[2]

These drugs also suppress the ability of immune cells to synthesize or respond to chemical mediators such as the cytokines that promote autoimmune responses.[19] Chemicals such as interleukin-1, tumor necrosis factor, type 1 interferon, and related substances normally mediate the communication between immune system cells such as T cells, B cells, and other lymphocytes.[31-34] By suppressing the synthesis and effects of these mediators, glucocorticoids interrupt cellular interaction and inhibit activation of key cellular components that cause the immune response. We discuss the effects of glucocorticoids on the immune response and the clinical applications of glucocorticoid-induced immunosuppression further in Chapter 37.

Other Effects of Glucocorticoids

Cortisol and similar glucocorticoids affect a variety of other tissues.[2] These hormones affect renal function by enhancing sodium and water reabsorption and by impairing the ability of the kidneys to excrete a water load. They alter central nervous system (CNS) function, with abnormal glucocorticoid levels (either too high or too low) producing changes in behavior and mood. Glucocorticoids alter the formed elements in the blood by facilitating an increase in erythrocytes, neutrophils, and platelets while decreasing the number of lymphocytes, eosinophils, monocytes, and basophils.

Adequate amounts of glucocorticoids are needed for normal cardiac and skeletal muscle function. Vascular reactivity diminishes and capillary permeability increases if glucocorticoids are not present. Clearly, these hormones are involved in regulating several diverse and important physiological functions.

CLINICAL USES OF GLUCOCORTICOIDS

Glucocorticoids are used in two primary situations: to evaluate and treat endocrine disorders and to help resolve the symptoms of various nonendocrine problems. The primary glucocorticoids used pharmacologically are either chemically identical to the naturally occurring hormones or they are synthetic analogs of cortisol (Table 29-1). The clinical choice of a particular agent depends on the problem being treated and the desired effect in each patient.

Glucocorticoids are available in various preparations corresponding to the specific route of administration. For instance, systemic preparations can be administered either orally or parenterally to treat systemic disorders, such as collagen diseases and adrenocortical insufficiency. In more localized problems, these agents may be applied directly to a specific area using other preparations (e.g., topical, ophthalmic). Glucocorticoids are sometimes injected into a specific tissue or anatomic space to treat a localized problem.

Table 29-1
THERAPEUTIC GLUCOCORTICOIDS: TYPE OF PREPARATION AVAILABLE

Generic Name	Common Trade Name(s)	Systemic	Topical	Inhalation	Ophthalmic	Otic	Nasal
Alclometasone	Aclovate		X				
Amcinonide	Cyclocort		X				
Beclomethasone	Beclovent, Vanceril, others			X			X
Betamethasone	Celestone, Diprolene, others	X	X				
Budesonide	Entocort, Pulmicort Turbuhaler, Rhinocort	X		X			X
Ciclesonide	Omnaris						X
Clobetasol	Dermovate, Temovate, others		X				
Clocortolone	Cloderm		X				
Cortisone	Cortone	X					
Desonide	DesOwen, Tridesilon, Verdeso, others		X				
Desoximetasone	Topicort		X				
Dexamethasone	Decadron, DexPak, others	X	X		X		
Diflorasone	Florone, Psorcon		X				
Difluprednate	Durezol				X		
Flunisolide	AeroBid, Nasalide			X			X
Fluocinolone	Fluolar, Synalar, others		X				
Fluocinonide	Fluocin, Lidex, others		X				
Fluorometholone	FML S.O.P., Fluor- Op, others				X		
Flurandrenolide	Cordran, Drenison		X				
Fluticasone	Cultivate, Flonase, Flovent Diskus		X	X			X
Halcinonide	Halog		X				
Halobetasol	Ultravate		X				

Continued

Table 29-1
THERAPEUTIC GLUCOCORTICOIDS: TYPE OF PREPARATION AVAILABLE—cont'd

Generic Name	Common Trade Name(s)	Systemic	Topical	Inhalation	Ophthalmic	Otic	Nasal
Hydrocortisone	Cortef, Dermacort, many others	X	X				
Loteprednol	Alrex, Lotemax				X		
Methylprednisolone	Medrol, others	X					
Mometasone	Elocon, Nasonex		X				X
Prednicarbate	Dermatop		X				
Prednisolone	Pediapred, Prelone, others	X			X		
Prednisone	Sterapred	X					
Rimexolone	Vexol				X		
Triamcinolone	Azmacort, Aristocort, Nasacort, others	X	X	X			X

Glucocorticoid Use in Endocrine Disorders

Glucocorticoids are administered systemically to help restore normal function in conditions of adrenal cortical hypofunction. Glucocorticoid replacement is instituted in both primary and secondary adrenal insufficiency. In primary insufficiency (Addison disease), glucocorticoid production is deficient because of the destruction of the adrenal cortex. In secondary insufficiency, adrenal cortex function is diminished because of other factors, such as a lack of adequate ACTH release from the anterior pituitary. Replacement therapy can also be initiated after the removal of the adrenals or pituitary gland because of disease and tumors. For instance, adrenalectomy or destruction of the pituitary to resolve adrenal cortical hypersecretion (Cushing syndrome) is typically followed by long-term glucocorticoid administration. Replacement therapy is needed to maintain optimum health whenever normal physiological function of the adrenal cortex is disrupted.

Glucocorticoids may be given for diagnostic purposes to evaluate hormonal disorders. Exogenous glucocorticoids (especially the synthetic hormones such as dexamethasone) are potent inhibitors of ACTH secretion from the anterior pituitary. By suppressing the secretion of ACTH, glucocorticoids can help determine whether an endocrine imbalance is influenced by ACTH secretion. Favorable changes in the endocrine profile during ACTH suppression indicate that ACTH and ACTH-related hormones have a role in mediating the abnormality.

Glucocorticoid Use in Nonendocrine Conditions

Glucocorticoids are used primarily for their anti-inflammatory and immunosuppressive effects to treat a long and diverse list of nonendocrine conditions. Some of the approved indications for glucocorticoid administration are listed in Table 29-2. Of particular interest to rehabilitation specialists is the use of these agents in treating collagen diseases and rheumatic disorders, including rheumatoid arthritis. These drugs are typically administered systemically via oral or parenteral routes in the long-term management of these conditions. Glucocorticoids can also be administered systemically to help manage inflammation in certain musculoskeletal injuries, including various types of tenosynovitis and myositis.

On the other hand, it may be advantageous to inject glucocorticoids directly into a specific tissue to help localize the effects of these drugs and minimize systemic side effects. Physicians can, for example, treat certain types of back and neck pain by injecting glucocorticoids into the epidural space.[35,36] Local glucocorticoid injections have been used to treat problems such as carpal tunnel syndrome.[37] Likewise, glucocorticoids may be injected directly into a joint (knee, shoulder, etc.) to treat severe acute inflammation that is isolated to a particular joint.[38-40] The repeated intra-articular administration of glucocorticoids is not advisable, however, because of their catabolic effect on supporting tissues (see "Adverse Effects of Glucocorticoids"). In addition, the repeated injection of glucocorticoids in and around tendons is not recommended because

Table 29-2
NONENDOCRINE DISORDERS TREATED WITH GLUCOCORTICOIDS

General Indication	Examples of Specific Disorders	Principal Desired Effect(s) of Glucocorticoids
Allergic disorders	Anaphylactic reactions, drug-induced allergic reactions, severe hay fever, serum sickness	Decreased inflammation
Collagen disorders	Acute rheumatic carditis, dermatomyositis, systemic lupus erythematosus	Immunosuppression
Dermatologic disorders	Alopecia areata, dermatitis (various forms), keloids, lichens, mycosis fungoides, pemphigus, psoriasis	Decreased inflammation
Gastrointestinal disorders	Crohn disease, ulcerative colitis	Decreased inflammation
Hematologic disorders	Autoimmune hemolytic anemia, congenital hypoplastic anemia, erythroblastopenia, thrombocytopenia	Immunosuppression
Nonrheumatic inflammation	Bursitis, tenosynovitis	Decreased inflammation
Neoplastic disease	Leukemias, lymphomas, nasal polyps, cystic tumors	Antilymphocytic effects
Neurological disease	Tuberculous meningitis, multiple sclerosis, myasthenia gravis	Decreased inflammation and immunosuppression
Neurotrauma	Brain surgery, closed head injury, certain brain tumors, spinal cord injury	Decreased edema;* inhibit free radical–induced neuronal damage
Ophthalmic disorders	Chorioretinitis, conjunctivitis, herpes zoster ophthalmicus, iridocyclitis, keratitis, optic neuritis	Decreased inflammation
Organ transplant	Transplantation of liver, kidney, heart, and so forth	Immunosuppression
Renal diseases	Nephrotic syndrome, membranous glomerulonephritis	Decreased inflammation
Respiratory disorders	Bronchial asthma, berylliosis, aspiration pneumonitis, symptomatic sarcoidosis, pulmonary tuberculosis	Decreased inflammation
Rheumatic disorders	Ankylosing spondylitis, psoriatic arthritis, rheumatoid arthritis, gouty arthritis, osteoarthritis	Decreased inflammation and immunosuppression

**Efficacy of glucocorticoid use in decreasing cerebral edema has not been conclusively proved.*

they can cause breakdown and rupture of these structures.[41,42] A general rule of thumb is to limit the number of glucocorticoid injections into a specific joint to four or fewer per year.[43]

As indicated in Table 29-2, glucocorticoids are generally used to control inflammation or suppress the immune system for relatively short periods of time, regardless of the underlying pathology. They can be extremely helpful and even lifesaving in the short-term control of severe inflammation and various allergic responses. The very fact that these drugs are successful in such a wide range of disorders illustrates that glucocorticoids do not cure the underlying problem. In a sense, they only treat a symptom of the original disease—that is, inflammation. This fact is important because the patient may appear to be improving, with decreased symptoms of inflammation, while the disease continues to worsen. Also, medical practitioners often administer glucocorticoids in fairly high dosages to capitalize on their anti-inflammatory and immunosuppressive effects. These high dosages may create serious adverse effects when given for prolonged periods.

ADVERSE EFFECTS OF GLUCOCORTICOIDS

The effectiveness and extensive clinical use of natural and synthetic glucocorticoids must be tempered by the serious side effects these agents produce. Some of the more common problems associated with glucocorticoid use are described below.

Adrenocortical Suppression

Adrenocortical suppression occurs because of the negative feedback effect of the administered glucocorticoids on the hypothalamic–anterior pituitary system and the adrenal glands.[44,45] Basically, the patient's normal production of glucocorticoids is shut down by the exogenous hormones. The magnitude and duration of this suppression are related to the dosage, route of administration, and duration of glucocorticoid therapy.[46,47] Some degree of adrenocortical suppression can even occur after a single large dose.[48] This suppression will become more pronounced as systemic administration is continued for longer periods. Also, topical glucocorticoid administration over an extensive area of the body (especially in infants) may provide enough systemic absorption to suppress adrenocortical function.[49]

Adrenocortical suppression can be a serious problem when glucocorticoid therapy is terminated. Patients who have experienced complete suppression will not be able to immediately resume production of glucocorticoids. Because abrupt withdrawal can be life-threatening, glucocorticoids must be withdrawn slowly by tapering the dose.[44] Likewise, patients may need to take small (physiological) doses of glucocorticoids temporarily to prevent an adrenal crisis while the adrenal hypothalamic-pituitary-adrenal system recovers from the suppression caused by prolonged or high doses of glucocorticoids.[46,49]

Drug-Induced Cushing Syndrome

In drug-induced Cushing syndrome, patients begin to exhibit many of the symptoms associated with the adrenocortical hypersecretion typical of naturally occurring Cushing syndrome.[44,49] These patients commonly exhibit symptoms of roundness and puffiness in the face, fat deposition and obesity in the trunk region, muscle wasting in the extremities, hypertension, osteoporosis, increased body hair (*hirsutism*), and glucose intolerance. These changes are all caused by the metabolic effects of the glucocorticoids. The adverse effects can be alleviated somewhat by reducing the glucocorticoid dosage. Some of the Cushing syndrome effects must often be tolerated, however, to allow the glucocorticoids to maintain a therapeutic effect (decreased inflammation or immunosuppression).

Breakdown of Supporting Tissues

Glucocorticoids exert a general catabolic effect not only on muscle (as described previously) but also on other tissues. Bone, ligaments, tendons, and skin are also subject to a wasting effect from prolonged glucocorticoid use. The exact mechanisms are complex and not well understood. Glucocorticoids appear to weaken these supporting tissues by inhibiting the genes responsible for production of collagen and other tissue components and by increasing the expression of substances that promote breakdown of bone, muscle, and so forth.[50,51] Glucocorticoids, for example, probably interfere with muscle protein synthesis by altering the muscle's ability to retain and use amino acids.[52] Thus, these drugs cause atrophy of skeletal muscle by increasing the rate of protein breakdown and decreasing the rate of protein synthesis.[50] In severe cases, glucocorticoids can induce a steroid myopathy that is characterized by proximal muscle weakness, which can affect ambulation and functional ability.[52,53] This type of myopathy is typically resolved by discontinuing the glucocorticoid, but symptoms may persist long after the drug has been withdrawn.[54]

Glucocorticoids also have negative effects on bone; loss of bone strength is considered one of the most common side effects of prolonged, systemic glucocorticoid administration.[55,56] Again, the exact reasons for these effects are unclear, but glucocorticoids seem to shift the balance of bone metabolism toward increased breakdown by stimulating osteoclast-induced bone resorption while inhibiting osteoblast-induced bone formation.[57] Glucocorticoids probably exert these effects on bone cells by suppressing the production of substances that stimulate bone formation (e.g., insulin-like growth factor-I) while increasing the expression of substances that promote bone loss (e.g., colony-stimulating factor-1, nuclear factor k-B ligand).[58,59] The result is loss of bone mineral content that can lead to osteoporosis and osteonecrosis, resulting in fractures in the hips, vertebral bodies, and elsewhere throughout the skeleton.[59]

The magnitude of the wasting effect caused by systemic glucocorticoids is dependent on many factors, including the patient's overall health and the duration and dosage of drug therapy. In addition, bone and muscle loss can also occur because of certain inflammatory and autoimmune diseases. For example, conditions such as rheumatoid arthritis and systemic lupus erythematosis may directly cause catabolic effects, or at least increase the likelihood of bone and muscle wasting due to inactivity caused by pain and fatigue.[24,60] Hence, there is greater concern for loss of muscle mass and bone mineral content when glucocorticoids are used to treat these conditions because of the combined catabolic effects of glucocorticoids and the underlying disease.

The potential for tissue breakdown must always be considered during the rehabilitation of patients taking these drugs, and therapists must be especially careful to avoid overstressing tissues that are weakened by the prolonged use of systemic glucocorticoids. Bone loss and risk of osteoporosis should be evaluated periodically in patients receiving long-term systemic glucocorticoids.[59] Patients with evidence of excessive bone loss can be treated with drugs such as the bisphosphonates (etidronate, pamidronate).[61] Estrogen replacement may also be helpful in minimizing bone loss in women receiving glucocorticoids, although the beneficial effects on bone mineral content must be balanced against the risks of estrogen replacement (e.g., cancer, cardiovascular disease; see Chapter 30).[62] Other interventions such as calcium supplements, vitamin D supplements, teriparatide, and calcitonin may help prevent bone loss in people receiving long-term glucocorticoid therapy.[61,63] The ability of various drugs to stabilize bone and prevent osteoporosis is addressed in Chapter 31.

Other Adverse Effects

Several other problems can occur during prolonged glucocorticoid use. Peptic ulcer may develop because of the breakdown of supporting proteins in the stomach wall or direct mucosal irritation by the drugs. An increased susceptibility to infection often occurs because of the immunosuppressive effect of glucocorticoids. These drugs may retard growth in children, primarily through an inhibitory effect on the growth plates in developing bone.[64] Glucocorticoids may also cause glaucoma by impairing the normal drainage of aqueous fluid from the eye, and cataract formation is associated with prolonged use.[65] Mood changes and even psychoses have been reported, but the reasons for these occurrences are not clear.[66,67] Glucocorticoids with some mineralocorticoid-like activity may cause hypertension because of sodium and water retention. Some of the newer synthetic drugs have fewer mineralocorticoid effects, however, and hypertension occurs less frequently with these. Finally, glucocorticoids alter glucose metabolism, and people with diabetes mellitus will have an increased risk of hyperglycemia, insulin resistance, and decreased control of blood glucose levels.[23,44]

DRUGS THAT INHIBIT ADRENOCORTICAL HORMONE BIOSYNTHESIS

Occasionally, the production of adrenal steroids must be inhibited because of adrenocortical hyperactivity. Several agents are available that block specific enzymes in the glucocorticoid biosynthetic pathway. Aminoglutethimide (Cytadren) inhibits the first step in adrenal corticoid synthesis by blocking the conversion of cholesterol to subsequent hormone precursors (see Fig. 29-1). Metyrapone (Metopirone) inhibits the hydroxylation reaction of several intermediate compounds in the adrenal corticoid pathway. Ketoconazole (Nizoral) is an antifungal drug that is used primarily to treat candidiasis and other local and systemic fungal infections (see Chapter 35). This agent also inhibits several enzymes responsible for steroid biosynthesis, and patients with Cushing disease may use high doses to suppress adrenocortical hormone production. Finally, the antineoplastic drug mitotane (Lysodren)—used for treating adrenal tumors (see Chapter 36)—can also reduce hyperactivity of the adrenal gland in endocrine disorders. Mitotane directly suppresses the adrenal gland, although the exact mechanism of this suppression is unclear.

These drugs may also temporarily resolve adrenal hypersecretion caused by increased pituitary ACTH release (Cushing syndrome of pituitary origin). However, surgical removal of the pituitary, or destruction of the pituitary through irradiation, is usually a more effective long-term solution to pituitary ACTH hypersecretion.[68] Practitioners also use metyrapone to test hypothalamic–anterior pituitary function, or more specifically, to evaluate the ability of the anterior pituitary to release ACTH. When this drug attenuates the production of adrenal glucocorticoids, the anterior pituitary should respond by secreting ACTH into the bloodstream. If ACTH response is too low, pituitary hypofunction is indicated. If ACTH response is exaggerated, pituitary hyperfunction or Cushing syndrome of pituitary origin is indicated.

MINERALOCORTICOIDS

The adrenal cortex also produces the steroid hormones known as *mineralocorticoids*. The principal mineralocorticoid in humans is aldosterone. Aldosterone is primarily involved in maintaining fluid and electrolyte balance in the body. This hormone works on the kidneys to increase sodium and water reabsorption and potassium excretion.

Regulation of Mineralocorticoid Secretion

Aldosterone release is regulated by several factors that are related to the fluid and electrolyte status in the body.[69] A primary stimulus for aldosterone release is increased levels of angiotensin II.[70] Angiotensin II is part of the renin-angiotensin system, which is concerned with maintaining blood pressure (see Chapter 21). Basically, a sudden fall in blood pressure initiates a chain of events that increases circulating levels of angiotensin II. Angiotensin II helps maintain blood pressure by vasoconstricting peripheral vessels. It (and probably also its metabolic by-product angiotensin III) helps exert a more prolonged antihypotensive effect by stimulating aldosterone secretion from the adrenal cortex. Aldosterone can then facilitate sodium and water retention, thus maintaining adequate plasma volume.

In addition to the angiotensin II effects, aldosterone secretion is regulated by increased plasma potassium levels.[69,70] Presumably, elevated plasma potassium serves as a stimulus to increase aldosterone release, thus causing increased potassium excretion and a return to normal plasma levels. Finally, there is evidence that ACTH may also play a role in aldosterone release. Although ACTH is primarily involved in controlling glucocorticoid secretion, this hormone may also stimulate mineralocorticoid release to some extent.[70]

Mechanism of Action and Physiological Effects of Mineralocorticoids

Aldosterone exerts its effects on the kidneys by binding to specific receptors in epithelial cells that line the distal tubule of the nephron.[71,72] These receptors have a high affinity for mineralocorticoid hormones. They also have a moderate affinity for many of the natural glucocorticoid hormones (e.g., cortisol) and a low affinity for the newer synthetic glucocorticoids, such as dexamethasone. This fact accounts for the finding that certain glucocorticoids exert some mineralocorticoid-like effects, whereas others have relatively minor effects on electrolyte and fluid balance.[1]

Mineralocorticoids are believed to increase sodium reabsorption by affecting sodium channels and sodium pumps on the epithelial cells lining the renal tubules.[71,73] Mineralocorticoids' ability to increase the expression of sodium channels is illustrated in Figure 29-5. These hormones enter the tubular epithelial cell, bind to receptors in the cell, and create an activated hormone-receptor complex.[74] This complex then travels to the nucleus to initiate transcription of mRNA units, which are translated into specific membrane-related proteins.[1] The proteins either create or help open sodium pores on the cell membrane, thus allowing sodium to leave the tubule and enter the epithelial cell by passive diffusion.[74] Sodium is then actively transported out of the cell and reabsorbed into the bloodstream. Water reabsorption is increased as water follows the sodium movement back into the bloodstream. As sodium is reabsorbed, potassium is secreted by a sodium-potassium exchange, thus increasing potassium excretion.

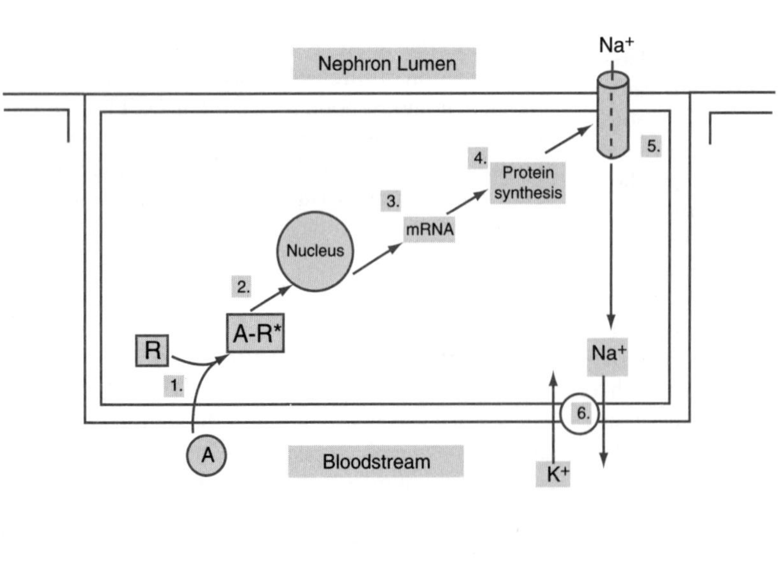

Figure 29-5
Effect of aldosterone on renal tubule cells. (*1*) Aldosterone (A) enters the cell and binds to a cytosolic receptor (R), creating an activated hormone-receptor complex (A–R). (*2*) A–R complex travels to the cell's nucleus, where it induces mRNA synthesis. (*3*) mRNA units undergo translation in the cytosol. (*4*) Specific proteins are synthesized that increase membrane permeability to sodium (Na^+). (*5*) Na^+ leaves the nephron lumen and enters the cell down an electrochemical gradient. (*6*) Na^+ is actively reabsorbed into the body, and potassium (K^+) is actively secreted from the bloodstream by the cellular Na^+-K^+ pump.

In addition to their effects on the synthesis of membrane sodium channels, mineralocorticoids also have a more rapid and immediate effect on sodium reabsorption.[71,75] In a situation analogous to glucocorticoids, certain effects may be mediated because mineralocorticoids bind to a different set of receptors located on the cell membrane. These membrane receptors could produce more rapid and direct effects on sodium and water reabsorption that do not involve nuclear activation and changes in mRNA transcription.[76] At this point, however, efforts to identify a specific mineralocorticoid receptor on the cell membrane remain questionable, although certain rapid effects of aldosterone may be mediated by a G protein–coupled receptor (GPR30) located on the membrane of vascular tissues and other cells.[77,78] Regardless of the exact mechanisms, the effects of mineralocorticoids (like the glucocorticoids discussed earlier) seem to occur in two phases: a rapid phase that is mediated by non-nuclear mechanisms and a delayed but prolonged phase that is mediated by intracellular receptors binding to the cell's nucleus and increasing the transcription of specific proteins.[75] The two phases of mineralocorticoid action both play a role in the physiological action of these hormones, and future research should help to define how these actions can be affected by various drugs and diseases.

In addition to its normal role in controlling fluid and electrolyte balance, abnormal aldosterone production can have detrimental effects on the cardiovascular system. It has long been understood that increased aldosterone production can promote renal sodium and water retention, thus leading to hypertension and heart failure.[79] It is now recognized, however, that mineralocorticoid receptors exist in many other tissues throughout the body and that increased aldosterone production from the adrenal cortex can cause other systemic abnormalities by affecting these extrarenal receptors.[80] Likewise, there is some evidence that aldosterone can be produced locally within the brain, heart, and other tissues, although the physiological significance to local aldosterone production remains unclear.[81]

Regardless of whether aldosterone is produced locally or reaches specific tissues through the systemic circulation, excessive aldosterone influence can certainly affect other tissues that contain mineralocorticoid receptors. For example, mineralocorticoid receptors exist in the brain, and these receptors are normally involved in the central control of salt and water balance. Abnormal activation of these receptors may lead to systemic changes associated with hypertension. Furthermore, there is considerable evidence that excess aldosterone production is associated with metabolic syndrome, a condition characterized by increased hypertension, insulin resistance, hyperlipidemia, and increased abdominal fat storage (see Chapter 21).[82,83] These widespread cardiovascular and metabolic changes indicate that aldosterone affects many tissues throughout the body.

On a cellular level, excess or prolonged aldosterone production can cause inflammation, hypertrophy, and fibrosis of cardiac, vascular, and other tissues, thus leading to detrimental changes in these tissues that can lead to cardiovascular problems and perhaps other diseases.[77,84] Hence, the aldosterone antagonist drugs (see below) may help control the detrimental effects of aldosterone, and they are gaining acceptance in the treatment of certain diseases such as hypertension, heart failure, and metabolic syndrome.[82]

Therapeutic Use of Mineralocorticoid Drugs

Patients frequently take drugs with mineralocorticoid-like activity (e.g., aldosterone agonists) as replacement therapy whenever their natural production of mineralocorticoids is impaired. Mineralocorticoid and glucocorticoid replacement is usually required in patients with chronic adrenocortical insufficiency (Addison disease), following adrenalectomy, and in other forms of adrenal cortex hypofunction.

Fludrocortisone (Florinef) is the primary aldosterone-like agent for replacement therapy. This compound is chemically classified as a glucocorticoid, but it has high levels of mineralocorticoid activity and is used exclusively as a mineralocorticoid. Fludrocortisone is administered orally.

Adverse Effects of Mineralocorticoid Agonists

The primary problem associated with mineralocorticoid agonists is hypertension. Because these drugs increase sodium and water retention, blood pressure may increase if the dosage is too high. Other adverse effects may include peripheral edema, weight gain, and hypokalemia. These problems are also caused by the effects of these drugs on electrolyte and fluid balance and are usually resolved by adjusting the dosage.

Mineralocorticoid Antagonists

The mineralocorticoid antagonists used clinically include spironolactone (Aldactone) and eplerenone (Inspra). These drugs are competitive antagonists of the aldosterone receptor—that is, they bind to the receptor but do not activate it. When bound to the receptor, these drugs block the effects of endogenous mineralocorticoids (aldosterone) by preventing the aldosterone from binding to renal cells and other tissues. Consequently, spironolactone and eplerenone antagonize the normal physiological effects of aldosterone, resulting in increased sodium and water excretion and decreased potassium excretion.

Physicians administer spironolactone and eplerenone primarily as diuretics when treating hypertension and heart failure. These drugs are classified as potassium-sparing diuretics because they help increase sodium and water excretion without increasing the excretion of potassium (see Chapter 21). Spironolactone is also used to help diagnose hyperaldosteronism. The patients take the drug for several days to antagonize the effects of excessive aldosterone production. When the drug is discontinued, serum potassium levels will decrease sharply if hyperaldosteronism is present—that is, plasma potassium levels will fall when aldosterone is again permitted to increase potassium excretion.

As indicated above, mineralocorticoid antagonists, such as spironolactone and eplerenone, can help decrease the detrimental effects of aldosterone on the kidneys, heart, vasculature, and other tissues.[85] By blocking aldosterone receptors in cardiac and vascular cells, these drugs prevent adverse cellular changes (fibrosis, hypertrophy) that can contribute to hypertension, heart failure, and other cardiovascular diseases.[77,86] Likewise, these drugs may prevent abnormal systemic changes associated with metabolic syndrome.[82] Clinical studies continue to clarify how these drugs can be best used as part of the pharmacological regimen for patients with cardiovascular dysfunction.[85,87]

Mineralocorticoid antagonists may cause an increase in plasma potassium levels (hyperkalemia), which could be life-threatening if prolonged or severe.[88] Spironolactone can also interfere with the function of the endogenous sex hormones, thereby producing side effects such as increased body hair, deepening of the voice, decreased libido, menstrual irregularities, and breast enlargement in men. However, it appears that eplerenone has a lower incidence of these sexual side effects, and it may preferentially suppress mineralocorticoid function without also affecting the sex hormones.[89] Finally, mineralocorticoid antagonists can cause gastrointestinal disturbances (diarrhea, stomach pain, gastric ulcers), and spironolactone can also cause CNS effects (e.g., drowsiness, lethargy, confusion, headache).

Special Concerns for Rehabilitation Patients

Adrenal steroids play an important role in the pharmacological management of many patients seen in rehabilitation. Physicians often treat systemic conditions such as rheumatoid arthritis, ankylosing spondylitis, and lupus erythematosus with glucocorticoid drugs (see Table 29-2). More localized musculoskeletal conditions, such as acute bursitis and tenosynovitis, may also be treated for short periods with glucocorticoids. Because these conditions are often being treated simultaneously in a rehabilitation setting, therapists must be especially cognizant of the effects and implications of glucocorticoids.

The primary aspect of glucocorticoid administration that concerns therapists is the catabolic effect of these hormones on supporting tissues. As discussed previously, glucocorticoids cause a general breakdown in muscle, bone, skin, and other collagenous structures. The glucocorticoid-induced catabolism of these tissues can be even greater than expected in the presence of other contributing factors such as inactivity, poor nutrition, and the effects of aging. For instance, a certain amount of osteoporosis would be expected in an elderly, sedentary woman with rheumatoid arthritis. The use of glucocorticoids, however, may greatly accelerate

Special Concerns for Rehabilitation Patients (Continued)

the bone dissolution in such a patient, even when the drugs are used for relatively limited periods.[55]

Therapists can help attenuate some of the catabolic effects of these drugs. Strengthening activities help maintain muscle mass and prevent severe wasting of the musculotendinous unit.[90-92] Various strengthening and weight-bearing activities may also reduce bone loss to some extent. In general, any activity that promotes mobility and ambulation will be beneficial during and after glucocorticoid therapy. Therapists must use caution, however, to avoid injuring structures that are weakened by glucocorticoid use. The load placed on the musculoskeletal system must be sufficient to evoke a therapeutic response but not so excessive that musculoskeletal structures are damaged. The difference between therapeutic stress and harmful stress may be rather small in some patients taking glucocorticoids; therapists must use sound clinical judgment when developing and implementing exercise routines for these patients. Because glucocorticoids also cause thinning and wasting of skin, therapists should make extra efforts to prevent skin breakdown in patients on prolonged glucocorticoid therapy.

Other aspects of prolonged adrenocorticoid administration also concern physical therapists and occupational therapists. Therapists should be aware of the sodium- and water-retaining properties of both glucocorticoids and mineralocorticoids. When used in acute situations or in long-term replacement therapy, both groups of adrenal steroids may cause hypertension. Therapists should routinely monitor blood pressure in patients taking either type of agent. Because of their immunosuppressive effects, glucocorticoids increase patients' susceptibility to infection. Therapists must be especially cautious about exposing these patients to any possible sources of infection. Finally, therapists should be alert for any other signs of toxicity to adrenal steroids, such as mood changes or psychoses. Therapists may recognize the early stages of such toxic reactions and prevent serious consequences by alerting medical staff.

CASE STUDY

ADRENOCORTICOSTEROIDS

Brief History. E.M. is a 58-year-old woman with a history of rheumatoid arthritis. She has involvement of many joints in her body, but her knees are especially affected by this disease. Her symptoms of pain, swelling, and inflammation are fairly well controlled by NSAIDs, but she does experience periods of exacerbation and remission. During periods of exacerbation, she receives physical therapy as an outpatient at a private practice. The therapy typically consists of heat, ultrasound, range of motion, and strengthening activities to both knees. During a recent exacerbation, her symptoms were more severe than usual, and she began to develop flexion contractures in both knees. The therapist suggested that she consult her physician. Upon noting the severe inflammation, the physician elected to inject both knees with a glucocorticoid agent. Methylprednisolone (Depo-Medrol) was injected into the knee joints, with each joint receiving 40 mg of the drug. The

Continued on following page

CASE STUDY (Continued)

patient was advised to continue physical therapy on a daily basis.

Problem/Influence of Medication. Glucocorticoid administration produced a dramatic decrease in the swelling and inflammation in both knees. The therapist considered initiating aggressive stretching activities to resolve the knee flexion contractures and restore normal range of motion.

1. *What possible negative effects can glucocorticoids have on joint tissues?*
2. *How long can the effects of a single injection affect E.M.'s joints?*
3. *How can the therapist increase joint movement without causing injury to the joint?*

See Appendix C, "Answers to Case Study Questions."

SUMMARY

The two principal groups of adrenal steroids are the glucocorticoids and mineralocorticoids. These hormones are synthesized from cholesterol within cells of the adrenal cortex. The primary glucocorticoid produced in humans is cortisol (hydrocortisone), and the primary mineralocorticoid is aldosterone. Glucocorticoids exert several effects, such as regulation of glucose metabolism, attenuation of the inflammatory response, and suppression of the immune system. Mineralocorticoids are involved primarily in the control of fluid and electrolyte balance.

Pharmacologically, natural and synthetic adrenal steroids are often used as replacement therapy to resolve a deficiency in adrenal cortex function. Patients also take glucocorticoids primarily for their anti-inflammatory and immunosuppressive effects on a diverse group of clinical problems. These agents can be extremely beneficial in controlling the symptoms of various rheumatic and allergic disorders. Prolonged glucocorticoid use, however, is limited by a number of serious effects, such as adrenocortical suppression and breakdown of muscle, bone, and other tissues. Physical therapists and occupational therapists should be especially aware of the potential side effects of glucocorticoids.

REFERENCES

1. Chrousos GP. Adrenocorticosteroids and adrenocortical antagonists. In: Katzung BG et al, eds. *Basic and Clinical Pharmacology.* 12th ed. New York: Lange Medical Books/McGraw-Hill; 2012.
2. Schimmer BP, Parker KL. ACTH, adrenal steroids, and pharmacology of the adrenal cortex. In: Brunton LL, et al, eds. *The Pharmacological Basis of Therapeutics* 12th ed. New York: McGraw-Hill; 2011.
3. Gallagher JP, Orozco-Cabal LF, Liu J, Shinnick-Gallagher P. Synaptic physiology of central CRH system. *Eur J Pharmacol.* 2008;583:215-225.
4. Stevens A, White A. ACTH: cellular peptide hormone synthesis and secretory pathways. *Results Probl Cell Differ.* 2010;50:63-84.
5. Yip CE, Stewart SA, Imran F, Clarke DB, et al. The role of morning basal serum cortisol in assessment of hypothalamic pituitary-adrenal axis. *Clin Invest Med.* 2013;36:E216-222.
6. Cutolo M, Buttgereit F, Straub RH. Regulation of glucocorticoids by the central nervous system. *Clin Exp Rheumatol.* 2011;29(suppl 68):S19-22.
7. Guarnieri DJ, Brayton CE, Richards SM, et al. Gene profiling reveals a role for stress hormones in the molecular and behavioral response to food restriction. *Biol Psychiatry.* 2012;71:358-365.
8. Herman JP, McKlveen JM, Solomon MB, et al. Neural regulation of the stress response: glucocorticoid feedback mechanisms. *Braz J Med Biol Res.* 2012;45:292-298.
9. Marik PE. Glucocorticoids in sepsis: dissecting facts from fiction. *Crit Care.* 2011;15:158.
10. Poll EM, Gilsbach JM, Hans FJ, Kreitschmann-Andermahr I. Blunted serum and enhanced salivary free cortisol concentrations in the chronic phase after aneurysmal subarachnoid haemorrhage—is stress the culprit? *Stress.* 2013;16:153-162.
11. Barrett EJ. Organization of endocrine control. In: Boron WF, Boulpaep EL, eds. *Medical Physiology: A Cellular and Molecular Approach.* 2nd ed. New York: Elsevier/Saunders; 2012.

12. Vandevyver S, Dejager L, Tuckermann J, Libert C. New insights into the anti-inflammatory mechanisms of glucocorticoids: an emerging role for glucocorticoid-receptor-mediated transactivation. *Endocrinology*. 2013;154:993-1007.
13. Strehl C, Spies CM, Buttgereit F. Pharmacodynamics of glucocorticoids. *Clin Exp Rheumatol*. 2011;29(suppl 68):S13-18.
14. Heitzer MD, Wolf IM, Sanchez ER, et al. Glucocorticoid receptor physiology. *Rev Endocr Metab Disord*. 2007;8:321-330.
15. Carlberg C, Seuter S. Dynamics of nuclear receptor target gene regulation. *Chromosoma*. 2010;119:479-484.
16. Goldminz AM, Au SC, Kim N, et al. NF-κB: an essential transcription factor in psoriasis. *J Dermatol Sci*. 2013;69:89-94.
17. Newton R, Holden NS. Separating transrepression and transactivation: a distressing divorce for the glucocorticoid receptor? *Mol Pharmacol*. 2007;72:799-809.
18. Ayroldi E, Cannarile L, Migliorati G, et al. Mechanisms of the anti-inflammatory effects of glucocorticoids: genomic and nongenomic interference with MAPK signaling pathways. *FASEB J*. 2012;26:4805-4820.
19. Flammer JR, Rogatsky I. Minireview: glucocorticoids in autoimmunity: unexpected targets and mechanisms. *Mol Endocrinol*. 2011;25:1075-1086.
20. Rogatsky I, Ivashkiv LB. Glucocorticoid modulation of cytokine signaling. *Tissue Antigens*. 2006;68:1-12.
21. Groeneweg FL, Karst H, de Kloet ER, Joëls M. Mineralocorticoid and glucocorticoid receptors at the neuronal membrane, regulators of nongenomic corticosteroid signalling. *Mol Cell Endocrinol*. 2012;350:299-309.
22. Levin ER. Rapid signaling by steroid receptors. *Am J Physiol Regul Integr Comp Physiol*. 2008;295:R1425-1430.
23. Kwon S, Hermayer KL. Glucocorticoid-induced hyperglycemia. *Am J Med Sci*. 2013;345:274-277.
24. Choy E. Understanding the dynamics: pathways involved in the pathogenesis of rheumatoid arthritis. *Rheumatology*. 2012; 51(suppl 5):v3-11.
25. Bouazzaoui A, Spacenko E, Mueller G, et al. Steroid treatment alters adhesion molecule and chemokine expression in experimental acute graft-vs.-host disease of the intestinal tract. *Exp Hematol*. 2011;39:238-249.
26. Fernandez-Borja M, van Buul JD, Hordijk PL. The regulation of leucocyte transendothelial migration by endothelial signalling events. *Cardiovasc Res*. 2010;86:202-210.
27. Wright HL, Moots RJ, Bucknall RC, Edwards SW. Neutrophil function in inflammation and inflammatory diseases. *Rheumatology*. 2010;49:1618-1631.
28. Yazid S, Norling LV, Flower RJ. Anti-inflammatory drugs, eicosanoids and the annexin A1/FPR2 anti-inflammatory system. *Prostaglandins Other Lipid Mediat*. 2012;98:94-100.
29. Chen L, Lv F, Pei L. Annexin 1: a glucocorticoid-inducible protein that modulates inflammatory pain. *Eur J Pain*. 2014;18:338-347.
30. Parente L, Solito E. Annexin 1: more than an anti-phospholipase protein. *Inflamm Res*. 2004;53:125-132.
31. Chu WM. Tumor necrosis factor. *Cancer Lett*. 2013;328:222-225.
32. Theofilopoulos AN, Gonzalez-Quintial R, Lawson BR, et al. Sensors of the innate immune system: their link to rheumatic diseases. *Nat Rev Rheumatol*. 2010;6:146-156.
33. Weber A, Wasiliew P, Kracht M. Interleukin-1 (IL-1) pathway. *Sci Signal*. 2010;3(105):cm1.
34. Wahren-Herlenius M, Dörner T. Immunopathogenic mechanisms of systemic autoimmune disease. *Lancet*. 2013;382: 819-831.
35. Stout A. Epidural steroid injections for cervical radiculopathy. *Phys Med Rehabil Clin N Am*. 2011;22:149-159.
36. Valat JP, Rozenberg S. Local corticosteroid injections for low back pain and sciatica. *Joint Bone Spine*. 2008;75:403-407.
37. Ly-Pen D, Andréu JL, Millán I, et al. Comparison of surgical decompression and local steroid injection in the treatment of carpal tunnel syndrome: 2-year clinical results from a randomized trial. *Rheumatology*. 2012;51:1447-1454.
38. Cheng OT, Souzdalnitski D, Vrooman B, Cheng J. Evidence-based knee injections for the management of arthritis. *Pain Med*. 2012;13:740-753.
39. Gialanella B, Prometti P. Effects of corticosteroids injection in rotator cuff tears. *Pain Med*. 2011;12:1559-1565.
40. Yavuz U, Sökücü S, Albayrak A, Oztürk K. Efficacy comparisons of the intraarticular steroidal agents in the patients with knee osteoarthritis. *Rheumatol Int*. 2012;32:3391-3396.
41. Gyuricza C, Umoh E, Wolfe SW. Multiple pulley rupture following corticosteroid injection for trigger digit: case report. *J Hand Surg Am*. 2009;34:1444-1448.
42. Zhang J, Keenan C, Wang JH. The effects of dexamethasone on human patellar tendon stem cells: implications for dexamethasone treatment of tendon injury. *J Orthop Res*. 2013;31:105-110.
43. Cole BJ, Schumacher HR Jr. Injectable corticosteroids in modern practice. *J Am Acad Orthop Surg*. 2005;13:37-46.
44. Lansang MC, Hustak LK. Glucocorticoid-induced diabetes and adrenal suppression: how to detect and manage them. *Cleve Clin J Med*. 2011;78:748-756.
45. Reddy P. Clinical approach to adrenal insufficiency in hospitalised patients. *Int J Clin Pract*. 2011;65:1059-1066.
46. Gordijn MS, Gemke RJ, van Dalen EC, et al. Hypothalamic-pituitary-adrenal (HPA) axis suppression after treatment with glucocorticoid therapy for childhood acute lymphoblastic leukaemia. *Cochrane Database Syst Rev*. 2012;5:CD008727.
47. Schwartz RH, Neacsu O, Ascher DP, Alpan O. Moderate dose inhaled corticosteroid-induced symptomatic adrenal suppression: case report and review of the literature. *Clin Pediatr*. 2012;51:1184-1190.
48. Elston MS, Conaglen HM, Hughes C, et al. Duration of cortisol suppression following a single dose of dexamethasone in healthy volunteers: a randomised double-blind placebo-controlled trial. *Anaesth Intensive Care*. 2013;41:596-601.
49. Tempark T, Phatarakijnirund V, Chatproedprai S, et al. Exogenous Cushing's syndrome due to topical corticosteroid application: case report and review literature. *Endocrine*. 2010;38: 328-334.
50. Schakman O, Kalista S, Barbé C, Loumaye A, Thissen JP. Glucocorticoid-induced skeletal muscle atrophy. *Int J Biochem Cell Biol*. 2013;45:2163-2172.
51. Shimizu N, Yoshikawa N, Ito N, et al. Crosstalk between glucocorticoid receptor and nutritional sensor mTOR in skeletal muscle. *Cell Metab*. 2011;13:170-182.
52. Pereira RM, Freire de Carvalho J. Glucocorticoid-induced myopathy. *Joint Bone Spine*. 2011;78:41-44.
53. Minetto MA, Lanfranco F, Motta G, et al. Steroid myopathy: some unresolved issues. *J Endocrinol Invest*. 2011;34:370-375.
54. Hanaoka BY, Peterson CA, Horbinski C, Crofford LJ. Implications of glucocorticoid therapy in idiopathic inflammatory myopathies. *Nat Rev Rheumatol*. 2012;8:448-457.
55. Bultink IE, Baden M, Lems WF. Glucocorticoid-induced osteoporosis: an update on current pharmacotherapy and future directions. *Expert Opin Pharmacother*. 2013;14:185-197.

56. den Uyl D, Bultink IE, Lems WF. Advances in glucocorticoid-induced osteoporosis. *Curr Rheumatol Rep.* 2011;13:233-240.
57. Mitra R. Adverse effects of corticosteroids on bone metabolism: a review. *PM&R.* 2011;3:466-471.
58. Olney RC. Mechanisms of impaired growth: effect of steroids on bone and cartilage. *Horm Res.* 2009;72(suppl 1):30-35.
59. Weinstein RS. Glucocorticoid-induced osteoporosis and osteonecrosis. *Endocrinol Metab Clin North Am.* 2012;41:595-611.
60. Bultink IE, Vis M, van der Horst-Bruinsma IE, Lems WF. Inflammatory rheumatic disorders and bone. *Curr Rheumatol Rep.* 2012;14:224-230.
61. Rizzoli R, Adachi JD, Cooper C, et al. Management of glucocorticoid-induced osteoporosis. *Calcif Tissue Int.* 2012;91: 225-243.
62. Rozenberg S, Vandromme J, Antoine C. Postmenopausal hormone therapy: risks and benefits. *Nat Rev Endocrinol.* 2013;9: 216-227.
63. Miller PD, Derman RJ. What is the best balance of benefits and risks among anti-resorptive therapies for postmenopausal osteoporosis? *Osteoporos Int.* 2010;21:1793-1802.
64. Lui JC, Baron J. Effects of glucocorticoids on the growth plate. *Endocr Dev.* 2011;20:187-193.
65. Carli L, Tani C, Querci F, et al. Analysis of the prevalence of cataracts and glaucoma in systemic lupus erythematosus and evaluation of the rheumatologists' practice for the monitoring of glucocorticoid eye toxicity. *Clin Rheumatol.* 2013;32:1071-1073.
66. Dubovsky AN, Arvikar S, Stern TA, Axelrod L. The neuropsychiatric complications of glucocorticoid use: steroid psychosis revisited. *Psychosomatics.* 2012;53:103-115.
67. Ross DA, Cetas JS. Steroid psychosis: a review for neurosurgeons. *J Neurooncol.* 2012;109:439-447.
68. Losa M, Picozzi P, Redaelli MG, et al. Pituitary radiotherapy for Cushing's disease. *Neuroendocrinology.* 2010;92(suppl 1):107-110.
69. Beuschlein F. Regulation of aldosterone secretion: from physiology to disease. *Eur J Endocrinol.* 2013;168:R85-93.
70. Hattangady NG, Olala LO, Bollag WB, Rainey WE. Acute and chronic regulation of aldosterone production. *Mol Cell Endocrinol.* 2012;350:151-162.
71. Dooley R, Harvey BJ, Thomas W. Non-genomic actions of aldosterone: from receptors and signals to membrane targets. *Mol Cell Endocrinol.* 2012;350:223-234.
72. Yang J, Fuller PJ. Interactions of the mineralocorticoid receptor—within and without. *Mol Cell Endocrinol.* 2012;350:196-205.
73. Schild L. The epithelial sodium channel and the control of sodium balance. *Biochim Biophys Acta.* 2010;1802:1159-1165.
74. Soundararajan R, Pearce D, Ziera T. The role of the ENaC-regulatory complex in aldosterone-mediated sodium transport. *Mol Cell Endocrinol.* 2012;350:242-247.
75. Williams JS. Evolving research in nongenomic actions of aldosterone. *Curr Opin Endocrinol Diabetes Obes.* 2013;20:198-203.
76. Wendler A, Albrecht C, Wehling M. Nongenomic actions of aldosterone and progesterone revisited. *Steroids.* 2012;77: 1002-1006.
77. Briet M, Schiffrin EL. Vascular actions of aldosterone. *J Vasc Res.* 2013;50:89-99.
78. Gros R, Ding Q, Davis M, et al. Delineating the receptor mechanisms underlying the rapid vascular contractile effects of aldosterone and estradiol. *Can J Physiol Pharmacol.* 2011;89:655-663.
79. Xanthakis V, Vasan RS. Aldosterone and the risk of hypertension. *Curr Hypertens Rep.* 2013;15:102-107.
80. Hawkins UA, Gomez-Sanchez EP, Gomez-Sanchez CM, Gomez-Sanchez CE. The ubiquitous mineralocorticoid receptor: clinical implications. *Curr Hypertens Rep.* 2012;14:573-580.
81. MacKenzie SM, Connell JM, Davies E. Non-adrenal synthesis of aldosterone: a reality check. *Mol Cell Endocrinol.* 2012;350:163-167.
82. Ronconi V, Turchi F, Appolloni G, et al. Aldosterone, mineralocorticoid receptor and the metabolic syndrome: role of the mineralocorticoid receptor antagonists. *Curr Vasc Pharmacol.* 2012;10:238-246.
83. Sowers JR, Whaley-Connell A, Epstein M. Narrative review: the emerging clinical implications of the role of aldosterone in the metabolic syndrome and resistant hypertension. *Ann Intern Med.* 2009;150:776-783.
84. Nguyen Dinh Cat A, Jaisser F. Extrarenal effects of aldosterone. *Curr Opin Nephrol Hypertens.* 2012;21:147-156.
85. Guichard JL, Clark D 3rd, Calhoun DA, Ahmed MI. Aldosterone receptor antagonists: current perspectives and therapies. *Vasc Health Risk Manag.* 2013;9:321-331.
86. Young MJ. Targeting the mineralocorticoid receptor in cardiovascular disease. *Expert Opin Ther Targets.* 2013;17:321-331.
87. Funder JW. Mineralocorticoid receptor antagonists: emerging roles in cardiovascular medicine. *Integr Blood Press Control.* 2013;6: 129-138.
88. Roscioni SS, de Zeeuw D, Bakker SJ, Lambers Heerspink HJ. Management of hyperkalaemia consequent to mineralocorticoid-receptor antagonist therapy. *Nat Rev Nephrol.* 2012;8:691-699.
89. Abuannadi M, O'Keefe JH. Review article: eplerenone: an underused medication? *J Cardiovasc Pharmacol Ther.* 2010;15: 318-325.
90. Barel M, Perez OA, Giozzet VA, et al. Exercise training prevents hyperinsulinemia, muscular glycogen loss and muscle atrophy induced by dexamethasone treatment. *Eur J Appl Physiol.* 2010;108:999-1007.
91. LaPier TK. Glucocorticoid-induced muscle atrophy. The role of exercise in treatment and prevention. *J Cardiopulm Rehabil.* 1997;17:76-84.
92. Seene T, Kaasik P. Role of exercise therapy in prevention of decline in aging muscle function: glucocorticoid myopathy and unloading. *J Aging Res.* 2012;2012:172492.

CHAPTER 30

Male and Female Hormones

The principal functions of male and female hormones are to control reproductive function and secondary sexual characteristics in their respective gender groups. Male hormones, such as testosterone, are usually referred to collectively as *androgens*. The female hormones consist of two principal groups: the estrogens (e.g., estradiol) and the progestins (e.g., progesterone). Androgens, estrogens, and progestins are classified as steroid hormones; their chemical structure is similar to those of the other primary steroid groups, the glucocorticoids and mineralocorticoids (see Chapter 29).

Male and female hormones are produced primarily in the gonads. Androgens are synthesized in the testes in the male. In the female, the ovaries are the main sites of estrogen and progestin production. As discussed in Chapter 29, small amounts of sex-related hormones are also produced in the adrenal cortex in both sexes, which accounts for the fact that low testosterone levels are seen in females, and males produce small quantities of estrogen. However, under normal conditions, the amounts of sex-related hormones produced by the adrenal cortex are usually too small to produce significant physiological effects.

In this chapter, we first discuss the physiological role of the male hormones and the pharmacological use of natural and synthetic androgens. We then address the physiological and pharmacological characteristics of the female hormones. There are several aspects of male and female hormones that should concern you as a physical therapist or occupational therapist. Rehabilitation patients may use these agents for approved purposes, such as female hormones as contraceptives. These agents may also be used for illicit reasons, such as the use of male hormones to enhance athletic performance. Hence, you should be aware of the therapeutic and potential toxic effects of these drugs.

ANDROGENS

Source and Regulation of Androgen Synthesis

In adult males, testosterone is the principal androgen produced by the testes.[1,2] Testosterone is synthesized by Leydig cells located in the interstitial space between the seminiferous tubules (Fig. 30-1). The seminiferous tubules are the convoluted ducts within the testes in which sperm production (spermatogenesis) takes place. Testosterone produced by the Leydig cells exerts a direct effect on the seminiferous tubules, as well as systemic effects on other physiological systems (see "Physiological Effects of Androgens").

Production of testosterone by the Leydig cells is regulated by the pituitary gonadotropins luteinizing hormone (LH) and follicle-stimulating hormone (FSH).[1] LH and FSH appear to control spermatogenesis, as shown in Figure 30-1. LH is the primary hormone that stimulates testosterone production. LH released from the anterior pituitary binds to receptors on the surface of Leydig cells and directly stimulates testosterone synthesis.[3,4] FSH is also released from the anterior pituitary; this hormone primarily affects the Sertoli cells that line the seminiferous tubules and are responsible for the

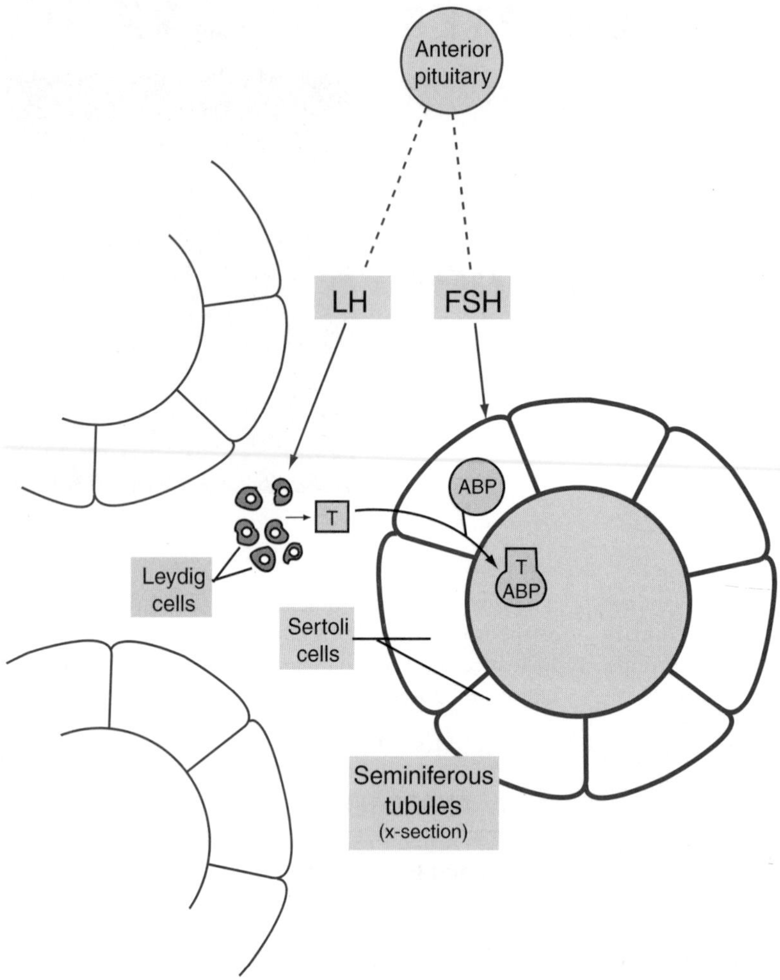

Figure ■ 30-1
Effects of pituitary gonadotropins on spermatogenesis. Luteinizing hormone (LH) stimulates testosterone (T) production from Leydig cells. Follicle-stimulating hormone (FSH) acts primarily on Sertoli cells to increase synthesis of androgen-binding protein (ABP). ABP appears to bind with T and facilitate transport into the seminiferous tubule, where spermatogenesis takes place.

development and maturation of normal sperm.[5,6] FSH stimulates the growth and function of Sertoli cells, and it induces Sertoli cells to produce several products that influence spermatogenesis and androgen function. For example, FSH increases the expression of a polypeptide known as androgen-binding protein (ABP), which helps concentrate testosterone within the seminiferous tubules and helps transport testosterone to the epididymis.[7] FSH may also affect Leydig cell function indirectly by increasing the production of other chemical messengers from the Sertoli cells that enhance differentiation and function of Leydig cells.[6]

Therefore, both pituitary gonadotropins are required for optimal androgen function. LH acts on the Leydig cells to stimulate testosterone synthesis, whereas FSH acts on the Sertoli cells to stimulate their function and help testosterone reach target tissues within the seminiferous tissues. Other hormones may also play a synergistic role in steroidogenesis in the male. For instance, growth hormone, thyroid hormones, insulin-like growth factor 1, and prolactin may also affect the functions of Leydig and Sertoli cells, thereby influencing the production and effects of testosterone.[8,9]

Release of the pituitary gonadotropins (LH, FSH) is regulated by gonadotropin-releasing hormone (GnRH) from the hypothalamus.[10,11] A classic negative feedback system exists between the GnRH/pituitary gonadotropins and testosterone synthesis. Increased plasma levels of testosterone inhibit the release of GnRH, LH, and FSH, thus maintaining testosterone levels within a relatively finite range. In addition, testosterone production is fairly tonic in normal men. Fluctuations may occur in the amount of testosterone produced over a given period, and androgen production tends to diminish slowly as part of normal aging.[12] Androgen production, however, does not correspond to a regular monthly cycle similar to hormonal production in women—that is, testosterone is produced more or less constantly, whereas female hormones are typically produced according to the stages of the menstrual cycle (see "Estrogen and Progesterone").

Physiological Effects of Androgens

Testosterone and other androgens are involved in the development of the sexual characteristics in males and in the stimulation of spermatogenesis. These two primary effects are described below.

Development of Male Characteristics

The influence of testosterone on sexual differentiation begins in utero. In the fetus, the testes produce small amounts of testosterone that affect the development of the male reproductive organs. Androgen production then remains relatively unimportant until puberty. At the onset of puberty, a complex series of hormonal events stimulates the testes to begin to synthesize significant amounts of testosterone. The production of testosterone brings about the development of most of the physical characteristics associated with men. Most notable are increased body hair, increased skeletal muscle mass, voice change, and maturation of the external genitalia.

These changes are all caused by the effect of androgenic steroids on their respective target tissues. Like other steroids, androgens exert their primary effects by entering the target cell and binding to a cytoplasmic receptor.[13,14] The activated steroid-receptor complex then travels to the cell's nucleus, where it binds to specific chromatin units. Protein synthesis increases through the transcription/translation of RNA by binding the activated complex to DNA gene segments. The proteins produced then cause a change in cellular function, which is reflected as one of the maturational effects of the androgens. For instance, testosterone increases protein synthesis in skeletal muscle, thus increasing muscle mass at the onset of puberty. Increased muscle mass as it relates to androgen abuse in athletes is discussed in more detail under "Androgen Abuse" later in this chapter.

Role in Spermatogenesis

As discussed previously, androgens are essential for the production and development of normal sperm.[1,15] LH serves as the primary stimulus to increase androgen production from Leydig cells. Testosterone enters the tubules to directly stimulate the production of sperm through an effect on protein synthesis within the tubule cells. FSH must also be present in the testes to facilitate testosterone transport into the Sertoli cells and to work synergistically with testosterone to allow full growth and maturation of developing sperm.[6]

CLINICAL USE OF ANDROGENS

Androgens and their synthetic derivatives are approved for administration in several clinical situations, ranging from common replacement therapy to rare hereditary disorders.

Replacement Therapy

Patients take testosterone and other androgens as replacement therapy when their endogenous production of testosterone is impaired. Such conditions include removal of the testes (orchiectomy), various intrinsic forms of testicular failure (cryptorchidism, orchitis), and problems in the endocrine regulation of testosterone production, such as lack of LH production and other forms of hypogonadism.[16,17]

Because androgen production also diminishes slowly with aging, relatively small or physiological doses of androgens have been used to replace the age-related decline in endogenous production in some older men.[18,19] This type of replacement has been reported to produce beneficial effects on body composition, strength, bone mineralization, glucose metabolism, mood, libido, and other characteristics associated with normal androgen production.[18,20] The primary concern, however, is that androgens can increase prostate growth and perhaps increase the risk of prostate cancer in susceptible older men.[21,22] Hence, researchers continue to evaluate androgen replacement as a therapeutic option in certain men who are experiencing an excessive decline in androgen production during aging.[22,23] Future studies should help clarify how these hormones might be used to promote optimal health in older men.[19,24]

Catabolic States

Androgens can be administered for their anabolic properties in conditions where there is substantial muscle catabolism and protein loss.[25,26] Such conditions include chronic infections, severe traumas, severe burns, and recovery from extensive surgeries.[25,27] However, the use of androgens in these situations is somewhat controversial. Physicians do not typically administer these agents as a primary treatment, but as adjuncts to more conventional treatments such as dietary supplementation and exercise.

Physiological dosages of androgens may also maintain or increase lean body mass and bone density in men who are infected with HIV. Men with HIV infection may have muscle wasting because of low testosterone production combined with the catabolic effects of this infection and subsequent anti-HIV therapies (see Chapter 34).[28,29] The effects of this treatment have not been overwhelmingly successful; only modest increases in lean body mass were seen in some studies.[30] However, larger (supraphysiological) dosages of androgens, such as oxandrolone, have been reported to produce beneficial effects on muscle mass and strength in men with HIV infection, especially if drug therapy is combined with resistance training.[31]

Delayed Puberty

Androgens administered on a short-term basis in selected adolescent males can mimic the characteristics normally associated with the onset of puberty (increased body mass, deepening voice, etc.).[32] These drugs are typically used when puberty is anticipated to occur spontaneously but at a relatively late date—that is, when puberty is not delayed because of some pathological condition.

Breast Cancer

Androgens may be used to treat a limited number of hormone-sensitive tumors, such as certain cases of breast cancer in women. However, other drugs, such as the antiestrogens, have largely replaced the use of androgens in such cancers. We discuss the role of various hormones in the treatment of cancer in more detail in Chapter 36.

Anemia

Testosterone and similar compounds are potent stimulators of erythropoietin synthesis from the kidneys and other tissues.[33] Erythropoietin, in turn, stimulates production of red blood cell synthesis in bone marrow. However, pharmacologists have developed erythropoietin-stimulating agents, such as darbepoetin and epoetin, to more directly treat anemia that occurs secondary to renal disease, cancer chemotherapy, and other anemic conditions.[34] Nonetheless, physicians may administer androgens as an adjunct to erythropoietin-stimulating agents to increase red blood cell production in certain patients with severe or recalcitrant anemia.[33]

Hereditary Angioedema

Hereditary angioedema is characterized by a defect in the control of clotting factors that ultimately leads to increased vascular permeability.[35] Loss of vascular fluid from specific capillary beds causes localized edema in various tissues such as the skin, upper respiratory tract, and gastrointestinal (GI) tract. Certain androgens act on the liver to restore production of several clotting factors and to increase production of a glycoprotein, inhibiting the initial stages of the clotting sequence that leads to increased vascular permeability.[36] Hence, androgens are typically given prophylactically to decrease the frequency and severity of angioedema attacks.

Specific Agents

The agents listed in Table 30-1 are the principal androgens approved for clinical use. Patients usually take the specific agents orally or intramuscularly, as indicated, to replace endogenous androgen production or to treat various medical problems such as catabolic states and anemias. Androgens can also be classified according to their relative androgenic and anabolic properties—that is, certain androgens are given primarily to mimic male sexual characteristics (androgenic effects), whereas other androgens are given primarily to enhance tissue metabolism (anabolic effects; see Table 30-1). This distinction is not absolute, however, because all compounds given to produce anabolism will also produce some androgenic effects. Many other androgenic and anabolic steroids exist and can be acquired relatively easily on the black market by individuals engaging in androgen abuse (see "Androgen Abuse").

Table 30-1
CLINICAL USE OF ANDROGENS

Generic Name	Trade Name(s)	Primary Indication(s)	Routes of Administration
Danazol	Cyclomen, Danocrine	Endometriosis, benign fibrocystic disease, hereditary angioedema	Oral
Fluoxymesterone	Android-F, Halotestin	Androgen deficiency; breast cancer in women; delayed puberty in boys	Oral
Methyltestosterone	Android, Oreton, Testred, Virilon, others	Androgen deficiency; breast cancer in women; delayed puberty in boys	Oral
Nandrolone	Generic	Anemia of renal insufficiency	Intramuscular
Oxandrolone	Oxandrin	Catabolic states	Oral
Oxymetholone	Anadrol	Anemia	Oral
Testosterone buccal system	Striant	Androgen deficiency	Buccal
Testosterone cypionate injection	Depo-Testosterone	Androgen deficiency	Intramuscular
Testosterone enanthate injection	Delatestryl	Androgen deficiency; breast cancer in women; delayed puberty in boys	Intramuscular
Testosterone implants	Testopel pellets	Androgen deficiency; delayed puberty in boys	Subcutaneous
Testosterone gel	AndroGel, Testim, Testoderm	Androgen deficiency	Transdermal
Testosterone transdermal system	Androderm	Androgen deficiency	Transdermal

Adverse Effects of Clinical Androgen Use

The adverse effects of androgens are related to the dose and duration of their use; problems are seen more frequently during prolonged androgen administration at relatively high doses. The primary problems are the masculinizing effects of these drugs.[37,38] In women, androgen administration can produce hirsutism, hoarseness or deepening of the voice, and changes in the external genitalia (enlarged clitoris). Irregular menstrual periods and acne may also occur in women undergoing androgen therapy. In men, these drugs may produce bladder irritation, breast swelling and soreness, and frequent or prolonged erections. When used in children, androgens may cause accelerated sexual maturation and impairment of normal bone development due to premature closure of epiphyseal plates. Consequently, these drugs are used very cautiously in children.

In adults, most of the adverse effects are reversible, and symptoms will diminish once the agent is discontinued. However, a few effects—such as vocal changes in females—may persist even after the drugs are withdrawn. Skeletal changes are irreversible, and permanent growth impairment may occur if these drugs are used in children.

Androgens may also increase the risk of prostate cancer, especially in older men who are susceptible to this disease.[21] Other side effects of long-term, high-dose androgen use include liver damage and hepatic carcinoma. Hypertension may occur because of the salt-retaining and water-retaining effects of these drugs, and androgens can adversely affect plasma lipids (i.e., increased total cholesterol and decreased levels of high-density lipoproteins). Although these hepatic and cardiovascular problems may occur during therapeutic androgen use, their incidence is even more prevalent when extremely large doses are used to enhance athletic performance (see "Androgen Abuse").

Antiandrogens

Antiandrogens inhibit the synthesis or effects of endogenous androgen production.[39] These agents can be helpful in illnesses such as prostate cancer and other conditions aggravated by excessive androgen production.[40,41] Specific antiandrogens affect endogenous male hormones in several different ways. Finasteride (Propecia, Proscar) and dutasteride (Avodart) inhibit the conversion of testosterone to dihydrotestosterone. Dihydrotestosterone accelerates the growth and development of the prostate gland; these antiandrogens may be helpful in attenuating this effect in conditions such as benign prostate hypertrophy. Flutamide (Eulexin), bicalutamide (Casodex), and nilutamide (Anandron, Nilandron) act as antagonists (blockers) of the cellular androgen receptor; these drugs are used to decrease hirsutism in women or to help treat prostate cancer.

Advanced prostate cancer is also treated with several drugs that mimic or block the effects of GnRH. GnRH analogs include goserelin (Zoladex), leuprolide (Lupron, others), and nafarelin (Synarel). When first administered, these agents cause an increase in pituitary LH release, which in turn stimulates testicular androgen production. However, continued administration of GnRH analogs desensitizes pituitary GnRH receptors, thus decreasing LH and testosterone production from the pituitary and testes, respectively.[42] Newer agents, such as abarelix (Plenaxis) and degarelix (Firmagon), directly antagonize (block) the GnRH receptor on the pituitary.[43] These drugs are especially helpful in certain patients because they will cause a more direct and immediate decrease in LH production compared to the GnRH analogs.

ANDROGEN ABUSE

The use of androgens or anabolic steroids to increase athletic performance is controversial and concerning. It has been known for some time that certain athletes have been self-administering large doses of androgens in an effort to increase muscle size and strength. Typically, androgen use is associated with athletes involved in strength and power activities such as weight lifting and bodybuilding and in certain sports such as football, baseball, and track and field. Androgen abuse, however, has infiltrated many aspects of athletic competition at both the amateur and professional levels. There also appears to be a contingent of men, women, and adolescents who are not athletes who take anabolic steroids to increase lean body mass to simply appear more muscular.[44,45]

There are many well-publicized cases where top athletes in various sports have tested positive for androgen abuse or admitted to using anabolic steroids.[46] Also, researchers have documented that anabolic steroid abuse is occurring among the general athletic population, including younger athletes.[47,48] A comprehensive survey of male high school students, for example, indicated that over 6 percent had taken anabolic steroids at least once in their lifetime.[49] The studies reveal that androgen abuse is one of the major problems affecting the health and welfare of athletes of various ages and athletic pursuits.

Athletes engaging in androgen abuse usually obtain these drugs from various illicit but readily available sources.[50] These agents include testosterone, synthetic analogs of testosterone, and precursors that are converted to anabolic substances within the body (Table 30-2). In addition, several different androgens are often taken simultaneously for a combined dose that is 10 to 100 times greater than the therapeutic dose.[51] This "stacking" of different anabolic steroids often consists of combining oral and injectable forms

Table 30-2
EXAMPLES OF ANABOLIC ANDROGENS THAT ARE ABUSED BY ATHLETES

Generic Name	Trade Name
Orally Active Androgens	
Chlorodehydromethyltestosterone	Turinabol
Fluoxymesterone	Halotestin
Methandrostenolone	Dianabol
Methyl testosterone	Android
Oxandrolone	Anavar
Oxymetholone	Anadrol
Stanozolol	Winstrol
Androgens Administered by Intramuscular Injection	
Boldenone	Equipoise
Drostanolone	Masteron
Methenolone	Primobolan
Nandrolone decanoate	Deca-Durabolin
Stanozolol	Winstrol-V
Testosterone cypionate	
Testosterone enanthate	
Testosterone propionate	
Testosterone suspension	

Adapted from: Parkinson AB, Evans NA. Anabolic androgenic steroids: a survey of 500 users. Med Sci Sports Exerc. 2006;38:644-651.

of these drugs. Athletes often self-administer these drugs in cycles that last between 7 and 14 weeks, and the dosage of each drug is progressively increased during the cycle. An example of a dosing cycle using stacked anabolic steroids is shown in Table 30-3.

To help control anabolic steroid abuse, many sporting federations have instituted drug testing at the time of a specific competition. To prevent detection, an athlete will employ a complex pattern of high-dosage androgen administration followed with washout periods. Washouts are scheduled a sufficient amount of time prior to the competition in order to eliminate the drug from the body before testing. The practice of planned schedules can be negated to some extent through randomized drug testing that subjects the athlete to testing at any point in the training period and at the time of the competition.[52]

Two primary questions usually arise concerning anabolic steroids: Do these agents really enhance athletic performance, and what are the adverse effects of androgen abuse? Definitive answers to these questions are difficult because of the illicit nature of androgen abuse and because of the ethical and legal problems of administering large doses of androgens to healthy athletes as part of controlled research studies. The effects of androgens on athletic performance and the potential adverse effects of these drugs are discussed briefly here.

Effects of Androgens on Athletic Performance

There is little doubt that androgens can promote skeletal muscle growth and increase strength in people who do not synthesize meaningful amounts of endogenous androgens (e.g., women, prepubescent males). The question has often been whether large amounts of exogenous androgens can increase muscle size, strength, and athletic performance in healthy men. In general, it appears that athletic men taking androgens during strength training may experience greater increments in lean body mass and muscle strength than athletes training without androgens.[53,54] The extent of the increase, however, will vary considerably depending on the dosage and type of androgens used.[53]

It also remains unclear what magnitude of any strength gains can be directly attributed to anabolic steroids. For instance, the anabolic effects of steroids cannot be isolated easily from the other factors that produce increments in strength and muscle size (e.g., weight training). In particular, androgens appear to increase aggressiveness, and individuals taking these drugs may train longer and more intensely than athletes who are not taking them.[55] Consequently, strength increments in the athlete taking androgens may be brought about by the enhanced quality and quantity of training rather than as a direct effect of anabolic steroids on muscle protein synthesis.

Thus, the effects of androgens on athletic performance in men remain unclear. It seems probable that high dosages of androgens would increase muscle size and strength, which might ultimately translate to improved athletic performance.[54] However, we may never know the exact ergogenic effects of these drugs in men because of the illicit nature of androgen abuse and the ethical problems involved in performing clinical studies of these drugs in humans.[53]

Table 30-3
EXAMPLE OF A STEROID DOSING CYCLE USED DURING ANDROGEN ABUSE*

Drug Name	Eight-Week Dosage (mg) Regimen							
	1	2	3	4	5	6	7	8
Testosterone cypionate	200	400	600	1,200	2,400	4,200	4,200	4,200
Nandrolone (Deca-Durabolin)	100	100	100	200	400	600	600	600
Oxymetholone (Anadrol)	100	150	200	250	300	500	750	1,000
Methandrostenolone	25	30	35	50	60	75	100	125 (Dianabol)
Methandrostenolone (Dianabol injectable)	25	25	50	50	100	100	100	100
Oxandrolone (Anavar)	25	30	35	50	50	50	50	50

**This regimen was used by a bodybuilder who went through three cycles each year for 8 years. The subject also reported taking 600 mg of testosterone per week between cycles. This subject ultimately developed avascular necrosis in both femoral heads.*

Source: Pettine KA. Association of anabolic steroids and avascular necrosis of femoral heads. Am J Sports Med. 1991;19:96-98, with permission.

Adverse Effects of Androgen Abuse

Virtually any drugs that are taken at extremely high dosages can be expected to produce serious side effects. Exactly how harmful androgen abuse is in an athletic population remains somewhat uncertain.[44,56] The illicit nature of androgen abuse and the various dosage regimens have made it difficult to determine the precise incidence and type of adverse effects.[53,56] Also, the long-term effects of androgen abuse may not be known for some time; pathologies may not be fully realized until several years after the drugs are discontinued.[44,45]

People who abuse anabolic steroids often use additional performance-enhancing interventions (growth hormone, blood doping, etc.) and are also likely to abuse other drugs, including alcohol, opioids, and cocaine.[44,57] Hence, some adverse effects may be attributed to these other substances and illicit behaviors. Nonetheless, there is considerable evidence, often in the form of individual reports and case studies, that androgen abuse can have severe and possibly fatal consequences. Some of the more common adverse effects are presented below. Further discussion of the potential adverse effects in athletes can be found in several reviews listed at the end of this chapter.[56,58,59]

High doses of androgens can produce liver damage, including the formation of hepatic tumors and peliosis hepatis (blood-filled cysts within the liver).[60,61] In some individuals, these liver abnormalities have proved fatal. Androgens can also produce detrimental changes in cardiac structure and function that result in cardiomyopathy, ischemic heart disease, arrhythmias, and heart failure.[59,62,63] Furthermore, these hormones pose additional cardiovascular risks by producing unfavorable changes in blood lipid profiles, such as decreased high-density lipoprotein cholesterol levels.[59,64] These effects on plasma lipids predispose the athlete to atherosclerotic lesions and subsequent vessel occlusion, and specific cases of stroke and myocardial infarction in athletes using androgens have been attributed to the atherogenic effects of these drugs.[59,64] Androgens also cause hypertension because of direct effects on the myocardium and because of the salt- and water-retaining properties of these drugs.[65] Problems with glucose metabolism brought about by insulin resistance have also been reported.[66]

Androgens can affect bone metabolism, and avascular necrosis of the femoral heads has been documented in a weight lifter using these drugs.[67] Androgens also accelerate closure of epiphyseal plates and can lead to impaired skeletal growth in young children. This effect on skeletal development is important because athletes may begin to self-administer anabolic steroids at a relatively young age (i.e., prior to age 16).[48] As previously mentioned, androgens may produce behavioral changes, including increased aggression, leading to radical mood swings and violent episodes in some individuals.[68,69]

Androgens can produce changes in reproductive function and secondary sexual characteristics. In males, high levels of androgens act as negative feedback and lead to testicular atrophy and impaired sperm production.[58] Infertility in males may result because of an inability to form sperm (azoospermia).[58,70] In females, androgens produce certain masculinizing effects and may also impair the normal female reproductive (menstrual) cycle, as discussed earlier. Some changes in male and female sexual and reproductive function appear to be reversible, but changes such as male infertility and azoospermia may take 4 months or longer to return to normal, and in some cases may be irreversible.[70,71] Other effects, such as vocal changes in females, may likewise be permanent.

In summary, anabolic steroids may produce some ergogenic benefits in a limited subset of athletes, but rather serious consequences may occur. Nonetheless, athletes may be so driven to succeed that they disregard the adverse effects. Also, athletes may suspect that their competitors are using steroids and feel that they must also take these drugs to remain competitive. Health-care professionals can discourage androgen abuse by informing athletes and nonathletes that the risks of androgen abuse exceed any potential benefits.[48,72]

ESTROGEN AND PROGESTERONE

In women, the ovaries produce two major categories of steroid hormones: estrogens and progestins. The primary estrogen produced in humans is estradiol, and the primary progestin is progesterone. For simplicity, the terms *estrogen* and *progesterone* will be used to indicate these two primary forms of female hormones. Small amounts of male hormones (androgens) are also produced by the ovaries. Androgens may play a role in the development of some secondary sexual characteristics in the female during puberty, such as increased body hair and growth spurts. Nonetheless, the hormones exerting the major influence on sexual development and reproduction in the female are estrogen and progesterone.

Effects of Estrogen and Progesterone on Sexual Maturation

Estrogen and progesterone play a primary role in promoting sexual differentiation in the developing female fetus. These hormones also become important in completing female sexual maturation during puberty.

At the onset of puberty, a complex series of hormonal events stimulates the ovaries to begin producing estrogen and progesterone. Ovarian production of these hormones initiates the maturation of reproductive function and development of secondary sexual characteristics in the female.

Estrogen is the principal hormone that initiates the growth and development of the female reproductive system during puberty. Changes in the external genitalia and maturation of the internal reproductive organs (e.g., uterus, oviducts, vagina) are primarily brought about by the influence of estrogen. Estrogen also produces several other characteristic changes in females, such as breast development, deposition of subcutaneous fat stores, and changes in the skeletal system (e.g., closure of epiphyseal plates, widening of the pelvic girdle). Progesterone is less important in sexual maturation and is involved to a greater extent in facilitating and maintaining pregnancy.

Regulation and Effects of Hormonal Synthesis During the Menstrual Cycle

In the nonpregnant, postpubescent female, production of estrogen and progesterone is not tonic in nature but follows a pattern or cycle of events commonly referred to as the *menstrual cycle.* The menstrual cycle usually occurs over a 28-day period. The primary function of this cycle is to stimulate the ovaries to produce an ovum that is available for fertilization, while simultaneously preparing the endometrium of the uterus for implantation of the ovum, should fertilization occur (Fig. 30-2). The cycle is characterized by several specific phases and events that we briefly outline below. A more detailed description of the regulation of female reproduction can be found in several sources listed at the end of this chapter.[73-75]

Follicular Phase

The first half of the menstrual cycle is influenced by hormonal release from a developing ovarian follicle, hence the term *follicular phase*. In the follicular phase, the anterior pituitary releases FSH, which stimulates the maturation of several follicles within the ovary. Usually, one such follicle undergoes full maturation and ultimately yields an ovum. The developing follicle also begins to secrete increasing amounts of estrogen during the follicular phase. Estrogen produced by the ovarian follicle causes proliferation and thickening of the endometrial lining of the uterus. The follicular phase is also referred to as the *proliferative phase*. Endometrial vascularization is increased, and glandular structures begin to develop in the uterine wall. The uterine glands, however, do not begin to function (secrete mucus) to any great extent during the follicular phase.

Ovulation

Just prior to the cycle's midpoint, the anterior pituitary secretes a sudden, large burst of LH. A smaller burst of FSH secretion also occurs around the midpoint of the cycle (see Fig. 30-2). The LH surge is the primary impetus for ovulation. During ovulation, the mature follicle ruptures, releasing the ovum from the ovary. At this point, the ovum should begin to travel toward the uterus via the fallopian tubes. The ruptured follicle remains in the ovary and continues to play a vital role in the reproductive cycle. After releasing the ovum, the follicle becomes infiltrated with lipids and is referred to as the *corpus luteum* (yellow body). The role of the corpus luteum is described next.

Luteal Phase

The corpus luteum governs the events in the second half of the menstrual cycle, which is called the *luteal phase*. In response to the residual effects of the LH-FSH surge, the corpus luteum continues to grow and develop for approximately 1 week after ovulation. During this time, the corpus luteum secretes both estrogen and progesterone. The combined effects of estrogen and progesterone cause further thickening in the uterine lining, as well as an increase in the vascularization and glandular secretion of the endometrium. During the luteal phase, progesterone is the primary stimulus that causes the uterine glands to fully develop and secrete a mucus that provides a favorable environment for implantation of the fertilized egg. Hence, the luteal phase is also referred to as the *secretory phase* because of the enhanced function of the uterine glands.

Corpus Luteum Regression and Termination of the Cycle

If the egg is not fertilized or implantation does not occur, the corpus luteum begins to regress, primarily because of a lack of continued support for the corpus

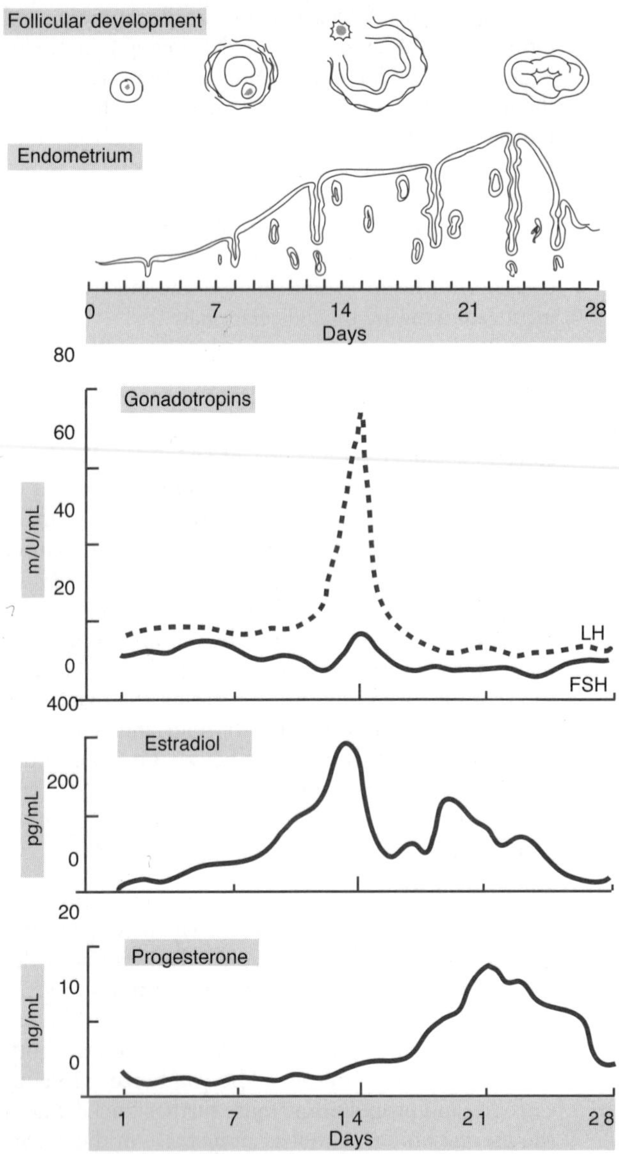

Figure ■ 30-2
The menstrual cycle, showing changes in follicular development, uterine endometrium, pituitary gonadotropins (LH, FSH), and ovarian hormones. *(From: Katzung BG. Basic and Clinical Pharmacology. 9th ed. New York: Lange Medical Books/McGraw-Hill; 2004: 662. Adapted with permission of the McGraw-Hill Companies.)*

luteum from the pituitary gonadotropins (i.e., LH, FSH). Because the corpus luteum regresses, it can no longer produce adequate amounts of estrogen and progesterone to maintain the endometrium of the uterus. Consequently, the endometrium begins to slough off, creating the menstrual bleeding that typifies the female reproductive cycle. The onset of menstrual bleeding marks the end of one reproductive cycle and the beginning of the next.

In summary, the menstrual cycle is primarily regulated by the interaction between pituitary and ovarian hormones. Also, hormones from the hypothalamus play a role in controlling female reproduction through their effects on LH and FSH release from the anterior pituitary.[73] A complex series of positive and negative feedback mechanisms controls the cyclic release of various female hormones.[73,74] For instance, increased estrogen secretion toward the end of the follicular phase signals the hypothalamus to release gonadotropin-releasing hormone, which in turn triggers the LH surge that causes ovulation. This sequence of events is considered an example of positive feedback because increased levels of estrogen act on the hypothalamic-pituitary axis to facilitate the release of hormones that cause ovulation. Conversely, secretion of the pituitary gonadotropins (i.e., LH, FSH) is inhibited toward the latter part of the luteal phase, presumably because the sustained production of estrogen and progesterone ultimately results in negative feedback on the pituitary and hypothalamus.

Pharmacological intervention can take advantage of these complex feedback systems in certain situations. Most notable is the use of estrogen and progesterone as hormonal contraceptives. By altering the normal control between pituitary and ovarian hormones and uterine function, preparations containing these two steroids are an effective means of birth control. The pharmacological use of female hormones is discussed in more detail in "Pharmacological Use of Estrogen and Progesterone."

Female Hormones in Pregnancy and Parturition

Estrogen and progesterone also play a significant role in pregnancy and childbirth. For successful implantation and gestation of the fertilized egg to occur, synthesis of these two steroids must be maintained to prevent the onset of menstruation. As just mentioned, menstruation begins when the corpus luteum is no longer able to produce sufficient estrogen and progesterone to sustain the endometrium. When fertilization does occur, however, some hormonal response must transpire to maintain steroid production from the corpus luteum and to ensure that the endometrium remains ready for implantation. This response is caused by the release of human chorionic gonadotropin (HCG) from the fertilized ovum. HCG, which is structurally and functionally similar to LH, takes over the role of LH and rescues the corpus luteum from destruction.[76] The corpus luteum then continues to produce steroids (especially progesterone), which maintain the uterine lining in a suitable state for implantation and gestation of the fertilized egg.

Eventually, the corpus luteum does begin to degenerate between the 9th and 14th week of gestation. By that point, the placenta has assumed estrogen and progesterone production. Generally speaking, maternal progesterone helps to maintain the uterus and placenta throughout the rest of the pregnancy. Progesterone also increases the growth and development of the maternal mammary glands in preparation for lactation. Although the role of estrogen is less clear, increased estrogen production may play a pivotal part in setting the stage for parturition. Clearly, both steroids are needed for normal birth and delivery.

PHARMACOLOGICAL USE OF ESTROGEN AND PROGESTERONE

The most frequent and prevalent use of the female hormones is in contraceptive preparations (see "Hormonal Contraceptives"). The other primary indications for estrogen and progesterone are to replace endogenous hormone production and to moderate the effects of endogenous hormones on the growth and function of reproductive and other tissues. Specific clinical conditions that may be resolved by estrogen and progesterone are addressed here. The use of estrogen and progesterone replacement therapy in women after menopause is also briefly reviewed.

Conditions Treated With Estrogen and Progesterone

Specific clinical conditions that may be resolved by estrogen and progesterone include the following:

Osteoporosis. There is little doubt that estrogens are essential in preventing and treating postmenopausal osteoporosis.[77–79] Women receiving hormone replacements with estrogen are able to maintain or increase bone mineral density. Estrogen replacement is often associated with a decreased incidence of vertebral fractures and other osteoporosis-related problems.[78,80,81] Estrogen can also be combined with other interventions such as physical activity, calcium supplements, vitamin D supplements, and other medications to provide optimal protection against osteoporosis following menopause (see Chapter 31).[82,83]

Hypogonadism. Estrogens, or a combination of estrogen and progesterone, may be used to treat abnormally low ovarian function. Appropriate use of these hormones induces the uterine changes and cyclic bleeding associated with the normal female reproductive cycle.

Failure of ovarian development. Occasionally, the ovaries fail to undergo normal development because of hypopituitarism or other disorders. Estrogens may be given at the time of puberty to encourage development of secondary sexual characteristics (e.g., breast development).

Menstrual irregularities. Various problems with normal menstruation are treated by estrogen and progesterone. These hormones are used either separately or are combined to resolve amenorrhea, dysmenorrhea, and other types of functional uterine bleeding that are caused by a hormonal imbalance.

Endometriosis. Endometriosis is characterized by growths of uterine-like tissue that occur at various locations within the pelvic cavity. Progesterone and estrogen-progesterone combinations help suppress bleeding from these tissues and may help shrink the size of these growths.

Carcinoma. Estrogen can help treat metastatic breast cancer in men and postmenopausal women. Advanced prostate cancer in men may also respond to estrogen treatment. Progesterone is helpful in treating uterine cancer and several other types of metastases, such as breast, renal, and endometrial carcinoma.

Use of Hormone Replacement Therapy Following Menopause

As indicated earlier, estrogen and progesterone can be administered to replace endogenous hormone production and to help resolve problems related to hormonal deficiencies. This strategy, known commonly as *hormone replacement therapy* (HRT), can be especially important following menopause—either when the female reproductive cycle ceases and the associated cyclic production of the ovarian hormones ends or for women who have had an ovariectomy.

Postmenopausal HRT, however, remains somewhat controversial because of the potential risks associated with replacement of both estrogen and progesterone, or the replacement of only estrogen (see "Adverse Effects of Estrogen and Progesterone"). There has been extensive research on this topic, and a detailed review of clinical studies on HRT is not possible here. This section is instead a brief summary of the possible benefits and risks of HRT in women after menopause.

There is no question that HRT, primarily in the form of estrogen replacement, can have positive effects on bone mineralization in women after menopause. This idea was addressed earlier in "Osteoporosis," in the list of "Conditions Treated With Estrogen and Progesterone." Certain women can also use HRT to control perimenopausal and postmenopausal symptoms such as atrophic vaginitis and atrophic dystrophy of the vulva. HRT can also limit vasomotor effects, such as hot flashes.[84–87]

Observational studies originally suggested that HRT might also improve plasma lipid profile and possibly reduce the risk of cardiovascular disease in postmenopausal women. However, certain randomized controlled trials refuted this idea and indicated that HRT may increase the risk of stroke and thromboembolic disease.[88] On the other hand, the timing of HRT may influence its effects on cardiovascular disease in postmenopausal women. Specifically, HRT may help decrease coronary heart disease in women who are under 60 years old and when HRT is initiated within 10 years of reaching menopause.[89] Women should be evaluated individually to determine if the cardiovascular benefits of HRT clearly outweigh any cardiovascular or other risks associated with HRT (see "Adverse Effects of Estrogen and Progesterone").[90,91] Research in this area will certainly continue to clarify whether HRT can help decrease cardiac morbidity and mortality in certain postmenopausal women.[92]

It has also been suggested that HRT may offer some protection against cognitive decline in conditions such as Alzheimer disease and other forms of dementia.[93] Estrogen may, for example, have several neuroprotective effects, including the ability to enhance synaptic plasticity and transmission in the hippocampus, sustain neuronal mitochondrial function, and inhibit other biochemical factors that cause neuronal degeneration in Alzheimer disease.[94-96]

The exact clinical effects of HRT on cognition and dementia remain controversial. For example, the original Women's Health Initiative (WHI) study—a large, randomized controlled trial—suggested that estrogen replacement may increase the incidence of dementia in older postmenopausal women.[97] In contrast, other studies of HRT in younger postmenopausal women (under age 60) indicated either no effect or slight benefits on memory and cognition.[98]

Recent studies also suggested that the specific type of hormonal formulation may influence the effects of HRT on cognitive function. In particular, combining conjugated equine estrogens with a progestin (medroxyprogesterone acetate) may negatively affect certain cognitive indicators such as verbal memory, whereas unopposed use of conjugated equine estrogen may have neither a positive nor negative effect on cognition in younger postmenopausal women.[99] In fact, there is some evidence that the progesterone component of certain HRT regimens may be a more important factor in possible impairment of cognition and memory.[98] This idea makes sense when one considers that progesterone typically antagonizes the neuroprotective effects of estrogen in areas of the brain related to memory, such as the hippocampus.[94] Additional studies are needed to determine the exact relationship between hormone replacement therapy and cognitive function and dementia in older women.

Specific Agents

Therapeutically used types of estrogens and progestins are listed in Tables 30-4 and 30-5, respectively. Both types of hormones can be administered in their natural form (estradiol and progesterone), and several synthetic derivatives of each type are also available. Most of the drugs listed in the tables are available as oral preparations to treat many conditions conveniently. These hormones may also be administered transdermally via patches, creams, or gels; the transdermal route may offer certain advantages, such as decreased side effects and fewer liver problems.[100,101] Certain preparations can be administered locally to the vagina via suppositories, tablets, creams, and rings. Vaginal administration can be helpful in treating local problems (postmenopausal dryness, vaginal atrophy) or dysfunction of the endometrium of the uterus.[102,103] Finally, several preparations are also available for injection, and parenteral routes may be required in some situations, such as severe uterine bleeding.

Table 30-4
CLINICAL USE OF ESTROGENS

Generic Name	Trade Name(s)	Primary Indication(s)
Estradiol	Estrace, Femtrace, Gynodiol	Estrogen replacement, antineoplastic, prevention of osteoporosis
Conjugated estrogens	Cenestin, Enjuvia, Premarin	Estrogen replacement, antineoplastic, prevention of osteoporosis, prevention of abnormal uterine bleeding
Esterified estrogens	Estratab, Menest	Estrogen replacement, antineoplastic, prevention of osteoporosis
Estropipate	Ogen, Ortho-Est	Estrogen replacement, prevention of osteoporosis

Adverse Effects of Estrogen and Progesterone

Cardiovascular disease is a primary risk factor during estrogen and progesterone therapy. Higher doses or prolonged exposure to estrogen has been associated with serious cardiovascular problems, including myocardial infarction, stroke, and thromboembolism.[104,105] These problems are significant when men take relatively large doses for the treatment of breast and prostate cancer. Cardiovascular disease, however, can also occur in women receiving estrogen or estrogen combined with progesterone as hormone replacement therapy. As indicated earlier in this chapter, increased risk of stroke was documented in older postmenopausal women who were treated with

Table 30-5
CLINICAL USE OF PROGESTINS

Generic Name	Trade Name(s)	Primary Indication(s)
Etonogestrel (implant)	Implanon	Contraceptive
Hydroxyprogesterone	Hylutin, Prodrox, others	Amenorrhea, dysfunctional uterine bleeding
Hydroxyprogesterone caproate	Makena	Maintain pregnancy and decrease risk of preterm birth
Levonorgestrel	Mirena, Skyla	Contraception
Medroxyprogesterone	Cycrin, Provera, others	Secondary amenorrhea, dysfunctional uterine bleeding, breast or endometrial carcinoma
Megestrol	Megace	Breast or endometrial carcinoma, anorexia/cachexia associated with AIDS
Norethindrone	Aygestin, Micronor, others	Secondary amenorrhea, dysfunctional uterine bleeding, endometriosis
Progesterone	Gesterol, Prometrium, others	Secondary amenorrhea, dysfunctional uterine bleeding, support of embryo implantation and early pregnancy

estrogen compared to a placebo during a large randomized controlled trial (the WHI study).[106] On the other hand, the risk of cardiovascular disease appears to be relatively low when moderate doses are administered to relatively younger women (under age 60) within 10 years after the onset of menopause.[106] Likewise, administration via the transdermal route may be associated with a lower risk of cardiovascular problems.[104] Nonetheless, the risk of cardiovascular disease should be considered in all individuals receiving estrogen, and practitioners should prescribe estrogen carefully in people who might have other cardiovascular risk factors such as atherosclerosis, hypertension, and so forth.[91]

The primary problems associated with progesterone also involve abnormal blood clotting, which may lead to thrombophlebitis, pulmonary embolism, and cerebral infarction.[77,107] Progesterone may alter the normal menstrual cycle, leading to unpredictable changes in the bleeding pattern. The adverse effects of progesterone, however, will vary depending on the exact type of progesterone administered.[107,108]

Hormonal therapies are also associated with an increased risk of certain cancers, but the carcinogenic potential of estrogen and progesterone replacement is not completely clear. Estrogen replacement, for example, may increase the risk of ovarian and endometrial cancers in certain postmenopausal women, but this risk seems to depend on many other factors, including the patient's age, additional cancer risks, prolonged use of estrogen, and concomitant use of progesterone.[109,110]

Certain breast cancers are estrogen sensitive, and estrogen replacement is contraindicated in women with these cancers. However, the risk of developing new breast cancer during hormone therapy is difficult to determine. Some evidence suggests that HRT (estrogen combined with progesterone) may slightly increase the risk of breast cancer.[111] Other reports, including the WHI, suggest that estrogen alone in postmenopausal women does not increase the risk of breast cancer and may even confer a slight reduction in the risk of such cancers.[112] Researchers continue to investigate the exact relationship between various hormone regimens and specific types of cancer and to identify situations where these hormones might be helpful or harmful in people at risk for cancer.

Finally, therapeutic use of estrogen and progesterone may cause nausea, which is usually transient. Swelling of the feet and ankles may also occur because of sodium and water retention.

OTHER DRUGS THAT AFFECT ESTROGEN AND PROGESTERONE ACTIVITY

It is sometimes helpful to stimulate only certain types of estrogen receptors or to block the effects of estrogen and progesterone on specific tissues. Drug strategies that exert such effects include the selective estrogen receptor modulators, antiestrogens, and antiprogestins.

Selective Estrogen Receptor Modulators

Selective estrogen receptor modulators (SERMs) bind to and activate estrogen receptors on certain tissues while blocking the effects of estrogen on other tissues.[113,114] Specifically, these agents activate estrogen receptors on bone and vascular tissues (including plasma lipid receptors) while acting as estrogen antagonists (blockers) on uterine and breast tissues. SERMs therefore have the obvious advantage of producing favorable effects on bone mineralization and cardiovascular function while reducing the potential carcinogenic effects of estrogen on breast and uterine tissues.

Tamoxifen (Nolvadex, Tamofen, others) was the first SERM developed for clinical use; this drug is approved for the prevention and treatment of breast cancer because it has strong antiestrogen effects on breast tissues. The anticancer effect is achieved while simultaneously stimulating other estrogen receptors that help maintain bone mineral density and improve cardiovascular function and plasma lipid profiles.[113] Tamoxifen, however, does not completely block estrogen receptors on uterine tissues and may actually stimulate endometrial proliferation and increase the incidence of uterine cancers.[114,115] However, this agent may lower the risk factors associated with cardiovascular disease (plasma lipid profile, vascular reactivity), but the risk of venous thromboembolism may be increased somewhat.[115] Tamoxifen can also produce symptoms that mimic estrogen withdrawal (hot flashes, vaginitis), especially when it is first administered to women. These symptoms often diminish with continued use. Toremifene (Fareston) is structurally and functionally similar to tamoxifen and is approved for treating breast cancer in postmenopausal women.

Raloxifene (Evista) was the second SERM developed for clinical use, and it is used primarily to prevent and treat osteoporosis in older women. This drug stimulates estrogen receptors on bone and can increase vertebral bone density and reduce the risk of vertebral fractures in postmenopausal women.[116,117] Unlike tamoxifen, raloxifene blocks estrogen receptors on breast *and* uterine tissues and may therefore inhibit breast cancer without increasing the risk of endometrial cancers.[115,118] Raloxifene is therefore also used to reduce the risk of breast and uterine cancers, especially in women with osteoporosis who are at high risk for developing invasive breast cancers.

Raloxifene may cause several bothersome side effects, including hot flashes, joint or muscle pain, depression, insomnia, and GI disturbances. More serious problems with raloxifene may be indicated by symptoms such as chest pain, flulike syndrome, leg cramping, venous thromboembolism, skin rash, and cystitis or urinary tract infections.

Pharmacologists are currently working on other SERMS that mimic the beneficial effects of estrogen while minimizing or even reducing the carcinogenic effects of estrogen on other tissues. As researchers develop newer agents, SERMs may have an expanded role in the treatment of various diseases and perhaps provide a safer and more effective method of estrogen replacement.[113]

Antiestrogens

In addition to the SERMs, a limited number of drugs directly antagonize all the effects of estrogen and are considered to be true antiestrogens. These antiestrogens appear to bind to estrogen receptors in the cytosol but do not cause any subsequent changes in cellular function. Hence, these drugs block the effects of estrogen by occupying the estrogen receptor and preventing estrogen from exerting a response.

Women sometimes receive the antiestrogen Clomiphene (Clomid, Serophene) to treat infertility.[119,120] The mechanism of clomiphene as a fertility drug is somewhat complex. Relatively high levels of estrogen normally produce an inhibitory or negative feedback effect on the release of pituitary gonadotropins (LH and FSH). As an antiestrogen, clomiphene blocks this inhibitory effect, thus facilitating gonadotropin release.[120] Increased gonadotropins (especially LH) promote ovulation, thus improving the chance of fertilization. The primary adverse effects associated with clomiphene are vascular hot flashes. Enlarged ovaries may also occur because of the stimulatory effect of increased gonadotropin release.

More recently, a pharmaceutical company introduced fulvestrant (Faslodex) as an antiestrogen. This drug binds to and blocks estrogen receptors and may also result in the receptors' degradation.[121,122] Hence, fulvestrant treats estrogen-sensitive breast cancers.[121,123] The patient receives a monthly intramuscular injection and some redness and irritation can occur at the injection site. Other common side effects include GI symptoms (nausea, vomiting, loss of appetite) and vasomotor symptoms (hot flashes).

Antiprogestins

Agents that specifically block progesterone receptors were first developed in the early 1980s.[124] The primary clinical application of these drugs is the termination of pregnancy; these drugs can induce abortion during the early stages of gestation. Because progesterone is largely responsible for sustaining the placenta and fetus, the blockade of progesterone receptors in the uterus negates the effects of this hormone, with subsequent detachment of the placenta and loss of placental hormones such as human chorionic gonadotropin. Detachment of the placenta from the uterine lining results in loss of the fetus and termination of the pregnancy.

The primary antiprogestin is mifepristone, known also as RU486.[125] This drug must be administered orally during the first 7 weeks of pregnancy, with abortion typically occurring within the next 2 to 3 days. To stimulate uterine contraction and ensure complete expulsion of the detached embryo, a prostaglandin analog such as misoprostol or prostaglandin E_1 is typically administered orally or intravaginally 24 to 48 hours after mifepristone administration.[126] This regimen of mifepristone followed by a prostaglandin agent is successful in terminating pregnancy in approximately 95 percent of cases.[127]

When used to induce abortion, the primary physical side effects of mifepristone are excessive uterine bleeding and cramping, although these side effects may be related more to the use of prostaglandins following mifepristone treatment.[128] The chance of incomplete abortion must also be considered, and a follow-up physician visit approximately 2 weeks after administration is needed to ensure that the pregnancy was fully terminated.

Mifepristone has received considerable attention worldwide because of its use to terminate pregnancy. The drug may likewise be useful as a "morning after" pill to prevent conception after unprotected sex (see "Types of Contraceptive Preparations").[129] Mifepristone may have potential as a contraceptive drug because it prevents ovulation and blocks the effects of progesterone on endometrial proliferation and vascularization, thus rendering the endometrium less favorable for implantation of the fertilized egg. The drug, however, is not widely used as a contraceptive because the effects are somewhat unpredictable, and specific doses must be administered to achieve certain contraceptive effects.[124]

However, mifepristone may also have other beneficial effects that are related to its ability to block progesterone receptors. For example, it can decrease pain and bleeding caused by benign uterine fibroid growths (leiomyomas), and it can also treat endometriois.[124,130] In addition to its effects on progesterone receptors, mifepristone can also block cellular glucocorticoid receptors. This drug can therefore be used to treat conditions caused by excessive glucocorticoid production (Cushing syndrome).[131,132] In fact, mifepristone is marketed in the United States under the trade name Korlym and is approved only for preventing hyperglycemia caused by excess cortisol production in Cushing syndrome or other conditions that increase glucocorticoid synthesis. Mifepristone may therefore have several clinical applications beyond its primary use in terminating pregnancy, and it will be interesting to see if this drug will ultimately be accepted as a common treatment for other conditions related to progesterone and glucocorticoids.

HORMONAL CONTRACEPTIVES

During the 1960s, the Food and Drug Administration (FDA) approved oral contraceptives containing estrogens and progestins for use in preventing pregnancy. The introduction of these birth control pills provided a relatively easy and effective method of contraception. Today, oral contraceptives are taken routinely by many women of child-bearing age, and they are among the most commonly prescribed medications in the United States and throughout the world.[133,134] Hormonal alternatives to oral contraceptives are also gaining popularity, and administration of various compounds by injection, transdermal patch, subcutaneous implants, vaginal inserts, and intrauterine devices are now available.

Types of Contraceptive Preparations

The most common form of hormonal preparation is the "birth control pill," which typically contains a fixed amount of estrogen and progesterone in each dose. Examples of some common estrogen-progestin contraceptives are listed in Table 30-6. When taken appropriately, these preparations appear to be 99 to 100 percent effective in preventing pregnancy.[135] Typically, the contraceptive pill is taken each day for 3 weeks, beginning at the onset of menstruation. This intake is followed by 1 week in which either no pill or a "blank" pill that lacks the hormones is taken. For convenience and improved adherence, these preparations are usually packaged in some form of dispenser that encourages the user to remember to take one pill each day.

More recently, a variation on the length of the oral contraceptive cycle was introduced in which women take the active form of the pill for 84 days and then take a 7-day placebo.[136,137] This provides a 3-month cycle before menstruation, thus reducing the number of menstrual periods to only 4 per year. These long cycle regimens seem to be as effective as the more traditional (monthly) cycle regimens, although the longer cycles may cause more unscheduled bleeding or "spotting," especially during the first few cycles.[137] Still, long cycle regimens may be preferred by some women because they offer the convenience of fewer periods and menstrual symptoms (cramps, etc.).[136]

Contraceptive hormones can also be administered via nonoral routes. A contraceptive patch containing ethinyl estradiol (an estrogen) and norelgestromin (a progestin) applied to the skin once a week allows the slow, transdermal administration of the hormones.[138] A vaginal ring is also available as an alternative to the oral contraceptive pill.[139] This ring typically contains estrogen and progesterone, which are released slowly into the vagina and local tissues following insertion. The ring is inserted vaginally for 3 weeks and then removed for 1 week to allow menstruation (i.e., it mimics the normal uterine cycle).[139] Transdermal patches and vaginal rings are similar to oral contraceptives in terms of effectiveness and side effects.[140] The primary advantages of the nonoral routes are increased convenience and adherence to the contraceptive regimen; the use of patches or a vaginal ring can be very helpful in women who sometimes forget to take a pill every day.[139,140]

Other versions of oral contraceptives are available that contain only a progestin (norethindrone, norgestrel; see Table 30-6). These "minipills" were developed to avoid the adverse effects normally attributed to

Table 30-6
HORMONAL CONTRACEPTIVES*

Estrogen Component	Progestin Component	Common Trade Name(s)
Oral Contraceptives		
Ethinyl estradiol	Desogestrel	Desogen, Mircette, Ortho-Cept, others
Ethinyl estradiol	Drospirenone	Yasmin, Yaz
Ethinyl estradiol	Ethynodiol diacetate	Demulen, Zovia
Ethinyl estradiol	Levonorgestrel	Alesse, Levlen, Nordette, Triphasil, others
Ethinyl estradiol	Norethindrone	Brevicon, Femcon FE, Loestrin, Ortho-Novum, many others
Ethinyl estradiol	Norgestimate	Ortho-Cyclen, Sprintec, others
Ethinyl estradiol	Norgestrel	Lo/Ovral, Ovral
Mestranol	Norethindrone	Genora 1/50, Norinyl 1+50, Ortho-Novum 1/50, others
None	Norethindrone	Micronor, Nor-QD
None	Norgestrel	Ovrette
Nonoral Contraceptives		
Ethinyl estradiol	Norelgestromin	Ortho Evra (transdermal patch)
Ethinyl estradiol	Etonogestrel	NuvaRing (vaginal ring)
None	Levonorgestrel	Norplant system (intrauterine device)
	Medroxyprogesterone	Depo-Provera (intramuscular injection)
Emergency Contraception		
None	Levonorgestrel	Plan B
None	Ulipristal	Ella

**Doses of estrogen and progesterone and sequence of each dose vary according to the specific product.*

estrogen. Progestin-only minipills are somewhat less attractive as an oral contraceptive because these preparations are only about 97 to 98 percent effective and because they tend to cause irregular and unpredictable menstrual cycles. Pharmacologists originally developed an implantable form of a progestin-only preparation (Norplant), whereby small, semipermeable tubes containing levonorgestrel were inserted subcutaneously in the arm.[141] This method of progestin delivery was discontinued in the United States and many other countries because of relatively poor contraceptive effectiveness and unacceptable side effects. However, there is a form of progesterone (medroxyprogesterone acetate, Depo-Provera) that can be administered by deep intramuscular injection every 12 weeks.[142] Also, an intrauterine device that slowly releases a progestin within the uterus is available.[143] These implantable and injectable forms of progesterone offer alternatives to women who cannot tolerate estrogen-progesterone pills or who have difficulty adhering to traditional oral contraceptive regimens.

Oral contraceptives that contain various hormones are sometimes used as "emergency" contraceptives after sexual intercourse, especially in specific situations such as rape or unprotected sex. Traditionally, these emergency interventions, or "morning-after pills," consisted of a high dose of a natural or synthetic estrogen, a progestin such as levonorgestrel, or estrogen combined with a progestin (e.g., ethinyl estradiol combined with norgestrel). The exact mechanism of these morning-after pills is not known, but they appear to somehow interfere with ovulation or make the endometrium less favorable for implantation.[144,145] As indicated earlier, some countries allow the use of the progesterone receptor blocker mifepristone for emergency contraception because it inhibits ovulation and blocks progesterone receptors in the uterus, thereby negating the effects of progesterone on the endometrium and developing placenta.[129]

At the present time, a preparation containing levonorgestrel (Plan B) is marketed in the United States as an emergency contraceptive and can be obtained without a prescription (see Table 30-6). In addition, the FDA has approved ulipristal (Ella) as a prescription method for emergency contraception.[146,147] This drug is a selective progesterone receptor modulator; it activates certain progesterone receptors while blocking or inhibiting other progesterone receptors.[148] Ulipristal probably exerts its primary contraceptive effects by inhibiting the progesterone receptors that affect ovulation and endometrial function, thereby reducing the chance that an egg will be released or have a suitable environment for implantation in the uterus.[144,148] Hence, several options exist for preventing pregnancy after sexual intercourse. Although these pills can be helpful in emergency situations, they are not meant to be an alternative to the regular methods of pharmacological contraception described earlier.

Mechanism of Contraceptive Action

Hormonal contraceptives exert their effects primarily by inhibiting ovulation and impairing the normal development of the uterine endometrium.[138,149] As discussed previously, the normal menstrual cycle is governed by the complex interaction between endogenous ovarian hormones and the pituitary gonadotropins. High levels of estrogen and progesterone in the bloodstream act as negative feedback and inhibit the release of LH and FSH from the anterior pituitary. Hormonal contraceptives maintain fairly high plasma levels of estrogen and progestin, thus limiting the release of LH and FSH through this negative feedback system. Because ovulation is normally caused by the midcycle LH surge (see Fig. 30-2), inhibition of LH release prevents ovulation. This event prevents an ovum from being made available for fertilization.

The estrogen and progestin supplied by the contraceptive also affect the development of the uterine lining. These hormones promote a certain amount of growth and proliferation of the uterine endometrium. The endometrium, however, does not develop to quite the same extent or in quite the same manner as it would if it were controlled by normal endogenous hormonal release. Consequently, the endometrial environment is less than optimal for implantation, even if ovulation and fertilization should take place. Also, there is an increase in the thickness and viscosity of the mucous secretions in the uterine cervix, thus impeding the passage of sperm through the cervical region, which adds to these preparations' contraceptive efficacy.

Through the effects on the endometrium, contraceptive regimens can be used to mimic a normal menstrual flow. When the contraceptive hormones are withdrawn, the endometrium undergoes a sloughing similar to that in the normal cycle. Of course, the endometrium is being regulated by the exogenous hormones rather than the estrogen and progesterone normally produced by the ovaries. Still, this method of administration and withdrawal can produce a more or less normal pattern of uterine activity, with the exception that chances of conception are dramatically reduced.

Adverse Effects of Hormonal Contraceptives

Although hormonal contraceptives provide an easy and effective means of birth control, their use has been limited somewhat by potentially serious side effects. In particular, contraceptive medications have been associated with cardiovascular problems such as venous thrombosis, ischemic stroke, and myocardial infarction.[150,151] Cardiovascular risks were certainly more prevalent in the original or "first-generation" versions of oral contraceptives, where these products contained relatively higher amounts of estrogen and different forms of progestins compared to more modern products.[135,152]

Over the years, the estrogen-progestin combinations in oral contraceptives have been modified so that they are safer and better tolerated than their predecessors but are still able to provide excellent contraceptive effects.[133,153,154] For example, the risk of certain cardiovascular problems, such as myocardial infarction and ischemic stroke, seem to be substantially lower than in the past.[151] Risk of venous thromboembolism is also relatively lower with the more modern forms of oral contraceptives, but this risk seems to vary greatly depending on the amount of estrogen and type of progestin in each product.[155,156] In particular, the progesterone component seems to be an important factor influencing the risk of venous thromboembolism, with some of the newest products (third- and fourth-generation oral contraceptives) containing a type of progestin that may actually have a higher risk of venous thrombosis than earlier (second-generation) oral contraceptives.[155]

Clearly, oral contraceptives have some potential to impair normal hemostasis and lead to venous thromboembolism and arterial thrombosis.[150,152] This risk is relatively modest if estrogen-progesterone preparations are taken by relatively healthy young women.[157] Likewise, the incidence of cardiovascular problems depends to some extent on whether the user has other risk factors associated with cardiovascular disease (hyperlipidemia, hypertension, smoking cigarettes, personal history of venous or arterial thrombosis, etc.).[158] Hence, each woman should be evaluated before being prescribed a hormonal contraceptive, and selection of a product should be based on any potential risk factors that might increase the chance of venous or arterial thrombosis.[157,158]

There has been some indication that hormonal contraceptives may lead to certain forms of cancer. Some early versions of the pill were believed to cause tumors of the endometrium of the uterus. Early forms that were sequential in nature may have caused this effect—that is, they provided only estrogen for the first half of the menstrual cycle and estrogen combined with progesterone for the second half. However, the newer combined forms that supply both hormones throughout the cycle do not appear to increase the risk of uterine cancer. In fact, it appears that modern forms of oral contraceptives actually *decrease* the risk of endometrial cancer, as well as prevent other forms of cancer, including ovarian.[159,160]

The carcinogenic properties of hormonal contraceptives have not been totally ruled out, however. The effects on breast cancer remain controversial, and the possibility exists that certain subgroups of women may have an increased risk of breast cancer, depending on factors such as how long they used the pill, their age, genetic predisposition, and so forth.[161,162] There is also considerable evidence that prolonged use of oral contraceptives (more than 8 years) may increase the risk of liver cancer.[161,163] Nonetheless, the overall incidence of cancer in women taking oral contraceptives is relatively low. Women who are concerned about the risk of specific cancers should consult their physician and discuss possible ways to minimize these risks.

Hormonal contraceptives can cause several other less serious but bothersome side effects. Problems such as nausea, loss of appetite, abdominal cramping, headache, dizziness, weight gain, and fatigue are fairly common. These symptoms are often transient and may diminish following continued use.

The serious risks associated with hormonal contraceptives have diminished considerably since their initial appearance on the market, but these drugs are not without some hazards. In general, it is a good policy to reserve this form of birth control for relatively young, healthy women who do not smoke cigarettes or have other risk factors for cardiovascular disease. Avoiding continuous, prolonged administration to diminish the risk of liver cancer may also be prudent. Finally, any increase in the other side effects associated with hormonal contraceptives, such as headache and abdominal discomfort, should be carefully evaluated to rule out a more serious underlying problem.

CASE STUDY

MALE AND FEMALE HORMONES

Brief History. S.K., a 32-year-old woman, sustained a whiplash injury during a motor vehicle accident. She was undergoing physical therapy as an outpatient for management of neck pain, decreased cervical range of motion, and cervicogenic headaches. The patient took an oral muscle relaxant (carisoprodol) for the neck pain and an over-the-counter acetaminophen product as needed. During the initial examination/evaluation, the therapist queried the patient about other medications, and the patient reported taking an oral contraceptive containing an estrogen (ethinyl estradiol, 0.05 mg) and a progestin (norgestrel, 0.5 mg). This contraceptive facilitated traditional monthly cycles (3 weeks of the active pill, 1 week of placebo); she had been taking this product continuously for the past 11 years. The patient also smoked cigarettes, and she had recently increased cigarette use following the neck injury.

Continued on following page

CASE STUDY (Continued)

Problem/Influence of Medication. Approximately 2 weeks after beginning treatment (i.e., during the fourth therapy session), the patient reported an increase in headache pain. This finding surprised the therapist because the patient's neck pain and cervical function had been steadily improving. Upon further examination, the patient also reported a dull ache and tightness in the right calf, which was exacerbated by active and passive ankle dorsiflexion. Her calf appeared slightly swollen and was tender to palpation. She also mentioned having leg cramps for the last night or two when trying to fall asleep.

1. ***What concerns should the therapist have about this patient's recent symptoms?***
2. ***What should the therapist do about these concerns?***
3. ***What additional medical interventions might be considered in this case?***

See Appendix C, "Answers to Case Study Questions."

Special Concerns for Rehabilitation Patients

Therapists should be cognizant of the adverse effects related to the estrogens, progesterones, and androgens so that they may help recognize problems related to these compounds. For instance, therapists should routinely monitor blood pressure during therapeutic administration of the sex hormones. These compounds tend to promote salt and water retention (mineralocorticoid-like properties), which may promote hypertension.

Therapists can play an important role in educating patients about the dangers of androgen abuse. Physical therapists who treat athletes are in an excellent position to serve as a source of information about anabolic steroids. Therapists should advise athletes about the potential side effects, such as liver, cardiovascular, and reproductive abnormalities. Therapists can also monitor blood pressure in athletes who appear to be using androgenic steroids. This interaction may help prevent a hypertensive crisis and may illustrate to the athlete the harmful effects of these drugs.

SUMMARY

The male hormones are the androgens, and the female hormones are the estrogens and progestins. These steroid hormones are primarily involved in the control of reproduction and sexual maturation. Male and female hormones also serve several important pharmacological functions. These agents are often used as replacement therapy to resolve deficiencies in endogenous endocrine function. Androgens and estrogens and/or progestins are administered for a variety of other therapeutic reasons, including the control of some neoplastic diseases. Estrogens and progestins are administered extensively to women as effective contraceptive agents. Finally, athletes sometimes use androgens in high doses in an attempt to increase muscle strength and performance. Although these drugs may produce increments in muscle strength in some individuals, the dangers of using high doses of anabolic steroids outweigh any potential ergogenic benefits.

REFERENCES

1. Page ST. Physiologic role and regulation of intratesticular sex steroids. *Curr Opin Endocrinol Diabetes Obes*. 2011;18:217-223.
2. Ye L, Su ZJ, Ge RS. Inhibitors of testosterone biosynthetic and metabolic activation enzymes. *Molecules*. 2011;16:9983-10001.
3. Chen H, Ge RS, Zirkin BR. Leydig cells: From stem cells to aging. *Mol Cell Endocrinol*. 2009;306:9-16.
4. Midzak AS, Chen H, Papadopoulos V, Zirkin BR. Leydig cell aging and the mechanisms of reduced testosterone synthesis. *Mol Cell Endocrinol*. 2009;299:23-31.
5. Loss ES, Jacobus AP, Wassermann GF. Rapid signaling responses in Sertoli cell membranes induced by follicle stimulating hormone and testosterone: calcium inflow and electrophysiological changes. *Life Sci*. 2011;89:577-583.
6. Walker WH, Cheng J. FSH and testosterone signaling in Sertoli cells. *Reproduction*. 2005;130:15-28.
7. Hammond GL. Diverse roles for sex hormone-binding globulin in reproduction. *Biol Reprod*. 2011;85:431-441.
8. Griffeth RJ, Carretero J, Burks DJ. Insulin receptor substrate 2 is required for testicular development. *PLoS One*. 2013;8:e62103.
9. Maggi M, Buvat J, Corona G, et al. Hormonal causes of male sexual dysfunctions and their management (hyperprolactinemia, thyroid disorders, GH disorders, and DHEA). *J Sex Med*. 2013;10:661-677.
10. Maeda K, Ohkura S, Uenoyama Y, et al. Neurobiological mechanisms underlying GnRH pulse generation by the hypothalamus. *Brain Res*. 2010;1364:103-115.
11. Matsumoto AM, Bremner WJ. Testicular disorders. In: Melmed S, et al, eds. *Williams Textbook of Endocrinology*. 12th ed. Philadelphia, PA: Saunders/Elsevier; 2011.
12. Angelopoulou R, Lavranos G, Manolakou P, Katsiki E. Fertility in the aging male: molecular pathways in the anthropology of aging. *Coll Antropol*. 2013;37:657-661.
13. Bennett NC, Gardiner RA, Hooper JD, et al. Molecular cell biology of androgen receptor signalling. *Int J Biochem Cell Biol*. 2010;42:813-827.
14. Ni L, Llewellyn R, Kesler CT, et al. Androgen induces a switch in the androgen receptor from cytoplasmic retention to nuclear import. *Mol Cell Biol*. 2013;33:4766-4778.
15. Wang RS, Yeh S, Tzeng CR, Chang C. Androgen receptor roles in spermatogenesis and fertility: lessons from testicular cell-specific androgen receptor knockout mice. *Endocr Rev*. 2009;30:119-132.
16. Basaria S. Male hypogonadism. *Lancet*. 2014;383:1250-1263.
17. King TF, Hayes FJ. Long-term outcome of idiopathic hypogonadotropic hypogonadism. *Curr Opin Endocrinol Diabetes Obes*. 2012;19:204-210.
18. Corona G, Rastrelli G, Maggi M. Diagnosis and treatment of late-onset hypogonadism: systematic review and meta-analysis of TRT outcomes. *Best Pract Res Clin Endocrinol Metab*. 2013;27:557-579.
19. Cunningham GR. Andropause or male menopause? Rationale for testosterone replacement therapy in older men with low testosterone levels. *Endocr Pract*. 2013;19:847-852.
20. Strollo F, Strollo G, Morè M, et al. Low-intermediate dose testosterone replacement therapy by different pharmaceutical preparations improves frailty score in elderly hypogonadal hyperglycaemic patients. *Aging Male*. 2013;16:33-37.
21. Corona G, Vignozzi L, Sforza A, Maggi M. Risks and benefits of late onset hypogonadism treatment: an expert opinion. *World J Mens Health*. 2013;31:103-125.
22. Staerman F, Léon P. Andropause (androgen deficiency of the aging male): diagnosis and management. *Minerva Med*. 2012; 103:333-342.
23. Biundo B. Treatment options for male hypogonadism. *Int J Pharm Compd*. 2013;17:28-38.
24. Zirkin BR, Tenover JL. Aging and declining testosterone: past, present, and hopes for the future. *J Androl*. 2012;33:1111-1118.
25. Gullett NP, Hebbar G, Ziegler TR. Update on clinical trials of growth factors and anabolic steroids in cachexia and wasting. *Am J Clin Nutr*. 2010;91:1143S-1147S.
26. Woerdeman J, de Ronde W. Therapeutic effects of anabolic androgenic steroids on chronic diseases associated with muscle wasting. *Expert Opin Investig Drugs*. 2011;20:87-97.
27. Maggio M, Nicolini F, Cattabiani C, et al. Effects of testosterone supplementation on clinical and rehabilitative outcomes in older men undergoing on-pump CABG. *Contemp Clin Trials*. 2012;33:730-738.
28. Blick G. Optimal diagnostic measures and thresholds for hypogonadism in men with HIV/AIDS: comparison between 2 transdermal testosterone replacement therapy gels. *Postgrad Med*. 2013;125:30-39.
29. Blick G, Khera M, Bhattacharya RK, et al. Testosterone replacement therapy in men with hypogonadism and HIV/AIDS: results from the TRiUS registry. *Postgrad Med*. 2013;125: 19-29.
30. Johns K, Beddall MJ, Corrin RC. Anabolic steroids for the treatment of weight loss in HIV-infected individuals. *Cochrane Database Syst Rev*. 2005;4:CD005483.
31. Orr R, Fiatarone Singh M. The anabolic androgenic steroid oxandrolone in the treatment of wasting and catabolic disorders: review of efficacy and safety. *Drugs*. 2004;64:725-750.
32. Ambler GR. Androgen therapy for delayed male puberty. *Curr Opin Endocrinol Diabetes Obes*. 2009;16:232-239.
33. Shahani S, Braga-Basaria M, Maggio M, Basaria S. Androgens and erythropoiesis: past and present. *J Endocrinol Invest*. 2009;32:704-716.
34. Hörl WH. Differentiating factors between erythropoiesis-stimulating agents: an update to selection for anaemia of chronic kidney disease. *Drugs*. 2013;73:117-130.
35. Xu YY, Buyantseva LV, Agarwal NS, et al. Update on treatment of hereditary angioedema. *Clin Exp Allergy*. 2013;43:395-405.
36. Banerji A, Sloane DE, Sheffer AL. Hereditary angioedema: a current state-of-the-art review, V: attenuated androgens for the treatment of hereditary angioedema. *Ann Allergy Asthma Immunol*. 2008;100(suppl 2):S19-22.
37. de Ronde W. Hyperandrogenism after transfer of topical testosterone gel: case report and review of published and unpublished studies. *Hum Reprod*. 2009;24:425-428.
38. Eliakim A, Cale-Benzoor M, Klinger-Cantor B, et al. A case study of virilizing adrenal tumor in an adolescent female elite tennis player—insight into the use of anabolic steroids in young athletes. *J Strength Cond Res*. 2011;25:46-50.
39. Mohler ML, Coss CC, Duke CB 3rd, et al. Androgen receptor antagonists: a patent review (2008-2011). *Expert Opin Ther Pat*. 2012;22:541-565.
40. Menon MP, Higano CS. Enzalutamide, a second generation androgen receptor antagonist: development and clinical applications in prostate cancer. *Curr Oncol Rep*. 2013;15:69-75.

41. Reismann P, Likó I, Igaz P, et al. Pharmacological options for treatment of hyperandrogenic disorders. *Mini Rev Med Chem.* 2009;9:1113-1126.
42. Limonta P, Manea M. Gonadotropin-releasing hormone receptors as molecular therapeutic targets in prostate cancer: current options and emerging strategies. *Cancer Treat Rev.* 2013;39: 647-663.
43. Van Poppel H, Klotz L. Gonadotropin-releasing hormone: an update review of the antagonists versus agonists. *Int J Urol.* 2012;19:594-601.
44. Kanayama G, Pope HG Jr. Illicit use of androgens and other hormones: recent advances. *Curr Opin Endocrinol Diabetes Obes.* 2012;19:211-219.
45. Melnik BC. Androgen abuse in the community. *Curr Opin Endocrinol Diabetes Obes.* 2009;16:218-223.
46. Fitch KD. Androgenic-anabolic steroids and the Olympic Games. *Asian J Androl.* 2008;10:384-390.
47. Basaria S. Androgen abuse in athletes: detection and consequences. *J Clin Endocrinol Metab.* 2010;95:1533-1543.
48. Kerr JM, Congeni JA. Anabolic-androgenic steroids: use and abuse in pediatric patients. *Pediatr Clin North Am.* 2007;54: 771-785.
49. Rosenfield C. The use of ergogenic agents in high school athletes. *J Sch Nurs.* 2005;21:333-339.
50. Cordaro FG, Lombardo S, Cosentino M. Selling androgenic anabolic steroids by the pound: identification and analysis of popular websites on the Internet. *Scand J Med Sci Sports.* 2011;21:e247-259.
51. Hall RC, Hall RC. Abuse of supraphysiologic doses of anabolic steroids. *South Med J.* 2005;98:550-555.
52. Thevis M, Kuuranne T, Geyer H, Schänzer W. Annual banned-substance review: analytical approaches in human sports drug testing. *Drug Test Anal.* 2013;5:1-19.
53. Hartgens F, Kuipers H. Effects of androgenic-anabolic steroids in athletes. *Sports Med.* 2004;34:513-554.
54. Lippi G, Franchini M, Banfi G. Biochemistry and physiology of anabolic androgenic steroids doping. *Mini Rev Med Chem.* 2011;11:362-373.
55. Cunningham RL, Lumia AR, McGinnis MY. Androgenic anabolic steroid exposure during adolescence: ramifications for brain development and behavior. *Horm Behav.* 2013;64:350-356.
56. Turillazzi E, Perilli G, Di Paolo M, et al. Side effects of AAS abuse: an overview. *Mini Rev Med Chem.* 2011;11:374-389.
57. Dodge T, Hoagland MF. The use of anabolic androgenic steroids and polypharmacy: a review of the literature. *Drug Alcohol Depend.* 2011;114:100-109.
58. de Souza GL, Hallak J. Anabolic steroids and male infertility: a comprehensive review. *BJU Int.* 2011;108:1860-1865.
59. Vanberg P, Atar D. Androgenic anabolic steroid abuse and the cardiovascular system. *Handb Exp Pharmacol.* 2010;195:411-457
60. Modlinski R, Fields KB. The effect of anabolic steroids on the gastrointestinal system, kidneys, and adrenal glands. *Curr Sports Med Rep.* 2006;5:104-109.
61. Socas L, Zumbado M, Pérez-Luzardo O, et al. Hepatocellular adenomas associated with anabolic androgenic steroid abuse in bodybuilders: a report of two cases and a review of the literature. *Br J Sports Med.* 2005;39:e27.
62. Montisci M, El Mazloum R, Cecchetto G, et al. Anabolic androgenic steroids abuse and cardiac death in athletes: morphological and toxicological findings in four fatal cases. *Forensic Sci Int.* 2012;217:e13-18.
63. Nascimento JH, Medei E. Cardiac effects of anabolic steroids: hypertrophy, ischemia and electrical remodelling as potential triggers of sudden death. *Mini Rev Med Chem.* 2011;11:425-429.
64. Achar S, Rostamian A, Narayan SM. Cardiac and metabolic effects of anabolic-androgenic steroid abuse on lipids, blood pressure, left ventricular dimensions, and rhythm. *Am J Cardiol.* 2010;106:893-901.
65. Higgins JP, Heshmat A, Higgins CL. Androgen abuse and increased cardiac risk. *South Med J.* 2012;105:670-674.
66. Geraci MJ, Cole M, Davis P. New onset diabetes associated with bovine growth hormone and testosterone abuse in a young body builder. *Hum Exp Toxicol.* 2011;30:2007-2012.
67. Pettine KA. Association of anabolic steroids and avascular necrosis of femoral heads. *Am J Sports Med.* 1991;19:96-98.
68. Beaver KM, Vaughn MG, Delisi M, Wright JP. Anabolic-androgenic steroid use and involvement in violent behavior in a nationally representative sample of young adult males in the United States. *Am J Public Health.* 2008;98:2185-2187.
69. Oberlander JG, Henderson LP. The Sturm und Drang of anabolic steroid use: angst, anxiety, and aggression. *Trends Neurosci.* 2012;35:382-392.
70. Moretti E, Collodel G, La Marca A, et al. Structural sperm and aneuploidies studies in a case of spermatogenesis recovery after the use of androgenic anabolic steroids. *J Assist Reprod Genet.* 2007;24:195-198.
71. Boregowda K, Joels L, Stephens JW, Price DE. Persistent primary hypogonadism associated with anabolic steroid abuse. *Fertil Steril.* 2011;96:e7-8.
72. Kersey RD, Elliot DL, Goldberg L, et al. National Athletic Trainers' Association position statement: anabolic-androgenic steroids. *J Athl Train.* 2012;47:567-588.
73. Berga S, Naftolin F. Neuroendocrine control of ovulation. *Gynecol Endocrinol.* 2012;28(suppl 1):9-13.
74. Henriet P, Gaide Chevronnay HP, Marbaix E. The endocrine and paracrine control of menstruation. *Mol Cell Endocrinol.* 2012;358:197-207.
75. Jabbour HN, Kelly RW, Fraser HM, Critchley HO. Endocrine regulation of menstruation. *Endocr Rev.* 2006;27:17-46.
76. Cole LA. Biological functions of hCG and hCG-related molecules. *Reprod Biol Endocrinol.* 2010;8:102.
77. de Villiers TJ, Stevenson JC. The WHI: the effect of hormone replacement therapy on fracture prevention. Climacteric. 2012;15:263-266.
78. Eriksen EF. Hormone replacement therapy or SERMS in the long term treatment of osteoporosis. Minerva Ginecol. 2012;64:207-221.
79. Marjoribanks J, Farquhar C, Roberts H, Lethaby A. Long term hormone therapy for perimenopausal and postmenopausal women. Cochrane Database Syst Rev. 2012;7:CD004143.
80. Bowring CE, Francis RM. National Osteoporosis Society's Position statement on hormone replacement therapy in the prevention and treatment of osteoporosis. Menopause Int. 2011;17: 63-65.
81. Gallagher JC, Levine JP. Preventing osteoporosis in symptomatic postmenopausal women. Menopause. 2011;18:109-118.
82. Christenson ES, Jiang X, Kagan R, Schnatz P. Osteoporosis management in post-menopausal women. Minerva Ginecol. 2012;64:181-194.
83. Lin JT, Lane JM. Nonpharmacologic management of osteoporosis to minimize fracture risk. Nat Clin Pract Rheumatol. 2008;4:20-25.

84. Archer DF, Sturdee DW, Baber R, et al. Menopausal hot flushes and night sweats: where are we now? *Climacteric*. 2011; 14:515-528.
85. Davey DA. Update: estrogen and estrogen plus progestin therapy in the care of women at and after the menopause. *Womens Health*. 2012;8:169-189.
86. Langer RD. Efficacy, safety, and tolerability of low-dose hormone therapy in managing menopausal symptoms. *J Am Board Fam Med*. 2009;22:563-573.
87. Lynch C. Vaginal estrogen therapy for the treatment of atrophic vaginitis. *J Womens Health*. 2009;18:1595-1606.
88. Main C, Knight B, Moxham T, et al. Hormone therapy for preventing cardiovascular disease in post-menopausal women. *Cochrane Database Syst Rev*. 2013;4:CD002229.
89. Hodis HN, Mack WJ. The timing hypothesis and hormone replacement therapy: a paradigm shift in the primary prevention of coronary heart disease in women. Part 1: comparison of therapeutic efficacy. *J Am Geriatr Soc*. 2013;61:1005-1010.
90. Manson JE. The role of personalized medicine in identifying appropriate candidates for menopausal estrogen therapy. *Metabolism*. 2013;62(suppl 1):S15-19.
91. Shoupe D. Individualizing hormone-therapy according to cardiovascular risk. *Minerva Med*. 2012;103:343-352.
92. de Villiers TJ, Gass ML, Haines CJ, et al. Global consensus statement on menopausal hormone therapy. *Climacteric*. 2013; 16:203-204.
93. Henderson VW. Action of estrogens in the aging brain: dementia and cognitive aging. *Biochim Biophys Acta*. 2010;1800: 1077-1083.
94. Baudry M, Bi X, Aguirre C. Progesterone-estrogen interactions in synaptic plasticity and neuroprotection. *Neuroscience*. 2013;239:280-294.
95. Mukai H, Kimoto T, Hojo Y, et al. Modulation of synaptic plasticity by brain estrogen in the hippocampus. *Biochim Biophys Acta*. 2010;1800:1030-1044.
96. Yao J, Brinton RD. Estrogen regulation of mitochondrial bioenergetics: implications for prevention of Alzheimer's disease. *Adv Pharmacol*. 2012;64:327-371.
97. Shumaker SA, Legault C, Rapp SR, et al. Estrogen plus progestin and the incidence of dementia and mild cognitive impairment in postmenopausal women: the Women's Health Initiative Memory Study: a randomized controlled trial. *JAMA*. 2003;289:2651-2662.
98. Maki PM. Minireview: effects of different HT formulations on cognition. *Endocrinology*. 2012;153:3564-3570.
99. Maki PM, Henderson VW. Hormone therapy, dementia, and cognition: the Women's Health Initiative 10 years on. *Climacteric*. 2012;15:256-262.
100. Mueck AO. Postmenopausal hormone replacement therapy and cardiovascular disease: the value of transdermal estradiol and micronized progesterone. *Climacteric*. 2012;15(suppl 1):11-17.
101. Studd J. Treatment of premenstrual disorders by suppression of ovulation by transdermal estrogens. *Menopause Int*. 2012;18:65-67.
102. Nappi RE, Albani F, Chiovato L, Polatti F. Local estrogens for quality of life and sexuality in postmenopausal women with cardiovascular disease. *Climacteric*. 2009;12(suppl 1): 112-116.
103. Panay N, Maamari R. Treatment of postmenopausal vaginal atrophy with 10-μg estradiol vaginal tablets. *Menopause Int*. 2012;18:15-19.
104. Archer DF, Oger E. Estrogen and progestogen effect on venous thromboembolism in menopausal women. *Climacteric*. 2012;15: 235-240.
105. Sandset PM. Mechanisms of hormonal therapy related thrombosis. *Thromb Res*. 2013;131(suppl 1):S4-7.
106. Henderson VW, Lobo RA. Hormone therapy and the risk of stroke: perspectives 10 years after the Women's Health Initiative trials. *Climacteric*. 2012;15:229-234.
107. Bernstein P, Pohost G. Progesterone, progestins, and the heart. *Rev Cardiovasc Med*. 2010;11:228-236.
108. Stanczyk FZ, Hapgood JP, Winer S, Mishell DR Jr. Progestogens used in postmenopausal hormone therapy: differences in their pharmacological properties, intracellular actions, and clinical effects. *Endocr Rev*. 2013;34:171-208.
109. Furness S, Roberts H, Marjoribanks J, Lethaby A. Hormone therapy in postmenopausal women and risk of endometrial hyperplasia. *Cochrane Database Syst Rev*. 2012;8:CD000402.
110. Ulrich LS. Endometrial cancer, types, prognosis, female hormones and antihormones. *Climacteric*. 2011;14:418-425.
111. Santen RJ, Allred DC, Ardoin SP, et al. Postmenopausal hormone therapy: an Endocrine Society scientific statement. *J Clin Endocrinol Metab*. 2010;95(suppl 1):s1-s66.
112. Lobo RA. Where are we 10 years after the Women's Health Initiative? *J Clin Endocrinol Metab*. 2013;98:1771-1180.
113. Maximov PY, Lee TM, Jordan VC. The discovery and development of selective estrogen receptor modulators (SERMs) for clinical practice. *Curr Clin Pharmacol*. 2013;8:135-155.
114. Silverman SL. New selective estrogen receptor modulators (SERMs) in development. *Curr Osteoporos Rep*. 2010;8:151-153.
115. Nelson HD, Smith ME, Griffin JC, Fu R. Use of medications to reduce risk for primary breast cancer: a systematic review for the U.S. Preventive Services Task Force. *Ann Intern Med*. 2013;158:604-614.
116. D'Amelio P, Isaia GC. The use of raloxifene in osteoporosis treatment. *Expert Opin Pharmacother*. 2013;14:949-956.
117. Ko SS, Jordan VC. Treatment of osteoporosis and reduction in risk of invasive breast cancer in postmenopausal women with raloxifene. *Expert Opin Pharmacother*. 2011;12:657-674.
118. Hadji P. The evolution of selective estrogen receptor modulators in osteoporosis therapy. *Climacteric*. 2012;15:513-523.
119. Brown J, Farquhar C, Beck J, et al. Clomiphene and antioestrogens for ovulation induction in PCOS. *Cochrane Database Syst Rev*. 2009;4:CD002249.
120. Wilkes S, Murdoch A. Ovulation induction with clomifene: a primary care perspective. *J Fam Plann Reprod Health Care*. 2012;38: 48-52.
121. Al-Mubarak M, Sacher AG, Ocana A, et al. Fulvestrant for advanced breast cancer: a meta-analysis. *Cancer Treat Rev*. 2013; 39:753-758.
122. Krell J, Januszewski A, Yan K, Palmieri C. Role of fulvestrant in the management of postmenopausal breast cancer. *Expert Rev Anticancer Ther*. 2011;11:1641-1652.
123. Scott SM, Brown M, Come SE. Emerging data on the efficacy and safety of fulvestrant, a unique antiestrogen therapy for advanced breast cancer. *Expert Opin Drug Saf*. 2011;10:819-826.
124. Spitz IM. Mifepristone: where do we come from and where are we going? Clinical development over a quarter of a century. *Contraception*. 2010;82:442-452.
125. Im A, Appleman LJ. Mifepristone: pharmacology and clinical impact in reproductive medicine, endocrinology and oncology. *Expert Opin Pharmacother*. 2010;11:481-488.

126. Shaw KA, Topp NJ, Shaw JG, Blumenthal PD. Mifepristone-misoprostol dosing interval and effect on induction abortion times: a systematic review. *Obstet Gynecol*. 2013;121:1335-1347.
127. Raymond EG, Shannon C, Weaver MA, Winikoff B. First-trimester medical abortion with mifepristone 200 mg and misoprostol: a systematic review. *Contraception*. 2013;87:26-37.
128. Wedisinghe L, Elsandabesee D. Flexible mifepristone and misoprostol administration interval for first-trimester medical termination. *Contraception*. 2010;81:269-274.
129. Broekhuizen FF. Emergency contraception, efficacy and public health impact. *Curr Opin Obstet Gynecol*. 2009;21:309-312.
130. Tristan M, Orozco LJ, Steed A, et al. Mifepristone for uterine fibroids. *Cochrane Database Syst Rev*. 2012;8:CD007687.
131. Fleseriu M, Molitch ME, Gross C, et al. A new therapeutic approach in the medical treatment of Cushing's syndrome: glucocorticoid receptor blockade with mifepristone. *Endocr Pract*. 2013;19:313-326.
132. Morgan FH, Laufgraben MJ. Mifepristone for management of Cushing's syndrome. *Pharmacotherapy*. 2013;33:319-329.
133. Burkman R, Bell C, Serfaty D. The evolution of combined oral contraception: improving the risk-to-benefit ratio. *Contraception*. 2011;84:19-34.
134. Christin-Maitre S. History of oral contraceptive drugs and their use worldwide. *Best Pract Res Clin Endocrinol Metab*. 2013;27:3-12.
135. Bitzer J. Oral contraceptives in adolescent women. *Best Pract Res Clin Endocrinol Metab*. 2013;27:77-89.
136. Cremer M, Phan-Weston S, Jacobs A. Recent innovations in oral contraception. *Semin Reprod Med*. 2010;28:140-146.
137. Shrader SP, Dickerson LM. Extended- and continuous-cycle oral contraceptives. *Pharmacotherapy*. 2008;28:1033-1040.
138. Sitruk-Ware R, Nath A, Mishell DR Jr. Contraception technology: past, present and future. *Contraception*. 2013;87:319-330.
139. Brache V, Payán LJ, Faundes A. Current status of contraceptive vaginal rings. *Contraception*. 2013;87:264-272.
140. Lopez LM, Grimes DA, Gallo MF, et al. Skin patch and vaginal ring versus combined oral contraceptives for contraception. *Cochrane Database Syst Rev*. 2013;4:CD003552.
141. Sivin I. Risks and benefits, advantages and disadvantages of levonorgestrel-releasing contraceptive implants. *Drug Saf*. 2003;26:303-335.
142. Roy G. Injectable contraception. *Semin Reprod Med*. 2010;28:126-132.
143. Bahamondes L, Bahamondes MV, Monteiro I. Levonorgestrel-releasing intrauterine system: uses and controversies. *Expert Rev Med Devices*. 2008;5:437-445.
144. Gemzell-Danielsson K, Berger C, P G L L. Emergency contraception—mechanisms of action. *Contraception*. 2013;87:300-308.
145. Lalitkumar PG, Berger C, Gemzell-Danielsson K. Emergency contraception. *Best Pract Res Clin Endocrinol Metab*. 2013;27:91-101.
146. Martinez AM, Thomas MA. Ulipristal acetate as an emergency contraceptive agent. *Expert Opin Pharmacother*. 2012;13:1937-1942.
147. Snow SE, Melillo SN, Jarvis CI. Ulipristal acetate for emergency contraception. *Ann Pharmacother*. 2011;45:780-786.
148. Sullivan JL, Bulloch MN. Ulipristal acetate: a new emergency contraceptive. *Expert Rev Clin Pharmacol*. 2011;4:417-427.
149. Levin ER, Hammes SR. Estrogens and progestins. In: Brunton LL, et al, eds. *The Pharmacological Basis of Therapeutics*. 12th ed. New York: McGraw-Hill; 2011.
150. Lidegaard Ø, Løkkegaard E, Jensen A, Skovlund CW, Keiding N. Thrombotic stroke and myocardial infarction with hormonal contraception. *N Engl J Med*. 2012;366:2257-2266.
151. Peragallo Urrutia R, Coeytaux RR, McBroom AJ, et al. Risk of acute thromboembolic events with oral contraceptive use: a systematic review and meta-analysis. *Obstet Gynecol*. 2013;122(Pt 1):380-389.
152. Plu-Bureau G, Hugon-Rodin J, Maitrot-Mantelet L, Canonico M. Hormonal contraceptives and arterial disease: an epidemiological update. *Best Pract Res Clin Endocrinol Metab*. 2013;27:35-45.
153. Bitzer J, Simon JA. Current issues and available options in combined hormonal contraception. *Contraception*. 2011;84:342-356.
154. Lawrie TA, Helmerhorst FM, Maitra NK, et al. Types of progestogens in combined oral contraception: effectiveness and side-effects. *Cochrane Database Syst Rev*. 2011;5:CD004861.
155. Rott H. Thrombotic risks of oral contraceptives. *Curr Opin Obstet Gynecol*. 2012;24:235-240.
156. Stegeman BH, de Bastos M, Rosendaal FR, et al. Different combined oral contraceptives and the risk of venous thrombosis: systematic review and network meta-analysis. *BMJ*. 2013;347:f5298.
157. Lalude OO. Risk of cardiovascular events with hormonal contraception: insights from the Danish cohort study. *Curr Cardiol Rep*. 2013;15:374.
158. Shufelt CL, Bairey Merz CN. Contraceptive hormone use and cardiovascular disease. *J Am Coll Cardiol*. 2009;53:221-231.
159. Havrilesky LJ, Moorman PG, Lowery WJ, et al. Oral contraceptive pills as primary prevention for ovarian cancer: a systematic review and meta-analysis. *Obstet Gynecol*. 2013;122:139-147.
160. Schindler AE. Non-contraceptive benefits of hormonal contraceptives. *Minerva Ginecol*. 2010;62:319-329.
161. Cibula D, Gompel A, Mueck AO, et al. Hormonal contraception and risk of cancer. *Hum Reprod Update*. 2010;16:631-650.
162. Hilakivi-Clarke L, de Assis S, Warri A. Exposures to synthetic estrogens at different times during the life, and their effect on breast cancer risk. *J Mammary Gland Biol Neoplasia*. 2013;18:25-42.
163. La Vecchia C, Bosetti C. Oral contraceptives and neoplasms other than breast and female genital tract. *Eur J Cancer Prev*. 2009;18:407-411.

CHAPTER 31

Thyroid and Parathyroid Drugs: Agents Affecting Bone Mineralization

In this chapter, we discuss the function and pharmacological aspects of two important endocrine structures: the thyroid and parathyroid glands. Hormones secreted from the thyroid gland are involved in controlling metabolism; they also work synergistically with other hormones to promote normal growth and development. The parathyroid glands are essential in regulating calcium homeostasis and are important in maintaining proper bone mineralization.

Problems in the function of the thyroid or parathyroid glands are often treated by pharmacological methods. It is important that you understand the pharmacological management of thyroid and parathyroid function so that you can adjust your therapies appropriately for patients with bone-healing disorders and other conditions caused by problems with these endocrine glands. The normal physiological function of the thyroid gland is covered first, followed by the types of drugs used to treat hyperthyroidism and hypothyroidism. The function of the parathyroid glands is covered next, with a discussion of the role of the parathyroid glands and other hormones in maintaining bone mineral homeostasis. The final section is an overview of the drugs used to regulate bone calcification.

HORMONES OF THE THYROID GLAND

The thyroid gland lies on either side of the trachea in the anterior neck region and consists of bilateral lobes connected by a central isthmus. The entire gland weighs approximately 15 to 20 g and receives a rich vascular supply and extensive innervation from the sympathetic nervous system.[1] The thyroid gland synthesizes two primary hormones: thyroxine and triiodothyronine.

Synthesis of Thyroid Hormones

The chemical structures of thyroxine and triiodothyronine are shown in Figure 31-1. Thyroid hormones are synthesized first by adding iodine to residues of the amino acid *tyrosine*. Addition of one iodine atom creates monoiodotyrosine, and the addition of a second iodine creates diiodotyrosine. Two of these iodinated tyrosines are then combined to complete the thyroid hormone. The combination of a monoiodotyrosine and a diiodotyrosine yields triiodothyronine, and the combination of two diiodotyrosines yields thyroxine.[1,2]

Because thyroxine contains four iodine residues, this compound is also called T_4. Likewise, triiodothyronine contains three iodine residues and is called T_3. There has been considerable discussion about which hormone exerts the primary physiological effects. Plasma levels of T_4 are much higher than T_3 levels, but T_3 may exert most of the physiological effects on various tissues, which suggests that T_4 is a precursor to T_3 and that the conversion of T_4 to T_3 occurs in peripheral tissues.[3] Regardless of which hormone ultimately affects cellular metabolism, both T_4 and T_3 are needed for normal thyroid function.

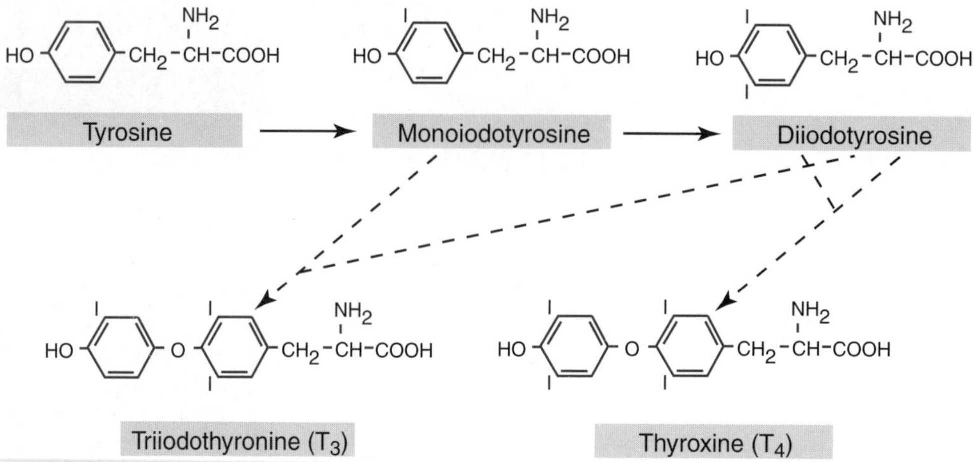

Figure ■ 31-1
Structure of the thyroid hormones triiodothyronine (T_3) and thyroxine (T_4). Addition of one iodine atom (I) to tyrosine produces monoiodotyrosine; addition of a second iodine atom produces diiodotyrosine. A monoiodotyrosine and diiodotyrosine combine to form triiodothyronine (T_3). Coupling of two diiodotyrosines forms thyroxine (T_4).

The primary steps in thyroid hormone biosynthesis are shown schematically in Figure 31-2. Thyroid follicle cells take up and concentrate iodide from the bloodstream—this is significant because there must be a sufficient amount of iodine in the diet to provide what is needed for thyroid hormone production.[4] Thyroid cells also manufacture a protein known as thyroglobulin (TGB), which contains tyrosine residues. The TGB molecule is manufactured within the follicle cell and stored in the central lumen of the thyroid follicle. During hormone synthesis, iodide is oxidized and covalently bonded to the tyrosine residues of the TGB molecule.[2] Two iodinated tyrosine residues combine within the TGB molecule to form T_4 (primarily), and smaller amounts of T_3 are also produced. At this point, the hormones are still incorporated within the large TGB molecule. The iodinated TGB molecule (TGB containing the iodinated tyrosines) is absorbed back

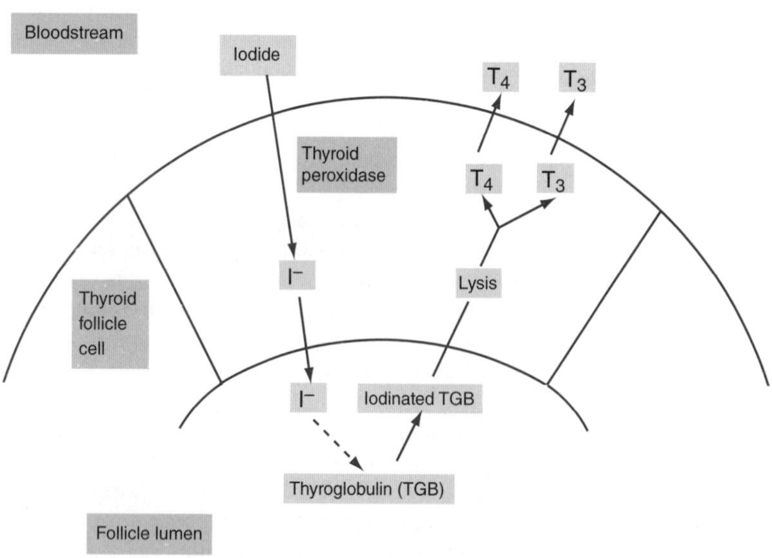

Figure ■ 31-2
Thyroid hormone biosynthesis. Iodide is taken into the follicle cell, where it is converted by thyroid peroxidase to an oxidized form of iodine (I^-). I^- is transported to the follicle lumen, where it is bonded to tyrosine residues of the thyroglobulin (TGB) molecule. Iodinated TGB is incorporated back into the cell, where it undergoes lysis to yield the thyroid hormones T_3 and T_4.

into the follicle cell, where the large molecule is lysed to yield thyroid hormones. The hormones are then secreted into the systemic circulation, where they can reach various target tissues.

Regulation of Thyroid Hormone Release

Thyroid hormone production is controlled by the hypothalamic-pituitary system (see Chapter 28). Thyrotropin-releasing hormone (TRH) from the hypothalamus stimulates the release of thyroid-stimulating hormone (TSH) from the anterior pituitary.[5,6] TSH then travels via the systemic circulation to the thyroid gland to stimulate the production of thyroxine and triiodothyronine.

Thyroid hormone release is subject to the negative feedback strategy that is typical of endocrine systems controlled by the hypothalamic-pituitary axis. Increased circulating levels of the thyroid hormones (T_4, T_3) serve to limit their own production by inhibiting TRH release from the hypothalamus and TSH release from the anterior pituitary.[5,7] This negative feedback control prevents peripheral levels of thyroid hormones from becoming excessively high.

Physiological Effects of Thyroid Hormones

Thyroid hormones affect a wide variety of peripheral tissues throughout the individual's life.[8,9] In some situations, these hormones exert a direct effect on cellular function (e.g., T_4 and T_3 appear to increase cellular metabolism by directly increasing oxidative enzyme activity). In other instances, thyroid hormones appear to play a permissive role in facilitating the function of other hormones. For instance, thyroid hormones must be present for growth hormone to function properly. They also affect central structures such as the hypothalamus, and certain effects of these hormones are mediated by their effects on the central nervous system (CNS) and autonomic nervous system.[10,11] The principal effects of the thyroid hormones are listed here:

Thermogenesis. T_4 and T_3 increase the basal metabolic rate and subsequent heat production from the body, which are important in maintaining adequate body temperature during exposure to cold environments. Increased thermogenesis is achieved by thyroid hormone stimulation of cellular metabolism in various tissues, such as skeletal muscle, cardiac muscle, and liver and kidney cells.

Growth and development. Thyroid hormones facilitate normal growth and development by stimulating the release of growth hormone and by enhancing the effects of growth hormone on peripheral tissues. Thyroid hormones also directly enhance the development of many physiological systems, especially the skeletal system and CNS. If thyroid hormones are not present, severe growth restriction and mental retardation (cretinism) ensue.

Cardiovascular effects. Thyroid hormones appear to increase heart rate and myocardial contractility, thus leading to an increase in cardiac output. It is unclear, however, if this occurrence is a direct effect of these hormones or if the thyroid hormones increase myocardial sensitivity to other hormones (norepinephrine and epinephrine).

Metabolic effects. Thyroid hormones affect energy substrate utilization in several ways. For instance, these hormones increase intestinal glucose absorption and increase the activity of several enzymes involved in carbohydrate metabolism. Thyroid hormones enhance lipolysis by increasing the response of fat cells to other lipolytic hormones. In general, these and other metabolic effects help to increase the availability of glucose and lipids for increased cellular activity.

Mechanism of Action of Thyroid Hormones

Thyroid hormones exert their primary effects by entering the cell and binding to specific receptors located within the cell's nucleus.[12,13] These thyroid hormone receptors act as DNA transcription factors that bind to specific DNA sequences regulating gene expression. When activated by the thyroid hormone, thyroid receptors induce transcription of specific DNA gene segments, which ultimately results in altered protein synthesis within the cell.[14,15] Most of the important physiological effects of the thyroid hormones are related to this alteration in cellular protein production. For instance, thyroid hormones may act through nuclear DNA transcription to stimulate the synthesis of a particular enzymatic protein. Such a protein may increase the transport of specific substances (e.g., amino acids, glucose, sodium) across the cell membrane, or the newly synthesized protein may be directly involved in a metabolic pathway (e.g., glycolysis or lipid oxidation).

Thyroid hormones may also cause certain effects that are not mediated by nuclear receptors and altered

DNA transcription. Certain "nongenomic" effects, for example, could be mediated by an effect of thyroid hormones on non-nuclear receptors located on the cell surface, in the cytoplasm, or in the mitochondria.[15,16] Thyroid hormones may also have a direct effect on immune system cells, and they may cause rapid changes in immune function that are unrelated to their effects on the cell's genome.[17] Although these nongenomic effects seem secondary to the effects mediated by nuclear thyroid receptors, researchers continue to investigate the nongenomic role of thyroid hormones in health and disease.

TREATMENT OF THYROID DISORDERS

Thyroid disorders can be divided into two primary categories: conditions that increase thyroid function (hyperthyroidism) and conditions that decrease thyroid function (hypothyroidism).[18] There are several different types of hyperthyroidism and hypothyroidism, depending on the apparent etiology, symptoms, and age of onset of each type (Table 31-1). The clinical manifestations of hyperthyroidism and hypothyroidism are listed in Table 31-2. Although we cannot review the causes and effects of all the various forms of thyroid dysfunction at this time, this topic is dealt with elsewhere extensively.[1,18-21]

From a pharmacotherapeutic standpoint, hyperthyroidism is treated with drugs that attenuate the synthesis and effects of thyroid hormones. Hypothyroidism is usually treated by thyroid hormone administration (replacement therapy). This section discusses the general aspects and more common forms of hyperthyroidism and hypothyroidism, along with the drugs used to resolve these primary forms of thyroid dysfunction.

Table 31-2
PRIMARY SYMPTOMS OF HYPERTHYROIDISM AND HYPOTHYROIDISM

Hyperthyroidism	Hypothyroidism
Nervousness	Lethargy/slow cerebration
Weight loss	Weight gain (in adult hypothyroidism)
Diarrhea	Constipation
Tachycardia	Bradycardia
Insomnia	Sleepiness
Increased appetite	Anorexia
Heat intolerance	Cold intolerance
Oligomenorrhea	Menorrhagia
Muscle wasting	Weakness
Goiter	Dry, coarse skin
Exophthalmos	Facial edema

Adapted from: Kuhn MA Thyroid and parathyroid agents. In: Kuhn MA, ed. Pharmacotherapeutics: A Nursing Process Approach. 4th ed. Philadelphia, PA: FA Davis; 1997.

Hyperthyroidism

Hyperthyroidism (thyrotoxicosis) results in the increased secretion of thyroid hormones. This condition may occur secondary to a number of conditions, including thyroid tumors and problems in the endocrine regulation of thyroid secretion—for example, excess TSH secretion.[20,22] Hyperthyroidism is usually associated with enlargement of the thyroid gland, or goiter. One of the more common causes of hyperthyroidism is diffuse toxic goiter (Graves disease). Graves disease is thought to be caused by a problem in the

Table 31-1
PRIMARY TYPES OF HYPERTHYROIDISM AND HYPOTHYROIDISM

Hyperthyroidism (Thyrotoxicosis)	Hypothyroidism (Hypothyroxinemia)
Primary hyperthyroidism Graves disease Thyroid adenoma/carcinoma Secondary hyperthyroidism Hyperthyroidism induced by excessive hypothalamic or pituitary stimulation	Primary hypothyroidism Genetic deficiency of enzymes that synthesize thyroid hormones Secondary hypothyroidism Hypothyroidism induced by hypothalamic or pituitary deficiencies Cretinism (childhood hypothyroidism) Myxedema (adult hypothyroidism) Other forms of hypothyroidism Hypothyroidism induced by peripheral insensitivity to thyroid hormones, inadequate hormone transport, other causes

immune system. Because of a genetic defect, antibodies are synthesized that directly stimulate the thyroid gland, resulting in exaggerated thyroid hormone production.[23,24] Other types of hyperthyroidism are characterized by different causes and pathophysiological features (see Table 31-1).[20,25]

The treatment of this condition often consists of ablation of the thyroid gland, accomplished by surgically removing the thyroid or by administering radioactive iodine. Physicians may also administer various pharmacological agents to manage hyperthyroidism in various situations.[22] These agents include antithyroid drugs, iodide, radioactive iodine, and beta-adrenergic blockers.

Antithyroid Agents

Antithyroid drugs, such as propylthiouracil (Propyl-Thyracil) and methimazole (Tapazole), directly inhibit thyroid hormone synthesis.[26,27] These drugs are typically used to control excessive thyroid hormone prior to surgical removal of the thyroid or destruction of the thyroid gland using radioactive iodine (see below). Antithyroid drugs work by inhibiting thyroid peroxidase (the enzyme that oxidizes iodide to enable it to bond to tyrosine residues) and by preventing the coupling of tyrosine residues within the thyroglobulin molecule (see Fig. 31-2).[26,28,29] Propylthiouracil also inhibits the effects of the thyroid hormones by blocking the conversion of T_4 to T_3 in peripheral tissues.[26] The most common adverse effects of antithyroid drugs are skin rash and itching, but this is usually mild and transient. Although serious problems involving formed blood elements (agranulocytosis and aplastic anemia) may occur, the incidence of such problems is relatively small. Finally, excessive inhibition of thyroid hormone synthesis from drug overdose may cause symptoms resembling hypothyroidism, such as lethargy and feeling cold.

Iodide

Relatively large dosages of iodide (exceeding 6 mg/d) cause a rapid and dramatic decrease in thyroid function.[30] In sufficient amounts, iodide inhibits virtually all the steps involved in thyroid hormone biosynthesis. For instance, high iodide levels limit the uptake of iodide into thyroid follicle cells, inhibit the formation of T_4 and T_3, and decrease the secretion of the completed hormones from the thyroid cell.

Although iodide is effective in treating hyperthyroidism for short periods, the effects of this drug begin to diminish after about 2 weeks of administration.[30] In addition, iodide may cause a severe hypersensitive reaction in susceptible individuals. Therefore, other agents such as antithyroid drugs and beta blockers have somewhat replaced the use of iodide. High doses of iodide, however, may be useful in limited situations to temporarily control symptoms of hyperthyroidism a week or so before the surgical removal of the thyroid.

In addition to treating hyperthyroidism, high doses of iodine can decrease the risk of thyroid cancer after exposure to radioactive fallout from nuclear disasters.[31,32] For example, after the nuclear reactor accidents in Chernobyl and Fukushima released radioactive iodine into the atmosphere and soil, people living in those areas took high doses of iodine to negate the effects of radioactive iodine on the thyroid gland. Iodine is converted to iodide in the GI tract before absorption into the body. Basically, high levels of stable (nonradioactive) iodide in the bloodstream will reduce the need for the thyroid gland to absorb additional (radioactive) iodide.[30]

Radioactive Iodine

A radioactive isotope of iodine (^{131}I) is often used to selectively destroy thyroid tissues in certain forms of hyperthyroidism, such as in Graves disease.[33,34] A specific oral dose of radioactive iodine rapidly sequesters within the thyroid gland. The isotope then begins to emit beta radiation, which selectively destroys the thyroid follicle cells. Essentially no damage occurs to surrounding tissues because the radioactivity is contained within the thyroid gland. Thus, administration of radioactive iodine is a simple, relatively safe method of permanently ablating the thyroid gland and reducing excess thyroid hormone function.[35] Radioactive iodine can, however, worsen the ophthalmopathy associated with hyperthyroidism, exacerbating eye symptoms such as inflammation, redness, swelling, and bulging of the eyes in some patients.[36,37] In addition, most patients who undergo radioactive destruction of the thyroid gland must typically be given thyroid hormones as replacement therapy.[30]

Beta-Adrenergic Blockers

Beta-adrenergic blockers are usually associated with the treatment of cardiovascular problems such as hypertension and angina pectoris (see Chapter 21). Beta blockers may also be helpful as adjuncts to other medications such as antithyroid drugs. Although these drugs do not directly lower plasma levels of thyroid hormones, they may help suppress symptoms such as tachycardia, palpitations, fever, and restlessness. Beta blockers may be especially helpful in severe, acute exacerbations of thyrotoxicosis (thyroid storm).[19,38-40] These drugs are administered preoperatively to control symptoms until a more permanent means of treating thyrotoxicosis (thyroidectomy) can be implemented.[41] Some beta blockers that are effective in thyrotoxicosis are acebutolol, atenolol, metoprolol, nadolol, oxprenolol, propranolol, sotalol, and timolol. See Chapter 20 for the pharmacology and adverse effects of these compounds.

Hypothyroidism

There are many forms of hypothyroidism, differing in their cause and age of onset (see Table 31-1). Severe adult hypothyroidism (myxedema) may occur idiopathically or may be caused by specific factors such as autoimmune lymphocytic destruction (Hashimoto disease). In the child, thyroid function may be congenitally impaired, and cretinism will result if this condition is untreated. Hypothyroidism may result at any age if the dietary intake of iodine is extremely low. Several other forms of hypothyroidism that have a genetic or familial basis also exist.[1]

The primary physiological effects of decreased thyroid function are listed in Table 31-2. Although enlargement of the thyroid gland (*goiter*) is usually associated with hyperthyroidism, goiter may also be present in some forms of hypothyroidism, albeit for different reasons. For instance, thyroid enlargement occurs during hypothyroidism when there is a lack of dietary iodine (endemic goiter). Under the influence of TSH, the thyroid manufactures large quantities of thyroglobulin. But thyroid hormone synthesis is incomplete, because no iodine is available to add to the tyrosine residues. If no thyroid hormones are produced, there is no negative feedback to limit the secretion of TSH. Consequently, the thyroid gland increases in size because of the unabated production of thyroglobulin.

Replacement of deficient thyroid hormones is essential for maintaining optimal health in adults with various forms of hypothyroidism.[42,43] The primary method of treatment is to administer natural thyroid hormones and synthetic analogs, such as preparations containing T_4 (levothyroxine), T_3 (liothyronine), or both. There has been considerable debate about whether a replacement regimen should consist of T_4 only or a combination of T_4 and T_3. Some studies suggested that combining both hormones does not provide additional benefits in certain physiological responses (e.g., body weight, lipid metabolism) compared to replacement using only T_4.[44] Some patients may benefit from a combination of T_4 and T_3, and a combined regimen may result in greater improvements in mood, psychometric skills, and perceived quality-of-life in these individuals.[42,45] Hence, each patient's needs will determine the ideal replacement regimen, and efforts should be made to find the optimal type and dose of thyroid hormones.

Administration of thyroid hormones is likewise important in infants and children with hypothyroidism because adequate amounts of these hormones are needed for normal physical and mental development.[46,47] Thyroid hormone replacement is also necessary following thyroidectomy or pharmacological ablation of the thyroid gland with radioactive iodine. Physicians may administer thyroid hormones to prevent and treat cancer of the thyroid gland and to prevent enlargement of the thyroid gland (goiter) caused by other drugs, such as lithium. Thyroid hormone maintenance may be beneficial in patients who are in the preliminary or subclinical phase of hypothyroidism. Some clinicians feel that administering these hormones in the early stages may prevent the disease from fully developing.[48]

Thyroid hormone preparations used clinically are listed in Table 31-3. Long-term administration of the hormones is usually a safe, effective means of maintaining optimal patient health. The primary problems associated with these agents occur with overdosage. Symptoms of excess drug levels are similar to the symptoms of hyperthyroidism (see Table 31-2). Decreasing the dosage or changing the medication resolves these symptoms.

Table 31-3
THYROID HORMONES USED TO TREAT HYPOTHYROIDISM

Generic Name	Trade Name(s)	Thyroid Hormone Content	Source
Levothyroxine	Levothroid, Synthroid, others	T_4	Synthetic
Liothyronine	Cytomel	T_3	Synthetic
Liotrix	Thyrolar	T_3 and T_4	Synthetic
Thyroid	Armour Thyroid, others	T_3 and T_4	Natural

PARATHYROID HORMONE

In humans, there are usually four parathyroid glands that are embedded on the posterior surface of the thyroid gland. Each parathyroid gland is a pea-sized structure weighing about 50 mg. Despite their diminutive size, parathyroids serve a vital role in controlling calcium homeostasis.[49] Because calcium is crucial in many physiological processes—including synaptic transmission, muscle contraction, and bone mineralization—the importance of parathyroid function is obvious. In fact, removal of the parathyroid glands results in convulsions and death because of inadequate plasma calcium levels. The parathyroids control calcium homeostasis through the synthesis and secretion of parathyroid hormone (PTH).

PTH—a polypeptide hormone—is synthesized within the cells of the parathyroid glands. The primary factor controlling the release of PTH is the amount of calcium in the bloodstream.[49] A calcium-sensing receptor located on the outer surface of the parathyroid cell membrane monitors plasma calcium levels.[50,51] A decrease in plasma calcium activates this receptor and causes increased release of PTH. As blood calcium levels increase, the receptor is inhibited, and PTH release is reduced.

The primary physiological effect of PTH is to increase blood calcium levels by altering calcium metabolism in three primary tissues: bone, kidney, and the GI tract[52,53] (Fig. 31-3). PTH directly affects skeletal tissues by increasing bone turnover, thus liberating calcium from skeletal stores.[53,54] High, sustained levels of PTH appear to enhance the development and action of cells (osteoclasts) that break down skeletal tissues.[54,55] Increased osteoclast activity degrades the collagen matrix within the bone, thus releasing calcium into the bloodstream. PTH also increases plasma calcium levels by increasing renal reabsorption of calcium. As renal calcium reabsorption increases, PTH produces a simultaneous increase in phosphate excretion by inhibiting phosphate reabsorption in the kidney. Thus, PTH produces a rise in plasma calcium that is accompanied by a decrease in plasma phosphate levels.[56]

PTH also helps increase the absorption of calcium from the GI tract. This effect appears to be caused by the interaction between PTH and vitamin D metabolism. Vitamin D is a steroidlike hormone obtained from dietary sources or synthesized in the skin from cholesterol derivatives in the presence of ultraviolet light. PTH increases the conversion of vitamin D to 1,25-dihydroxycholecalciferol (calcitriol) in the kidneys.[57] Calcitriol directly stimulates calcium absorption from the intestine.

Consequently, PTH and vitamin D, as well as several other endocrine factors, are all involved in controlling calcium levels for various physiological needs. How these hormones interact in controlling normal bone formation and resorption is of particular interest to rehabilitation specialists. The following section presents the regulation of bone mineral homeostasis and the principal hormones involved in this process.

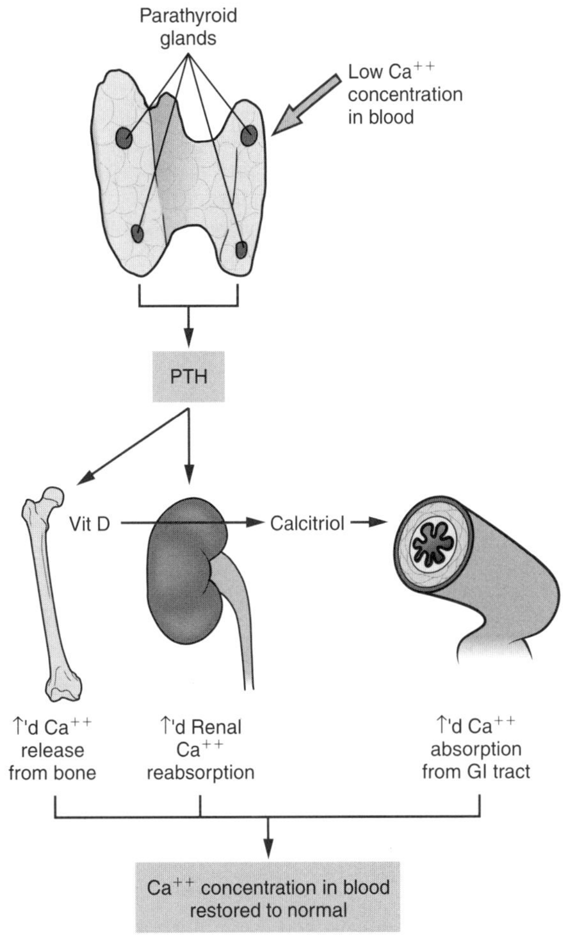

Figure ■ 31-3
Effects of parathyroid hormone (PTH) on calcium (Ca^{++}) metabolism. Low Ca^{++} concentration in the blood stimulates the parathyroid glands to release PTH. PTH affects Ca^{++} metabolism in the bone, kidney, and GI tract so that Ca^{++} concentration in the blood returns to normal.

REGULATION OF BONE MINERAL HOMEOSTASIS

Bone serves two primary functions: to provide a rigid framework for the body and to provide a readily available and easily interchangeable calcium pool.[58] To serve both functions simultaneously, an appropriate balance must exist between bone formation and bone resorption.[59] Bone resorption (breakdown) can supply calcium and other minerals for various physiological processes. Mineral release from bone, however, occurs at the expense of bone formation. The primary minerals that enable bone to maintain its rigidity are calcium and phosphate. Excessive release of these minerals from storage sites in bone will result in bone demineralization, and the skeletal system will undergo failure (i.e., fracture). In addition, bone is continually undergoing specific changes in its internal architecture. This process of remodeling allows bone to adapt to changing stresses and optimally resist applied loads.[60]

Bone, therefore, is a rather dynamic tissue that is constantly undergoing changes in mineral content and internal structure. The balance between bone resorption and formation is controlled by the complex interaction of local and systemic factors. In particular, several hormones regulate bone formation and help maintain adequate plasma calcium levels. The role of parathyroid hormone, vitamin D, and calcitonin in regulating bone mineral homeostasis is described below.

Parathyroid Hormone and Bone Formation

The role of the parathyroid gland and PTH in controlling calcium metabolism was previously discussed. A prolonged or continuous increase in the secretion of PTH increases blood calcium levels by several methods, including increased release of calcium from bone. High levels of PTH accelerate bone breakdown (catabolic effect) to mobilize calcium for other physiological needs.

However, normal or intermittent release of moderate amounts of PTH may actually enhance bone formation.[53,61] That is, PTH can stimulate osteoblast activity and promote an anabolic effect. Although early studies indicated that the anabolic effects of low or normal PTH levels seem limited to trabecular or cancellous bone, more recent evidence suggests that PTH also can enhance fracture healing in cortical bone.[62] If small, intermittent doses of PTH do increase certain types of bone formation, it may be possible to use this hormone to prevent or reverse bone demineralization in certain conditions, including osteoporosis (see later).[61] Therefore, PTH plays an important and complex role in regulating bone metabolism. A prolonged, continuous increase in PTH secretion favors bone breakdown, whereas normal (intermittent) PTH release encourages bone synthesis and remodeling.

Vitamin D

Vitamin D produces several metabolites that are important in bone mineral homeostasis.[63,64] In general, vitamin D derivatives such as 1,25 dihydroxyvitamin D_3 increase serum calcium and phosphate levels primarily by increasing intestinal calcium and phosphate absorption and, to a lesser extent, by decreasing renal calcium and phosphate excretion.[63,65] The effects of vitamin D metabolites on bone are somewhat complex. Under normal conditions, vitamin D generally enhances bone formation by increasing the supply of the two primary minerals needed for bone formation (calcium and phosphate).[64] Vitamin D also suppresses the synthesis and release of PTH from the parathyroid glands, an effect that tends to promote bone mineralization by limiting the catabolic effects of PTH.[66,67] However, if dietary levels of calcium are extremely low or if calcium absorption from the GI tract is impaired, the active form of vitamin D will increase bone resorption and decrease bone mineralization.[68] That is, vitamin D will liberate calcium from skeletal stores and help maintain plasma calcium levels in an acceptable range. Hence, vitamin D usually favors increased bone mineralization, but this effect may be reversed to help resolve a deficiency of plasma calcium.

Calcitonin

Calcitonin is secreted by cells located in the thyroid gland. These calcitonin-secreting cells (also known as *parafollicular* or *C cells*) are interspersed between follicles that produce thyroid hormones. Calcitonin generally has the opposite effects of high levels of PTH.[69] That is, the hormone lowers blood calcium by stimulating bone formation and increasing the incorporation of calcium into skeletal storage. The action of calcitonin also enhances the incorporation of phosphate into bone. Renal excretion of calcium and phosphate is increased by a direct effect of calcitonin on the kidneys, which further reduces the levels of these minerals in the bloodstream. The effects of calcitonin on bone mineral metabolism, however, are relatively minor compared with PTH, and endogenous production of calcitonin is not essential for normal bone mineral homeostasis.[70] In contrast, PTH is a much more dominant hormone, and the absence of PTH produces acute disturbances in calcium metabolism that result in death. Calcitonin does have an important therapeutic function, and pharmacological doses of calcitonin may be helpful in preventing bone loss in certain conditions (see "Pharmacological Control of Bone Mineral Homeostasis").

Other Hormones

A number of other hormones influence bone mineral content.[70] For example, estrogen, androgens, growth hormone, insulin, and the thyroid hormones generally enhance bone formation. On the other hand, glucocorticoids produce a catabolic effect on bone and other supporting tissues (see Chapter 29). Certain prostaglandins are also potent stimulators of bone resorption. Bone cells produce the protein fibroblast growth factor 23 (FGF23) that decreases bone mineralization by increasing renal phosphate excretion and inhibiting vitamin D biosynthesis.[71]

Thus, all of the hormones that influence bone metabolism interact to some extent in the regulation of bone formation and breakdown. Several other hormones can affect bone mineralization to some extent, but the effects of these other hormones are usually secondary to the more direct effects of PTH, vitamin D, and calcitonin. In addition, disturbances in any of these secondary endocrine systems may produce problems that are manifested in abnormal bone formation, including excess glucocorticoid activity and growth hormone deficiency.

PHARMACOLOGICAL CONTROL OF BONE MINERAL HOMEOSTASIS

Satisfactory control of the primary bone minerals is important in both acute and long-term situations. Blood calcium levels must be maintained within a limited range to ensure an adequate supply of free calcium for various physiological purposes. The normal range of total plasma calcium in adults is 8.5 to 10.4 mg/100 mL.[70] If plasma calcium levels fall to below 6 mg/100 mL, tetanic muscle convulsions quickly ensue. Excess plasma calcium (blood levels greater than 12 mg/100 mL) depresses nervous function, leading to sluggishness, lethargy, and possibly coma.

Chronic disturbances in calcium homeostasis can also produce problems in bone calcification. Likewise, various metabolic bone diseases and problems in bone metabolism can alter blood calcium levels, leading to hypocalcemia or hypercalcemia. Some of the more common metabolic diseases affecting bone mineralization are listed in Table 31-4.

Consequently, patients often must use pharmacological methods to help control bone mineral levels in their bloodstream and maintain adequate bone mineralization. The following sections discuss the specific drugs used to control bone mineralization and the clinical conditions in which they are used. A summary of these drugs is in Table 31-5.

Table 31-4
EXAMPLES OF METABOLIC BONE DISEASE

Disease	Pathophysiology	Primary Drug Treatment
Hypoparathyroidism	Decreased parathyroid hormone secretion; leads to impaired bone resorption and hypocalcemia	Calcium supplements, vitamin D
Hyperparathyroidism	Increased parathyroid hormone secretion, usually caused by parathyroid tumors; leads to excessive bone resorption and hypercalcemia	Usually treated surgically by partial or complete resection of the parathyroid gland
Osteoporosis	Generalized bone demineralization; often associated with effects of aging and hormonal changes in postmenopausal women	Calcium supplements, vitamin D, calcitonin, bisphosphonates, intermittent parathyroid hormone, estrogen, or SERMs (raloxifene) (see Chapter 30)
Rickets	Impaired bone mineralization in children; caused by a deficiency of vitamin D	Calcium supplements, vitamin D
Osteomalacia	Adult form of rickets	Calcium supplements, vitamin D
Paget disease	Excessive bone formation and resorption (turnover); leads to ineffective remodeling and structural abnormalities within the bone	Calcitonin, bisphosphonates

Continued

Table 31-4
EXAMPLES OF METABOLIC BONE DISEASE—cont'd

Disease	Pathophysiology	Primary Drug Treatment
Renal osteodystrophy	Chronic renal failure; induces complex metabolic changes resulting in excessive bone resorption	Vitamin D, calcium supplements
Gaucher disease	Excessive lipid storage in bone leads to impaired remodeling and excessive bone loss	No drugs are effective
Hypercalcemia of malignancy	Many forms of cancer accelerate bone resorption, leading to hypercalcemia	Calcitonin, bisphosphonates

SERMs = selective estrogen receptor modulators.

Table 31-5
DRUGS USED TO CONTROL BONE MINERAL HOMEOSTASIS

General Category	Examples*	Treatment Rationale and Principal Indications
Bisphosphonates	Alendronate (Fosamax) Etidronate (Didronel) Ibandronate (Boniva) Pamidronate (Aredia) Risedronate (Actonel) Zoledronic acid (Reclast, others)	Appear to block excessive bone resorption and formation Used to normalize bone turnover in conditions such as osteoporosis and Paget disease Prevent hypercalcemia resulting from excessive bone resorption in certain forms of cancer
Calcitonin	Human calcitonin (Fortical) Salmon calcitonin (Miacalcin)	Mimics the effects of endogenous calcitonin Increases bone formation in conditions such as Paget disease and osteoporosis Also used to lower plasma calcium levels in hypercalcemic emergencies
Calcium supplements	Calcium acetate (Eliphos, PhosLo) Calcium carbonate (Os-Cal 500, Tums, others) Calcium chloride Calcium citrate (Citracal) Calcium gluconate Calcium lactate (Ridactate) Tribasic calcium phosphate (Posture)	Provide an additional source of calcium to prevent calcium depletion and encourage bone formation in conditions such as osteoporosis, osteomalacia, rickets, and hypoparathyroidism
Estrogens	Conjugated estrogens (Premarin) Esterified estrogen (Menest) Estradiol (Estrace, Femtrace, others) Estropipate (Ogen, Ortho-Est) Raloxifene** (Evista)	Stabilize bone turnover and promote bone mineralization in women who lack endogenous estrogen production (e.g., following menopause or ovariectomy)
Vitamin D analogs	Calcitriol (Calcijex, Rocaltrol) Cholecalciferol (Replesta, vitamin D3, others) Doxercalciferol (Hectorol) Ergocalciferol (Calciferol, Drisdol, others) Paricalcitol (Zemplar)	Generally enhance bone formation by increasing the absorption and retention of calcium and phosphate in the body Useful in treating disorders caused by vitamin D deficiency, including hypocalcemia, hypophosphatemia, rickets, and osteomalacia
Others	Cinacalcet (Sensipar) Denosumab (Prolia) Teriparatide (Forteo)	Work by other mechanisms to stabilize bone turnover (see text for details about each drug).

**Common trade names are shown in parentheses.*
***Selective estrogen receptor modulator; see text and Chapter 30 for details.*

Calcium Supplements

Patients may take calcium preparations to ensure that adequate calcium levels are available in the body for various physiological needs, including bone formation. Specifically, the patients may use calcium supplements to help prevent bone loss in conditions such as osteoporosis, osteomalacia, rickets, and hypoparathyroidism (see Table 31-5). Calcium supplements, for example, are recommended in preventing and treating osteoporosis in postmenopausal women.[72,73] For optimal effects, calcium supplements are often combined with other bone mineralizing agents such as vitamin D (see the next section) and bisphosphonate drugs (see "Bisphosphonates").[74] The use of oral calcium supplements appears to be especially important in individuals who do not receive sufficient amounts of calcium in their diet.[58]

The dose of a calcium supplement should make up the difference between dietary calcium intake and established daily guidelines for each patient. The exact dose for a patient therefore depends on factors such as the amount of dietary calcium, age, gender, and hormonal and reproductive status (e.g., women who are pregnant, premenopausal, or postmenopausal).[58,75] For example, a woman who is postmenopausal and ingests 500 to 600 mg of dietary calcium per day would need a supplemental dosage of approximately 800 mg/d because the recommended dietary allowance (RDA) guideline for postmenopausal women is 1,200 to 1,500 mg/d.[76]

However, there is concern about the maximum dose of calcium supplement that can be administered safely. Certain guidelines, for example, suggest that no more than 500 mg of calcium should be administered at one time[77] and that daily calcium doses used to prevent fractures in adults should be limited to 1,000 mg/day or less in divided doses.[78] Although the total daily value is well below the maximum tolerated limit of 2,500 mg/day, daily calcium supplements above 1,000 mg/day do not seem to provide additional benefits in preventing fracture and may increase the risk of arterial calcification and cardiovascular disease.[79]

Clearly, the dosage of a calcium supplement must be determined by the specific needs of each individual. In addition to concerns about cardiovascular disease, excessive calcium doses may also produce symptoms of hypercalcemia, including constipation, drowsiness, fatigue, and headache. As hypercalcemia becomes more pronounced, confusion, irritability, cardiac arrhythmias, hypertension, nausea and vomiting, skin rashes, and pain in bones and muscle may occur. Hypercalcemia is a cause for concern because severe cardiac irregularities may prove fatal.

Vitamin D

As indicated earlier, vitamin D is a precursor for several compounds that tend to promote bone mineralization, primarily by increasing intestinal absorption of calcium and phosphate.[68] Metabolites of vitamin D and their pharmacological analogs are therefore used to increase blood calcium and phosphate levels and to enhance bone mineralization in conditions such as osteodystrophy, rickets, or other situations where people lack adequate amounts of vitamin D (see Table 31-5). Vitamin D analogs such as calcitriol can be combined with calcium supplements to help treat postmenopausal osteoporosis[75] and to treat bone loss caused by anti-inflammatory steroids (glucocorticoids; see Chapter 29).[80]

Like calcium supplements, there is considerable debate about the maximum safe daily dose of vitamin D. Currently, the recommended daily intake of vitamin D is 400 units in infants up to 1 year, 600 units in children and adults up to age 70, and 800 units in adults over age 70.[76] Some studies, however, suggest that daily intake of vitamin D should be much higher and that a daily adult allowance somewhere between 2,000 and 10,000 units per day may be tolerable and beneficial.[75] A primary concern is that vitamin D is a fat-soluble vitamin, and excessive doses can accumulate in the body, leading to toxicity. Early signs of vitamin D toxicity include headache, increased thirst, decreased appetite, metallic taste, fatigue, and GI disturbances (nausea, vomiting, constipation, diarrhea). Increased vitamin D toxicity is associated with hypercalcemia, high blood pressure, cardiac arrhythmias, renal failure, mood changes, and seizures. Vitamin D toxicity is a serious problem that can cause death from cardiac and renal failure. Hence, researchers continue to investigate the amount of daily vitamin D that will provide optimal benefits and minimal risk in a given individual.

Bisphosphonates

The bisphosphonates (also called *diphosphonates*) are a group of inorganic compounds that include alendronate (Fosamax), pamidronate (Aredia), and several similar agents (see Table 31-5). Although their exact mechanism is unclear, these compounds appear to adsorb directly into calcium crystals in the bone and reduce bone resorption by inhibiting osteoclast activity.[81,82] Patients with Paget disease often use bisphosphonates to help prevent exaggerated bone turnover and promote adequate mineralization.[83,84] These agents also inhibit abnormal bone formation in conditions such as heterotopic ossification[85] and maintain bone mineralization and prevent bone pain and fractures in cancers that metastasize to bone.[86,87] Bisphosphonates can also help prevent and treat bone loss during prolonged administration of anti-inflammatory steroids (glucocorticoids).[80,88]

Bisphosphonates have emerged as one of the primary treatments for osteoporosis, including osteoporosis associated with estrogen loss in postmenopausal women.[83,89–91] For men and women with osteoporosis, the use of these drugs can increase bone mineral density and reduce the risk of vertebral and nonvertebral fractures (e.g., hip fractures).[91-93] Bisphosphonates have become especially attractive in treating postmenopausal osteoporosis because they improve bone health in women without the risks associated with estrogen replacement (see "Estrogen Therapy"). Researchers continue to investigate optimal dosing regimens that take advantage of the beneficial effects of these drugs.[90]

Despite their beneficial effects on bone mineralization, bisphosphonates may cause local defects in bone metabolism that leads to death of bone tissue (osteonecrosis) of the jaw.[94,95] Although this problem is relatively rare, osteonecrosis of the jaw seems to occur more often in patients receiving these drugs intravenously, in patients with cancer, or during the concurrent use of other drugs such as glucocorticoids.[75,95] Likewise, bisphosphonates may lead to atypical (subtrochanteric) hip fractures in susceptible patients.[91] Hence, clinicians should be aware of the possibility of osteonecrosis of the jaw and other adverse skeletal reactions and should report any unexplained bone pain.

Bisphosphonates can also produce some relatively minor side effects, including GI disturbances such as nausea and diarrhea. In addition, patients should remain upright after taking a bisphosphonate so that the drug does not reflux into the esophagus and cause irritation (esophagitis). Specific agents may also be associated with certain side effects. Etidronate (Didronel), for example, can cause tenderness and pain over bony lesion sites in Paget disease, leading to fractures if excessive doses are taken for prolonged periods. Pamidronate (Aredia) may cause fever and localized pain and redness at the injection site, but these effects usually last for only a day or two.

Calcitonin

Calcitonin derived from synthetic sources can mimic the effects of the endogenous hormone. As described previously, endogenous calcitonin decreases blood calcium levels and promotes bone mineralization. Consequently, synthetically derived calcitonin is used to treat hypercalcemia and to decrease bone resorption in Paget disease.[96] Patients also use calcitonin to help prevent bone loss in a variety of other conditions, including osteoarthritis,[97] postmenopausal osteoporosis,[96] and glucocorticoid-induced osteoporosis.[98] Administration of calcitonin can reduce the risk of vertebral fractures but does not seem to be as effective as the bisphosphonates in reducing this risk.[99] Likewise, patients may soon become refractory to the effects of this drug—that is, the positive effects of calcitonin on bone may begin to diminish within a few days after starting treatment.[70] On the other hand, calcitonin may have an analgesic effect on bone pain that complements the drug's ability to promote bone healing, especially in acute vertebral fractures.[100] Hence, calcitonin may be a helpful adjunct for people with acute painful vertebral fractures or a suitable alternative for people with painful vertebral fractures who cannot tolerate other drugs such as bisphosphonates.[101]

At the present time, calcitonin must be administered parenterally, either by injection (intramuscular or subcutaneous) or by aerosolized versions that allow delivery in the form of nasal sprays.[102,103] Oral delivery of calcitonin is difficult because this hormone is absorbed poorly from the GI tract and because calcitonin is degraded by proteolytic enzymes in the stomach.[104] Nonetheless, researchers are making efforts to overcome these limitations, and an oral form of calcitonin is currently in development.[105,106]

Calcitonin is an effective and easy way to treat a variety of conditions that are characterized by increased bone resorption.[69,96] Calcitonin preparations used clinically are either identical to the human form of this hormone (Fortical) or chemically identical to salmon calcitonin (Miacalcin). Redness and swelling may occur locally when these agents are administered by injection. Other side effects include GI disturbances (e.g., stomach pain, nausea, vomiting, diarrhea), loss of appetite, and flushing or redness in the head, hands, and feet.

Estrogen Therapy

Estrogen is critical in maintaining adequate bone mineralization in women (the benefits and risks of estrogen replacement therapy were addressed in Chapter 30). There is little doubt that providing estrogen to women who lack endogenous estrogen production—that is, following menopause or ovariectomy—can help increase bone mineral content and reduce the risk of fractures.[107-109] Replacement of estrogen following menopause has been shown to be especially effective—this treatment can return the rate of bone formation and bone resorption to premenopausal levels.[110]

Research, however, has indicated that estrogen replacement is associated with substantial risks, including an increased incidence of cardiovascular disease and certain cancers (see Chapter 30).[111,112] The incidence of these problems is influenced by many factors such as the patient's age, time since menopause, dose and type of estrogen being administered, and other risk factors in each patient. As a result, estrogen replacement is no longer considered the cornerstone for the long-term management of women with postmenopausal osteoporosis.[113] Estrogen can be used on a limited basis to prevent osteoporosis in certain postmenopausal women with persistent vasomotor symptoms (i.e., hot flashes). That is, estrogen is useful for improving bone health while simultaneously treating the vasomotor symptoms in relatively younger women (under age 60) within 10 years after reaching menopause.[114,115] Candidates for this treatment must still be considered on a case-by-case basis to make sure they do not have an increased risk for cardiovascular disease or breast and uterine cancers.[115] Estrogen can also be combined with other treatments (e.g., calcium supplements, calcitonin, calcitriol, bisphosphonates) to promote optimal bone mineralization in suitable candidates.

Concerns about estrogen led to the development of estrogenlike compounds. These compounds activate estrogen receptors on certain tissues such as bone while blocking the effects of estrogen on breast and uterine tissues. The agents are known as *selective estrogen receptor modulators* (SERMs) because of their ability to preferentially activate certain estrogen receptors on certain types of tissue.[108,116] See Chapter 30 for more details of the pharmacology of SERMs.

The primary SERM used to prevent osteoporosis is raloxifene (Evista).[116,117] This drug binds to and activates estrogen receptors in bone, thus preventing bone loss and demineralization. At the same time, raloxifene blocks estrogen receptors on breast and uterine tissues, thereby preventing the excessive stimulation of receptors that might lead to the development of cancer. Raloxifene also promotes improvements in plasma lipid profiles but may increase the risk of venous thromboembolism.[117] Hence, SERMs such as raloxifene provide an alternative to traditional estrogen therapy when treating postmenopausal osteoporosis, and raloxifene may be especially useful in women with hyperlipidemia or those at risk for breast or uterine cancer.[117,118] Pharmacologists are working to develop other SERMs that will be effective in preventing osteoporosis while minimizing the risks associated with traditional estrogen replacement therapy.

Other Agents That Promote Bone Mineral Content

Several other innovative strategies are now available to improve bone mineralization. Researchers, for example, developed teriparatide (Forteo)—a synthetic form of human PTH—to treat severe cases of osteoporosis.[119-121] As indicated earlier, prolonged or continuous release of PTH increases bone resorption and breakdown, whereas intermittent doses of PTH may increase bone mineral density. Hence, small dosages of teriparatide (20 μg) administered daily by subcutaneous injection provide a burst of PTH activity.[122] Whereas other antiresorptive drugs (bisphosphonates, calcitonin, estrogens) can help stabilize bone turnover, teriparatide is the only currently available agent that can increase *new* bone formation (anabolic effect).[121] Teriparatide is therefore useful in patients who are at high risk of vertebral and nonvertebral fractures in conditions such as postmenopausal osteoporosis and glucocorticoid-induced osteoporosis.[123,124]

Another new strategy involves drugs that stimulate calcium receptors on the parathyroid gland, thereby inhibiting the release of PTH.[125] As indicated earlier, plasma calcium ions regulate the release of PTH by affecting calcium receptors on the parathyroid gland. An increase in plasma calcium inhibits release of PTH, and a decrease in plasma calcium stimulates PTH release. Drugs mimicking the effects of endogenous calcium (i.e., calcimimetics) can therefore reduce PTH release in people with parathyroid tumors or other conditions that cause prolonged, continuous release of PTH.[125,126] This effect helps prevent bone breakdown and the resulting increase in plasma calcium levels (hypercalcemia) that are associated with excessive PTH release. Cinacalcet (Sensipar) is the primary calcimimetic agent in clinical use; other calcimimetics and strategies for controlling bone mineral content may be forthcoming.

Finally, denosumab (Prolia) is a monoclonal antibody that binds to specific receptors on osteoclasts and inhibits the ability of endogenous chemicals to stimulate osteoclast activity.[127] As a result, osteoclast-induced bone resorption is inhibited, thus helping maintain bone mineral density.[128] Like teriparatide, denosumab must be administered by subcutaneous injection, thus limiting its practical use somewhat. Denosumab is therefore used primarily in postmenopausal women who are at high risk for fracture and who have not responded adequately to other antiosteoporosis treatments.[129,130]

Special Concerns for Rehabilitation Patients

Physical therapists and occupational therapists should generally be concerned about the potential side effects of the drugs discussed in this chapter. Excessive doses of drugs used to treat either hyperthyroidism or hypothyroidism tend to produce symptoms of the opposite disorder—that is, overdose of antithyroid drugs can produce signs of hypothyroidism, and vice versa. Therapists should be aware of the signs of thyroid dysfunction (see Table 31-2) and should watch for signs of inappropriate drug dosage. Therapists should also avoid using rehabilitation techniques that may exacerbate any symptoms of thyroid dysfunction. For instance, care must be taken not to overstress the cardiovascular system of a patient with decreased cardiac output and hypotension caused by hypothyroidism (see Table 31-2).

Likewise, physical therapists and occupational therapists should be aware of the potential adverse effects of the drugs that regulate calcium homeostasis. For instance, excessive doses of calcium supplements may alter cardiovascular function, resulting in cardiac arrhythmias. Therapists may help detect these arrhythmias while monitoring pulses or electrocardiogram (ECG) recordings. Finally, therapists can enhance the effects of bone-mineralizing drugs by employing exercise and weight-bearing activities to stimulate bone formation. In addition, certain modalities may enhance the effects of bone-mineralizing agents. In particular, ultraviolet light increases endogenous vitamin D biosynthesis, thus facilitating calcium absorption and bone formation (see the following case study).

CASE STUDY

AGENTS AFFECTING BONE MINERAL METABOLISM

Brief History. R.D. is a 74-year-old woman with a history of generalized bone demineralization caused by osteomalacia that was primarily brought on by poor diet; her total caloric intake and dietary levels of calcium and vitamin D have been very low. The patient is also rather reclusive, spending most of her time indoors. Consequently, she lacks any significant exposure to natural sunlight. To treat her osteomalacia, she was placed on a regimen of oral

CASE STUDY (Continued)

calcium supplements and vitamin D. However, she has been reluctant to take these supplements because they occasionally cause diarrhea. Recently, she sustained a fracture of the femoral neck during a fall. She was admitted to the hospital, and the fracture was stabilized by open reduction and internal fixation. The patient was referred to physical therapy for strengthening and pre-weight-bearing activities.

Problem/Influence of Medication. During the postoperative period, calcium and vitamin D supplements were reinstituted to facilitate bone formation. The patient soon began to experience bouts of diarrhea, apparently as a side effect of the vitamin D supplements. Consequently, the vitamin D supplements were withdrawn, and only the calcium supplement was continued. Because metabolic by-products of vitamin D accelerate the absorption of calcium from the GI tract, both agents should be administered together. This patient, however, was apparently unable to tolerate vitamin D (or its analogs), possibly because of hypersensitivity to these compounds.

1. ***Which physical agent might help stimulate vitamin D production in this patient?***
2. ***How can this physical agent affect bone metabolism?***
3. ***How can the therapist incorporate the physical agent into the comprehensive treatment for this patient?***

See Appendix C, "Answers to Case Study Questions."

SUMMARY

The thyroid and parathyroid glands serve several vital endocrine functions. The thyroid gland synthesizes and secretes the thyroid hormones T_3 and T_4. These hormones are important regulators of cellular metabolism and metabolic rate. Thyroid hormones also interact with other hormones to facilitate normal growth and development. The parathyroid glands control calcium homeostasis through the release of PTH. This hormone is crucial in maintaining normal blood calcium levels and in regulating bone formation and resorption. PTH also interacts with other hormones such as vitamin D and calcitonin in the control of bone mineral metabolism. Acute and chronic problems in thyroid and parathyroid function are often successfully treated with various pharmacological agents. Rehabilitation specialists should be aware of the general strategies for treating thyroid and parathyroid disorders and of the basic pharmacotherapeutic approach to these problems.

REFERENCES

1. Salvatore D, Davies TF, Schlumberger MJ, et al. Thyroid physiology and diagnostic evaluation of patients with thyroid disorders. In: Melmed S, et al, eds. *Williams Textbook of Endocrinology*. 12th ed. Philadelphia, PA: Saunders/Elsevier; 2011.
2. Mansourian AR. Metabolic pathways of tetraiodothyronine and triiodothyronine production by thyroid gland: a review of articles. *Pak J Biol Sci*. 2011;14:1-12.
3. Williams GR, Bassett JH. Deiodinases: the balance of thyroid hormone: local control of thyroid hormone action: role of type 2 deiodinase. *J Endocrinol*. 2011;209:261-272.
4. Pearce EN, Andersson M, Zimmermann MB. Global iodine nutrition: where do we stand in 2013? *Thyroid*. 2013;23:523-528.
5. Chiamolera MI, Wondisford FE. Minireview: thyrotropin-releasing hormone and the thyroid hormone feedback mechanism. *Endocrinology*. 2009;150:1091-1096.
6. Nikrodhanond AA, Ortiga-Carvalho TM, Shibusawa N, et al. Dominant role of thyrotropin-releasing hormone in the hypothalamic-pituitary-thyroid axis. *J Biol Chem*. 2006;281:5000-5007.
7. Costa-e-Sousa RH, Hollenberg AN. Minireview: The neural regulation of the hypothalamic-pituitary-thyroid axis. *Endocrinology*. 2012;153:4128-4135.
8. Song Y, Yao X, Ying H. Thyroid hormone action in metabolic regulation. *Protein Cell*. 2011;2:358-368.

9. Stathatos N. Thyroid physiology. *Med Clin North Am*. 2012;96: 165-173.
10. Alkemade A. Central and peripheral effects of thyroid hormone signaling in the control of energy metabolism. *J Neuroendocrinol.* 2010;22:56-63.
11. Warner A, Mittag J. Thyroid hormone and the central control of homeostasis. *J Mol Endocrinol.* 2012;49:R29-35.
12. Aranda A, Alonso-Merino E, Zambrano A. Receptors of thyroid hormones. *Pediatr Endocrinol Rev.* 2013;11:2-13.
13. Tata JR. The road to nuclear receptors of thyroid hormone. *Biochim Biophys Acta*. 2013;1830:3860-3866.
14. Boelen A, Kwakkel J, Fliers E. Thyroid hormone receptors in health and disease. *Minerva Endocrinol.* 2012;37:291-304.
15. Cheng SY, Leonard JL, Davis PJ. Molecular aspects of thyroid hormone actions. *Endocr Rev*. 2010;31:139-170.
16. Davis PJ, Davis FB, Mousa SA, et al. Membrane receptor for thyroid hormone: physiologic and pharmacologic implications. *Annu Rev Pharmacol Toxicol.* 2011;51:99-115.
17. De Vito P, Balducci V, Leone S, et al. Nongenomic effects of thyroid hormones on the immune system cells: new targets, old players. *Steroids*. 2012;77:988-995.
18. Gessl A, Lemmens-Gruber R, Kautzky-Willer A. Thyroid disorders. *Handb Exp Pharmacol.* 2012;214:361-386.
19. Klubo-Gwiezdzinska J, Wartofsky L. Thyroid emergencies. *Med Clin North Am.* 2012;96:385-403.
20. Seigel SC, Hodak SP. Thyrotoxicosis. *Med Clin North Am.* 2012;96:175-201.
21. Taylor PN, Razvi S, Pearce SH, Dayan CM. Clinical review: a review of the clinical consequences of variation in thyroid function within the reference range. *J Clin Endocrinol Metab.* 2013;98:3562-3571.
22. Franklyn JA, Boelaert K. Thyrotoxicosis. *Lancet*. 2012;379: 1155-1166.
23. Li H, Wang T. The autoimmunity in Graves disease. *Front Biosci.* 2013;18:782-787.
24. Orgiazzi J. Thyroid autoimmunity. *Presse Med.* 2012;41(P 2): e611-625.
25. Sharma M, Aronow WS, Patel L, et al. Hyperthyroidism. *Med Sci Monit.* 2011;17:RA85-91.
26. Manna D, Roy G, Mugesh G. Antithyroid drugs and their analogues: synthesis, structure, and mechanism of action. *Acc Chem Res*. 2013;46:2706-2715.
27. Weissel M. Propylthiouracil: clinical overview of its efficacy and its side effects more than 50 years after the introduction of its use in thyrostatic treatment. *Exp Clin Endocrinol Diabetes*. 2010;118:101-104.
28. Cooper DS. Antithyroid drugs. *N Engl J Med.* 2005;352: 905-917.
29. Roy G, Mugesh G. Bioinorganic chemistry in thyroid gland: effect of antithyroid drugs on peroxidase-catalyzed oxidation and iodination reactions. *Bioinorg Chem Appl.* 2006:23214.
30. Brent GA, Koenig RJ. Thyroid and anti-thyroid drugs. In: Brunton LL, et al, eds. *The Pharmacological Basis of Therapeutics*. 12th ed. New York: McGraw-Hill; 2011.
31. Hänscheid H, Reiners C, Goulko G, et al. Facing the nuclear threat: thyroid blocking revisited. *J Clin Endocrinol Metab.* 2011;96:3511-3516.
32. Reiners C, Schneider R. Potassium iodide (KI) to block the thyroid from exposure to I-131: current questions and answers to be discussed. *Radiat Environ Biophys*. 2013;52: 189-193.
33. Gurgul E, Sowinski J. Primary hyperthyroidism—diagnosis and treatment. Indications and contraindications for radioiodine therapy. *Nucl Med Rev Cent East Eur.* 2011;14:29-32.
34. Lubin E. Radioactive iodine 131I (RAI) treatment. The nearest to the "magic bullet" but should always be preceded by a risk assessment, especially in the pediatric patient. *Pediatr Endocrinol Rev*. 2011;9:415-416.
35. Sundaresh V, Brito JP, Wang Z, et al. Comparative effectiveness of therapies for Graves' hyperthyroidism: a systematic review and network meta-analysis. *J Clin Endocrinol Metab.* 2013;98:3671-3677.
36. Bartalena L. The dilemma of how to manage Graves hyperthyroidism in patients with associated orbitopathy. *J Clin Endocrinol Metab*. 2011;96:592-599.
37. Stan MN, Durski JM, Brito JP, et al. Cohort study on radioactive iodine-induced hypothyroidism: implications for Graves ophthalmopathy and optimal timing for thyroid hormone assessment. *Thyroid*. 2013;23:620-625.
38. Ozbilen S, Eren MA, Turan MN, Sabuncu T. The impact of carvedilol and metoprolol on serum lipid concentrations and symptoms in patients with hyperthyroidism. *Endocr Res.* 2012;37:117-123.
39. Tagami T, Yambe Y, Tanaka T, et al. Short-term effects of β-adrenergic antagonists and methimazole in new-onset thyrotoxicosis caused by Graves disease. *Intern Med.* 2012;51:2285-2290.
40. Nayak B, Burman K. Thyrotoxicosis and thyroid storm. *Endocrinol Metab Clin North Am*. 2006;35:663-686.
41. Langley RW, Burch HB. Perioperative management of the thyrotoxic patient. *Endocrinol Metab Clin North Am*. 2003;32: 519-534.
42. Biondi B, Wartofsky L. Combination treatment with T4 and T3: toward personalized replacement therapy in hypothyroidism? *J Clin Endocrinol Metab*. 2012;97:2256-2271.
43. Gaitonde DY, Rowley KD, Sweeney LB. Hypothyroidism: an update. *Am Fam Physician*. 2012;86:244-251.
44. Escobar-Morreale HF, Botella-Carretero JI, Escobar del Rey F, Morreale de Escobar G. REVIEW: treatment of hypothyroidism with combinations of levothyroxine plus liothyronine. *J Clin Endocrinol Metab*. 2005;90:4946-4954.
45. McDermott MT. Does combination T_4 and T_3 therapy make sense? *Endocr Pract.* 2012;18:750-757.
46. Carreón-Rodríguez A, Pérez-Martínez L. Clinical implications of thyroid hormones effects on nervous system development. *Pediatr Endocrinol Rev*. 2012;9:644-649.
47. Wit JM, Camacho-Hübner C. Endocrine regulation of longitudinal bone growth. *Endocr Dev.* 2011;21:30-41.
48. Khandelwal D, Tandon N. Overt and subclinical hypothyroidism: who to treat and how. *Drugs*. 2012;72:17-33.
49. Bringhurst FR, Demay MB, Kronenberg HM. Hormones and disorders of mineral metabolism. In: Melmed S, et al, eds. *Williams Textbook of Endocrinology*. 12th ed. Philadelphia, PA: Saunders/Elsevier; 2011.
50. Kumar R, Thompson JR. The regulation of parathyroid hormone secretion and synthesis. *J Am Soc Nephrol.* 2011;22: 216-224.
51. Ward DT, Riccardi D. New concepts in calcium-sensing receptor pharmacology and signalling. *Br J Pharmacol.* 2012;165: 35-48.
52. Boros S, Bindels RJ, Hoenderop JG. Active Ca(2+) reabsorption in the connecting tubule. *Pflugers Arch*. 2009;458:99-109.

53. Lombardi G, Di Somma C, Rubino M, et al. The roles of parathyroid hormone in bone remodeling: prospects for novel therapeutics. *J Endocrinol Invest*. 2011;34(suppl):18-22.
54. Silva BC, Costa AG, Cusano NE, et al. Catabolic and anabolic actions of parathyroid hormone on the skeleton. *J Endocrinol Invest*. 2011;34:801-810.
55. Bellido T, Saini V, Pajevic PD. Effects of PTH on osteocyte function. *Bone*. 2013;54:250-257.
56. Picard N, Capuano P, Stange G, et al. Acute parathyroid hormone differentially regulates renal brush border membrane phosphate cotransporters. *Pflugers Arch*. 2010;460:677-687.
57. Henry HL. Regulation of vitamin D metabolism. *Best Pract Res Clin Endocrinol Metab*. 2011;25:531-541.
58. Emkey RD, Emkey GR. Calcium metabolism and correcting calcium deficiencies. *Endocrinol Metab Clin North Am*. 2012;41: 527-556.
59. Marie PJ. Signaling pathways affecting skeletal health. *Curr Osteoporos Rep*. 2012;10:190-198.
60. Lee CS, Szczesny SE, Soslowsky LJ. Remodeling and repair of orthopedic tissue: role of mechanical loading and biologics: part II: cartilage and bone. *Am J Orthop*. 2011;40:122-128.
61. Esbrit P, Alcaraz MJ. Current perspectives on parathyroid hormone (PTH) and PTH-related protein (PTHrP) as bone anabolic therapies. *Biochem Pharmacol*. 2013;85:1417-1423.
62. Ellegaard M, Jørgensen NR, Schwarz P. Parathyroid hormone and bone healing. *Calcif Tissue Int*. 2010;87:1-13.
63. Lips P, van Schoor NM. The effect of vitamin D on bone and osteoporosis. *Best Pract Res Clin Endocrinol Metab*. 2011;25:585-591.
64. Yoshida T, Stern PH. How vitamin D works on bone. *Endocrinol Metab Clin North Am*. 2012;41:557-569.
65. Haussler MR, Whitfield GK, Kaneko I, et al. Molecular mechanisms of vitamin D action. *Calcif Tissue Int*. 2013;92:77-98.
66. Bienaimé F, Prié D, Friedlander G, Souberbielle JC. Vitamin D metabolism and activity in the parathyroid gland. *Mol Cell Endocrinol*. 2011;347:30-41.
67. Ritter CS, Armbrecht HJ, Slatopolsky E, Brown AJ. 25-Hydroxyvitamin D(3) suppresses PTH synthesis and secretion by bovine parathyroid cells. *Kidney Int*. 2006;70:654-659.
68. Lieben L, Carmeliet G. Vitamin D signaling in osteocytes: effects on bone and mineral homeostasis. *Bone*. 2013;54:237-243.
69. de Paula FJ, Rosen CJ. Back to the future: revisiting parathyroid hormone and calcitonin control of bone remodeling. *Horm Metab Res*. 2010;42:299-306.
70. Friedman PA. Agents affecting mineral ion homeostasis and bone turnover. In: Brunton LL, et al, eds. *The Pharmacological Basis of Therapeutics*. 12th ed. New York: McGraw-Hill; 2011.
71. Liao E. FGF23 associated bone diseases. *Front Med*. 2013;7: 65-80.
72. Lecart MP, Reginster JY. Current options for the management of postmenopausal osteoporosis. *Expert Opin Pharmacother*. 2011;12:2533-2552.
73. Nordin BE. The effect of calcium supplementation on bone loss in 32 controlled trials in postmenopausal women. *Osteoporos Int*. 2009;20:2135-2143.
74. Curtis JR, Safford MM. Management of osteoporosis among the elderly with other chronic medical conditions. *Drugs Aging*. 2012;29:549-564.
75. O'Connell MB, Vondracek SF. Osteoporosis and other metabolic bone diseases. In: DiPiro JT, et al, eds. *Pharmacotherapy: A Pathophysiologic Approach*. 8th ed. New York: McGraw-Hill; 2011.
76. Committee to Review Dietary Reference Intakes for Vitamin D and Calcium, Food and Nutrition Board, Institute of Medicine. Dietary Reference Intakes for Calcium and Vitamin D. Washington, DC: National Academy Press; 2010.
77. Straub DA. Calcium supplementation in clinical practice: a review of forms, doses, and indications. *Nutr Clin Pract*. 2007;22: 286-296.
78. Moyer VA; U.S. Preventive Services Task Force. Vitamin D and calcium supplementation to prevent fractures in adults: U.S. Preventive Services Task Force recommendation statement. *Ann Intern Med*. 2013;158:691-696.
79. Anderson JJ, Klemmer PJ. Risk of high dietary calcium for arterial calcification in older adults. *Nutrients*. 2013;5:3964-3974.
80. De Nijs RN. Glucocorticoid-induced osteoporosis: a review on pathophysiology and treatment options. *Minerva Med*. 2008;99: 23-43.
81. Drake MT, Cremers SC. Bisphosphonate therapeutics in bone disease: the hard and soft data on osteoclast inhibition. *Mol Interv*. 2010;10:141-152.
82. Russell RG. Bisphosphonates: the first 40 years. *Bone*. 2011;49: 2-19.
83. Hampson G, Fogelman I. Clinical role of bisphosphonate therapy. *Int J Womens Health*. 2012;4:455-469.
84. Reid IR. Pharmacotherapy of Paget's disease of bone. *Expert Opin Pharmacother*. 2012;13:637-646.
85. Vasileiadis GI, Sakellariou VI, Kelekis A, et al. Prevention of heterotopic ossification in cases of hypertrophic osteoarthritis submitted to total hip arthroplasty. Etidronate or indomethacin? *J Musculoskelet Neuronal Interact*. 2010;10:159-165.
86. Saylor PJ, Lee RJ, Smith MR. Emerging therapies to prevent skeletal morbidity in men with prostate cancer. *J Clin Oncol*. 2011;29:3705-3714.
87. Wong MH, Stockler MR, Pavlakis N. Bisphosphonates and other bone agents for breast cancer. *Cochrane Database Syst Rev*. 2012;2:CD003474.
88. Rizzoli R, Adachi JD, Cooper C, et al. Management of glucocorticoid-induced osteoporosis. *Calcif Tissue Int*. 2012;91: 225-243.
89. Das S, Crockett JC. Osteoporosis—a current view of pharmacological prevention and treatment. *Drug Des Devel Ther*. 2013;7:435-448.
90. Rizzoli R. Bisphosphonates for post-menopausal osteoporosis: are they all the same? *QJM*. 2011;104:281-300.
91. Khosla S, Bilezikian JP, Dempster DW, et al. Benefits and risks of bisphosphonate therapy for osteoporosis. *J Clin Endocrinol Metab*. 2012;97:2272-2282.
92. Migliore A, Broccoli S, Massafra U, et al. Ranking antireabsorptive agents to prevent vertebral fractures in postmenopausal osteoporosis by mixed treatment comparison meta-analysis. *Eur Rev Med Pharmacol Sci*. 2013;17:658-667.
93. Reginster JY. Antifracture efficacy of currently available therapies for postmenopausal osteoporosis. *Drugs*. 2011;71:65-78.
94. Beninati F, Pruneti R, Ficarra G. Bisphosphonate-related osteonecrosis of the jaws (Bronj). *Med Oral Patol Oral Cir Bucal*. 2013;18:e752-758.
95. Paiva-Fonseca F, Santos-Silva AR, Della-Coletta R, et al. Alendronate-associated osteonecrosis of the jaws: a review of the main topics. *Med Oral Patol Oral Cir Bucal*. 2014;19:e106-111.
96. Chesnut CH 3rd, Azria M, Silverman S, et al. Salmon calcitonin: a review of current and future therapeutic indications. *Osteoporos Int*. 2008;19:479-491.

97. Esenyel M, İçağasıoğlu A, Esenyel CZ. Effects of calcitonin on knee osteoarthritis and quality of life. *Rheumatol Int.* 2013; 33:423-427.
98. Fraser LA, Adachi JD. Glucocorticoid-induced osteoporosis: treatment update and review. *Ther Adv Musculoskelet Dis.* 2009;1:71-85.
99. Chen JS, Sambrook PN. Antiresorptive therapies for osteoporosis: a clinical overview. *Nat Rev Endocrinol.* 2011;8:81-91.
100. Knopp-Sihota JA, Newburn-Cook CV, Homik J, et al. Calcitonin for treating acute and chronic pain of recent and remote osteoporotic vertebral compression fractures: a systematic review and meta-analysis. *Osteoporos Int.* 2012;23:17-38.
101. Miller PD, Derman RJ. What is the best balance of benefits and risks among anti-resorptive therapies for postmenopausal osteoporosis? *Osteoporos Int.* 2010;21:1793-1802.
102. Hoyer H, Perera G, Bernkop-Schnürch A. Noninvasive delivery systems for peptides and proteins in osteoporosis therapy: a retroperspective. *Drug Dev Ind Pharm.* 2010;36:31-44.
103. Lee SL, Yu LX, Cai B, et al. Scientific considerations for generic synthetic salmon calcitonin nasal spray products. *AAPS J.* 2011;13:14-19.
104. Maricic MJ. Oral calcitonin. *Curr Osteoporos Rep.* 2012;10: 80-85.
105. Hamdy RC, Daley DN. Oral calcitonin. *Int J Womens Health.* 2012;4:471-479.
106. Henriksen K, Bay-Jensen AC, Christiansen C, Karsdal MA. Oral salmon calcitonin—pharmacology in osteoporosis. *Expert Opin Biol Ther.* 2010;10:1617-1629.
107. de Villiers TJ, Stevenson JC. The WHI: the effect of hormone replacement therapy on fracture prevention. *Climacteric.* 2012;15:263-266.
108. Eriksen EF. Hormone replacement therapy or SERMS in the long term treatment of osteoporosis. *Minerva Ginecol.* 2012;64:207-221.
109. Marjoribanks J, Farquhar C, Roberts H, Lethaby A. Long term hormone therapy for perimenopausal and postmenopausal women. *Cochrane Database Syst Rev.* 2012;7:CD004143.
110. Gambacciani M, Vacca F. Postmenopausal osteoporosis and hormone replacement therapy. *Minerva Med.* 2004;95:507-520.
111. Archer DF, Oger E. Estrogen and progestogen effect on venous thromboembolism in menopausal women. *Climacteric.* 2012;15: 235-240.
112. Henderson VW, Lobo RA. Hormone therapy and the risk of stroke: perspectives 10 years after the Women's Health Initiative trials. *Climacteric.* 2012;15:229-234.
113. Christenson ES, Jiang X, Kagan R, Schnatz P. Osteoporosis management in post-menopausal women. *Minerva Ginecol.* 2012;64:181-194.
114. Gallagher JC, Levine JP. Preventing osteoporosis in symptomatic postmenopausal women. *Menopause.* 2011;18:109-118.
115. Shoupe D. Individualizing hormone-therapy according to cardiovascular risk. *Minerva Med.* 2012;103:343-352.
116. Maximov PY, Lee TM, Jordan VC. The discovery and development of selective estrogen receptor modulators (SERMs) for clinical practice. *Curr Clin Pharmacol.* 2013;8: 135-155.
117. D'Amelio P, Isaia GC. The use of raloxifene in osteoporosis treatment. *Expert Opin Pharmacother.* 2013;14:949-956.
118. Ko SS, Jordan VC. Treatment of osteoporosis and reduction in risk of invasive breast cancer in postmenopausal women with raloxifene. *Expert Opin Pharmacother.* 2011;12:657-674.
119. Resmini G, Iolascon G. New insights into the role of teriparatide. *Aging Clin Exp Res.* 2011;23(suppl):30-32.
120. Silverman SL, Nasser K. Teriparatide update. *Rheum Dis Clin North Am.* 2011;37:471-477.
121. Uihlein AV, Leder BZ. Anabolic therapies for osteoporosis. *Endocrinol Metab Clin North Am.* 2012;41:507-525.
122. Blick SK, Dhillon S, Keam SJ. Spotlight on teriparatide in osteoporosis. *BioDrugs.* 2009;23:197-199.
123. Han SL, Wan SL. Effect of teriparatide on bone mineral density and fracture in postmenopausal osteoporosis: meta-analysis of randomised controlled trials. *Int J Clin Pract.* 2012;66:199-209.
124. Saag KG, Zanchetta JR, Devogelaer JP, et al. Effects of teriparatide versus alendronate for treating glucocorticoid-induced osteoporosis: thirty-six-month results of a randomized, double-blind, controlled trial. *Arthritis Rheum.* 2009;60: 3346-3355.
125. Nemeth EF, Shoback D. Calcimimetic and calcilytic drugs for treating bone and mineral-related disorders. *Best Pract Res Clin Endocrinol Metab.* 2013;27:373-384.
126. Messa P, Alfieri C, Brezzi B. Clinical utilization of cinacalcet in hypercalcemic conditions. *Expert Opin Drug Metab Toxicol.* 2011;7:517-528.
127. Moen MD, Keam SJ. Denosumab: a review of its use in the treatment of postmenopausal osteoporosis. *Drugs Aging.* 2011;28: 63-82.
128. Hanley DA, Adachi JD, Bell A, Brown V. Denosumab: mechanism of action and clinical outcomes. *Int J Clin Pract.* 2012;66: 1139-1146.
129. Josse R, Khan A, Ngui D, Shapiro M. Denosumab, a new pharmacotherapy option for postmenopausal osteoporosis. *Curr Med Res Opin.* 2013;29:205-216.
130. Sutton EE, Riche DM. Denosumab, a RANK ligand inhibitor, for postmenopausal women with osteoporosis. *Ann Pharmacother.* 2012;46:1000-1009.

CHAPTER 32

Pancreatic Hormones and the Treatment of Diabetes Mellitus

The pancreas functions uniquely as both an endocrine and an exocrine gland. The gland's exocrine role consists of excretion of digestive enzymes into the duodenum via the pancreatic duct. Pancreatic endocrine function consists of the secretion of two principal hormones—insulin and glucagon—into the bloodstream. Insulin and glucagon are involved primarily with the regulation of blood glucose. Insulin also plays a role in protein and lipid metabolism and is important in several aspects of growth and development. Problems with the production and function of insulin cause a fairly common and clinically significant disease known as **diabetes mellitus**.

This chapter reviews the normal physiological roles of the pancreatic hormones and describes the pathogenesis and treatment of diabetes mellitus (DM). Diabetes mellitus has many sequelae that influence patients' neuromuscular and cardiovascular functioning, and patients with this condition often undergo physical rehabilitation for problems related to these issues. Consequently, the nature of DM and its pharmacotherapeutic treatment are important to physical therapists and occupational therapists.

STRUCTURE AND FUNCTION OF THE ENDOCRINE PANCREAS

The cellular composition of the pancreas has been described in great detail in other sources.[1-3] The relevance of pancreatic structure to its endocrine function is reviewed briefly here. The bulk of the gland consists of acinar cells that synthesize and release pancreatic digestive enzymes (thereby providing the exocrine function). Interspersed within the acinar tissues are smaller clumps of tissue known as the *islets of Langerhans*. These islets contain cells that synthesize and secrete pancreatic hormones, thus constituting the endocrine portion of the gland.

The pancreatic islets consist of at least five primary cell types: alpha (A) cells, which produce glucagon; beta (B) cells, which produce insulin; delta (D) cells, which produce somatostatin; (F) cells, which produce pancreatic polypeptide; and epsilon (E) cells, which produce ghrelin.[4] As previously mentioned, this discussion will focus on the functions of insulin and glucagon. The exact physiological roles of the other pancreatic hormones are not entirely clear. Somatostatin, for example, is a polypeptide hormone that appears to affect several physiological systems, including the regulation of gastrointestinal (GI) absorption and motility. This hormone may inhibit the release of glucagon and insulin.[5] Somatostatin is also produced in other tissues, including the brain and GI tract, and it may affect many other neuroendocrine responses.[6,7]

Likewise, pancreatic ghrelin inhibits insulin release from beta cells, but ghrelin is also produced in the stomach and other tissues. This peptide helps regulate GI function, lipid metabolism, cardiovascular function, growth hormone release, and several other physiological functions that continue to be investigated.[8] The effects of the pancreatic polypeptide released from pancreatic F cells remain to be fully determined.[4] Future studies are needed to further clarify the physiological effects of somatostatin, ghrelin, and pancreatic polypeptide.

INSULIN

Insulin is a large polypeptide of 51 amino acids arranged in a specific sequence and configuration. The primary effect of insulin is to lower blood glucose levels by facilitating the entry of glucose into peripheral tissues. The effects of insulin on energy metabolism, specific aspects of insulin release, and insulin's mechanism of action are discussed here.

Effects of Insulin on Carbohydrate Metabolism

Following a meal, blood glucose sharply increases. Insulin is responsible for facilitating the movement of glucose out of the bloodstream and into the liver and other tissues, where it can be stored for future needs.[9,10] Most tissues in the body (including skeletal muscle cells) are relatively impermeable to glucose and require the presence of some sort of transport system, or carrier, to help convey the glucose molecule across the cell membrane.[11,12] The carrier-mediated transport of glucose into muscle cells is believed to be a form of facilitated diffusion (see Chapter 2). Insulin appears to directly stimulate this facilitated diffusion, resulting in a tenfold or greater increase in the rate of glucose influx.[13] The possible ways that insulin affects glucose transport on the cellular level are discussed later in "Cellular Mechanism of Insulin Action."

Insulin affects the uptake and use of glucose in the liver somewhat differently than in skeletal muscle and other tissues. Hepatic cells are relatively permeable to glucose, and glucose enters these cells quite easily, even when insulin is not present. Glucose, however, is also free to leave liver cells just as easily, unless it is trapped in the cells in some manner. Insulin stimulates the activity of the glucokinase enzyme, which phosphorylates glucose and subsequently traps the glucose molecule in the hepatic cell. Insulin also increases the activity of enzymes that promote glycogen synthesis and inhibits the enzymes that promote glycogen breakdown. Thus, the primary effect of insulin on the liver is to promote the sequestration of the glucose molecule and to increase the storage of glucose in the form of hepatic glycogen.

Effects of Insulin on Protein and Lipid Metabolism

Although insulin is normally associated with regulating blood glucose, this hormone also exerts significant effects on proteins and lipids. In general, insulin promotes storage of protein and lipid in muscle and adipose tissue, respectively.[14] Insulin encourages protein synthesis in muscle cells by stimulating amino acid uptake, increasing DNA/RNA activity related to protein synthesis, and inhibiting protein breakdown. In fat cells, insulin stimulates the synthesis of fatty acids and triglycerides (the primary form of lipid storage in the body), increases the uptake of triglycerides from the blood into adipose and muscle tissues, and inhibits the enzyme that breaks down stored lipids (i.e., hormone-sensitive lipase). Consequently, insulin is involved in carbohydrate, protein, and lipid metabolism; disturbances in insulin function in conditions like DM will affect the storage and use of all the primary energy substrates.

Cellular Mechanism of Insulin Action

Insulin exerts its effects first by binding to a receptor located on the surface membrane of target cells.[15] This receptor is a glycoprotein that is highly specific for insulin. The complete insulin receptor consists of two matching or paired units, with each unit consisting of an alpha and a beta subunit (Fig. 32-1). The alpha subunit is the binding site for insulin. The beta subunit appears to be an enzyme that functions as a tyrosine kinase, which means that it catalyzes the addition of phosphate groups to tyrosine residues within the beta subunit.[15,16] Thus, binding insulin to the alpha subunit causes the beta subunit to undergo *autophosphorylation*—that is, the receptor adds phosphate groups to itself. This autophosphorylation of the insulin receptor then initiates a series of biochemical changes within the cell.

The way that the insulin-receptor interaction triggers subsequent changes in cellular activity has been the subject of extensive research. Researchers have determined that the insulin receptor, when activated, begins to add phosphate molecules to other large intracellular proteins known as *insulin receptor substrates* (IRSs).[15,16] Although the exact details need to be elucidated, IRSs initiate changes in various metabolic pathways that ultimately result in increased glucose uptake, increased protein synthesis, and other changes in cell metabolism.[17,18] In particular, certain IRSs initiate the movement (translocation) of glucose transporters

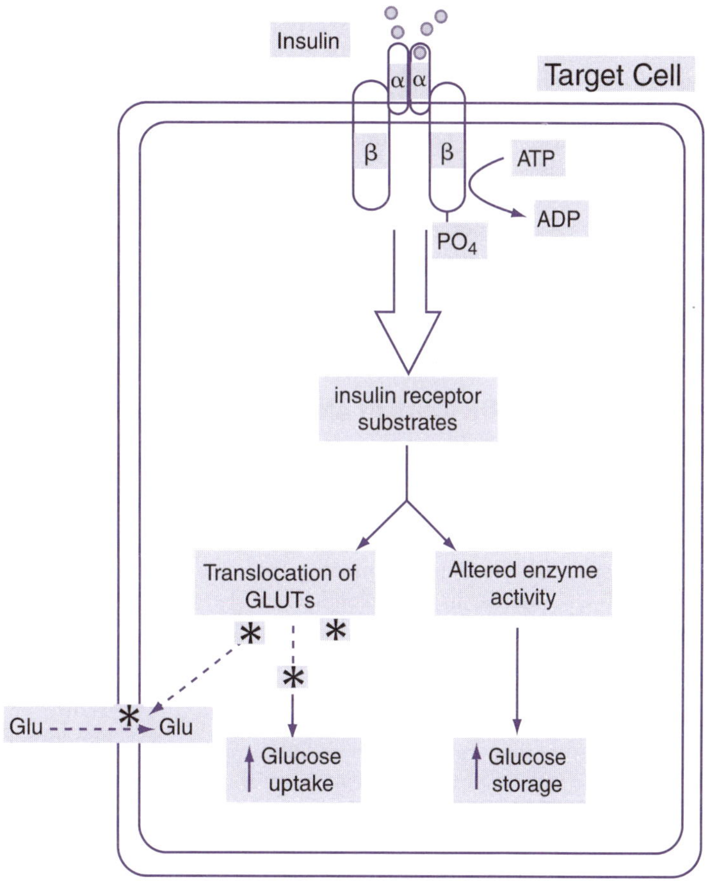

Figure ■ 32-1
Possible mechanism of insulin action on glucose metabolism in skeletal muscle cells. An insulin receptor located on the cell's surface consists of two alpha (α) and two beta (β) subunits. Binding of insulin to the α subunits causes addition of phosphate groups (PO_4) to the β subunits. This receptor autophosphorylation causes the activation of one or more insulin receptor substrates (IRSs), which promote translocation of glucose carriers (GLUTs) to the cell membrane, where they increase facilitated diffusion of glucose (Glu) into the cell. Activated IRSs also increase the activity of enzymes that promote glucose storage.

from intracellular storage sites to the cell membrane of skeletal muscle cells and other peripheral tissues (see Fig. 32-1). These glucose transporters are proteins that are synthesized and stored within the Golgi system of the cell. These proteins are likewise often referred to as glucose tranporter (GLUT) proteins, or simply GLUTs; several different forms of GLUTs exist, depending on the specific cell that is affected by insulin. Perhaps the most important GLUT protein is the GLUT4 subtype, which is the glucose transporter in muscle and fat cells.[9,11,13] By binding to the insulin receptor on the cell membrane, insulin ultimately causes GLUT4 proteins to travel to the cell membrane, where they can then promote the facilitated diffusion of glucose into the cell (see Fig. 32-1).

Consequently, we now have a fairly clear idea of how insulin binds to a specific receptor and exerts its effects on target cells. Knowledge of exactly how insulin interacts with target tissues is important because defects in receptor binding and problems in the subsequent postreceptor events may be responsible for some of the changes seen in certain forms of DM. The possible role of these receptor-mediated problems in diabetes is discussed later in "Type 2 Diabetes."

GLUCAGON

Glucagon is considered to be the hormonal antagonist of insulin.[19-21] The primary effect of glucagon is to increase blood glucose to maintain normal blood glucose levels and to prevent hypoglycemia.[22] Glucagon produces a rapid increase in glycogen breakdown (glycogenolysis) in the liver, thus liberating glucose into the bloodstream from hepatic glycogen stores.[23] Glucagon then stimulates a more prolonged increase in hepatic glucose production (gluconeogenesis). This gluconeogenesis sustains blood glucose levels even after hepatic glycogen has been depleted.[19]

Glucagon appears to exert its effects on liver cells by a classic adenyl cyclase–cyclic adenosine monophosphate (cAMP) second messenger system (see Chapter 4).[1] Glucagon binds to a specific receptor located on the hepatic cell membrane. This stimulates the activity of the adenyl cyclase enzyme that transforms adenosine triphosphate (ATP) into cAMP. Then cAMP acts as an intracellular second messenger that activates specific enzymes to increase glycogen breakdown and stimulate gluconeogenesis.

CONTROL OF INSULIN AND GLUCAGON RELEASE

An adequate level of glucose in the bloodstream is necessary to provide a steady supply of energy for certain tissues, especially the brain. Normally, fasting blood glucose (i.e., glucose in the bloodstream between meals) is maintained between 70 and 110 mg of glucose per 100 mL of blood.[19] A severe drop in blood glucose (i.e., hypoglycemia) is a potentially serious problem that can result in coma and death. Chronic elevations in blood glucose (hyperglycemia) have been implicated in producing pathological changes in neural and vascular structures. Consequently, insulin and glucagon play vital roles in controlling glucose levels, and the release of these hormones must be closely regulated.

The level of glucose in the bloodstream is the primary factor affecting pancreatic hormone release.[19,24] As blood glucose rises (e.g., following a meal), insulin secretion from pancreatic beta cells is increased. Insulin then promotes the movement of glucose out of the bloodstream and into various tissues, thus reducing plasma glucose back to normal levels. As blood glucose levels fall (e.g., during a sustained fast), glucagon is released from the alpha cells in the pancreas. Glucagon resolves this hypoglycemia by stimulating the synthesis and release of glucose from the liver.

The release of insulin and glucagon may also be governed by other energy substrates (e.g., lipids and amino acids), other hormones (e.g., thyroxine, cortisol, growth hormone, others), and autonomic neural control.[24-27] Nonetheless, the major factor influencing pancreatic hormone release is blood glucose concentration. Cells located in the pancreatic islets act as glucose sensors, directly monitoring plasma glucose levels in the blood reaching the pancreas. In particular, the beta cells or insulin-secreting cells act as the primary glucose sensors, and adequate control of insulin release seems to be a somewhat higher priority than the control of glucagon function.[19]

An important interaction between insulin and glucagon may also take place directly within the pancreas, and insulin appears to be the dominant hormone controlling this interaction.[28,29] When the beta cells sense an increase in blood glucose, they release insulin, which in turn inhibits glucagon release from the alpha cells. When insulin release diminishes, the inhibition of glucagon production is removed, and glucagon secretion is free to increase. This intra-islet regulation between insulin and glucagon is important during normal physiological function as well as in pathological conditions, such as the deficiency of insulin production characteristic of type 1 diabetes mellitus.[24] The effects of increased glucagon may contribute to some of the metabolic changes in DM (although the exact role of increased glucagon in DM remains controversial).[30]

Consequently, insulin and glucagon serve to maintain blood glucose within a finite range. If the endocrine portion of the pancreas is functioning normally, blood glucose levels remain remarkably constant, even in situations such as exercise and prolonged fasting. However, any abnormalities in pancreatic endocrine function can alter the regulation of blood glucose. In particular, problems associated with the production and effects of insulin can produce serious disturbances in glucose metabolism and several other metabolic problems. Problems in insulin production and function are characteristic of DM. The pathogenesis and treatment of this disease are presented in the following section.

DIABETES MELLITUS

DM is caused by insufficient insulin secretion or a decrease in the peripheral effects of insulin. This disease is characterized by a primary defect in the metabolism of carbohydrates and other energy substrates. These metabolic defects can lead to serious acute and chronic pathological changes. The term *diabetes mellitus* differentiates this disease from an unrelated disorder known as *diabetes insipidus*. Diabetes insipidus is caused by a lack of antidiuretic hormone (ADH) production or insensitivity to ADH. Consequently, the full term *diabetes mellitus* should be used when referring to the insulin-related disease. Most clinicians, however, refer to diabetes mellitus as simply "diabetes."

Diabetes mellitus is a common disease that affects approximately 24 million people in the United States.[31]

This disease is a serious problem in terms of increased morbidity and mortality. It is the leading cause of blindness in adults[32] and is responsible for one-third of all cases of end-stage renal disease.[33] It is also estimated that 71,000 lower-extremity amputations are performed annually because of complications related to DM.[31] Consequently, this disease affects the lives of many individuals.

DM is apparently not a single, homogeneous disease but rather a disease existing in two primary forms: type 1 and type 2.[31,34] In addition, other forms of DM exist, such as gestational diabetes (i.e., impaired glucose metabolism that occurs during pregnancy) and several genetic disorders that result in structural defects of the insulin molecule or the insulin receptor.[34] Most people with DM, however, are classified as having either type 1 or type 2 DM, according to the primary characteristics summarized in Table 32-1. Specific aspects of these two primary forms of DM are discussed in more detail below.

Type 1 Diabetes

Type 1 diabetes accounts for approximately 5 to 10 percent of the individuals with DM.[31] Patients with type 1 diabetes are unable to synthesize any appreciable amounts of insulin. There appears to be an almost total destruction of pancreatic beta cells in these individuals. Because of their inability to produce insulin, people with type 1 diabetes were previously referred to as having insulin-dependent diabetes mellitus (IDDM)—that is, administration of exogenous insulin is necessary for survival. The onset of type 1 diabetes is usually during childhood, so this form of diabetes has also been referred to as *juvenile diabetes*. Classic type 1 diabetes, however, can develop in people of all ages.[31] Hence, terms such as *IDDM* and *juvenile diabetes* are no longer commonly used, and *type 1 diabetes* is generally the preferred term for this disease. Patients with type 1 diabetes are typically close to normal body weight or slightly underweight.

The exact cause of type 1 diabetes is unknown, but there is considerable evidence that the beta cell destruction characteristic of this disease may be caused in many patients by an autoimmune reaction.[35,36] Specifically, a virus or some other antigen may trigger an autoimmune reaction that selectively destroys the insulin-secreting beta cells in susceptible individuals.[37,38] Certain patients' susceptibility to such viral-initiated immunodestruction may be due to genetic predisposition, environmental factors, or other factors that remain to be determined.[36,39,40] The idea that type 1 diabetes may have an autoimmune basis has led to the use of immunosuppressant agents in the early stages of this disease (see "Prevention of Type 1 Diabetes Mellitus: The Potential Role of Immune-Based Therapies").

Type 2 Diabetes

Type 2 diabetes, also known previously as *non-insulin-dependent diabetes mellitus* (NIDDM), accounts for 90 to 95 percent of people with DM.[31] This form of diabetes usually occurs in adults, especially in older individuals.[41] However, type 2 diabetes can also occur in young people, and there is concern that the incidence of this disease is increasing dramatically in children and adolescents.[42,43] Although the specific factors

Table 32-1
COMPARISON OF TYPE 1 AND TYPE 2 DIABETES MELLITUS

Characteristic	Type 1	Type 2
Age at onset	Usually before 20	Usually after 30
Type of onset	Abrupt; often severe	Gradual; usually subtle
Usual body weight	Normal	Overweight
Blood insulin	Markedly reduced	Normal or increased
Peripheral response to insulin	Normal	Decreased
Clinical management	Insulin and diet	Diet; insulin or oral antidiabetics if diet control alone is ineffective

Adapted from: Craighead JE. Diabetes. In: Rubin E, Farber JL, eds. Pathology. 3rd ed. Philadelphia, PA: Lippincott-Raven; 1999.

responsible for this disease are unknown, a genetic predisposition combined with poor diet, obesity, and lack of exercise all seem to contribute to the onset of type 2 diabetes.[42,44-46] Increased body weight is common in patients with type 2 diabetes.

Whereas insulin cannot be produced in type 1 diabetes, the problem in type 2 diabetes is somewhat more complex.[47] Type 2 diabetes is characterized by a combination of pancreatic beta cell dysfunction and decreased sensitivity of peripheral tissues to circulating insulin (i.e., insulin resistance).[47,48] For instance, tissues such as the skeletal muscle, adipose tissue, and the liver fail to respond adequately to insulin in the bloodstream.[49] Thus, peripheral uptake and use of glucose are blunted, even when insulin is present.

The exact cellular mechanisms responsible for insulin resistance are unknown. The resistance may be caused by a primary (intrinsic) defect at the target cell that results in a decreased response of the cell to insulin. The decreased insulin response most likely occurs because of changes in the way the cell responds *after* insulin binds to the surface receptor. Problems in postreceptor signaling—such as altered protein phosphorylation, impaired production of chemical mediators, and a lack of glucose transporters—have been suggested as intracellular events that could help explain insulin resistance.[50-52] Therefore, even though insulin binds to the receptor, the cellular response is inadequate. Hence, insulin resistance appears to be a complex phenomenon caused by changes in the cellular response to insulin at the tissue level. However, the exact defects in insulin receptor signaling and postreceptor function remain to be determined.

As indicated above, a defect in pancreatic beta cell function may also contribute to the manifestations of type 2 diabetes.[47] Beta cells may still be able to produce insulin, but these cells do not respond adequately to increased plasma glucose levels and other substances that normally cause insulin secretion after a meal.[53] That is, insulin release after a meal is not proportional to the increased glucose levels in the bloodstream, resulting in hyperglycemia. Moreover, repeated hyperglycemia seems to cause additional damage to beta cells, resulting in a further decrease in beta cell function and response to glucose.[54] Prolonged and repeated hyperglycemia seems to progressively decrease the size and number of functioning beta cells, ultimately resulting in the total loss of beta cells and insulin secretion.[53]

Furthermore, some evidence indicates that beta cell dysfunction precedes insulin resistance in skeletal muscle and other peripheral tissues and that disordered beta cell function is a key initiating factor in type 2 DM.[54] This idea suggests that the progression of type 2 DM may be caused by a vicious cycle where beta cell dysfunction causes disordered insulin secretion, which leads to repeated hyperglycemia, which in turn promotes peripheral insulin resistance and more hyperglycemia, which further increases beta cell dysfunction, and so on. Clearly, type 2 DM involves a complex interaction between inappropriate beta cell response and peripheral insulin resistance, and research continues to clarify how these factors interact with each other in the pathogenesis of type 2 DM.

Finally, insulin resistance is present in disease states other than type 2 DM. Patients with conditions such as hypertension, obesity, and certain hyperlipidemias are also found to have decreased tissue sensitivity to circulating insulin.[50,55,56] As discussed in Chapter 21, metabolic syndrome, or syndrome X, occurs when insulin resistance, high blood pressure, abdominal obesity, and hyperlipidemia occur simultaneously in the patient.[56-59] Although the causes of insulin resistance in this syndrome are not completely understood, they probably involve a complex series of changes at the systemic, cellular, and subcellular levels.[60,61] There is consensus, however, that therapeutic strategies for resolving insulin resistance should be considered an important part of the management of various conditions that exhibit this phenomenon.[57,62]

Effects and Complications of Diabetes Mellitus

The most common symptom associated with DM is a chronic elevation of blood glucose (hyperglycemia). This results from a relative lack of insulin-mediated glucose uptake and use by peripheral tissues. Hyperglycemia initiates several complex and potentially serious acute metabolic changes. For example, it is usually accompanied by increased glucose excretion by the kidneys (glycosuria). Glycosuria is caused by an inability of the kidneys to adequately reabsorb the excess amount of glucose reaching the nephron. Increased glucose excretion creates an osmotic force that promotes fluid and electrolyte excretion, thus leading to dehydration and electrolyte imbalance.[63] Also, the loss of glucose in the urine causes a metabolic shift toward the mobilization of fat and protein as an energy source. Increased use of fats and protein leads to the formation of acidic ketone bodies in the bloodstream. Excessive accumulation of ketones lowers plasma pH, producing acidosis (i.e., ketoacidosis), which can lead to coma and death.[64]

DM is associated with several other long-term complications involving vascular and neural structures. Perhaps the most devastating complications associated with this disease result from the development of abnormalities in small blood vessels (i.e., microangiopathy).[65,66] Small vessels may undergo a thickening of the basement membrane, which can progress to the point of vessel occlusion.[67,68] The progressive ischemia caused by small-vessel disease is particularly damaging to certain structures such as the retina (leading to blindness) and the kidneys (leading to nephropathy and renal failure).[67,69,70] Damage to cutaneous vessels results in poor wound healing that can lead to ulcer formation.[71] Problems with large blood vessels (i.e., macroangiopathy) can also occur in DM because of defects in the vascular endothelium and disordered lipid metabolism that leads to atherosclerosis.[72,73] Macroangiopathy is a principal contributing factor in hypertension, myocardial infarction, and cerebral vascular accident in diabetic patients. Finally, peripheral neuropathies are quite common among patients with poorly controlled DM.[74]

The neurovascular complications described previously are directly related to the severity and duration of hyperglycemia in diabetic patients.[75] Although the details are somewhat unclear, prolonged elevations in blood glucose may promote structural and functional changes in vascular endothelial cells and peripheral neurons. These cellular changes are ultimately responsible for the gross pathological abnormalities characteristic of poorly controlled DM.

Consequently, the primary goal in the treatment of both type 1 and type 2 DM is to control blood glucose levels. Maintenance of blood glucose at or close to normal levels—referred to as *tight glycemic control*—will prevent acute metabolic derangements and greatly reduce the risk of the chronic neurovascular complications associated with this disease.[75-77] The pharmacological agents used to treat DM are described in the next sections.

USE OF INSULIN IN DIABETES MELLITUS

Therapeutic Effects and Rationale for Use

Exogenous insulin is administered to replace normal pancreatic hormone production in all patients with type 1 DM and in some patients with type 2 DM. Exogenous insulin is crucial in maintaining normal glucose levels and proper metabolic function in patients with type 1 DM because beta cell function is essentially absent in these individuals. Without exogenous insulin, the general health of patients with type 1 DM is severely compromised, and they often succumb to the metabolic and neurovascular derangements associated with this disease.

Insulin may also be administered in some cases of type 2 diabetes to complement other drugs (oral antidiabetic agents) and to supplement endogenous insulin release.[78,79] Exogenous insulin can help make up the difference between the patient's endogenous hormone production and his or her specific insulin requirement. In particular, many patients with advanced cases of type 2 DM ultimately require supplemental insulin because other interventions (e.g., diet, exercise, other drugs) are not able to adequately control this disease.[80,81] Researchers continue to clarify how and when exogenous insulin can be used most effectively in people with type 2 DM.

Insulin Preparations

There are many different forms of insulin, depending on the chemical structure and the length of pharmacological effects of each compound (Table 32-2). In the past, insulin used in the treatment of DM was often derived from beef and pork insulin. These sources were obtained by extracting the hormone from the pancreas of the host animal. The animal forms of insulin were effective in controlling glucose metabolism in humans, even though pork insulin has one amino acid that is different from the human insulin sequence, and beef insulin differs from human insulin by 3 amino acids.[31] Because of the development of chemically manufactured human forms of insulin, animal sources are no longer produced in the United States.

Certain contemporary forms of insulin are identical to the structure and effects of human insulin. The hormone is produced through the use of cell cultures and recombinant DNA techniques.[31,82] However, this biosynthetically produced insulin must be administered by subcutaneous injection or other parenteral routes, and the effects of this exogenous insulin do not occur as rapidly as natural insulin released into the bloodstream from pancreatic beta cells—that is, absorption of exogenous insulin from subcutaneous injection sites does not mimic the normal release of endogenous insulin occurring after a meal.[82]

Researchers therefore used biosynthetic techniques to produce insulin analogs that are better able

Table 32-2
INSULIN PREPARATIONS

Type of Insulin	Effects (hr) Onset	Peak	Duration	Common Trade Names
Rapid Acting				
Aspart	0.25	0.6–0.8	3–5	NovoLog
Lispro	>0.5	0.5–1.5	2–5	Humalog
Glulisine	—	0.5–1.5	1–2.5	Apidra
Short-Acting				
Regular insulin	0.5–1	2–4	5–7	Humulin R Novolin R
Intermediate Acting				
Isophane insulin	3–4	6–12	18–28	Humulin N Novolin N
Long-Acting				
Glargine	2–5	5–24	18–24	Lantus
Detemir	3–4	3–14	6–24	Levemir
Insulin Mixtures				
75% protamine lispro/25% lispro	.25–.50	2.8	24	Humalog Mix 75/25
50% protamine lispro/50% lispro	.25–.50	2.8	24	Humalog Mix 50/50
70% protamine aspart/30% aspart	.25	1–4	18–24	NovoLog 70/30
70% NPH/30% regular insulin	.50	4–8	24	Humulin 50/50 Novolin 70/30
50% NPH/ 50% regular insulin	.50	4–8	24	Humulin 50/50

to mimic the absorption and effects of endogenously produced human insulin. By altering the amino acid sequence slightly, researchers discovered that certain biosynthetic insulins could be absorbed more rapidly than regular human insulin.[83] This idea resulted in the development of rapid-acting insulins such as insulin aspart, insulin glulisine, and insulin lispro (see Table 32-2).[83,84] These rapid-acting forms can be administered immediately before or after a meal to more closely approximate the time course of insulin effects following the sudden increase in blood glucose occurring after a meal.[85] In addition, studies are currently under way to develop ultra-rapid-acting forms of insulin that can provide even faster effects around mealtime.[86]

On the other hand, it is sometimes advantageous to administer forms of insulin that are absorbed more slowly and have a more prolonged effect than regular human insulin (see Table 32-2). These intermediate- or long-acting forms provide a sustained background (basal) level of insulin effects throughout the day or night. Intermediate-acting preparations are typically created by adding zinc and protamine to the insulin molecule; these preparations are known as neutral protamine Hagedorn (NPH) insulins.[87] These chemical modifications delay the absorption of the insulin molecule, thereby prolonging the effects and decreasing the need for frequent administration. In addition, pharmacologists have produced biosynthetic long-acting insulin glargine and insulin detemir by adding and substituting specific amino acids (glargine) or attaching fatty acids (detemir) to the regular insulin molecule.[87-89] Some patients prefer these long-acting preparations because they can be administered once each day to provide a steady basal level of insulin that results in more predictable effects with fewer incidences of side effects, such as hypoglycemia.[90] In addition, patients can use combinations of different preparations to manage DM in specific situations. For instance, a long-acting preparation can provide basal insulin effects, and a rapid-acting agent used around mealtime can provide optimal glycemic control.

Finally, several commercial preparations are now available that combine two forms of insulin in the same product. These preparations are sometimes called *biphasic insulins* because they combine a relatively rapid-acting form of insulin (phase 1—regular human insulin, aspart, or lispro) with a more prolonged intermediate or long-acting insulin (phase 2—NPH insulin).[91] The insulins can be combined in specific amounts, such as a 50:50 or 70:30 ratio of intermediate- to rapid-acting form, depending on the preparation (see Table 32-2). Products that combine two different forms of insulin can help provide optimal control of blood glucose levels while minimizing the number of injections needed to achieve this control.

Administration of Insulin

Insulin, a large polypeptide, is not suitable for oral administration. Even if the insulin molecule survived digestion by proteases in the stomach and small intestine, this compound is much too large to be absorbed through the GI wall. Consequently, insulin is usually administered through subcutaneous injection. Typically, a small syringe or a needle-tipped "pen" that contains a cartridge of a specific type of insulin can be set to inject a given amount of insulin. Insulin may also be administered by IV in emergency situations (e.g., diabetic coma).

Patients on long-term insulin therapy are usually trained to administer their own medication. In order to safely use insulin, it is important to provide adequate storage of the preparation, to maintain sterile syringes, to accurately measure the dose and fill the syringe, and to use a proper injection technique. Patients should rotate the sites of administration (e.g., abdomen, upper thighs, upper arms, back, and buttocks) to avoid local damage from repeated injection.

The optimal dosage of insulin varies greatly from patient to patient, as well as within each patient. Factors such as exercise and dietary modification can change the insulin requirements for each individual. Consequently, the dosage of insulin is often adjusted periodically by monitoring the patient's blood glucose level. Adjustment of insulin dosage in poorly controlled DM is usually done under the close supervision of a physician. However, many patients can make their own insulin adjustments based on periodic blood glucose measurement. Home glucose-monitoring devices permit patients to routinely check their own blood glucose levels. This process of glucose self-monitoring and insulin dosage adjustment permits optimal management of blood glucose levels on a day-to-day basis.

Insulin pumps were also developed as a more convenient and precise way to administer insulin. These pumps can deliver a continuous (background) infusion of insulin that can also be supplemented at mealtime by manually activating the pump. These pumps can be worn outside the body, with insulin administered subcutaneously through a small catheter and needle that is held in place by skin tape.[92,93] Insulin pumps are obviously much more convenient than using a hypodermic syringe to make multiple injections each day and avoid some of the problems of repeated subcutaneous injection. These pumps may also provide better control over blood glucose levels while reducing the risk of side effects such as severe hypoglycemia.[94,95]

Researchers are making progress toward developing small implantable pumps that can be placed surgically under the skin and programmed to release insulin as needed.[96,97] These implantable pumps could also monitor blood glucose electronically, thus creating a closed-loop system that monitors blood glucose and automatically releases insulin to return glucose levels back to the normal range.[97,98] This type of implantable pump system would essentially assume the normal role of pancreatic beta cells and provide an "artificial" pancreas for people with type 1 DM.[99] It will be interesting to see if the technology of such implantable pumps can be refined so that these pumps become commercially available.

Currently, the major drawback of insulin pumps is that they can malfunction, primarily because the catheter delivering insulin becomes occluded or obstructed.[100,101] Patients using insulin pumps must also monitor their glucose levels several times each day, and they must understand how to correctly use the pump to deliver the appropriate amount of insulin. Nonetheless, insulin pumps currently offer a convenient way to administer insulin, and technological improvements in these devices will continue to improve their safety and reliability.[92]

Researchers also considered alternative routes for administering insulin.[102] For example, they developed a form of insulin (Exubera) that can be administered by inhalation or nasal spray.[53] Unfortunately, this product was not commercially successful and was subsequently removed from the U.S. market.[102] It is not clear at the present time if other inhaled forms of insulin will be approved and marketed in the future.[103] Other modifications of the insulin molecule or use of gels and chemical enhancers can increase the permeability of insulin so that it can be administered through the skin (transcutaneously) or even via oral or buccal routes.[104-106] Researchers continue to explore technological and practical advancements in insulin delivery, and methods for administering insulin may be safer and more convenient in the future.

Intensive Insulin Therapy

As indicated previously, the ultimate goal in the treatment of DM is to maintain blood glucose in the normal physiological range as much as possible. To achieve this goal, an administration strategy known as *intensive insulin therapy* has been developed for persons who require exogenous insulin.[107] The idea of intensive insulin therapy is that the patient frequently monitors his or her blood glucose levels throughout the day and administers insulin as needed to maintain blood glucose in the appropriate range.[108]

One common way to achieve tight control is to administer an intermediate or long-acting insulin once each day to provide basal insulin effects between meals and then administer a bolus dose of regular or short-acting insulin around mealtime to deal with the sudden rise in blood sugar that occurs after eating.[31] This "basal-bolus" strategy can be implemented in many ways using various forms of insulin and some of the newer technologies such as insulin pens and pumps. Obviously, each basal-bolus regimen must be designed and adjusted based on the needs of each patient, and the patient's willingness to adhere to the regimen.

Patients, of course, must be motivated and committed to achieve adequate intensive insulin therapy. Intensive therapy may also be associated with a somewhat greater risk of severe hypoglycemia if the insulin dosage does not carefully match the patient's needs throughout the day.[109,110] Nonetheless, there is considerable evidence that this strategy reduces the long-term complications associated with poorly controlled DM, including a lower incidence of neuropathies, renal disease, and other complications related to microangiopathy.[107,109] Hence, intensive insulin therapy may be worth the extra effort if it prevents these devastating complications. As indicated earlier, technological advancements such as automatic (closed-loop) glucose sensing–insulin delivery systems may soon be available, and these devices could be instrumental in helping patients with DM achieve optimal glycemic control.[107,111]

Adverse Effects of Insulin Therapy

The primary problem associated with insulin administration is hypoglycemia.[110] Exogenous insulin may produce a dramatic fall in blood glucose levels because insulin lowers blood glucose. Hypoglycemia may occur during insulin therapy if the dose is higher than the patient's needs. Missing a meal or receiving a delayed meal may also precipitate hypoglycemia. During insulin treatment, insulin is not released exclusively after a meal, as it would be during normal function. Insulin administered from an exogenous source may be present in the bloodstream even if the patient fails to provide glucose by eating. Hence, insulin may reduce blood glucose below normal levels because of the lack of a periodic replenishment of blood glucose from dietary sources.

Strenuous physical activity may promote hypoglycemia during insulin therapy. Exercise generally produces an insulinlike effect, meaning that it accelerates the movement of glucose out of the bloodstream and into the peripheral tissues (skeletal muscle) where it is needed. The combined effects of exercise and insulin may produce an exaggerated decrease in blood glucose, thus leading to hypoglycemia. To avoid exercise-induced hypoglycemia, the insulin dose should be decreased proportionally depending on the type, intensity, and duration of the activity.[112] Careful measurement of blood glucose before and after exercise can help predict how much the insulin should be adjusted in each patient.

Initial symptoms of hypoglycemia include headache, fatigue, hunger, tachycardia, sweating, anxiety, and confusion. Symptoms progressively worsen as blood glucose continues to decrease, and severe hypoglycemia may lead to loss of consciousness, convulsions, and death. Consequently, early detection and resolution of hypoglycemia are imperative.[112,113] In the early stages, hypoglycemia can usually be reversed if the patient ingests foods containing glucose (soft drinks, fruit juice, glucose tablets, etc.). Typically, administration of the equivalent of 15 to 20 g of D-glucose is recommended to restore blood glucose in the early stages of hypoglycemia.[114]

Other problems that may be encountered are related to the immunological effects of insulin use—that is, insulin allergy.[115] Various forms of insulin may stimulate antibody production in susceptible patients, and these anti-insulin antibodies may cause an allergic reaction and a resistance to the exogenous insulin molecule. Although allergic reactions were more common from the animal forms of insulin, they can still occur with the biosynthetic insulins. Hence, this immunological response may be due to either the insulin molecule or to preservatives added to the insulin preparation.[115] Although most responses are fairly minor, any signs of allergic reactions, such as pulmonary symptoms (e.g., tightness in the throat and chest, wheezing, cough, dyspnea) or skin reactions (e.g., rash, pruritus, urticaria), should be reported immediately.

PRIMARY AGENTS IN TYPE 2 DIABETES

As indicated above, insulin can play a key role in managing glucose levels in certain patients with type 2 DM. In addition, considerable effort has been made to develop other agents that can help prevent hyperglycemia and provide long-term glycemic control in type 2 DM.[116,117] These antidiabetic drugs tend to be most effective if some endogenous insulin production is present but relatively inadequate and the peripheral tissues are resistant to the effects of the endogenous insulin. Most of these agents are therefore not effective for treating type 1 DM, but they can be used along with diet and exercise for the long-term management of type 2 DM.

Drugs used commonly in type 2 DM are often combined with one another or with insulin therapy to provide optimal glucose control in specific patients.[118,119] That is, drugs from the different classes discussed below will work together to control glucose. The drug combinations can be tailored to the specific needs of each patient, thereby providing better long-term outcomes.[118] Treatment of type 2 DM will undoubtedly continue to improve as more is learned about the best way to use existing drugs, and as other new antidiabetic agents become available.[117]

Nonetheless, the antidiabetic drugs addressed here do not offer a cure for type 2 DM, and their effectiveness varies considerably from patient to patient. Still, it appears that early and aggressive use of one or more of these agents can substantially reduce any complications associated with this disease. Likewise, many of these agents can be administered orally, thus providing a convenient method of drug administration. Antidiabetic drugs are grouped here by functional classes,[120] with a brief description of currently available agents in each class (Table 32-3).

Drugs That Stimulate Insulin Secretion and Supply

Sulfonylureas

Sulfonylureas comprise a fairly large group of oral agents used to treat people with type 2 DM. These drugs act directly on pancreatic beta cells and stimulate the release of insulin,[121,122] which is released directly into the hepatic portal vein and subsequently travels to the liver, inhibiting hepatic glucose production.[123] Increased plasma levels of insulin also help facilitate glucose entry into muscle and other peripheral tissues. The combined effects of decreased hepatic glucose production and increased glucose uptake by muscle helps lower blood sugar in many people with type 2 DM. These drugs seem to be most effective in people who are in the early stages of the disease and still have reasonable beta cell function.[31]

Specific sulfonylureas that are clinically used are listed in Table 32-3. These agents are all fairly similar chemically, but the effects of a given agent may vary from patient to patient because of genetic factors that influence drug pharmacokinetics and effects in each patient.[124] Hence, practitioners should try to find the most effective sulfonylurea in each patient.

The principal adverse effect of these drugs is hypoglycemia.[125,126] As with insulin therapy, hypoglycemia may be precipitated by sulfonylureas if the dose is excessive, if a meal is skipped, or if the patient increases his or her activity level. Consequently, patients should be observed for any indications of low blood glucose, such as anxiety, confusion, headache, and sweating.[125] Other side effects that may occur include heartburn, GI distress (e.g., nausea, vomiting, stomach pain, diarrhea), headache, dizziness, skin rashes, and hematologic abnormalities (e.g., leukopenia, agranulocytosis). These side effects are usually mild and transient but may require attention if they are severe or prolonged.

Meglitinides

Repaglinide (Prandin) and nateglinide (Starlix) are derived from a compound known as *meglitinide*. These drugs act like the sulfonylureas because they directly increase the release of insulin from pancreatic beta cells.[127,128] Both agents are relatively short acting and are typically used with other antidiabetic agents

Table 32-3
PRIMARY AGENTS USED IN TYPE 2 DIABETES MELLITUS

Classification and Examples*	Mechanism of Action and Effects	Primary Adverse Effects
Drugs That Stimulate Insulin Secretion and Supply		
Sulfonylureas Chlorpropamide (Diabinese) Glimepiride (Amaryl) Glipizide (Glucotrol) Glyburide (DiaBeta, Micronase) Tolazamide (Tolinase) Tolbutamide (Orinase)	Increase insulin secretion from pancreatic beta cells; increased insulin release helps reduce blood glucose by increasing glucose storage in muscle and by inhibiting hepatic glucose production.	Hypoglycemia is the most common and potentially serious side effect of the sulfonylureas; other bothersome effects (GI disturbances, headache, etc.) may occur, depending on the specific agent.
Meglitinides Repaglinide (Prandin) Nateglinide (Starlix)	Similar to the sulfonylureas	Hypoglycemia; bronchitis; upper respiratory tract infections; joint and back pain; GI disturbances; headache
Incretin-Based Therapies GLP-1 receptor agonists[†] exenatide (Byetta) liraglutide (Victoza) DPP-4 inhibitors[‡] linagliptin (Tradjenta) saxagliptin (Onglyza) sitagliptin (Januvia).	Mimic or prolong the effects of GLP-1, an endogenous peptide that enhances the release of insulin from pancreatic beta cells and generally increases the size and function of these cells.	GLP-1 receptor agonists can cause GI problems (nausea, vomiting, diarrhea) and pancreatitis. DPP-4 inhibitors are generally well tolerated but may cause mild hypoglycemia.
Insulin Sensitizers		
Biguanides Metformin (Glucophage)	Act directly on the liver to decrease hepatic glucose production; also increase sensitivity of peripheral tissues (muscle) to insulin	GI disturbances; lactic acidosis may also occur in rare cases, and this effect can be severe or fatal.
Thiazolidinediones Pioglitazone (Actos) Rosiglitazone (Avandia)	Similar to the biguanides (metformin)	Headache; dizziness; fatigue/weakness; back pain; rare but potentially severe cases of hepatic toxicity
Others		
Alpha-Glucosidase Inhibitors Acarbose (Precose) Miglitol (Glyset)	Inhibit sugar breakdown in the intestines and delay glucose absorption from the GI tract	GI disturbances
Amylin Analogs Pramlintide (Symlin)	Mimics the effects of amylin, an endogenous substance that limits the rise in blood glucose that occurs after eating by suppressing glucagon secretion, delaying gastric emptying, and promoting feelings of satiety. This drug can be used with insulin to control glucose levels and promote weight loss in type 1 and type 2 DM.	Nausea, vomiting, and loss of appetite are the primary side effects of this drug. Co-administration with insulin may also cause hypoglycemia.
Bile Acid Sequestrants Colesevelam (Welchol)	Binds to bile and glucose in the GI tract, thus limiting glucose absorption and reducing hyperglycemia after eating.	Some GI upset and constipation can occur.

**Examples include generic names with trade names listed in parentheses.*
† GLP-1: glucagon-like peptide 1
‡DPP4: dipeptidyl peptidase 4

to prevent hyperglycemia after a meal. The primary adverse effect of meglitinides is similar to the sulfonylureas; they may lower blood glucose too much, leading to hypoglycemia.[126]

Incretin-Based Therapies

Incretins are hormones released from the GI tract after eating a meal. These hormones help regulate the secretion and effects of endogenously produced insulin.[129,130] The primary incretins are glucagon-like peptide 1 (GLP-1) and glucose-dependent insulinotropic polypeptide (GIP). Both hormones increase the ability of blood glucose to stimulate insulin release from pancreatic beta cells.[131,132] GLP-1, however, can also improve the size and function of pancreatic beta cells, decrease glucagon release from pancreatic alpha cells, reduce appetite, and help promote weight loss.[132-134]

GLP-1 levels are often deficient in people with type 2 DM, whereas GIP levels are typically normal in this population.[31] Hence, researchers developed pharmacological strategies to mimic or enhance the effects of GLP-1. Two such strategies, GLP-1 receptor agonists and dipeptidyl peptidase 4 inhibitors, are addressed briefly here.

GLP-1 Receptor Agonists. GLP-1 receptor agonists mimic the effects of endogenously produced GLP-1. In particular, these hormones can increase insulin release in response to a rise in blood glucose—that is, GLP-1 receptor agonists sensitize pancreatic beta cells so that a relatively greater amount of insulin is released when these cells sense a rise in blood glucose.[131] As indicated above, GLP-1 also exerts several other beneficial effects, including suppression of glucagon secretion and weight loss.[132,134]

At the present time, exenatide (Byetta) and liraglutide (Victoza) are the primary GLP-1 agonists on the market. Evidence suggests that these agents can improve glycemic control and decrease body weight in people with type 2 DM.[133,135,136] These agents, however, cannot be taken orally and are usually administered via daily subcutaneous injections. GI problems (e.g., nausea, vomiting, diarrhea) are the primary side effects. Pancreatitis may also occur in certain patients. On the other hand, these drugs do not typically cause hypoglycemia, making them an attractive alternative to other antidiabetic agents. Efforts continue to be made to develop additional GLP-1 receptor agonists, and perhaps an oral form may be available someday.

Dipeptidyl Peptidase 4 Inhibitors. Incretin hormones are normally degraded by an enzyme known as *dipeptidyl peptidase 4* (DPP-4). Hence, drugs that inhibit this enzyme will prolong the effects of endogenously produced incretins, thus helping to promote the beneficial effects of these hormones on insulin release and glucose metabolism.[137,138] Several DPP-4 inhibitors are available, including linagliptin (Tradjenta), saxagliptin (Onglyza), and sitagliptin (Januvia). These drugs can be taken orally and can be taken alone or in combination with other pharmacological agents to help prevent hyperglycemia and manage glucose levels in people with type 2 DM. The drugs can cause mild hypoglycemia, especially when DPP-4 inhibitors are combined with other drugs, such as the sulfonylureas. Otherwise, DPP-4 inhibitors are fairly well tolerated.

Insulin Sensitizers

Metformin

Metformin (Glucophage) is classified chemically as a biguanide agent, and it acts on the liver to inhibit glucose production.[139] Metformin also increases the sensitivity of peripheral tissues to insulin, an effect that helps treat a fundamental problem in type 2 DM (i.e., decreased tissue sensitivity to insulin).[120,140] Although the exact mechanism of action on tissue sensitivity is not clear, metformin has emerged as one of the primary oral antidiabetic agents. This is often the cornerstone drug when combining several drugs for treatment.[118] Metformin may cause GI problems such as nausea, vomiting, and diarrhea, but these effects are often transient. Lactic acidosis may also occur in rare cases and may be serious. Patients taking metformin should be monitored for signs of lactic acidosis (i.e., confusion, lethargy, stupor, shallow rapid breathing, tachycardia), especially during exercise.

Thiazolidinediones

Rosiglitazone (Avandia) and pioglitazone (Actos) are members of a drug group called the *thiazolididinediones*.[120,141] These agents, also known as *glitazones*, work like metformin; they decrease hepatic glucose production and increase tissue sensitivity to insulin.[142] Thiazolidinediones, however, often take several months to achieve maximum benefit in lowering blood glucose levels.[31] Moreover, these drugs are associated with several side effects, including hepatic toxicity, lactic acidosis, edema, and weight gain. Likewise, pioglitazone and rosiglitazone may cause fractures of the arm, hands, and feet in women. Clinicians should therefore be alert for any unexplained pain that might indicate fractures in women taking these drugs.

Other Antidiabetics

Alpha-Glucosidase Inhibitors

Acarbose (Precose) and miglitol (Glyset) are characterized as alpha-glucosidase inhibitors because they inhibit enzymes that break down sugars in the GI tract.[143] This effect helps delay glucose absorption from the intestines, thereby slowing the entry of glucose into the bloodstream and allowing time for the beta cells to respond to hyperglycemia after a meal.[144] Hence, these drugs are used primarily as an adjunct to other drugs in people with type 2 DM. Acarbose and miglitol may cause some GI distress (e.g., diarrhea, abdominal pain, flatulence) but are otherwise well tolerated.

Amylin Analogs

Pramlintide (Symlin) is a synthetic analog of **amylin**, a substance produced endogenously by pancreatic beta cells.[145,146] Normally, amylin is released from beta cells along with insulin, and amylin produces several effects that help limit the rise in blood glucose that occurs after eating. These effects include suppression of glucagon secretion (which prevents glucagon from increasing hepatic glucose production), delayed gastric emptying (which slows the entry of glucose into the bloodstream), and increased feelings of satiety (which helps limit carbohydrate ingestion and may help promote weight loss).[145] Amylin levels, however, are decreased or absent in people with type 1 or type 2 DM.[31]

Hence, pramlintide was developed biosynthetically to mimic the effects of amylin, and it can be administered subcutaneously in people with type 1 or type 2 DM as an adjunct to insulin therapy.[146,147] That is, pramlintide can be administered at approximately the same time as mealtime bolus insulin doses, thus supplementing the effects of insulin and helping control postmeal hyperglycemia.

GI problems such as nausea, vomiting, and loss of appetite are the primary side effects of this drug. Hypoglycemia can also occur, but this probably occurs because pramlintide is administered with insulin, and excessive insulin causes the hypoglycemic response.[31]

Bile Acid Sequestrants

As discussed in Chapter 25, certain drugs are known as *bile acid sequestrants* because they attach to bile acids within the GI tract and increase the loss of bile acids in the feces. This action helps improve plasma cholesterol levels because cholesterol in the bloodstream is used to synthesize and replace the bile acids that are eliminated from the GI tract. One such agent, colesevelam (Welchol), also helps reduce blood glucose levels and prevent hyperglycemia following a meal.[148,149] Although the reasons for this effect are not clear, colesevelam probably binds to glucose in the GI tract, thus delaying glucose absorption.[31] Hence, people with type 2 DM can use colesevelam alone or as an adjunct to other antihyperglycemics to help control their glucose levels.[150] This drug is generally well tolerated, although some GI upset and constipation can occur.

PREVENTION OF TYPE 1 DIABETES MELLITUS: THE POTENTIAL ROLE OF IMMUNE-BASED THERAPIES

As indicated earlier, most cases of type 1 DM are caused by an autoimmune response that selectively attacks and destroys pancreatic beta cells in susceptible individuals. Drugs that suppress this autoimmune response may be helpful in limiting beta cell destruction, thereby decreasing the severity of this disease.[151,152] Researchers investigated several immunosuppressants as a way to potentially minimize beta cell loss from the autoimmune reactions underlying type 1 DM, including cyclosporine, azathioprine, cyclophosphamide, methotrexate, and glucocorticoids.[152] Although certain drugs such as cyclosporine showed some promise in blunting autoimmune beta cell destruction, clinical use was often limited because traditional immunosuppressants are notorious for producing rather severe side effects (see Chapter 37).[153] Likewise, there was concern that these drugs may negatively affect the developing immune system when administered to adolescent youths who typically begin to show signs of type 1 DM.[151,152]

More recently, efforts have been made to develop targeted therapies to prevent or reduce the autoimmune response underlying type 1 DM. For example, researchers have attempted to develop monoclonal antibodies that target specific antigens involved in the immune reaction underlying beta cell destruction.[153,154]

Monoclonal antibodies have been used successfully to blunt the autoimmune response in conditions such as rheumatoid arthritis (see Chapter 17), and a similar application might be possible in the early stages of type 1 DM. Likewise, it may be possible to manipulate the immune system by increasing the activity of regulatory T cells using chemical mediators such as interleukin-2.[155,156] Activation of such cells might counteract the destructive effects of other immune system components, thereby reducing or preventing beta cell loss in people at risk for type 1 DM.[157]

Unfortunately, clinical trials using antigen-specific and immunomodulatory interventions have not been overwhelmingly successful in preventing the onset of type 1 DM.[153,158] The lack of beneficial effects may be due to the fact that the immune responses that cause beta cell destruction are not fully understood, making it difficult to develop immunomodulatory strategies that specifically affect these responses. Nonetheless, efforts continue to be made to develop methods to control the autoimmune reactions associated with type 1 DM. Controlling immune responses is understandably a risky procedure. Hence, there is ongoing research to develop newer, less toxic antigen-specific and immunomodulating agents that could be useful in preventing the onset of type 1 DM in genetically susceptible individuals.[158] Agents that negate the autoimmune destruction of beta cells will hopefully be available someday, thereby providing a way to limit or even cure type 1 DM.[159]

NONPHARMACOLOGICAL INTERVENTION IN DIABETES MELLITUS

Dietary Management and Weight Reduction

Despite advancements in the pharmacological treatment of DM, the most important and effective factors in controlling types 1 and 2 DM center around lifestyle issues such as diet, physical activity, and maintaining a healthy body weight.[160-162] Total caloric intake and the percentage of calories from specific sources (i.e., carbohydrates, fats, or proteins) is important in controlling blood glucose. Also, weight loss is a significant factor in decreasing the patient's need for drugs such as insulin and other antidiabetic drugs.[163] By losing weight, a patient may reduce the amount of tissue that requires insulin, thereby reducing the need for exogenous drugs. Because obesity is quite prevalent in patients with type 2 DM, weight loss seems to be especially important in reducing drug requirements and improving overall health in these individuals.[164,165]

Exercise

Exercise appears to be beneficial in DM for several reasons. First, physical training may help facilitate weight loss, thus helping to decrease body mass and drug requirements.[165] Secondly, regular exercise appears to increase the sensitivity of peripheral tissues to insulin—that is, training helps overcome insulin resistance.[166-168] The exact reason for this effect is not clear. Finally, a program of physical training will improve general health and well-being, making patients with DM less susceptible to various problems, such as cardiovascular disease.[169,170] Of course, patients beginning a program of regular exercise should undergo a complete physical examination, and the frequency and intensity of the exercise should be closely monitored.

Tissue Transplants and Gene Therapy

A relatively new approach in treatment is the transplantation of tissues containing pancreatic beta cells into the pancreas of patients with type 1 DM.[171] The islet tissues containing functioning beta cells are harvested from adult, neonatal, or fetal pancreatic tissues. Other strategies induce stem cells to develop into insulin-producing cells that can be transplanted into the pancreas.[172,173] Agents that induce differentiation and growth of endogenous beta cells may likewise help sustain or increase beta cell mass in certain patients.[174,175] Alternatively, the entire pancreas can be transplanted from organ donors into patients with type 1 DM; this procedure may be done simultaneously with a kidney transplant in patients with diabetic nephropathy.[176,177] If successful, these tissue transplants can provide the patient with an endogenous source of insulin that will decrease or eliminate the need for insulin therapy. The success rates of these transplants are rising steadily, primarily because of improved surgical techniques and newer immunosuppressant agents and gene-based strategies that are available to prevent tissue rejection.[178,179]

Researchers are also investigating new molecular strategies that could reestablish insulin production and insulin sensitivity by transplanting insulin-related genes into the cells of patients.[180,181] These techniques basically attempt to either deliver insulin genes directly into patients' cells, create genetically altered cells that will produce or respond to insulin, or deliver genes that will enhance the survival of transplanted islet cells.[181,182] Although techniques such as tissue transplants and gene therapy are still relatively experimental, they may eventually be developed to provide a more permanent means of treating DM.

Special Concerns for Rehabilitation Patients

Patients often undergo rehabilitation for complications arising from DM. For instance, peripheral neuropathies may produce functional deficits that require physical therapy and occupational therapy. Small-vessel angiopathy may cause decreased peripheral blood flow, resulting in tissue ischemia, ulceration, and poor wound healing. This ischemia can lead to tissue necrosis and subsequent amputation, especially in the lower extremities. In advanced stages of DM, general debilitation combined with specific conditions (e.g., end-stage renal failure) creates multiple problems that challenge the individual's health. Consequently, rehabilitation specialists will be involved in the treatment of various sequelae of DM throughout the course of this disease.

Physical therapists and occupational therapists should be aware of the possibility that acute metabolic derangements exist in their patients who have DM. Therapists should realize that patients on insulin and oral hypoglycemic medications could experience episodes of hypoglycemia due to these drugs' exaggerated lowering of blood glucose. Hypoglycemia may be precipitated if the patient has not eaten or is engaging in relatively strenuous physical activity. Therapists must ensure that patients are maintaining a regular dietary schedule and have not skipped a meal prior to the therapy session. Furthermore, therapists should be especially alert for any signs of hypoglycemia during and after exercise. Therapists should note any changes in the patient that may signal the onset of hypoglycemia (e.g., confusion, fatigue, sweating, nausea). If these symptoms are observed, administration of a high-glucose snack is typically recommended to reverse these hypoglycemic symptoms. Therapists working with diabetic patients should have sources of glucose on hand, such as soft drinks, fruit juices, and tablets containing D-glucose.[114]

Physical therapists and occupational therapists may help reinforce the importance of patient involvement during the pharmacological management of DM. Therapists can question whether patients have been taking their medications on a routine basis. Regular administration of insulin is essential in preventing a metabolic shift toward ketone body production and subsequent ketoacidosis, especially in patients with type 1 DM. In addition, therapists can help explain that adequate control of blood glucose not only prevents acute metabolic problems but also seems to decrease the incidence of the neurovascular complications.

Finally, rehabilitation specialists can help engage patients in the nonpharmacological management of their disease. They can emphasize the importance of an appropriate diet and adequate physical activity in both type 1 and type 2 DM. Therapists may also play an important role in preventing the onset of diabetic foot ulcers and infection by educating the patient in proper skin care and footwear.

CASE STUDY

DIABETES MELLITUS

Brief History. W.S. is an 18-year-old woman who began experiencing problems with glucose metabolism following a viral infection when she was 12. She was subsequently diagnosed as having type 1 DM. Since then, her condition has been successfully managed by insulin administration combined with dietary control. Once-daily administration of intermediate-acting insulin combined with periodic administration of short-acting insulin usually provides optimal therapeutic effects. She is also very active athletically and was a member of her high school soccer team. She is entering her first year of college and is beginning preseason practice with the college's soccer team. The physical therapist who serves as the team's athletic trainer was apprised of her condition.

Problem/Influence of Medication. Exercise produces an insulinlike effect; it lowers blood glucose by facilitating the movement of glucose out of the bloodstream and into peripheral tissues. Because insulin also lowers blood glucose, the additive effects of insulin and exercise may produce profound hypoglycemia. As a result, a lower dosage of insulin is usually required on days that involve strenuous activity. The physical therapist was aware of this and other potential problems that could arise.

1. ***What instructions should the therapist give W.S. about monitoring and adjusting her blood glucose levels?***
2. ***What precautions should the therapist have in place during practices?***
3. ***How can the therapist help guard against any problems that might arise after practice?***

See Appendix C, "Answers to Case Study Questions."

SUMMARY

The islet cells of the pancreas synthesize and secrete insulin and glucagon. These hormones are important in regulating glucose uptake and use, as well as in other aspects of energy metabolism. Problems in the production and effects of insulin are typical of DM. This disease can be categorized into two primary forms: type 1, which is caused by an absolute deficiency of insulin, and type 2, which is caused by a decrease in peripheral insulin effects, combined with abnormal insulin release.

Administration of exogenous insulin is required in the treatment of type 1 DM. Patients with type 2 DM may be treated with insulin or with other antidiabetic drugs, depending on the severity of their disease. In both forms of DM, dietary control and adequate physical activity may help reduce the need for drug treatment and improve the patient's general health and well-being. Physical therapists and occupational therapists play an important role in helping treat the complications of DM and in promoting good patient adherence to disease management. Therapists must be cognizant of the potential problems that may occur when working with these patients (e.g., hypoglycemia) and should be able to recognize and deal with any problems before a medical emergency arises.

REFERENCES

1. Barrett EJ. The endocrine pancreas. In: Boron WF, Boulpaep EL, eds. *Medical Physiology*. 2nd ed. Philadelphia, PA: Elsevier Saunders; 2012.
2. In't Veld P, Marichal M. Microscopic anatomy of the human islet of Langerhans. *Adv Exp Med Biol*. 2010;654:1-19.
3. Steiner DJ, Kim A, Miller K, Hara M. Pancreatic islet plasticity: interspecies comparison of islet architecture and composition. *Islets*. 2010;2:135-145.
4. Youos JG. The role of α-, δ- and F cells in insulin secretion and action. *Diabetes Res Clin Pract*. 2011;93(suppl 1):S25-26.
5. Hauge-Evans AC, King AJ, Carmignac D, et al. Somatostatin secreted by islet delta-cells fulfills multiple roles as a paracrine regulator of islet function. *Diabetes*. 2009;58:403-411.
6. Corleto VD. Somatostatin and the gastrointestinal tract. *Curr Opin Endocrinol Diabetes Obes*. 2010;17:63-68.

7. Lin LC, Sibille E. Reduced brain somatostatin in mood disorders: a common pathophysiological substrate and drug target? *Front Pharmacol.* 2013;4:110.
8. Dezaki K, Yada T. Islet β-cell ghrelin signaling for inhibition of insulin secretion. *Methods Enzymol.* 2012;514:317-331.
9. Leto D, Saltiel AR. Regulation of glucose transport by insulin: traffic control of GLUT4. *Nat Rev Mol Cell Biol.* 2012;13: 383-396.
10. Moore MC, Coate KC, Winnick JJ, et al. Regulation of hepatic glucose uptake and storage in vivo. *Adv Nutr.* 2012;3:286-294.
11. Chen Y, Lippincott-Schwartz J. Insulin triggers direct trafficking to the cell surface of sequestered GLUT4 storage vesicles marked by Rab10. *Small GTPases.* 2013;4:193-197.
12. Mueckler M, Thorens B. The SLC2 (GLUT) family of membrane transporters. *Mol Aspects Med.* 2013;34:121-138.
13. Richter EA, Hargreaves M. Exercise, GLUT4, and skeletal muscle glucose uptake. *Physiol Rev.* 2013;93:993-1017.
14. Dimitriadis G, Mitrou P, Lambadiari V, et al. Insulin effects in muscle and adipose tissue. *Diabetes Res Clin Pract.* 2011;93(suppl 1): S52-59.
15. Hubbard SR. The insulin receptor: both a prototypical and atypical receptor tyrosine kinase. *Cold Spring Harb Perspect Biol.* 2013;5:a008946.
16. Copps KD, White MF. Regulation of insulin sensitivity by serine/threonine phosphorylation of insulin receptor substrate proteins IRS1 and IRS2. *Diabetologia.* 2012;55:2565-2582.
17. Boller S, Joblin BA, Xu L, et al. From signal transduction to signal interpretation: an alternative model for the molecular function of insulin receptor substrates. *Arch Physiol Biochem.* 2012;118:148-155.
18. Desbuquois B, Carré N, Burnol AF. Regulation of insulin and type 1 insulin-like growth factor signaling and action by the Grb10/14 and SH2B1/B2 adaptor proteins. *FEBS J.* 2013;280:794-816.
19. Cryer PE. Hypoglycemia. In: Melmed S, et al, eds. *Williams Textbook of Endocrinology.* 12th ed. Philadelphia, PA: Saunders/ Elsevier; 2011.
20. Gosmain Y, Masson MH, Philippe J. Glucagon: the renewal of an old hormone in the pathophysiology of diabetes. *J Diabetes.* 2013;5:102-109.
21. Heppner KM, Habegger KM, Day J, et al. Glucagon regulation of energy metabolism. *Physiol Behav.* 2010;100:545-548.
22. Ramnanan CJ, Edgerton DS, Kraft G, Cherrington AD. Physiologic action of glucagon on liver glucose metabolism. *Diabetes Obes Metab.* 2011;13(suppl 1):118-125.
23. Taborsky GJ Jr. The physiology of glucagon. *J Diabetes Sci Technol.* 2010;4:1338-1344.
24. Fu Z, Gilbert ER, Liu D. Regulation of insulin synthesis and secretion and pancreatic beta-cell dysfunction in diabetes. *Curr Diabetes Rev.* 2013;9:25-53.
25. Beaudry JL, Riddell MC. Effects of glucocorticoids and exercise on pancreatic β-cell function and diabetes development. *Diabetes Metab Res Rev.* 2012;28:560-573.
26. Ranawana V, Kaur B. Role of proteins in insulin secretion and glycemic control. *Adv Food Nutr Res.* 2013;70:1-47.
27. Thorens B. Brain glucose sensing and neural regulation of insulin and glucagon secretion. *Diabetes Obes Metab.* 2011;13(suppl 1): 82-88.
28. Barker CJ, Leibiger IB, Berggren PO. The pancreatic islet as a signaling hub. *Adv Biol Regul.* 2013;53:156-163.
29. Rutter GA, Hodson DJ. Minireview: intraislet regulation of insulin secretion in humans. *Mol Endocrinol.* 2013;27:1984-1995.
30. Unger RH, Cherrington AD. Glucagonocentric restructuring of diabetes: a pathophysiologic and therapeutic makeover. *J Clin Invest.* 2012;122:4-12.
31. Triplitt CL, Reasner CA. Diabetes mellitus. In: DiPiro JT, et al, eds. *Pharmacotherapy: A Pathophysiologic Approach.* 8th ed. New York: McGraw-Hill; 2011.
32. Tarr JM, Kaul K, Wolanska K, et al. Retinopathy in diabetes. *Adv Exp Med Biol.* 2012;771:88-106.
33. Rossing P, de Zeeuw D. Need for better diabetes treatment for improved renal outcome. *Kidney Int Suppl.* 2011;120:S28-32.
34. Maraschin Jde F. Classification of diabetes. *Adv Exp Med Biol.* 2012;771:12-19.
35. Boitard C. Pancreatic islet autoimmunity. *Presse Med.* 2012;41: e636-650.
36. Ting C, Bansal V, Batal I, et al. Impairment of immune systems in diabetes. *Adv Exp Med Biol.* 2012;771:62-75.
37. Galleri L, Sebastiani G, Vendrame F, et al. Viral infections and diabetes. *Adv Exp Med Biol.* 2012;771:252-271.
38. Grieco FA, Sebastiani G, Spagnuolo I, et al. Immunology in the clinic review series; focus on type 1 diabetes and viruses: how viral infections modulate beta cell function. *Clin Exp Immunol.* 2012;168:24-29.
39. La Torre D. Immunobiology of beta-cell destruction. *Adv Exp Med Biol.* 2012;771:194-218.
40. Nokoff N, Rewers M. Pathogenesis of type 1 diabetes: lessons from natural history studies of high-risk individuals. *Ann N Y Acad Sci.* 2013;1281:1-15.
41. Kaul K, Tarr JM, Ahmad SI, et al. Introduction to diabetes mellitus. *Adv Exp Med Biol.* 2012;771:1-11.
42. Caprio S. Development of type 2 diabetes mellitus in the obese adolescent: a growing challenge. *Endocr Pract.* 2012;18:791-795.
43. Springer SC, Silverstein J, Copeland K, et al. Management of type 2 diabetes mellitus in children and adolescents. *Pediatrics.* 2013;131:e648-664.
44. Inadera H. Developmental origins of obesity and type 2 diabetes: molecular aspects and role of chemicals. *Environ Health Prev Med.* 2013;18:185-197.
45. Karam JG, McFarlane SI. Update on the prevention of type 2 diabetes. *Curr Diab Rep.* 2011;11:56-63.
46. Ntzani EE, Kavvoura FK. Genetic risk factors for type 2 diabetes: insights from the emerging genomic evidence. *Curr Vasc Pharmacol.* 2012;10:147-155.
47. Schofield CJ, Sutherland C. Disordered insulin secretion in the development of insulin resistance and type 2 diabetes. *Diabet Med.* 2012;29:972-979.
48. Soumaya K. Molecular mechanisms of insulin resistance in diabetes. *Adv Exp Med Biol.* 2012;771:240-251.
49. Abdul-Ghani MA. Type 2 diabetes and the evolving paradigm in glucose regulation. *Am J Manag Care.* 2013;19(suppl):S43-50.
50. Buse JB, Polonsky KS, Burant CF. Type 2 diabetes mellitus. In: Melmed S, et al, eds. *Williams Textbook of Endocrinology.* 12th ed. Philadelphia, PA: Saunders/Elsevier; 2011.
51. Karlsson HK, Zierath JR. Insulin signaling and glucose transport in insulin resistant human skeletal muscle. *Cell Biochem Biophys.* 2007;48:103-113.
52. Muntoni S, Muntoni S. Insulin resistance: pathophysiology and rationale for treatment. *Ann Nutr Metab.* 2011;58:25-36.
53. Powers AC, D'Alessio D. Endocrine pancreas and pharmacology of diabetes mellitus and hypoglycemia. In: Brunton LL, et al, eds. *The Pharmacological Basis of Therapeutics.* 12th ed. New York: McGraw-Hill; 2011.

54. Campbell RK. Fate of the beta-cell in the pathophysiology of type 2 diabetes. *J Am Pharm Assoc.* 2009;49(suppl 1):S10-15.
55. Klop B, Elte JW, Cabezas MC. Dyslipidemia in obesity: mechanisms and potential targets. *Nutrients.* 2013;5:1218-1240.
56. Roberts CK, Hevener AL, Barnard RJ. Metabolic syndrome and insulin resistance: underlying causes and modification by exercise training. *Compr Physiol.* 2013;3:1-58.
57. Cerezo C, Segura J, Praga M, Ruilope LM. Guidelines updates in the treatment of obesity or metabolic syndrome and hypertension. *Curr Hypertens Rep.* 2013;15:196-203.
58. Nikolopoulou A, Kadoglou NP. Obesity and metabolic syndrome as related to cardiovascular disease. *Expert Rev Cardiovasc Ther.* 2012;10:933-939.
59. Weiss R, Bremer AA, Lustig RH. What is metabolic syndrome, and why are children getting it? *Ann N Y Acad Sci.* 2013;1281:123-140.
60. Khoo MC, Oliveira FM, Cheng L. Understanding the metabolic syndrome: a modeling perspective. *IEEE Rev Biomed Eng.* 2013;6:143-155.
61. Murphy R, Carroll RW, Krebs JD. Pathogenesis of the metabolic syndrome: insights from monogenic disorders. *Mediators Inflamm.* 2013;2013:920214.
62. Goldberg RB, Mather K. Targeting the consequences of the metabolic syndrome in the Diabetes Prevention Program. *Arterioscler Thromb Vasc Biol.* 2012;32:2077-2090.
63. Westphal SA, Childs RD, Seifert KM, et al. Managing diabetes in the heat: potential issues and concerns. *Endocr Pract.* 2010;16:506-511.
64. Wilson V. Diagnosis and treatment of diabetic ketoacidosis. *Emerg Nurse.* 2012;20:14-18.
65. Schalkwijk CG, Miyata T. Early- and advanced non-enzymatic glycation in diabetic vascular complications: the search for therapeutics. *Amino Acids.* 2012;42:1193-1204.
66. Tsilibary EC. Microvascular basement membranes in diabetes mellitus. *J Pathol.* 2003;200:537-546.
67. Durham JT, Herman IM. Microvascular modifications in diabetic retinopathy. *Curr Diab Rep.* 2011;11:253-264.
68. Roy S, Ha J, Trudeau K, Beglova E. Vascular basement membrane thickening in diabetic retinopathy. *Curr Eye Res.* 2010;35:1045-1056.
69. Barot M, Gokulgandhi MR, Patel S, Mitra AK. Microvascular complications and diabetic retinopathy: recent advances and future implications. *Future Med Chem.* 2013;5:301-314.
70. Eleftheriadis T, Antoniadi G, Pissas G, et al. The renal endothelium in diabetic nephropathy. *Ren Fail.* 2013;35:592-599.
71. Game FL, Hinchliffe RJ, Apelqvist J, et al. A systematic review of interventions to enhance the healing of chronic ulcers of the foot in diabetes. *Diabetes Metab Res Rev.* 2012;28(suppl 1):119-141.
72. Calkin AC, Allen TJ. Diabetes mellitus-associated atherosclerosis: mechanisms involved and potential for pharmacological invention. *Am J Cardiovasc Drugs.* 2006;6:15-40.
73. D'Souza A, Hussain M, Howarth FC, et al. Pathogenesis and pathophysiology of accelerated atherosclerosis in the diabetic heart. *Mol Cell Biochem.* 2009;331:89-116.
74. Pasnoor M, Dimachkie MM, Kluding P, Barohn RJ. Diabetic neuropathy part 1: overview and symmetric phenotypes. *Neurol Clin.* 2013;31:425-445.
75. Bianchi C, Miccoli R, Del Prato S. Hyperglycemia and vascular metabolic memory: truth or fiction? *Curr Diab Rep.* 2013;13:403-410.
76. Dailey G. Early and intensive therapy for management of hyperglycemia and cardiovascular risk factors in patients with type 2 diabetes. *Clin Ther.* 2011;33:665-678.
77. Dokun AO. Lessons learned from glycemia control studies. *Curr Diab Rep.* 2010;10:133-138.
78. King A. Integrating advances in insulin into clinical practice: advances in insulin formulations. *J Fam Pract.* 2013;62(suppl insulin):S9-17.
79. Retnakaran R, Zinman B. Short-term intensified insulin treatment in type 2 diabetes: long-term effects on β-cell function. *Diabetes Obes Metab.* 2012;14(suppl 3):161-166.
80. Maria Rotella C, Pala L, Mannucci E. Role of insulin in the type 2 diabetes therapy: past, present and future. *Int J Endocrinol Metab.* 2013;11:137-144.
81. Philis-Tsimikas A. Initiating basal insulin therapy in type 2 diabetes: practical steps to optimize glycemic control. *Am J Med.* 2013;126(suppl 1):S21-27.
82. Tibaldi JM. Evolution of insulin development: focus on key parameters. *Adv Ther.* 2012;29:590-619.
83. Sheldon B, Russell-Jones D, Wright J. Insulin analogues: an example of applied medical science. *Diabetes Obes Metab.* 2009;11:5-19.
84. Roach P. New insulin analogues and routes of delivery: pharmacodynamic and clinical considerations. *Clin Pharmacokinet.* 2008;47:595-610.
85. Home PD. The pharmacokinetics and pharmacodynamics of rapid-acting insulin analogues and their clinical consequences. *Diabetes Obes Metab.* 2012;14:780-788.
86. Krasner A, Pohl R, Simms P, et al. A review of a family of ultra-rapid-acting insulins: formulation development. *J Diabetes Sci Technol.* 2012;6:786-796.
87. Owens DR. Insulin preparations with prolonged effect. *Diabetes Technol Ther.* 2011;13(suppl 1):S5-14.
88. Jensen MG, Hansen M, Brock B, Rungby J. Differences between long-acting insulins for the treatment of type 2 diabetes. *Expert Opin Pharmacother.* 2010;11:2027-2035.
89. Keating GM. Insulin detemir: a review of its use in the management of diabetes mellitus. *Drugs.* 2012;72:2255-2287.
90. Abrahamson MJ. Basal insulins: pharmacological properties and patient perspectives. *Prim Care Diabetes.* 2010;4(suppl 1):S19-23.
91. Søeborg T, Rasmussen CH, Mosekilde E, Colding-Jørgensen M. Bioavailability and variability of biphasic insulin mixtures. *Eur J Pharm Sci.* 2012;46:198-208.
92. Ejaz S, Wilson T. Managing type 1 diabetes—a journey from starvation to insulin pump. *Minerva Endocrinol.* 2013;38:123-131.
93. Pickup J. Insulin pumps. *Int J Clin Pract Suppl.* 2011;170:16-19.
94. Didangelos T, Iliadis F. Insulin pump therapy in adults. *Diabetes Res Clin Pract.* 2011;93(suppl 1):S109-113.
95. Valla V. Continuous subcutaneous insulin infusion (CSII) pumps. *Adv Exp Med Biol.* 2012;771:414-419.
96. Ricotti L, Assaf T, Dario P, Menciassi A. Wearable and implantable pancreas substitutes. *J Artif Organs.* 2013;16:9-22.
97. Weinzimer SA. Closed-loop artificial pancreas: current studies and promise for the future. *Curr Opin Endocrinol Diabetes Obes.* 2012;19:88-92.
98. Schaepelynck P, Darmon P, Molines L, et al. Advances in pump technology: insulin patch pumps, combined pumps and glucose sensors, and implanted pumps. *Diabetes Metab.* 2011;37(suppl 4):S85-93.

99. Bequette BW. Challenges and recent progress in the development of a closed-loop artificial pancreas. *Annu Rev Control.* 2012;36:255-266.
100. Pickup JC, Yemane N, Brackenridge A, Pender S. Nonmetabolic complications of continuous subcutaneous insulin infusion: a patient survey. *Diabetes Technol Ther.* 2014;16:145-149.
101. Wheeler BJ, Donaghue KC, Heels K, Ambler GR. Family perceptions of insulin pump adverse events in children and adolescents. *Diabetes Technol Ther.* 2014;16:204-207.
102. Heinemann L. New ways of insulin delivery. *Int J Clin Pract Suppl.* 2010;166:29-40.
103. Heinemann L. New ways of insulin delivery. *Int J Clin Pract Suppl.* 2011;170:31-46.
104. Chaturvedi K, Ganguly K, Nadagouda MN, Aminabhavi TM. Polymeric hydrogels for oral insulin delivery. *J Control Release.* 2013;165:129-138.
105. Fonte P, Araújo F, Reis S, Sarmento B. Oral insulin delivery: how far are we? *J Diabetes Sci Technol.* 2013;7:520-531.
106. Selam JL. Evolution of diabetes insulin delivery devices. *J Diabetes Sci Technol.* 2010;4:505-513.
107. Switzer SM, Moser EG, Rockler BE, Garg SK. Intensive insulin therapy in patients with type 1 diabetes mellitus. *Endocrinol Metab Clin North Am.* 2012;41:89-104.
108. Golden SH, Sapir T. Methods for insulin delivery and glucose monitoring in diabetes: summary of a comparative effectiveness review. *J Manag Care Pharm.* 2012;18(suppl):S1-17.
109. Giordano C. Insulin therapy: unmet needs and new perspectives. *Minerva Endocrinol.* 2013;38:95-102.
110. McCall AL. Insulin therapy and hypoglycemia. *Endocrinol Metab Clin North Am.* 2012;41:57-87.
111. Moser EG, Morris AA, Garg SK. Emerging diabetes therapies and technologies. *Diabetes Res Clin Pract.* 2012;97:16-26.
112. Kourtoglou GI. Insulin therapy and exercise. *Diabetes Res Clin Pract.* 2011;93(suppl 1):S73-77.
113. Shafiee G, Mohajeri-Tehrani M, Pajouhi M, Larijani B. The importance of hypoglycemia in diabetic patients. *J Diabetes Metab Disord.* 2012;11:17.
114. Living with diabetes: blood glucose control. Available at www.diabetes.org.
115. Ghazavi MK, Johnston GA. Insulin allergy. *Clin Dermatol.* 2011;29:300-305.
116. Cuny T, Guerci B, Cariou B. New avenues for the pharmacological management of type 2 diabetes: an update. *Ann Endocrinol.* 2012;73:459-468.
117. Guthrie RM. Evolving therapeutic options for type 2 diabetes mellitus: an overview. *Postgrad Med.* 2012;124:82-89.
118. Erlich DR, Slawson DC, Shaughnessy A. Diabetes update: new drugs to manage type 2 diabetes. *FP Essent.* 2013;408:20-24.
119. Han S, Iglay K, Davies MJ, et al. Glycemic effectiveness and medication adherence with fixed-dose combination or coadministered dual therapy of antihyperglycemic regimens: a meta-analysis. *Curr Med Res Opin.* 2012;28:969-977.
120. McGill JB. Pharmacotherapy in type 2 diabetes: a functional schema for drug classification. *Curr Diabetes Rev.* 2012;8:257-267.
121. Seino S. Cell signalling in insulin secretion: the molecular targets of ATP, cAMP and sulfonylurea. *Diabetologia.* 2012;55:2096-2108.
122. Seino S, Takahashi H, Takahashi T, Shibasaki T. Treating diabetes today: a matter of selectivity of sulphonylureas. *Diabetes Obes Metab.* 2012;14(suppl 1):9-13.
123. Dube S, Errazuriz I, Cobelli C, et al. Assessment of insulin action on carbohydrate metabolism: physiological and non-physiological methods. *Diabet Med.* 2013;30:664-670.
124. Aquilante CL. Sulfonylurea pharmacogenomics in type 2 diabetes: the influence of drug target and diabetes risk polymorphisms. *Expert Rev Cardiovasc Ther.* 2010;8:359-372.
125. Ahrén B. Avoiding hypoglycemia: a key to success for glucose-lowering therapy in type 2 diabetes. *Vasc Health Risk Manag.* 2013;9:155-163.
126. Inkster B, Zammitt NN, Frier BM. Drug-induced hypoglycaemia in type 2 diabetes. *Expert Opin Drug Saf.* 2012;11:597-614.
127. Guardado-Mendoza R, Prioletta A, Jiménez-Ceja LM, et al. The role of nateglinide and repaglinide, derivatives of meglitinide, in the treatment of type 2 diabetes mellitus. *Arch Med Sci.* 2013;9:936-943.
128. Scott LJ. Repaglinide: a review of its use in type 2 diabetes mellitus. *Drugs.* 2012;72:249-272.
129. Drucker DJ. Incretin action in the pancreas: potential promise, possible perils, and pathological pitfalls. *Diabetes.* 2013;62:3316-3323.
130. Namba M, Katsuno T, Kusunoki Y, et al. New strategy for the treatment of type 2 diabetes mellitus with incretin-based therapy. *Clin Exp Nephrol.* 2013;17:10-15.
131. Koole C, Pabreja K, Savage EE, et al. Recent advances in understanding GLP-1R (glucagon-like peptide-1 receptor) function. *Biochem Soc Trans.* 2013;41:172-179.
132. Morales J. The pharmacologic basis for clinical differences among GLP-1 receptor agonists and DPP-4 inhibitors. *Postgrad Med.* 2011;123:189-201.
133. Gallwitz B. GLP-1 agonists and dipeptidyl-peptidase IV inhibitors. *Handb Exp Pharmacol.* 2011;203:53-74.
134. Mudaliar S, Henry RR. Effects of incretin hormones on beta-cell mass and function, body weight, and hepatic and myocardial function. *Am J Med.* 2010;123(suppl):S19-27.
135. Shyangdan DS, Royle P, Clar C, et al. Glucagon-like peptide analogues for type 2 diabetes mellitus. *Cochrane Database Syst Rev.* 2011;10:CD006423.
136. Vilsbøll T, Christensen M, Junker AE, et al. Effects of glucagon-like peptide-1 receptor agonists on weight loss: systematic review and meta-analyses of randomised controlled trials. *BMJ.* 2012;344:d7771.
137. Karagiannis T, Paschos P, Paletas K, et al. Dipeptidyl peptidase-4 inhibitors for treatment of type 2 diabetes mellitus in the clinical setting: systematic review and meta-analysis. *BMJ.* 2012;344:e1369.
138. Kountz D. The dipeptidyl peptidase (DPP)-4 inhibitors for type 2 diabetes mellitus in challenging patient groups. *Adv Ther.* 2013;30:1067-1085.
139. Viollet B, Foretz M. Revisiting the mechanisms of metformin action in the liver. *Ann Endocrinol.* 2013;74:123-129.
140. Wong AK, Symon R, AlZadjali MA, et al. The effect of metformin on insulin resistance and exercise parameters in patients with heart failure. *Eur J Heart Fail.* 2012;14:1303-1310.
141. Barnett AH. Redefining the role of thiazolidinediones in the management of type 2 diabetes. *Vasc Health Risk Manag.* 2009;5:141-151.
142. Derosa G, Tinelli C, Maffioli P. Effects of pioglitazone and rosiglitazone combined with metformin on body weight in people with diabetes. *Diabetes Obes Metab.* 2009;11:1091-1099.

143. Standl E, Schnell O. Alpha-glucosidase inhibitors 2012—cardiovascular considerations and trial evaluation. *Diab Vasc Dis Res*. 2012;9:163-169.
144. Wu QL, Liu YP, Lu JM, et al. Efficacy and safety of acarbose chewable tablet in patients with type 2 diabetes: a multicentre, randomized, double-blinded, double-dummy positive controlled trial. *J Evid Based Med*. 2012;5:134-138.
145. Singh-Franco D, Robles G, Gazze D. Pramlintide acetate injection for the treatment of type 1 and type 2 diabetes mellitus. *Clin Ther*. 2007;29:535-562.
146. Younk LM, Mikeladze M, Davis SN. Pramlintide and the treatment of diabetes: a review of the data since its introduction. *Expert Opin Pharmacother*. 2011;12:1439-1451.
147. Lee NJ, Norris SL, Thakurta S. Efficacy and harms of the hypoglycemic agent pramlintide in diabetes mellitus. *Ann Fam Med*. 2010;8:542-549.
148. Brunetti L, Campbell RK. Clinical efficacy of colesevelam in type 2 diabetes mellitus. *J Pharm Pract*. 2011;24:417-425.
149. Ooi CP, Loke SC. Colesevelam for type 2 diabetes mellitus. *Cochrane Database Syst Rev*. 2012;12:CD009361.
150. Rosenstock J, Rigby SP, Ford DM, et al. The glucose and lipid effects of colesevelam as monotherapy in drug-naïve type 2 diabetes. *Horm Metab Res*. 2014;46:348-353.
151. Chatenoud L, You S, Okada H, et al. 99th Dahlem conference on infection, inflammation and chronic inflammatory disorders: immune therapies of type 1 diabetes: new opportunities based on the hygiene hypothesis. *Clin Exp Immunol*. 2010;160:106-112.
152. von Herrath M, Peakman M, Roep B. Progress in immune-based therapies for type 1 diabetes. *Clin Exp Immunol*. 2013;172:186-202.
153. Coppieters KT, Harrison LC, von Herrath MG. Trials in type 1 diabetes: Antigen-specific therapies. *Clin Immunol*. 2013;149:345-355.
154. Chatenoud L, Warncke K, Ziegler AG. Clinical immunologic interventions for the treatment of type 1 diabetes. *Cold Spring Harb Perspect Med*. 2012;2:8.
155. Battaglia M, Roncarolo MG. Immune intervention with T regulatory cells: past lessons and future perspectives for type 1 diabetes. *Semin Immunol*. 2011;23:182-194.
156. Long SA, Buckner JH, Greenbaum CJ. IL-2 therapy in type 1 diabetes: "trials" and tribulations. *Clin Immunol*. 2013;149:324-331.
157. Castro CN, Barcala Tabarrozi AE, Noguerol MA, et al. Disease-modifying immunotherapy for the management of autoimmune diabetes. *Neuroimmunomodulation*. 2010;17:173-176.
158. Chen W, Xie A, Chan L. Mechanistic basis of immunotherapies for type 1 diabetes mellitus. *Transl Res*. 2013;161:217-229.
159. Gupta S. Immunotherapies in diabetes mellitus type 1. *Med Clin North Am*. 2012;96:621-634.
160. Gillett M, Royle P, Snaith A, et al. Non-pharmacological interventions to reduce the risk of diabetes in people with impaired glucose regulation: a systematic review and economic evaluation. *Health Technol Assess*. 2012;16:1-236.
161. Schellenberg ES, Dryden DM, Vandermeer B, et al. Lifestyle interventions for patients with and at risk for type 2 diabetes: a systematic review and meta-analysis. *Ann Intern Med*. 2013;159:543-551.
162. Shrestha P, Ghimire L. A review about the effect of life style modification on diabetes and quality of life. *Glob J Health Sci*. 2012;4:185-190.
163. Kumar AA, Palamaner Subash Shantha G, Kahan S, et al. Intentional weight loss and dose reductions of anti-diabetic medications—a retrospective cohort study. *PLoS One*. 2012; 7:e32395.
164. Gregg EW, Chen H, Wagenknecht LE, et al. Association of an intensive lifestyle intervention with remission of type 2 diabetes. *JAMA*. 2012;308:2489-2496.
165. Khazrai YM, Defeudis G, Pozzilli P. Effect of diet on type 2 diabetes mellitus: a review. *Diabetes Metab Res Rev*. 2014; 30(suppl 1):24-33.
166. Li J, Zhang W, Guo Q, et al. Duration of exercise as a key determinant of improvement in insulin sensitivity in type 2 diabetes patients. *Tohoku J Exp Med*. 2012;227:289-296.
167. McCormack SE, McCarthy MA, Harrington SG, et al. Effects of exercise and lifestyle modification on fitness, insulin resistance, skeletal muscle oxidative phosphorylation and intramyocellular lipid content in obese children and adolescents. *Pediatr Obes*. 2014;9:281-291.
168. Winnick JJ, Sherman WM, Habash DL, et al. Short-term aerobic exercise training in obese humans with type 2 diabetes mellitus improves whole-body insulin sensitivity through gains in peripheral, not hepatic insulin sensitivity. *J Clin Endocrinol Metab*. 2008;93:771-778.
169. Peiris C. Supervised aerobic and resistance exercise improves glycaemic control and modifiable cardiovascular risk factors in people with type 2 diabetes mellitus. *J Physiother*. 2011;57:126.
170. Wang CC, Reusch JE. Diabetes and cardiovascular disease: changing the focus from glycemic control to improving long-term survival. *Am J Cardiol*. 2012;110(suppl):58B-68B.
171. Hatziavramidis DT, Karatzas TM, Chrousos GP. Pancreatic islet cell transplantation: an update. *Ann Biomed Eng*. 2013;41:469-476.
172. Chhabra P, Brayman KL. Stem cell therapy to cure type 1 diabetes: from hype to hope. *Stem Cells Transl Med*. 2013;2:328-336.
173. Dave S. Extrinsic factors promoting insulin producing cell-differentiation and insulin expression enhancement-hope for diabetics. *Curr Stem Cell Res Ther*. 2013;8:471-483.
174. Brun T, Gauthier BR. A focus on the role of Pax4 in mature pancreatic islet beta-cell expansion and survival in health and disease. *J Mol Endocrinol*. 2008;40:37-45.
175. Mellado-Gil JM, Cobo-Vuilleumier N, Gauthier BR. Islet β-cell mass preservation and regeneration in diabetes mellitus: four factors with potential therapeutic interest. *J Transplant*. 2012;2012:230870.
176. Dhanireddy KK. Pancreas transplantation. *Gastroenterol Clin North Am*. 2012;41:133-142.
177. Tavakoli A, Liong S. Pancreatic transplant in diabetes. *Adv Exp Med Biol*. 2012;771:420-437.
178. Boggi U, Vistoli F, Egidi FM, et al. Transplantation of the pancreas. *Curr Diab Rep*. 2012;12:568-579.
179. Scalea JR, Cooper M. Current concepts in the simultaneous transplantation of kidney and pancreas. *J Intensive Care Med*. 2012;27:199-206.
180. Sanlioglu AD, Altunbas HA, Balci MK, et al. Insulin gene therapy from design to beta cell generation. *Expert Rev Mol Med*. 2012;14:e18.
181. Tudurí E, Bruin JE, Kieffer TJ. Restoring insulin production for type 1 diabetes. *J Diabetes*. 2012;4:319-331.
182. Hughes A, Jessup C, Drogemuller C, et al. Gene therapy to improve pancreatic islet transplantation for type 1 diabetes mellitus. *Curr Diabetes Rev*. 2010;6:274-284.

SECTION

8

Chemotherapy of Infectious and Neoplastic Diseases

CHAPTER 33

Treatment of Infections I: Antibacterial Drugs

This chapter and the next two address drugs used to treat infections caused by pathogenic microorganisms and parasites. Microorganisms such as bacteria, viruses, and protozoa, as well as larger multicellular parasites, frequently invade human tissues and are responsible for various afflictions, ranging from mild and annoying symptoms to life-threatening diseases. Often, the body's natural defense mechanisms are unable to deal with these pathogenic invaders, and pharmacological treatment is essential in resolving infections and promoting recovery. The development of drugs to treat infection represent one of the most significant advances in medical history, and these agents are among the most important and widely used pharmacological agents throughout the world.

Drugs used to treat infectious diseases share a common goal of **selective toxicity**, meaning they must selectively kill or attenuate the growth of the pathogenic organism without causing excessive damage to the host (human) cells. In some cases, the pathogenic organism may have some distinctive structural or biochemical feature that allows the drug to selectively attack the invading cell. For instance, drugs that capitalize on certain differences in membrane structure, protein synthesis, or other unique aspects of cellular metabolism in the pathogenic organism will be effective and safe anti-infectious agents. Of course, *selective toxicity* is a relative term, because all of the drugs discussed in the following chapters exert some adverse effects on human tissues. However, these drugs generally impair function much more in the pathogenic organism than in human tissues.

Several other general terms are also used to describe the drugs. Agents used against small, unicellular organisms (e.g., bacteria, viruses) are often referred to as *antimicrobial drugs*. Another common term for antimicrobial agents is *antibiotics*, indicating that these substances are used to kill other living organisms (i.e., anti-*bios*, or *life*). To avoid confusion, this text classifies and identifies the antimicrobial agents according to the primary type of infectious organism they are used to treat—that is, whether they are antibacterial, antiviral, antifungal, and so on. This chapter focuses on drugs that treat bacterial infections. Drugs for treating and preventing viral infections are presented in Chapter 34, followed by the pharmacological management of other parasitic infections (i.e., antifungal, antiprotozoal, and anthelmintic drugs) in Chapter 35.

Because infectious disease represents one of the most common forms of illness, many patients undergoing physical rehabilitation may be taking one or more of these drugs. Physical therapists and occupational therapists will undoubtedly deal with patients on a routine basis who are undergoing chemotherapy for infectious disease. Patients can, for example, develop infections following joint replacements and other surgeries. These infections must be treated effectively to allow full recovery and enable the patient to progress during physical rehabilitation. Infections in the respiratory tract, kidneys, gastrointestinal (GI) tract, and other organs and tissues must also be resolved so that the patient can fully engage in exercise and other rehabilitation interventions.

On the other hand, anti-infectious agents may have side effects that impair neuromusculoskeletal function and the function of other physiological systems, thus limiting the patient's response to physical rehabilitation. Rehabilitation specialists also work closely with patients for extended periods of time, so clinicians must be careful about spreading infections from one patient to another. The pharmacotherapeutic management of infectious disease that is presented in Chapters 33 through 35 should therefore be of interest to all rehabilitation specialists.

BACTERIA: BASIC CONCEPTS

Bacterial Structure and Function

Bacteria are unicellular microorganisms, ranging in size from approximately 1 to 10 μm in diameter.[1] Bacteria are distinguished from other microorganisms by several features, including a rigid cell wall that surrounds the bacterial cell and the lack of a true nuclear membrane (i.e., the genetic material within the bacterial cell is not confined by a distinct membrane).[1,2] Bacteria usually contain the basic subcellular organelles needed to synthesize proteins and maintain cellular metabolism, including ribosomes, enzymes, and cytoplasmic storage granules. Bacteria, however, must depend on some kind of nourishing medium to provide metabolic substrates to maintain function. Hence, these microorganisms often invade human tissues to gain access to a supply of amino acids, sugars, and other substances.

Pathogenic Effects of Bacteria

Bacterial infections can be harmful to host organisms in several ways.[1-3] First, bacteria multiply, competing with host (human) cells for essential nutrients. Bacteria also may directly harm human cells by releasing toxic substances. Moreover, bacteria may cause an immune response that will ultimately damage human tissues along with the invading bacteria.

Of course, not all bacteria in the human body are harmful. For example, certain bacteria in the GI system inhibit the growth of other microorganisms and assist in the digestion of food and synthesis of certain nutrients. In addition, many bacteria that enter the body are adequately dealt with by normal immunologic responses.

However, the invasion of pathogenic bacteria can lead to severe infections and death, especially if the patient's immune system is compromised or the body's endogenous defense mechanisms are unable to combat the infection. In some cases, bacteria may establish growth areas or colonies that remain innocuous for extended periods. However, this colonization may begin to proliferate and become a health threat when the patient succumbs to some other disorder or illness. Consequently, the chance of severe, life-threatening infections is especially high in individuals who are debilitated or have some immune system defect.

Bacterial Nomenclature and Classification

Bacteria are usually named according to their genus and species; these names are identified in italics.[4] For instance, *Escherichia coli* refers to bacteria from the *Escherichia* genus and *coli* species. According to this nomenclature, the genus is capitalized and refers to bacteria with common genetic, morphological, and biochemical characteristics. The species name is not capitalized and often refers to some physical, pathogenic, or other characteristic of the species. For example, *Streptococcus pyogenes* refers to bacteria from the *Streptococcus* genus that are commonly associated with pyogenic or pus-producing characteristics.

Because of diverse bacterial genera, bacteria are often categorized according to common characteristics, such as the shape and histological staining of the bacterial cell.[4,5] For example, *gram-positive cocci* refers to spherical bacteria (cocci) that retain the discoloration of a particular staining technique (e.g., Gram staining). However, development of a comprehensive taxonomy that neatly categorizes all bacteria is difficult because of the diverse morphological and biochemical characteristics of the various bacterial families and genera.

For the purpose of this chapter, the bacteria are categorized according to the criteria outlined in Table 33-1. This classification scheme does not fully identify all of the various characteristics of the many bacterial families; it is used here only to categorize bacteria according to the use of antibacterial agents, which are discussed later in this chapter under "Specific Antibacterial Agents."

Table 33-1
TYPES OF BACTERIA

Type	Principal Features	Common Examples
Gram-positive bacilli	Generally rod-shaped; retain color when treated by Gram's method	*Bacillus anthracis, Clostridium tetani*
Gram-negative bacilli	Rod-shaped; do not retain color by Gram's method	*Escherichia coli, Klebsiella pneumoniae, Pseudomonas aeruginosa*
Gram-positive cocci	Generally spherical or ovoid in shape; retain color by Gram's method	*Staphylococcus aureus, Streptococcus pneumoniae*
Gram-negative cocci	Spherical or ovoid; do not retain color by Gram's method	*Neisseria gonorrhoeae* (gonococcus), *Neisseria meningitidis* (meningococcus)
Acid-fast bacilli	Rod-shaped; retain color of certain stains even when treated with acid	*Mycobacterium leprae, Mycobacterium tuberculosis*
Spirochetes	Slender; spiral shape; able to move about without flagella (intrinsic locomotor ability)	Lyme disease agent; *Treponema pallidum* (syphilis)
Actinomycetes	Thin filaments that stain positively by Gram's method	*Actinomyces israelii;* Nocardia
Others		
Mycoplasmas	Spherical; lack the rigid, highly structured cell wall found in most bacteria	*Mycoplasma pneumoniae*
Rickettsiae	Small; gram-negative bacteria	*Rickettsia typhi, Rickettsia rickettsii*

SPECTRUM AND ACTIVITY OF ANTIBACTERIAL DRUGS

Spectrum of Antibacterial Activity

Some drugs are effective against a variety of bacteria; these are usually referred to as *broad-spectrum agents*. For example, a drug such as tetracycline is considered to have a broad spectrum of activity because it is effective against many gram-negative, gram-positive, and other types of bacteria. In contrast, a drug such as isoniazid is specific for the bacillus that causes tuberculosis (i.e., *Mycobacterium tuberculosis*), and its spectrum of activity is relatively narrow. Hence, the antibacterial spectrum is one property of an antibacterial drug that determines the clinical applications of that agent. Other factors, including patient tolerance, bacterial resistance, and physician preference, also influence the selection of a particular drug for a particular condition. The clinical use of antibacterial drugs relative to specific bacterial pathogens is discussed in "Clinical Use of Antibacterial Drugs: Relationship to Specific Bacterial Infections."

Bactericidal Versus Bacteriostatic Activity

Antibacterial drugs are usually classified as either bactericidal or bacteriostatic, depending on their mechanism of action. The term *bactericidal* refers to drugs that typically kill or destroy bacteria. In contrast, drugs that do not actually kill bacteria but limit their growth and proliferation are referred to as *bacteriostatic*. In addition, the classification of whether a drug is bactericidal or bacteriostatic may depend on the drug dosage. For instance, drugs such as erythromycin exhibit bacteriostatic activity at lower doses but are bactericidal at higher doses.

BASIC MECHANISMS OF ANTIBACTERIAL DRUGS

As mentioned previously, antibacterial and other antimicrobial drugs must be selectively toxic to the infectious microorganism, without causing excessive damage to human cells. Drugs that exert selective toxicity against bacteria generally employ one of the mechanisms shown in Figure 33-1. These mechanisms include:

- inhibition of bacterial cell wall synthesis and function;
- inhibition of bacterial protein synthesis;
- inhibition of bacterial DNA/RNA function.

The details of these mechanisms, along with the reasons why each mechanism is specific for bacterial (versus human) cells, are discussed next.

Inhibition of Bacterial Cell Wall Synthesis and Function

Penicillin, cephalosporins, and several other commonly used drugs exert antibacterial effects by inhibiting the synthesis of bacterial cell walls.[6,7] These drugs are selectively toxic because the bacterial cell walls differ considerably from those of their mammalian counterparts. The membrane surrounding most bacterial cells (with the exception of the *Mycoplasma* genus) is a relatively rigid, firm structure.[7] This rigidity appears to be essential in constraining the high osmotic pressure within the bacterial cell.[8,9] This behavior contrasts with the relatively supple, flexible membrane encompassing the mammalian cell.

The increased rigidity of bacterial cell walls is caused by the presence of protein-polysaccharide structures known as *peptidoglycans*.[8,10] Peptidoglycan units (also known as *mureins*) are cross-linked to one another within the cell wall in such a way as to provide a remarkable amount of rigidity and firmness to the cell. If these peptidoglycans are not present, the bacterial membrane will lack integrity and will cause altered function and impaired homeostasis within the bacterial cell. Also, the lack of adequate membrane cytoarchitecture appears to initiate a suicidal autolysis, whereby bacterial hydrolases released from lysosomes begin to break down the cell wall, thus further contributing to destruction of the microorganism.[11]

Consequently, drugs that cause inadequate production of peptidoglycans or other structural components within the cell wall may produce a selective bactericidal effect. Also, a limited number of antibacterial agents directly punch holes in the bacterial cell membrane, destroying the selective permeability and separation of internal from external environment, which is crucial for the life of the microorganism.[12] These agents include the polymyxin antibiotics (e.g., polymyxin B, colistin); these cationic compounds are attracted to negatively charged phospholipids in the bacterial cell membrane. The selectivity of these agents for bacterial cell membranes may be due to a greater attraction to certain bacterial phospholipids, as opposed to human cell membrane phospholipids. In any event, these drugs penetrate and disrupt the architecture and integrity of the surface membrane. In essence, the drugs act as detergents that break apart the phospholipid bilayer, creating gaps and leaks in the bacterial cell membrane.[12] The loss of cell membrane integrity leads to rapid death of the bacteria.

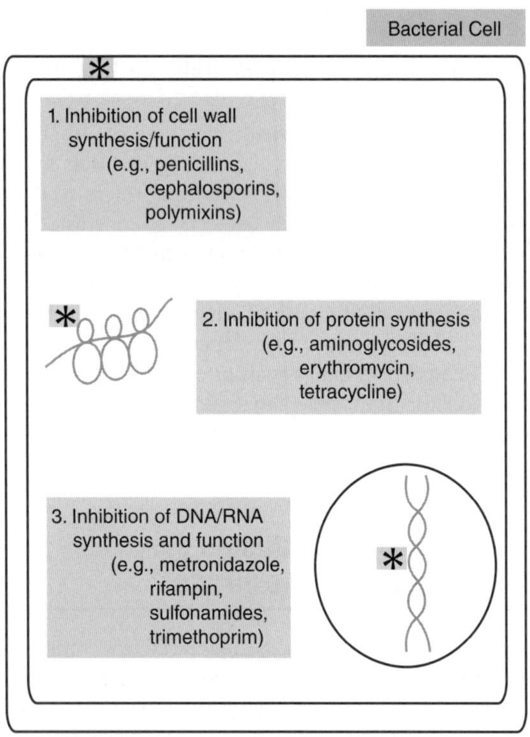

Figure ■ 33-1
Primary sites of antibacterial drug action on bacterial cells.

Inhibition of Bacterial Protein Synthesis

Bacteria, like most living organisms, must continually synthesize specific proteins to carry out various cellular functions, including enzymatic reactions and membrane transport. A fairly large and well-known group of antibacterial agents works by inhibiting or impairing the synthesis of these bacterial proteins. The drugs in this group include the aminoglycosides (e.g., gentamicin, streptomycin), erythromycin, the tetracyclines, and several other agents.[13,14]

Generally, drugs that inhibit bacterial protein synthesis enter the bacterial cell and bind to specific ribosomal subunits.[13,15,16] These drugs have a much greater affinity for bacterial ribosomes than for human ribosomes, hence their relative specificity in treating bacterial infections. Binding of the drug to the ribosome either blocks protein synthesis or causes the ribosome to misread the messenger RNA (mRNA) code, resulting in the production of meaningless or nonsense proteins.[14] The lack of appropriate protein production impairs bacterial cell membrane transport and metabolic function, resulting in retarded growth or death of the bacteria.

Inhibition of Bacterial DNA/RNA Synthesis and Function

As in any cell, bacteria must be able to replicate their genetic material to reproduce and function normally. An inability to produce normal DNA and RNA will prohibit the bacteria from mediating continued growth and reproduction. Drugs that exert their antibacterial activity by directly or indirectly interfering with the structure, synthesis, and function of DNA and RNA in susceptible bacteria include the fluoroquinolones, sulfonamides, and several other agents.[17] These drugs are able to selectively impair bacterial DNA/RNA function because they have a greater affinity for bacterial genetic material and enzymes related to bacterial DNA/RNA synthesis.

Several antibacterial drugs inhibit bacterial nucleic acid synthesis by inhibiting the production of folic acid.[17,18] Folic acid serves as an enzymatic cofactor in several reactions, including synthesis of bacterial nucleic acids and certain essential amino acids. The pathway for synthesis of these folic acid cofactors is illustrated in Figure 33-2. Certain antibacterial drugs block specific steps in the folate pathway, thus impairing the production of this enzymatic cofactor and ultimately impairing the production of nucleic acids and other essential metabolites. Examples of drugs that exert antibacterial effects by this mechanism are trimethoprim and the sulfonamide drugs (e.g., sulfadiazine, sulfamethoxazole).[17]

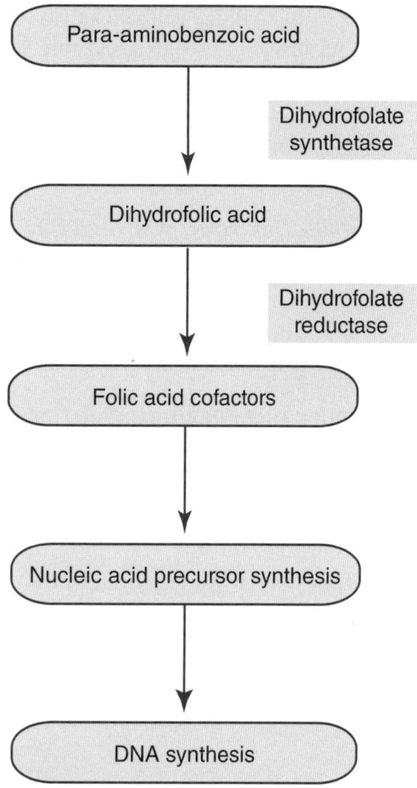

Figure ■ 33-2
Folic acid metabolism in bacterial cells. Certain antibacterial drugs (e.g., sulfonamides and trimethoprim) inhibit the dihydrofolate synthetase and reductase enzymes, thus interfering with DNA biosynthesis.

SPECIFIC ANTIBACTERIAL AGENTS

Considering the vast number of antibacterial drugs, this chapter cannot explore the pharmacokinetic and pharmacological details of each individual agent. For the purposes of this chapter, the major groups of antibacterial drugs are categorized according to the basic modes of antibacterial action that were previously discussed (inhibition of cell wall synthesis, etc.). Pertinent aspects of each group's actions, uses, and potential side effects are briefly discussed. For a more detailed description of any specific agent, see one of the current drug indexes, such as *Davis's Drug Guide for Rehabilitation Professionals.*

ANTIBACTERIAL DRUGS THAT INHIBIT BACTERIAL CELL WALL SYNTHESIS AND FUNCTION

The first group of antibacterial drugs discussed here are those that impair the construction and function of the bacterial cell membrane. The clinical use and specific aspects of penicillins, cephalosporins, carbapenems, and other drugs in this group (Table 33-2) are presented below.

Penicillins

Penicillin, the first antibiotic, was originally derived from mold colonies of the *Penicillium* fungus during the early 1940s. Currently, there are several forms of natural and semisynthetic penicillins (see Table 33-2). These agents have a chemical structure and mode of action similar to the cephalosporin drugs and several other agents. Collectively, the penicillins and these other drugs are known as *beta-lactam antibiotics* because they share a common structure known as a *beta-lactam* ring.[19]

Penicillin and other beta-lactam agents exert their effects by binding to specific enzymatic proteins

Table 33-2
DRUGS THAT INHIBIT BACTERIAL CELL MEMBRANE SYNTHESIS

Penicillins	Cefixime (Suprax)
Natural penicillins	Cefoperazone (Cefobid)
Penicillin G (Wycillin, others)	Cefotaxime (Claforan)
Penicillin V (Beepen-VK, Pen-Vee, others)	Cefpodoxime (Banan, Vantin)
Penicillinase-resistant penicillins	Ceftazidime (Fortaz, Tazicef, others)
Cloxacillin (Cloxapen, Novo-Cloxin, others)	Ceftibuten (Cedax)
Dicloxacillin (Dycill, Dynapen, Pathocil)	Ceftizoxime (Cefizox)
Nafcillin (Nallpen, Unipen)	Ceftriaxone (Rocephin)
Oxacillin (Bactocill)	***Fourth-generation cephalosporins***
Aminopenicillins	Cefepime (Maxipime)
Amoxicillin (Amoxil, Wymox, others)	Ceftaroline (Teflaro)
Ampicillin (Omnipen, Polycillin, others)	**Carbapenems**
Extended-spectrum penicillins	Aztreonam (Azactam)
Piperacillin (generic)	Doripenem (Doribax)
Ticarcillin (Ticar)	Ertapenem (Invanz)
Cephalosporins	Imipenem/cilastatin (Primaxin)
First-generation cephalosporins	Meropenem (Merrem I.V.)
Cefadroxil (Duricef)	**Other Agents**
Cefazolin (Ancef, Kefzol)	Bacitracin (Baci-IM, Bacitracin ointment)
Cephalexin (Keflex, others)	Colistin (Coly-Mycin S)
Second-generation cephalosporins	Cycloserine (Seromycin)
Cefaclor (Ceclor, Raniclor)	Ethambutol (Myambutol)
Cefotetan (Cefotan)	Fosfomycin (Monurol)
Cefoxitin (Mefoxin)	Polymyxin B (generic)
Cefprozil (Cefzil)	Vancomycin (Vancocin, others)
Cefuroxime (Ceftin, Zinacef)	**Penicillin and Beta-Lactamase Combinations**
Third-generation cephalosporins	Ampicillin and sulbactam (Unasyn)
Cefdinir (Omnicef)	Piperacillin and tazobactam (Zosyn)
Cefditoren (Spectracef)	Ticarcillin and clavulanate (Timentin)

within the bacterial cell wall. These enzymatic proteins, known as *penicillin-binding proteins* (PBPs), are responsible for the normal synthesis and organization of the bacterial cell wall. In particular, PBPs help manufacture the peptidoglycans, which are essential for normal membrane structure and function.[20,21] Penicillins and other beta-lactam drugs attach to the PBPs and inhibit their function.[7,22] Thus, construction of the bacterial cell wall is impaired, and the cell dies from the membrane's inability to serve as a selective barrier and to contain the high internal osmotic pressure of the bacterial cell.

Classification and Use of Penicillins

As indicated in Table 33-2, penicillins can be classified according to their chemical background, spectrum of antibacterial activity, or pharmacokinetic features.[7] The naturally occurring penicillins (i.e., penicillin G and V) can be administered orally but have a relatively narrow antibacterial spectrum. Some semisynthetic penicillins (e.g., amoxicillin, ampicillin) have a broader antibacterial spectrum and may be administered either orally or parenterally, depending on the specific agent.

Certain strains of bacteria contain an enzyme known as a *penicillinase* or beta-lactamase. This enzyme destroys natural and some semisynthetic penicillins, rendering these drugs ineffective in bacteria containing this enzyme. Researchers developed penicillinase-resistant forms of semisynthetic penicillin to overcome the destruction by the penicillinase (see Table 33-2).

Discussing all the clinical applications of the penicillins goes well beyond the scope of this chapter. These agents are a mainstay in the treatment of infection and remain the drugs of choice in a diverse array of clinical disorders (see Table 33-5 in "Clinical Use of Antibacterial Drugs"). Clearly, these agents continue to be one of the most important and effective antibacterial regimens currently available.

Adverse Effects

One of the primary problems with penicillin drugs is the potential for allergic reactions.[23] Hypersensitivity to penicillin is exhibited by skin rashes, hives, itching, and difficulty breathing. In some individuals, these reactions may be minor and may not represent a true allergic reaction.[24] Actual penicillin hypersensitivity, however, may be severe and lead to an anaphylactic reaction (i.e., severe bronchoconstriction and cardiovascular collapse). Likewise, some skin reactions associated with penicillin allergy can be severe and life-threatening, including toxic-epidermal necrosis and Steven-Johnson syndrome.[25]

During prolonged administration, penicillin drugs may also cause central nervous system (CNS) problems (e.g., confusion, hallucinations) and certain blood disorders, such as hemolytic anemia and thrombocytopenia. Other relatively minor side effects of penicillin drugs include GI problems such as nausea, vomiting, and diarrhea.

Cephalosporins

The cephalosporin drugs, which are also classified as beta-lactam antibiotics, exert their bactericidal effects in a manner similar to that of the penicillins (i.e., inhibition of PBPs, resulting in inadequate peptidoglycan production).[7] Generally, the cephalosporins serve as alternative agents to penicillins if the penicillin drugs are ineffective or poorly tolerated by the patient. Cephalosporins may also be the drugs of choice in certain types of urinary tract infections (see Table 33-5).

Cephalosporins can be subdivided into first-, second-, third-, and fourth-generation groups, according to their spectrum of antibacterial activity (see Table 33-2). First-generation cephalosporins, which are generally effective against gram-positive cocci, may also be used against some gram-negative bacteria. Second-generation cephalosporins are also effective against gram-positive cocci, but they are somewhat more effective than first-generation agents against gram-negative bacteria. Third-generation cephalosporins have the broadest spectrum of effectiveness against gram-negative bacteria, but they have limited effects on gram-positive cocci. Fourth-generation agents have the broadest antibacterial spectrum of the cephalosporins, and they are effective against gram-positive and gram-negative organisms (see Table 33-5).

Adverse Effects

In some patients, cephalosporins may cause an allergic reaction similar to the penicillin hypersensitivity described previously. A cross-sensitivity often exists: a patient who is allergic to penicillin drugs will also display hypersensitivity to cephalosporin agents. Other principal adverse effects of cephalosporins include GI problems, such as stomach cramps, diarrhea, nausea, and vomiting.

Carbapenems

Carbapenems are a third category of beta-lactam antibacterial agents (see Table 33-2).[26] That is, these drugs also contain a beta-lactam ring but have slightly different chemical constituents compared to the penicillins and cephalosporins. Carbapenems act similarly to other beta-lactam agents; they bind to penicillin-binding proteins and inhibit the synthesis and structure of the cell membrane in susceptible bacteria.[27]

Carbapenem agents tend to have a somewhat broader spectrum of activity compared to the penicillins and cephalosporins (see Table 33-5).[7] Specifically, carbapenems tend to affect a variety of aerobic gram-positive or gram-negative bacteria, as well as some anaerobic bacterial strains.[28] An exception is aztreonam, which is a carbapenem that may be useful against serious infections caused by certain gram-negative bacilli (e.g., *Enterobacter aerogenes* and *Pseudomonas aeruginosa*) but is not effective against gram-positive or anaerobic bacteria. Also, imipenem is a carbapenem that is typically administered with cilastatin. This agent enhances the bactericidal effects of imipenem by inhibiting metabolic inactivation of imipenem within the kidneys, even though cilastatin does not exhibit any antibacterial activities by itself.[7]

Adverse Effects

As is the case with other beta-lactam drugs, carbapenems can cause hypersensitivity (allergic) reactions, which can be severe in susceptible individuals.[25] CNS abnormalities such as confusion, tremors, and seizures may also occur with certain carbapenems, especially in patients who have a preexisting seizure disorder or if the drug dosage is too high, based on the patient's body weight.[29] Other side effects include chest pain, GI problems (e.g., nausea, diarrhea), headache, and fever.

Other Agents That Inhibit Bacterial Cell Wall Synthesis

Bacitracin

Bacitracin refers to a group of polypeptide antibiotics that have similar chemical and pharmacological properties. These compounds inhibit bacterial cell wall synthesis by inhibiting the incorporation of amino acids and nucleic acid precursors into the bacterial cell wall. Bacitracin compounds, which have a broad range of antibacterial activity, are effective against many gram-positive bacilli and gram-positive cocci, as well as several other microorganisms. Bacitracin is usually applied topically to prevent and treat infection in superficial skin wounds and certain ophthalmic infections. Commercial preparations containing bacitracin may also contain other antibiotics, such as neomycin and polymyxin B. The primary problem associated with bacitracin is local hypersensitivity, as indicated by skin rashes and itching.

Colistin

Colistin (also known as *colistimethate* or *polymyxin E*) is similar to polymyxin B (see below) in terms of pharmacological mechanism and antibacterial effects.[12] Colistin is used primarily in combination with other agents (e.g., neomycin and hydrocortisone) to treat local infections of the external auditory canal. Adverse effects are relatively rare during the local and topical use of colistin. This drug can also be administered systemically to patients with gram-negative infections that are resistant to other agents.[12] Systemic administration, however, increases the likelihood of serious adverse effects, such as nephrotoxicity.[30]

Cycloserine

Cycloserine inhibits bacterial wall synthesis by interfering with the final stage of peptidoglycan synthesis (i.e., the addition of two units of the amino acid D-alanine). Cycloserine, which is similar in structure to D-alanine, competitively inhibits the enzyme that adds the final D-alanine units onto the peptidoglycan structures. Cycloserine is considered a broad-spectrum antibiotic but is used primarily as an adjunct in the treatment of tuberculosis. The primary adverse effect of this drug is CNS toxicity, which may occur during prolonged use at relatively high dosages.

Ethambutol

Ethambutol (Myambutol) inhibits an enzyme (arabinosyl transferase III) that synthesizes a key structural component (arabinogalactan) of the cell wall of mycobacteria.[31] Hence, cell wall integrity is compromised, resulting in death of these microorganisms. Ethambutol is primarily effective against *M. tuberculosis* infections and is a secondary agent in the treatment of tuberculosis.[32] Adverse effects associated with this drug include joint pain, nausea, skin rash and itching, and CNS abnormalities (e.g., dizziness, confusion, hallucinations).

Fosfomycin (Monurol)

This drug inhibits an enzyme (phosphoenolpyruvate synthetase) that helps synthesize a key membrane component found only in certain bacteria.[33] Loss of this membrane component impairs the integrity of the cell membrane, resulting in cell death. The drug has a broad antibacterial spectrum against gram-positive and gram-negative bacteria and is used primarily to treat urinary tract infections caused by susceptible microorganisms.[33] Fosfomycin is generally well tolerated, although some GI distress (e.g., nausea, diarrhea) can occur.

Polymyxin B

Polymyxin antibiotics are cationic compounds that are attracted to negatively charged phospholipids in the bacterial cell membrane. These drugs penetrate and disrupt the architecture and integrity of the surface membrane. Essentially, polymyxins act as detergents that break apart the phospholipid bilayer, which creates gaps in the bacterial cell wall, leading to the subsequent destruction of the bacteria.[12]

Polymyxin B is effective against many gram-negative bacteria, including *E. coli*, *Klebsiella*, and *Salmonella*. Systemic administration of this drug, however, is often associated with extreme nephrotoxicity. Hence, this agent is used primarily for the treatment of local, superficial infections of the skin, eyes, and mucous membranes. When applied topically for these conditions, adverse reactions are relatively rare. Polymyxin B is often combined with other antibiotics such as bacitracin and neomycin in commercial topical preparations.

Vancomycin

Vancomycin appears to bind directly to bacterial cell wall precursors such as D-alanine and to impair the incorporation of these precursors into the cell wall.[34] Vancomycin is effective against gram-positive bacilli and cocci and primarily serves as an alternative to the penicillins in treating a variety of infections, including certain bacterial strains that are resistant to the penicillins (see Table 33-5).[35] The emergence of bacteria that are resistant to vancomycin has generated concern about the continued use of this drug (see "Resistance to Antibacterial Drugs").[36] The primary adverse effects associated with vancomycin include hypersensitivity (e.g., skin rashes), a bitter or unpleasant taste in the mouth, and GI disturbances (e.g., nausea and vomiting). Vancomycin also has the potential to cause nephrotoxicity and ototoxicity.

Use of Beta-Lactamase Inhibitors

A primary problem in using penicillins, cephalosporins, and other beta-lactam antibiotics is that certain bacteria produce enzymes known as **beta-lactamases**.[37] These beta-lactamase enzymes bind to the beta-lactam drug and destroy it before it can exert an antibacterial effect. Bacteria that produce these beta-lactamase enzymes are therefore resistant to penicillin and other beta-lactam antibacterial drugs (see "Resistance to Antibacterial Drugs").[37,38] Fortunately, several drugs are available that inhibit these beta-lactamase enzymes,[39,40] including clavulanate, sulbactam, and tazobactam. Beta-lactamase inhibitors are typically combined with a specific type of penicillin or other beta-lactam agent to treat infections caused by bacteria that produce beta-lactamase enzymes.[40,41] The beta-lactamase inhibitor prevents the enzymes from destroying the penicillin, thus allowing the penicillin to remain intact and effective against the bacterial infection.

Some common combinations of penicillins and specific beta-lactamase inhibitors were listed in Table 33-2. Administration of these drug combinations may produce side effects that are caused primarily by the penicillin component such as headache, GI problems, and allergic reactions. Nonetheless, combining a beta-lactamase inhibitor with a penicillin can be an effective way of treating bacterial infections that might otherwise be resistant to traditional antibacterial therapy.

DRUGS THAT INHIBIT BACTERIAL PROTEIN SYNTHESIS

As discussed previously, a large and well-known group of antibacterial agents works by inhibiting or impairing the synthesis of bacterial proteins. Without appropriate protein production, bacterial cell membrane transport and metabolic function is impaired, resulting in retarded growth or death of the bacteria. This section presents the drugs in this group, including the aminoglycosides (e.g., gentamicin, streptomycin), erythromycin, the tetracyclines, and several other agents (Table 33-3).[13,14]

Aminoglycosides

The aminoglycosides include streptomycin, gentamicin, neomycin, and similar agents (see Table 33-3).

Table 33-3
DRUGS THAT INHIBIT BACTERIAL PROTEIN SYNTHESIS

Aminoglycosides
Amikacin (Amikin)
Gentamicin (Garamycin, others)
Kanamycin (Kantrex)
Neomycin (Neo-Fradin)
Streptomycin (generic)
Tobramycin (Nebcin, TOBI)
Macrolides
Azithromycin (Zithromax, Zmax)
Clarithromycin (Biaxin)
Erythromycin (Eryc, E-Mycin, many others)
Tetracyclines
Demeclocycline (Declomycin)
Doxycycline (Monodox, Vibramycin, others)
Minocycline (Minocin)
Tetracycline (Achromycin V, Sumycin, others)
Tigecycline* (Tygacil)
Other Agents
Chloramphenicol (Chloromycetin)
Clindamycin (Cleocin, Dalacin, others)
Ethionamide (Trecator)
Lincomycin (Lincocin, Lincorex, others)
Linezolid (Zyvox)
Quinupristin and Dalfopristin (Synercid)
Telithromycin (Ketek)

**Derived from tetracycline, this drug is classified chemically as a glycycline.*

These agents bind irreversibly to certain parts of bacterial ribosomes and cause several changes in protein synthesis, including alterations in the ribosome's ability to read the mRNA genetic code.[13,14] This misreading results in the improper synthesis of proteins that control specific aspects of cell function, such as membrane structure and permeability.[42] The lack of normal cell proteins leads to the bacterial cell's death.

Antibacterial Spectrum and General Indications

Aminoglycosides have a very broad spectrum of antibacterial activity and are effective against many aerobic gram-negative bacteria, including *E. coli*, *Pseudomonas*, and *Salmonella*.[42] Aminoglycosides are active against some aerobic gram-positive bacteria, such as certain species of *Staphylococcus*, and many anaerobic bacteria. Consequently, aminoglycosides are used to treat a variety of tissue and wound infections (see Table 33-5).

Adverse Effects

Aminoglycoside use is limited somewhat by problems with toxicity.[43] Nephrotoxicity, as indicated by bloody urine, acute renal tubular necrosis, and so on, is one of the more common and serious adverse effects.[44,45] Ototoxicity, as indicated by dizziness and ringing or fullness in the ears, may also occur. This effect can be irreversible in severe cases.[46,47] Toxicity may occur more frequently in certain individuals, such as patients with liver or kidney failure or in elderly patients. To reduce the risk of toxicity, drug levels in the bloodstream must be periodically monitored so dosages can be adjusted for individual patients. Other adverse effects include hypersensitivity (e.g., skin rashes, itching) in susceptible individuals.

Erythromycin and Other Macrolides

Erythromycin and its chemical derivatives (i.e., azithromycin, clarithromycin) comprise a group of agents known as *macrolide antibiotics*.[48] These drugs inhibit bacterial protein synthesis by binding to specific parts of the 50S ribosome in susceptible bacteria (*50S* refers to the sedimentation [S] coefficient used to differentiate and characterize ribosomal subunits during centrifugation).[15] This binding impairs protein synthesis primarily by interfering with the function of transfer RNA (tRNA) at the ribosome. Erythromycin, for example, inhibits the movement of tRNA units at their binding sites on the ribosome.[49] Normally, the tRNAs bring amino acids to the ribosome, where the amino acids are linked together to form proteins. Erythromycin and other macrolides inhibit tRNA movement on the ribosome, thereby impairing amino acid delivery and impairing elongation of the polypeptide chain. These drugs may also block the exit site (polypeptide tunnel) on the ribosome so that the polypeptide chain cannot undergo further modification after this chain has been synthesized.[14,50]

Antibacterial Spectrum and General Indications

Erythromycin and the other macrolides exhibit a very broad spectrum of antibacterial activities and are active against many gram-positive bacteria, as well as some gram-negative bacteria. These agents are often used as the primary or alternative drug in a variety of clinical conditions (see Table 33-5). Macrolides may be especially useful in patients who are allergic to penicillin.

These agents may produce other beneficial effects that complement their antibacterial properties. For example, they seem to have anti-inflammatory effects, especially in diseases associated with airway inflammation.[51,52] Hence, these drugs may be particularly useful in treating certain airway infections in people with cystic fibrosis or other respiratory disorders associated with infection and inflammation in airway tissues.[51,53]

Adverse Effects

When erythromycin is given in high (bactericidal) dosages, GI distress is a common problem; for example, stomach cramps, nausea, vomiting, and diarrhea may occur. Hence, erythromycin is usually given in doses that only impair the growth of bacteria (bacteriostatic doses). Some of the newer macrolides (e.g., clarithromycin, dirithromycin) may be somewhat safer and produce fewer side effects than erythromycin.[54,55] However, various degrees of allergic reactions—ranging from mild skin rashes to acute anaphylaxis—may occur when macrolides are used in susceptible individuals. Likewise, these drugs may cause liver toxicity (e.g., drug-induced hepatitis, liver failure) in some patients, and certain macrolides (e.g., clarithromycin, erythromycin, telithromycin) may cause cardiac arrhythmias in patients with risk factors that predispose them to cardiac irregularities (electrolyte imbalances, latent arrhythmias, other pro-arrhythmic drugs).[55]

Tetracyclines

Tetracycline and tetracycline derivatives (see Table 33-3) inhibit protein synthesis by binding to several components of the ribosomal apparatus in susceptible bacteria.[13,55] Hence, these drugs may cause misreading of the mRNA code and may impair the formation of peptide bonds at the bacterial ribosome. Thus, tetracyclines are very effective in preventing bacterial protein synthesis.

Antibacterial Spectrum and General Indications

Tetracyclines are active against a variety of bacteria, including many gram-positive and gram-negative bacteria, and other bacterial microorganisms (e.g., Rickettsia, spirochetes).[55,56] Their use as a broad-spectrum antibiotic has diminished somewhat, however, because of the development of tetracycline-resistant bacterial strains (see "Resistance to Antibacterial Drugs").

Some of the newer tetracycline-like drugs, such as tigecycline (a drug classified chemically as a glycycline agent that is derived from minocycline), can overcome bacterial strains that are resistant to the traditional drugs.[57] Currently, tetracyclines are used to treat specific infections relating to such bacilli as *Chlamydia*, *Rickettsia*, and certain spirochetes (see Table 33-5). Tetracyclines may also be used as alternative agents in treating bacterial strains that are resistant to other drugs, such as chloramphenicol, streptomycin, and various penicillins.

Tetracyclines also seem to have anti-inflammatory, neuroprotective, and immunomodulating effects.[58,59] Although the exact reasons for these effects are unclear, these drugs may protect cells from damage caused by harmful enzymes and free radicals.[56] Researchers are investigating the administration of tetracyclines on an experimental basis to treat various conditions other than bacterial infections, including Parkinson disease, cancer, dermatological conditions (rosacea), and cardiovascular disease.[58]

Adverse Effects

GI distress (e.g., nausea, vomiting, diarrhea) may be a problem with tetracycline use. Hypersensitivity reactions such as rashes may also occur, as well as an increase in skin sensitivity to ultraviolet light (photosensitivity).[60] Tetracyclines may affect bone growth by influencing cells associated with bone remodeling (osteoblasts, osteoclasts) and their precursors.[61,62] Although these drugs may impair bone formation somewhat in premature infants, tetracyclines may actually have a positive effect on bone resorption in adults and may stabilize bone loss in conditions such as rheumatoid arthritis, osteoporosis, and periodontal (gum) disease.[62,63] Tetracyclines, however, also cause discoloration of teeth, bone, and skin, which may be permanent if these drugs are used in high doses for prolonged periods.[64-66] As mentioned previously, development of tetracycline-resistant strains and resulting superinfections may be a serious problem during tetracycline therapy.

Other Agents That Inhibit Bacterial Protein Synthesis

Chloramphenicol

Chloramphenicol (Chloromycetin) is a synthetically produced agent that exerts antibacterial effects similar to those of erythromycin—that is, it binds to the 50S subunit of bacterial ribosomes and inhibits peptide bond formation. Chloramphenicol is a broad-spectrum antibiotic that is active against many gram-negative and gram-positive bacteria. The drug is administered systemically to treat serious infections such as typhoid fever, *Haemophilus* infections such as osteomyelitis, rickettsial infections such as Rocky Mountain spotted fever, and certain forms of meningitis. Chloramphenicol may also be administered topically to treat various skin, eye, and ear infections.

The most serious problem associated with chloramphenicol is the potential for bone marrow aplasia, which can lead to aplastic anemia and possibly death.[67,68] Chloramphenicol is also associated with other blood dyscrasias, such as agranulocytosis and thrombocytopenia. Because of these risks, chloramphenicol is not typically used as a first-choice drug but is reserved for severe infections that do not respond to other antibacterials or situations where safer drugs are contraindicated (e.g., patients are allergic to other medications).[67]

Clindamycin and Lincomycin

Clindamycin (Cleocin, others) is derived from lincomycin (Lincocin, Lincorex). Both drugs are similar in structure and function to erythromycin and inhibit protein synthesis by binding to the 50S ribosomal subunit of susceptible bacteria. These agents are effective against most gram-positive bacteria and some gram-negative microorganisms.[55] Typically, clindamycin and lincomycin are reserved as alternative drugs (rather than primary agents) in the treatment of local and systemic infections; these agents may be especially useful if patients are unable to tolerate either penicillin or erythromycin. The principal adverse effects associated with these drugs include GI distress (e.g., nausea, diarrhea, colitis) and various allergic reactions, ranging from mild skin rashes to anaphylactic shock.

Ethionamide

Ethionamide (Trecator-SC) appears to inhibit bacterial protein synthesis, but the exact mechanism of action is unknown. The drug may act in a manner similar to that of some of the other drugs discussed previously in this section (binding to bacterial ribosomes), or it may mediate its effect by some other means. Ethionamide is effective against *M. tuberculosis* and is used primarily as a secondary agent when first-choice antituberculosis drugs are ineffective. GI distress (e.g., nausea, vomiting) is the most frequent problem encountered with ethionamide use. CNS disorders (drowsiness, mental depression, etc.) and severe orthostatic hypotension may also occur.

Linezolid

Linezolid (Zyvox) binds to a specific site on the bacterial ribosome and inhibits protein synthesis in many gram-positive bacteria, including staphylococci, streptococci, and enterococci. Hence, this drug is commonly used to treat pneumonia caused by *S. aureus* or *S. pneumoniae* and other susceptible skin and soft tissue infections. Common side effects include GI problems (e.g., nausea, diarrhea), with more serious blood dyscrasias (e.g., anemia, leukopenia, thrombocytopenia) occurring in some patients during prolonged drug administration.

Quinupristin and Dalfopristin

Quinupristin and dalfopristin are combined in the same product (Synercid) for the treatment of certain gram-positive bacteria, such as staphylococci and some enterococcal strains. These agents bind to the bacterial ribosome at slightly different sites and work together to prevent the formation of bacterial polypeptide chains. Treatments are administered via IV infusion; primary side effects include pain, irritation, and thrombophlebitis at the infusion site. Other side effects include muscle and joint pain and GI disturbances (e.g., nausea, vomiting, diarrhea).

Telithromycin

Telithromycin (Ketek) is the first agent from a new class of drugs known as *ketolide antibacterials*.[69] The drug is derived from erythromycin but is altered structurally so that it is able to overcome certain forms of bacterial resistance. Telithromycin acts by binding to the bacterial ribosome and inhibiting protein synthesis. It has an antibacterial spectrum similar to erythromycin but is typically reserved for gram-negative strains that are resistant to other agents. The drug may cause severe hepatotoxicity in some patients, and patients taking the drug should be monitored for signs of hepatitis and liver failure (e.g., yellow skin or eyes, abdominal pain, fever, sore throat, malaise, weakness, facial edema).[69] Other side effects include GI disturbances (e.g., nausea, vomiting, diarrhea) and cardiac arrhythmias in susceptible patients.

DRUGS THAT INHIBIT BACTERIAL DNA/RNA SYNTHESIS AND FUNCTION

Drugs can exert their antibacterial activity by directly or indirectly interfering with the structure, synthesis, and function of DNA and RNA in susceptible bacteria. This section presents fluoroquinolones, sulfonamides, and several other agents (Table 33-4).

Aminosalicylic Acid

Aminosalicylic acid (Paser, PAS) exerts its effects in a manner similar to the sulfonamide drugs—it is structurally similar to para-aminobenzoic acid (PABA) and inhibits folic acid synthesis by competing with PABA in tuberculosis bacteria. This drug is used as an adjunct to the primary antitubercular agents, isoniazid and rifampin. Adverse effects are fairly common with aminosalicylic acid use and include GI problems, hypersensitivity reactions, and blood dyscrasias (e.g., agranulocytosis, thrombocytopenia).

Table 33-4
DRUGS THAT INHIBIT BACTERIAL DNA/RNA SYNTHESIS AND FUNCTION

Fluoroquinolones
Besifloxacin (Besivance)
Ciprofloxacin (Cipro, Proquin XR)
Gemifloxacin (Factive)
Levofloxacin (Levaquin)
Moxifloxacin (Avelox)
Norfloxacin (Noroxin)
Ofloxacin (Floxin)
Rifamycins
Rifabutin (Mycobutin)
Rifampin (Rifadin, Rimactane, Rofact)
Rifapentine (Priftin)
Sulfonamides
Silver sulfadiazine (Silvadene, others)
Sulfadiazine (generic)
Sulfisoxazole (Gantrisin, others)
Others
Aminosalicylic acid (Paser)
Clofazimine (Lamprene)
Dapsone (Aczone, Avlosulfon)
Metronidazole (Flagyl, Protostat, others)
Mupirocin (Bactroban)
Trimethoprim (Primsol, Proloprim, Trimpex)
Trimethoprim/Sulfamethoxazole (Bactrim, Sulfatrim, others)

Clofazimine

Although the exact mechanism of clofazimine (Lamprene) is unclear, the drug appears to bind directly to bacterial DNA in susceptible microorganisms. Drug binding may prevent the double-stranded DNA helix from unraveling to allow replication of the DNA genetic code. An inability to replicate its genetic material will prevent the bacteria from undergoing mitosis.

Clofazimine is effective against *Mycobacterium leprae* and is used primarily as an adjunct in the treatment of leprosy (Hansen's disease). During clofazimine therapy, many patients experience problems with red to brownish black discoloration of the skin. Although this discoloration is reversible, it may take several months to years before skin color returns to normal. Other adverse effects include abdominal pain, nausea, vomiting, and rough, scaly skin.

Dapsone

Dapsone (Avlosulfon) belongs to a class of chemical agents known as the *sulfones*. Dapsone is especially effective against *M. leprae* and is used with rifampin as the primary method of treating leprosy. Dapsone appears to exert its antibacterial effects in a manner similar to that of the sulfonamide drugs; it impairs folic acid synthesis by competing with PABA in bacterial cells. Primary adverse effects associated with dapsone include peripheral motor weakness, hypersensitivity reactions (skin rashes, itching), fever, and blood dyscrasias, such as hemolytic anemia.

Fluoroquinolones

The fluoroquinolone antibiotics include ciprofloxacin (Cipro), levofloxacin (Levaquin), and similar drugs with a *-floxacin* suffix (see Table 33-4). These drugs inhibit two specific enzymes—DNA-gyrase and topoisomerase IV—that affect DNA function in certain bacteria.[70,71] DNA-gyrase is responsible for controlling the amount of DNA winding (supercoiling) in bacterial cells. Topoisomerase IV enzymatically separates two new DNA strands that form during bacterial cell division. Fluoroquinolones inhibit these enzymes, thereby impairing the normal DNA structure and function that is needed for cell growth and replication.[70,71]

Fluoroquinolones are effective against a wide range of gram-positive and gram-negative aerobic bacteria and are especially useful in urinary tract infections caused by *E. coli*, *Klebsiella*, *Proteus*, and *Enterobacter aerogenes*.[17,72] Other indications include the treatment of GI infections, respiratory infections, osteomyelitis, and certain sexually transmitted diseases (e.g., gonorrhea).[17,73] A specific agent, ciprofloxacin (Cipro), is particularly effective against anthrax infections, and this drug received considerable attention as an intervention against bioterrorist activities that use anthrax.[74] Primary adverse effects include CNS toxicity, manifested by visual disturbances, headache, and dizziness. GI distress (e.g., nausea, vomiting, diarrhea) and allergic reactions (e.g., skin rashes, itching) may also occur.[75] These drugs produce photosensitivity and increase the skin's sensitivity to ultraviolet light.[76] Rare but potentially serious cases of nephrotoxicity may occur in certain patients.[77]

Finally, these drugs may cause tendon pain and inflammation (tendinopathy) that can be severe and can ultimately lead to tendon rupture in some patients.[78] Tendinopathy seems to occur most commonly in the Achilles tendon, but other tendons such as the patellar, quadriceps, biceps, supraspinatus, and wrist extensor tendons may also be affected.[79,80] Although the overall incidence of tendinopathy is fairly low, patients may be more susceptible if they are older, have renal failure, are taking glucocorticoids, or have a history of fluoroquinolone-induced tendinopathy.[78,81] Although all of the fluoroquinolones can potentially cause tendinopathy, the risk of tendon damage seems highest with ofloxacin.[78] Hence, complaints of pain in any tendon should be carefully evaluated in patients taking fluoroquinolones, and the affected tendon(s) should not be exercised until the cause of tendinopathy can be determined. If it seems that fluoroquinolones are causing tendinopathy, these drugs should be discontinued, and efforts should be made to protect the tendon from excessive stress until the tendinopathy is resolved.

Metronidazole

The exact mechanism of metronidazole (Flagyl, Protostat, others) is not fully understood. This drug appears to be incorporated into bacterial cells, where it undergoes chemical reduction. Apparently, the reduced metabolite of metronidazole interacts with bacterial DNA and causes it to lose its characteristic double-helix structure. This leads to the disintegration of DNA molecules and loss of the ability to replicate and carry out normal genetic functions. Further details of this bactericidal effect remain to be determined.

Metronidazole is effective against most anaerobic bacteria and is useful in treating serious infections caused by *Bacteroides* and *Fusobacterium*. Metronidazole is also effective against certain protozoa and is discussed in Chapter 35 with regard to its antiprotozoal effects. Common side effects associated with metronidazole include GI distress (e.g., nausea, diarrhea), allergic reactions (such as rashes), and CNS symptoms (e.g., confusion, dizziness, mood changes). This drug may also cause peripheral neuropathies as indicated by numbness and tingling in the hands and feet.

Mupirocin

Mupirocin (Bactroban) inhibits a specific enzyme responsible for tRNA synthesis in susceptible bacteria. Topical administration of this drug is effective for treating skin infections caused by *Staphylococcus aureus* or *Streptococcus pyogenes*. Likewise, mupirocin can be administered by nasal spray to treat local colonization of *S. aureus* in the nasal mucosa. This delivery method may be especially helpful in preventing systemic infection in individuals such as health-care workers who are exposed to an outbreak of resistant strains of *S. aureus*. Local/topical administration is well tolerated, although some irritation of the skin may occur during topical use, and cough and respiratory irritation can occur when mupirocin is administered by nasal spray.

Rifamycins

Rifampin (Rifadin, Rimactane) and similar agents such as rifabutin (Mycobutin) and rifapentine (Priftin) directly impair DNA replication by binding to and inhibiting the DNA-dependent RNA polymerase enzyme in susceptible bacteria. This enzyme initiates the replication of genetic material by generating the formation of RNA strands from the DNA template. By inhibiting this enzyme, rifamycins block RNA chain synthesis and subsequent replication of the nucleic acid code in bacterial cells.

Rifampin is effective against many gram-negative and gram-positive bacteria and is often used to treat tuberculosis and leprosy. Typically, this drug is combined with another agent—for example, rifampin plus dapsone for leprosy, or rifampin plus isoniazid for tuberculosis—to increase effectiveness and to prevent the development of resistance to rifampin. Rifampin is also used in combination with erythromycin to treat Legionnaire disease and certain forms of meningitis (see Table 33-5). Rifabutin is used primarily to treat mycobacterium avian complex, and rifapentine is combined with other agents to treat pulmonary tuberculosis.

Common adverse effects of rifamycins include GI distress (e.g., nausea, vomiting, stomach cramps) and various hypersensitivity reactions (e.g., rashes and fever). Disturbances in liver function have also been noted, and serious hepatic abnormalities may occur in patients with preexisting liver disease.

Sulfonamides

The sulfonamides include sulfadiazine, sulfisoxazole, and similar agents (see Table 33-4). These agents interfere with bacterial nucleic acid production by disrupting folic acid synthesis in susceptible bacteria. Sulfonamide drugs are structurally similar to PABA, which is the substance used in the first step of folic acid synthesis in certain types of bacteria (see Fig. 33-2). These drugs either directly inhibit the enzyme responsible for PABA utilization or become a substitute for PABA, which results in the abnormal synthesis of folic acid. In either case, folic acid synthesis is reduced, and bacterial nucleic acid synthesis is impaired.

Sulfonamides have the potential to be used against a wide variety of bacteria, including gram-negative and gram-positive bacilli and cocci. However, the development of resistance in various bacteria has limited the use of these drugs. Currently, sulfonamides are used systemically to treat certain urinary tract infections and infections caused by *Nocardia* bacteria. Sulfonamides may also be applied topically to treat vaginal infections, ophthalmic conditions, and other local infections. Sulfadiazine, combined with silver nitrate, forms silver sulfadiazine, which is often applied topically to control bacterial infection in burns.[82,83]

The problems encountered most frequently with sulfonamide drugs include GI distress, increased skin sensitivity to ultraviolet light, and allergic reactions. Serious disturbances in the formed blood elements, including blood dyscrasias such as agranulocytosis and hemolytic anemia, may also occur during systemic sulfonamide therapy.

Trimethoprim

Trimethoprim (Proloprim, Trimpex) interferes with the bacterial folic acid pathway by inhibiting the dihydrofolate reductase enzyme in susceptible bacteria (see Fig. 33-2). This enzyme converts dihydrofolic acid to tetrahydrofolic acid during the biosynthesis of folic acid cofactors. By inhibiting this enzyme, trimethoprim directly interferes with the production of folic acid cofactors, and subsequent production of vital bacterial nucleic acids is impaired.

Trimethoprim is effective against several gram-negative bacilli, including *E. coli*, *Enterobacter*, *Proteus mirabilis*, and *Klebsiella*. Patients use trimethoprim primarily to treat urinary tract infections caused by these and other susceptible bacteria (see Table 33-5). Trimethoprim is frequently used in combination with the sulfonamide drug sulfamethoxazole.[17,84] Primary adverse effects associated with trimethoprim include headache, skin rashes and itching, decreased appetite, an unusual taste in the mouth, and GI problems (e.g., nausea, vomiting, diarrhea). Trimethoprim may also cause excessively high levels of potassium in the blood (hyperkalemia), especially in older adults.[85]

OTHER ANTIBACTERIAL DRUGS

Several other antibacterial drugs work by mechanisms that are either unknown or are different from the classical antibacterial mechanisms described previously. These drugs are discussed individually here.

Capreomycin

Capreomycin (Capastat) is used as an adjunct or alternative drug for the treatment of tuberculosis. The drug's mechanism of action is unknown. The primary problems associated with this drug include ototoxicity and nephrotoxicity.

Daptomycin

Daptomycin (Cubicin) is unique in that it binds to the cell membrane of susceptible bacteria and depolarizes the cell. Loss of membrane polarity results in a general inhibition of cell function and subsequent death of the bacterium. Physicians prescribe daptomycin primarily to treat skin infections caused by certain staphylococcal, streptococcal, and enterococcal bacteria. Because of its unique mechanism of action, daptomycin may also be helpful in treating strains that are resistant to more traditional antibacterial drugs. Primary side effects include GI problems (e.g., nausea, constipation, diarrhea), and higher doses may cause myopathy and neuropathy in some patients.

Isoniazid

Isoniazid (INH, Laniazid, Nydrazid, others) is one of the primary drugs used to prevent and treat tuberculosis.[86,87] Likewise, patients often take this drug in combination with other agents such as pyrazinamide, rifampin, and ethambutol to receive effective treatment and overcome resistant strains of tubercular mycobacteria.[88] Isoniazid enters these bacteria where it activates and changes chemically to produce several metabolites that inhibit enzymes involved in bacterial cell wall structure and nucleic acid biosynthesis. Adverse reactions to isoniazid are common, however, and patients may develop disorders such as hepatitis and peripheral neuropathies.

Methenamine

Methenamine (Hiprex, Mandelamine, Urex) exerts antibacterial properties in a unique fashion. In an acidic environment, this drug decomposes into formaldehyde and ammonia. Formaldehyde is bactericidal to almost all bacteria, and bacteria do not develop resistance to the toxin. This mechanism enables methenamine to be especially useful in treating urinary tract infections, because the presence of this drug in acidic urine facilitates the release of formaldehyde at the site of infection (i.e., within the urinary tract). Use of methenamine is safe, although high doses are associated with GI upset and problems with urination (e.g., bloody urine or pain while urinating).

Nitrofurantoin

Bacterial enzymes reduce nitrofurantoin (Furadantin, Macrodantin, others) into a metabolite that is toxic to the bacterial cell. This toxic metabolite inhibits bacterial metabolic function by interfering with ribosomal function and other molecules involved in energy production and utilization in the bacterial cell. Nitrofurantoin is primarily used to treat urinary tract infections caused by a number of gram-negative and some gram-positive bacteria. Adverse effects associated with this drug include GI distress (e.g., nausea, vomiting, diarrhea) and neurotoxicity (as indicated by headache, numbness, and excessive fatigue). Acute pneumonitis (as indicated by coughing, chills, fever, and difficulty in breathing) may also occur soon after nitrofurantoin is initiated. This pneumonitis appears to be a direct chemical effect of the drug and usually disappears within hours after the drug is withdrawn.

Pyrazinamide

Pyrazinamide is used primarily as an adjunct to other drugs in treating tuberculosis. This drug's mechanism of action against *M. tuberculosis* is not fully understood but may involve activation to a toxic metabolite when exposed to acidic conditions in or around the site of bacterial infections. Problems associated with pyrazinamide include hepatotoxicity and lower-extremity joint pain.

CLINICAL USE OF ANTIBACTERIAL DRUGS: RELATIONSHIP TO SPECIFIC BACTERIAL INFECTIONS

Medical practitioners have an incredible array of antibacterial agents at their disposal to treat bacterial infections. As mentioned previously, selection of a particular agent is based on the effectiveness of the drug against a range or spectrum of different bacteria. The clinical application of antibacterial drugs according to their effectiveness against specific bacteria is summarized in Table 33-5.

As this table indicates, various antibacterial drugs can serve as either the primary or the alternative agents against specific bacterial infections. The actual selection of an antibacterial agent is often highly variable, depending on the particular patient, the type and location of

Table 33-5
TREATMENT OF COMMON BACTERIAL INFECTIONS*

Bacillus	Common Disease(s)	Primary Agent(s)	Alternative Agent(s)
Gram-Positive Bacilli			
Bacillus anthracis	Anthrax; pneumonia	Ciprofloxacin; a tetracycline[d]	Amoxicillin; clindamycin; erythromycin; imipenem; penicillin G; levofloxacin
Bacillus cereus	Foodborne illnesses	Vancomycin	Clindamycin; imipenem or meropenem
Clostridium difficile	Antibiotic-associated colitis	Metronidazole	Vancomycin
Clostridium perfringens	Gas gangrene	Penicillin G ± clindamycin	Cefazolin; clindamycin; doxycycline; metronidazole; a carbapenem[b]
Corynebacterium diphtheria	Diphtheria	Erythromycin	Penicillin G
Listeria monocytogenes	Listeriosis (meningitis, brain abcess, other CNS infections)	Ampicillin ± an aminoglycoside[a]	Trimethoprim-sulfamethoxazole
Gram-Negative Bacilli			
Acinetobacter species	Infections in various tissues; hospital-acquired infections	A carbapenem[b] ± an aminoglycoside[a]	Ciprofloxacin; colistin; doxycycline; trimethoprim-sulfamethoxazole; tigecycline; ampicillin/sulbactam; piperacillin/tazobactam; ticarcillin/clavulanate
Enterobacter species	Urinary tract and other infections	A carbapenem[b] or cefepime ± an aminoglycoside[a]	Aztreonam; ciprofloxacin; levofloxacin; third-generation cephalosporin; tigecycline; trimethoprim-sulfamethoxazole; piperacillin/tazobactam; ticarcillin/clavulanate
Escherichia coli	Meningitis	Cefotaxime; ceftriaxone; meropenem	—
Escherichia coli	Bacteremia; other systemic infections	Cefotaxime; ceftriaxone	A carbapenem[b]; a fluoroquinolone[c]; ampicillin/sulbactam; piperacillin/tazobactam; ticarcillin/clavulanate
Escherichia coli	Urinary tract infections	Ampicillin; doxycycline; cephalexin; amoxicillin/clavulanate	An aminoglycoside[a]; a fluoroquinolone[c]; a first-generation cephalosporin; nitrofurantoin
Haemophilus influenza	Meningitis	Ceftriaxone or cefotaxime	Chloramphenicol; meropenem
Haemophilus influenza	Otitis media; pneumonia; sinusitis	Amoxicillin, ampicillin, or amoxicillin-clavulanate	Azithromycin; clarithromycin; cefuroxime; a fluoroquinolone[c]; a tetracycline[d]; trimethoprim-sulfamethoxazole
Klebsiella pneumonia	Pneumonia; urinary tract infection	Cefotaxime; ceftriaxone; cefepime; ceftazidime	An aminoglycoside[a]; a carbapenem[b]; a fluoroquinolone[c]; piperacillin/tazobactam; ticarcillin/clavulanate; tigecycline; trimethoprim-sulfamethoxazole
Legionella pneumophila	Legionnaires' disease	Azithromycin; a fluoroquinolone[c]; erythromycin ± rifampin	Clarithromycin; doxycycline; erythromycin; trimethoprim-sulfamethoxazole
Pasteurella multocida	Abscesses; bacteremia; meningitis; wound infections (animal bites)	Penicillin G, ampicillin, amoxicillin	Ceftriaxone; doxycycline; piperacillin/tazobactam; ticarcillin/clavulanate; trimethoprim-sulfamethoxazole
Proteus mirabilis	Urinary tract and other infections	Ampicillin	An aminoglycoside[a]; a carbapenem[b]; a cephalosporin; chloramphenicol; a fluoroquinolone[c]; piperacillin/tazobactam; ticarcillin/clavulanate; trimethoprim-sulfamethoxazole

Continued

Table 33-5
TREATMENT OF COMMON BACTERIAL INFECTIONS*—cont'd

Bacillus	Common Disease(s)	Primary Agent(s)	Alternative Agent(s)
Pseudomonas aeruginosa	Bacteremia; pneumonia	Cefepime; ceftazidime; an carbapenem[b]; an aminoglycoside[a] ; piperacillin/tazobactam; ticarcillin/clavulanate	Aztreonam; colistin; ciprofloxacin; levofloxacin
Pseudomonas aeruginosa	Urinary tract infection	An aminoglycoside[a]	Ciprofloxacin; levofloxacin
Salmonella typhi	Bacteremia; paratyphoid fever; typhoid fever	Ceftriaxone; cefotaxime; ciprofloxacin; levofloxacin	Trimethoprim-sulfamethoxazole
Serratia marcescens	Various opportunistic and hospital-acquired infections	Ceftriaxone; cefotaxime; cefepime; ciprofloxacin; levofloxacin	Aztreonam; a carbapenem[b]; piperacillin/tazobactam; ticarcillin/clavulanate; trimethoprim-sulfamethoxazole
Gram-Positive Cocci			
Enterococcus faecalis	Endocarditis or other serious infection (bacteremia)	Ampicillin or penicillin G + gentamicin or streptomycin	Vancomycin + gentamicin or streptomycin; linezolid; daptomycin; telavancin; tigecycline
Enterococcus faecalis	Urinary tract infection	Ampicillin; amoxicillin	Fosfomycin; nitrofurantoin
Staphylococcus aureus	Abscesses; bacteremia; cellulitis; endocarditis; osteomyelitis; pneumonia; others	If methicillin-sensitive: nafcillin or oxacillin	First-generation cephalosporin; clindamycin; erythromycin; trimethoprim-sulfamethoxazole; a penicillin + a penicillinase inhibitor
		If hospital-acquired methicillin-resistant: vancomycin ± gentamicin or rifampin	Daptomycin; linezolid; telavancin; tigecycline; trimethoprim-sulfamethoxazole; quinupristin-dalfopristin
		If community-acquired methicillin-resistant: clindamycin; doxycycline; trimethoprim-sulfamethoxazole	Daptomycin; linezolid; telavancin; tigecycline; vancomycin
Streptococcus pneumonia	Arthritis; otitis; pneumonia; sinusitis	If penicillin sensitive: ampicillin or penicillin G or V	A first-generation cephalosporin; erythromycin; azithromycin; clarithromycin; doxycycline; a carbapenem[b]; a fluoroquinolone[c]; trimethoprim-sulfamethoxazole
		If penicillin resistant: drug selection depends on specific resistant strain	Vancomycin ± rifampin; cefotaxime; ceftriaxone; a fluoroquinolone[c]
Streptococcus (viridians group)	Bacteremia; endocarditis	Penicillin G ± gentamicin	Azithromycin; cefotaxime; ceftriaxone; clarithromycin; erythromycin; telavancin; vancomycin ± gentamicin
Gram-Negative Cocci			
Moraxella catarrhalis	Otitis; pneumonia; sinusitis	Amoxicillin/clavulanate; ampicillin/sulbactam	A cephalosporin; azithromycin; clarithromycin; doxycycline; erythromycin; trimethoprim-sulfamethoxazole
Neisseria gonorrhoeae (gonococcus)	Arthritis-dermatitis syndrome; genital infections	Ceftriaxone; cefotaxime; cefpodoxime	Cefixime, a fluoroquinolone[c]
Neisseria meningitidis (meningococcus)	Meningitis	Penicillin G	Cefotaxime; ceftriaxone; chloramphenicol; a fluoroquinolone[c]

Table 33-5
TREATMENT OF COMMON BACTERIAL INFECTIONS*—cont'd

Bacillus	Common Disease(s)	Primary Agent(s)	Alternative Agent(s)
Spirochetes			
Borrelia burgdorferi	Lyme disease	Amoxicillin; doxycycline; ceftriaxone; cefuroxime	Azithromycin; cefotaxime; clarithromycin; penicillin G (high dose)
Treponema pallidum	Syphilis	Penicillin G	Ceftriaxone; doxycycline
Other Microorganisms			
Chlamydia pneumonia	Pneumonia	Doxycycline	Azithromycin; clarithromycin; erythromycin; a fluoroquinolone[c]
Chlamydia trachomatis	Blennorrhea; lymphogranuloma venereum; nonspecific urethritis; trachoma	Azithromycin; doxycycline	Amoxicillin; erythromycin; levofloxacin; ofloxacin
Mycoplasma pneumoniae	"Atypical" pneumonia	Azithromycin, clarithromycin, erythromycin, a fluoroquinolone[c]	Doxycycline

**Selection of primary or alternative agents varies depending on the identification of specific bacterial strains and the presence or absence of resistance to each drug. Drug selection will also be influenced by other factors such as the patient's age, comorbidities, drug allergies, pregnancy, and its possible interactions with other medications.*

a. Aminoglycosides: amikacin, gentamicin, netilmicin, tobramycin
b. Carbapenems: imipenem, meropenem, doripenem, ertapenem
c. Fluoroquinolones: besifloxacin, ciprofloxacin, gemifloxacin, levofloxacin, moxifloxacin, norfloxacin, ofloxacin
d. Tetracyclines: demeclocycline, doxycycline, minocycline, tetracycline, tigecycline

the infection, the experience of the physician, and many other factors.

RESISTANCE TO ANTIBACTERIAL DRUGS

One of the most serious problems of antibacterial therapy is the potential for development of strains of bacteria that are resistant to one or more antibacterial agents.[89,90] Certain bacterial strains have a natural or acquired defense mechanism against specific antibacterial drugs. This enables the strain to survive the effects of the drug and continue to grow and reproduce similar resistant strains, thus representing a genetic selection process in which only the resistant strains survive the drug. If other drugs are not effective against the resistant strain, or if cross-resistance to several antibacterial drugs occurs, the resistant bacteria become especially dangerous because of their immunity from antibacterial chemotherapy.[90]

Bacterial resistance can occur because of several mechanisms[91-93] (Fig. 33-3). Certain bacterial strains may be able to enzymatically destroy the antibacterial drug. The best example is the beta-lactamase enzyme found in bacteria resistant to beta-lactam drugs (penicillins and cephalosporins).[37,93] As previously discussed, bacteria containing this enzyme can destroy certain penicillin and cephalosporin drugs, thus rendering the drug ineffective against these strains.

Resistance may also occur because the bacterial cell modifies or masks the site where the antibacterial drug typically binds on or within the cell. For instance, penicillins, aminoglycosides, vancomycin, and other drugs must bind to membrane proteins, intracellular proteins, ribosomes, and the like to exert their effect. The bacterial cell may mutate and acquire differences in the affinity of these binding sites, thus decreasing the drug's effectiveness.[21,94] Bacteria may also develop resistance through genetic mutations that change the enzymes targeted by certain drugs. For example, fluoroquinolones, rifampin, and other drugs that normally inhibit enzymes responsible for bacterial DNA/RNA function will be ineffective if enzymes and metabolic pathways are modified within resistant bacteria.[95,96]

Resistance can likewise occur if the drug's ability to penetrate the bacterial cell is reduced. Most drugs must first penetrate the cell membrane and then enter the bacterial cell to exert their bactericidal effects.

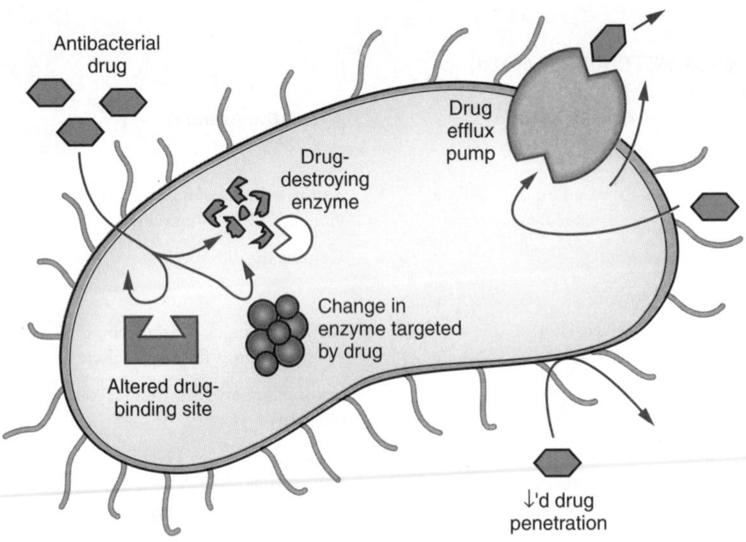

Figure ■ 33-3
Primary bacterial mutations that result in resistance to antibacterial drugs.

Specific bacteria that have a natural or acquired opposition to drug penetration render drugs such as aminoglycosides or other agents useless, thus leading to the development of resistant strains.[97,98] Certain bacteria also develop drug efflux pumps that expel the drug from the bacterial cell, thus rendering the drug ineffective.[97,99] These pumps are a common way that bacteria develop resistance to tetracyclines and several other antimicrobial agents.[99,100] Consequently, a number of factors may be responsible for mediating the formation of bacterial resistance to penicillins, cephalosporins, aminoglycosides, tetracyclines, and other antibacterial agents.

Antibacterial resistance is typically categorized according to the name of the drug and the associated resistant bacterial strain. For example, some of the best known and most important types of resistance include vancomycin-resistant *Staphylococcus aureus* (VRSA), methicillin-resistant *S. aureus* (MRSA), vancomycin-resistant *Enterococcus* (VRE), and penicillin-resistant *Streptococcus pneumoniae* (PRSP).[36,101,102] Even though a resistant organism may be linked to a specific drug by name, the organism is typically resistant to other drugs as well (multidrug resistance).[90,103]

Development of resistant bacteria is understandably a very serious problem in contemporary drug therapy.[90] A progressive increase in the number of resistant bacterial strains is especially problematic in developing countries and in certain clinical situations such as long-term care facilities.[104-106] To limit the development of resistant strains, antibacterial drugs should be used judiciously and not overused, a concept referred to commonly as *antibiotic stewardship*.[107,108] For instance, it is often worthwhile to perform culture and sensitivity tests on sputum, blood, and other body fluids to identify the pathogenic bacteria. Identification leads to the use of more selective agents. Administering selective agents as opposed to broad-spectrum antibiotics may help attenuate and kill resistant strains more effectively, thus limiting the spread of their resistance.[109, 110] The selective use of current antibacterial drugs, combined with the development of new agents that overcome bacterial resistance, will be essential in helping control the problem of bacterial resistance.[90]

Special Concerns for Rehabilitation Patients

Patients undergoing physical therapy and occupational therapy will be taking antibacterial drugs for any number of reasons, including the prevention or treatment of infection in conditions relating directly to the rehabilitation program. For example, bone infections (osteomyelitis), infections sustained from trauma and various wounds, and infections following joint replacement and other types of surgery require antibacterial therapy. In addition, therapists are often involved in administering topical antibacterial agents, such as sulfadiazine to patients with burns. Other types of infection that are not directly related to rehabilitation (e.g., urinary tract infection, pneumonia) are also very common, occurring frequently in hospitalized patients and in those receiving outpatient physical therapy and occupational therapy. Consequently, therapists will be working routinely with patients who are receiving antibacterial treatment.

Therapists should generally be aware of the possible adverse effects of antibacterial drugs. Many of these agents have the potential to cause hypersensitivity reactions, including skin rashes, itching, and respiratory difficulty (such as wheezing). Therapists may recognize the onset of such reactions when working with these patients. Other common side effects, including GI problems (e.g., nausea, vomiting, diarrhea), are usually not serious but may be bothersome if they continually interrupt therapy. Therapists may have to alter the time of the rehabilitation session to work around these effects, especially if GI and similar side effects tend to occur at a specific time of the day (e.g., early morning, late afternoon).

Certain agents may have adverse effects that directly interact with specific rehabilitation treatments. In particular, tetracyclines, sulfonamides, and fluoroquinolones (ciprofloxacin, norfloxacin, etc.) cause increased skin sensitivity to ultraviolet light. This problem is obvious if the therapist is administering ultraviolet treatments. Therapists must be especially careful to establish an accurate minimal erythemal dosage to ultraviolet light. Therapists should also be prepared to adjust the ultraviolet light treatments in accordance with changes in the dosage of the antibacterial drug.

Finally, therapists play a vital role in preventing the spread of bacterial and other infections. Therapists must maintain appropriate sterile technique when dealing with open wounds. Adequate sterilization of whirlpools with strong disinfectants is also critical in preventing the spread of infection from patient to patient in a rehabilitation setting. Therapists must also recognize the importance of hand washing in preventing the spread of infection and must not neglect to wash their own hands between patients.

CASE STUDY

ANTIBACTERIAL DRUGS

Brief History. P.M. is a 40-year-old computer programmer/analyst and recreational runner. She typically runs 15 to 20 miles each week and occasionally competes in local 5- and 10-kilometer road races. Recently, she began to experience increased urinary frequency and a burning sensation while urinating and suspected she may have a urinary tract infection (UTI). She visited her physician, who confirmed the infection and prescribed a short course of oral ciprofloxacin (Cipro), 100 mg every 12 hours for

Continued on following page

CASE STUDY (Continued)

3 days. Several days later, she began to experience pain and stiffness in her left Achilles tendon. She had been steadily increasing her weekly mileage in preparation for a half-marathon and assumed her tendon pain was related to her increased training. She made an appointment with a physical therapist who had treated her running injuries in the past, including an episode of left Achilles tendinopathy that occurred several years ago.

Problem/Influence of Medication. The physical therapist performed a thorough evaluation, including a review of P.M.'s medications. P.M. mentioned that she had recently taken ciprofloxacin for her UTI.

1. ***Why should the therapist be concerned about the effects of ciprofloxacin on P.M.'s Achilles tendon?***

2. ***What should the therapist do in this situation?***

See Appendix C, "Answers to Case Study Questions."

SUMMARY

Antibacterial drugs are used to prevent and treat infection in a variety of clinical situations. Some drugs are effective against a limited number of bacteria (narrow-spectrum), whereas other agents may be used against a relatively wide variety of bacterial pathogens (broad-spectrum). Specific agents may exert their antibacterial effects by preventing bacterial cell wall synthesis and function or by inhibiting either bacterial protein synthesis or bacterial DNA/RNA synthesis and function. Although most bacterial infections can be effectively treated with one or more agents, the development of bacterial strains that are resistant to drug therapy continues to be a serious problem. Rehabilitation specialists will routinely treat patients receiving antibacterial drugs for conditions that are directly or indirectly related to the need for physical therapy and occupational therapy. Therapists should be cognizant of the potential side effects of these drugs and should know how these drugs may interfere with specific physical therapy and occupational therapy procedures.

REFERENCES

1. Ryan KJ, Drew WL. The nature of bacteria. In: Ryan KJ, Ray CG, eds. *Sherris Medical Microbiology*. 5th ed. New York: McGraw-Hill; 2010.
2. McAdam AJ, Sharpe AH. Infectious diseases. In: Kumar V, Abbas AK, Fausto N, Aster JC, eds. *Pathologic Basis of Disease*. 8th ed. New York: Elsevier Saunders; 2010.
3. Navarro-Garcia F, Elias WP. Autotransporters and virulence of enteroaggregative *E. coli*. *Gut Microbes*. 2011;2:13-24.
4. DiRita VJ. Introduction to the pathogenic bacteria. In: Engleberg NC, DiRita V, Dermody TS, eds. *Schaechter's Mechanisms of Microbial Disease*. 5th ed. Philadelphia, PA: Lippincott Williams and Wilkins; 2013.
5. Murphy EC, Frick IM. Gram-positive anaerobic cocci—commensals and opportunistic pathogens. *FEMS Microbiol Rev*. 2013;37:520-553.
6. Goo KS, Sim TS. Designing new β-lactams: implications from their targets, resistance factors and synthesizing enzymes. *Curr Comput Aided Drug Des*. 2011;7:53-80.
7. Petri WA. Penicillins, cephalosporins, and other beta-lactam antibiotics. In: Brunton L, et al, eds. *The Pharmacological Basis of Therapeutics*. 12th ed. New York: McGraw-Hill; 2011.
8. Desmarais SM, De Pedro MA, Cava F, Huang KC. Peptidoglycan at its peaks: how chromatographic analyses can reveal bacterial cell wall structure and assembly. *Mol Microbiol*. 2013;89:1-13.
9. Vollmer W, Bertsche U. Murein (peptidoglycan) structure, architecture and biosynthesis in *Escherichia coli*. *Biochim Biophys Acta*. 2008;1778:1714-1734.
10. Lovering AL, Safadi SS, Strynadka NC. Structural perspective of peptidoglycan biosynthesis and assembly. *Annu Rev Biochem*. 2012;81:451-478.
11. van Heijenoort J. Peptidoglycan hydrolases of *Escherichia coli*. *Microbiol Mol Biol Rev*. 2011;75:636-663.
12. Velkov T, Roberts KD, Nation RL, et al. Pharmacology of polymyxins: new insights into an 'old' class of antibiotics. *Future Microbiol*. 2013;8:711-724.
13. Lambert T. Antibiotics that affect the ribosome. *Rev Sci Tech*. 2012;31:57-64.
14. McCoy LS, Xie Y, Tor Y. Antibiotics that target protein synthesis. *Wiley Interdiscip Rev RNA*. 2011;2:209-232.

15. Kannan K, Mankin AS. Macrolide antibiotics in the ribosome exit tunnel: species-specific binding and action. *Ann N Y Acad Sci*. 2011;1241:33-47.
16. Wilson DN. On the specificity of antibiotics targeting the large ribosomal subunit. *Ann N Y Acad Sci.* 2011;1241:1-16.
17. Petri WA. Sulfonamides, trimethoprim-sulfamethoxazole, quinolones, and agents for urinary tract infections. In: Brunton L, et al, eds. *The Pharmacological Basis of Therapeutics*. 12th ed. New York: McGraw-Hill; 2011.
18. Sharma M, Chauhan PM. Dihydrofolate reductase as a therapeutic target for infectious diseases: opportunities and challenges. *Future Med Chem*. 2012;4:1335-1365.
19. Tahlan K, Jensen SE. Origins of the β-lactam rings in natural products. *J Antibiot*. 2013;66:401-410.
20. Zapun A, Noirclerc-Savoye M, Helassa N, Vernet T. Peptidoglycan assembly machines: the biochemical evidence. *Microb Drug Resist*. 2012;18:256-260.
21. Zervosen A, Sauvage E, Frère JM, et al. Development of new drugs for an old target: the penicillin binding proteins. *Molecules*. 2012;17:12478-12505.
22. Schneider T, Sahl HG. An oldie but a goodie—cell wall biosynthesis as antibiotic target pathway. *Int J Med Microbiol.* 2010;300:161-169.
23. Chang C, Mahmood MM, Teuber SS, Gershwin ME. Overview of penicillin allergy. *Clin Rev Allergy Immunol.* 2012;43:84-97.
24. Lagacé-Wiens P, Rubinstein E. Adverse reactions to β-lactam antimicrobials. *Expert Opin Drug Saf.* 2012;11:381-399.
25. Torres MJ, Blanca M. The complex clinical picture of beta-lactam hypersensitivity: penicillins, cephalosporins, monobactams, carbapenems, and clavams. *Med Clin North Am.* 2010;94:805-820.
26. Breilh D, Texier-Maugein J, Allaouchiche B, et al. Carbapenems. *J Chemother.* 2013;25:1-17.
27. Papp-Wallace KM, Endimiani A, Taracila MA, Bonomo RA. Carbapenems: past, present, and future. *Antimicrob Agents Chemother*. 2011;55:4943-4960.
28. El-Gamal MI, Oh CH. Current status of carbapenem antibiotics. *Curr Top Med Chem*. 2010;10:1882-1897.
29. Miller AD, Ball AM, Bookstaver PB, et al. Epileptogenic potential of carbapenem agents: mechanism of action, seizure rates, and clinical considerations. *Pharmacotherapy*. 2011;31: 408-423.
30. Vaara M. Polymyxins and their novel derivatives. *Curr Opin Microbiol.* 2010;13:574-581.
31. Rombouts Y, Brust B, Ojha AK, et al. Exposure of mycobacteria to cell wall-inhibitory drugs decreases production of arabinoglycerolipid related to Mycolyl-arabinogalactan-peptidoglycan metabolism. *J Biol Chem.* 2012;287:11060-11069.
32. Zumla A, Nahid P, Cole ST. Advances in the development of new tuberculosis drugs and treatment regimens. *Nat Rev Drug Discov.* 2013;12:388-404.
33. Michalopoulos AS, Livaditis IG, Gougoutas V. The revival of fosfomycin. *Int J Infect Dis.* 2011;15:e732-739.
34. Nailor MD, Sobel JD. Antibiotics for gram-positive bacterial infections: vancomycin, teicoplanin, quinupristin/dalfopristin, oxazolidinones, daptomycin, dalbavancin, and telavancin. *Infect Dis Clin North Am*. 2009;23:965-982.
35. Vandecasteele SJ, De Vriese AS, Tacconelli E. The pharmacokinetics and pharmacodynamics of vancomycin in clinical practice: evidence and uncertainties. *J Antimicrob Chemother.* 2013;68:743-748.
36. Cattoir V, Leclercq R. Twenty-five years of shared life with vancomycin-resistant enterococci: is it time to divorce? *J Antimicrob Chemother.* 2013;68:731-742.
37. Gutkind GO, Di Conza J, Power P, Radice M. β-lactamase-mediated resistance: a biochemical, epidemiological and genetic overview. *Curr Pharm Des.* 2013;19:164-208.
38. Babic M, Hujer AM, Bonomo RA. What's new in antibiotic resistance? Focus on beta-lactamases. *Drug Resist Updat.* 2006;9:142-156.
39. Biondi S, Long S, Panunzio M, Qin WL. Current trends in β-lactam based β-lactamases inhibitors. *Curr Med Chem.* 2011;18:4223-4236.
40. Watkins RR, Papp-Wallace KM, Drawz SM, Bonomo RA. Novel β-lactamase inhibitors: a therapeutic hope against the scourge of multidrug resistance. *Front Microbiol.* 2013;4:392.
41. Shlaes DM. New β-lactam-β-lactamase inhibitor combinations in clinical development. *Ann N Y Acad Sci.* 2013;1277:105-114.
42. MacDougall C, Chambers HF. Aminoglycosides. In: Brunton L, et al, eds. *The Pharmacological Basis of Therapeutics.* 12th ed. New York: McGraw-Hill; 2011.
43. Karasawa T, Steyger PS. Intracellular mechanisms of aminoglycoside-induced cytotoxicity. *Integr Biol.* 2011;3:879-886.
44. Lopez-Novoa JM, Quiros Y, Vicente L, et al. New insights into the mechanism of aminoglycoside nephrotoxicity: an integrative point of view. *Kidney Int.* 2011;79:33-45.
45. Quiros Y, Vicente-Vicente L, Morales AI, et al. An integrative overview on the mechanisms underlying the renal tubular cytotoxicity of gentamicin. *Toxicol Sci.* 2011;119:245-256.
46. Warchol ME. Cellular mechanisms of aminoglycoside ototoxicity. *Curr Opin Otolaryngol Head Neck Surg.* 2010;18:454-458.
47. Xie J, Talaska AE, Schacht J. New developments in aminoglycoside therapy and ototoxicity. *Hear Res.* 2011;281:28-37.
48. Ying L, Tang D. Recent advances in the medicinal chemistry of novel erythromycin-derivatized antibiotics. *Curr Top Med Chem.* 2010;10:1441-1469.
49. McCusker KP, Fujimori DG. The chemistry of peptidyltransferase center-targeted antibiotics: enzymatic resistance and approaches to countering resistance. *ACS Chem Biol.* 2012;7: 64-72.
50. Kannan K, Vázquez-Laslop N, Mankin AS. Selective protein synthesis by ribosomes with a drug-obstructed exit tunnel. *Cell.* 2012;151:508-520.
51. Cameron EJ, McSharry C, Chaudhuri R, et al. Long-term macrolide treatment of chronic inflammatory airway diseases: risks, benefits and future developments. *Clin Exp Allergy.* 2012;42: 1302-1312.
52. Zarogoulidis P, Papanas N, Kioumis I, et al. Macrolides: from in vitro anti-inflammatory and immunomodulatory properties to clinical practice in respiratory diseases. *Eur J Clin Pharmacol.* 2012;68:479-503.
53. Southern KW, Barker PM, Solis-Moya A, Patel L. Macrolide antibiotics for cystic fibrosis. *Cochrane Database Syst Rev.* 2012;11:CD002203.
54. Gutiérrez-Castrellón P, Mayorga-Buitron JL, Bosch-Canto V, et al. Efficacy and safety of clarithromycin in pediatric patients with upper respiratory infections: a systematic review with meta-analysis. *Rev Invest Clin.* 2012;64:126-135.
55. MacDougall C, Chambers HF. Protein synthesis inhibitors and miscellaneous antibacterial agents. In: Brunton L, et al, eds. *The Pharmacological Basis of Therapeutics.* 12th ed. New York: McGraw-Hill; 2011.

56. Griffin MO, Fricovsky E, Ceballos G, Villarreal F. Tetracyclines: a pleitropic family of compounds with promising therapeutic properties. Review of the literature. *Am J Physiol Cell Physiol.* 2010;299:C539-548.
57. Stein GE, Babinchak T. Tigecycline: an update. *Diagn Microbiol Infect Dis.* 2013;75:331-336.
58. Bahrami F, Morris DL, Pourgholami MH. Tetracyclines: drugs with huge therapeutic potential. *Mini Rev Med Chem.* 2012;12:44-52.
59. Griffin MO, Ceballos G, Villarreal FJ. Tetracycline compounds with non-antimicrobial organ protective properties: possible mechanisms of action. *Pharmacol Res.* 2011;63:102-107.
60. Drucker AM, Rosen CF. Drug-induced photosensitivity: culprit drugs, management and prevention. *Drug Saf.* 2011;34: 821-837.
61. Cheng W, Yue Y, Fan W, et al. Effects of tetracyclines on bones: an ambiguous question needs to be clarified. *Pharmazie.* 2012;67:457-459.
62. Kinugawa S, Koide M, Kobayashi Y, et al. Tetracyclines convert the osteoclastic-differentiation pathway of progenitor cells to produce dendritic cell-like cells. *J Immunol.* 2012;188: 1772-1781.
63. Payne JB, Golub LM. Using tetracyclines to treat osteoporotic/osteopenic bone loss: from the basic science laboratory to the clinic. *Pharmacol Res.* 2011;63:121-129.
64. Johnston S. Feeling blue? Minocycline-induced staining of the teeth, oral mucosa, sclerae and ears—a case report. *Br Dent J.* 2013;215:71-73.
65. Kerbleski GJ, Hampton TT, Cornejo A. Black bone disease of the foot: a case study and review of literature demonstrating a correlation of long-term minocycline therapy and bone hyperpigmentation. *J Foot Ankle Surg.* 2013;52:239-241.
66. Sánchez AR, Rogers RS 3rd, Sheridan PJ. Tetracycline and other tetracycline-derivative staining of the teeth and oral cavity. *Int J Dermatol.* 2004;43:709-715.
67. Civljak R, Giannella M, Di Bella S, Petrosillo N. Could chloramphenicol be used against ESKAPE pathogens? A review of in vitro data in the literature from the 21st century. *Expert Rev Anti Infect Ther.* 2014;12:249-264.
68. Wiest DB, Cochran JB, Tecklenburg FW. Chloramphenicol toxicity revisited: a 12-year-old patient with a brain abscess. *J Pediatr Pharmacol Ther.* 2012;17:182-188.
69. Zuckerman JM, Qamar F, Bono BR. Review of macrolides (azithromycin, clarithromycin), ketolids (telithromycin) and glycylcyclines (tigecycline). *Med Clin North Am.* 2011;95: 761-791.
70. Collin F, Karkare S, Maxwell A. Exploiting bacterial DNA gyrase as a drug target: current state and perspectives. *Appl Microbiol Biotechnol.* 2011;92:479-497.
71. Pommier Y, Leo E, Zhang H, Marchand C. DNA topoisomerases and their poisoning by anticancer and antibacterial drugs. *Chem Biol.* 2010;17:421-433.
72. Sharma PC, Jain A, Jain S. Fluoroquinolone antibacterials: a review on chemistry, microbiology and therapeutic prospects. *Acta Pol Pharm.* 2009;66:587-604.
73. Bolon MK. The newer fluoroquinolones. *Infect Dis Clin North Am.* 2009;23:1027-1051.
74. Sweeney DA, Hicks CW, Cui X, et al. Anthrax infection. *Am J Respir Crit Care Med.* 2011;184:1333-1341.
75. Liu HH. Safety profile of the fluoroquinolones: focus on levofloxacin. *Drug Saf.* 2010;33:353-369.
76. Sailer E, Kamarachev J, Boehler A, et al. Persistent photodamage following drug photosensitization in a lung-transplant recipient. *Photodermatol Photoimmunol Photomed.* 2011;27: 213-215.
77. Bird ST, Etminan M, Brophy JM, et al. Risk of acute kidney injury associated with the use of fluoroquinolones. *CMAJ.* 2013;185:E475-482.
78. Stephenson AL, Wu W, Cortes D, Rochon PA. Tendon injury and fluoroquinolone use: a systematic review. *Drug Saf.* 2013. [Epub ahead of print]
79. Sode J, Obel N, Hallas J, Lassen A. Use of fluoroquinolone and risk of Achilles tendon rupture: a population-based cohort study. *Eur J Clin Pharmacol.* 2007;63:499-503.
80. Stinner DJ, Orr JD, Hsu JR. Fluoroquinolone-associated bilateral patellar tendon rupture: a case report and review of the literature. *Mil Med.* 2010;175:457-459.
81. Wise BL, Peloquin C, Choi H, et al. Impact of age, sex, obesity, and steroid use on quinolone-associated tendon disorders. *Am J Med.* 2012;125:1228.
82. Lloyd EC, Rodgers BC, Michener M, Williams MS. Outpatient burns: prevention and care. *Am Fam Physician.* 2012;85:25-32.
83. Miller AC, Rashid RM, Falzon L, et al. Silver sulfadiazine for the treatment of partial-thickness burns and venous stasis ulcers. *J Am Acad Dermatol.* 2012;66:e159-165.
84. Bodro M, Paterson DL. Has the time come for routine trimethoprim-sulfamethoxazole prophylaxis in patients taking biologic therapies? *Clin Infect Dis.* 2013;56:1621-1628.
85. Antoniou T, Gomes T, Mamdani MM, et al. Trimethoprim-sulfamethoxazole induced hyperkalaemia in elderly patients receiving spironolactone: nested case-control study. *BMJ.* 2011;343:d5228.
86. Lobue P, Menzies D. Treatment of latent tuberculosis infection: an update. *Respirology.* 2010;15:603-622.
87. Sia IG, Wieland ML. Current concepts in the management of tuberculosis. *Mayo Clin Proc.* 2011;86:348-361.
88. Dooley KE, Mitnick CD, Ann DeGroote M, et al. Old drugs, new purpose: retooling existing drugs for optimized treatment of resistant tuberculosis. *Clin Infect Dis.* 2012;55:572-581.
89. Livermore DM. Fourteen years in resistance. *Int J Antimicrob Agents.* 2012;39:283-294.
90. Paphitou NI. Antimicrobial resistance: action to combat the rising microbial challenges. *Int J Antimicrob Agents.* 2013; 42(suppl):S25-28.
91. Martinez M, Silley P. Antimicrobial drug resistance. *Handb Exp Pharmacol.* 2010;199:227-264.
92. Rice LB. Mechanisms of resistance and clinical relevance of resistance to β-lactams, glycopeptides, and fluoroquinolones. *Mayo Clin Proc.* 2012;87:198-208.
93. Talbot GH. β-Lactam antimicrobials: what have you done for me lately? *Ann N Y Acad Sci.* 2013;1277:76-83.
94. Long KS, Vester B. Resistance to linezolid caused by modifications at its binding site on the ribosome. *Antimicrob Agents Chemother.* 2012;56:603-612.
95. Tenover FC. Mechanisms of antimicrobial resistance in bacteria. *Am J Med.* 2006;119(suppl 1):S3-10; discussion S62-70.
96. Tupin A, Gualtieri M, Roquet-Banères F, et al. Resistance to rifampicin: at the crossroads between ecological, genomic and medical concerns. *Int J Antimicrob Agents.* 2010;35:519-523.
97. Fernández L, Hancock RE. Adaptive and mutational resistance: role of porins and efflux pumps in drug resistance. *Clin Microbiol Rev.* 2012;25:661-681.

98. Giedraitienė A, Vitkauskienė A, Naginienė R, Pavilonis A. Antibiotic resistance mechanisms of clinically important bacteria. *Medicina*. 2011;47:137-146.
99. Soto SM. Role of efflux pumps in the antibiotic resistance of bacteria embedded in a biofilm. *Virulence*. 2013;4:223-229.
100. Sun Y, Cai Y, Liu X, et al. The emergence of clinical resistance to tigecycline. *Int J Antimicrob Agents*. 2013;41:110-116.
101. Gould IM. Treatment of bacteraemia: meticillin-resistant *Staphylococcus aureus* (MRSA) to vancomycin-resistant *S. aureus* (VRSA). *Int J Antimicrob Agents*. 2013;42(suppl):S17-21.
102. Rennie RP. Current and future challenges in the development of antimicrobial agents. *Handb Exp Pharmacol*. 2012;211:45-65.
103. Lynch JB. Multidrug-resistant tuberculosis. *Med Clin North Am*. 2013;97:553-579.
104. Diene SM, Rolain JM. Investigation of antibiotic resistance in the genomic era of multidrug-resistant Gram-negative bacilli, especially *Enterobacteriaceae*, *Pseudomonas* and *Acinetobacter*. *Expert Rev Anti Infect Ther*. 2013;11:277-296.
105. Johnson AP, Woodford N. Global spread of antibiotic resistance: the example of New Delhi metallo-β-lactamase (NDM)-mediated carbapenem resistance. *J Med Microbiol*. 2013;62(Pt 4):499-513.
106. van Buul LW, van der Steen JT, Veenhuizen RB, et al. Antibiotic use and resistance in long term care facilities. *J Am Med Dir Assoc*. 2012;13:568.e1-13.
107. Goff DA. Antimicrobial stewardship: bridging the gap between quality care and cost. *Curr Opin Infect Dis*. 2011;24(suppl 1):S11-20.
108. Tamma PD, Cosgrove SE. Antimicrobial stewardship. *Infect Dis Clin North Am*. 2011;25:245-260.
109. Lynch TJ. Choosing optimal antimicrobial therapies. *Med Clin North Am*. 2012;96:1079-1094.
110. Pulcini C, Gyssens IC. How to educate prescribers in antimicrobial stewardship practices. *Virulence*. 2013;4:192-202.

CHAPTER 34

Treatment of Infections II: Antiviral Drugs

A virus is one of the smallest microorganisms, consisting of only a nucleic acid core surrounded by a protein shell.[1] Several types of viruses commonly infect human cells and are responsible for a diverse range of pathologies. Viral infections extend from relatively mild disorders such as the common cold to serious, life-threatening conditions such as AIDS. Viruses are somewhat unique in that they must rely totally on the metabolic processes of the host (human) cell to function.[2] Hence, the pharmacological treatment of viral infections is complex, because it is often difficult to selectively destroy the virus without also destroying human cells.

This chapter describes the basic characteristics of viruses and the relatively limited number of drugs that can act selectively as antiviral agents. A brief discussion of methods of preventing viral infections (antiviral vaccines) follows. The chapter ends with a discussion of the current methods of treating a specific viral-induced disease—AIDS.

You will often treat patients who are in the active stages of a viral infection, as well as those suffering from the sequelae of viral disorders, such as gastroenteritis, encephalitis, and influenza. Such infections can be very debilitating, and you can play a role in maintaining and restoring the patient's strength and functional abilities during and after antiviral treatments. Certain viruses such as polioviruses can have devastating effects on neuromuscular function, and much of the historical basis of physical rehabilitation was developed during the polio epidemics of the 1940s and 1950s. Fortunately, antiviral drugs and vaccines have been instrumental in controlling or even eradicating certain viral infections. However, other viruses remain difficult to treat pharmacologically, and there is still a need for effective vaccines against many viruses, including HIV. Antiviral drug research is a very dynamic and rapidly changing area of pharmacology, and you should stay abreast of developments in this area to enrich your own knowledge and serve as a reliable source of information for your patients. Hence, you should understand pharmacotherapeutic treatment and prophylaxis of viral infections.

VIRAL STRUCTURE AND FUNCTION

Classification of Viruses

Viruses are classified according to several criteria, including physical, biochemical, and pathogenic characteristics.[1,2] The classifications of some of the more common viruses affecting humans, and their associated diseases, are listed in Table 34-1. The table shows that viruses can be divided into two categories, depending on the type of genetic material contained in the virus (DNA or RNA viruses). Families within each major subdivision are classified according to physical characteristics (e.g., configuration of the genetic material, shape of the virus capsule) and other functional criteria.

Table 34-1
CLASSIFICATION OF COMMON VIRUSES AFFECTING HUMANS

Virus Family	Virus	Type of Infection
DNA Viruses		
Adenoviridae	Adenovirus, types 1–33	Respiratory tract and eye infections
Hepatitis B	Hepatitis B virus	Hepatitis B
Herpesviridae	Cytomegalovirus	Cytomegalic inclusion disease (i.e., widespread involvement of virtually any organ, especially the brain, liver, lung, kidney, intestine)
	Epstein-Barr virus	Infectious mononucleosis
	Herpes simplex, types 1 and 2	Local infections of oral, genital, and other mucocutaneous areas; systemic infections
	Varicella-zoster virus	Chicken pox; herpes zoster (shingles); other systemic infections
Poxviridae	Smallpox virus	Smallpox
RNA Viruses		
Coronaviridae	Coronavirus	Upper respiratory tract infection
Flaviviridae	Hepatitis C virus	Hepatitis C
Orthomyxoviridae	Influenza virus, types A and B	Influenza
Paramyxoviridae	Measles virus	Measles virus
	Mumps virus	Mumps
	Respiratory syncytial virus	Respiratory tract infection in children
Picornaviridae	Hepatitis A virus	Hepatitis A
	Polioviruses	Poliomyelitis
	Rhinovirus, types 1–89	Common cold
Retroviridae	HIV	AIDS
Rhabdoviridae	Rabies virus	Rabies
Togaviridae	Alphavirus	Encephalitis
	Rubella virus	Rubella

Characteristics of Viruses

Viruses are somewhat unique in structure and function as compared with other microorganisms. The basic components of viral microorganisms are illustrated in Figure 34-1. A virus essentially consists of a core of viral DNA or RNA.[1,3] The genetic core is surrounded by a protein shell, or *capsid*. This structure—the capsid enclosing the nucleic acid core—is referred to as the *nucleocapsid*. The shape and size of the nucleocapsid will vary, depending on the specific virus in question. In some viruses, the nucleocapsid is also surrounded by a viral membrane, or envelope, which is composed of glycoproteins extending outward from a lipid bilayer.

The virus, however, does not contain any of the cellular components necessary to replicate itself or synthesize proteins and other macromolecules—that is, the virus lacks ribosomes, endoplasmic reticulum, and so on.[1] The virus contains only the genetic code (viral genome) that will produce additional viruses. To replicate itself, the virus must rely on the biochemical machinery of the host cell.[2,3] In essence, the virus invades the host cell, takes control of the cell's metabolic function, and uses its macromolecular-synthesizing apparatus to crank out new viruses. The

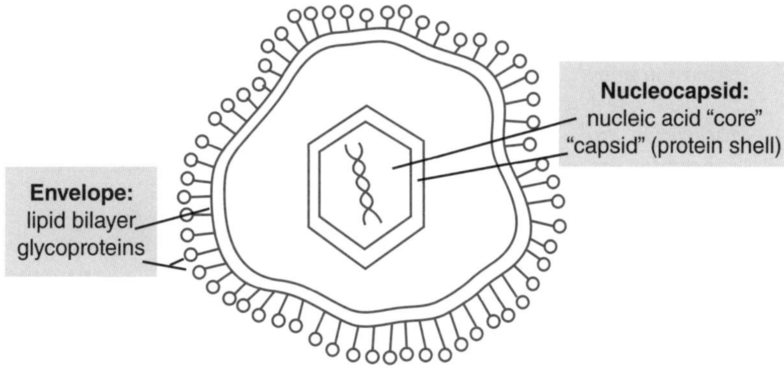

Figure ■ 34-1
Basic components of a virus. Note the relative lack of most cellular organelles (ribosomes, endoplasmic reticulum, etc.).

specific steps in the viral replication process are presented next.

Viral Replication

Self-replication of a virus occurs in several distinct steps:[1,3] adsorption, penetration and uncoating, biosynthesis, and maturation and release (Fig. 34-2).

Adsorption. Initially, the virus attaches or adsorbs to the surface of the host cell. Most viruses are attracted to the host cell because of the interaction between proteins on the outer surface of the virus and receptorlike proteins on the host-cell membrane. The interaction of the virus with these surface proteins causes the virus to adhere to the outer surface of the host-cell membrane.

Penetration and uncoating. The virus enters the host cell either by passing directly through the cell membrane or by fusing with the host-cell membrane and releasing the viral genetic material into the host cell. Once inside the host cell, its proteolytic enzymes usually remove any coating that remains on the virus.

Biosynthesis. When viral genetic material is released within the host cell, the virus takes control of the cell's molecular synthesizing machinery to initiate the biosynthesis of new viral enzymes and proteins. Different viruses exert their effects on the host cell in different ways, but many viruses control the host cell through a direct effect on the cell's nucleus. Some viruses, including the virus that causes AIDS, actually insert their genetic material directly into the host cell's DNA, thereby becoming integrated within the genetic control of the infected cell.

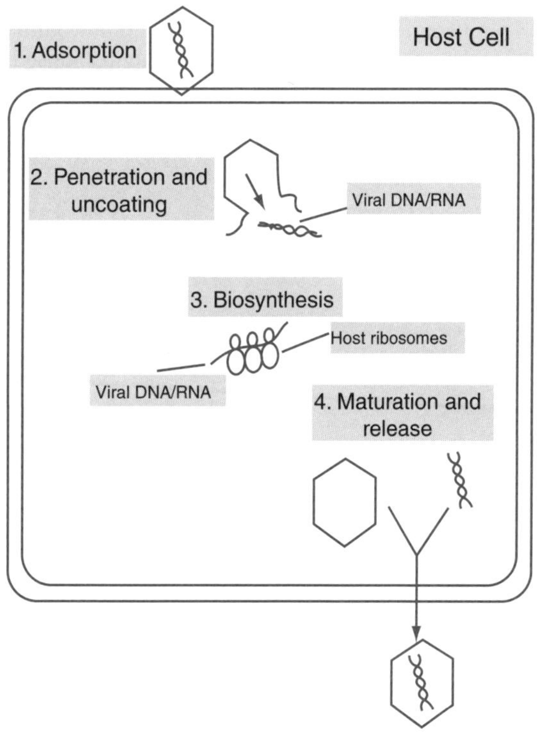

Figure ■ 34-2
Basic sequence of viral replication.

Regardless of the exact mechanism of infection, the virus essentially commands the cell to synthesize the enzymes that produce more copies of viral DNA or RNA and to synthesize structural proteins that will ultimately form new viral shells or capsids. Thus, the virus uses the biosynthetic machinery as well as the structural components and nutrients of the cell (amino acids, nucleic acids, etc.) to replicate itself. In addition, the virus often incapacitates the infected cell so that the infected cell cannot carry out its normal physiological activities.

Maturation and release. The component parts of the virus (the genetic core and surrounding shell) are assembled into mature viruses and released from the host cell. In some cases, the virus is released by a process of exocytosis, leaving the host cell relatively intact (although still infected with the original virus). Alternatively, the host cell may simply be destroyed (undergo lysis), thus releasing the viral offspring. Lysis of the host cell results in the release of the virus and the death of the cell and may stimulate the production of inflammatory mediators (prostaglandins, kinins, etc.), which create a hypersensitivity response.

The steps involved in viral replication are important pharmacologically because antiviral drugs may interrupt this process at one or more of the steps. The specific agents currently used as antiviral drugs and their pharmacodynamic aspects are discussed next.

SPECIFIC ANTIVIRAL DRUGS

As indicated earlier, there are a relatively limited number of FDA-approved drugs that can act selectively as antiviral agents (Tables 34-2 and 34-3). This section briefly discusses the antiviral efficacy, clinical use, mechanism of action, and adverse effects of these agents.

Table 34-2
ANTIVIRAL DRUGS*

Generic Name	Trade Name(s)	Principal Indication(s)
Acyclovir	Zovirax	Treatment of initial and recurrent herpesvirus infections (especially herpes simplex–related infections)
Adefovir	Hepsera	Chronic hepatitis B infections
Amantadine	Symadine, Symmetrel	Prevention and treatment of influenza A infections (also used as an antiparkinsonism drug; see Chapter 10)
Cidofovir	Vistide	Treatment of cytomegalovirus (CMV) retinitis in immunocompromised patients
Docosanol	Abreva	Topical treatment of recurrent herpes simplex infections (cold sores)
Entecavir	Baraclude	Chronic hepatitis B infection
Famciclovir	Famvir	Treatment and suppression of herpesvirus infections, including herpes simplex (genital herpes) and herpes zoster (shingles)
Foscarnet	Foscavir	Treatment of CMV infections in immunocompromised patients
Ganciclovir	Cytovene	Treatment of CMV retinitis in immunocompromised patients; also used to prevent CMV infection after organ transplants
Imiquimod	Aldara	Topical treatment for warts caused by condylomata acuminate
Oseltamivir	Tamiflu	Prevention and treatment of influenza A and B infections
Palivizumab	Synagis	Prevention of respiratory tract disease in children and premature infants at high risk for respiratory syncytial virus (RSV) infection
Penciclovir	Denavir	Topical treatment of recurrent herpes simplex infections (cold sores)
Ribavirin	Virazole	Treatment of severe viral pneumonia caused by respiratory syncytial virus in infants and young children
Rimantadine	Flumadine	Prevention and treatment of influenza A infections
Telbivudine	Tyzeka	Chronic hepatitis B infection
Trifluridine	Viroptic	Local (ophthalmic) administration for treatment of herpes simplex keratitis and keratoconjunctivitis

Table 34-2
ANTIVIRAL DRUGS*—cont'd

Generic Name	Trade Name(s)	Principal Indication(s)
Valacyclovir	Valtrex	Treatment of initial and recurrent herpesvirus infections, including herpes simplex (genital herpes) and herpes zoster (shingles)
Valganciclovir	Valcyte	Treatment of cytomegalovirus (CMV) retinitis in immunocompromised patients; also used to prevent CMV infection after organ transplants
Zanamivir	Relenza	Prevention and treatment of influenza A and B infections

**Antivirals in this table are targeted for infections other than HIV. Drugs used to treat HIV infection are listed in Table 34-3.*

Acyclovir and Valacyclovir

Acyclovir (Zovirax) and its precursor (prodrug) valacyclovir are effective against herpesvirus infections, especially those involving herpes simplex types I and II.[4-6] Acyclovir is one of the principal drugs used to treat genital herpes and herpes simplex–related infections in other mucosal and cutaneous areas (lips and face).[7-9] Acyclovir is also effective against other members of the herpesvirus family, including the varicella-zoster and Epstein-Barr virus.[5,10] This agent may be useful for treating varicella-zoster–related infections such as herpes zoster and chickenpox. Epstein-Barr virus infections, including infectious mononucleosis, may also respond to acyclovir. Acyclovir is available as a topical cream to treat cutaneous and mucosal infections. The drug can also be administered systemically, either orally or intravenously in severe, acute infections.

Valacyclovir (Valtrex) is the precursor or "prodrug" of acyclovir.[5,11] When administered orally, valacyclovir is converted to acyclovir in the intestinal tract and liver. This conversion typically results in the eventual appearance of higher levels of acyclovir in the bloodstream, because valacyclovir is absorbed more readily from the gastrointestinal (GI) tract than acyclovir.[12] Thus, oral administration of valacyclovir is a more effective way to achieve the therapeutic effects of acyclovir.[13]

Mechanism of Action

Acyclovir is taken into virus-infected cells and converted to acyclovir triphosphate by an enzyme known as *viral thymidine kinase*.[14] The activated (phosphorylated) drug directly inhibits the function of the viral DNA polymerase enzyme, thus impairing the replication of viral genetic material. The virus also incorporates the drug into viral DNA strands, which halts further production of DNA because of the presence of a false nucleic acid.[15]

The antiviral specificity of acyclovir is due to the drug's higher affinity for viral DNA polymerase rather than the analogous enzyme in human cells.[15] Also, the first step in the phosphorylation of acyclovir is greatly accelerated in virus-infected cells versus healthy cells. Hence, the amount of the phosphorylated form of acyclovir is much greater in the cells that really need it—that is, cells infected with the virus.

Adverse Effects

Topical application of acyclovir may produce local irritation of cutaneous and mucosal tissues. Prolonged systemic administration of acyclovir or valacyclovir may cause headaches, dizziness, skin rashes, and GI problems (e.g., nausea, vomiting, diarrhea).

Amantadine and Rimantadine

Amantadine (Symmetrel) and rimantadine (Flumadine) are used in the prevention and treatment of infections caused by the influenza A virus.[16] When administered prophylactically, they appear to be approximately 70 to 90 percent effective in preventing influenza A infections.[17] These drugs are therefore given to individuals who may have been exposed to influenza A and to high-risk patients, such as the elderly or those with cardiopulmonary problems and other diseases. As discussed in Chapter 10, amantadine is also effective in alleviating some of the motor abnormalities of Parkinson disease. As an anti-Parkinson drug, amantadine may block the effects of excitatory neurotransmitters in the basal ganglia, thus exerting effects that are quite different from its antiviral effects. These drugs are typically administered orally, either in capsule form or in a syrup preparation.

Table 34-3
AGENTS USED TO INHIBIT HIV REPLICATION

Generic Name	Trade Name(s)
Nucleoside Reverse Transcriptase Inhibitors (NRTIs)	
Abacavir	Ziagen
Didanosine	Videx
Emtricitabine	Emtriva
Lamivudine	Epivir
Stavudine	Zerit
Tenofovir	Viread
Zidovudine	Retrovir
Nonnucleoside Reverse Transcriptase Inhibitors (NNRTIs)	
Delavirdine	Rescriptor
Efavirenz	Sustiva
Etravirine	Intelence
Nevirapine	Viramune
Protease Inhibitors	
Amprenavir	Agenerase
Atazanavir	Reyataz
Darunavir	Prezista
Fosamprenavir	Lexiva
Indinavir	Crixivan
Lopinavir	Kaletra*
Nelfinavir	Viracept
Ritonavir	Norvir
Saquinavir	Fortovase, Invirase
Tipranavir	Aptivus
HIV Entry Inhibitors	
Enfuvirtide	Fuzeon
Maraviroc	Selzentry
Integrase Inhibitors	
Dolutegravir	Tivicay
Elvitegravir	Stribild**
Raltegravir	Isentress

**Trade name for a combination of lopinavir and low-dose ritonavir.*

***Trade name for a combination of elvitegravir with cobicistat, emtricitabine, tenofovir*

Amantadine and rimantadine are also administered to individuals already infected with influenza A to lessen the effects of this infection; these drugs usually decrease the severity and duration of flu symptoms if drug therapy is initiated when symptoms first appear.[17] However, certain strains of influenza have developed resistance to these drugs; hence, their clinical usefulness in treating active influenza infections has declined somewhat in recent years.[17,18]

Mechanism of Action

Amantadine and rimantadine block an ion channel (the M2 protein) on the surface of the influenza virus.[19,20] This action inhibits one of the first steps of viral replication by impairing the ability of the virus to shed its capsid and release viral nucleic acid within the host cell. These drugs may also interfere with the assembly of viral components, thus inhibiting one of the final steps in the replication process.[17] This dual inhibitory effect on the early and late steps of viral replication accounts for the drugs' antiviral effectiveness.

Adverse Effects

Amantadine and rimantadine may produce central nervous system (CNS) symptoms such as confusion, loss of concentration, mood changes, nervousness, dizziness, and light-headedness. These symptoms may be especially problematic in elderly patients. Excessive doses of amantadine and rimantadine may increase the severity of these CNS symptoms, and overdose may cause seizures.

Cidofovir

Cidofovir (Vistide) is used primarily to treat cytomegalovirus (CMV) retinitis in people with AIDS.[21,22] When used clinically, the drug is often combined with probenecid, an agent that inhibits renal excretion of cidofovir, thereby providing higher plasma levels of this antiviral agent.[23] Cidofovir may also be helpful in other types of CMV infections, but use is somewhat limited because of renal toxicity and other toxic side effects (see below).

Mechanism of Action

Cidofovir works like acyclovir and ganciclovir; these drugs inhibit viral DNA replication by inhibiting DNA polymerase activity and by halting elongation of viral DNA chains.[24]

Adverse Effects

Cidofovir may cause nephrotoxicity, especially at higher doses. This drug may also decrease the number of neutrophilic leukocytes, resulting in neutropenia and related symptoms such as fever, chills, and sore throat. Other side effects include headache and GI disturbances (e.g., anorexia, nausea, diarrhea).

Docosanol

Docosanol (Abreva) is applied topically to treat recurrent outbreaks of orofacial herpes lesions caused by herpes virus simplex.[25] This drug is available as an over-the-counter product.

Mechanism of Action

Docosanol does not inactivate the herpes virus but appears to act on the host (human) cells so that the virus cannot adsorb to the surface of the cell. As such, it must be applied early in the course of outbreaks before the virus has a chance to cause substantial lesions.

Adverse Effects

Patients using topical docosanol may experience headache and some local skin irritation.

Dolutegravir, Elvitegravir, and Raltegravir

Pharmacologists developed dolutegravir (Tivicay) and raltegravir (Isentress) to treat HIV infection.[26] These drugs are typically used as an adjunct to other anti-HIV drugs, especially when more conventional agents have failed to adequately prevent viral replication.[27] The FDA also approved a third agent in this category—elvitegravir—as part of a multi-ingredient product for treating HIV infection. Elvitegravir is combined in the same pill with other antivirals (cobicistat, emtricitabine, tenofovir) and marketed under the trade name Stribild.[28] Dolutegravir, raltegravir, and elvitegravir target an enzyme known as *HIV integrase* (see below); hence, these drugs are often referred to as *integrase inhibitors*. The use of these drugs in the comprehensive treatment of HIV infection is addressed in more detail in the "Inhibition of HIV Proliferation in Infected Individuals" section.

Mechanism of Action

As indicated, dolutegravir, elvitegravir, and raltegravir inhibit the HIV integrase enzyme.[26] This enzyme is required for HIV to splice its viral DNA into the host cell (human) chromosome. If this enzyme is inhibited, HIV cannot integrate its genetic code into the host cell DNA and cannot command the host cell to synthesize new viral components.

Adverse Effects

The most common side effects of integrase inhibitors include headache, fever, and GI problems (e.g., nausea, vomiting, abdominal pain). Other problems such as myopathy, lipodystrophy, blood dyscrasias (e.g., anemia, neutropenia), and immune system disorders have been reported, but serious adverse effects are relatively rare with these drugs.

Enfuvirtide and Maraviroc

Enfuvirtide (Fuzeon) is the first approved drug that limits the ability of HIV to enter host cells.[29,30] Enfuvirtide is typically added to other agents (**reverse transcriptase** inhibitors, **protease** inhibitors) in patients who do not respond adequately to traditional anti-HIV treatment. This drug is effective against HIV type 1 but not against HIV type 2 (types of HIV are addressed in "HIV and the Treatment of AIDS").[31]

Enfuvirtide must be administered parenterally by subcutaneous injection, and it is associated with frequent and potentially serious side effects (see below). Likewise, some strains of HIV-1 have developed resistance to this drug through binding site mutations that render the drug ineffective.[31] Hence, pharmacologists developed other HIV entry inhibitors such as maraviroc (Selzentry; see later). Researchers are continuing their investigations to create new entry inhibitors that act in different ways to impair HIV entry into human cells.[30]

Mechanism of Action

As indicated, enfuvirtide and maraviroc inhibit the ability of HIV to bind to and enter susceptible host cells such as CD4 lymphocytes. These drugs actually bind to specific components on the outer glycoprotein envelope of the virus, thereby retarding the ability of the virus to change its shape in preparation for adsorbing to the surface of the host cell. If the virus cannot attach to host cells, the risk of infection is reduced.

Adverse Effects

Enfuvirtide must be administered by subcutaneous injection, and local pain and irritation occurs at the injection site in most patients. Other common side effects include GI distress (e.g., nausea, diarrhea, loss of appetite) and immune complex reactions that can cause an allergic response and possibly lead to other infections (e.g., pneumonia, herpes simplex). Maraviroc, which is administered orally, can sometimes cause allergic reactions and hepatotoxicity, but serious adverse reactions seem to be fairly rare.

Famciclovir and Penciclovir

Penciclovir (Denavir) is similar to acyclovir in terms of its antiviral effects and clinical indications. However, penciclovir is absorbed poorly from the GI tract. This drug is primarily administered topically to treat recurrent herpes simplex infections of the lips and face (cold sores).[32]

Famciclovir (Famvir) is the precursor (prodrug) to penciclovir; the drug is converted to penciclovir following oral administration.[33] This situation is analogous to the relationship between acyclovir and valacyclovir, where it is advantageous to administer the prodrug because it will be absorbed more completely and will ultimately result in higher plasma levels of the drug's active form. Hence, famciclovir is administered orally to treat infections related to herpes simplex (e.g., genital herpes) and varicella zoster (e.g., herpes zoster).[33,34] However, the actual antiviral effects of famciclovir occur because this drug is converted to penciclovir within the body.

Mechanism of Action

Penciclovir acts like acyclovir—that is, the drug is activated (phosphorylated) within virus-infected cells, where it subsequently inhibits viral DNA synthesis and viral replication. As indicated, famciclovir exerts its antiviral effects after being converted to penciclovir in vivo.

Adverse Effects

Topical application of penciclovir may cause some skin reactions (e.g., rashes, irritation) at the application site, but the incidence of these reactions is fairly low. Systemic (oral) administration of famciclovir is generally well tolerated, with only minor side effects such as headache, dizziness, and GI disturbances (e.g., nausea, diarrhea).

Foscarnet

Foscarnet (Foscavir) is primarily given to treat CMV retinitis in patients with AIDS.[22,35,36] This agent may also help control other infections in patients with a compromised immune system, including serious CMV infections (e.g., pneumonia, GI infections) and some herpesvirus infections (e.g., herpes simplex, varicella-zoster).

Mechanism of Action

Foscarnet works somewhat like acyclovir and ganciclovir—that is, it inhibits the DNA polymerase enzyme necessary for viral DNA replication. Foscarnet differs from these other antiviral drugs, however, in that it does not require phosphorylation (activation) by enzymes such as viral thymidine kinase. Certain strains of viruses are thymidine-kinase deficient, meaning that they lack the enzyme needed to activate antiviral agents such as acyclovir and ganciclovir. Hence, patients with these particular viruses who do not respond to acyclovir or ganciclovir often use foscarnet.

Adverse Effects

The primary problem associated with foscarnet is impaired renal function, including acute tubular necrosis. Hematological disorders (e.g., anemia, granulocytopenia, leukopenia), GI disturbances (e.g., cramps, nausea, vomiting), and CNS toxicity (e.g., confusion, dizziness, seizures) may also occur during foscarnet treatment.

Ganciclovir and Valganciclovir

Ganciclovir (Cytovene, Vitrasert) is given primarily to patients with AIDS to treat problems related to CMV infection, including CMV retinitis, polyradiculopathy, and other systemic CMV infections.[21,36,37] Valganciclovir (Valcyte) is the precursor (prodrug) form that is converted to ganciclovir within the body. Ganciclovir and similar agents (acyclovir and valacyclovir; see earlier) can also help reduce the risk of CMV infection in people receiving solid organ transplants such as kidney transplants.[38]

Mechanism of Action

Ganciclovir, like acyclovir, inhibits viral DNA replication by inhibiting DNA polymerase activity and by halting elongation of viral DNA chains.

Adverse Effects

The most serious problems associated with ganciclovir include anemia, granulocytopenia, thrombocytopenia, and related hematologic disorders. Ganciclovir may also cause GI disturbances (e.g., nausea, loss of appetite) and CNS disturbances (e.g., mood changes, nervousness, tremor, seizures).

Imiquimod

Imiquimod (Aldara) is applied topically to treat condylomata acuminate infections that cause genital and perianal warts.[39,40] It is also beneficial for treating certain skin conditions, such as actinic keratoses of the face and scalp and in certain cases of superficial basal cell carcinoma.

Mechanism of Action

Although the details are unclear, imiquimod enhances the local production of interferons, tumor necrosis factor-alpha, and possibly other cytokines that produce antiviral responses. Hence, this drug does not act directly on the virus but instead modulates the host (human) immune responses that have antiviral effects.

Adverse Effects

Some local skin irritation and blistering can occur when imiquimod is applied topically.

Trifluridine

Trifluridine (Viroptic) is administered with eyedrops to treat local eye infections associated with herpes simplex virus—that is, herpes virus–related keratitis and keratoconjunctivitis.[41]

Mechanism of Action

This drug impairs viral DNA synthesis by inhibiting the enzymes that incorporate a specific nucleotide (thymidine) into viral DNA. The drug also substitutes itself for thymidine in the viral DNA sequence, thus creating a false DNA code that is ineffective in promoting viral replication.

Adverse Effects

Some local redness and irritation of the eye may develop during local/topical application of trifluridine, but serious adverse effects are rare.

Oseltamivir and Zanamivir

Oseltamivir (Tamiflu) and Zanamivir (Relenza) are effective against influenza virus types A and B. These drugs can reduce the duration and severity of flu symptoms if the drug is administered within 48 hours after symptoms first appear.[42,43] These drugs can also be taken prophylactically to reduce the risk of getting the flu, especially in people who are at high risk (older adults, people with respiratory disorders) or in cases where an individual is exposed to a family member or someone else with the flu.[44]

Mechanism of Action

Oseltamivir and zanamivir inhibit a specific enzyme (neuraminidase) that the influenza virus uses to complete its biosynthesis and release. By inhibiting this enzyme, these drugs impair a key step in viral replication and reduce the ability of the virus to infect other respiratory cells.

Adverse Effects

Oral administration of oseltamivir can cause GI disturbances (e.g., nausea, vomiting) and CNS problems such as confusion, agitation, delirium, and seizures. Zanamivir can cause similar CNS problems and is also associated with bronchospasm and reduced opening of the airway. Zanamivir is administered by inhalation. The adverse effects on the airway can be quite severe in people with bronchoconstrictive disease (e.g., asthma, chronic obstructive pulmonary disease), so the drug should probably be avoided in these individuals.

Protease Inhibitors

These drugs inhibit an enzyme known as *HIV protease*. This enzyme is needed to manufacture specific HIV proteins, including enzymes such as the HIV reverse transcriptase enzyme and structural proteins that comprise the HIV molecule.[45,46] By inhibiting this enzyme, protease inhibitors prevent the synthesis and maturation of HIV, thus helping to prevent HIV replication and progression of HIV-related disease.[46] The protease inhibitors currently available include atazanavir (Reyataz), fosamprenavir (Lexiva), indinavir (Crixivan), lopinavir (Kaletra; the trade name for lopinavir combined with ritonavir), nelfinavir (Viracept), ritonavir (Norvir), saquinavir (Fortovase, Invirase), and tipranavir (Aptivus) (see Table 34-3).

Physicians often incorporate protease inhibitors into the comprehensive treatment of people with HIV infection (see "HIV and the Treatment of AIDS").

In addition, a specific protease inhibitor can be combined with a low dose of ritonavir—a process known as *protease-inhibitor boosting*.[47,48] Ritonavir inhibits the hepatic breakdown of the other (primary) protease drug, thereby allowing the primary drug to exert better therapeutic effects at a lower dose.[48]

Mechanism of Action

Protease inhibitors bind to the HIV protease and prevent this enzyme from acting on HIV substrates.[49] This effect negates the ability of the protease enzyme to cleave polypeptide precursors from larger, polypeptide chains.[50] If these precursors are not available for the manufacture of HIV proteins, the virus cannot fully develop.[50] Treatment with protease inhibitors therefore results in the manufacture of incomplete and noninfectious fragments of HIV rather than the mature virus.[46]

Adverse Effects

Protease inhibitors may cause alterations in fat deposition in the body (lipodystrophy)—fat deposits atrophy in the limbs, but excess fat is deposited in the abdomen.[51,52] Blood lipids may also be adversely affected, resulting in increased plasma cholesterol, increased triglycerides, and decreased high-density lipoproteins.[53] Protease inhibitors may also cause other metabolic disturbances, including insulin resistance.[51,54] These drug-induced problems create a metabolic syndrome that can increase the patient's risk of cardiovascular disease.[55,56] The extent of these metabolic problems depends on several factors, including the specific protease inhibitor, other anti-HIV medications that are also being administered, and the characteristics of each patient.[57] Other side effects include diarrhea, headache, and fatigue.[50]

Reverse Transcriptase Inhibitors

Reverse transcriptase inhibitors (RTIs) are used to inhibit the replication and proliferation of HIV type I (HIV-1). These agents act on a specific enzyme (HIV reverse transcriptase) and inhibit a key step in HIV replication.[58,59] Although RTIs do not eliminate the virus from infected cells, they are often effective in reducing HIV proliferation and the spread of HIV to noninfected cells.[50] These drugs are therefore beneficial in preventing or delaying the progression of HIV and AIDS. The use of RTIs in treating HIV infection is discussed in more detail later in this chapter.

Zidovudine (Retrovir), also known generically as *azidothymidine* or *AZT*, was the first RTI approved for treating people infected with HIV.[59] The FDA has subsequently approved other zidovudine-like drugs; currently available agents include abacavir (Ziagen), didanosine (Videx), emtricitabine (Emtriva), lamivudine (Epivir), stavudine (Zerit), and tenofovir (Viread).[49] These RTIs can also be subclassified as nucleoside reverse transcriptase inhibitors (NRTIs) because they share a common chemical background (see Table 34-3).

More recently, pharmacologists have developed RTIs that are chemically distinct from zidovudine and other NRTIs (see Table 34-3). These agents are known as *nonnucleoside reverse transcriptase inhibitors* (NNRTIs) and include drugs such as delavirdine (Rescriptor), efavirenz (Sustiva), etravirine (Intelence), and nevirapine (Viramune).[49,60] These drugs also inhibit the reverse transcriptase enzyme but act at a different site on the enzyme than do their NRTI counterparts.

Therefore, several types of RTIs are available that can help prevent HIV replication and inhibit the proliferation and spread of the virus to noninfected cells. Although these drugs do not kill HIV, RTIs are the cornerstone of treatment for preventing the progression of HIV disease.[61] Use of the various RTIs in combination with each other and with other anti-HIV drugs is discussed in more detail in "HIV and the Treatment of AIDS," later in this chapter.

Mechanism of Action

RTIs impair HIV replication by inhibiting the reverse transcriptase enzyme that is needed to convert viral RNA to viral DNA (Fig. 34-3). Zidovudine and the other NRTIs enter viral-infected cells, where they are progressively phosphorylated (activated) by various intracellular enzymes.[50,62] The phosphorylated version of the drug then acts as a false nucleic acid, competing with the real nucleic acid (thymidine) for incorporation into growing viral DNA strands. This competition slows down the reverse transcriptase enzyme because the enzyme cannot handle the false nucleic acid (the drug) as easily as the real nucleic acid (thymidine). Even if the reverse transcriptase is successful in incorporating the drug into viral DNA strands, this action prematurely terminates DNA strand synthesis because a false nucleic acid has been added to the viral DNA instead of the real nucleic acid.

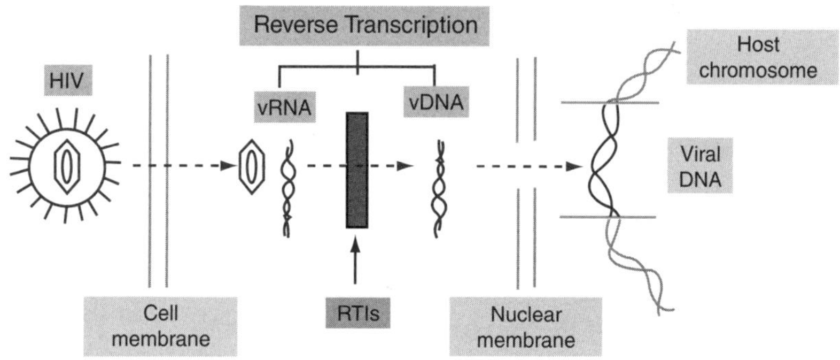

Figure ■ 34-3
Schematic illustration of HIV replication and the site of action of the reverse transcriptase inhibitors (RTIs). These drugs interfere with the process of reverse transcription by inhibiting the enzyme that converts viral RNA (vRNA) to viral DNA (vDNA).

The nonnucleoside RTIs such as delavirdine directly inhibit the reverse transcriptase enzyme by binding to the enzyme's active (catalytic) site and preventing this enzyme from converting viral RNA to viral DNA.[58,63] Thus, these agents offer an alternative way to impair reverse transcriptase function and prevent viral replication.

Adverse Effects

RTIs are associated with several bothersome side effects, and certain agents can also cause potentially serious problems. The most common problems associated with zidovudine are blood dyscrasias, such as anemia and granulocytopenia. Other symptoms may include fever, chills, nausea, diarrhea, dizziness, headache, and excessive fatigue. NRTI drugs may also cause myopathy, as indicated by skeletal muscle tenderness, weakness, and atrophy.[64] Likewise, peripheral neuropathies, liver dysfunction, and lactic acidosis may also occur, especially when NRTIs such as abacavir, didanosine, stavudine, and tenofovir are administered in higher doses.[65,66] These adverse neuromuscular and metabolic effects are probably due to the toxic effects of these drugs on mitochondrial function in various tissues.[66] However, considering that these drugs are often used in severely immunocompromised patients (such as patients with AIDS), adverse neuromuscular effects may be also be caused by other sequelae of AIDS in addition to the drug's effects. Hence, neuromuscular problems are seen frequently in patients with advanced cases of HIV infection and AIDS.

Other effects associated with NRTIs include pancreatitis, CNS toxicity (e.g., headache, irritability, insomnia), and GI disturbances (e.g., nausea, diarrhea). Abacavir can cause an allergic (hypersensitivity) reaction in genetically susceptible people, as indicated by symptoms such as fever, joint and muscle pain, skin rashes, abdominal pain, nausea, diarrhea, and vomiting.[67] In severe cases, this allergic reaction can progress to anaphylactic shock and possibly death.

Skin rashes are the most common side effect of the NNRTIs, and some agents such as efavirenz and etravirine may cause nervous system symptoms such as headache, dizziness, confusion, and insomnia.[65]

Ribavirin

Ribavirin (Virazole, others) is active against several RNA and DNA viruses, including respiratory syncytial virus (RSV).[68] Clinically, this drug is effective for treating severe RSV pneumonia in infants and young children[69] and RSV in certain adult populations, including the elderly, people with cardiopulmonary problems, and people with a compromised immune system.[68,70] Ribavirin may also be useful as a secondary agent in the treatment of influenza A and B in young adults. The combination of ribavirin and interferons (see "Interferons," later) is often the treatment of choice in chronic hepatitis C infection.[71,72]

For the treatment of RSV, ribavirin is typically administered through inhalation; this drug is suspended in an aerosol form and administered to the patient by a mechanical aerosol generator and a ventilation mask, mouthpiece, or hood. Ribavirin can also be administered orally to treat hepatitis or influenza.

Mechanism of Action

The mechanism of action of this drug is not fully understood. Ribavirin appears to impair viral messenger RNA (mRNA) synthesis, probably by selectively inhibiting enzymes responsible for RNA replication.[17]

Inadequate viral mRNA production leads to impaired viral protein synthesis, which ultimately curtails viral replication.

Adverse Effects

Ribavirin produces relatively few adverse effects when administered by inhalation. Most of the drug's action is confined to local pulmonary tissues, and severe systemic effects are rare. One adverse effect that may occur is local irritation of the eyes (conjunctivitis), due to the direct contact of aerosol with the eyes. This occurrence may be a problem if the drug is administered via some sort of hood or tent that encloses the patient's entire head. Systemic administration can cause breakdown of red blood cells (hemolytic anemia), but this effect is usually reversed when the drug is discontinued or a lower dose is administered.

VIRAL RESISTANCE

As discussed in the last chapter, certain bacteria can develop strategies that render them resistant to drug therapy. This is true for other microorganisms, including most types of virus. Viruses can mutate and alter their structural or functional characteristics so that previously effective drugs will be unable to control specific viral infections adequately. It is beyond the scope of this chapter to address all the resistant viral strains and how these strains acquired resistance against antiviral drugs. Viral resistance, like bacterial resistance, is a growing concern. Efforts should be made to limit the indiscriminate or inappropriate use of antiviral drugs and to contain the spread of resistant viruses. Developing methods to overcome viral resistance using new drugs or different drug combinations is also a critical area of laboratory and clinical research.

INTERFERONS

Interferons are a group of proteins that produce several beneficial pharmacological and physiological effects.[73-75] These agents were first recognized as endogenous substances that exert nonspecific antiviral activity—that is, interferons are synthesized as part of the immune response to viral infection, and these substances enable healthy cells to resist infection from a wide array of viruses.[76,77] Interferons produce other beneficial effects, including the control of cell differentiation, the limiting of excessive cell proliferation, and the modification of certain immune processes.[78,79]

Interferons are grouped into three major classes, depending on their structure and how they affect receptors on specific cells.[73] These classes are commonly identified as type I interferons (which contain the alpha and beta interferons), type II (gamma) interferons, and type III (lambda) interferons. Each major type can also be subclassified into specific agents, such as interferon alpha-2a, interferon gamma-1b, and so forth. All three major types of interferons share the ability to control viral infections to some extent, but certain interferons seem more effective when controlling certain viral infections. Specific types of interferons and their pharmacological indications are summarized in Table 34-4.

The potential role of interferons as therapeutic drugs has generated considerable interest in the field of pharmacology. By using recombinant DNA techniques and cell tissue cultures, specific interferons can be synthesized to treat viral diseases and other problems. The rationale is that exogenously administered interferons will produce antiviral and other beneficial effects in a manner similar to their endogenously produced counterparts. Some of the pertinent aspects of interferon action and clinical applications are presented below.

Synthesis and Cellular Effects of Interferons

Virtually all of the body's cells are capable of producing interferons, and these substances serve as an early step in preventing the virus from infecting healthy cells.[80,81] The basic sequence of events in the cellular production and antiviral action of interferons is illustrated in Figure 34-4. Cells that have been infected by a virus produce interferons that are subsequently released from the infected cell. These interferons then travel to noninfected cells, where they bind to specific receptors located on the surface of the healthy cells. Binding of the interferon then activates signaling pathways in the healthy cell to manufacture antiviral proteins. In particular, the healthy cell is directed to synthesize enzymes that inhibit viral mRNA and protein synthesis.[82,83] Thus, even if the virus does penetrate into the healthy cell, it cannot replicate because of an inability to synthesize viral proteins.

The manner in which interferons control cell growth and proliferation is not fully understood.

Table 34-4
TYPES OF INTERFERONS

Type and Subtype	Specific Agents*	Primary Indications
Type I		
Alpha	Alphacon-1 (Infergen)	Chronic hepatitis C
	Peginterferon alfa 2-a (Pegasys)	Chronic hepatitis B and C
	Alfa-2b (Intron A)	Hairy cell leukemia; Kaposi sarcoma (AIDS related); chronic hepatitis B and C; condyloma acuminatum; malignant melanoma
	Peginterferon alfa 2-b (Pegintron)	Chronic hepatitis C
	Alfa-n3 (Alferon N)	Condyloma acuminatum
Beta	Beta-1A (Avonex, Rebif)	Multiple sclerosis
	Beta-1B (Betaseron, Extavia)	Multiple sclerosis
Type II		
Gamma	Gamma-1b (Actimmune)	Chronic granulomatous disease; osteopetrosis

**Specific agents are synthesized using recombinant DNA or other biosynthetic techniques to mimic the effects of naturally occurring type I or type II interferons. Agents that mimic type III (lambda) interferons are still in development.*

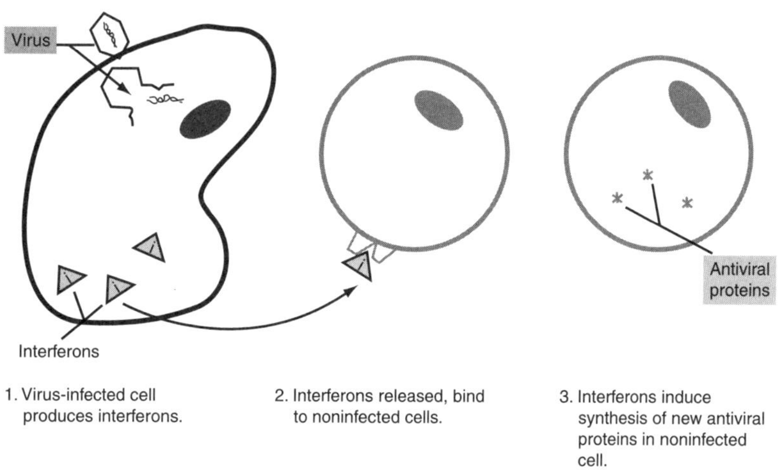

Figure ■ 34-4
Antiviral effects of interferons.

Interferons may limit excessive cell division by controlling specific gene segments in normal and cancerous cells.[79,84] In particular, interferons may activate signaling pathways that promote the synthesis of proteins that limit abnormal cell proliferation and encourage programmed cell death (apoptosis) in cancerous and precancerous tissues.[85] Interferons may also limit cancer growth by activating certain aspects of the immune system, including increased activity of natural killer cells and other cytotoxic cells that attack cancerous tissues.[79,84] Hence, interferons have proved effective in controlling several forms of cancer (see Table 34-4). The use of these agents as anticancer drugs is discussed in more detail in Chapter 36.

Pharmacological Applications of Interferons

When interferons were first discovered, there was a great deal of optimism about their use as antiviral agents. Although early clinical trials with interferons were somewhat disappointing, their use as antiviral agents gained acceptance as more was learned about the three primary types and subtypes of interferons.

We now realize that interferons cannot be used interchangeably as antiviral drugs but that certain types of interferons can be administered to treat specific viruses (see Table 34-4). For example, type I (alpha) interferons have been instrumental in the treatment of chronic hepatitis B and C infections.[73,86] That is, standard treatment of hepatitis C typically consists of alpha interferons combined with other antivirals such as ribavirin, boceprevir, and telaprevir.[87] However, preliminary studies suggest that type III (lambda) interferons may be also be effective in hepatitis infections and could serve as an alternative for patients who fail to respond to type I interferons.[88] Specific alpha interferons can also be injected locally to treat certain forms of viral-induced warts such as condylomata acuminate infections (see Table 34-4). The clinical use of interferons as antiviral drugs should continue to increase as more is learned about various interferons and other factors influencing their effectiveness.[89]

As mentioned, interferons also help control abnormal cell proliferation, and these drugs are approved for use in certain cancers. Interferons are often part of the treatment for specific leukemias, lymphomas, and several other forms of cancer (see Table 34-4). Interferon use in cancer chemotherapy is discussed in more detail in Chapter 36.

Finally, certain interferons may decrease exacerbations of multiple sclerosis (MS).[90,91] Specifically, interferon beta-1a (Avonex, Rebif) and interferon beta-1b (Betaseron) may help reduce the incidence and severity of relapses in exacerbating-remitting MS.[73,92] This effect seems to occur because these beta interferons modulate several aspects of the autoimmune response that initiates the pathological changes associated with MS.[93] Although the details are unclear, it appears that type I interferons can reduce the activity of macrophages, lymphocytes, and other immune system components that are responsible for the autoimmune destruction of glial cells and neuronal structures in patients with MS.

Adverse Effects of Interferons

Interferons may cause flulike symptoms, including fever, sweating, chills, muscle aches, and general malaise. Other side effects such as loss of appetite, nausea, vomiting, diarrhea, and unusual tiredness can also occur, depending on the type of interferon and the dosage. Interferons may also cause behavioral side effects such as depression, presumably because these drugs inhibit serotonin activity in the brain.[94,95] When interferons are administered by intramuscular or subcutaneous injection, some irritation may develop around the injection site. Finally, the immune system may produce anti-interferon antibodies, especially when interferons are administered for prolonged periods.[96] These antibodies can neutralize the interferons, thus decreasing their effectiveness in controlling viral infections and other conditions such as cancer and MS.

CONTROL OF VIRAL INFECTION WITH VACCINES

Vaccines can be administered to healthy individuals to provide them with immunity from certain viral infections. The vaccines prevent viral infection by stimulating the endogenous production of immune factors that will selectively destroy the invading virus. A vaccine acts as an antigen that induces the immune system to generate virus-specific antibodies. The vaccine, however, does not cause any appreciable viral infection because it contains a virus that has been modified in some way so that it retains its antigenic properties but lacks the ability to produce infection. For example, vaccines typically consist of a whole virus or part of the virus (viral particle or fragment) that has been completely inactivated (killed vaccines) or partially inactivated (live attenuated vaccines).[97] Thus, most antiviral vaccinations are accomplished by administering small amounts of the modified virus.

In general, it is somewhat easier to develop vaccines that prevent viral infection than to develop drugs that destroy the virus once it has infected human cells. This notion is reasonable when one considers that the virus is essentially coexisting with the host cell. As indicated previously, there are currently only a limited number of drugs that are able to selectively inhibit the virus without harming the host cell. A more practical strategy is to use vaccines to enable the body to destroy the virus before an infection is established.

At present, vaccines are available for several serious viral infections, including polio, smallpox, rabies, measles, mumps, rubella, hepatitis A and B, and influenza. In some situations, vaccination against certain viral infections is routine. For instance, schoolchildren must periodically show evidence of polio, measles, and other vaccinations according to state and local laws. In other cases, vaccines are administered prior to potential exposure to the virus or in high-risk groups. Influenza vaccinations, for example, are often recommended before seasonal influenza outbreaks for all individuals 6 months of age or older.[98]

Although vaccines exist for many serious viral infections, there are some drawbacks. Some vaccines are only partially effective, and viral infection still occurs in a significant percentage of vaccinated individuals. Other vaccines, especially killed vaccines, often require periodic readministration (boosters) to help maintain antiviral immunity. In addition, certain types of viruses still lack an effective vaccination. For example, no vaccine is currently approved for HIV.[99,100] Hence, the improvement of existing vaccines and the development of new vaccines remain two of the more important aspects of antiviral chemotherapy.[101]

HIV AND THE TREATMENT OF AIDS

HIV is a member of the retrovirus family (see Table 34-1).[50] It impairs the function of certain cells in the immune system such as CD4+ (T-helper) lymphocytes.[102,103] Destruction of immune system components often leads to a severe immunocompromised state. When immune function deteriorates beyond a certain point (typically less than 200 CD4 lymphocytes per microliter), these patients are said to have AIDS. The HIV virus exists in at least two forms: HIV-1 and HIV-2. Both forms of the virus are capable of causing AIDS, but HIV-1 is more prevalent, and HIV-2 infection is less likely to progress to AIDS.[104] Hence, HIV-1 is also referred to informally as the "AIDS virus." Because there is currently no effective way to kill the AIDS virus in humans, there is no cure for AIDS.

AIDS is a life-threatening disorder because the patient's immune system is unable to control invasive microorganisms or abnormal cell proliferation.[105,106] In particular, patients with AIDS often suffer from severe viral infections (e.g., CMV, various herpesvirus infections), bacterial infections (e.g., *Mycobacterium tuberculosis*), fungal infections (e.g., *Pneumocystis jiroveci*), and infections caused by various other microbes and parasites. Patients with AIDS also develop relatively unusual neoplastic diseases, such as Kaposi sarcoma.

Considerable neuromuscular involvement also occurs in patients with AIDS.[107] Peripheral neuropathies, myopathies, and various CNS manifestations (dementia, other psychological manifestations) can occur directly from HIV infection or secondarily, due to some other opportunistic infection.[108,109] Likewise, peripheral neuropathies are a common side effect of certain anti-HIV drugs (didanosine, stavudine, others),[66,110] and myopathies are a side effect of zidovudine therapy.[111] Patients with HIV often have painful symptoms such as joint pain, back pain, and pain related to neuropathies and myopathies.[107] Hence, HIV disease can often be regarded as a degenerative neuromuscular disorder from the standpoint of a rehabilitation professional. Therapists can use exercise and other interventions to help improve function and decrease pain in patients with HIV infection and AIDS.[112-114]

Individuals who are infected with HIV may remain asymptomatic for several years before developing the full-blown clinical picture of AIDS. Even people exposed to HIV who do not initially develop AIDS carry the virus for the rest of their lives and are thus capable of transmitting the virus to others. Transmission of HIV from one individual to another occurs primarily through intimate sexual contact and through sharing IV needles. Transfusions of blood from HIV-infected donors are also a potential source of HIV transmission. Hence, practicing safe sex, not sharing needles, and improving blood-screening techniques are crucial in preventing the transmission of HIV and the subsequent risk of developing AIDS.

The treatment of patients with AIDS and individuals infected by HIV is continually being modified as new drugs become available and more information is gained about the nature of the AIDS virus. Currently, the pharmacological management of patients infected with HIV consists of two principal strategies: (1) controlling the proliferation and effects of HIV in infected individuals and (2) treating and preventing various opportunistic infections that can overwhelm the compromised immune system in patients with AIDS. The pharmacological methods used to accomplish these principal strategies are presented here.

Inhibition of HIV Proliferation in Infected Individuals

No drugs are currently available that selectively kill HIV in humans, hence the lack of a cure for this viral infection. Nonetheless, several antiviral drugs can inhibit the replication of this virus, thus decreasing the morbidity and mortality of HIV infection. These drugs are usually specific for the HIV-1 form of the virus, because HIV-1 is more prevalent in people infected by HIV. The pharmacological strategies for inhibiting

HIV proliferation are summarized in Figure 34-5 and are discussed briefly here.

Zidovudine (Retrovir, AZT) was the first drug approved as an anti-HIV agent,[59] followed by agents that act like zidovudine to prevent HIV replication. These drugs include abacavir (Ziagen), didanosine (Videx), emtricitabine (Emtriva), lamivudine (Epivir), stavudine (Zerit), and tenofovir (Viread) (see Table 34-3). As discussed earlier in *Specific Antiviral Drugs*, zidovudine and similar drugs are classified as NRTIs because they share a common mechanism of action (see Fig. 34-3); that is, these drugs inhibit the reverse transcriptase enzyme that HIV uses to synthesize viral DNA from viral RNA. This action impairs one of the early steps in viral replication, thus slowing the progression of HIV infection and the development of AIDS.

Protease inhibitors were the second major breakthrough in the pharmacological treatment of HIV infection. These agents are typically identified by generic names containing an *-avir* suffix. Protease inhibitors currently available include atazanavir (Reyataz), darunavir (Prezista), fosamprenavir (Lexiva), indinavir (Crixivan), lopinavir (Kaletra; combination with Ritonavir), nelfinavir (Viracept), ritonavir (Norvir), saquinavir (Fortovase, Invirase), and tipranavir (Aptivus). As indicated earlier, these drugs impair the HIV protease enzyme that is responsible for several steps in HIV replication. Like the NRTIs, these drugs do not kill the virus but can slow its replication and prevent the spread of HIV to noninfected cells.

The third strategy developed to inhibit HIV replication is the NNRTIs. These drugs include delavirdine (Rescriptor), efavirenz (Sustiva), etravirine (Intelence), and nevirapine (Viramune). Like their nucleoside counterparts, NNRTIs also inhibit the reverse transcriptase enzyme's ability to perform one of the initial steps in HIV replication. The NNRTIs, however, directly inhibit the active (catalytic) site on this enzyme, whereas zidovudine and other NRTIs serve as false substrates that take the place of the substance (thymidine) normally acted on by this enzyme (see "Mechanism of Action" in the "Reverse Transcriptase Inhibitors" section). Hence, NNRTIs provide another way to impair one of the key steps in HIV replication, and patients can use these drugs along with other agents (NRTIs, protease inhibitors) to provide optimal benefits in

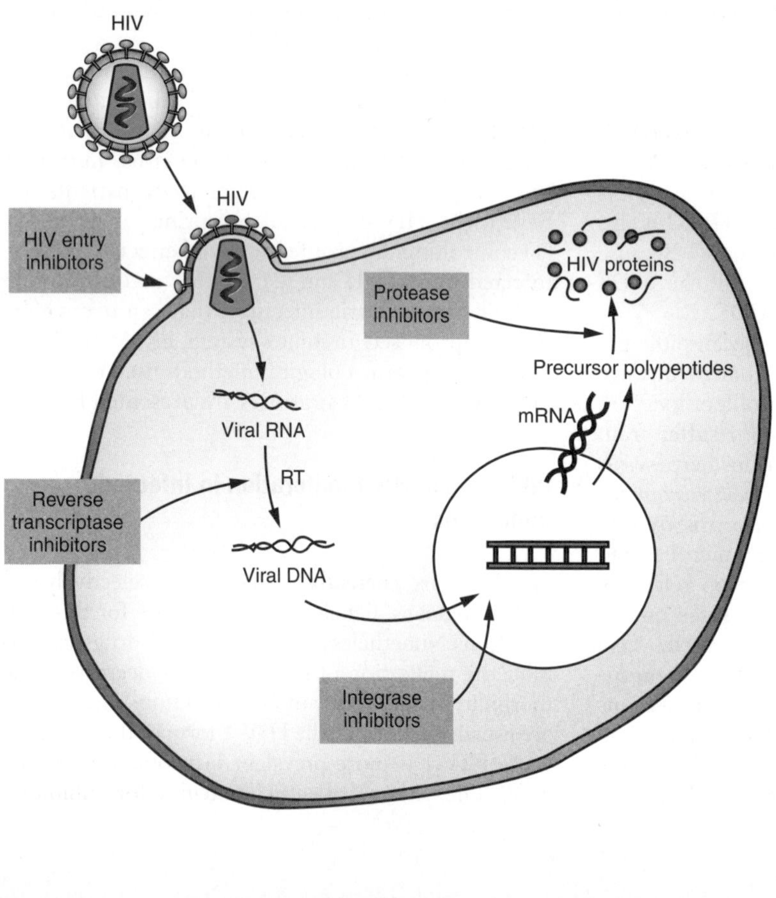

Figure ■ 34-5
Primary anti-HIV drug strategies.

preventing HIV replication and proliferation (see the next section).

One of the newer strategies against HIV infection are drugs known as *HIV entry inhibitors*. These drugs include enfuvirtide (Fuzeon) and maraviroc (Selzentry). They impair the virus's ability to attach to the host cell's surface, thereby inhibiting HIV entry into susceptible lymphocytes. If the virus cannot enter the cell, it cannot infect that cell or begin the process of viral replication.

Finally, drugs known as *integrase inhibitors* have been developed as part of the treatment of HIV. These drugs inhibit a key enzyme (HIV integrase) that enables HIV to splice its viral DNA into the host cell (human) chromosome. By inhibiting this enzyme, these drugs limit the ability of HIV to integrate its genetic code into the host cell DNA, thus preventing the virus from inducing the host cell to manufacture new viral components. Integrase inhibitors that are currently available include raltegravir (Isentress) and dolutegravir (Tivicay). As indicated earlier, elvitegravir is a third integrase inhibitor, and this drug is combined in the same pill with other antivirals (e.g., cobicistat, emtricitabine, tenofovir) and marketed under the trade name Stribild. Researchers are developing other integrase inhibitors, which may reach the market in the near future.

The arsenal of anti-HIV agents has therefore grown steadily since the development of the first anti-HIV drug (zidovudine). In addition, other drugs and strategies that inhibit HIV infection continue to be explored.[115,116] As more is learned about the structure and function of this virus, pharmacologists can develop drugs that impair specific steps in the absorption and replication of HIV in human cells. If clinical trials using these other drugs are favorable, they may also be approved for future use in individuals infected with HIV.

Anti-HIV Drug Combinations: Use of Highly Active Antiretroviral Therapy

Several anti-HIV drugs are often administered simultaneously to provide optimal inhibition of HIV replication and proliferation. The idea of combining several agents is referred to as *highly active antiretroviral therapy*, or HAART.[117] HAART often involves the simultaneous use of at least three anti-HIV agents.[50] For example, a typical HAART strategy for the initial treatment of HIV infection involves the use of two nucleoside RTIs and one nonnucleoside RTI.[50,117] The HAART therapy, however, can involve many variations of the specific drug combinations. Other drugs such as a protease inhibitor, HIV entry inhibitor, or integrase inhibitor can be added to, or substituted for, the RTIs to achieve optimal antiviral effects.[118,119] The exact number and types of drugs used during HAART are selected based on the specific needs of each patient. Moreover, HAART regimens are continually being revised as new drugs reach the market or problems arise with existing strategies.

Regardless of the exact drugs used, there is ample evidence that HAART can successfully delay the progression of HIV disease in people infected with the virus. In many cases, strict adherence to HAART regimens can reduce the viral load (i.e., the amount of viral RNA present in the bloodstream) to levels that are undetectable with current testing procedures.[120] This does not mean that HAART has successfully eliminated the virus from the infected host or that the person infected with HIV has been cured. Even if HAART successfully reduces evidence of the virus in the plasma, the virus can be sequestered into T cells and other tissue "reservoirs" so that viral components cannot be detected in the bloodstream.[121] Still, HAART regimens can prevent the progression of HIV infection and help sustain immune function by allowing increases in the number of functioning CD4 lymphocytes.[122] The use of HAART is therefore associated with a substantial reduction in the incidence of AIDS and with improved clinical outcomes (fewer infections, decreased cancers, prolonged survival) in people who are infected with HIV.[118,123,124]

HAART regimens are, however, associated with several problems and limitations. A certain percentage of people with HIV do not respond adequately to HAART—that is, HAART may not be very successful in producing a sustained and complete reduction in viral load in up to 20 percent of patients receiving these regimens.[125] The lack of effectiveness may be a consequence of poor adherence to the HAART regimen. Adherence to HAART is often difficult because of the potential for side effects with these drugs and because of difficulties in remembering the complicated dosage regimens associated with taking three or more agents.[126,127] Resistance to anti-HIV drugs can also develop,[128,129] especially if there is poor adherence to HAART regimens.[130,131] As mentioned earlier, HAART does not completely eliminate the virus from the infected host, because some of the viral components remain sequestered within tissues, where they remain hidden from HAART drugs.[121] Finally, the simultaneous use of several drugs during HAART increases the risk for drug-drug interactions, increases the likelihood of metabolic disorders that affect lipid and glucose metabolism, and may cause toxicity to the liver, kidneys, and other organs.[132-134]

Nonetheless, HAART can suppress HIV disease in many people who are infected with this virus. Drug combinations can be used successfully for the long-term management of HIV disease, and they offer hope that people with HIV do not have to progress inexorably toward AIDS and death. Researchers continue to find the best way to combine existing agents and to incorporate new agents into a comprehensive and successful regimen for people infected with HIV.

HIV Vaccines

An HIV vaccine has not yet been successfully developed and approved for use in the United States. As indicated earlier, vaccines are typically an altered form of the original virus that is administered to stimulate the immune system, so the immune system can recognize and destroy the virus if a person is exposed to it. Creation of an HIV vaccine is understandably a complicated endeavor, given the complexity of this virus and its tendency to evolve and mutate into different types of HIV.[135] Nonetheless, the development of a safe, effective vaccine remains the best pharmacological method for dealing with the spread of the virus, especially in underdeveloped nations that continue to experience a rise in the incidence of HIV and AIDS.[99,100]

Hence, efforts continue to develop an HIV vaccine that will produce adequate immunity from HIV infection without severe untoward side effects.[136,137] There is concern, however, that a successful vaccine may be very difficult to produce.[99,100] For example, development of an HIV vaccine that is not 100 percent effective might give recipients a false sense of security—that is, a vaccine that confers only partial immunity (e.g., a 50 to 75 percent reduction in the risk of contracting HIV) might encourage the recipient to forgo other precautions, such as safe sex, not sharing IV needles, and so forth. Likewise, the question arises about whether a single vaccine will be successful in providing immunity from all the various HIV strains and subtypes.[137] An HIV vaccine is urgently needed and would undoubtedly be received as one of the most important pharmacological advancements of our time. But the development of such a vaccine may be delayed until we have a better understanding of HIV and how to best modify it into a successful vaccine.

We must therefore remember that zidovudine and other drugs currently available for treating HIV are not curative and may be helpful only in delaying or reducing AIDS-related deaths. A cure for AIDS, if possible, will take several years or even several decades before becoming a reality. As with many viruses, developing a vaccine against the AIDS virus is somewhat easier than making a drug that selectively destroys HIV. The development of an HIV vaccine, however, is probably still years away. Until a vaccine is developed, preventing transmission of HIV remains the best method of controlling the spread of AIDS.

Management of Opportunistic Infections

If HIV infection is not treated successfully, the body is open to infection from various other microorganisms. These infections are known commonly as *opportunistic infections* because microorganisms take advantage of the chance to infect people who lack normal immune defenses.[138,139] Fortunately, newer anti-HIV drugs and the use of HAART regimens have reduced the risk of opportunistic infections.[140] Hence, the best prevention against opportunistic infections is aggressive anti-HIV treatment that promotes T lymphocyte survival and helps maintain a functioning immune system.[141] Still, some patients are prone to opportunistic infections, including patients who are newly diagnosed with HIV infection, patients who develop resistance to anti-HIV drugs, or patients who cannot otherwise tolerate or adhere to HAART regimens.[129,142] Opportunistic infections are still a major cause of illness and death in areas of the world where HAART regimens are unavailable or unaffordable (i.e., developing countries).[143]

Because of a virtual lack of immunologic defenses, patients with AIDS often succumb to a variety of opportunistic infections.[106] Essentially, these patients simply do not have the ability to fight off various viral, bacterial, and other microbial invaders.[144] Consequently, much of the pharmacological approach to the treatment of AIDS is associated with trying to curtail various infections by using the respective antimicrobial drugs that are currently available.

It is beyond the scope of this chapter to give a detailed description of the pharmacological treatment of all the possible opportunistic infections that occur in patients with AIDS. Some of the more common types of opportunistic infections and the drugs commonly used to treat them are listed in Table 34-5 as examples. Early recognition of infectious symptoms is crucial in helping initiate drug therapy before the infection becomes uncontrollable.[144] Because patients with AIDS essentially lack endogenous defense systems, drug therapy must often be continued indefinitely, or the infection will recur. On the other hand, successful implementation or reinstitution of HAART strategies can restore immune function in certain patients, and drugs for opportunistic infections can sometimes be discontinued.[145] Nonetheless, strategies for dealing with various infections are constantly changing, and drug therapy for HIV and opportunistic infections will surely be modified as new antimicrobial agents are developed and new evidence is provided about how these agents can be used in various infections.

Table 34-5
TREATMENT OF OPPORTUNISTIC INFECTIONS IN PATIENTS WITH AIDS

Organism	Type of Infection	Drug Treatment*
Viral infections		
Cytomegalovirus	Pneumonia; hepatitis; chorioretinitis; involvement of many other organs	Ganciclovir ± valganciclovir
Herpes simplex	Unusually severe vesicular and necrotizing lesions of mucocutaneous areas (mouth, pharynx) and GI tract	Acyclovir, famciclovir, or valacyclovir
Varicella-zoster	Painful, vesicular eruption of skin according to dermatomal boundaries (shingles)	Acyclovir, famciclovir, or valacyclovir
Bacterial Infections		
Mycobacterium avium complex	Involvement of bone marrow, reticuloendothelial tissues	Clarithromycin plus ethambutol ± rifabutin
Mycobacterium tuberculosis	Tuberculosis	Isoniazid plus pyridoxine; if isoniazid resistant, other agents selected depending on *Mycobacterium* strain
Salmonella	Enterocolitis and bacteremia	Ciprofloxacin
Fungal Infections		
Candida	Inflammatory lesions in oropharyngeal region and esophagitis	Oral infections: fluconazole or nystatin; esophageal infections: fluconazole or itraconazole
Coccidioides	Primarily affects lungs but may disseminate to other tissues	Amphotericin B followed by fluconazole
Cryptococcus	Meningoencephalitis	Amphotericin B plus flucytosine, followed by fluconazole
Histoplasma capsulatum	Affects various tissues, including lungs, lymphatics, and mucocutaneous tissues; also causes blood dyscrasias (anemias, leucopenia)	Amphotericin B followed by itraconazole
Pneumocystis jiroveci	Pneumonia	Trimethoprim-sulfamethoxazole, pentamidine, or atovaquone
Protozoal Infections		
Toxoplasma	CNS infections (cerebral degeneration, meningoencephalitis)	Pyrimethamine and sulfadiazine

**Choice of specific drugs varies according to disease status, presence of other infections, and so forth. Pharmacotherapeutic rationale is also constantly changing as new agents are developed and tested.*

Special Concerns for Rehabilitation Patients

The major significance of antiviral drugs to rehabilitation specialists and other health-care professionals is the potential for controlling or eliminating infectious disease at present and in the future. Currently, only a few drugs can effectively resolve viral infections in humans. Nonetheless, the development of new antiviral agents and the improved use of existing compounds such as the interferons are exciting and important areas of pharmacology. In addition, viral prophylaxis through vaccination has virtually eliminated some types of serious infections, and the possibility of new and improved antiviral vaccines may enhance the health and welfare of patients throughout the world.

Consequently, physical therapists and occupational therapists should keep abreast of advances in treating and preventing viral infections. Health-care professionals can serve as a reliable source of information for their patients. This notion is especially true for the AIDS crisis, which promises to be a major health issue for some time.

In addition, viral infections may produce pain and other symptoms that can be treated by physical rehabilitation. In particular, chronic HIV infection and the drug therapy for this disorder can both produce neuromuscular problems such as myopathy and peripheral neuropathy.[107,146] Neuromuscular impairments can occur at any stage in the disease process, but they become especially problematic in advanced cases of HIV infection or when this disease progresses to AIDS.[146] Hence, therapists can use massage and various physical agents to help decrease pain[112] and can implement aerobic and resistive exercise programs to help maintain muscle strength and function.[147] These interventions can be invaluable in helping maintain quality of life in people with HIV infection and AIDS.

CASE STUDY

ANTIVIRAL DRUGS

Brief History. R.K. is a 28-year-old man who was infected with HIV after sharing hypodermic syringes with a fellow drug abuser. He began a pharmacological regimen of highly active antiretroviral therapy, consisting of two reverse transcriptase inhibitors (zidovudine [Retrovir], 600 mg/d and didanosine [Videx], 400 mg/d) and one protease inhibitor (indinavir [Crixivan], 2,400 mg/d). This regimen was quite successful in controlling HIV replication and proliferation. During a recent examination, his viral load was so low that it was not detectable by current blood tests. He was reminded that he was not cured and that the virus was still present in his body. Nonetheless, the patient began to lapse into periods of noncompliance and frequently failed to take his medications according to the proper dosing schedule. As a result, HIV proliferated and suppressed his immune function to the point where he was considered to have developed AIDS. Recently, he developed a fever and respiratory infection due to *Pneumocystis jiroveci* pneumonia. He was admitted to the hospital and treated with a combination of pentamidine and trimethoprim-sulfamethoxazole. The patient

CASE STUDY (Continued)

also exhibited muscular weakness and began to develop burning pain in both lower extremities. The weakness and pain were attributed to radiculopathy caused by infection of peripheral nerves by HIV or by some other opportunistic infection. The physical therapy department was consulted to determine what could be done to alleviate the neuropathic pain and dysfunction.

1. *How can the therapist intervene to reduce R.K.'s pain and improve his functional ability?*
2. *Given this patient's lack of adherence to anti-HIV drugs, what is the likely outcome in this case?*

See Appendix C, "Answers to Case Study Questions."

SUMMARY

Viruses present a unique problem in terms of the pharmacological treatment of infectious disease. These microorganisms rely totally on the metabolic function of host (human) cells to function and replicate more viruses. Hence, there are currently only a limited number of effective antiviral agents that selectively kill or attenuate the virus without seriously harming the human cells. Viruses can acquire resistance to previously effective drugs by mutating and altering their structural or functional characteristics. Developing and administering antiviral vaccines that stimulate the immunity of the host to specific viral infections is often more practical. In the future, the development of new antiviral agents and vaccines may help treat and eliminate viral infections that currently pose a serious health threat.

REFERENCES

1. Ahmad N, Ray CG, Drew WL. The nature of viruses. In: Ryan KJ, Ray CG, eds. *Sherris Medical Microbiology.* 5th ed. New York: McGraw-Hill; 2010.
2. McAdam AJ, Sharpe AH. Infectious diseases. In: Kumar V, Abbas AK, Fausto N, Aster JC, eds. *Pathologic Basis of Disease.* 8th ed. New York: Elsevier Saunders; 2010.
3. Dermody TS, Bergelson JM. Biology of viruses. In: Engleberg NC, DiRita V, Dermody TS, eds. *Schaechter's Mechanisms of Microbial Disease.* 5th ed. Philadelphia, PA: Lippincott Williams and Wilkins; 2013.
4. Chayavichitsilp P, Buckwalter JV, Krakowski AC, Friedlander SF. Herpes simplex. *Pediatr Rev.* 2009;30:119-129.
5. Field HJ, Vere Hodge RA. Recent developments in anti-herpesvirus drugs. *Br Med Bull.* 2013;106:213-249.
6. Vere Hodge RA, Field HJ. Antiviral agents for herpes simplex virus. *Adv Pharmacol.* 2013;67:1-38.
7. Rahimi H, Mara T, Costella J, et al. Effectiveness of antiviral agents for the prevention of recurrent herpes labialis: a systematic review and meta-analysis. *Oral Surg Oral Med Oral Pathol Oral Radiol.* 2012;113:618-627.
8. Roett MA, Mayor MT, Uduhiri KA. Diagnosis and management of genital ulcers. *Am Fam Physician.* 2012;85:254-262.
9. Usatine RP, Tinitigan R. Nongenital herpes simplex virus. *Am Fam Physician.* 2010;82:1075-1082.
10. Andrei G, Snoeck R. Advances in the treatment of varicella-zoster virus infections. *Adv Pharmacol.* 2013;67:107-168.
11. Vigil KJ, Chemaly RF. Valacyclovir: approved and off-label uses for the treatment of herpes virus infections in immunocompetent and immunocompromised adults. *Expert Opin Pharmacother.* 2010;11:1901-1913.
12. Yang B, Smith DE. Significance of peptide transporter 1 in the intestinal permeability of valacyclovir in wild-type and PepT1 knockout mice. *Drug Metab Dispos.* 2013;41:608-614.
13. Kimberlin DW, Jacobs RF, Weller S, et al. Pharmacokinetics and safety of extemporaneously compounded valacyclovir oral suspension in pediatric patients from 1 month through 11 years of age. *Clin Infect Dis.* 2010;50:221-228.
14. Piret J, Boivin G. Resistance of herpes simplex viruses to nucleoside analogues: mechanisms, prevalence, and management. *Antimicrob Agents Chemother.* 2011;55:459-472.
15. Razonable RR. Antiviral drugs for viruses other than human immunodeficiency virus. *Mayo Clin Proc.* 2011;86:1009-1026.
16. Ison MG. Clinical use of approved influenza antivirals: therapy and prophylaxis. *Influenza Other Respir Viruses.* 2013;7(suppl 1): 7-13.
17. Acosta EP, Flexner C. Antiviral agents (nonretroviral). In: Brunton L, et al, eds. *The Pharmacological Basis of Therapeutics.* 12th ed. New York: McGraw-Hill; 2011.
18. Bearman GM, Shankaran S, Elam K. Treatment of severe cases of pandemic (H1N1) 2009 influenza: review of antivirals and adjuvant therapy. *Recent Pat Antiinfect Drug Discov.* 2010;5:152-156.
19. Cady SD, Schmidt-Rohr K, Wang J, et al. Structure of the amantadine binding site of influenza M2 proton channels in lipid bilayers. *Nature.* 2010;463:689-692.

20. Pielak RM, Chou JJ. Flu channel drug resistance: a tale of two sites. *Protein Cell.* 2010;1:246-258.
21. Ahmed A. Antiviral treatment of cytomegalovirus infection. *Infect Disord DrugTargets.* 2011;11:475-503.
22. Vadlapudi AD, Vadlapatla RK, Mitra AK. Current and emerging antivirals for the treatment of cytomegalovirus (CMV) retinitis: an update on recent patents. *Recent Pat Antiinfect Drug Discov.* 2012;7:8-18.
23. Hsu V, de LT Vieira M, Zhao P, et al. Towards quantitation of the effects of renal impairment and probenecid inhibition on kidney uptake and efflux transporters, using physiologically based pharmacokinetic modelling and simulations. *Clin Pharmacokinet.* 2014;53:283-293.
24. Andrei G, De Clercq E, Snoeck R. Drug targets in cytomegalovirus infection. *Infect Disord Drug Targets.* 2009;9:201-222.
25. Treister NS, Woo SB. Topical n-docosanol for management of recurrent herpes labialis. *Expert Opin Pharmacother.* 2010;11: 853-860.
26. Métifiot M, Marchand C, Pommier Y. HIV integrase inhibitors: 20-year landmark and challenges. *Adv Pharmacol.* 2013;67: 75-105.
27. Messiaen P, Wensing AM, Fun A, et al. Clinical use of HIV integrase inhibitors: a systematic review and meta-analysis. *PLoS One.* 2013;8:e52562.
28. Karmon SL, Markowitz M. Next-generation integrase inhibitors: where to after raltegravir? *Drugs.* 2013;73:213-228.
29. Haqqani AA, Tilton JC. Entry inhibitors and their use in the treatment of HIV-1 infection. *Antiviral Res.* 2013;98:158-170.
30. Tan JJ, Ma XT, Liu C, et al. The current status and challenges in the development of fusion inhibitors as therapeutics for HIV-1 infection. *Curr Pharm Des.* 2013;19:1810-1817.
31. Joly V, Jidar K, Tatay M, Yeni P. Enfuvirtide: from basic investigations to current clinical use. *Expert Opin Pharmacother.* 2010;11:2701-2713.
32. Hasler-Nguyen N, Shelton D, Ponard G, et al. Evaluation of the in vitro skin permeation of antiviral drugs from penciclovir 1% cream and acyclovir 5% cream used to treat herpes simplex virus infection. *BMC Dermatol.* 2009;9:3.
33. Mubareka S, Leung V, Aoki FY, Vinh DC. Famciclovir: a focus on efficacy and safety. *Expert Opin Drug Saf.* 2010;9:643-658.
34. Bader MS. Herpes zoster: diagnostic, therapeutic, and preventive approaches. *Postgrad Med.* 2013;125:78-91.
35. De Clercq E. Antiviral drugs in current clinical use. *J Clin Virol.* 2004;30:115-133.
36. Carmichael A. Cytomegalovirus and the eye. *Eye.* 2012;26: 237-240.
37. You DM, Johnson MD. Cytomegalovirus infection and the gastrointestinal tract. *Curr Gastroenterol Rep.* 2012;14:334-342.
38. Razonable RR. Management strategies for cytomegalovirus infection and disease in solid organ transplant recipients. *Infect Dis Clin North Am.* 2013;27:317-342.
39. A Gaspari A, Tyring SK, Rosen T. Beyond a decade of 5% imiquimod topical therapy. *J Drugs Dermatol.* 2009;8:467-474.
40. Grossberg AL, Gaspari AA. Topical antineoplastic agents in the treatment of mucocutaneous diseases. *Curr Probl Dermatol.* 2011;40:71-82.
41. Skevaki CL, Galani IE, Pararas MV, et al. Treatment of viral conjunctivitis with antiviral drugs. *Drugs.* 2011;71:331-347.
42. Clark NM, Lynch JP 3rd. Influenza: epidemiology, clinical features, therapy, and prevention. *Semin Respir Crit Care Med.* 2011;32:373-392.
43. Smith JR, Ariano RE, Toovey S. The use of antiviral agents for the management of severe influenza. *Crit Care Med.* 2010;38(suppl):e43-51.
44. Jackson RJ, Cooper KL, Tappenden P, et al. Oseltamivir, zanamivir and amantadine in the prevention of influenza: a systematic review. *J Infect.* 2011;62:14-25.
45. Lee SK, Potempa M, Swanstrom R. The choreography of HIV-1 proteolytic processing and virion assembly. *J Biol Chem.* 2012;287:40867-40874.
46. Qiu X, Liu ZP. Recent developments of peptidomimetic HIV-1 protease inhibitors. *Curr Med Chem.* 2011;18:4513-4537.
47. Hornberger J, Simpson K, Shewade A, et al. Broadening the perspective when assessing evidence on boosted protease inhibitor-based regimens for initial antiretroviral therapy. *Adv Ther.* 2010;27:763-773.
48. Hull MW, Montaner JS. Ritonavir-boosted protease inhibitors in HIV therapy. *Ann Med.* 2011;43:375-388.
49. De Clercq E. The nucleoside reverse transcriptase inhibitors, nonnucleoside reverse transcriptase inhibitors, and protease inhibitors in the treatment of HIV infections (AIDS). *Adv Pharmacol.* 2013;67:317-358.
50. Flexner C. Antiretroviral agents and treatment of HIV infection. In: Brunton L, et al, eds. *The Pharmacological Basis of Therapeutics.* 12th ed. New York: McGraw-Hill; 2011.
51. Anuurad E, Bremer A, Berglund L. HIV protease inhibitors and obesity. *Curr Opin Endocrinol Diabetes Obes.* 2010;17:478-485.
52. Caron-Debarle M, Lagathu C, Boccara F, et al. HIV-associated lipodystrophy: from fat injury to premature aging. *Trends Mol Med.* 2010;16:218-229.
53. Souza SJ, Luzia LA, Santos SS, Rondó PH. Lipid profile of HIV-infected patients in relation to antiretroviral therapy: a review. *Rev Assoc Med Bras.* 2013;59:186-198.
54. Hruz PW. Molecular mechanisms for insulin resistance in treated HIV-infection. *Best Pract Res Clin Endocrinol Metab.* 2011;25:459-468.
55. Garg H, Joshi A, Mukherjee D. Cardiovascular complications of HIV infection and treatment. *Cardiovasc Hematol Agents Med Chem.* 2013;11:58-66.
56. Villarroya F, Domingo P, Giralt M. Drug-induced lipotoxicity: lipodystrophy associated with HIV-1 infection and antiretroviral treatment. *Biochim Biophys Acta.* 2010;1801:392-399.
57. Dubé MP, Cadden JJ. Lipid metabolism in treated HIV Infection. *Best Pract Res Clin Endocrinol Metab.* 2011;25:429-442.
58. Menéndez-Arias L, Betancor G, Matamoros T. HIV-1 reverse transcriptase connection subdomain mutations involved in resistance to approved non-nucleoside inhibitors. *Antiviral Res.* 2011;92:139-149.
59. Sierra-Aragón S, Walter H. Targets for inhibition of HIV replication: entry, enzyme action, release and maturation. *Intervirology.* 2012;55:84-97.
60. Usach I, Melis V, Peris JE. Non-nucleoside reverse transcriptase inhibitors: a review on pharmacokinetics, pharmacodynamics, safety and tolerability. *J Int AIDS Soc.* 2013;16:1-14.
61. Shey MS, Kongnyuy EJ, Alobwede SM, Wiysonge CS. Co-formulated abacavir-lamivudine-zidovudine for initial treatment of HIV infection and AIDS. *Cochrane Database Syst Rev.* 2013;3:CD005481.
62. Bazzoli C, Jullien V, Le Tiec C, et al. Intracellular pharmacokinetics of antiretroviral drugs in HIV-infected patients, and their correlation with drug action. *Clin Pharmacokinet.* 2010;49: 17-45.

63. Monroe JI, El-Nahal WG, Shirts MR. Investigating the mutation resistance of nonnucleoside inhibitors of HIV-RT using multiple microsecond atomistic simulations. *Proteins*. 2014;82:130-144.
64. Margolis AM, Heverling H, Pham PA, Stolbach A. A review of the toxicity of HIV medications. *J Med Toxicol*. 2014;10:26-39.
65. Abers MS, Shandera WX, Kass JS. Neurological and psychiatric adverse effects of antiretroviral drugs. *CNS Drugs*. 2014;28:131-145.
66. Leung GP. Iatrogenic mitochondriopathies: a recent lesson from nucleoside/nucleotide reverse transcriptase inhibitors. *Adv Exp Med Biol*. 2012;942:347-369.
67. Martin MA, Kroetz DL. Abacavir pharmacogenetics—from initial reports to standard of care. *Pharmacotherapy*. 2013;33:765-775.
68. Chu HY, Englund JA. Respiratory syncytial virus disease: prevention and treatment. *Curr Top Microbiol Immunol*. 2013;372:235-258.
69. Krilov LR. Respiratory syncytial virus disease: update on treatment and prevention. *Expert Rev Anti Infect Ther*. 2011;9:27-32.
70. Hynicka LM, Ensor CR. Prophylaxis and treatment of respiratory syncytial virus in adult immunocompromised patients. *Ann Pharmacother*. 2012;46:558-566.
71. Flori N, Funakoshi N, Duny Y, et al. Pegylated interferon-α2a and ribavirin versus pegylated interferon-α2b and ribavirin in chronic hepatitis C: a meta-analysis. *Drugs*. 2013;73:263-277.
72. Ilyas JA, Vierling JM. An overview of emerging therapies for the treatment of chronic hepatitis C. *Med Clin North Am*. 2014;98:17-38.
73. George PM, Badiger R, Alazawi W, et al. Pharmacology and therapeutic potential of interferons. *Pharmacol Ther*. 2012;135:44-53.
74. Hertzog P, Forster S, Samarajiwa S. Systems biology of interferon responses. *J Interferon Cytokine Res*. 2011;31:5-11.
75. Reyes-Vázquez C, Prieto-Gómez B, Dafny N. Interferon modulates central nervous system function. *Brain Res*. 2012;1442:76-89.
76. Chevaliez S, Pawlotsky JM. Interferons and their use in persistent viral infections. *Handb Exp Pharmacol*. 2009;189:203-241.
77. Sedger LM. microRNA control of interferons and interferon induced anti-viral activity. *Mol Immunol*. 2013;56:781-793.
78. Biggioggero M, Gabbriellini L, Meroni PL. Type I interferon therapy and its role in autoimmunity. *Autoimmunity*. 2010;43:248-254.
79. Wang BX, Rahbar R, Fish EN. Interferon: current status and future prospects in cancer therapy. *J Interferon Cytokine Res*. 2011;31:545-552.
80. Malmgaard L. Induction and regulation of IFNs during viral infections. *J Interferon Cytokine Res*. 2004;24:439-454.
81. Schoggins JW, Rice CM. Interferon-stimulated genes and their antiviral effector functions. *Curr Opin Virol*. 2011;1:519-525.
82. Haller O, Kochs G. Human MxA protein: an interferon-induced dynamin-like GTPase with broad antiviral activity. *J Interferon Cytokine Res*. 2011;31:79-87.
83. Zhao C, Collins MN, Hsiang TY, Krug RM. Interferon-induced ISG15 pathway: an ongoing virus-host battle. *Trends Microbiol*. 2013;21:181-186.
84. Bracarda S, Eggermont AM, Samuelsson J. Redefining the role of interferon in the treatment of malignant diseases. *Eur J Cancer*. 2010;46:284-297.
85. Kotredes KP, Gamero AM. Interferons as inducers of apoptosis in malignant cells. *J Interferon Cytokine Res*. 2013;33:162-170.
86. Degasperi E, Viganò M, Aghemo A, et al. PegIFN-α2a for the treatment of chronic hepatitis B and C: a 10-year history. *Expert Rev Anti Infect Ther*. 2013;11:459-474.
87. Pawlotsky JM. Hepatitis C virus: standard-of-care treatment. *Adv Pharmacol*. 2013;67:169-215.
88. Donnelly RP, Dickensheets H, O'Brien TR. Interferon-lambda and therapy for chronic hepatitis C virus infection. *Trends Immunol*. 2011;32:443-450.
89. Scagnolari C, Antonelli G. Antiviral activity of the interferon α family: biological and pharmacological aspects of the treatment of chronic hepatitis C. *Expert Opin Biol Ther*. 2013;13:693-711.
90. McGraw CA, Lublin FD. Interferon beta and glatiramer acetate therapy. *Neurotherapeutics*. 2013;10:2-18.
91. Thouvenot E, Carlander B, Camu W. Subcutaneous IFN-β1a to treat relapsing-remitting multiple sclerosis. *Expert Rev Neurother*. 2012;12:1283-1291.
92. Minagar A. Current and future therapies for multiple sclerosis. *Scientifica*. 2013;2013:249101.
93. Karussis D. Immunotherapy of multiple sclerosis: the state of the art. *BioDrugs*. 2013;27:113-148.
94. Sockalingam S, Links PS, Abbey SE. Suicide risk in hepatitis C and during interferon-alpha therapy: a review and clinical update. *J Viral Hepat*. 2011;18:153-160.
95. Udina M, Castellví P, Moreno-España J, et al. Interferon-induced depression in chronic hepatitis C: a systematic review and meta-analysis. *J Clin Psychiatry*. 2012;73:1128-1138.
96. Farrell RA, Marta M, Gaeguta AJ, Souslova V, Giovannoni G, Creeke PI. Development of resistance to biologic therapies with reference to IFN-β. *Rheumatology*. 2012;51:590-599.
97. Mollica A, Stefanucci A, Costante R. Strategies for developing tuberculosis vaccines: emerging approaches. *Curr Drug Targets*. 2013;14:938-951.
98. Monto AS. Seasonal influenza and vaccination coverage. *Vaccine*. 2010;28(suppl 4):D33-44.
99. Schiffner T, Sattentau QJ, Dorrell L. Development of prophylactic vaccines against HIV-1. *Retrovirology*. 2013;10:72.
100. Watkins DI. Update on progress in HIV vaccine development. *Top Antivir Med*. 2012;20:30-31.
101. Finco O, Rappuoli R. Designing vaccines for the twenty-first century society. *Front Immunol*. 2014;5:12.
102. Chowdhury A, Silvestri G. Host-pathogen interaction in HIV infection. *Curr Opin Immunol*. 2013;25:463-469.
103. Naif HM. Pathogenesis of HIV infection. *Infect Dis Rep*. 2013;5(suppl 1):e6.
104. Nyamweya S, Hegedus A, Jaye A, et al. Comparing HIV-1 and HIV-2 infection: lessons for viral immunopathogenesis. *Rev Med Virol*. 2013;23:221-240.
105. Carr ER. HIV- and AIDS-associated cancers. *Clin J Oncol Nurs*. 2013;17:201-204.
106. Chang CC, Crane M, Zhou J, et al. HIV and co-infections. *Immunol Rev*. 2013;254:114-142.
107. Harrison TB, Smith B. Neuromuscular manifestations of HIV/AIDS. *J Clin Neuromuscul Dis*. 2011;13:68-84.
108. Kamerman PR, Wadley AL, Cherry CL. HIV-associated sensory neuropathy: risk factors and genetics. *Curr Pain Headache Rep*. 2012;16:226-236.
109. Schütz SG, Robinson-Papp J. HIV-related neuropathy: current perspectives. *HIV AIDS*. 2013;5:243-251.

110. Gutierrez Mdel M, Mateo MG, Vidal F, Domingo P. The toxicogenetics of antiretroviral therapy: the evil inside. *Curr Med Chem*. 2011;18:209-219.
111. Teener JW. Inflammatory and toxic myopathy. *Semin Neurol*. 2012;32:491-499.
112. Hillier SL, Louw Q, Morris L, et al. Massage therapy for people with HIV/AIDS. *Cochrane Database Syst Rev*. 2010;1:CD007502.
113. O'Brien K, Nixon S, Tynan AM, Glazier R. Aerobic exercise interventions for adults living with HIV/AIDS. *Cochrane Database Syst Rev*. 2010;8:CD001796.
114. O'Brien K, Tynan AM, Nixon S, Glazier RH. Effects of progressive resistive exercise in adults living with HIV/AIDS: systematic review and meta-analysis of randomized trials. *AIDS Care*. 2008;20:631-653.
115. Arribas JR, Eron J. Advances in antiretroviral therapy. *Curr Opin HIV AIDS*. 2013;8:341-349.
116. Miyamoto F, Kodama EN. Novel HIV-1 fusion inhibition peptides: designing the next generation of drugs. *Antivir Chem Chemother*. 2012;22:151-158.
117. Jayaweera D, Dilanchian P. New therapeutic landscape of NNRTIs for treatment of HIV: a look at recent data. *Expert Opin Pharmacother*. 2012;13:2601-2612.
118. Boyd MA, Hill AM. Clinical management of treatment-experienced, HIV/AIDS patients in the combination antiretroviral therapy era. *Pharmacoeconomics*. 2010;28(suppl 1):17-34.
119. Taiwo B, Murphy RL, Katlama C. Novel antiretroviral combinations in treatment-experienced patients with HIV infection: rationale and results. *Drugs*. 2010;70:1629-1642.
120. Hull MW, Montaner J. Antiretroviral therapy: a key component of a comprehensive HIV prevention strategy. *Curr HIV/AIDS Rep*. 2011;8:85-93.
121. Rouzioux C, Richman D. How to best measure HIV reservoirs? *Curr Opin HIV AIDS*. 2013;8:170-175.
122. Miró JM, Manzardo C, Pich J, et al. Immune reconstitution in severely immunosuppressed antiretroviral-naive HIV type 1-infected patients using a nonnucleoside reverse transcriptase inhibitor-based or a boosted protease inhibitor-based antiretroviral regimen: three-year results (the Advanz Trial): a randomized, controlled trial. *AIDS Res Hum Retroviruses*. 2010;26:747-757.
123. Boyd MA. Improvements in antiretroviral therapy outcomes over calendar time. *Curr Opin HIV AIDS*. 2009;4:194-199.
124. Gatell JM. When and why to start antiretroviral therapy? *J Antimicrob Chemother*. 2010;65:383-385.
125. Low A, Markowitz M. Predictors of response to highly active antiretroviral therapy. *AIDS Read*. 2006;16:425-436.
126. Esté JA, Cihlar T. Current status and challenges of antiretroviral research and therapy. *Antiviral Res*. 2010;85:25-33.
127. Mills EJ, Nachega JB, Bangsberg DR, et al. Adherence to HAART: a systematic review of developed and developing nation patient-reported barriers and facilitators. *PLoS Med*. 2006;3:e438.
128. Cortez KJ, Maldarelli F. Clinical management of HIV drug resistance. *Viruses*. 2011;3:347-378.
129. Tang MW, Shafer RW. HIV-1 antiretroviral resistance: scientific principles and clinical applications. *Drugs*. 2012;72:e1-25.
130. Emamzadeh-Fard S, Fard SE, SeyedAlinaghi S, Paydary K. Adherence to anti-retroviral therapy and its determinants in HIV/AIDS patients: a review. *Infect Disord Drug Targets*. 2012;12:346-356.
131. Gardner EM, Hullsiek KH, Telzak EE, et al. Antiretroviral medication adherence and class-specific resistance in a large prospective clinical trial. *AIDS*. 2010;24:395-403.
132. Calza L. Renal toxicity associated with antiretroviral therapy. *HIV Clin Trials*. 2012;13:189-211.
133. Jones M, Núñez M. Liver toxicity of antiretroviral drugs. *Semin Liver Dis*. 2012;32:167-176.
134. Lake JE, Currier JS. Metabolic disease in HIV infection. *Lancet Infect Dis*. 2013;13:964-975.
135. Ndung'u T, Weiss RA. On HIV diversity. *AIDS*. 2012;26:1255-1260.
136. Haynes BF, McElrath MJ. Progress in HIV-1 vaccine development. *Curr Opin HIV AIDS*. 2013;8:326-332.
137. Stephenson KE, Barouch DH. A global approach to HIV-1 vaccine development. *Immunol Rev*. 2013;254:295-304.
138. Kaplan JE, Benson C, Holmes KK, et al. Guidelines for prevention and treatment of opportunistic infections in HIV-infected adults and adolescents: recommendations from CDC, the National Institutes of Health, and the HIV Medicine Association of the Infectious Diseases Society of America. *MMWR Recomm Rep*. 2009;58(RR-4):1-207.
139. Luetkemeyer AF, Havlir DV, Currier JS. Complications of HIV disease and antiretroviral therapy. *Top Antivir Med*. 2012;20:48-60.
140. Wilson EM, Sereti I. Immune restoration after antiretroviral therapy: the pitfalls of hasty or incomplete repairs. *Immunol Rev*. 2013;254:343-354.
141. Okoye AA, Picker LJ. CD4(+) T-cell depletion in HIV infection: mechanisms of immunological failure. *Immunol Rev*. 2013;254:54-64.
142. Sarmento-Castro R, Vasconcelos C, Aguas MJ, et al. Virologic suppression in treatment-experienced patients after virologic rebound or failure of therapy. *Curr Opin HIV AIDS*. 2011;6(suppl 1):S12-20.
143. Vella S, Schwartländer B, Sow SP, et al. The history of antiretroviral therapy and of its implementation in resource-limited areas of the world. *AIDS*. 2012;26:1231-1241.
144. Lawn SD, Harries AD, Wood R. Strategies to reduce early morbidity and mortality in adults receiving antiretroviral therapy in resource-limited settings. *Curr Opin HIV AIDS*. 2010;5:18-26.
145. Cossarini F, Spagnuolo V, Gianotti N, et al. Management of HIV infection after triple class failure. *New Microbiol*. 2013;36:23-39.
146. Robinson-Papp J, Simpson DM. Neuromuscular diseases associated with HIV-1 infection. *Muscle Nerve*. 2009;40:1043-1053.
147. Gomes Neto M, Ogalha C, Andrade AM, Brites C. A systematic review of effects of concurrent strength and endurance training on the health-related quality of life and cardiopulmonary status in patients with HIV/AIDS. *Biomed Res Int*. 2013;2013:319524.

CHAPTER 35

Treatment of Infections III: Antifungal and Antiparasitic Drugs

Humans are susceptible to infection by a number of parasitic species of fungi, protozoa, and helminths (worms). Although some types of parasitic infections are limited or unknown in developed nations such as the United States, parasitic infections generally represent the most common form of disease worldwide. These infections are especially prevalent in tropical and subtropical environments and in impoverished areas of the world where sanitation and hygiene are inadequate. In addition, the incidence of serious fungal and other parasitic infections has been increasing in industrialized nations because of the increased susceptibility of immunocompromised patients to these infections, such as patients with AIDS or those receiving immunosuppressant drugs after organ transplantation.[1-3] Hence, the effective pharmacological treatment of these infections remains an important topic in the global management of disease.

The pharmacological treatment of parasitic infections is a complex and extensive topic. In this limited space, it is difficult to describe the many species of each parasite, all the diseases caused by parasites, and the chemical methods currently available to selectively destroy various fungi, protozoa, and helminths in humans. Consequently, this chapter briefly reviews the general aspects of the three types of parasites, followed by the primary drugs used to treat specific fungal, protozoal, and helminthic infections. Certain infections such as superficial fungal infections that cause athlete's foot and similar conditions are quite common, and clinicians may be involved in helping treat and prevent these infections. As indicated above, more serious fungal and parasitic infections can occur in patients who are immunocompromised or in locations where patients are exposed to these infections. The drugs used in these more serious infections can be quite toxic and cause adverse effects that impact rehabilitation procedures. This discussion will therefore acquaint physical therapists and occupational therapists with these infections and will address the positive and negative aspects of the chemotherapeutic techniques and agents administered to treat these problems.

ANTIFUNGAL AGENTS

Fungi are plantlike microorganisms that exist ubiquitously throughout the soil and air and in plants and animals. Fungi are abundant in nature (over 200,000 species have been identified), and approximately 200 species can cause infections in humans.[4,5] A disease caused by fungal infection is also referred to as a **mycosis**. Some fungal infections are relatively local or superficial, affecting cutaneous and mucocutaneous tissue. Examples of common superficial fungal infections include the tinea (ringworm) infections that cause problems such as athlete's foot. Common mucocutaneous fungal infections include candidiasis and yeast infections of vaginal tissues. Other fungal infections are deeper or more systemic. For instance, fungal infections may affect the lungs, central nervous system (CNS), or other tissues and organs throughout the body.[6-8]

Often, fungal infections are relatively innocuous because they can be destroyed by the body's normal immune defense mechanisms. However, some infections require pharmacological treatment, especially if the patient's endogenous defense mechanisms are compromised in some way. For instance, patients undergoing immunosuppressive drug treatment (see Chapter 37) or receiving other anti-infectious drugs may develop systemic fungal infections. In addition, diseases that attack the immune system, such as AIDS, leave the patient vulnerable to severe fungal infections (see Chapter 34). Fungal infections that are relatively easy to treat in the immunocompetent person may become invasive and life-threatening in those who lack adequate immune function.[6,9] Hence, there is a significant need for effective systemic antifungal agents in specific high-risk patients.

Certain drugs can be administered systemically to treat common fungal infections in various tissues (Table 35-1). Other agents are more toxic; their use is limited to local or topical application for fungal infections in the skin and mucous membranes (Table 35-2). Antifungal drugs typically impair fungal cells by disrupting membrane function, impairing RNA and protein synthesis, or inhibiting mitosis (Fig. 35-1). The use of systemic and topical antifungal agents is addressed in more detail in the following sections.

Table 35-1
USE OF SYSTEMIC ANTIFUNGAL AGENTS IN INVASIVE AND DISSEMINATED MYCOSES*

Type of Infection	Principal Sites of Infection	Principal Agent(s)	Secondary/Alternative Agent(s)
Aspergillosis	Lungs, other organs, body orifices	Voriconazole, amphotericin B	Caspofungin, itraconazole
Blastomycosis	Lungs, skin; may disseminate to other tissues	Amphotericin B	Itraconazole, ketoconazole
Candidiasis	Intestinal tract, skin, mucous membranes (mouth, pharynx, vagina)	Amphotericin B, fluconazole, voriconazole	Caspofungin, anidulafungin, micafungin, ketoconazole
Coccidioidomycosis	Lungs, skin, subcutaneous tissues; may form disseminated lesions throughout the body	Fluconazole, itraconazole	Amphotericin B
Cryptococcosis	Lungs, meninges, other tissues	Amphotericin B, fluconazole	Flucytosine, itraconazole
Histoplasmosis	Lungs, spleen	Amphotericin B, itraconazole	Ketoconazole
Tinea (ringworm) infections	Skin, subcutaneous tissues	Griseofulvin, itraconazole, terbinafine	Fluconazole, ketoconazole

**Drugs indicated here are administered systemically (orally, intravenously) to treat widespread or invasive fungal infections. Some of these agents are also available in topical preparations, especially in the treatment of candidiasis and tinea infections in the skin and mucocutaneous tissues. Selection of a specific drug or preparation will also depend on patient-specific factors, such as immune function, age, pregnancy, and identification of resistant fungal species.*

Table 35-2
TOPICAL ANTIFUNGALS

Generic Name	Trade Name	Type of Preparation	Primary Indication(s)
Azoles			
Butoconazole	Gynezole-1; Mycelex-3	Vaginal cream	Vulvovaginal candidiasis
Clotrimazole	Gyne-Lotrimin; FemCare; others	Vaginal cream; vaginal tablets	Vulvovaginal candidiasis
	Mycelex Troches	Lozenges	Oropharyngeal candidiasis
	Cruex; Lotriderm; others	Cream; solution	Cutaneous candidiasis, tinea (ringworm) infections
Econazole	Spectazole	Cream	Cutaneous candidiasis, tinea (ringworm) infections

Table 35-2
TOPICAL ANTIFUNGALS—cont'd

Generic Name	Trade Name	Type of Preparation	Primary Indication(s)
Miconazole	Monistat; Vagistat-3	Vaginal cream; vaginal suppositories	Vulvovaginal candidiasis
	Micazole; Monistat-Derm; others	Cream; lotion; powder; ointment; solution	Cutaneous candidiasis, tinea (ringworm) infections
Oxiconazole	Oxistat	Cream; lotion	Tinea (ringworm) infections
Sulconazole	Exelderm	Cream; solution	Tinea (ringworm) infections
Terconazole	Terazol	Vaginal cream; vaginal suppositories	Vulvovaginal candidiasis
Tioconazole	Monistat 1 Day; Vagistat-1	Vaginal ointment	Vulvovaginal candidiasis
Other Topical Agents			
Butenafine	Lotrimin Ultra; Mentax	Cream	Tinea (ringworm) infections
Ciclopirox	Loprox, Penlac, others	Cream; lotion; gel; shampoo; nail lacquer	Tinea (ringworm) infections; onychomycosis
Naftifine	Naftin	Cream; gel	Tinea (ringworm) infections
Nystatin	Mycostatin; Nilstat; others	Lozenges; oral suspension; tablets	Oropharyngeal candidiasis
	Mycostatin; Nyaderm; Nystop	Cream; ointment; powder	Cutaneous and mucocutaneous candidiasis
	Mycostatin	Vaginal tablets	Vulvovaginal candidiasis
Sertaconazole	Ertaczo	Cream	Tinea pedis
Tolnaftate	Podactin; Tinactin; others	Aerosol powder; aerosol solution; cream; powder; solution	Tinea (ringworm) infections

Note: Drugs listed here are only available in topical or local preparations. Certain systemic agents listed in Table 35-1 can also be applied locally to treat various superficial fungal infections.

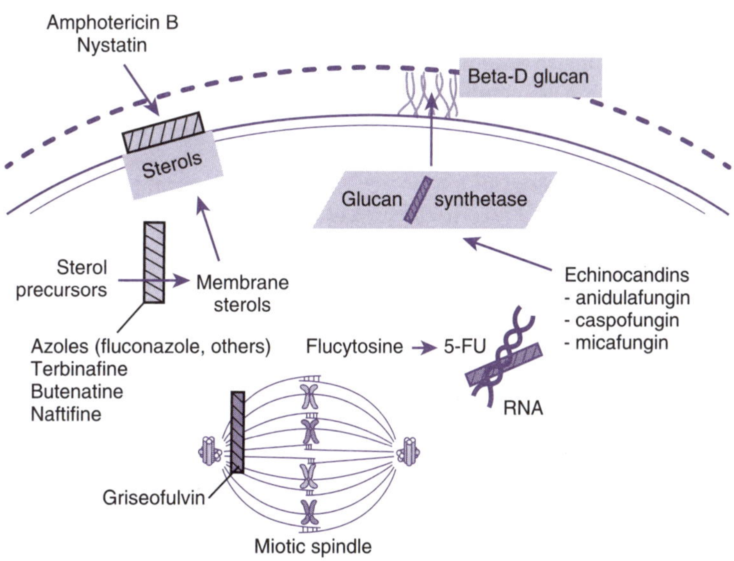

Figure ■ 35-1
Mechanism of action of primary antifungal drugs. Amphotericin B and nystatin bind to membrane sterols and disrupt the integrity and function of the fungal cell membrane. Azole drugs, terbinafine, and similar drugs inhibit enzymes responsible for membrane sterol synthesis. Echinocandins inhibit the synthesis of beta-d-glucan polysaccharides that support the fungal cell membrane. Flucytosine is converted to 5-fluorouracil (5-FU), which is then incorporated into fungal RNA, where it disrupts protein synthesis. Griseofulvin binds to the mitotic spindle to impair fungal cell division.

Systemic Antifungal Agents

The antifungal agents that can be administered systemically by oral or intravenous routes are often used to treat invasive (deep) fungal infections in the body. They can also be administered systemically to treat more superficial infections that have disseminated over a large area of the skin or subcutaneous tissues. The clinical use, mechanism of action, and potential adverse effects of these drugs are addressed here.

Amphotericin B

Clinical Use. Amphotericin B (Amphocin, Fungizone) is one of the primary drugs used to treat severe systemic fungal infections.[10] This drug is often chosen to treat the systemic infections and meningitis caused by *Candida*, *Cryptococcus*, and several other species of pathogenic fungi (see Table 35-1). Amphotericin is also effective against certain protozoal infections such as leishmaniasis.[11] Typically, this drug is administered by slow IV infusion. Local and topical administration may also be used to treat limited infections caused by susceptible fungi.

Several newer forms of amphotericin B (Abelcet, AmBisome, Amphotec) are encapsulated in small lipid spheres (liposomes) and then injected slowly by IV infusion.[12,13] The lipid-based preparations appear to deliver higher doses of amphotericin B to the site of fungal infections more directly than the older forms.[13] Clinical studies suggest that these lipid forms can therefore be used to treat serious fungal infections while reducing the risk of nephrotoxicity and other side effects.[13,14]

Mechanism of Action. Amphotericin B appears to work by binding to specific steroidlike lipids (sterols) located in the cell membrane of susceptible fungi.[15] This binding causes increased permeability in the cell membrane, leading to a leaky membrane and loss of cellular components.

Adverse Effects. The effectiveness of amphotericin B against serious systemic fungal infections is tempered somewhat by a high incidence of side effects.[13,16] Most patients experience problems such as headache, fever, muscle and joint pain, muscle weakness, and gastrointestinal (GI) distress (e.g., nausea, vomiting, stomach pain or cramping). As indicated, nephrotoxicity may also occur in some patients, but the use of the lipid-based formulations of this drug may reduce this risk. Considering the life-threatening nature of some fungal infections such as meningitis, certain side effects of amphotericin B must often be tolerated while the drug exerts its antifungal actions.

Fluconazole

Clinical Use. Fluconazole (Diflucan) can be administered orally to treat systemic and localized infections caused by the *Candida* species of fungus.[17,18] This drug, for example, can be used in disseminated candida infections in the bloodstream and in infections in the oropharyngeal region, vulvovaginal area, finger/toenail beds (onychomycosis), and other localized sites, including deep candida infections in bone and other structures.[19-21] Fluconazole can also be used to prevent candida infections in premature infants who are at risk for developing systemic fungal infections.[22] Fluconazole is effective in treating other mycoses such as cryptococcal meningitis and may help prevent recurrence of cryptococcal infections in patients with AIDS. Fluconazole is somewhat less toxic than more traditional agents such as amphotericin B and can be administered orally, which is an advantage over amphotericin B.

However, fluconazole may not be as effective as other antifungals in treating certain types of deep, systemic fungal infections in severely ill patients.[23] Hence, this drug remains a standard for the prevention and treatment of uncomplicated candida infections, but other agents may need to be considered in certain patients or if fungal resistance to fluconazole has been identified.[18,24]

Mechanism of Action. Fluconazole and similar agents (itraconazole, ketoconazole) inhibit certain enzymes in fungal cells that are responsible for the synthesis of important sterols.[25,26] A deficiency of these sterols results in impaired membrane function and other metabolic abnormalities within the fungal cell. Fluconazole also directly damages the fungal membrane by destroying certain membrane components such as triglycerides and phospholipids. Loss of normal membrane structure and function results in the destruction of the fungus.

Adverse Effects. Hepatotoxicity is the most serious adverse effect of fluconazole; this drug should be used cautiously in patients with impaired liver function. Some patients may also exhibit severe skin reactions, including exfoliative dermatitis and Stevens-Johnson syndrome. Other common side effects include headache and GI disturbances (e.g., abdominal pain, nausea, vomiting).

Flucytosine

Clinical Use. The antifungal spectrum of flucytosine (Ancobon) is limited primarily to the *Candida* and *Cryptococcus* species.[4] This drug is used systemically to treat endocarditis, urinary tract infections, and the presence of fungi in the bloodstream (fungemia) during candidiasis. Flucytosine is also beneficial for treating meningitis and severe pulmonary infections caused by *cryptococcosis*. This drug is often combined with amphotericin B to provide optimal effects and to decrease the chance of fungal resistance.[27]

Mechanism of Action. Flucytosine is incorporated into susceptible fungi, where it undergoes enzymatic conversion to fluorouracil,[4] which acts as an antimetabolite during RNA synthesis in the fungus. Fluorouracil is incorporated into RNA chains but acts as a false nucleic acid. This event ultimately impairs protein synthesis, thus disrupting the normal function of the fungus.

Adverse Effects. Flucytosine may cause hepatotoxicity and may also impair bone marrow function, resulting in anemia, leukopenia, and several other blood dyscrasias.[28] This drug may also produce severe GI disturbances, including nausea, vomiting, diarrhea, and loss of appetite.

Griseofulvin

Clinical Use. Griseofulvin (Fulvicin, Grisactin, others) is used primarily in the treatment of common fungal infections of the skin known as tinea, or ringworm.[29,30] For example, individuals take this drug to treat fungal infections of the feet (tinea pedis, or "athlete's foot"), infections in the groin area (tinea cruris, or "jock rash"), and similar infections of the skin, nails, and scalp. Griseofulvin is administered orally.

Mechanism of Action. Griseofulvin enters susceptible fungal cells and binds to the mitotic spindle during cell division.[31] This binding impairs the mitotic process, thus directly inhibiting the ability of the cell to replicate itself.

Adverse Effects. Common side effects of griseofulvin include headaches—which may be severe—and GI disturbances (e.g., nausea, vomiting, diarrhea). Some individuals may exhibit hypersensitivity to this drug, as evidenced by skin rashes. Skin photosensitivity (increased reaction to ultraviolet light) may also occur.

Itraconazole

Clinical Use. Itraconazole (Sporanox) is an azole antifungal agent that is effective against many systemic fungal infections.[32] For example, this drug is used to treat blastomycosis and histoplasmosis infections in the lungs and other tissues, especially in patients with a compromised immune system.[33,34] Itraconazole may also be used as the primary or alternative treatment for other fungal infections, such as aspergillosis, chromomycosis, coccidioidomycosis, and various infections caused by the *Candida* species. Like fluconazole, itraconazole can be administered orally and can be given intravenously in severe systemic infections.[32]

Mechanism of Action. Itraconazole works like fluconazole and similar azoles. These drugs disrupt membrane function of the fungal cell by inhibiting the synthesis of key membrane components such as sterols and by directly damaging other membrane components such as phospholipids. Impaired membrane function leads to metabolic abnormalities and subsequent death of the fungal cell.

Adverse Effects. Side effects associated with itraconazole include headache, GI disturbances (nausea, vomiting), and skin rash.

Ketoconazole

Clinical Use. Ketoconazole (Nizoral) is effective against a variety of superficial and deep fungal infections, but toxic effects limit the systemic use of this drug (see below).[4] Nonetheless, it can be administered orally to selected patients to treat pulmonary and systemic infections in candidiasis, coccidioidomycosis, histoplasmosis, and several other types of deep fungal infections. Oral administration is sometimes used to treat tinea infections of the skin, scalp, and other body areas. Ketoconazole, however, is available in topical preparations, and its primary use is the treatment of tinea infections and other relatively localized infections, including certain vaginal infections. This drug also inhibits several enzymes responsible for steroid biosynthesis, and high doses may be used to suppress adrenocortical hormone production in Cushing's disease (see Chapter 29).

Mechanism of Action. Ketoconazole selectively inhibits certain enzymes that are responsible for the synthesis of important sterols in fungal cells.[35] A deficiency of sterols results in impaired membrane function and other metabolic abnormalities within the fungal cell. At higher concentrations, ketoconazole may also directly disrupt the cell membrane, resulting in the destruction of the fungus.

Adverse Effects. GI disturbances (e.g., nausea, vomiting, stomach pain) are the most common adverse effects when ketoconazole is administered systemically. Some degree of hepatotoxicity may occur, and severe or even fatal hepatitis has been reported on rare occasions. In large, prolonged dosages, this drug may also impair testosterone and adrenocorticosteroid synthesis, resulting in breast tenderness and enlargement (gynecomastia) and decreased sex drive in some men. Because of these side effects, other drugs such as itraconazole have largely replaced systemic use of ketoconazole.

Echinocandins

Clinical Use. Echinocandins comprise a relatively new group of antifungals that includes drugs such as anidulafungin (Eraxis), caspofungin (Cancidas), and micafungin (Mycamine).[36,37] These drugs are administered intravenously to treat severe esophageal and abdominal infections caused by *Candida*. Physicians also administer caspofungin to treat patients with systemic aspergillosis infections who cannot tolerate other drugs, such as amphotericin B or fluconazole.[38] Other echinocandin drugs are currently being developed, and their use may be expanded in the future if newer agents reach the market.

Mechanism of Action. These drugs inhibit the glucan synthase enzyme that is responsible for the biosynthesis of beta-D-glucan—a component of the fungal cell membrane.[37] Loss of this membrane component disrupts the integrity of the fungal cell wall, resulting in death of the fungus.

Adverse Effects. Primary side effects of caspofungin and micafungin include GI disturbances (e.g., nausea, vomiting) and headache. Severe allergic reactions (anaphylaxis) can also occur in rare incidences. Anidulafungin is associated with diarrhea, dyspnea, hypotension, and skin reactions (rash, hives). Some local irritation may also occur at the injection site when these drugs are administered intravenously.

Terbinafine

Clinical Use. Terbinafine (Lamisil) is effective against a broad spectrum of fungi and can be administered systemically to treat various fungal infections in the toenails and fingernails (onychomycosis).[39] Oral administration of this drug may also be useful in treating ringworm infections such as tinea corporis, tinea capitis (ringworm of the scalp), and tinea cruris, especially if these infections do not respond to topical treatment. Terbinafine is likewise available in creams and solutions for topical treatment of various tinea infections, including tinea pedis and tinea versicolor.

Mechanism of Action. Terbinafine inhibits a specific enzyme (squalene epoxidase) that is responsible for sterol synthesis in the fungal cell membrane. This action impairs cell wall synthesis, with subsequent loss of cell membrane function and integrity. Inhibition of this enzyme causes squalene to accumulate in the fungal cell, which can also impair cell function and lead to death of the fungus.

Adverse Effects. Systemic administration of terbinafine may cause a hypersensitivity reaction (e.g., skin rashes, itching) and GI problems such as nausea, vomiting, and diarrhea. This drug may also cause a change or loss of taste, an effect that may last several weeks after the drug is discontinued. Topical administration is generally well tolerated, although signs of local irritation (e.g., itching, redness, peeling skin) may indicate a need to discontinue this drug.

Voriconazole

Clinical Use. Voriconazole (Vfend) is similar chemically to other azole antifungals such as fluconazole. This drug has a broad antifungal spectrum and is administered systemically to treat aspergillosis and other serious fungal infections caused by *Scedosporium apiospermum* and *Fusarium*.[40]

Mechanism of Action. Voriconazole inhibits sterol biosynthesis in fungal cell membranes.[26] That is, this drug acts like fluconazole and similar agents to impair membrane synthesis, which results in membrane integrity loss and death of the fungal cell.

Adverse Effects. Skin rashes and vision disturbances (e.g., blurred vision, seeing bright spots) are common during voriconazole administration, but these side effects are usually transient and fairly uneventful. Serious problems, such as liver toxicity and cardiac arrhythmias, may occur in susceptible patients.

Topical Antifungal Agents

As mentioned earlier, certain antifungals are too toxic to be administered systemically. However, patients can apply these drugs topically to treat fungal infections in the skin (dermatophytosis), including tinea infections such as tinea pedis and tinea cruris.[29,41] These drugs can also be applied locally to treat *Candida* infections in the mucous membranes of the mouth, pharynx, and vagina. The primary topical antifungals are listed in Table 35-2 and are addressed briefly below.

Topical Azole Antifungals

Clinical Use. Azole antifungals that are administered topically include clotrimazole, miconazole, and other topical agents (see Table 35-2). These drugs are related to the systemic azoles (fluconazole, itraconazole, ketoconazole; see earlier) and share a common chemical background, mechanism of action, and antifungal spectrum. The topical azoles, however, are too toxic for systemic use and are therefore restricted to local application. Nonetheless, these drugs are valuable in controlling fungal infections in the skin and mucocutaneous tissues (see Table 35-2). For example, azoles such as butoconazole, clotrimazole, miconazole, terconazole, and tioconazole can be applied via creams, ointments, and suppositories to treat vaginal *Candida* infections. Other agents such as econazole, oxiconazole, and sulconazole can be applied via creams, solutions, or powders to treat tinea infections that cause athlete's foot (tinea pedis) and jock rash (tinea cruris). Certain azoles can also be applied locally via lozenges or elixirs (syrups) to treat oral candidiasis infections that occur in patients with a compromised immune system (see Table 35-2). Hence, these agents are beneficial for treating local mycoses that occur in a variety of clinical situations.

Mechanism of Action. Like the systemic azoles, clotrimazole and other topical antifungal azoles work by inhibiting the synthesis of key components of the fungal cell membrane—that is, these drugs impair production of membrane sterols, triglycerides, and phospholipids.[25] Loss of these components results in the membrane's inability to maintain intracellular homeostasis, leading to death of the fungus.

Adverse Effects. There are relatively few side effects when these drugs are applied locally. GI distress (e.g., cramps, diarrhea, vomiting) can occur if azole lozenges are swallowed. Other problems associated with topical use include local burning or irritation of the skin or mucous membranes.

Other Topical Agents

Clinical Use. Other topical antifungals include butenafine (Mentax), ciclopirox (Lorox, others), naftifine (Naftin), tolnaftate (Aftate, Tinactin, others), and nystatin (Mycostatin, Nilstat, others) (see Table 35-2). Nystatin has a wide spectrum of activity against various fungi but is not used to treat systemic infections because it is not absorbed from the GI tract. Therefore, nystatin is administered via several topical preparations to treat cutaneous, oropharyngeal, or vaginal candidiasis. Topical and local (oropharyngeal) use of nystatin is especially important in treating candidiasis in immunocompromised patients, including those with AIDS.[42]

Topical naftifine, tolnaftate, ciclopirox, and butenafine are used primarily to treat local and superficial cases of tinea infection such as tinea pedis and tinea cruris. These agents are found in several over-the-counter products.

Mechanism of Action. Nystatin exerts its antifungal effects in a manner similar to that of amphotericin B—that is, it binds to sterols in the cell membrane, which causes an increase in membrane permeability and a loss of cellular homeostasis. Naftifine and butenafine inhibit a fungal enzyme (squalene epoxidase) that is responsible for the synthesis of a key membrane component (ergosterol), resulting in the loss of membrane integrity and death of the fungus. Ciclopirox impairs several aspects of DNA, RNA, and protein synthesis in the fungal cell, probably by inhibiting specific aspects of intracellular transport and signaling. Tolnaftate appears to stunt the growth of fungal cell bodies, but the exact mechanism of this drug is unknown.

Adverse Effects. Nystatin is generally well tolerated when applied locally. Systemic absorption through mucous membranes may cause some GI disturbances (e.g., nausea, vomiting, diarrhea), but these side effects are generally mild and transient. Topical use of butenafine, ciclopirox, naftifine, and tolnaftate is likewise safe, although local burning and irritation of the skin may occur in some individuals.

ANTIPROTOZOAL AGENTS

Protozoa are single-celled organisms that represent the lowest division of the animal kingdom. Several thousand species of protozoa exist in nature, and certain protozoa pose a serious threat of parasitic infection in humans.[43]

Malaria is a relatively common disease caused by protozoal infection; its source is one of several species of a parasite known as *plasmodia*. Although this disease has been virtually eliminated in North America and Europe, malaria remains a primary health problem throughout many other parts of the world.[44] Individuals who live in these areas, as well as those traveling to parts of the world where malaria is prevalent, must often undergo antimalarial chemotherapy. Hence, drugs that prevent and treat malaria are extremely important.

In addition to malaria, several other serious infections may occur in humans due to parasitic invasion by protozoa.[45] Severe intestinal infections produced by various protozoa (e.g., dysentery) occur quite frequently, especially in areas where contaminated food and drinking water are prevalent. Protozoal infestation may also cause infections in tissues such as the liver, heart, lungs, brain, and other organs. Individuals with a compromised immune system may be especially susceptible to these intestinal and extraintestinal infections.[2,46,47]

The primary agents used to treat protozoal infections are listed in Tables 35-3 and 35-4. The drugs that are primarily used to treat and prevent malaria are discussed first, followed by drugs that are used to treat other types of protozoal infections (intestinal and extraintestinal infections).

Antimalarial Agents

Chloroquine

Clinical Use. Historically, chloroquine (Aralen) has been one of the primary antimalarial drugs.[48] This drug provides a safe, effective, and relatively inexpensive method for treating malaria and is also administered routinely to individuals who are traveling to areas of the world where they may be exposed to malaria infection.[49] Resistance to this drug, however, has emerged in many regions where malaria is prevalent.[50] That is, the parasite that causes this disease (the *Plasmodium* amoeba) has developed mechanisms that render this drug ineffective. If individuals encounter these chloroquine-resistant strains, they must use other antimalarial drugs such as quinine or artemisinin derivatives (see Table 35-3).[50]

Chloroquine is also used for the treatment of conditions other than malaria. This drug is effective

Table 35-3
TREATMENT OF MALARIA

Plasmodium Species	Type of Infection or Resistance	Primary Agent(s)	Adjunctive/Alternative Agent(s)
P. malariae; P. falciparum	Chloroquine-sensitive	Chloroquine	—
P. vivax; P. ovale	Uncomplicated infections	Chloroquine followed by primaquine	Artemisinin derivatives
P. falciparum	Uncomplicated, chloroquine-resistant	Artemether plus lumefantrine (Coartem)	Mefloquine; quinine; atovaquone plus proguanil; other artemisinin combinations
P. falciparum	Complicated or severe	Quinidine or artemisinin derivatives	Mefloquine; Pyrimethamine-sulfadoxine; Antibacterials (e.g., clindamycin, doxycycline, or tetracycline)

Table 35-4
TREATMENT OF OTHER PROTOZOAL INFECTIONS

Type of Infection	Principal Site(s) of Infection	Primary Agent(s)	Alternative/Secondary Agent(s)
Amebiasis	Intestinal tract; liver; lungs	Metronidazole, tinidazole	Iodoquinol; antibacterials (paromomycin, tetracycline)
Balantidiasis	Lower GI tract	Tetracycline	Metronidazole
Giardiasis	Small intestine	Metronidazole, tinidazole	Albendazole; paromomycin; nitazoxanide
Leishmaniasis	Skin; mucocutaneous tissues; viscera	Amphotericin B, sodium stibogluconate	Pentamidine; paromomycin
Trichomoniasis	Vagina; genitourinary tract	Metronidazole	Tinidazole
Toxoplasmosis	Lymph nodes; many organs and tissues	Pyrimethamine-sulfadiazine (see antimalarial drugs); other antibacterials (clindamycin)	Trimethoprim-sulfamethoxazole ± another agent (azithromycin, clarithromycin, atovaquone, or dapsone)
Trypanosomiasis (Chagas disease; African sleeping sickness)	Heart; brain; many other organs	Early stages: pentamidine; suramin Later stages: melarsoprol	Nifurtimox

against other types of protozoal infections such as amebiasis and may be used with iodoquinol or emetine to treat infections in the liver and pericardium. As discussed in Chapter 16, chloroquine is effective in rheumatoid disease and is used in the treatment of conditions such as rheumatoid arthritis and systemic lupus erythematosus. However, the reasons why this antiprotozoal agent is also effective against rheumatoid disease are unclear. Chloroquine is administered orally.

Mechanism of Action. Although the exact mechanism is unknown, chloroquine may impair metabolic and digestive function in the protozoa by becoming concentrated within subcellular vacuoles and raising their pH.[51] This effect may inhibit the ability of the parasite to digest hemoglobin from the blood of the host erythrocytes. Impaired hemoglobin digestion leads to the accumulation of toxic heme by-products in the protozoa, which subsequently leads to its death.[51] Chloroquine may also bind directly to DNA within susceptible parasites and inhibit DNA/RNA function and subsequent protein synthesis. The ability to impair protein synthesis may contribute to the antiprotozoal actions of this drug.

Adverse Effects. The most serious problem associated with chloroquine is the possibility of toxicity to the retina and subsequent visual disturbances. This issue is usually insignificant, however, when this drug is used for short periods in relatively low doses (see Chapter 16). Other relatively mild side effects may occur, including GI distress (e.g., nausea, vomiting, stomach cramps, diarrhea), behavior and mood changes (e.g., irritability, confusion, nervousness, depression), and skin disorders (e.g., rashes, itching, discoloration).

Hydroxychloroquine

Hydroxychloroquine (Plaquenil) is derived chemically from chloroquine and is similar to it in clinical use, mechanism of action, and adverse effects. Hydroxychloroquine does not have any distinct therapeutic advantages over chloroquine, but it may be substituted in certain individuals who do not respond well to chloroquine.

Mefloquine

Clinical Use. Mefloquine (Lariam) has emerged as one of the most important antimalarial agents.[52] This drug is especially important in the prevention and treatment of malaria that is resistant to traditional antimalarial drugs, such as chloroquine and quinine.[53] Mefloquine is often the drug of choice for antimalarial prophylaxis, especially in areas of the world where chloroquine-resistant strains of malaria are common.[52] Mefloquine can be used alone, but combining this drug with other antimalarials such as an artemisinin derivative may provide more effective treatment against malaria.[54]

Mechanism of Action. Although the drug's exact mechanism of action is unknown, mefloquine may exert antimalarial effects similar to chloroquine—that is, it inhibits hemoglobin digestion in malarial parasites, thus causing heme by-products to accumulate to toxic levels within the protozoa and cause its death.[51]

Adverse Effects. Mefloquine is safe and well tolerated when used at moderate doses to prevent malarial infection. At higher doses, such as those used to treat infection, mefloquine may cause dizziness, headache, fever, joint and muscle pain, and GI problems (e.g., abdominal pain, nausea, vomiting, diarrhea). These side effects, however, may be difficult to distinguish from the symptoms associated with malaria. Although rare, neuropsychiatric symptoms such as confusion, psychosis, and seizures may occur, especially when this drug is used at higher dosages for prolonged periods.[52]

Primaquine

Clinical Use. Primaquine is typically used to treat the relapses of specific forms of malaria[55] and is generally administered in acute or severe exacerbations or when other drugs (chloroquine, mefloquine) are ineffective in suppressing malarial attacks. Primaquine may also be used to fully eradicate any hidden (latent) plasmodium parasites and prevent the onset of malaria in individuals who are especially at risk because of prolonged exposure to the disease.[56] This drug is administered orally.

Mechanism of Action. Primaquine appears to impair DNA function in susceptible parasites. The exact manner in which this occurs is unknown.

Adverse Effects. GI distress (e.g., nausea, vomiting, abdominal pain), headache, and visual disturbances may occur during primaquine therapy. A more serious side effect, acute hemolytic anemia, may occur in patients who have a specific deficiency in the glucose-6-phosphate dehydrogenase enzyme. This enzymatic deficiency is genetic and is more common in certain individuals of African, Mediterranean, and Asian descent; hence there is an increased risk of hemolytic anemia in these groups.[57] People with specific cases of this enzyme deficiency should be identified so that alternative antimalarial drugs can be used.[58]

Pyrimethamine

Clinical Use. When used alone, pyrimethamine (Daraprim) is only of minor use in treating and preventing malaria. However, its antimalarial effectiveness is increased dramatically by combining it with the antibacterial drug sulfadoxine.[59] The combination of these two drugs (known commercially as Fansidar) has been used to prevent or treat certain forms of chloroquine-resistant malaria (see Table 35-3).[60] Regrettably, resistance to pyrimethamine/sulfadoxine treatment has also increased to the point where this drug combination is no longer effective for the routine treatment of malaria in many areas.[61] Still, intermittent doses of pyrimethamine/sulfadoxine can be given to pregnant women in parts of Africa. This treatment may reduce the risk of the mother contracting malaria, thus improving birth weight and infant survival in the newborn child.[62]

Pyrimethamine/sulfadoxine may also be combined with other antimalarials such as artemisinin derivatives, but these regimens should only be used if the malarial parasites are not resistant to the specific drugs in the regimen.[63] Pyrimethamine can also be combined with a sulfonamide drug such as dapsone, sulfadiazine, or sulfamethoxazole to treat protozoal infections that cause toxoplasmosis or fungal infections that cause *Pneumocystis* pneumonia. These agents are administered orally.

Mechanism of Action. Pyrimethamine blocks the production of folic acid in susceptible protozoa by inhibiting the function of the dihydrofolate reductase enzyme. Folic acid helps catalyze the production of nucleic and amino acids in these parasites. Therefore, this drug ultimately impairs nucleic acid and protein synthesis by interfering with folic acid production. The action of sulfadoxine and other sulfonamide antibacterial agents was discussed in Chapter 33. These agents also inhibit folic acid synthesis in certain bacterial and protozoal cells.

Adverse Effects. The incidence and severity of side effects from pyrimethamine-sulfadoxine are related to the dosage and duration of therapy. Toxicity is fairly common when these drugs are given in high dosages for prolonged periods, and adverse effects include GI disturbances (e.g., vomiting, stomach cramps, loss of appetite), blood dyscrasias (e.g., agranulocytosis, leukopenia, thrombocytopenia), CNS abnormalities (e.g., tremors, ataxia, seizures), and hypersensitivity reactions (e.g., skin rashes, anaphylaxis, liver dysfunction). As indicated above, resistance may also occur during repeated use, and this drug strategy may be ineffective in certain strains of malaria that have already developed resistant mechanisms. Hence, pyrimethamine-sulfadoxine is usually administered on a very limited basis, such as a single dose at the onset of malarial symptoms or intermittent doses to prevent malaria in pregnant women.

Quinine

Clinical Use. Quinine is one of the oldest forms of antimalarial chemotherapy; people were obtaining the drug from the bark of certain South American trees as early as the 1600s.[64] Although quinine was the principal method of preventing and treating malaria for many years, the use of this drug has diminished somewhat because it is relatively toxic and expensive to produce.[60] Hence, quinine, as a routine drug, has largely been replaced by newer, safer agents such as mefloquine and artemisinin derivatives. Quinine, however, remains one of the most effective antimalarial drugs, and it is currently used to treat severe malaria that is resistant to other drugs.[64] Quinine sulfate is administered orally, and quinine dihydrochloride is administered by slow IV infusion.

Mechanism of Action. The exact mechanism of quinine is not known. This drug probably exerts antimalarial effects similar to those of chloroquine—that is, inhibition of hemoglobin digestion and subsequent accumulation of toxic heme by-products that lead to death in susceptible protozoa.[65]

Adverse Effects. Quinine is associated with many adverse effects involving several primary organ systems. This drug may produce disturbances in the CNS (e.g., headache, visual disturbances, ringing in the ears), GI system (e.g., nausea, vomiting, abdominal pain), and cardiovascular system (e.g., cardiac arrhythmias). Problems with hypersensitivity, blood disorders, liver dysfunction, and hypoglycemia may also occur in some individuals.

Other Antimalarials: Use of Artemisinin Derivatives

Clinical Use. Artemisinin derivatives are naturally occurring compounds that appear to be effective against many forms of the protozoa that cause malaria.[66] These drugs consist of the parent compound (artemisinin) and several products that can be synthesized from artemisinin such as artesunate, artemether, and dihydroartemisinin.[67] These agents are all structurally similar; hence, we can use the term *artemisinin derivative* to collectively describe this group.[60] However, used alone, these agents are ineffective in completely eliminating the *Plasmodium* parasite. Their antimalarial effects, however, are greatly increased by combining an artemisinin drug with a "partner" drug such as mefloquine, piperaquine, lumefantrine, or pyrimethamine/sulfadoxine (see Table 35-3). This strategy, known commonly as *artemisinin-based combination therapy* (ACT), is one of the primary methods for treating malaria throughout the world.[68,69] However, resistance to artemisinin derivatives and ACTs has started to emerge in some areas, and there is concern that this treatment will be rendered ineffective if resistance becomes more widespread.[50,70] Still, at the present time, ACT remains a common strategy that physicians use to treat malaria. Researchers are continuing their efforts to develop new artemisinin derivatives and explore specific drug combinations that prevent or overcome resistant forms of malaria.

Mechanism of Action. Although there is considerable debate about the exact way that artemisinin derivatives affect protozoal cells, these drugs appear to work by a two-step process occurring within the malarial parasite.[71] In the first step, the drug is activated when it is cleaved by the heme-iron component within the protozoa. This cleavage forms a highly reactive free radical that, in the second step, reacts with and destroys essential protozoal proteins, including mitochondrial enzymes and ion transport proteins.[72] Destruction of these proteins results in the loss of cellular function and subsequent death of the protozoa.

Adverse Effects. Artemisinin derivatives and their use in ACTs appear to be relatively safe. There are some concerns that these drugs can be neurotoxic, but much of the information about neurotoxicity and other adverse effects has been obtained from animal studies.[73] Large-scale human studies on drug toxicity have generally been favorable, but it is sometimes difficult to differentiate drug-related side effects from the symptoms of severe malaria.[60] Hence, efforts continue to identify possible adverse reactions when these drugs are used for the long-term control of malaria and their level of safety when used in specific populations, such as children and pregnant women.[74,75]

Drugs Used to Treat Protozoal Infections in the Intestines and Other Tissues

Atovaquone

Clinical Use. Atovaquone (Mepron) is used primarily to treat the protozoon that causes toxoplasmosis and the fungus that causes pneumocystis pneumonia in immunocompromised patients.[76,77] This drug is not typically the primary treatment for pneumocystis but is often reserved for patients who cannot tolerate more traditional treatments using sulfamethoxazole and trimethoprim (see Chapter 34) or pentamidine (see later in this section). Atovaquone can also be used to prevent and treat certain cases of malaria, and its antimalarial effects seem especially useful when combined with proguanil.[78]

Mechanism of Action. Atovaquone appears to selectively inhibit electron transport in susceptible microorganisms.[79] This inhibition directly decreases production of ATP in the microorganism and may interfere with nucleic acid synthesis, ultimately resulting in death of the parasite.

Adverse Effects. Atovaquone may cause side effects such as fever, skin rash, cough, headache, and GI problems (e.g., nausea, vomiting, diarrhea).

Iodoquinol

Clinical Use. Iodoquinol (Diquinol, Yodoxin, others) is used primarily to treat protozoal infections within the intestinal tract,[80] and it is often combined with a second tissue amebicide, which kills protozoa at extraintestinal sites. For instance, iodoquinol may be combined with metronidazole to ensure the destruction of parasites throughout the body. Iodoquinol is usually administered orally. Because iodoquinol is relatively toxic, the routine use of this drug has been replaced somewhat by other agents such as paromomycin, which may be a bit safer.

Mechanism of Action. The mechanism of action of iodoquinol as an amebicide is unknown.

Adverse Effects. Iodoquinol is neurotoxic and may produce optic and peripheral neuropathies when administered in large dosages for prolonged periods. Problems with muscle weakness and ataxia may also occur because of the neurotoxic effects of this drug. Other adverse effects include GI distress (e.g., nausea, vomiting, cramps) and various skin reactions (e.g., rashes, itching, discoloration), but these effects are relatively mild and transient.

Metronidazole and Tinidazole

Clinical Use. Metronidazole (Flagyl, Protostat, others) is effective against a broad spectrum of protozoa and is often the primary agent used against protozoal infections in intestinal and extraintestinal tissues.[81] Metronidazole is often the drug of choice for treating several intestinal infections (e.g.., amebiasis, giardiasis) and amebic abscesses in other tissues such as the liver. Metronidazole is also the primary drug used to treat trichomoniasis, a sexually transmitted protozoal disease affecting the vagina and male genitourinary tract.[81]

As indicated in Chapter 33, metronidazole has bactericidal effects and is used in certain gram-negative bacterial infections. This drug may be administered orally or intravenously. Other agents are available that are structurally and functionally similar to metronidazole. Tinidazole (Tindamax), for example, can be used in cases where metronidazole is not tolerated or is ineffective.[82]

Mechanism of Action. The exact mechanism of action of metronidazole and tinidazole is not known. It is believed that these drugs are reduced chemically within the parasitic cell to a metabolite that impairs nucleic acid and DNA synthesis.[45] The exact nature of this metabolite and other features of its cytotoxic effects remain to be determined.

Adverse Effects. GI disturbances, including nausea, vomiting, diarrhea, stomach pain, and an unpleasant taste in the mouth, are relatively common with metronidazole and tinidazole. Other adverse effects such as hypersensitivity reactions, peripheral neuropathy, hematologic abnormalities, and genitourinary problems have been reported, but their incidence is relatively low.

Nitazoxanide

Clinical Use. Nitazoxanide (Alinia) is used primarily to treat diarrhea caused by intestinal *Cryptosporidium* and *Giardia* infections.[83] This drug is administered orally and is approved for use in adults and children aged 1 or older.

Mechanism of Action. Nitazoxanide appears to inhibit electron transport in susceptible protozoa, thus inhibiting energy metabolism in these parasites. This drug may have other antiprotozoal effects that remain to be determined.

Adverse Effects. This drug is generally well tolerated. GI disturbances (e.g., vomiting, diarrhea) and headache have been reported, but these effects may be due to the intestinal infection rather than the drug.

Paromomycin

Clinical Use. Paromomycin (Humatin) is an aminoglycoside antibacterial (see Chapter 33) that is used primarily to treat mild to moderate intestinal infections (amebiasis).[82] This drug may also be used as an adjunct to other amebicides during the treatment of more severe protozoal infections. Paromomycin is also effective against some bacteria and tapeworms and may be used as a secondary agent in certain bacterial or helminthic infections. This drug is administered orally.

Mechanism of Action. Paromomycin acts selectively on protozoa within the intestinal lumen and destroys these parasites by a direct toxic effect.

Adverse Effects. Paromomycin is not absorbed from the intestine to any great extent, so adverse effects are fairly limited. Nonetheless, problems with GI distress (e.g., nausea, vomiting, abdominal pain) may occur, as this drug exerts amebicidal effects within the intestine.

Pentamidine

Clinical Use. Pentamidine (NebuPent, Pentam, others) is effective against several types of extraintestinal protozoal infections, including certain forms of trypanosomiasis (African sleeping sickness) and visceral infections caused by *Leishmania* protozoa. Typically, pentamidine is reserved as a secondary agent in treating these infections and is used when the principal drug in each case is not available or is tolerated poorly (see Table 35-4). This drug is also effective in preventing or treating *Pneumocystis* infections in immunocompromised patients with HIV infection and AIDS.[76] Pentamidine is usually administered by slow IV infusion to treat *Pneumocystis* infections but can be administered by oral inhalation to prevent these infections in patients with decreased immune function.[84]

Mechanism of Action. The exact mechanism of this drug is not clear, and pentamidine may affect different parasites in different ways. Some possible antiprotozoal actions of this drug include the inhibition of protein and nucleic acid synthesis, cellular metabolism, and oxidative phosphorylation in susceptible parasites.

Adverse Effects. The primary adverse effect of systemic pentamidine administration is renal toxicity. Renal function may be markedly impaired in some patients, but kidney function usually returns to normal when the drug is withdrawn. Pentamidine is also associated with pancreatitis, although this problem may be due to the underlying HIV infection or other drugs used to manage HIV. Other adverse effects include hypotension, hypoglycemia, GI distress, blood dyscrasias (e.g., leukopenia, thrombocytopenia), and local pain and tenderness at the site of injection. Adverse effects are reduced substantially when the drug is given by inhalation, and this method of administration is desirable when pentamidine is used to prevent *Pneumocystis* pneumonia in patients with HIV.

Other Antiprotozoal Drugs

Several additional agents are available to treat intestinal and extraintestinal infections caused by various protozoa. These agents include melarsoprol, nifurtimox, sodium stibogluconate, and suramin. The use and distribution of these drugs, however, is quite different from the agents described previously. In the United States, these additional drugs are usually available only from the Centers for Disease Control and Prevention (CDC), in Atlanta, Georgia. At the request of the physician, the CDC dispenses the drug to the physician, who then provides the agent to the patient.

Clinical applications of individual drugs in this category are indicated in Table 35-4. In general, these drugs are reserved for some of the more serious or rare types of protozoal infections, which is why the CDC controls their distribution. As might be expected, adverse side effects of these drugs are quite common, but these agents may be lifesaving in some of the more severe infections. The references at the end of this chapter provide sources for more information about specific agents in this group.[4]

ANTHELMINTICS

Infection from helminths, or parasitic worms, is the most common form of disease in the world.[85,86] There are several types of worms that may invade and subsist from human tissues.[87] Common examples include tapeworms (cestodes), roundworms (nematodes), and flukes (trematodes).[43,87] Worms can enter the body by various routes but often are ingested as eggs in contaminated food and water. Once in the body, the eggs hatch, and adult worms ultimately lodge in various tissues, especially the digestive tract. Some types (e.g., flukes) may also lodge in blood vessels such as the hepatic portal vein. Depending on the species, adult worms may range from a few millimeters to several meters in length. The adult worms steal nutrients from their human host and may begin to obstruct the intestinal lumen or other ducts if they reproduce in sufficient numbers.

Some of the common **anthelmintics** used to kill the basic types of worms in humans are listed in Table 35-5. These agents are often very effective; a single oral dose is usually sufficient to selectively destroy the parasite. This section presents brief descriptions of the basic pharmacological effects and possible adverse effects of the primary anthelmintic agents. Several authors have also extensively reviewed the pharmacological treatment of helminthic infections.[85,88-90]

Albendazole

Albendazole (Albenza) is primarily used to treat infections caused by the larval form of certain

Table 35-5
TREATMENT OF COMMON HELMINTHIC INFECTIONS

Parasite	Primary Agent(s)	Secondary Agent(s)
Roundworms (Nematodes)		
Ascariasis (roundworm)	Albendazole; mebendazole; pyrantel pamoate	Ivermectin; piperazine citrate
Filariasis	Albendazole; diethylcarbamazine; ivermectin	—
Hookworm	Albendazole; mebendazole	Ivermectin; thiabendazole
Pinworm	Albendazole; mebendazole; pyrantel pamoate	—
Trichinosis	Albendazole; mebendazole	Thiabendazole
Tapeworms (Cestodes)		
Beef tapeworm	Niclosamide; praziquantel	Mebendazole
Pork tapeworm	Albendazole; praziquantel	Niclosamide
Fish tapeworm	Niclosamide; praziquantel	—
Flukes (Trematodes)		
Blood flukes	Praziquantel	Oxamniquine
Fluke infections in other organs	Praziquantel	—

cestodes (tapeworms). These infections often cause cysts (hydatid disease) in the liver, lungs, and other tissues; albendazole is used as an adjunct to the surgical removal of these cysts or as the primary treatment if these cysts are inoperable. This drug is also effective against many GI roundworms and hookworms and is typically used as a secondary agent if other anthelmintics are not effective in treating these infections.

Albendazole exerts its anthelmintic effects by acting on the intestinal cells of the parasitic worms and by inhibiting their glucose uptake and glycogen storage. This effect ultimately leads to lack of energy production, degeneration of intracellular components, and subsequent death of the parasite. Albendazole is usually well tolerated when used for short-term treatment of infections in GI or other tissues. Long-term treatment for conditions such as hydatid disease may result in abnormal liver function tests (e.g., increased serum aminotransferase activity); liver function should therefore be monitored periodically to prevent hepatotoxicity if the patient uses this drug for extended periods.

Diethylcarbamazine

Diethylcarbamazine (Hetrazan) is used to treat certain roundworm infections of the lymphatics and connective tissues, including loiasis, onchocerciasis, and *Bancroft filariasis*. This agent immobilizes immature roundworms (microfilariae) and facilitates the destruction of these microfilariae by the body's immune system. Diethylcarbamazine is also effective against the adult forms of certain roundworms, but the mechanism of this anthelmintic action against mature nematodes is not known.

Side effects associated with diethylcarbamazine include headache, malaise, weakness, and loss of appetite. More severe reactions (e.g., fever, acute inflammatory response) may also occur following diethylcarbamazine use, but these may be caused by the release of antigenic substances from the dying roundworms rather than from the drug itself.

Ivermectin

Ivermectin (Stromectol) is the primary treatment for filarial nematode infections (onchocerciasis) that invade ocular tissues and cause loss of vision (river blindness). Ivermectin may also be used in filarial infections in other tissues (e.g., lymphatics, skin). This drug is a secondary agent for treating intestinal nematodes such as strongyloidosis.

Ivermectin binds to chloride ion channels in parasitic nerve and muscle cells, thereby increasing membrane permeability to chloride. Increased intracellular chloride results in hyperpolarization of nerve and muscle tissues, which results in paralysis and death of the parasite. Ivermectin is well tolerated during short-term use in mild-to-moderate infections. Administration in more severe infections may cause swollen or tender lymph glands, fever, skin rash, itching, and joint and muscle pain, but these reactions may be caused by the death of the infectious parasites rather than by the drug itself.

Mebendazole

Mebendazole (Vermox) is effective against many types of roundworms and a few tapeworms that parasitize humans. Like albendazole, this drug selectively damages the worms' intestinal cells, thus inhibiting the uptake and intracellular transport of glucose and other nutrients into these parasites. This activity leads to the destruction of the epithelial lining and subsequent death of the parasite. Mebendazole is a relatively safe drug, although some mild, transient GI problems may occur.

Praziquantel

Praziquantel (Biltricide) is one of the most versatile and important anthelmintic agents and is the drug of choice in treating all major trematode (fluke) infections and several common types of tapeworm infections (see Table 35-5). This drug's exact mechanism of action is unknown. Praziquantel may stimulate muscular contraction of the parasite, resulting in a type of spastic paralysis, which causes the worm to lose its hold on intestinal or vascular tissue. At higher concentrations, this drug may initiate destructive changes in the integument of the worm, allowing the host defense mechanisms (e.g., enzymes, phagocytes) to destroy the parasite. Praziquantel is associated with several frequent side effects, including GI problems (e.g., abdominal pain, nausea, vomiting), CNS effects (e.g., headache, dizziness), and mild hepatotoxicity. These effects can usually be tolerated for the relatively short time that the drug is in effect.

Pyrantel Pamoate

Pyrantel pamoate (Antiminth, others) is one of the primary agents used in several types of roundworm and pinworm infections (see Table 35-5). This drug stimulates acetylcholine release and inhibits acetylcholine breakdown at the neuromuscular junction, thus producing a prolonged state of excitation and muscular contraction that causes spastic paralysis of the worm. The worm is unable to retain its hold on the intestinal tissue and can be expelled from the digestive tract by normal bowel movements. This drug is generally well tolerated, with only occasional problems of mild GI disturbances.

Thiabendazole

Thiabendazole (Mintezol) is often used in trichinosis and several other types of roundworm infections (see Table 35-5). The anthelmintic mechanism of this drug is not fully understood, but selective inhibition of certain key metabolic enzymes in susceptible parasites is probable. Although thiabendazole is quite effective, its use has declined somewhat in favor of less toxic agents such as mebendazole. The most common side effects associated with this drug involve GI distress, such as nausea, vomiting, loss of appetite. Allergic reactions (e.g., skin rash, itching, chills) may also occur in some individuals.

Other Anthelmintics

Several other agents such as niclosamide, oxamniquine, and piperazine have been used to treat helminth infections. These agents, however, are no longer available for use in humans in the United States and have generally been replaced by other drugs that are safer and more effective. These drugs may still be used in other countries, and some are reserved for use in veterinary settings. More information about these drugs can be found in other sources.[85,91]

Special Concerns for Rehabilitation Patients

The drugs discussed in this chapter are relevant because they relate largely to specific groups of patients that therapists will see in a rehabilitation setting. Therapists working in sports physical therapy may deal frequently with topical antifungal agents in the treatment of cutaneous ringworm infections. For instance, physical therapists and athletic trainers may be responsible for recognizing and helping treat tinea pedis, tinea cruris, and similar infections. Therapists and trainers can make sure the drugs are being applied in the proper fashion and as directed by the physician. Therapists may also play a crucial role in preventing the spread of these infections by educating athletes about how to prevent transmission among team members (e.g., not sharing towels and combs).

Physical therapists and occupational therapists working with patients who have AIDS will frequently encounter patients taking systemic antifungal and antiprotozoal drugs. The use of these agents is critical in controlling parasitic infections in patients with AIDS and other individuals with a compromised or deficient immune system.

Finally, the drugs discussed in this chapter will have particular importance to therapists working in or traveling to parts of the world where parasitic infections remain a primary health problem and source of human suffering. Therapists involved in the Peace Corps or similar organizations will routinely treat patients taking these drugs. Also, therapists working in these areas may be taking some of the drugs themselves, such as the prophylactic antimalarial agents chloroquine and mefloquine. Hence, therapists should be aware of the pharmacology and potential side effects of these agents, both in their patients and in themselves. Of course, therapists working in North America should know that individuals who have returned from or have immigrated from certain geographic areas may carry various fungal and parasitic infections and that these patients will also require chemotherapy using the drugs discussed in this chapter.

CASE STUDY

ANTIFUNGAL DRUGS

Brief History. A physical therapist working with a college football team was taping a team member's ankle when he noticed redness and inflammation between the athlete's toes. The athlete reported that the redness and itching had developed within the last few days and was becoming progressively worse. The therapist suspected a cutaneous fungal infection (probably tinea pedis) and reported this information to the team physician.

Influence of Medication. The physician prescribed a topical antifungal preparation containing 2 percent miconazole (Monistat-Derm). The athlete was instructed to apply this preparation to the affected area twice daily for the next 4 weeks.

1. ***What additional instructions can the therapist give the athlete about administering the antifungal agent?***
2. ***What can the therapist do to reduce the chance of teammates getting this infection?***

See Appendix C, "Answers to Case Study Questions."

SUMMARY

This chapter presented three general groups of drugs that are used to treat infection caused by specific microorganisms in humans. Antifungal drugs are used against local or systemic infections caused by pathogenic fungi. Antiprotozoal agents are used to prevent and treat protozoal infections such as malaria, severe intestinal infection (dysentery), and infections in other tissues and organs. Anthelmintic drugs are used against parasitic worms (tapeworm, roundworm, etc.), which may infect the human intestinal tract and other tissues. Although the use of some of these agents is relatively limited in the United States, these drugs tend to be some of the most important agents in controlling infection and improving health on a worldwide basis. In addition, some of these agents are effective for treating opportunistic fungal and protozoal infections in patients who have AIDS and others with compromised immune systems. Physical therapists and occupational therapists may be involved with treating specific groups of patients taking these drugs, including patients with AIDS and patients located in geographic areas where these types of infections are prevalent.

REFERENCES

1. Galimberti R, Torre AC, Baztán MC, Rodriguez-Chiappetta F. Emerging systemic fungal infections. *Clin Dermatol.* 2012;30:633-650.
2. Marcos LA, Gotuzzo E. Intestinal protozoan infections in the immunocompromised host. *Curr Opin Infect Dis.* 2013;26:295-301.
3. Vijayan VK, Kilani T. Emerging and established parasitic lung infestations. *Infect Dis Clin North Am.* 2010;24:579-602.
4. Bennett JE. Antifungal agents. In: Brunton L, et al, eds. *The Pharmacological Basis of Therapeutics.* 12th ed. New York: McGraw-Hill; 2011.
5. Ryan KJ. The nature of fungi. In: Ryan KJ, Ray CG, eds. *Sherris Medical Microbiology.* 5th ed. New York: McGraw-Hill; 2010.
6. Garcia-Vidal C, Viasus D, Carratalà J. Pathogenesis of invasive fungal infections. *Curr Opin Infect Dis.* 2013;26:270-276.
7. Raman Sharma R. Fungal infections of the nervous system: current perspective and controversies in management. *Int J Surg.* 2010;8:591-601.
8. Smith JA, Kauffman CA. Pulmonary fungal infections. *Respirology.* 2012;17:913-926.
9. Brown GD, Denning DW, Gow NA, et al. Hidden killers: human fungal infections. *Sci Transl Med.* 2012;4:165.
10. Lacerda JF, Oliveira CM. Diagnosis and treatment of invasive fungal infections focus on liposomal amphotericin B. *Clin Drug Investig.* 2013;33(suppl 1):S5-14
11. Balasegaram M, Ritmeijer K, Lima MA, et al. Liposomal amphotericin B as a treatment for human leishmaniasis. *Expert Opin Emerg Drugs.* 2012;17:493-510.

12. Bassetti M, Aversa F, Ballerini F, et al. Amphotericin B lipid complex in the management of invasive fungal infections in immunocompromised patients. *Clin Drug Investig*. 2011;31:745-758.
13. Hamill RJ. Amphotericin B formulations: a comparative review of efficacy and toxicity. *Drugs*. 2013;73:919-934.
14. Klepser M. The value of amphotericin B in the treatment of invasive fungal infections. *J Crit Care*. 2011;26:e1-10.
15. Cohen BE. Amphotericin B membrane action: role for two types of ion channels in eliciting cell survival and lethal effects. *J Membr Biol*. 2010;238:1-20.
16. Laniado-Laborín R, Cabrales-Vargas MN. Amphotericin B: side effects and toxicity. *Rev Iberoam Micol*. 2009;26:223-227.
17. Lass-Flörl C. Triazole antifungal agents in invasive fungal infections: a comparative review. *Drugs*. 2011;71:2405-2419.
18. Mikulska M, Del Bono V, Ratto S, Viscoli C. Occurrence, presentation and treatment of candidemia. *Expert Rev Clin Immunol*. 2012;8:755-765.
19. Gupta AK, Drummond-Main C, Paquet M. Evidence-based optimal fluconazole dosing regimen for onychomycosis treatment. *J Dermatolog Treat*. 2013;24:75-80.
20. Pienaar ED, Young T, Holmes H. Interventions for the prevention and management of oropharyngeal candidiasis associated with HIV infection in adults and children. *Cochrane Database Syst Rev*. 2010;11:CD003940.
21. Ray A, Ray S, George AT, Swaminathan N. Interventions for prevention and treatment of vulvovaginal candidiasis in women with HIV infection. *Cochrane Database Syst Rev*. 2011;8: CD008739.
22. Castagnola E, Jacqz-Aigrain E, Kaguelidou F, et al. Fluconazole use and safety in the nursery. *Early Hum Dev*. 2012;88(suppl 2): S11-15.
23. Sinnollareddy M, Peake SL, Roberts MS, et al. Pharmacokinetic evaluation of fluconazole in critically ill patients. *Expert Opin Drug Metab Toxicol*. 2011;7:1431-1440.
24. Bassetti M, Mikulska M, Viscoli C. Bench-to-bedside review: therapeutic management of invasive candidiasis in the intensive care unit. *Crit Care*. 2010;14:244.
25. Sgherri C, Porta A, Castellano S, et al. Effects of azole treatments on the physical properties of Candida albicans plasma membrane: a spin probe EPR study. *Biochim Biophys Acta*. 2014;1838 (Pt B):465-473.
26. Warrilow AG, Martel CM, Parker JE, et al. Azole binding properties of Candida albicans sterol 14-alpha demethylase (CaCYP51). *Antimicrob Agents Chemother*. 2010;54:4235-4245.
27. Brizendine KD, Baddley JW, Pappas PG. Pulmonary cryptococcosis. *Semin Respir Crit Care Med*. 2011;32:727-734.
28. Meletiadis J, Chanock S, Walsh TJ. Defining targets for investigating the pharmacogenomics of adverse drug reactions to antifungal agents. *Pharmacogenomics*. 2008;9:561-584.
29. Kelly BP. Superficial fungal infections. *Pediatr Rev*. 2012;33: e22-37.
30. Meadows-Oliver M. Tinea capitis: diagnostic criteria and treatment options. *Dermatol Nurs*. 2009;21:281-286.
31. Panda D, Rathinasamy K, Santra MK, Wilson L. Kinetic suppression of microtubule dynamic instability by griseofulvin: implications for its possible use in the treatment of cancer. *Proc Natl Acad Sci USA*. 2005;102:9878-9883.
32. Lestner J, Hope WW. Itraconazole: an update on pharmacology and clinical use for treatment of invasive and allergic fungal infections. *Expert Opin Drug Metab Toxicol*. 2013;9:911-926.
33. López-Martínez R, Méndez-Tovar LJ. Blastomycosis. *Clin Dermatol*. 2012;30:565-572.
34. McKinsey DS, McKinsey JP. Pulmonary histoplasmosis. *Semin Respir Crit Care Med*. 2011;32:735-744.
35. Heeres J, Meerpoel L, Lewi P. Conazoles. *Molecules*. 2010;15: 4129-4188.
36. Emri T, Majoros L, Tóth V, Pócsi I. Echinocandins: production and applications. *Appl Microbiol Biotechnol*. 2013;97: 3267-3284.
37. Sucher AJ, Chahine EB, Balcer HE. Echinocandins: the newest class of antifungals. *Ann Pharmacother*. 2009;43:1647-1657.
38. Yuan X, Wang R, Bai CQ, et al. Caspofungin for prophylaxis and treatment of fungal infections in adolescents and adults: a meta-analysis of randomized controlled trials. *Pharmazie*. 2012;67: 267-273.
39. Van Duyn Graham L, Elewski BE. Recent updates in oral terbinafine: its use in onychomycosis and tinea capitis in the US. *Mycoses*. 2011;54:e679-685.
40. Mikulska M, Novelli A, Aversa F, et al. Voriconazole in clinical practice. *J Chemother*. 2012;24:311-327.
41. Rotta I, Ziegelmann PK, Otuki MF, et al. Efficacy of topical antifungals in the treatment of dermatophytosis: a mixed-treatment comparison meta-analysis involving 14 treatments. *JAMA Dermatol*. 2013;149:341-349.
42. Pankhurst CL. Candidiasis (oropharyngeal). *Clin Evid*. 2013; 2013:1304.
43. McAdam AJ, Sharpe AH. Infectious diseases. In: Kumar V, Abbas AK, Fausto N, Aster JC, eds. *Pathologic Basis of Disease*. 8th ed. New York: Elsevier Saunders; 2010.
44. Garcia LS. Malaria. *Clin Lab Med*. 2010;30:93-129.
45. Phillips MA, Stanley SL. Chemotherapy of protozoal infections: amebiasis, giardiasis, trichomoniasis, trypanosomiasis, leishmaniasis, and other protozoal infections. In: Brunton L, et al, eds. *The Pharmacological Basis of Therapeutics*. 12th ed. New York: McGraw-Hill; 2011.
46. Bern C. Chagas disease in the immunosuppressed host. *Curr Opin Infect Dis*. 2012;25:450-457.
47. Saporito L, Giammanco GM, De Grazia S, Colomba C. Visceral leishmaniasis: host-parasite interactions and clinical presentation in the immunocompetent and in the immunocompromised host. *Int J Infect Dis*. 2013;17:e572-576.
48. Krafts K, Hempelmann E, Skórska-Stania A. From methylene blue to chloroquine: a brief review of the development of an antimalarial therapy. *Parasitol Res*. 2012;111:1-6.
49. Steinhardt LC, Magill AJ, Arguin PM. Review: malaria chemoprophylaxis for travelers to Latin America. *Am J Trop Med Hyg*. 2011;85:1015-1024.
50. Noedl H. The need for new antimalarial drugs less prone to resistance. *Curr Pharm Des*. 2013;19:266-269.
51. Wunderlich J, Rohrbach P, Dalton JP. The malaria digestive vacuole. *Front Biosci*. 2012;4:1424-1448.
52. Schlagenhauf P, Adamcova M, Regep L, et al. The position of mefloquine as a 21st century malaria chemoprophylaxis. *Malar J*. 2010;9:357.
53. Douglas NM, John GK, von Seidlein L, et al. Chemotherapeutic strategies for reducing transmission of Plasmodium vivax malaria. *Adv Parasitol*. 2012;80:271-300.
54. Sinclair D, Zani B, Donegan S, et al. Artemisinin-based combination therapy for treating uncomplicated malaria. *Cochrane Database Syst Rev*. 2009;3:CD007483.

55. Hill DR, Baird JK, Parise ME, et al. Primaquine: report from CDC expert meeting on malaria chemoprophylaxis I. *Am J Trop Med Hyg.* 2006;75:402-415.
56. Fernando D, Rodrigo C, Rajapakse S. Primaquine in vivax malaria: an update and review on management issues. *Malar J.* 2011;10:351.
57. Howes RE, Battle KE, Satyagraha AW, et al. G6PD deficiency: global distribution, genetic variants and primaquine therapy. *Adv Parasitol.* 2013;81:133-201.
58. von Seidlein L, Auburn S, Espino F, et al. Review of key knowledge gaps in glucose-6-phosphate dehydrogenase deficiency detection with regard to the safe clinical deployment of 8-aminoquinoline treatment regimens: a workshop report. *Malar J.* 2013;12:112.
59. Hwang J, Bitarakwate E, Pai M, et al. Chloroquine or amodiaquine combined with sulfadoxine-pyrimethamine for uncomplicated malaria: a systematic review. *Trop Med Int Health.* 2006;11:789-799.
60. Vinetz JM, Clain J, Bounnkeuka, et al. Chemotherapy of malaria. In: Brunton L, et al, eds. *The Pharmacological Basis of Therapeutics.* 12th ed. New York: McGraw-Hill; 2011.
61. Abdul-Ghani R, Farag HF, Allam AF. Sulfadoxine-pyrimethamine resistance in Plasmodium falciparum: a zoomed image at the molecular level within a geographic context. *Acta Trop.* 2013;125:163-190.
62. Kayentao K, Garner P, van Eijk AM, et al. Intermittent preventive therapy for malaria during pregnancy using 2 vs 3 or more doses of sulfadoxine-pyrimethamine and risk of low birth weight in Africa: systematic review and meta-analysis. *JAMA.* 2013;309:594-604.
63. Nosten F, White NJ. Artemisinin-based combination treatment of falciparum malaria. *Am J Trop Med Hyg.* 2007;77 (suppl):181-192.
64. Achan J, Talisuna AO, Erhart A, et al. Quinine, an old anti-malarial drug in a modern world: role in the treatment of malaria. *Malar J.* 2011;10:144.
65. Sullivan DJ. Plasmodium drug targets outside the genetic control of the parasite. *Curr Pharm Des.* 2013;19:282-289.
66. Barbacka K, Baer-Dubowska W. Searching for artemisinin production improvement in plants and microorganisms. *Curr Pharm Biotechnol.* 2011;12:1743-1751.
67. Chaturvedi D, Goswami A, Saikia PP, et al. Artemisinin and its derivatives: a novel class of anti-malarial and anti-cancer agents. *Chem Soc Rev.* 2010;39:435-454.
68. Jelinek T. Artemisinin based combination therapy in travel medicine. *Travel Med Infect Dis.* 2013;11:23-28.
69. Sinclair D, Gogtay N, Brand F, Olliaro P. Artemisinin-based combination therapy for treating uncomplicated Plasmodium vivax malaria. *Cochrane Database Syst Rev.* 2011;7:CD008492.
70. O'Brien C, Henrich PP, Passi N, Fidock DA. Recent clinical and molecular insights into emerging artemisinin resistance in Plasmodium falciparum. *Curr Opin Infect Dis.* 2011;24:570-577.
71. Meunier B, Robert A. Heme as trigger and target for trioxane-containing antimalarial drugs. *Acc Chem Res.* 2010;43: 1444-1451.
72. Li J, Zhou B. Biological actions of artemisinin: insights from medicinal chemistry studies. *Molecules.* 2010;15:1378-1397.
73. Efferth T, Kaina B. Toxicity of the antimalarial artemisinin and its derivatives. *Crit Rev Toxicol.* 2010;40:405-421.
74. Agnandji ST, Kurth F, Bélard S, et al. Current status of the clinical development and implementation of paediatric artemisinin combination therapies in Sub-Saharan Africa. *Wien Klin Wochenschr.* 2011;123(suppl 1):7-9.
75. Manyando C, Kayentao K, D'Alessandro U, et al. A systematic review of the safety and efficacy of artemether-lumefantrine against uncomplicated Plasmodium falciparum malaria during pregnancy. *Malar J.* 2012;11:141.
76. Porollo A, Meller J, Joshi Y, et al. Analysis of current antifungal agents and their targets within the Pneumocystis carinii genome. *Curr Drug Targets.* 2012;13:1575-1585.
77. Pyrgos V, Shoham S, Roilides E, Walsh TJ. Pneumocystis pneumonia in children. *Paediatr Respir Rev.* 2009;10:192-198.
78. Nixon GL, Moss DM, Shone AE, et al. Antimalarial pharmacology and therapeutics of atovaquone. *J Antimicrob Chemother.* 2013;68:977-985.
79. Barton V, Fisher N, Biagini GA, et al. Inhibiting Plasmodium cytochrome bc1: a complex issue. *Curr Opin Chem Biol.* 2010;14: 440-446.
80. Marie C, Petri WA Jr. Amoebic dysentery. *Clin Evid.* 2013;2013.
81. Moya IA, Su Z, Honek JF. Current and future perspectives on the chemotherapy of the parasitic protozoa Trichomonas vaginalis and Entamoeba histolytica. *Future Med Chem.* 2009;1:619-643.
82. Stover KR, Riche DM, Gandy CL, Henderson H. What would we do without metronidazole? *Am J Med Sci.* 2012;343:316-319.
83. Wright SG. Protozoan infections of the gastrointestinal tract. *Infect Dis Clin North Am.* 2012;26:323-339.
84. Castro JG, Morrison-Bryant M. Management of Pneumocystis jirovecii pneumonia in HIV infected patients: current options, challenges and future directions. *HIV AIDS.* 2010;2:123-134.
85. McCarthy J, Loukas A, Hotez PJ. Chemotherapy of helminth infections. In: Brunton L, et al, eds. *The Pharmacological Basis of Therapeutics.* 12th ed. New York: McGraw-Hill; 2011.
86. Engleberg C. Intestinal helminths. In: Engleberg NC, DiRita V, Dermody TS, eds. *Schaechter's Mechanisms of Microbial Disease.* 5th ed. Philadelphia, PA: Lippincott Williams & Wilkins; 2013.
87. Ray CG, Plorde JJ. Pathogenic parasites. In: Ryan KJ, Ray CG, eds. *Sherris Medical Microbiology.* 5th ed. New York: McGraw-Hill; 2010.
88. Geary TG, Woo K, McCarthy JS, et al. Unresolved issues in anthelmintic pharmacology for helminthiases of humans. *Int J Parasitol.* 2010;40:1-13.
89. Katiyar D, Singh LK. Filariasis: current status, treatment and recent advances in drug development. *Curr Med Chem.* 2011;18:2174-2185.
90. Rana AK, Misra-Bhattacharya S. Current drug targets for helminthic diseases. *Parasitol Res.* 2013;112:1819-1831.
91. Page SW. Antiparasitic drugs. In: Maddison JE, Page SW, Church DB, eds. *Small Animal Clinical Pharmacology.* Philadelphia, PA: Saunders Elsevier; 2008.

CHAPTER 36

Cancer Chemotherapy

Cancer encompasses a group of diseases that are marked by rapid, uncontrolled cell proliferation and a conversion of normal cells to a more primitive and undifferentiated state.[1,2] Large tumors, or *neoplasms*, may form from excessive cell proliferation. Although some types of tumors are well contained (benign), malignant tumors continue to proliferate within local tissues and can possibly spread (metastasize) to other tissues in the body. The term *cancer* specifically refers to the malignant forms of neoplastic disease, which can often be fatal, as tumors invade and destroy tissues throughout the body. However, benign tumors can also be life-threatening; for example, a large benign tumor may produce morbidity and mortality by obstructing the intestinal tract or by pressing on crucial central nervous system (CNS) structures. Cancer cells, however, are unique in their progressive invasion of local tissues and their ability to metastasize to other tissues.[1]

Cancer ranks second to cardiovascular disease as the leading cause of death in the United States.[3] There are many different types of cancer, and malignancies are classified by the location and the type of tissue from which the cancer originated.[1] For instance, cancers arising from certain epithelial tissues (e.g., skin, gastrointestinal lining) are labeled as *carcinomas;* cancers arising from connective tissues (e.g., bone, striated muscle) are labeled as *sarcomas*. In addition, cancers associated with the formed blood elements are connoted by the suffix *-emia* (e.g., *leukemia* is the cancerous proliferation of leukocytes). Many other descriptive terms are used to describe various malignancies, and certain forms of cancer are often named after a specific person (e.g., Hodgkin disease, Wilms' tumor). It is beyond the scope of this chapter to describe all the various types of malignancies. You may want to consult a pathology text or similar reference for more information about the location and morphology of particular forms of cancer.[1,2,4]

The exact cause of many cases of neoplastic disease is unknown. However, a great deal has been learned about possible environmental, viral, genetic, and other elements, or **carcinogens,** that may cause or increase a person's susceptibility to various types of cancer. Conversely, certain positive lifestyles, including adequate exercise, a high-fiber diet, and the avoidance of tobacco products, may be crucial in preventing certain forms of cancer. Of course, routine checkups and early detection play a vital role in reducing cancer mortality.

When cancer is diagnosed, three primary treatment modalities are available: surgery, radiation treatment, and cancer chemotherapy. The purpose of this chapter is to describe the basic rationale of cancer chemotherapy and to provide an overview of the drugs that are currently available to treat specific forms of cancer. You may routinely work with patients undergoing cancer chemotherapy. For reasons that will become apparent in this chapter, these drugs tend to produce toxic effects that directly influence physical therapy and occupational therapy procedures. Therefore, this chapter should provide you with a better understanding of the pharmacodynamic principles and beneficial effects, as well as the reasons for the potential adverse effects of these important drugs.

GENERAL PRINCIPLES

Cytotoxic Strategy

The basic strategy of anticancer drugs is to limit cell proliferation by killing or attenuating the growth of the cancerous cells. However, the pharmacological treatment of cancer represents a unique and perplexing problem. Although cancer cells have become more primitive and have lost much of their normal appearance, they are still human cells that have simply gone wild. In addition, they cannot be easily destroyed without also causing some harm to healthy human tissue. The concept of selective toxicity becomes more difficult to achieve when using anticancer drugs in contrast to drugs that attack foreign invaders and parasites, such as antibacterial drugs or antifungal drugs (see Chapters 33 through 35). Most traditional anticancer drugs lack specificity—that is, these drugs impair function in noncancerous tissues as well as in cancerous cells.[5,6]

Hence, most anticancer drugs rely on the basic strategy of inhibiting DNA/RNA synthesis and function or on directly inhibiting cell division (mitosis). Cancerous cells have a greater need to replicate their genetic material and thus undergo mitosis at a much higher rate than most noncancerous cells. Therefore, the anticancer drugs will affect cancerous cells to a greater extent. On the other hand, researchers have been making considerable effort to develop chemotherapeutic agents that somehow target only the cancer cells, thus reducing the toxicity to healthy cells.[7] The strategies of specific traditional and newer targeted therapies are addressed later in this chapter.

Cell-Cycle–Specific Versus Cell-Cycle–Nonspecific Drugs

Antineoplastic drugs are sometimes classified as either cell-cycle specific or cell-cycle nonspecific.[8] Cancer cells and most normal cells typically undergo a life cycle that can be divided into several distinct phases: a nondividing (quiescent) state (G_0), a pre-DNA synthesis phase (G_1), a period of DNA synthesis (S), a post-DNA synthesis phase (G_2), and the period of actual cell division or mitosis (M) (Fig. 36-1).[9,10] Cell-cycle–specific drugs exert their effects only when the cancer cell is in a certain phase. For instance, most antimetabolites (cytarabine, methotrexate, others) act when the cell is in the S phase. Other drugs are classified as cell-cycle–nonspecific because they exert antineoplastic effects on the cell regardless of the cell cycle's phase. Examples of cell-cycle–nonspecific agents include most alkylating agents and antineoplastic antibiotics.

The significance of cell-cycle–specificity or nonspecificity is obvious. Cell-cycle–specific drugs will be effective only in cells that are progressing through the cell cycle—that is, cells that are not remaining in the nondividing (G_0) phase. Cell-cycle–nonspecific agents have a more general effect and should inhibit replication in all the cells that the drug reaches.

Concepts of Growth Fraction and Cell Kill

Cancer cells are not all uniform in their rate of replication and proliferation. In any given tumor or type of disseminated cancer, certain cells do not proliferate, while other cells reproduce at variable rates. The term *growth fraction* refers to the percentage of proliferating cells relative to total neoplastic cell population.[1] The cells in the growth fraction are more susceptible to antineoplastic drugs because these cells must synthesize and replicate their genetic material. Fortunately, these are the cells that must be killed to prevent the cancer from spreading. In addition, the growth fraction typically *decreases* as a tumor gets larger—that is, the percentage of cells that are actively dividing starts to decline as the tumor gets larger because blood flow and nutrient supply to the tumor cannot sustain extremely rapid tumor growth.

The *cell kill hypothesis* is based on the idea that each round of chemotherapy will kill a certain percentage of cancerous cells.[1] Thus, if a chemotherapy regimen kills 90 percent of tumor cells, 10 percent of the tumor cells will survive each round of chemotherapy. According to this theory, the chemotherapeutic regimen can never completely eliminate the tumor because some percentage of cells will remain alive after each round of treatment. Nonetheless, if chemotherapy can reduce the tumor to a certain size (typically less than 10,000 cells), the body's endogenous defense mechanisms (i.e., cytotoxic immune responses) can deal with the remaining cancerous tissues, and the disease is considered to be in remission.[1]

Concepts such as growth fraction and cell kill illustrate an obvious but important point: early detection and aggressive chemotherapy are essential in successfully treating cancer. There is a greater chance of survival if several rounds of chemotherapy are instituted in fairly rapid succession when the tumor is small and a large proportion of the cells are actively dividing. Consider, for example, a tumor that has 10 million cells. If the first round of chemotherapy kills 90 percent of the cancerous

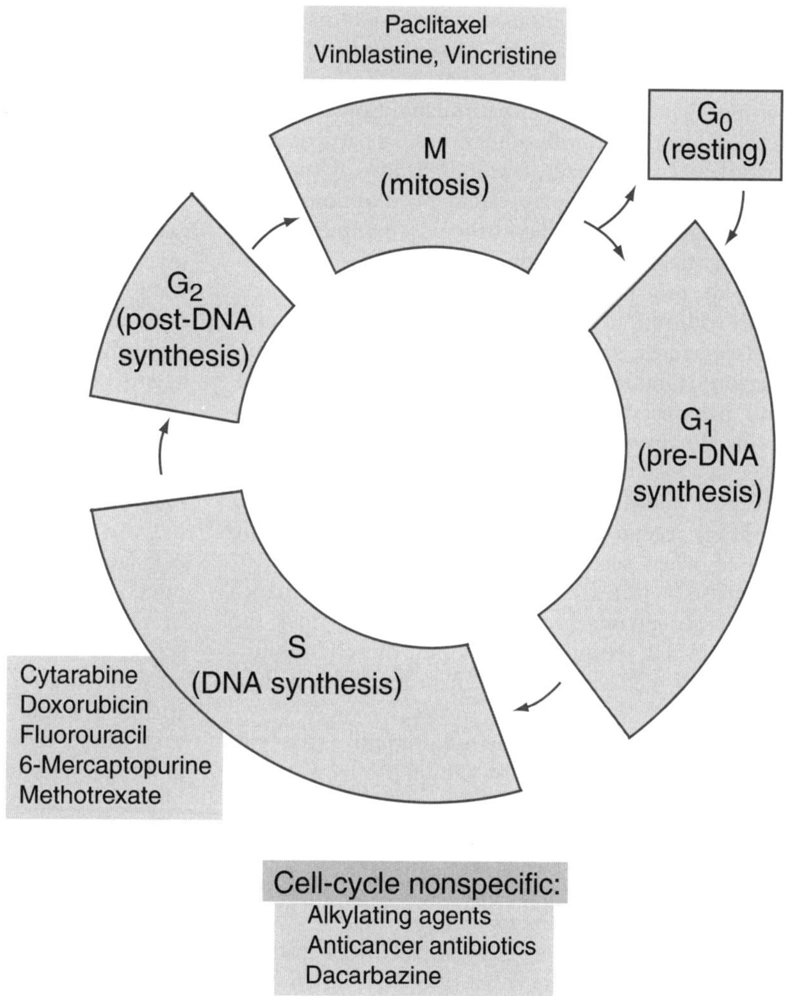

Figure ■ 36-1
Phases of the cell cycle. Examples of cell-cycle–specific drugs are listed next to the phase of the cycle they act on. Examples of cell-cycle–nonspecific drugs are listed below the figure.

cells, 1 million cells will survive. A second round will kill 90 percent of the remaining cells, leaving 100,000 cells, and a third round will kill 90 percent of those cells, leaving 10,000 cancerous cells. Thus, three rounds of chemotherapy could successfully reduce the tumor to a size that might enable the body's endogenous systems to control the remaining cancerous tissues.

Prevalence and Management of Adverse Effects

Because antineoplastic agents often impair replication of normal tissues, these drugs are generally associated with several common and relatively severe adverse effects. Normal human cells must often undergo controlled mitosis to sustain normal function. This is especially true for certain tissues such as hair follicles, bone marrow, immune system cells, and epithelial cells in the skin and gastrointestinal (GI) tract. Most cancer chemotherapy agents will also affect these tissues to some extent. In fact, the primary reason for most of the common adverse effects (e.g., hair loss, anemia, nausea) is that normal cells are also experiencing the same toxic changes as the tumor cells. The cancer cells, however, tend to suffer these toxic effects to a greater extent because of their increased rate of replication and cell division. Still, healthy cells often exhibit some toxic effects, even at the minimum effective doses of the chemotherapeutic agents.

Consequently, antineoplastic drugs typically have a very low therapeutic index compared with drugs that are used to treat less serious disorders (see Chapter 1). Considering that cancer is usually life-threatening, these toxic effects must be expected and tolerated during chemotherapeutic treatments. Some side effects can be treated with other drugs. In particular, GI disturbances (e.g., nausea, vomiting, loss of appetite) may be relieved to some extent by traditional antiemetic agents such as glucocorticoids (dexamethasone) or drugs that block dopamine receptors (e.g., metoclopramide, prochlorperazine).[11,12]

In addition, there are newer antiemetic and antinausea agents, such as dolasetron (Anzemet), granisetron (Granisol, Kytril), ondansetron (Zofran), and palonosetron (Aloxi), to treat chemotherapy-induced nausea and vomiting (CINV). These newer agents, which block a specific type of CNS serotonin receptor known as the 5-hydroxytryptamine type 3 ($5\text{-}HT_3$) receptor, reduce the nausea and vomiting caused when serotonin binds to that receptor.[13,14] Likewise, newer agents, such as aprepitant (Emend) and fosaprepitant (Emend for injection), block the neurokinin-1 receptor in the CNS, thereby inhibiting CINV mediated by other neuropeptides such as substance P.[15-17]

Some patients may elect to use alternative strategies such as medical marijuana or natural products such as ginger to help control CINV. Use of these alternative strategies is somewhat controversial, however, and the evidence of their effectiveness is generally not on par with some of the newer treatments such as the $5\text{-}HT_3$ and neurokinin-1 receptor antagonists.[18,19] Nonetheless, several drugs are now available that patients undergoing chemotherapy can use alone or in combination to prevent or reduce the severity of CINV. These drugs are often essential in helping improve the patient's quality of life.[14,20]

Other forms of supportive care can also be helpful in improving the quality of life and functional status of patients with cancer. Analgesics (see Chapters 14 and 15) are often needed to help patients cope with cancer pain and to make the rigors of chemotherapy treatment more tolerable.[21,22] Physicians can administer a variety of other medications to treat a patient's specific symptoms, such as anemia, cough, weight loss, and constipation.[23-25] Support from medical, nursing, and other health-care providers (including physical therapists and occupational therapists) can likewise help immeasurably in reassuring the patient that chemotherapy-induced side effects are normal—and even necessary—for the cancer chemotherapy drugs to exert their antineoplastic effects.

SPECIFIC ANTICANCER DRUGS

Drugs used against cancer can be classified by their chemical structure, source, or mechanism of action. The primary groups of antineoplastic drugs are the alkylating agents, antimetabolites, anticancer antibiotics, antimicrotubule agents, topoisomerase inhibitors, antineoplastic hormones, targeted/biological therapies, platinum coordination complexes, and several other miscellaneous drug groups and individual agents. The principal antineoplastic medications are presented below.

Alkylating Agents

Alkylating agents exert their primary cytotoxic effects by inducing binding within DNA strands and by preventing DNA function and replication.[26] Essentially, the drug causes cross-links to be formed between the strands of the DNA double helix or within a single DNA strand (Fig. 36-2). In either case, these cross-links effectively tie up the DNA molecule, eliminating the ability of the DNA double helix to untwist. If the DNA double helix cannot unravel, the genetic code of the cell cannot be reproduced, and cell reproduction is arrested. In addition, cross-linking within the double helix impairs cellular protein synthesis because the DNA double helix cannot unwind to allow formation of messenger RNA strands. The cell therefore cannot synthesize vital cellular proteins (enzymes, transport proteins, etc.). Alkylating agents likewise initiate a process of cell death (apoptosis) by disrupting DNA function, in which several degradative enzymes (nucleases, proteases) are released and begin to destroy the cell.[27]

Alkylating agents are so named because they typically generate a chemical alkyl group on one of the bases, such as guanine in the DNA chain. This alkyl group acts as the bridge that ultimately links two bases in the DNA molecule (see Fig. 36-2). The bonds formed by this cross-linking are strong and resistant to breakage. Thus, the DNA double helix remains tied up for the cell's life. Alkylating agents may interact with other DNA components and can disrupt other aspects of DNA function, but it is the cross-linking within DNA strands that accounts for their primary cytotoxic effects.

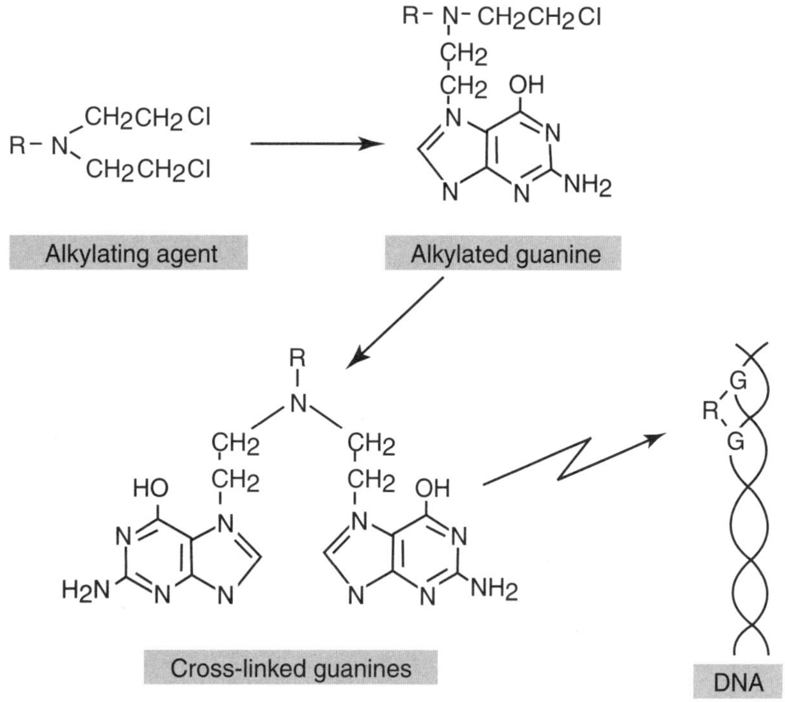

Figure ■ 36-2
Mechanism of action of anticancer alkylating agents. The alkylating agent (R) causes alkylation of guanine nucleotides located in the DNA strand. Cross-links are then formed between two alkylated guanines, thus creating strong bonds between or within the DNA strands that inhibit DNA function and replication.

Anticancer drugs that work primarily as alkylating agents are listed in Table 36-1. As indicated, these agents represent one of the largest categories of anticancer drugs and are used to treat a variety of leukemias, carcinomas, and other neoplasms. Common side effects of alkylating agents are also listed in Table 36-1. As previously discussed, most of these adverse effects are caused by the effect of the alkylating agent on DNA replication in normal, healthy tissues.

Antimetabolites

Cells are able to synthesize genetic material (DNA, RNA) from endogenous metabolites known as *purine and pyrimidine nucleotides* (Fig. 36-3). Certain anticancer drugs are structurally similar to these endogenous metabolites and compete with these compounds during DNA/RNA biosynthesis. These drugs are therefore called antimetabolites because they interfere with the normal metabolites during cellular biosynthesis.[8,28]

Antimetabolites can impair the biosynthesis of genetic material in two primary ways.[1] First, the drug may be incorporated directly into the genetic material, thus forming a fake and nonfunctional genetic product. This effect would be like baking a cake but substituting an inappropriate ingredient (salt) for a normal ingredient (sugar). Obviously, the product would not work very well (or taste very good). The second manner in which antimetabolites may impair DNA/RNA biosynthesis is by occupying the enzymes that synthesize various components of the genetic material.

These enzymes do not recognize the difference between the antimetabolite drug and the normal metabolite and waste their time trying to convert the antimetabolite into a normal metabolic product. The enzyme, however, cannot effectively act on the drug, so the normal metabolic products are not formed. Methotrexate, for example, is a common antimetabolite that mimics folic acid.[29] Folic acid is an important cofactor that helps catalyze specific enzymatic reactions during DNA biosynthesis. Because methotrexate only imitates the real folic acid, these enzymatic reactions are inhibited, resulting in decreased DNA synthesis.

Hence, antimetabolites either mimic the active ingredients or other constituents needed for DNA synthesis and replication. In either case, the cell's ability to synthesize normal DNA and RNA is impaired, and the cell cannot replicate its genetic material or carry

Table 36-1
ALKYLATING AGENTS

Generic Name	Trade Name	Primary Antineoplastic Indication(s)*	Common Adverse Effects
Altretamine	Hexalen, Hexastat	Ovarian cancer	GI distress (nausea, vomiting, loss of appetite); blood disorders (anemia, leukopenia, thrombocytopenia); CNS neurotoxicity (seizures, unusual tiredness, dizziness, confusion, depression, anxiety); peripheral neuropathies
Bendamustine	Treanda	Chronic lymphocytic leukemia	Blood disorders (anemia, leukopenia, neutropenia, thrombocytopenia); GI distress (nausea, vomiting); fever; metabolic imbalances (hyperkalemia, hyperphosphatemia, hypocalcemia) caused by release of electrolytes from dying cancer cells (tumor lysis syndrome)
Busulfan	Busulfex, Myleran	Chronic myelogenous leukemia	Blood disorders (anemia, leukopenia, thrombocytopenia); GI distress (nausea, vomiting, diarrhea, others); CNS neurotoxicity (seizures, unusual tiredness, dizziness, confusion, depression, anxiety); bladder irritation; hair loss; cardiotoxicity; pulmonary toxicity; metabolic disorders (hyperuricemia, fatigue, weight loss, other symptoms); muscle and joint pain; fever; allergic reactions
Carmustine	BCNU, BiCNU, Gliadel	Primary brain tumors; Hodgkin disease; non-Hodgkin lymphomas; multiple myeloma	Blood disorders (thrombocytopenia, leukopenia); GI distress (nausea, vomiting); hepatotoxicity; pulmonary toxicity
Chlorambucil	Leukeran	Chronic lymphocytic leukemia; Hodgkin disease; malignant lymphoma	Blood disorders (leukopenia, thrombocytopenia, anemia); skin rashes/itching; pulmonary toxicity
Cyclophosphamide	Cytoxan, Neosar	Acute and chronic lymphocytic leukemia; acute and chronic myelocytic leukemia; carcinoma of ovary, breast; Hodgkin disease; non-Hodgkin lymphomas; multiple myeloma	Blood disorders (anemia, leukopenia, thrombocytopenia); GI distress (nausea, vomiting, loss of appetite); bladder irritation; hair loss; cardiotoxicity; pulmonary toxicity
Dacarbazine	DTIC-Dome	Malignant melanoma; refractory Hodgkin lymphomas	GI distress (nausea, vomiting, loss of appetite); blood disorders (anemia, leukopenia, thrombocytopenia); liver toxicity; anaphylactoid reactions
Ifosfamide	IFEX	Testicular cancer	Blood disorders (leukopenia, thrombocytopenia); CNS effects (agitation, confusion, dizziness, hallucinations, somnolence); urotoxicity; GI distress (nausea, vomiting); hair loss
Lomustine	CCNU, CeeNU	Brain tumors; Hodgkin disease	Blood disorders (anemia, leukopenia, thrombocytopenia); GI disorders (nausea, vomiting)
Mechlorethamine	Mustargen, nitrogen mustard	Bronchogenic carcinoma; chronic leukemia; Hodgkin disease; non-Hodgkin lymphomas	Blood disorders (anemia, leukopenia, thrombocytopenia); GI distress (nausea, vomiting); CNS effects (seizures, headache, dizziness, convulsions); tissue necrosis and local irritation at injection site
Melphalan	Alkeran	Ovarian carcinoma; multiple myeloma	Blood disorders (leukopenia, thrombocytopenia); skin rashes/itching; anaphylactoid reactions
Procarbazine	Matulane, Natulan	Hodgkin disease	Blood disorders (leukopenia, thrombocytopenia); GI distress (nausea, vomiting); CNS toxicity (seizures, mood changes, confusion, incoordination, motor problems); respiratory toxicity (cough, pleural effusion)
Temozolomide	Temodar	Astrocytoma and glioblastoma that have not responded to other treatments	Blood disorders (leukopenia, thrombocytopenia); GI distress (nausea, vomiting); seizures; fatigue; headache
Thiotepa	Thioplex	Carcinoma of breast, ovary, and bladder	Blood disorders (anemia, leukopenia, thrombocytopenia)

**Only the indications listed in the U.S. product labeling are included here. Many anticancer drugs are used for additional types of neoplastic disease.*

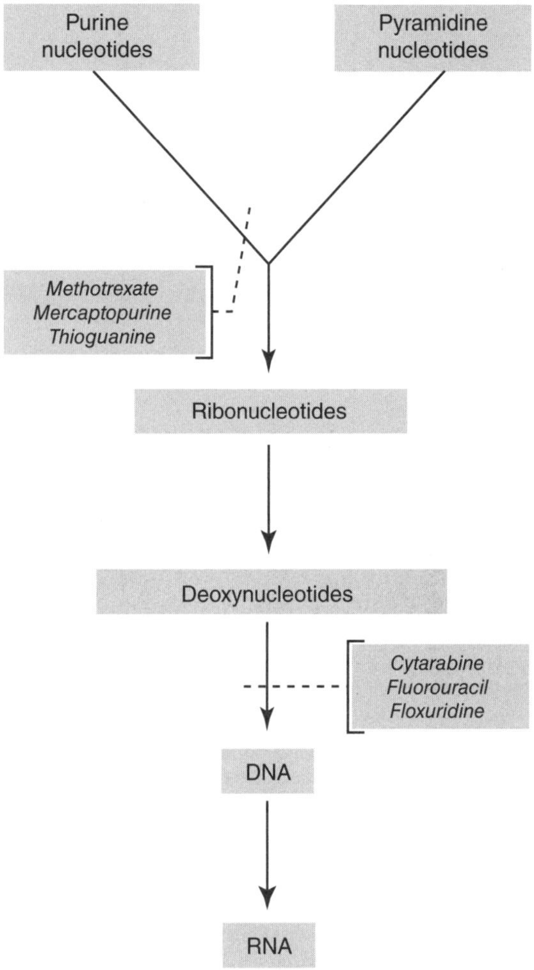

Figure ■ 36-3
Sites of anticancer antimetabolite action. Various drugs interfere with DNA/RNA production by inhibiting nucleic acid biosynthesis at specific sites, indicated by the dashed lines.

out normal protein synthesis because of a lack of functional DNA and RNA.

Cancer chemotherapeutic agents that act as antimetabolites and the principal neoplastic diseases for which they are indicated are listed in Table 36-2. As stated previously, these drugs interrupt cellular pathways that synthesize DNA and RNA; the primary sites where specific antimetabolites interrupt these pathways are indicated in Figure 36-3. As with most anticancer drugs, these agents are especially toxic to cells that have a large growth fraction and undergo extensive replication. These cells have a great need to synthesize nucleic acids—hence the preferential effect of antimetabolites on these cells.

Anticancer Antibiotics

Several anticancer drugs are chemically classified as antibiotics but are usually reserved for neoplastic diseases because of their relatively high toxicity (Table 36-3). The exact mechanism of action for these antibiotics to exert antineoplastic effects is still being investigated. These drugs may act directly on DNA by becoming intercalated (inserted) between base pairs in the DNA strand. This insertion would cause a general disruption or even lysis of the DNA strand, thus preventing DNA replication and RNA synthesis.[30,31]

Alternatively, these antibiotics may act in other ways, including having direct inhibitory effects on DNA-related enzymes such as topoisomerase type II enzyme. This enzyme is normally responsible for regulating DNA replication, and inhibition by certain anticancer antibiotics disrupts DNA synthesis, resulting in breaks in the DNA molecule.[1,32] In this regard, anticancer antibiotics may work in a manner similar to the topoisomerase inhibitors discussed below. Regardless of their exact mechanism, these agents play a role in the treatment of several neoplastic diseases.

Antimicrotubule Agents

During cell replication, the mitotic apparatus must function at a specific time and rate to direct the cell to divide into two new (daughter) cells. Likewise, the mitotic apparatus contains certain microtubules that are important in guiding the mitotic apparatus and allowing this apparatus to orchestrate cell division. Hence, several anticancer drugs are available that bind to these microtubules and alter the function of the mitotic apparatus (Table 36-4).[33] Certain agents known as the *vinca alkaloids* (e.g., vinblastine, vincristine, vinorelbine) inhibit the formation of the mitotic apparatus, whereas others known as the *taxanes* (e.g., docetaxel, paclitaxel) inhibit breakdown of these microtubules, thereby creating a stable but nonfunctional mitotic apparatus.[34,35] In either situation, these drugs disrupt the normal function of the mitotic apparatus and prevent the cell from dividing and proliferating. In fact, when the cell attempts to divide, the nuclear material becomes disrupted and dispersed throughout the cytosol. This effect causes direct damage to the chromosomes, leading to subsequent cell dysfunction and death.

Table 36-2
ANTIMETABOLITES

Generic Name	Trade Name	Primary Antineoplastic Indication(s)*	Common Adverse Effects
Azacitidine	Vidaza	Chronic myelomonocytic leukemia	Blood disorders (anemia, neutropenia, thrombocytopenia); GI distress (constipation, nausea, vomiting, diarrhea); hepatotoxicity; unusual tiredness; fever; anaphylactoid reactions
Capecitabine	Xeloda	Breast cancer, colorectal cancer	Blood disorders (anemia, neutropenia, thrombocytopenia); GI distress (abdominal pain, constipation, nausea, vomiting, diarrhea); dermatitis; stomatitis; unusual tiredness; headache; muscle and joint pain
Cladribine	Leustatin	Hairy cell leukemia	Blood disorders (anemia, neutropenia, thrombocytopenia); fever; infection; GI distress (loss of appetite, nausea, vomiting); skin rash; headache; unusual tiredness; respiratory toxicity (cough, dyspnea)
Clofarabine	Clolar	Acute lymphoblastic leukemia	Blood disorders (anemia, neutropenia, thrombocytopenia); infection; cardiotoxicity (tachycardia, pericardial effusion); GI distress (nausea, vomiting); hepatotoxicity; metabolic imbalances (hyperkalemia, hyperphosphatemia, hypocalcemia) caused by release of electrolytes from dying cancer cells (tumor lysis syndrome)
Cytarabine	Ara-C, Cytosar-U, DepoCyt	Several forms of acute and chronic leukemia; non-Hodgkin lymphomas	Blood disorders (anemia, leukopenia, thrombocytopenia); GI distress (nausea, vomiting); skin rash; hair loss
Floxuridine	FUDR	Carcinoma of the GI tract and liver	Blood disorders (anemia, leukopenia, thrombocytopenia); GI disorders (nausea, vomiting, diarrhea, loss of appetite); skin disorders (discoloration, rash, hair loss)
Fludarabine	Fludara	Chronic lymphocytic leukemia	Blood disorders (anemia, leukopenia, thrombocytopenia); infection; respiratory toxicity (cough, pneumonia); GI distress (nausea, vomiting, diarrhea, GI bleeding); skin rash; unusual tiredness; hair loss
Fluorouracil	Adrucil, Efudex, Fluoroplex, 5-FU	Carcinoma of colon, rectum, stomach, pancreas, and breast	GI distress (loss of appetite, nausea, vomiting); blood disorders (anemia, leukopenia, thrombocytopenia); skin disorders (rash, hair loss)
Gemcitabine	Gemzar	Carcinoma of the pancreas; non-small cell lung cancer, breast cancer, ovarian cancer	Blood disorders (anemia, leukopenia, neutropenia, thrombocytopenia); cardiovascular toxicity (arrhythmias, myocardial infarction, stroke, edema); respiratory toxicity (dyspnea, bronchospasm); fever; skin rash; hematuria; GI distress (nausea, vomiting, diarrhea); hepatotoxicity
Mercaptopurine	Purinethol	Acute lymphocytic and myelogenous leukemia; chronic myelocytic leukemia	Blood disorders (anemia, leukopenia, thrombocytopenia); GI distress (nausea, loss of appetite); hepatotoxicity
Methotrexate	Generic (when used for cancer)	Acute lymphocytic leukemia; meningeal leukemia; carcinoma of head and neck region, lung; non-Hodgkin lymphomas	Blood disorders (anemia, leukopenia, thrombocytopenia); GI distress (including ulceration of GI tract); skin disorders (rashes, photosensitivity, hair loss); hepatotoxicity; CNS effects (headaches, drowsiness, fatigue); nephropathy
Nelarabine	Arranon	T-cell acute lymphoblastic leukemia or T-cell lymphoblastic lymphoma	Blood disorders (anemia, leukopenia, neutropenia, thrombocytopenia); severe neurological events
Pemetrexed	Alimta	Mesothelioma; non-small cell lung cancer	Blood disorders (anemia, leukopenia, thrombocytopenia); GI distress (nausea, vomiting, constipation, others); fever; infection; skin reactions (rash, desquamation)

Table 36-2
ANTIMETABOLITES—cont'd

Generic Name	Trade Name	Primary Antineoplastic Indication(s)*	Common Adverse Effects
Pentostatin	Nipent	Hairy cell leukemia	Blood disorders (anemia, leukopenia, thrombocytopenia); anaphylactoid reactions; CNS toxicity (unusual tiredness, anxiety, confusion, headache); respiratory toxicity (pneumonia, cough, dyspnea); muscle pain; GI distress (nausea, vomiting, diarrhea, others); hepatotoxicity; skin reactions (rash, itching)
Pralatrexate	Folotyn	Peripheral T-cell lymphoma	Blood disorders (anemia, neutropenia, thrombocytopenia); GI distress (nausea, mucositis); respiratory toxicity (cough, dyspnea); unusual tiredness; fever/sepsis
Thioguanine	Lanvis	Acute nonlymphocytic leukemia	Blood disorders (anemia, leukopenia, thrombocytopenia); GI distress (nausea, vomiting); hepatotoxicity

**Only the indications listed in the U.S. product labeling are included here. Many anticancer drugs are used for additional types of neoplastic disease.*

Table 36-3
ANTICANCER ANTIBIOTICS

Generic Name	Trade Name	Primary Antineoplastic Indication(s)*	Common Adverse Effects
Bleomycin	Blenoxane	Carcinoma of head, neck, cervical region, skin, penis, vulva, and testicle; Hodgkin disease; non-Hodgkin lymphomas	Pulmonary toxicity (interstitial pneumonitis); skin disorders (rash, discoloration); mucosal lesions; fever; GI distress; anaphylactoid reactions
Dactinomycin	Cosmegen	Carcinoma of testicle and endometrium; carcinosarcoma of kidney (Wilms' tumor); Ewing sarcoma; rhabdomyosarcoma	Blood disorders (anemia, leukopenia, thrombocytopenia); GI distress (nausea, vomiting, loss of appetite); mucocutaneous lesions; skin disorders (rash, acne, hair loss); local irritation at injection site
Daunorubicin	Cerubidine, DaunoXome	Several forms of acute leukemia	Blood disorders (anemia, leukopenia, thrombocytopenia); cardiotoxicity (arrhythmias, congestive heart failure); GI distress (nausea, vomiting, GI tract ulceration); allergic reactions; fever; peripheral neuropathies; back, joint, and muscle pain; hair loss
Doxorubicin	Adriamycin RDF, Rubex, others	Acute leukemias; carcinoma of bladder, breast, ovary, thyroid, and other tissues; Hodgkin disease; non-Hodgkin lymphomas; several sarcomas	Similar to daunorubicin
Epirubicin	Ellence	Axillary tumor after breast cancer resection	Similar to daunorubicin
Idarubicin	Idamycin	Acute myelogenous leukemia	Similar to daunorubicin
Mitomycin	MitoExtra, Mutamycin	Carcinoma of stomach and pancreas	Blood disorders (leukopenia, thrombocytopenia); GI distress (nausea, vomiting, GI irritation and ulceration); nephrotoxicity; pulmonary toxicity
Mitoxantrone	Novantrone	Carcinoma of the prostate; acute nonlymphocytic leukemia	Blood disorders (anemia, leukopenia, thrombocytopenia); GI distress (nausea, vomiting, diarrhea, abdominal pain); respiratory toxicity (cough, dyspnea); CNS toxicity (seizures, headache); cardiotoxicity (arrhythmias, congestive heart failure); fever; hair loss
Streptozocin	Zanosar	Pancreatic carcinoma	Nephrotoxicity; hepatotoxicity; GI distress (nausea, vomiting); blood disorders (anemia, leukopenia, thrombocytopenia); local irritation at injection site

**Only the indications listed in the U.S. product labeling are included here. Many anticancer drugs are used for additional types of neoplastic disease.*

Table 36-4
ANTIMICROTUBULE AGENTS

Generic Name	Trade Name	Primary Antineoplastic Indication(s)*	Common Adverse Effects
Cabazitaxel	Jevtana	Refractory prostate cancer	Blood disorders (anemia, leukopenia, neutropenia); GI distress (nausea, vomiting, diarrhea, others); cardiopulmonary toxicity (arrhythmias, hypotension); renal toxicity; peripheral neuropathies; muscle and joint pain; anaphylactoid reactions; fever; hair loss
Docetaxel	Taxotere	Breast cancer; refractory or inoperable non-small cell lung cancer, prostate cancer, or squamous cell carcinoma of the head and neck	Blood disorders (anemia, leukopenia, neutropenia); GI distress (nausea, vomiting, diarrhea); cardiopulmonary toxicity (arrhythmias, pericardial effusion, pulmonary edema, peripheral edema); muscle and joint pain; anaphylactoid reactions; skin problems (rashes, hair loss)
Ixabepilone	Ixempra	Refractory or advanced breast cancer	Blood disorders (anemia, leukopenia, neutropenia); GI distress (nausea, vomiting, diarrhea, abdominal pain, others); renal toxicity; peripheral neuropathies; muscle and joint pain; skin reactions (rashes, itching, hair loss)
Paclitaxel	Onxol, Taxol	Carcinoma of the breast, ovaries; Kaposi sarcoma; non-small cell lung cancer	Blood disorders (anemia, leukopenia, neutropenia); GI distress (nausea, vomiting, diarrhea); cardiopulmonary toxicity (arrhythmias, pericardial effusion, pulmonary edema, peripheral edema); muscle and joint pain; anaphylactoid reactions; skin problems (rashes, hair loss)
Vinblastine	Velban, Velbe	Carcinoma of breast, testes, other tissues; Hodgkin disease; non-Hodgkin lymphomas; Kaposi sarcoma	Blood disorders (anemia, leukopenia, thrombocytopenia); GI distress (nausea, vomiting); hair loss; neurotoxicity (peripheral neuropathies, CNS disorders); hair loss; local irritation at injection site
Vincristine	Oncovin, Vincasar PFS	Acute lymphocytic leukemia; neuroblastoma; Wilms' tumor; Hodgkin disease; non-Hodgkin lymphomas; Ewing sarcoma, other tumors	Similar to vinblastine
Vinorelbine	Navelbine	Non-small cell lung cancer	Similar to vinblastine

**Only the indications listed in the U.S. product labeling are included here. Many anticancer drugs are used for additional types of neoplastic disease.*

Topoisomerase Inhibitors

Drugs classified as topoisomerase inhibitors include etoposide, irinotecan, teniposide, and topotecan (Table 36-5). These drugs inhibit specific enzymes known as *topoisomerase enzymes*, which are necessary for normal DNA replication.[36] Etoposide and teniposide inhibit the topoisomerase I form of this enzyme, and irinotecan and topotecan inhibit the topoisomerase II form. Inhibition of these enzymes causes a break in both strands of the DNA double helix, which leads to DNA destruction and cell death.[37]

Anticancer Hormones

Several forms of cancer are referred to as *hormone sensitive* because they tend to be exacerbated by certain hormones and attenuated by others. In particular, adrenocorticosteroids (see Chapter 29) and the sex hormones (i.e., androgens, estrogens, progesterone; see Chapter 30) may influence the proliferation of certain tumors. Hence, drugs that either mimic or block (antagonize) the effects of these hormones may be useful in treating certain hormone-sensitive forms of cancer.[38,39] Hormonal anticancer drugs are typically used as adjuvant therapy—that is, they are used in conjunction with surgery, radiation treatment, and other anticancer drugs.

The primary drugs that inhibit neoplasms via hormonal mechanisms are listed in Table 36-6. In some cases, these drugs work by direct inhibitory effects on cancerous cells (e.g., adrenocorticoid suppression of lymphocyte function) or by negative feedback mechanisms that decrease the endogenous hormonal stimulation of the tumor (e.g., gonadotropin-releasing hormones). In other cases, drugs can directly block the

Table 36-5
TOPOISOMERASE INHIBITORS

Generic Name	Trade Name	Primary Antineoplastic Indication(s)*	Common Adverse Effects
Etoposide	VePesid, VP-16	Carcinoma of lung, testes	Blood disorders (anemia, leukopenia, thrombocytopenia); GI distress (nausea, vomiting, diarrhea, others); severe allergic reactions; neurotoxicity (peripheral neuropathies, CNS effects); skin reactions (hair loss, rashes, itching)
Irinotecan	Camptosar	Colorectal cancer	Blood disorders (anemia, leukopenia, neutropenia); dyspnea; GI distress (nausea, vomiting, diarrhea, constipation, others); respiratory toxicity (coughing, rhinitis, dyspnea); CNS toxicity (dizziness, headache, insomnia); fever; skin reactions (hair loss, rashes)
Teniposide	Vumon, VM-26	Acute lymphoblastic leukemia	Blood disorders (anemia, leukopenia, neutropenia, thrombocytopenia); mucositis; GI distress (nausea, vomiting, diarrhea); hypersensitivity reaction
Topotecan	Hycamtin	Ovarian cancer; small lung cell carcinoma	Blood disorders (anemia, leukopenia, thrombocytopenia); GI distress (abdominal pain, loss of appetite, nausea, vomiting, diarrhea, constipation); dyspnea; hair loss

**Only the indications listed in the U.S. product labeling are included here. Many anticancer drugs are used for additional types of neoplastic disease.*

Table 36-6
ANTICANCER HORMONES

Types of Hormones	Primary Antineoplastic Indications(s)*	Common Adverse Effects
Adrenocorticosteroids Prednisone Prednisolone Others	Acute and chronic lymphocytic leukemia; Hodgkin disease; non-Hodgkin lymphoma; multiple myeloma; breast cancer	Adrenocortical suppression; general catabolic effect on supporting tissues (see Chapter 29)
Androgens Fluoxymesterone Testosterone Other testosterone derivatives	Advanced, inoperable breast cancer in postmenopausal women	Masculinization in women (see Chapter 30)
Antiandrogens Bicalutamide Flutamide Nilutamide	Inhibits the cellular uptake and effects of androgens in advanced, metastatic prostate cancer	Nausea; vomiting; diarrhea; decreased sex drive
Aromatase inhibitors Anastrozole Exemestane Letrozole	Inhibits estrogen biosynthesis to reduce the effects of estrogen in estrogen-sensitive breast cancer	Nausea; vomiting; dizziness; hot flashes; joint and muscle pain; dyspnea; (generally well tolerated relative to other antineoplastic hormones; side effects vary, depending on the specific drug)
Estrogens Diethylstilbestrol Estradiol Other estrogen derivatives	Advanced, inoperable breast cancer in selected men and postmenopausal women; advanced, inoperable prostate cancer in men	Cardiovascular complications (including stroke and heart attack, especially in men); many other adverse effects (see Chapter 30)
Antiestrogens Fulvestrant Tamoxifen Toremifene	Acts as an estrogen antagonist to decrease the recurrence of cancer following mastectomy or to reduce tumor growth in advanced stages of breast cancer	Nausea; vomiting; hot flashes (generally well tolerated relative to other antineoplastic hormones)
Progestins Hydroxyprogesterone Medroxyprogesterone Megestrol	Carcinoma of the breast and endometrium; advanced prostate cancer; advanced renal cancer	Menstrual irregularities; hyperglycemia; edema; mood changes; unusual tiredness; abdominal pain/cramps

Continued

Table 36-6
ANTICANCER HORMONES—cont'd

Types of Hormones	Primary Antineoplastic Indications(s)*	Common Adverse Effects
Gonadotropin-releasing hormone drugs Abarelix Goserelin Leuprolide Triptorelin	Works by negative feedback mechanisms to inhibit testosterone or estrogen production; used primarily in advanced prostate cancer or breast cancer	Hot flashes; bone pain; CNS effects (headache, dizziness); GI disturbances (nausea, vomiting)

**Only the indications listed in the U.S. product labeling are included here. Many anticancer drugs are used for additional types of neoplastic disease.*

effects of the endogenous hormone and prevent that hormone from stimulating specific tumors. In particular, androgen receptor blockers (flutamide, others) can treat prostate cancer by blocking the effects of testosterone on the prostate gland.[40,41]

Estrogen receptor blockers (fulvestrant, tamoxifen) can likewise help prevent and treat breast and uterine cancers that are stimulated by estrogen.[42] Fulvestrant is a true estrogen receptor antagonist or blocker that binds to estrogen receptors but fails to activate these receptors and ultimately results in downregulation and degradation of estrogen receptors.[43] As indicated in Chapter 30, tamoxifen and similar drugs (raloxifene, toremifene) are classified as a selective estrogen receptor modulators (SERMs), meaning that these drugs block estrogen receptors on certain tissues (breast, uterus) while stimulating other estrogen receptors in bone, cardiovascular tissues, skin, and so forth.[44]

In contrast to estrogen blockers, **aromatase** inhibitors such as anastrozole (Arimidex), letrozole (Femara), and exemestane (Aromasin) can decrease estrogen production in breast and other tissues by inhibiting the aromatase enzyme that is responsible for estrogen biosynthesis.[45] That is, these agents do not block estrogen receptors but instead reduce estrogen production, thereby decreasing the influence of estrogen on breast tumors.[45,46] Hence, several options are now available for controlling hormone-sensitive cancers that are responsive to estrogen and androgens in women and men, respectively. Refer to Chapter 30 for more details about the effects of androgens, estrogens, and their respective receptor-blocking agents.

Targeted and Biological Therapies

Certain anticancer drugs are classified as "targeted" therapies because they attempt to seek out and inhibit biochemical characteristics that are unique to the cancer cell. Similarly, certain agents are known as *biological therapies* or *biological response modifiers* because they encourage the body's immune system to fight cancerous cells. Targeted and biological therapies offer the potential advantage of impairing function in the cancer cells with minimal effects on healthy human cells. These therapies include the monoclonal antibodies, cytokines (interferons, interleuklin-2), and tyrosine kinase inhibitors (Table 36-7).

Monoclonal Antibodies

Monoclonal antibodies are one of the primary ways to target specific cancer cells.[47,48] Basically, these drugs are manufactured using cell cloning techniques that produce an antibody that is specific for an antigen on the surface of a particular type of cancer cell (see Table 36-7). When administered, the monoclonal antibody is attracted directly to the cancer cell, without any appreciable effect on healthy tissues—that is, healthy cells lack the antigen that is present on the cancerous cell and should therefore remain unaffected by the drug. Once it has reached the cancerous cell, the monoclonal antibody exerts several complex effects that can limit cell function, inhibit mitosis, and possibly result directly in the cell's death.[49] Some monoclonal agents may also function as biological response modifiers in that they bind to the antigen on the cancer cell and enhance the ability of cytotoxic T lymphocytes or other immune system components to attack the tumor.[50,51] Finally, monoclonal antibodies can be linked to other anticancer drugs or radioactive substances (antibody-drug conjugates), thus delivering these substances directly to the cancer cells that contain the appropriate antigen.[52,53]

Hence, monoclonal antibodies are one of the most exciting and promising anticancer strategies, and development of anticancer antibodies continues to be an

Table 36-7
TARGETED AND BIOLOGICAL THERAPIES

Drug(s)	Primary Antineoplastic Indication(s)*	Common Adverse Effects
Monoclonal Antibodies		
Alemtuzumab (Campath)	Chronic lymphocytic leukemia	Blood disorders (anemia, leukopenia, neutropenia, thrombocytopenia); GI distress (abdominal pain, constipation); respiratory toxicity (bronchospasm, cough, dyspnea); infection
Bevacizumab (Avastin)	Colorectal carcinoma; inoperable advanced non-small cell lung cancer	Cardiovascular toxicity (hemorrhage, blood pressure changes, arterial thrombosis, heart failure); poor wound healing
Cetuximab (Erbitux)	Colorectal carcinoma; head and neck cancer	GI distress (nausea, vomiting, diarrhea, others); pulmonary embolism; skin reactions (itching, dermatitis); fever
Gemtuzumab (Mylotarg)	Acute myeloid leukemia	GI distress (nausea, vomiting, diarrhea); metabolic imbalances (hyperkalemia, hyperphosphatemia, hypocalcemia) caused by release of electrolytes from dying cancer cells (tumor lysis syndrome); skin rash
Ibritumomab (Zevalin)	Non-Hodgkin lymphoma	Blood disorders (anemia, leukopenia, thrombocytopenia); GI distress (abdominal pain, constipation); respiratory toxicity (bronchospasm, cough, dyspnea); anaphylactoid reactions; joint pain; anxiety; dizziness
Ofatumumab (Arzerra)	Chronic lymphocytic leukemia	Blood disorders (anemia, neutropenia, thrombocytopenia); intestinal obstruction; infections; progressive multifocal leukoencephalopathy
Panitumumab Vectibix	Colorectal cancer	GI distress (abdominal pain, nausea, vomiting, constipation, others); respiratory toxicity (pulmonary fibrosis, cough); ocular toxicity; skin reactions (rashes, exfoliative dermatitis)
Rituximab (Rituxan)	Non-Hodgkin lymphoma	Blood disorders (anemia, neutropenia, thrombocytopenia); GI distress (nausea, vomiting, diarrhea); cardiovascular toxicity (arrhythmias, hypotension, peripheral edema); metabolic imbalances (hyperkalemia, hyperphosphatemia, hypocalcemia) caused by release of electrolytes from dying cancer cells (tumor lysis syndrome); anaphylactoid reactions; skin reactions (rashes, flushing); fever
Tositumomab (Bexxar)	Non-Hodgkin lymphoma	Blood disorders (anemia, neutropenia, thrombocytopenia); GI distress (abdominal pain, nausea, vomiting, diarrhea); muscle and joint pain; peripheral neuropathies; muscle and joint pain
Trastuzumab (Herceptin)	Breast cancer	GI distress (abdominal pain, nausea, vomiting, diarrhea); cardiovascular toxicity (arrhythmia, heart failure, hypertension); respiratory toxicity (pulmonary fibrosis, pneumonitis, pulmonary edema); skin rashes; anaphylactoid reactions; fever; infection
Cytokines		
Interferons Interferon alfa-2b (Intron-A)	Hairy-cell leukemia; Kaposi sarcoma; malignant melanoma; follicular non-Hodgkin lymphoma	Blood disorders (anemia, leukopenia, thrombocytopenia); cardiovascular toxicity (arrhythmias, ischemia); neuropsychiatric effects; GI distress (nausea, vomiting, diarrhea, colitis, others); flulike syndrome (mild fever, chills, malaise)
Interleukin-2 aldesleukin (Proleukin)	Renal carcinoma	Blood disorders (anemia, eosinophilia, leukopenia, thrombocytopenia); cardiovascular toxicity (arrhythmias, hypotension, cardiac arrest, heart failure, stroke); pulmonary toxicity (dyspnea, pulmonary congestion, apnea, respiratory failure); renal toxicity; electrolyte imbalances; GI distress (nausea, vomiting, diarrhea); skin reactions (itching, exfoliative dermatitis)
Tyrosine Kinase Inhibitors		
Erlotinib (Tarceva)	Non-small cell lung cancer	GI distress (nausea, vomiting, diarrhea); interstitial lung disease; skin rashes
Gefitinib (Iressa)	Non-small cell lung cancer	Pulmonary toxicity; GI distress (nausea, vomiting, diarrhea); allergic reactions; skin reactions (rash, itching, acne)

Continued

Table 36-7
TARGETED AND BIOLOGICAL THERAPIES—cont'd

Drug(s)	Primary Antineoplastic Indication(s)*	Common Adverse Effects
Imatinib (Gleevec)	Chronic myeloid leukemia; acute lymphoblastic leukemia; GI stromal tumors; others	GI distress (nausea, vomiting, diarrhea, constipation); blood disorders (anemia, neutropenia, thrombocytopenia, hemorrhage); hepatotoxicity; respiratory toxicity (cough, dyspnea, pneumonia); joint and muscle pain; skin reactions (rash, itching, petechiae); fever
Sorafenib (Nexavar)	Renal cellular carcinoma; hepatocellular carcinoma	GI distress (nausea, vomiting, diarrhea, constipation, others); blood disorders (anemia, leukopenia, thrombocytopenia, hemorrhage); cardiovascular toxicity (hypertension, myocardial ischemia); CNS toxicity (depression, fatigue, weakness); joint and muscle pain; peripheral neuropathies; skin reactions (rash, itching, exfoliative dermatitis, others)
Sunitinib (Sutent)	GI stromal tumor; advanced renal cell carcinoma	GI distress (nausea, vomiting, diarrhea, others); blood disorders (anemia, neutropenia, thrombocytopenia, hemorrhage); cardiovascular toxicity (hypertension, peripheral edema, thrombosis); joint and muscle pain; peripheral neuropathies; skin reactions (rash, itching, exfoliative dermatitis, others)

**Only the indications listed in the U.S. product labeling are included here. Many anticancer drugs are used for additional types of neoplastic disease.*

important area of research. New antibodies that selectively inhibit or kill cancer cells with minimal or no effects on healthy tissues will undoubtedly be available in the future.[48,54]

Certain monoclonal antibodies, such as bevacizumab (Avastin), can also be used as **angiogenesis** inhibitors—that is, these agents inhibit the formation of new blood vessels in growing tumors.[55,56] Because tumors often need a rich vascular supply to grow and proliferate, angiogenesis inhibitors can literally starve the tumor of oxygen and nutrients.[55,57] Bevacizumab binds specifically to vascular endothelial growth factor (VEGF) and prevents it from stimulating the formation of blood vessels in the tumor.[56,58] Hence, this intervention can be used along with other more traditional anticancer drugs to treat specific cancers, such as advanced colorectal cancer. Other strategies to prevent angiogenesis are currently being developed, and various types of angiogenesis inhibitors may be forthcoming.[57]

Cytokines

Cytokines, such as the interferons and interleukin-2, are small proteins that play an important role in modulating immune responses. Their role as potential biological anticancer drugs is based on their ability to stimulate the immune mechanisms that normally deal with abnormal cell proliferation.

The chemistry and pharmacology of the interferons were discussed in Chapter 34. These peptide compounds exert several beneficial effects, including antiviral and antineoplastic activity. However, the exact mechanism of action for interferons to impair cancerous cell growth is not clear. It is possible that interferons affect several aspects of tumor growth, including the activation of cytotoxic immune cells (natural killer cells) and the activation of signaling pathways in the cancer cell that help retard cell division and bring about programmed death (apoptosis) of cancerous tissues.[59,60] Regardless of their exact mechanism, these agents are effective in treating certain types of leukemias, lymphomas, Kaposi sarcoma, and cancer in other organs and tissues (see Table 36-7).[61,62]

Interleukin-2 (IL-2) is an endogenous cytokine that normally exerts a number of beneficial immunologic responses. In particular, IL-2 stimulates the growth and differentiation of T-cell lymphocytes and natural killer cells that are toxic for tumor cells.[63,64] Hence, IL-2 is now synthesized using recombinant DNA techniques so that this agent can be used to treat cancers such as renal cancer and malignant melanoma (see Table 36-7). Research continues to identify the antineoplastic role of interleukins, interferons, and other cytokines, as well as to define how these agents can be used alone or in combination to treat various forms of cancer.[60,65]

Tyrosine Kinase Inhibitors

As discussed in Chapter 4, the tyrosine kinase enzyme, found in many cells, is responsible for transmitting signals from the cell membrane to other functional components throughout the cell. In certain types of cancer, defective function of tyrosine kinases leads to abnormal cell function and proliferation.[66] Hence, drugs that inhibit tyrosine kinase activity will be especially useful in some cancers.[67,68] Several tyrosine kinase drugs are currently available, including erlotinib (Tarceva), gefitinib (Iressa), imatinib (Gleevec), and other agents with a *-nib* suffix (see Table 36-7). These drugs are gaining acceptance as a part of the treatment of certain leukemias, as well as cancers affecting other tissues such as the lungs, stomach, and pancreas. Use of specific drugs is likewise dependent on certain cellular receptors that control tyrosine kinase activity and cell-signaling pathways in each type of cancer. Nonetheless, researchers continue to explore strategies that affect abnormal tyrosine kinase activity, and more information about optimal use of tyrosine kinase inhibitors will surely be forthcoming.

Platinum Coordination Complexes

Platinum coordination complexes used to treat cancer include cisplatin, carboplatin, and oxaliplatin (Table 36-8). These drugs, which contain platinum, are also known as *heavy metal compounds*.[69,70] Platinum coordination complex drugs act like the alkylating agents; they form strong cross-links between and within DNA strands, thereby preventing DNA translation and replication. The chemical nature of these cross-links, however, involves the platinum component of the drug rather than actual formation of an alkyl side group. Platinum coordination compounds are especially important as part of the treatment of certain epithelial cancers, including testicular cancer, ovarian cancer, bladder cancer, and others.[69,71,72]

Aspirin and Other NSAIDs

Considerable evidence exists that aspirin and similar NSAIDs can prevent colorectal cancer and might also decrease malignancies in other tissues such as the stomach, esophagus, breast, prostate, and lungs.[73,74] This effect seems to be related to the duration of treatment, with increased protection occurring in people who use aspirin on a regular basis for several years.[75] Although the exact reason for this anticancer effect is unknown, recent evidence suggests that aspirin's anticancer effects are due to platelet inhibition.[74,76] That is, platelet activation may enhance the growth of certain tumors, and aspirin can inhibit this platelet-induced cell proliferation, probably by inhibiting thromboxane biosynthesis. As addressed in Chapters 15 and 25, aspirin potently inhibits the production of thromboxanes (a type of prostaglandin) that normally activate platelets during hemostasis. This explains the use of low-dose aspirin therapy in preventing platelet-induced arterial thrombosis in heart attack and ischemic stroke. Hence, aspirin's antitumor effects are likely due to similar platelet inhibition in tumor cells or precancerous tissues.[74,76] In addition, the COX-2 form of the cyclooxygenase enzyme seems to be prevalent in certain tumors, and inhibition of this enzyme using COX-2 selective drugs may ultimately provide optimal results in certain cancers.[77] More information will surely be

Table 36-8
PLATINUM COORDINATION COMPLEXES

Drug	Primary Antineoplastic Indication(s)*	Common Adverse Effects
Carboplatin (Paraplatin)	Carcinoma of the ovaries	Blood disorders (anemia, leukopenia, neutropenia, thrombocytopenia); GI distress (nausea, vomiting, diarrhea, abdominal pain); anaphylactoid reactions; peripheral neuropathies
Cisplatin (Platinol)	Carcinoma of bladder, ovaries, testicles, and other tissues	Blood disorders (anemia, leukopenia, thrombocytopenia); nephrotoxicity; GI distress (nausea, vomiting, diarrhea); neurotoxicity (cranial and peripheral nerves); anaphylactoid reactions
Oxaliplatin (Eloxatin)	Colorectal cancer	Blood disorders (anemia, leukopenia, neutropenia, thrombocytopenia); GI distress (nausea, vomiting, diarrhea, abdominal pain); respiratory toxicity (pulmonary fibrosis, cough, dyspnea); anaphylactoid reactions; peripheral neuropathies

**Only the indications listed in the U.S. product labeling are included here. Many anticancer drugs are used for additional types of neoplastic disease.*

forthcoming about how aspirin and other NSAIDs can help prevent specific types of cancer.

Miscellaneous Agents

Certain chemotherapy agents do not fall into one of the categories addressed above. These miscellaneous drugs are listed in Table 36-9 and are described briefly in the following sections.

Arsenic Trioxide

Arsenic is a heavy metal that can exert toxic, poisonous effects. Therapeutic dosages of arsenic trioxide (Trisenox), however, may limit the growth of certain leukemias such as acute promyelocytic leukemia.[78] Because of its

Table 36-9
MISCELLANEOUS ANTINEOPLASTIC DRUGS

Drug	Primary Antineoplastic Indication(s)*	Common Adverse Effects
Arsenic trioxide (Trisenox)	Acute promyelocytic leukemia	Blood disorders (anemia, neutropenia, thrombocytopenia, others); GI distress (abdominal pain, constipation); cardiac arrhythmias; respiratory toxicity (hypoxia, dyspnea, pleural effusion); muscle and joint pain
Asparaginase (Elspar, Kidrolase)	Acute lymphocytic leukemia	GI distress (nausea, vomiting, abdominal pain); hepatic toxicity; pancreatitis; delayed hemostasis; CNS toxicity (fatigue, mood changes, seizures); GI distress (nausea, vomiting); anaphylactoid reactions
Bortezomib (Velcade)	Multiple myeloma	Blood disorders (anemia, neutropenia, thrombocytopenia, hemorrhage); GI distress (nausea, vomiting, diarrhea, constipation); hypotension; peripheral neuropathies; fever
Denileukin Diftitox (Ontak)	Cutaneous T-cell lymphomas	Blood disorders (anemia, leukopenia, thrombocytopenia); GI distress (nausea, vomiting, diarrhea); cardiovascular toxicity (edema, chest pain, hypotension, arrhythmias, thrombosis); respiratory toxicity (cough, dyspnea, rhinitis); skin reactions (rash, itching); acute allergic reactions; joint and muscle pain; flulike symptoms; infection
Estramustine (Emcyt)	Prostate cancer	Cardiovascular toxicity (thromboembolism, edema, hypertension); blood disorders (leukopenia, thrombocytopenia); thrombosis; GI distress (nausea, diarrhea, vomiting)
Histone deacetylase inhibitors Vorinostat (Zolinza) Romidepsin (Istodax)	Cutaneous T-cell lymphoma	Blood disorders (anemia, leukopenia, thrombocytopenia); GI distress (nausea, vomiting, abdominal pain); ECG changes
Hydroxyurea (Droxia, Hydrea, Mylocel)	Carcinoma of the ovaries, head/neck region, other tissues; chronic myelogenous leukemia; melanomas	Blood disorders (primarily leukopenia); GI distress (nausea, vomiting, diarrhea, loss of appetite, GI tract irritation and ulceration); skin reactions (rash, hair loss, itching)
Mitotane (Lysodren)	Suppresses adrenal gland; used primarily to treat adrenocortical carcinoma	GI distress (nausea, vomiting, diarrhea, loss of appetite); CNS toxicity (lethargy, fatigue, mood changes); muscle and joint pain; skin rashes
Thalidomide (Thalomid)	Multiple myeloma	Peripheral neuropathy; dizziness; drowsiness; skin rash; contraindicated in pregnant women because of teratogenic potential
Retinoids Tretinoin (Vesanoid) Alitretinoin (Panretin) Bexarotene (Targretin)	Acute promyelocytic leukemia	Cardiovascular toxicity (arrhythmias, edema, blood pressure abnormalities, phlebitis; peripheral edema, coagulation disorders); CNS toxicity (seizures, depression, anxiety, confusion, others); renal insufficiency; GI distress (abdominal distention, bleeding, nausea, vomiting, others); muscle pain; paresthesias; contraindicated in pregnant women because of teratogenic potential

**Only the indications listed in the U.S. product labeling are included here. Many anticancer drugs are used for additional types of neoplastic disease.*

potential toxicity, arsenic trioxide is not usually an initial treatment but is reserved for patients who relapse or who are resistant to other treatments. Although the exact mechanism of action is unclear, this drug apparently induces several cytotoxic effects by directly damaging DNA and proteins that regulate DNA synthesis and replication.

Asparaginase

Asparaginase is an enzyme that converts the amino acid asparagine into aspartic acid and ammonia. Most normal cells are able to synthesize sufficient amounts of asparagine to function properly. Some tumor cells (especially certain leukemic cells) must rely on extracellular sources for a supply of asparagine. By breaking down asparagine in the bloodstream and extracellular fluid, asparaginase (Elspar) deprives tumor cells of their source of asparagine, thus selectively impairing cell metabolism in these cells.[79] Asparaginase is used primarily in the treatment of acute lymphocytic leukemia (see Table 36-9).

Bortezomib

Bortezomib (Velcade) inhibits proteasome activity in mammalian cells.[80] Mammalian proteasome is responsible for degrading certain cellular proteins affecting cell function and division. By prolonging the activity of these proteins, bortezomib brings about complex changes in cell function that lead to cell dysfunction and death. Certain types of cancer, such as multiple myeloma, are more sensitive to impaired proteasome regulation, hence the use of this drug in these cancers.

Denileukin Diftitox

Denileukin Diftitox (Ontak) is formulated by combining interleukin-2 with diphtheria toxin.[81] Certain leukemia and lymphoma cells have a surface receptor that has a high affinity for interleukin-2, thus attracting this drug directly to these cells. Upon binding with the receptor, the diphtheria toxin component of the drug inhibits cellular protein synthesis, which ultimately results in cell death. This drug is used primarily to treat recurrent cutaneous T-cell lymphoma.

Estramustine

Estramustine (Emcyt) is a chemical combination of mechlorethamine (an alkylating agent) and estrogen. It is not clear how this drug exerts antineoplastic effects. The beneficial effects of this drug are probably not related to any alkylating effects. Rather, they may be the direct result of its estrogenic component or its inhibitory effect on the microtubules that comprise the mitotic apparatus.[82] This drug is typically used for the palliative treatment of advanced prostate cancer.[83]

Histone Deacetylase Inhibitors

Vorinostat (Zolinza) and romidepsin (Istodax) are relatively new drugs that work by inhibiting the histone deacetylase enzyme.[84,85] This enzyme is normally responsible for modifying the proteins (histones) that wrap DNA tightly to form chromatin within the cell's nucleus. By inhibiting this enzyme, these drugs can help correct excessive removal of acetyl groups (deacetylation) from amino acid residues, thereby normalizing gene transcription and cell proliferation in certain cancers such as cutaneous T-cell lymphoma.[86]

These drugs also represent a new anticancer strategy known as *epigenetic modification*. Certain cancers may be caused by modification of the DNA molecule by factors other than a defect in the actual nucleotide sequence that comprises DNA.[87] That is, abnormal activity of the cancerous cell is caused by the addition or removal of chemical constituents such as acetyl or methyl groups to the proteins surrounding the DNA molecule. As indicated above, excess deacetylation is one type of abnormal epigenetic modification that causes certain cancers, and drugs are now available that can normalize deacetylation and inhibit these cancers. Efforts continue to identify other cancers that are caused by defective epigenetic modifications, and drugs that correct these modifications will hopefully be forthcoming.

Hydroxyurea

It is believed that hydroxyurea (Hydrea) impairs DNA synthesis by inhibiting a specific enzyme (ribonucleoside reductase) involved in synthesizing nucleic acid precursors.[88] The uses of hydroxyurea are listed in Table 36-9.

Mitotane

Although the exact mechanism of this drug is unknown, mitotane (Lysodren) selectively inhibits adrenocortical function. This agent is used exclusively to treat inoperable carcinoma of the adrenal cortex.[89]

Thalidomide and Lenalidomide

Thalidomide (Thalomid) was originally developed as a sedative and antinausea drug but was withdrawn from the market because it caused severe birth defects when administered to pregnant women. However, it has reemerged as a potential treatment for cancers such as multiple myeloma.[90,91] Likewise, lenalidomide (Revlimid), a derivative of thalidomide, may also be helpful in treating multiple myeloma. Although the exact reasons for the anticancer effects of these drugs are not clear, thalidomide and lenalidomide exert a number of complex effects on immune function, including the suppression of tumor necrosis factor alpha.[90,92] These drugs also inhibit angiogenesis and may therefore limit the growth of solid tumors by inhibiting vascularization and nutrient supply.[92]

Retinoids

Tretinoin (Vesanoid), also known as *all-trans-retinoic acid*, is derived from vitamin A (retinol).[93] Other retinoids include alitretinoin (Panretin) and bexarotene (Targretin). These drugs are not cytotoxic, but it may help cells differentiate and replicate at a more normal rate. However, the exact way that these agents affect cell differentiation is not known. Tretinoin is used primarily to treat certain forms of leukemia.[93] Bexarotene is used is administered systemically to treat cutaneous T-cell lymphoma,[94] and alitretinoin is typically administered topically to treat cutaneous lesions in Kaposi sarcoma.[95]

COMBINATION CHEMOTHERAPY

Frequently, several different anticancer drugs are administered simultaneously. This process of combination chemotherapy increases the chance of successfully treating the cancer because of the additive and synergistic effect of each agent. Often, different types of anticancer drugs are combined in the same regimen to provide optimal results.[96-99] For instance, a particular drug regimen may include an alkylating agent, an antineoplastic antibiotic, a hormonal agent, or some other combination of anticancer drugs.

Some common anticancer drug combinations and the types of cancer in which they are used are listed in Table 36-10. These drug combinations are often indicated by an acronym of the drug names. For instance, *FAC* indicates a regimen of fluorouracil, doxorubicin (Adriamycin), and cyclophosphamide. These abbreviations are used to summarize drug therapy in a patient's medical chart, so therapists should be aware of the more common chemotherapy combinations.

Table 36-10
FREQUENTLY USED COMBINATION CHEMOTHERAPY REGIMENS

Chemotherapeutic Regimen*	Components of Regimen	Primary Indication
ABVD	Doxorubicin (**A**driamycin), **B**leomycin (Blenoxane), **V**inblastine (Velban), **D**acarbazine (DTIC)	Hodgkin lymphoma
BEP	**B**leomycin, **E**toposide, cis**P**latin	Testicular cancer
CEF	**C**yclophosphamide, **E**pirubicin, **F**luorouracil	Breast cancer
R-CHOP	**R**ituximab, **C**yclophosphamide (Cytoxan), doxorubicin,** vincristine (**O**ncovin), **P**rednisone	Chronic lymphocytic leukemia; non-Hodgkin lymphoma
CMF	**C**yclophosphamide (Cytoxan), **M**ethotrexate, **F**luorouracil	Breast cancer
FAC	**F**luorouracil, doxorubicin (**A**driamycin), **C**yclophosphamide (Cytoxan)	Breast cancer
FEC	**F**luorouracil, **E**pirubicin, **C**yclophosphamide	Breast cancer
FOLFOX	**FOL**inic acid, **F**luorouracil, **OX**aliplatin	Colorectal cancer
PCb	**P**aclitaxel, **C**ar**b**oplatin	Lung cancer
PCV	**P**rocarbazine, lomustine (**C**CNU), **V**incristine	Brain cancer
VAD	**V**incristine, doxorubicin (**A**driamycin), **D**examethasone	Multiple myeloma

**A few examples of commonly used regimens are listed here. Many other combinations are used clinically, and regimens are often tailored for the needs of each patient.*

***The H in this regimen refers to hydroxydaunorubicin, the chemical synonym for doxorubicin.*

USE OF ANTICANCER DRUGS WITH OTHER TREATMENTS

Cancer chemotherapy is only one method of treating neoplastic disease. The other primary weapons in the anticancer arsenal are surgery and radiation treatment.[100-102] The choice of one or more of these techniques depends primarily on the patient, the type of cancer, and the tumor location. In many situations, chemotherapy may be the primary or sole form of treatment in neoplastic disease, especially for certain advanced or inoperable tumors or in widely disseminated forms of cancer, such as leukemia or lymphoma.[1,103,104] In other situations, chemotherapy is used in combination with other techniques, such as an adjuvant to surgery and radiation treatment.[101,102,105] Primary examples of adjuvant cancer chemotherapy include using anticancer drugs following a mastectomy or surgical removal of other carcinomas.[106-109] Alternatively, chemotherapeutic agents can be administered prior to a more aggressive surgical or radiation treatment. This technique, known commonly as *neoadjuvant therapy*, can help control or reduce the cancerous growth so that the nondrug intervention is more successful in eliminating the cancer.[110,111]

Whether anticancer drugs are used as the primary treatment or as adjuvant therapy, a common general strategy is upheld. All reasonable means of dealing with the cancer must be employed as early as possible to achieve a total cell kill. Cancer is not the type of disease in which a wait-and-see approach can be used. The general strategy is more aligned with the idea that a barrage of anticancer modalities (i.e., surgery, radiation, and a combination of several different antineoplastic drugs) may be necessary to achieve a successful outcome. In addition, a multimodal approach (combining chemotherapy with radiation or using several drugs simultaneously) may produce a synergistic effect between these modalities. For instance, certain drugs may sensitize cancer cells to radiation treatment.[112,113] Likewise, several drugs working together may increase the antineoplastic effects of one another through a synergistic cytotoxic effect.[114,115]

SUCCESS OF ANTICANCER DRUGS

Various forms of cancer exhibit a broad spectrum of response to antineoplastic medications. Some forms of cancer (choriocarcinoma, Wilms' tumor) can be cured in more than 90 percent of affected patients. In other neoplastic disorders, chemotherapy may not cure the disease but may succeed in mediating remission and prolonging survival in a large patient percentage. Of course, other factors such as early detection and the concomitant use of other interventions (surgery, radiation) will greatly influence the success of chemotherapy drugs.

However, certain forms of cancer do not respond well to treatment. For example, once the cancer has spread (metastasized) to distant sites in the body, most cancers are difficult to cure by current chemotherapeutic methods or by any other type of treatment.[1,116] In addition, some of the most common forms of adult neoplastic disease are difficult to treat with anticancer drugs. As indicated in Table 36-11, the number of deaths associated with colorectal, prostate, and breast

Table 36-11
INCIDENCE AND MORTALITY OF THE LEADING FORMS OF CANCER IN WOMEN AND MEN

Type/Site of Cancer	Number of New Cases*	Number of Deaths*
Women		
Breast	232,670	40,000
Colon and rectum	65,000	24,040
Leukemia	22,280	10,050
Lung and bronchus	108,210	72,330
Lymphoma	36,650	9,030
Ovary	21,980	14,270
Pancreas	22,890	19,420
Uterine cervix	12,360	4,020
Uterine corpus	52,630	8,590
Men		
Colon and rectum	71,830	26,270
Esophagus	14,660	12,450
Leukemia	30,100	14,040
Liver and bile duct	24,600	15,870
Lung and bronchus	116,000	86,930
Lymphoma	43,340	11,140
Pancreas	23,530	20,170
Prostate	233,000	29,480
Urinary system	97,420	20,610

Source: The American Cancer Society Department of Epidemiology and Surveillance Research.

**Estimates for 2014.*

cancer is unacceptably high, and the mortality rate for lung cancer and pancreatic cancer is well over 90 percent in both men and women.

Exactly why some forms of cancer are more difficult to treat pharmacologically than others remains unclear. Differences in the biochemistry, genetics, and location of certain cancer cells may make them less sensitive to the toxic effects of anticancer drugs.[1] Resistance to anticancer drugs (see "Resistance to Anticancer Drugs") may also explain why certain cancers respond poorly to chemotherapy. Consequently, investigations of how to improve the efficacy of existing agents and the development of new anticancer drugs remain the major foci in pharmacological research. Some of the primary strategies in improving cancer chemotherapy are discussed later in "Future Perspectives."

RESISTANCE TO ANTICANCER DRUGS

As indicated previously, certain cancers do not respond well to cancer chemotherapy. A primary reason is that cancers may develop resistance to a broad range of chemotherapeutic agents (multiple drug resistance), thus rendering these drugs ineffective in treating the cancer.[117-119]

Cancers can become resistant to drugs through several different mechanisms. One common mechanism occurs when the cancer cell synthesizes a glycoprotein that acts as a drug efflux pump.[120] The glycoprotein pump is inserted into the cancer cell's membrane and effectively expels different types of anticancer drugs from the cancer cell before the drugs have a chance to exert cytotoxic effects. Cancer cells can induce drug resistance through the production of enzymes and specific substances (e.g., glutathione, glutathione-*S*-transferases) that inactivate anticancer drugs within the cancer cell.[121,122] Cells can also develop mechanisms that repair DNA damaged by anticancer drugs such as the alkylating agents and platinum complex drugs.[123] Likewise, many anticancer drugs must bind to a specific receptor on or within the cancer cell; these cells can develop drug resistance by modifying the structure or function of these receptors so that the drug is unable to bind to the receptor.[124] Cancer cells are therefore capable of developing several methods for self-preservation against a broad range of cytotoxic drugs.

Hence, researchers are exploring various strategies to prevent or overcome multiple-drug resistance during cancer chemotherapy. These strategies include altering the dosage, timing, delivery methods, and sequence of administration of different medications.[125-127] Use of these strategies, along with the development of new anticancer agents that do not cause resistance (see "Future Perspectives"), should help increase the effectiveness of chemotherapy in certain types of cancer.

FUTURE PERSPECTIVES

Researchers are also investigating several new strategies to increase the effectiveness and decrease the toxicity of anticancer drugs.[128-130] As discussed previously, most of the traditional drugs are toxic not only to tumor cells but also to normal cells. If the drug can be delivered or targeted specifically for tumor cells, it will produce a more selective effect. One way to accomplish this targeting is by creating monoclonal antibodies that are attracted specifically to an antigen or some other structural feature on the tumor cell (see the section "Targeted and Biological Therapies"). These antibodies can then directly inhibit function in the tumor cell, sensitize the cell to anticancer immune responses, or deliver another drug directly to the cancer cell. Hence, use of monoclonal antibodies as targeted therapies has emerged as a primary way to treat specific cancers, and researchers will undoubtedly continue to improve on this strategy as a principal way to focus drugs on cancerous tissues with minimal effects on healthy cells.[131,132]

Drugs may likewise be delivered more effectively to cancerous cells by using other techniques. As addressed in Chapter 2, advances in nanotechnology enable pharmacologists to attach the drugs to very small particles, which can deliver the drugs to selected tissues, including cancer cells.[133,134] Some drugs can likewise be encapsulated in a microsphere or liposome that increases the attraction and penetration into the cancerous tissues and then causes the drugs to be retained exclusively in those tissues.[135,136] Variations on these nanotechnology techniques and other delivery methods continue to be explored to increase effectiveness while decreasing the toxicity of anticancer drugs.

As addressed earlier in the chapter, important advances have been made in understanding how the body's immune system can be recruited to help prevent and treat certain cancers. If the body's immune system recognizes the cancer cell as an invader, then various endogenous immune responses can be initiated to combat the cancerous cells. Hence, researchers are looking into various strategies to help stimulate this immunologic response or modify the cancer cells to increase their antigenic properties and expose these cells to immune attack.[137-139] Likewise, anticancer vaccines exist for specific types of cancer, whereby the immune system can be sensitized to search out and destroy cancerous cells before they can develop into serious cancers.[140,141] Anticancer immunotherapies continue to be an intense area of research, and new immune strategies that affect specific cancers will surely be forthcoming.

Other unique strategies under development will involve selectively impairing the chemistry or metabolism of cancerous tissues. As indicated earlier, drugs already in use that employ this strategy include bevacizumab, which acts as an angiogenesis inhibitor that restricts the formation of new blood vessels in developing tumors. This effect can limit tumor growth and promote the death of cancerous cells by starving the tumor of oxygen and nutrients, without producing excessive effects on healthy tissues that do not need to rapidly generate new blood vessels.[55,56] Other strategies attempt to capitalize on an enzymatic or signaling pathway that is unique to the cancer cell. Examples include the tyrosine kinase inhibitors (imatinib, gefitinib, others) that inhibit abnormal tyrosine kinase activity in certain cancerous cells (see "Tyrosine Kinase Inhibitors" above).[66] As more is learned about the unique aspects of cancer cell metabolism, other agents will be developed that selectively impair the biochemistry of the cancer cell with minimal effects on the metabolism and function of normal cells.

Additionally, strategies are emerging to administer drugs that can protect healthy cells from the more traditional anticancer agents.[142,143] An example is the possible use of antioxidants or free-radical scavengers that reduce chemotherapy-induced damage to healthy cells.[144,145] These strategies, however, must be used cautiously because protection of healthy cells may also enable the cancer cells to be more resistant to the toxic effects of chemotherapeutic drugs.[146] Protective interventions are therefore complex, but future research may be able to identify ways to protect healthy cells while still maintaining cytotoxic effects on cancerous tissues.

Finally, important advances have been made in tailoring cancer chemotherapy to the individual characteristics of each patient's tumor. This idea, known commonly as *personalized oncology*, is based on first understanding the specific genetic and metabolic function of the cancer cells in each patient and then designing drug therapy to selectively attack those cells.[147,148] Personalized interventions can provide the most appropriate anticancer drugs to each patient, thus maximizing the therapeutic potential of these drugs. The ability of personalized oncology to provide optimal effects will continue to expand as more is learned about the biology of specific cancer cells.

In summary, a number of new strategies are currently being implemented or explored that selectively affect cancer cells and help eliminate cancerous tissues in specific patients. Increased knowledge about the nature of cancer, combined with a better understanding of the endogenous control of cell replication, may ultimately provide drugs that are safe and effective in curing all forms of cancer.

Special Concerns for Rehabilitation Patients

The adverse side effects of antineoplastic drugs will have a significant effect on physical therapy and occupational therapy. These drugs are routinely associated with a number of severe toxic effects, including GI problems, blood disorders, and profound fatigue. In addition, neurotoxic effects may occur with many cancer chemotherapy agents, including peripheral neuropathies and CNS abnormalities (e.g., convulsions, ataxia, confusion, anxiety). In terms of physical rehabilitation, these side effects are typically a source of frustration to both the patient and the therapist. On some days, the patient undergoing cancer chemotherapy will simply not be able to tolerate even a relatively mild rehabilitation session. This reality can be especially demoralizing to patients who want to try to overcome the disease and actively

Continued on following page

Special Concerns for Rehabilitation Patients (Continued)

participate in therapy as much as possible. Physical therapists and occupational therapists must take into account the debilitating nature of these drugs and be sensitive to the needs of the patient on a day-to-day basis. At certain times, the therapist must simply back off in trying to encourage active participation from the patient. Therapists, however, can often be particularly helpful in providing psychological support to patients undergoing antineoplastic drug treatment. They can reassure the patient that the side effects of these drugs are usually transient and that there will be better days when rehabilitation can be resumed.

Therapists may also be helpful in treating other problems associated with neoplastic disease. In particular, they may be involved in reducing the severe pain typically associated with many forms of cancer. Therapists can use transcutaneous electric nerve stimulation (TENS) or other physical agents as a nonpharmacological means to attenuate pain. Other physical interventions such as massage can also be invaluable in helping decrease the pain and anxiety that often occur in people receiving cancer chemotherapy. These approaches may reduce the need for pain medications, thus reducing the chance that these drugs will cause additional adverse effects and drug interactions with anticancer agents. The therapeutic and psychological support physical therapists and occupational therapists can offer play a vital and immeasurable role in improving the patient's quality of life.

CASE STUDY

CANCER CHEMOTHERAPY

Brief History. R.J. is a 57-year-old woman who was diagnosed with metastatic breast cancer 1 year ago, at which time she underwent a modified radical mastectomy followed by treatment with antineoplastic drugs. The cancer, however, had evidently metastasized to other tissues, including bone. She recently developed pain in the lumbosacral region, which was attributed to metastatic skeletal lesions in the lower lumbar vertebrae. She was admitted to the hospital to pursue a course of radiation treatment to control pain and minimize bony destruction at the site of the skeletal lesion. Her current pharmacological regimen consists of an antineoplastic antimetabolite (doxorubicin) and an antiestrogen (tamoxifen). She was also given a combination of opioid and nonopioid analgesics (codeine and aspirin) to help control pain. Physical therapy was initiated to help control pain and maintain function in this patient.

Problem/Influence of Medication. The patient began to experience an increase in GI side effects, including nausea, vomiting, loss of appetite, and epigastric pain. The patient, however, experienced adequate pain relief from the aspirin-codeine combination and was reluctant to consider alternative medications. The persistent nausea and loss of appetite had a general debilitating effect on her, and the physical therapist was having difficulty engaging her in an active general conditioning program.

1. *Why does R.K.'s drug regimen contribute to her GI problems?*
2. *How might the therapist intervene to help decrease the patient's pain and reduce the need for analgesic medications?*

See Appendix C, "Answers to Case Study Questions."

SUMMARY

Antineoplastic drugs typically limit excessive growth and proliferation of cancer cells by impairing DNA synthesis and function or by directly limiting cell division (mitosis). To replicate at a rapid rate, cancer cells must synthesize rather large quantities of DNA and RNA and continually undergo mitosis. Hence, cancer cells tend to be affected by antineoplastic drugs to a somewhat greater extent than normal cells. Normal cells, however, are also frequently affected by these drugs, resulting in a high incidence of side effects. Currently, cancer chemotherapy is effective in reducing and even curing many neoplastic diseases. However, other forms of cancer are much more difficult to treat pharmacologically. Several strategies are available to target the antineoplastic drug directly for cancer cells or enhance biological and immune responses that can fight the cancer. Increased use of these targeted and biological strategies may improve the efficacy and safety of anticancer agents. Rehabilitation specialists should be aware of the general debilitating nature of traditional chemotherapy regimens, and therapists must be prepared to adjust their treatment based on the ability of the patient to tolerate the adverse effects of cancer chemotherapy.

REFERENCES

1. Medina PJ, Shord SS. Cancer treatment and chemotherapy. In: DiPiro JT, et al, eds. *Pharmacotherapy: A Pathophysiologic Approach*. 8th ed. New York: McGraw-Hill; 2011.
2. Stricker TP, Kumar V. Neoplasia. In: Kumar V et al, eds. *Robbins and Contran Pathologic Basis of Disease*. 8th ed. Philadelphia, PA: Saunders/Elsevier; 2010.
3. Chu E, Sartorelli AC. Cancer chemotherapy. In: Katzung BG, ed. *Basic and Clinical Pharmacology*. 12th ed. New York: Lange Medical Books/McGraw Hill; 2012.
4. Moasser MM. Neoplasia. In: McPhee SJ, Hammer GD, eds. *Pathophysiology of Disease*. 6th ed. New York: McGraw-Hill; 2010.
5. Dunn KB, Heffler M, Golubovskaya VM. Evolving therapies and FAK inhibitors for the treatment of cancer. *Anticancer Agents Med Chem*. 2010;10:722-734.
6. Kaestner P, Bastians H. Mitotic drug targets. *J Cell Biochem*. 2010;111:258-265.
7. Park SR, Davis M, Doroshow JH, Kummar S. Safety and feasibility of targeted agent combinations in solid tumours. *Nat Rev Clin Oncol*. 2013;10:154-168.
8. Chabner BA. General principles of cancer chemotherapy. In: Brunton L, et al, eds. *The Pharmacological Basis of Therapeutics*. 12th ed. New York: McGraw-Hill; 2011.
9. Bertoli C, Skotheim JM, de Bruin RA. Control of cell cycle transcription during G1 and S phases. *Nat Rev Mol Cell Biol*. 2013;14:518-528.
10. Suryadinata R, Sadowski M, Sarcevic B. Control of cell cycle progression by phosphorylation of cyclin-dependent kinase (CDK) substrates. *Biosci Rep*. 2010;30:243-255.
11. Barbour SY. Corticosteroids in the treatment of chemotherapy-induced nausea and vomiting. *J Natl Compr Canc Netw*. 2012;10:493-499.
12. Wickham R. Evolving treatment paradigms for chemotherapy-induced nausea and vomiting. *Cancer Control*. 2012;19(suppl):3-9.
13. Billio A, Morello E, Clarke MJ. Serotonin receptor antagonists for highly emetogenic chemotherapy in adults. *Cochrane Database Syst Rev*. 2010;CD006272.
14. Grunberg SM, Slusher B, Rugo HS. Emerging treatments in chemotherapy-induced nausea and vomiting. *Clin Adv Hematol Oncol*. 2013;11(suppl 1):1-18.
15. Aapro MS, Schmoll HJ, Jahn F, et al. Review of the efficacy of aprepitant for the prevention of chemotherapy-induced nausea and vomiting in a range of tumor types. *Cancer Treat Rev*. 2013;39:113-117.
16. dos Santos LV, Souza FH, Brunetto AT, et al. Neurokinin-1 receptor antagonists for chemotherapy-induced nausea and vomiting: a systematic review. *J Natl Cancer Inst*. 2012;104:1280-1292.
17. Ruhlmann CH, Herrstedt J. Fosaprepitant for the prevention of chemotherapy-induced nausea and vomiting. *Expert Rev Anticancer Ther*. 2012;12:139-150.
18. Marx WM, Teleni L, McCarthy AL, et al. Ginger (Zingiber officinale) and chemotherapy-induced nausea and vomiting: a systematic literature review. *Nutr Rev*. 2013;71:245-254.
19. Todaro B. Cannabinoids in the treatment of chemotherapy-induced nausea and vomiting. *J Natl Compr Canc Netw*. 2012;10:487-492.
20. Basch E, Prestrud AA, Hesketh PJ, et al. Antiemetics: American Society of Clinical Oncology clinical practice guideline update. *J Clin Oncol*. 2011;29:4189-4198.
21. Lee SK, Dawson J, Lee JA, et al. Management of cancer pain: 1. Wider implications of orthodox analgesics. *Int J Gen Med*. 2014;7:49-58.
22. Mercadante S. Cancer pain. *Curr Opin Support Palliat Care*. 2013;7:139-143.
23. Molassiotis A, Bailey C, Caress A, et al. Interventions for cough in cancer. *Cochrane Database Syst Rev*. 2010;9:CD007881.
24. Suzuki H, Asakawa A, Amitani H, et al. Cancer cachexia—pathophysiology and management. *J Gastroenterol*. 2013;48:574-594.
25. Vansteenkiste J, Wauters I, Elliott S, et al. Chemotherapy-induced anemia: the story of darbepoetin alfa. *Curr Med Res Opin*. 2013;29:325-337.
26. Puyo S, Montaudon D, Pourquier P. From old alkylating agents to new minor groove binders. *Crit Rev Oncol Hematol*. 2014;89:43-61.
27. Osawa T, Davies D, Hartley JA. Mechanism of cell death resulting from DNA interstrand cross-linking in mammalian cells. *Cell Death Dis*. 2011;2:e187.
28. Hagner N, Joerger M. Cancer chemotherapy: targeting folic acid synthesis. *Cancer Manag Res*. 2010;2:293-301.
29. Visentin M, Zhao R, Goldman ID. The antifolates. *Hematol Oncol Clin North Am*. 2012;26:629-648.
30. Pang B, Qiao X, Janssen L, et al. Drug-induced histone eviction from open chromatin contributes to the chemotherapeutic effects of doxorubicin. *Nat Commun*. 2013;4:1908.

31. Yang F, Teves SS, Kemp CJ, Henikoff S. Doxorubicin, DNA torsion, and chromatin dynamics. *Biochim Biophys Acta.* 2014;1845: 84-89.
32. Pommier Y, Leo E, Zhang H, Marchand C. DNA topoisomerases and their poisoning by anticancer and antibacterial drugs. *Chem Biol.* 2010;17:421-433.
33. Marzo I, Naval J. Antimitotic drugs in cancer chemotherapy: promises and pitfalls. *Biochem Pharmacol.* 2013;86:703-710.
34. Morris PG, Fornier MN. Microtubule active agents: beyond the taxane frontier. *Clin Cancer Res.* 2008;14:7167-7172.
35. Perez EA. Microtubule inhibitors: differentiating tubulin-inhibiting agents based on mechanisms of action, clinical activity, and resistance. *Mol Cancer Ther.* 2009;8:2086-2095.
36. Chen SH, Chan NL, Hsieh TS. New mechanistic and functional insights into DNA topoisomerases. *Annu Rev Biochem.* 2013;82:139-170.
37. Pommier Y. Drugging topoisomerases: lessons and challenges. *ACS Chem Biol.* 2013;8:82-95.
38. Chiuri VE, Lorusso V. Which patients with estrogen receptor-positive early breast cancer should be treated with adjuvant chemotherapy? *Oncology.* 2009;77(suppl 1):18-22.
39. Massard C, Fizazi K. Targeting continued androgen receptor signaling in prostate cancer. *Clin Cancer Res.* 2011;17:3876-3883.
40. Ahmed A, Ali S, Sarkar FH. Advances in androgen receptor targeted therapy for prostate cancer. *J Cell Physiol.* 2014;229: 271-276.
41. Rathkopf D, Scher HI. Androgen receptor antagonists in castration-resistant prostate cancer. *Cancer J.* 2013;19:43-49.
42. McDonnell DP, Wardell SE. The molecular mechanisms underlying the pharmacological actions of ER modulators: implications for new drug discovery in breast cancer. *Curr Opin Pharmacol.* 2010;10:620-628.
43. Krell J, Januszewski A, Yan K, Palmieri C. Role of fulvestrant in the management of postmenopausal breast cancer. *Expert Rev Anticancer Ther.* 2011;11:1641-1652.
44. Cuzick J, Sestak I, Bonanni B, et al. Selective oestrogen receptor modulators in prevention of breast cancer: an updated meta-analysis of individual participant data. *Lancet.* 2013;381: 1827-1834.
45. Lønning PE, Eikesdal HP. Aromatase inhibition 2013: clinical state of the art and questions that remain to be solved. *Endocr Relat Cancer.* 2013;20:R183-201.
46. Litton JK, Arun BK, Brown PH, Hortobagyi GN. Aromatase inhibitors and breast cancer prevention. *Expert Opin Pharmacother.* 2012;13:325-331.
47. Dienstmann R, Markman B, Tabernero J. Application of monoclonal antibodies as cancer therapy in solid tumors. *Curr Clin Pharmacol.* 2012;7:137-145.
48. Sliwkowski MX, Mellman I. Antibody therapeutics in cancer. *Science.* 2013;341:1192-1198.
49. Xin L, Cao J, Cheng H, et al. Human monoclonal antibodies in cancer therapy: a review of recent developments. *Front Biosci.* 2013;18:765-772.
50. Fournier P, Schirrmacher V. Bispecific antibodies and trispecific immunocytokines for targeting the immune system against cancer: preparing for the future. *BioDrugs.* 2013;27:35-53.
51. Maher J, Adami AA. Antitumor immunity: easy as 1, 2, 3 with monoclonal bispecific trifunctional antibodies? *Cancer Res.* 2013;73:5613-5617.
52. Flygare JA, Pillow TH, Aristoff P. Antibody-drug conjugates for the treatment of cancer. *Chem Biol Drug Des.* 2013;81:113-121.
53. Teicher BA, Chari RV. Antibody conjugate therapeutics: challenges and potential. *Clin Cancer Res.* 2011;17:6389-6397.
54. Marcucci F, Bellone M, Rumio C, Corti A. Approaches to improve tumor accumulation and interactions between monoclonal antibodies and immune cells. *MAbs.* 2013;5:34-46.
55. Al-Husein B, Abdalla M, Trepte M, et al. Antiangiogenic therapy for cancer: an update. *Pharmacotherapy.* 2012;32:1095-1111.
56. Pavlidis ET, Pavlidis TE. Role of bevacizumab in colorectal cancer growth and its adverse effects: a review. *World J Gastroenterol.* 2013;19:5051-5060.
57. Konno H, Yamamoto M, Ohta M. Recent concepts of antiangiogenic therapy. *Surg Today.* 2010;40:494-500.
58. Fakih M. The evolving role of VEGF-targeted therapies in the treatment of metastatic colorectal cancer. *Expert Rev Anticancer Ther.* 2013;13:427-438.
59. Kotredes KP, Gamero AM. Interferons as inducers of apoptosis in malignant cells. *J Interferon Cytokine Res.* 2013;33:162-170.
60. Li Q, Kawamura K, Tada Y, et al. Novel type III interferons produce anti-tumor effects through multiple functions. *Front Biosci.* 2013;18:909-918.
61. Ishitsuka K, Tsukasaki K, Tamura K. Interferon alfa and antiretroviral agents: a treatment option for adult T-cell leukemia/lymphoma. *Drugs Today.* 2011;47:615-623.
62. Régnier-Rosencher E, Guillot B, Dupin N. Treatments for classic Kaposi sarcoma: a systematic review of the literature. *J Am Acad Dermatol.* 2013;68:313-331.
63. Antony GK, Dudek AZ. Interleukin 2 in cancer therapy. *Curr Med Chem.* 2010;17:3297-3302.
64. Liao W, Lin JX, Leonard WJ. Interleukin-2 at the crossroads of effector responses, tolerance, and immunotherapy. *Immunity.* 2013;38:13-25.
65. Amedei A, Prisco D, D'Elios MM. The use of cytokines and chemokines in the cancer immunotherapy. *Recent Pat Anticancer Drug Discov.* 2013;8:126-142.
66. Zheng Y, Tyner AL. Context-specific protein tyrosine kinase 6 (PTK6) signalling in prostate cancer. *Eur J Clin Invest.* 2013;43: 397-404.
67. Robinson KW, Sandler AB. EGFR tyrosine kinase inhibitors: difference in efficacy and resistance. *Curr Oncol Rep.* 2013;15: 396-404.
68. Tsai CJ, Nussinov R. The molecular basis of targeting protein kinases in cancer therapeutics. *Semin Cancer Biol.* 2013;23: 235-242.
69. Cimino GD, Pan CX, Henderson PT. Personalized medicine for targeted and platinum-based chemotherapy of lung and bladder cancer. *Bioanalysis.* 2013;5:369-391.
70. Monneret C. Platinum anticancer drugs. From serendipity to rational design. *Ann Pharm Fr.* 2011;69:286-295.
71. Ng JS, Low JJ, Ilancheran A. Epithelial ovarian cancer. *Best Pract Res Clin Obstet Gynaecol.* 2012;26:337-345.
72. Rosa DD, Medeiros LR, Edelweiss MI, et al. Adjuvant platinum-based chemotherapy for early stage cervical cancer. *Cochrane Database Syst Rev.* 2012;6:CD005342.
73. Bosetti C, Rosato V, Gallus S, et al. Aspirin and cancer risk: a quantitative review to 2011. *Ann Oncol.* 2012;23:1403-1415.
74. Sostres C, Gargallo CJ, Lanas A. Aspirin, cyclooxygenase inhibition and colorectal cancer. *World J Gastrointest Pharmacol Ther.* 2014;5:40-49.
75. Din FV, Theodoratou E, Farrington SM, et al. Effect of aspirin and NSAIDs on risk and survival from colorectal cancer. *Gut.* 2010;59:1670-1679.

76. Dovizio M, Bruno A, Tacconelli S, Patrignani P. Mode of action of aspirin as a chemopreventive agent. *Recent Results Cancer Res.* 2013;191:39-65.
77. Kraus S, Naumov I, Arber N. COX-2 active agents in the chemoprevention of colorectal cancer. *Recent Results Cancer Res.* 2013;191:95-103.
78. Lengfelder E, Hofmann WK, Nowak D. Impact of arsenic trioxide in the treatment of acute promyelocytic leukemia. *Leukemia.* 2012;26:433-442.
79. Rizzari C, Conter V, Star_ J, et al. Optimizing asparaginase therapy for acute lymphoblastic leukemia. *Curr Opin Oncol.* 2013;25(suppl 1):S1-9.
80. Romano A, Conticello C, Di Raimondo F. Bortezomib for the treatment of previously untreated multiple myeloma. *Immunotherapy.* 2013;5:327-352.
81. Lansigan F, Stearns DM, Foss F. Role of denileukin diftitox in the treatment of persistent or recurrent cutaneous T-cell lymphoma. *Cancer Manag Res.* 2010;2:53-59.
82. Mohan R, Panda D. Kinetic stabilization of microtubule dynamics by estramustine is associated with tubulin acetylation, spindle abnormalities, and mitotic arrest. *Cancer Res.* 2008;68:6181-6189.
83. Ravery V, Fizazi K, Oudard S, et al. The use of estramustine phosphate in the modern management of advanced prostate cancer. *BJU Int.* 2011;108:1782-1786.
84. Giannini G, Cabri W, Fattorusso C, Rodriquez M. Histone deacetylase inhibitors in the treatment of cancer: overview and perspectives. *Future Med Chem.* 2012;4:1439-1460.
85. Iwamoto M, Friedman EJ, Sandhu P, et al. Clinical pharmacology profile of vorinostat, a histone deacetylase inhibitor. *Cancer Chemother Pharmacol.* 2013;72:493-508.
86. Kavanaugh SM, White LA, Kolesar JM. Vorinostat: a novel therapy for the treatment of cutaneous T-cell lymphoma. *Am J Health Syst Pharm.* 2010;67:793-797.
87. Campbell RM, Tummino PJ. Cancer epigenetics drug discovery and development: the challenge of hitting the mark. *J Clin Invest.* 2014;124:64-69.
88. Saban N, Bujak M. Hydroxyurea and hydroxamic acid derivatives as antitumor drugs. *Cancer Chemother Pharmacol.* 2009;64:213-221.
89. De Francia S, Ardito A, Daffara F, et al. Mitotane treatment for adrenocortical carcinoma: an overview. *Minerva Endocrinol.* 2012;37:9-23.
90. Castelli R, Cannavò A, Conforti F, et al. Immunomodulatory drugs in multiple myeloma: from molecular mechanisms of action to clinical practice. *Immunopharmacol Immunotoxicol.* 2012;34:740-753.
91. Watanabe R, Tokuhira M, Kizaki M. Current approaches for the treatment of multiple myeloma. *Int J Hematol.* 2013;97:333-344.
92. Kumar N, Sharma U, Singh C, Singh B. Thalidomide: chemistry, therapeutic potential and oxidative stress induced teratogenicity. *Curr Top Med Chem.* 2012;12:1436-1455.
93. Connolly RM, Nguyen NK, Sukumar S. Molecular pathways: current role and future directions of the retinoic acid pathway in cancer prevention and treatment. *Clin Cancer Res.* 2013;19:1651-1659.
94. Pileri A, Delfino C, Grandi V, Pimpinelli N. Role of bexarotene in the treatment of cutaneous T-cell lymphoma: the clinical and immunological sides. *Immunotherapy.* 2013;5:427-433.
95. Rhoads J. Alitretinoin (Panretin) gel 0.1%. *J Assoc Nurses AIDS Care.* 2001;12:86-91.
96. Bekaii-Saab T, Wu C. Seeing the forest through the trees: A systematic review of the safety and efficacy of combination chemotherapies used in the treatment of metastatic colorectal cancer. *Crit Rev Oncol Hematol.* 2014;91:9-35.
97. Kelly CM, Buzdar AU. Using multiple targeted therapies in oncology: considerations for use, and progress to date in breast cancer. *Drugs.* 2013;73:505-515.
98. McLaughlin P. Management options for follicular lymphoma: observe; R-CHOP; B-R; others? *Clin Lymphoma Myeloma Leuk.* 2011;11(suppl 1):S91-95.
99. Munzone E, Curigliano G, Burstein HJ, et al. CMF revisited in the 21st century. *Ann Oncol.* 2012;23:305-311.
100. Fokas E, Weiss C, Rödel C. The role of radiotherapy in the multimodal management of esophageal cancer. *Dig Dis.* 2013;31:30-37.
101. Weber GF, Rosenberg R, Murphy JE, et al. Multimodal treatment strategies for locally advanced rectal cancer. *Expert Rev Anticancer Ther.* 2012;12:481-494.
102. Yang H, Diao LQ, Shi M, et al. Efficacy of intensity-modulated radiotherapy combined with chemotherapy or surgery in locally advanced squamous cell carcinoma of the head-and-neck. *Biologics.* 2013;7:223-229.
103. Copeland A, Younes A. Current treatment strategies in Hodgkin lymphomas. *Curr Opin Oncol.* 2012;24:466-474.
104. Gupta AA, Yao X, Verma S, et al. Sarcoma Disease Site Group and the Gynecology Cancer Disease Site Group. Systematic chemotherapy for inoperable, locally advanced, recurrent, or metastatic uterine leiomyosarcoma: a systematic review. *Clin Oncol.* 2013;25:346-355.
105. Mitra A, Khoo V. Adjuvant therapy after radical prostatectomy: clinical considerations. *Surg Oncol.* 2009;18:247-254.
106. Balduzzi A, Leonardi MC, Cardillo A, et al. Timing of adjuvant systemic therapy and radiotherapy after breast-conserving surgery and mastectomy. *Cancer Treat Rev.* 2010;36:443-450.
107. Kirkwood JM, Tarhini A, Sparano JA, et al. Comparative clinical benefits of systemic adjuvant therapy for paradigm solid tumors. *Cancer Treat Rev.* 2013;39:27-43.
108. Mascaux C, Shepherd FA. Adjuvant chemotherapy after pulmonary resection for lung cancer. *Thorac Surg Clin.* 2013;23:401-410.
109. Smaglo BG, Pishvaian MJ. Postresection chemotherapy for pancreatic cancer. *Cancer J.* 2012;18:614-623.
110. Gampenrieder SP, Rinnerthaler G, Greil R. Neoadjuvant chemotherapy and targeted therapy in breast cancer: past, present, and future. *J Oncol.* 2013;2013:732047.
111. Lou DY, Fong L. Neoadjuvant therapy for localized prostate cancer: examining mechanism of action and efficacy within the tumor. *Urol Oncol.* 2014. [Epub ahead of print]
112. Linkous AG, Yazlovitskaya EM. Novel radiosensitizing anticancer therapeutics. *Anticancer Res.* 2012;32:2487-2499.
113. Palacios DA, Miyake M, Rosser CJ. Radiosensitization in prostate cancer: mechanisms and targets. *BMC Urol.* 2013;13:4.
114. Mato AR, Feldman T, Goy A. Proteasome inhibition and combination therapy for non-Hodgkin's lymphoma: from bench to bedside. *Oncologist.* 2012;17:694-707.
115. Stiborová M, Eckschlager T, Poljaková J, et al. The synergistic effects of DNA-targeted chemotherapeutics and histone deacetylase inhibitors as therapeutic strategies for cancer treatment. *Curr Med Chem.* 2012;19:4218-4238.

116. Rossi A, Torri V, Garassino MC, et al. The impact of personalized medicine on survival: comparisons of results in metastatic breast, colorectal and non-small-cell lung cancers. *Cancer Treat Rev.* 2014;40:485-494.
117. Holohan C, Van Schaeybroeck S, Longley DB, Johnston PG. Cancer drug resistance: an evolving paradigm. *Nat Rev Cancer.* 2013;13:714-726.
118. Lavi O, Gottesman MM, Levy D. The dynamics of drug resistance: a mathematical perspective. *Drug Resist Updat.* 2012;15: 90-97.
119. Lippert TH, Ruoff HJ, Volm M. Current status of methods to assess cancer drug resistance. *Int J Med Sci.* 2011;8:245-253.
120. Wu CP, Hsieh CH, Wu YS. The emergence of drug transporter-mediated multidrug resistance to cancer chemotherapy. *Mol Pharm.* 2011;8:1996-2011.
121. Backos DS, Franklin CC, Reigan P. The role of glutathione in brain tumor drug resistance. *Biochem Pharmacol.* 2012;83: 1005-1012.
122. Singh S, Khan AR, Gupta AK. Role of glutathione in cancer pathophysiology and therapeutic interventions. *J Exp Ther Oncol.* 2012;9:303-316.
123. Salehan MR, Morse HR. DNA damage repair and tolerance: a role in chemotherapeutic drug resistance. *Br J Biomed Sci.* 2013;70:31-40.
124. Vadlapatla RK, Vadlapudi AD, Pal D, Mitra AK. Mechanisms of drug resistance in cancer chemotherapy: coordinated role and regulation of efflux transporters and metabolizing enzymes. *Curr Pharm Des.* 2013;19:7126-7140.
125. Matsuo K, Lin YG, Roman LD, Sood AK. Overcoming platinum resistance in ovarian carcinoma. *Expert Opin Investig Drugs.* 2010;19:1339-1354.
126. Palakurthi S, Yellepeddi VK, Vangara KK. Recent trends in cancer drug resistance reversal strategies using nanoparticles. *Expert Opin Drug Deliv.* 2012;9:287-301.
127. Yunos NM, Beale P, Yu JQ, Huq F. Synergism from sequenced combinations of curcumin and epigallocatechin-3-gallate with cisplatin in the killing of human ovarian cancer cells. *Anticancer Res.* 2011;31:1131-1140.
128. Jang M, Kim SS, Lee J. Cancer cell metabolism: implications for therapeutic targets. *Exp Mol Med.* 2013;45:e45.
129. Khan KH, Blanco-Codesido M, Molife LR. Cancer therapeutics: targeting the apoptotic pathway. *Crit Rev Oncol Hematol.* 2014;90:200-219.
130. Yap TA, Omlin A, de Bono JS. Development of therapeutic combinations targeting major cancer signaling pathways. *J Clin Oncol.* 2013;31:1592-1605.
131. Leone Roberti Maggiore U, Bellati F, Ruscito I, et al. Monoclonal antibodies therapies for ovarian cancer. *Expert Opin Biol Ther.* 2013;13:739-764.
132. Prenen H, Vecchione L, Van Cutsem E. Role of targeted agents in metastatic colorectal cancer. *Target Oncol.* 2013;8:83-96.
133. Gao Y, Xie J, Chen H, et al. Nanotechnology-based intelligent drug design for cancer metastasis treatment. *Biotechnol Adv.* 2013. [E pub ahead of print]
134. Minko T, Rodriguez-Rodriguez L, Pozharov V. Nanotechnology approaches for personalized treatment of multidrug resistant cancers. *Adv Drug Deliv Rev.* 2013;65:1880-1895.
135. Hyodo K, Yamamoto E, Suzuki T, et al. Development of liposomal anticancer drugs. *Biol Pharm Bull.* 2013;36:703-707.
136. Kroon J, Metselaar JM, Storm G, van der Pluijm G. Liposomal nanomedicines in the treatment of prostate cancer. *Cancer Treat Rev.* 2014;40:578-584.
137. Darcy PK, Neeson P, Yong CS, Kershaw MH. Manipulating immune cells for adoptive immunotherapy of cancer. *Curr Opin Immunol.* 2014;27C:46-52.
138. Kershaw MH, Devaud C, John LB, et al. Enhancing immunotherapy using chemotherapy and radiation to modify the tumor microenvironment. *Oncoimmunology.* 2013;2:e25962.
139. Park JH, Brentjens RJ. Immunotherapies in CLL. *Adv Exp Med Biol.* 2013;792:241-257.
140. Aranda F, Vacchelli E, Eggermont A, et al. Peptide vaccines in cancer therapy. *Oncoimmunology.* 2013;2:e26621.
141. Guo C, Manjili MH, Subjeck JR, et al. Therapeutic cancer vaccines: past, present, and future. *Adv Cancer Res.* 2013;119:421-475.
142. Ocean AJ, Vahdat LT. Chemotherapy-induced peripheral neuropathy: pathogenesis and emerging therapies. *Support Care Cancer.* 2004;12:619-625.
143. Pabla N, Dong Z. Curtailing side effects in chemotherapy: a tale of PKC_ in cisplatin treatment. *Oncotarget.* 2012;3:107-111.
144. Sahin K, Sahin N, Kucuk O. Lycopene and chemotherapy toxicity. *Nutr Cancer.* 2010;62:988-995.
145. Tabassum A, Bristow RG, Venkateswaran V. Ingestion of selenium and other antioxidants during prostate cancer radiotherapy: a good thing? *Cancer Treat Rev.* 2010;36:230-234.
146. Lawenda BD, Kelly KM, Ladas EJ, et al. Should supplemental antioxidant administration be avoided during chemotherapy and radiation therapy? *J Natl Cancer Inst.* 2008;100:773-783.
147. Gonzalez-Angulo AM, Hennessy BT, Mills GB. Future of personalized medicine in oncology: a systems biology approach. *J Clin Oncol.* 2010;28:2777-2783.
148. Kalia M. Personalized oncology: recent advances and future challenges. *Metabolism.* 2013;62(suppl 1):S11-14.

CHAPTER 37

Immunomodulating Agents

The immune system is responsible for controlling the body's response to various types of injury and for defending the body from invading pathogens, including bacteria, viruses, and other parasites.[1,2] The importance of this system in maintaining health is illustrated by the devastating effects that can occur in people who lack adequate immune function, such as patients with AIDS. The use of drugs to modify immune responses, or immunomodulating agents, is therefore an important area of pharmacology. For example, it may be helpful to augment immune function if a person's immune system is not functioning adequately. By contrast, it is sometimes necessary to suppress immune function pharmacologically to prevent immune-mediated injury to certain tissues or organs. Following organ transplants and tissue grafts, the immune system may cause the rejection of tissues transplanted from other donors (allografts) or from other sites in the patient's body (autografts).[3,4] Likewise, immunosuppression may be helpful when the immune system causes damage to the body's tissues. Such conditions are often referred to as *autoimmune diseases.* Clinical disorders such as rheumatoid arthritis, multiple sclerosis, and systemic lupus erythematosus (SLE) are now recognized as having an autoimmune basis.[5,6]

This chapter begins with a brief overview of the immune response, followed by the drugs that are currently available to suppress or stimulate this response. Immunosuppressive drugs, or **immunosuppressants,** can prevent the rejection of transplants or treat specific diseases caused by an autoimmune response. Clearly, these drugs must be used very cautiously because too much suppression of the immune system will increase a patient's susceptibility to infection from foreign pathogens.[7] Likewise, these drugs are rather toxic and often cause several adverse effects to the kidneys, lungs, musculoskeletal system, and other tissues. Nonetheless, immunosuppressive agents are often lifesaving because of their ability to prevent and treat organ rejection and to decrease immune-mediated tissue damage in other diseases. The group of drugs that increase immune function, or immunostimulants, is rather small and the clinical use of immunostimulants is limited when compared with the indications for immunosuppressive drugs. However, the development and use of immunostimulants is an exciting area of pharmacology, and some insight into the therapeutic use of these drugs is provided.

Physical therapists and occupational therapists may be involved in the rehabilitation of patients who have received organ transplants, skin grafts, or similar procedures that necessitate the use of immunosuppressant drugs. Rehabilitation specialists also treat patients with autoimmune disorders or immunodeficiency syndromes that affect the musculoskeletal system; these patients are also likely to be taking immunomodulating drugs. Hence, this chapter will provide therapists with knowledge about the pharmacology of these drugs and how their effects and side effects can affect physical rehabilitation.

OVERVIEW OF THE IMMUNE RESPONSE

One of the primary responsibilities of the immune system is to protect the body from bacteria, viruses, and other foreign pathogens. The immune response consists of two primary components: innate and adaptive (acquired) immunity.[1] Innate immunity involves specific cells (leukocytes) that are present at birth and provide a relatively rapid and nonselective defense against foreign invaders and pathogens throughout the individual's lifetime.[8] Adaptive immunity primarily involves certain lymphocytes (T and B) that develop slowly but retain the ability to recognize specific invading microorganisms and to initiate specific steps to attack and destroy the invading cell.[9]

The innate and adaptive branches of the immune response are both needed for optimal immune function, and the two interact extensively.[1] The adaptive response's ability to recognize and deal with foreign pathogens likewise involves an incredibly complex interaction between various cellular and chemical (humoral) components.[10,11] A detailed description of the intricacies of how these components work together is beyond the scope of this chapter. Many aspects of the immune response are still being investigated. An overview of key cellular and humoral elements that mediate acquired immunity is illustrated in Figure 37-1, and these elements are described briefly as the following steps:

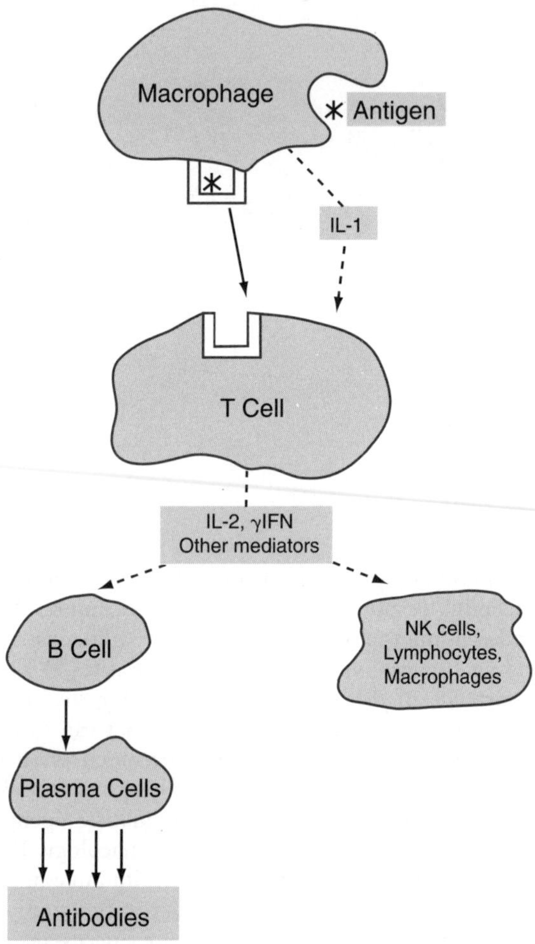

Figure ■ 37-1
A schematic diagram of some of the key cellular and humoral elements involved in the acquired immune response. Macrophages engulf and process antigens and present these antigens to T lymphocytes (T cells). Macrophages also stimulate T-cell function by releasing interleukin-1 (IL-1). T cells synthesize and release humoral factors, including interleukin-2 (IL-2), gamma interferon (γ IFN), and other mediators. These mediators activate other lymphocytes (B cells) and cause these cells to differentiate into plasma cells, which produce various antibodies. T-cell–derived mediators also stimulate the activity of other immune system cells, such as natural killer (NK) cells, other cytotoxic lymphocytes, and other macrophages.

1. *Antigen ingestion, processing, and presentation.* An invading substance (antigen) is engulfed by phagocytes such as macrophages and other antigen-presenting cells (APCs) such as dendritic cells.[12-14] The APCs process the antigen by forming a complex between the antigen and specific membrane proteins known as *major histocompatibility complex (MHC) proteins*. The antigen-MHC complex is placed on the surface of the APC, where it can be presented to other lymphocytes such as the T cells. The APCs also synthesize and release chemical mediators such as interleukin-1 (IL-1) and other cytokines, which act on other immune cells (T cells) to amplify these cells' response to immune mediators.
2. *Antigen recognition and T-cell activation.* Lymphocytes derived from thymic tissues (hence the term *T cell*) recognize the antigen-MHC complex that is presented to the T cell on the macrophage surface. This recognition activates certain T cells (T-helper cells), which begin to synthesize and release several chemical mediators known as **lymphokines.**[15,16] Lymphokines are cytokines and chemokines derived from activated T lymphocytes and include mediators such as interleukin-2 (IL-2), other interleukins, gamma interferon, B-cell growth and differentiation factors, and other chemicals that stimulate

the immune system.[17,18] Certain T cells (T-killer cells) are also activated by APC presentation and directly destroy targeted antigens.

3. *Proliferation, amplification, and recruitment.* T cells continue to replicate and proliferate, thus producing more lymphokines, which further amplifies the T-cell effects. These lymphokines also recruit lymphocytes derived from bone marrow—that is, B cells.[19] Under the direction of IL-1 and other lymphokines, B cells proliferate and differentiate into plasma cells. Plasma cells ultimately release specific antibodies known as *immunoglobulins* (IgG, IgA, IgM, etc.). Likewise, T-cell and macrophage-derived lymphokines recruit additional cellular components, including other macrophages, cytotoxic lymphocytes (natural killer, or NK, cells), and various cells that can participate in the destruction of the foreign antigen.

Clearly, the immune response is an intricate sequence of events that involves a complex interaction between a number of cellular and humoral components. The overview provided here is just a brief summary of how some of the primary components participate in mediating acquired immunity. The references at the end of this chapter provide sources for more information on this topic.[1,17,18,20]

PHARMACOLOGICAL SUPPRESSION OF THE IMMUNE RESPONSE

Drugs are used to suppress the immune system for two basic reasons. First, the immune response is often attenuated pharmacologically following the transplantation of organs or tissues to prevent the rejection of these tissues.[21,22] Sometimes, organs and other tissues can be attacked by the recipient's immune system, even if these tissues appear to be cross-matched between donor and recipient. This rejection is often caused by membrane proteins on the donor tissue that are recognized as antigens by the host's immune system.[23] Hence, drugs that suppress the cellular and chemical response to these membrane proteins can help prevent them from destroying the transplanted tissues and causing additional injury to the host's tissues.

Often, several different types of immunosuppressants are used together in fairly high doses to prevent or treat transplant rejection.[24,25] For instance, a glucocorticoid such as betamethasone is often administered with nonsteroidal drugs such as cyclosporine and tacrolimus to provide optimal success and viability of the transplant. Of course, giving several powerful drugs at high doses often causes unpleasant or even toxic side effects. These effects must often be tolerated, however, considering the limited number of organs available for transplantation and the need to ensure the survival of the transplant as much as possible.

A second major indication for these drugs is to limit immune-mediated damage to the body's tissues—that is, suppression of an autoimmune response.[26] Autoimmune responses occur when the immune system loses the ability to differentiate the body's own tissues from foreign or pathogenic tissues.[27] Exactly what causes this defect in immune recognition is often unclear, but prior exposure to some pathogen such as a virus may activate the immune response in a way that causes the immune system to mistakenly attack normal tissues while trying to destroy the virus. This autoimmune activation may remain in effect even after the original pathogen has been destroyed, thus leading to chronic immune-mediated injury to the body's tissues.

Autoimmune responses seem to be the underlying basis for many diseases, including rheumatoid arthritis, diabetes mellitus, myasthenia gravis, SLE, scleroderma, polymyositis/dermatomyositis, and several other disorders.[27-29] It is not exactly clear what factors cause autoimmune responses or why certain individuals are more prone to autoimmune-related diseases. Nonetheless, drugs that suppress the immune system can limit damage to various other tissues, and these drugs may produce dramatic improvements in patients with diseases that are caused by an autoimmune response.

SPECIFIC IMMUNOSUPPRESSIVE AGENTS

Drugs commonly used to suppress the immune system are listed in Table 37-1; the pharmacology of specific agents follows.

Azathioprine

Clinical Use. Azathioprine (Imuran) is a cytotoxic agent that is structurally and functionally similar to certain anticancer drugs, such as mercaptopurine.[30,31] Azathioprine is primarily used to prevent the rejection of transplanted organs, especially in patients with kidney transplants. Individuals may also take azathioprine

Table 37-1
COMMON IMMUNOSUPPRESSIVE AGENTS

		Primary Indications*	
Generic Name	**Trade Name(s)**	**Prevention or Treatment of Transplant Rejection**	**Diseases That Have an Autoimmune Response**
Antibodies	Names vary according to specific lymphocyte targets (see Table 37-2)	Bone marrow; other organ transplants (see Table 37-2)	Idiopathic thrombocytic purpura; other hemolytic disorders
Azathioprine	Imuran	Kidney; heart; liver; pancreas	Rheumatoid arthritis; inflammatory bowel disease; myasthenia gravis; systemic lupus erythematosus (SLE); others
Cyclophosphamide	Cytoxan; Neosar	Bone marrow; other organ transplants	Rheumatoid arthritis; multiple sclerosis; SLE; dermatomyositis; glomerulonephritis; hematologic disorders
Cyclosporine	Neoral; Sandimmune	Kidney; liver; heart; lung; pancreas; bone marrow	Psoriasis; rheumatoid arthritis; nephrotic syndrome
Everolimus	Zortress	Kidney	Rheumatoid arthritis
Glucocorticoids	See text for listing	Heart; kidney; liver; bone marrow	Multiple sclerosis; rheumatoid arthritis; SLE; inflammatory bowel disease; hemolytic disorders; others
Methotrexate	Folex; Rheumatrex	—	Rheumatoid arthritis; psoriasis
Mycophenolate mofetil	CellCept	Heart; kidney	—
Sirolimus	Rapamune	Kidney; heart; liver	Rheumatoid arthritis; psoriasis; SLE
Sulfasalazine	Azulfidine; others	—	Rheumatoid arthritis; inflammatory bowel disease
Tacrolimus	Prograf	Liver; kidney; heart; lung; pancreas	Uveitis
Temsirolimus	Torisel	—	Renal cell carcinoma

**Indications vary considerably and many indications listed here are not in the U.S. product labeling for each drug; optimal use of these drugs alone or in combination with each other continues to be investigated.*

to suppress immune responses in a wide range of other conditions, such as SLE, dermatomyositis, inflammatory myopathy, hepatic disease, myasthenia gravis, and ulcerative colitis. As presented in Chapter 16, azathioprine is also used as an antiarthritic disease–modifying agent.

Mechanism of Action. Although the exact mechanism of azathioprine is unknown, this drug probably interferes with DNA synthesis in cells mediating the immune response. Azathioprine appears to act like the antimetabolite drugs used in cancer chemotherapy (see Chapter 36). The cell normally uses various endogenous substances, such as purines, as ingredients during DNA synthesis. Azathioprine is structurally similar to these purines, and it acts as a false ingredient that competes with the naturally occurring substances to slow down and disrupt DNA synthesis. Impaired nucleic acid synthesis slows down the replication of lymphocytes and other key cellular components that direct the immune response. Thus, azathioprine directly limits cellular proliferation through this inhibitory effect on DNA synthesis and ultimately limits the production of humoral components (antibodies) produced by these cells.

Adverse Effects. The primary side effects of azathioprine are related to suppression of bone marrow function, including leukopenia, megaloblastic anemia, and similar blood dyscrasias. Other side effects include skin rash and gastrointestinal (GI) distress (e.g., appetite loss, nausea, vomiting); hepatic dysfunction can also occur when higher doses are used.

Cyclophosphamide

Clinical Use. Cyclophosphamide (Cytoxan, Neosar) is an anticancer alkylating agent that is commonly used in a variety of neoplastic disorders (see Chapter 36). This drug may also be helpful in suppressing the immune response in certain autoimmune diseases, such as multiple sclerosis, SLE, and rheumatoid arthritis.[7] High doses of cyclophosphamide are used to prevent tissue rejection in patients receiving bone marrow transplants and other organ transplants.

Mechanism of Action. As an anticancer alkylating agent, cyclophosphamide causes the formation of strong cross-links between strands of DNA and RNA, thus inhibiting DNA/RNA replication and function (see "Alkylating Agents" in Chapter 36). Cyclophosphamide probably exerts immunosuppressant effects in a similar manner—that is, it inhibits DNA and RNA function in lymphocytes and other key cells, thus limiting the rapid proliferation of these cells during the immune response.

Adverse Effects. Cyclophosphamide is used very cautiously as an immunosuppressant because of the possibility of severe side effects, including carcinogenic effects during long-term use. Other side effects include hematologic disorders (e.g., leukopenia, thrombocytopenia), cardiotoxicity, nephrotoxicity, and pulmonary toxicity.

Cyclosporine

Clinical Use. Cyclosporine (Neoral, Sandimmune) is one of the primary medications used to suppress immune function following organ transplantation.[24,32] This medication can be used alone or combined with glucocorticoids, mycophenolate mofetil, and other immunosuppressants to prevent the rejection of a kidney, lung, liver, heart, pancreas, and other organ transplants. Cyclosporine is used to a somewhat lesser extent in treating autoimmune diseases, but it may be helpful in conditions such as psoriasis, rheumatoid arthritis, inflammatory bowel disease, autoimmune hepatitis, and glomerulonephritis.[33-36]

Although cyclosporine is one of the most effective immunosuppressants, the traditional form of this drug is associated with unpredictable absorption from the GI tract and potentially severe side effects, such as nephrotoxicity and neurotoxicity.[37,38] In a newer form of cyclosporine (Neoral, Gengraf), the drug is modified into microemulsion capsules that disperse more easily within the GI tract, thereby enabling the drug to be absorbed in a more predictable fashion.[39] The microemulsion form of cyclosporine appears to be safer because it is not as toxic to the kidneys and other tissues as is the regular formulation.[40] Hence, this microemulsion formulation is often the optimal way to administer cyclosporine following organ transplantation or other situations requiring immunosuppression.[18]

Mechanism of Action. Cyclosporine and tacrolimus (see below) are known as *calcineurin inhibitors* because they inhibit a specific protein (calcineurin) in lymphoid tissues.[41,42] Calcineurin normally removes a phosphate molecule from a specific nuclear transcription factor, thus enabling this factor to enter the nucleus of T cells and activate genes that produce cytokines such as interleukin-2. By inhibiting calcineurin, cyclosporine ultimately suppresses T-cell activation, thus limiting the ability of T cells to produce other chemical mediators that promote immune cell activity (see Fig. 37-1).[18,42] Hence, cyclosporine is one of the premier immunosuppressants because of its relative selectivity for T cells and its inhibition of a key component of the immune response.[43] This relatively specific inhibition is often advantageous when compared with other nonselective drugs, such as azathioprine, cyclophosphamide, and glucocorticoids, which inhibit virtually all the cells and chemical mediators involved in the immune response.

Adverse Effects. The primary problem associated with cyclosporine is nephrotoxicity, which can range from mild, asymptomatic cases to severe kidney dysfunction, which requires discontinuation of the drug.[38,44] Hypertension is also a common adverse effect, especially when cyclosporine is used for prolonged periods.[45] Other problems include neurotoxicity, gingival hyperplasia, hair growth (hirsutism), and increased infections. These problems, however, tend to be less severe with cyclosporine than with other less-selective immunosuppressants.

Glucocorticoids

Clinical Use. As described in Chapter 29, glucocorticoids are powerful anti-inflammatory and immunosuppressive drugs. Glucocorticoids exert a rather nonspecific inhibition of virtually all aspects of cell- and chemical-mediated immunity, thus enabling these drugs to be used in a variety of situations when it is necessary to suppress immune function. Hence, these drugs are a mainstay in preventing transplant rejection and in treating various diseases associated with an autoimmune response.[46-48] Glucocorticoids commonly used as immunosuppressants include the following:

- Betamethasone (Celestone)
- Cortisone (Cortone)
- Dexamethasone (Decadron, others)
- Hydrocortisone (Cortef)
- Methylprednisolone (Medrol)
- Prednisolone (Pediapred, Prelone, others)
- Prednisone (Deltasone, others)
- Triamcinolone (Aristocort, others)

Mechanism of Action. Although their exact mechanism of immunosuppression is unclear, glucocorticoids probably interrupt the immune response by a complex effect at the genomic level of various immune cells.[49,50] These drugs enter immune system cells, where they bind to a cytoplasmic receptor. The drug-receptor complex then migrates to the cell's nucleus, where it acts directly on specific immunoregulatory genes. In particular, glucocorticoids influence the expression of cytokines and other chemicals that orchestrate the immune response—that is, they inhibit the transcription of messenger RNA units that are normally translated into immunostimulatory signals, such as interleukin-1, gamma interferon, and other substances. These signals activate the cells responsible for mediating the immune response. Hence, these drugs disrupt the production of chemical signals that activate and control various immune system cellular components. For more details about how glucocorticoids exert their effects on various cells and tissues, see Chapter 29.

Adverse Effects. The immunosuppressive effects of glucocorticoids are balanced by several side effects. As described in Chapter 29, glucocorticoids typically produce a catabolic effect on collagenous tissues, and the breakdown of muscle, bone, skin, and various other tissues is a common adverse effect. Glucocorticoids also produce other side effects, including hypertension, adrenocortical suppression, growth retardation in children, an increased chance of infection, glaucoma, decreased glucose tolerance, and gastric ulcer. These side effects can be especially problematic when glucocorticoids are used to prevent transplant rejection because these drugs are often given in high dosages for extended periods.

To lessen the side effects, glucocorticoids are typically combined with other nonsteroidal immunosuppressants, such as cyclosporine, azathioprine, or immunosuppressive antibodies, so that synergistic effects can be obtained and immunosuppression can be achieved with relatively low doses of each drug.[18,51] In addition, efforts are often made to progressively decrease the glucocorticoid dose so that immunosuppression is achieved by using the lowest possible dose. In some cases, the glucocorticoid may even be withdrawn during maintenance immunosuppressive therapy, and nonsteroidal drugs (cyclosporine, tacrolimus, mycophenolate mofetil) are used to provide long-term immunosuppression following organ transplantation.[51]

Methotrexate

Clinical Use. Methotrexate (Folex, Rheumatrex) was originally developed as an anticancer agent (see Chapter 36), but this drug is also used in certain noncancerous conditions that have an autoimmune component.[52,53] For example, methotrexate is commonly used as a disease-modifying drug in rheumatoid arthritis (see Chapter 16). Methotrexate is also approved for use in psoriasis. This agent has only mild immunosuppressive effects, however, and is not typically used to treat organ transplants or other conditions that require more extensive immunosuppression.

Mechanism of Action. The pharmacology of methotrexate is described in Chapter 36. This drug acts as an antimetabolite that interferes with the production of DNA and RNA precursors in rapidly proliferating cells. This interference produces a general inhibition of the replication of lymphocytes inherent in the immune response.

Adverse Effects. The major problems associated with methotrexate include hepatic and pulmonary toxicity. These problems are dose-related, however, and serious adverse effects tend to occur less frequently at doses used for immunosuppression than at those used for anticancer treatment.

Mycophenolate Mofetil

Clinical Use. Mycophenolate mofetil (CellCept) is primarily used to prevent or treat organ rejection following cardiac and renal transplantation. This drug is typically combined with other immunosuppressants (cyclosporine, glucocorticoids) to provide optimal immunosuppression in patients receiving these transplant types.[18,54] Mycophenolate mofetil may also be useful in suppressing the immune response associated with autoimmune conditions, such as SLE and autoimmune hepatitis.[55,56]

Mechanism of Action. Mycophenolate mofetil inhibits a specific enzyme (inosine monophosphate dehydrogenase) that is responsible for the synthesis of DNA precursors in T and B lymphocytes.[57] Because these lymphocytes cannot synthesize adequate amounts of DNA, their ability to replicate and proliferate is impaired, thus blunting the immune response. This drug may also inhibit lymphocyte attraction and adhesion to the vascular endothelium, thereby impairing the lymphocytes' ability to migrate to the site of the foreign (transplanted) tissues and to infiltrate these tissues from the bloodstream.[18]

Adverse Effects. The primary adverse effects associated with mycophenolate mofetil are blood disorders (e.g., anemia, leukopenia, neutropenia) and GI problems (e.g., abdominal pain, nausea, vomiting, heartburn, diarrhea, constipation).[54] Other side effects include chest pain, cough, dyspnea, muscle pain, weakness, and cardiovascular problems (e.g., hypertension, arrhythmias).

Sulfasalazine

Clinical Use. Sulfasalazine (Azulfidine, others) has unique properties, with some antibacterial characteristics similar to sulfonamide drugs (see Chapter 33) and some anti-inflammatory characteristics similar to the salicylates (see Chapter 15). This drug is primarily used to suppress the immune response associated with rheumatoid arthritis and inflammatory bowel disease.[58]

Mechanism of Action. The exact mechanism of this drug in immune-related disorders is not fully understood. Sulfasalazine may affect key components in the immune system, including suppression of NK cells. Other effects may be related to the drug's breakdown into active metabolites, including sulfapyridine and mesalamine, which exert antibiotic and anti-inflammatory effects, respectively.

Adverse Effects. The primary side effects include headache, blood dyscrasias (e.g., agranulocytosis, anemia, thrombocytopenia), increased sensitivity to ultraviolet light, and hypersensitivity reactions (e.g., fever, skin rash, itching). Hypersensitivity can be severe or even fatal in susceptible individuals.

Sirolimus and other mTOR Inhibitors

Clinical Use. Certain drugs affect immune function by inhibiting a key enzyme known as *mammalian target of rapamycin* (mTOR; see "Mechanism of Action" below). The primary mTOR inhibitor is sirolimus (Rapamune), which is an antibiotic that also has substantial immunosuppressant effects. Everolimus (Zortress) and temsirolimus (Torisel) are sirolimus analogs that are also classified as mTOR inhibitors. These drugs were approved originally to treat renal cell cancer but may also be successful in suppressing immune responses. Sirolimus and its analogs are used primarily to prevent organ rejection in people with solid organ transplants (kidney, heart, etc.).[59-61] Sirolimus and other mTOR inhibitors can be especially beneficial following kidney transplants because they help prevent organ rejection without adversely affecting glomerular filtration and other aspects of the kidney function.[59,60] Likewise, these drugs are often used preferentially in patients with renal dysfunction instead of more nephrotoxic drugs (e.g., cyclosporine, tacrolimus).[62,63]

To provide optimal immunosuppressant effects, mTOR inhibitors are typically combined with glucocorticoids or other immunosuppressants. These drugs also exert several other beneficial effects, including the ability to inhibit smooth muscle proliferation in blood vessel walls. For this reason, sirolimus and everolimus are sometimes incorporated into drug-eluting stents—a supportive tubular structure (stent) is placed in the lumen of a partially occluded artery, and the drug is released slowly from the stent to help reduce vessel occlusion.[64,65]

Mechanism of Action. Unlike other immunosuppressants (e.g., cyclosporine, tacrolimus), sirolimus and its analogs do not interfere directly with cytokine production. As indicated above, these drugs inhibit the function of mTOR.[66,67] This enzyme plays a key role in signaling pathways that promote the growth and proliferation of T and B cells.[68,69] By inhibiting mTOR, these drugs cause cell division to stop at a specific stage (G1), thereby limiting the ability of these cells to mount an attack on transplanted tissues.[67]

Adverse Effects. Sirolimus and its analogs may cause blood lipid disorders, including hypercholesterolemia and hypertriglyceridemia, and may also impair wound healing.[70,71] Other side effects include blood disorders (e.g., anemia, leukopenia, thrombocytopenia), diarrhea, skin rash, joint and muscle pain, and hypertension.[70]

Tacrolimus

Clinical Use. Tacrolimus (Prograf) is similar to cyclosporine in immunosuppressive effects, but this drug is approximately 10 to 100 times more potent than cyclosporine.[72] Tacrolimus may also be somewhat less toxic than cyclosporine and other immunosuppressants, although serious side effects may still occur at higher doses (see "Adverse Effects" below). Tacrolimus is used primarily to prevent rejection of kidney and liver transplants.[73,74] This drug may also be useful in preventing or treating the rejection of other organs and tissues, including heart, lung, pancreas, and bone marrow transplants.[74-76] Topical preparations of tacrolimus or an analogous drug known as pimecrolimus (Elidel) can also be used to treat skin disorders such as atopic dermatitis.[77]

Mechanism of Action. Tacrolimus acts like cyclosporine by binding to a specific protein (calcineurin) in lymphoid tissues and ultimately inhibiting the production of key cytokines such as IL-2.[72] IL-2 plays a critical role in the immune response because this substance promotes the growth and proliferation of activated T lymphocytes and other immune cells, such as NK cells (see Fig. 37-1). This binding provides a somewhat more selective inhibition of immune function than other drugs that exert a general or nonselective inhibition of the immune response.

Adverse Effects. Common side effects of tacrolimus include GI disturbances (e.g., cramps, nausea, diarrhea, constipation), weakness, fever, and skin rashes and itching. More serious problems include renal and central nervous system (CNS) toxicity (e.g., headache, anxiety, nervousness, seizures).[44,78] Tacrolimus is also associated with problems with glucose metabolism (e.g., hyperglycemia, glucose intolerance) and can cause diabetes mellitus in certain individuals.[79]

Other Methods of Immunosuppression

Immunosuppressant Antibodies and Fusion Proteins

A rather selective method of suppressing immune function makes use of antibodies and other proteins that interact with specific immune system cells and interfere with the cell's function (Table 37-2).[72,80,81] For example, antibodies such as Rho(D) immunoglobulin are used routinely to suppress immune response in mothers who have been exposed to a fetus's incompatible blood type. This immunosuppression prevents the mother from developing antibodies that will be passed on to the fetus or to a fetus in a subsequent pregnancy, thus blocking the production of maternal antibodies that can attack the fetus's blood and cause a potentially fatal condition known as *hemolytic anemia of the newborn*.[82] The immunosuppressive antibodies can be obtained from animal sources and cell culture techniques (monoclonal antibodies).

Researchers have also developed antibodies that are very selective for antigens located on the surface of specific T cells and other lymphocytes; these antibodies inhibit cell function or cause destruction of the cell.[18] Anti–T-cell antibodies are primarily used to help prevent or treat rejection of organ and bone marrow transplants (see Table 37-2).[83,84]

Other synthesized antibodies inhibit the effects of a specific cytokine or other chemical signal that normally activates immune cells. For example, agents have been developed that block the interleukin-2 receptor, thus preventing interleukin-2 from activating T lymphocytes.[85,86] These anti-interleukin-2 receptor agents, such as basiliximab (Simulect) and daclizumab (Zenapax), may be helpful in reducing the incidence of acute transplant rejection.[86] Antibodies seem to be especially useful in the initial (induction) phase of antirejection treatment because these drugs can delay or supplant the use of more toxic immunosuppressants, such as the glucocorticoids and calcineurin inhibitors (cyclosporine and tacrolimus).[87,88]

Agents also are available that block the receptor for interlukin-1, which is another proinflammatory cytokine that plays a key role in rheumatoid arthritis and in certain inherited inflammatory diseases categorized as cryopyrin-associated periodic syndromes (CAPS).[89,90] Hence, antibodies that block the interleukin-1 receptor on immune cells can reduce activation of these cells and help control the inflammatory responses in rheumatoid arthritis and CAPS. Clinical interleukin-1 receptor antagonists are listed in Table 37-2.

Exogenous antibodies, such as adalimumab (Humira), etanercept (Enbrel), and infliximab (Remicade), bind directly to tumor necrosis factor alpha (TNF-alpha), thereby preventing this cytokine from causing damage to joints and other tissues. These anti-TNF-alpha drugs are therefore helpful in autoimmune diseases such as rheumatoid arthritis; their pharmacology is addressed in more detail in Chapter 16.

Finally, the use of fusion proteins is another strategy for affecting specific immune functions. Fusion proteins can help impair T-cell activation in specific diseases. Normally, T cells require activation by two signals from the antigen-presenting cell (APC), a process known as *co-stimulation*. The first signal is provided by the major histocompatibility complex that is present on the surface of the APC, and the second (co-stimulatory) signal is from another surface molecule

Table 37-2
ANTIBODIES AND FUSION PROTEINS USED AS IMMUNOSUPPRESSANTS*

Generic Name	Trade Name	Primary Indication(s)
Interleukin-1 Receptor Antagonists		
Anakinra	Kineret	Rheumatoid arthritis
Canakinumab	Ilaris	Cryopyrin-associated periodic syndromes (CAPS), including familial cold autoinflammatory syndrome (FCAS) and Muckle-Wells syndrome (MWS)
Rilonacept	Arcalyst	Similar to canakinumab
Interleukin-2 Receptor Antagonists		
Basiliximab	Simulect	Prevention of acute rejection of kidney transplants
Daclizumab	Zenapax	Prevention of acute rejection of kidney transplants
Tumor Necrosis Factor-Alpha Inhibitors		
Adalimumab	Humira	Rheumatoid arthritis
Etanercept	Enbrel	Rheumatoid arthritis; ankylosing spondylitis; psoriatic arthritis; plaque psoriasis
Infliximab	Remicade	Rheumatoid arthritis; ulcerative colitis
Fusion Proteins		
Abatacept	Orencia	Rheumatoid arthritis
Alefacept	Amevive	Plaque psoriasis
Belatacept	Nulojix	Prevention of rejection of kidney transplants
Miscellaneous Antibodies		
Antithymocyte globulin	—	Treatment of rejection of kidney, heart, liver, lung, pancreas, and bone marrow transplants
Efalizumab	Raptiva	Plaque psoriasis
Muromonab-CD3 monoclonal antibody	Orthoclone OKT3	Acute rejection of heart, liver, and kidney transplants
Rh_O(D) immune globulin	BayRho-D, RhoGAM, others	Prevention of Rh hemolytic disease of the newborn

**Agents listed here are used primarily to prevent transplant rejection and to control immune responses in specific autoimmune diseases. Antibodies used in cancer are addressed in Chapter 36. Antibodies used in rheumatoid arthritis are addressed in more detail in Chapter 16.*

on the APC. Both signals from the APC are transmitted to the T cell through specific receptors on the T cell, and both signals must be present for T-cell activation. Fusion proteins basically block the receptor on the T cell that receives the second (co-stimulatory) signal, hence suppressing T-cell activation.

Fusion proteins are usually synthesized using recombinant DNA techniques and other biosynthetic tools.[18] Several fusion proteins such as abatacept (Orencia), alefacept (Amevive), and belatacept (Nulojix) are currently approved for treating various conditions that require immunosuppression (see Table 37-2). Other fusion proteins are in development, and these drugs may provide an effective strategy for modifying immune responses in specific diseases.

In summary, immunosuppressant antibodies and fusion proteins continue to gain acceptance as a method for preventing rejection of transplanted tissues and for treating various autoimmune diseases.[80,81] The references at the end of this chapter provide sources for more information on the use of specific agents in specific disorders.[18,72]

Miscellaneous Immunosuppressants

A variety of other agents with cytotoxic effects can suppress the immune system. These drugs include chlorambucil (Leukeran), mercaptopurine (Purinethol), vinblastine (Velban), and vincristine (Oncovin, Vincasar).[72] These agents are similar to methotrexate; they exert cytotoxic effects that interfere with the proliferation of immune system cellular components. The pharmacology of these drugs, which are used primarily as anticancer agents, is described in more detail in Chapter 36. Their use as immunosuppressants has generally declined in favor of drugs that have a more selective and strategic effect on immune function. Nonetheless, these drugs may be helpful in certain autoimmune disorders or in preventing the rejection of tissue and organ transplants in specific situations.

Thalidomide can also be used as an immunosuppressant in treating dermatological manifestations of SLE[91,92] and as an alternative agent in preventing graft-versus-host disease following bone marrow transplant.[93] This drug was originally developed as a sedative but was later discovered to cause severe birth defects when administered to women during pregnancy. Nonetheless, thalidomide may help blunt immunological responses by regulating the genes that express tumor necrosis factor-alpha.[94] Decreased production of this factor results in diminished activation of neutrophils and other immune components, thereby reducing the severity of immunologic reactions. Because of thalidomide's potential adverse effects, derivatives of thalidomide such as lenalidomide and pomalidomide have been developed, but the use of these derivatives as immunosuppressants remains to be fully determined. Hence, thalidomide's immunomodulatory effects and the potential use of thalidomide derivatives continue to be investigated, and use of these drugs in specific diseases may be modified in the future.

IMMUNOSTIMULANTS

A number of agents can suppress the immune system. However, there has been considerable interest in developing pharmacological methods to modify or even stimulate immune function in specific situations. In particular, agents that have a positive immunomodulating effect could be beneficial to patients with compromised immune function (such as those with AIDS or certain cancers) or chronic infections.[18,95] Development of immunostimulants is understandably a complex and potentially dangerous proposition. Excessive or incorrect immune activation could trigger a myriad of problems that resemble autoimmune diseases. Likewise, it may be difficult to selectively stimulate certain aspects of the immune system to treat a specific problem without also causing a more widespread and systemic immunologic response. Nonetheless, a few strategies are currently available to modify or stimulate immune function in a limited number of situations.

Bacille Calmette-Guérin

Clinical Use. Bacille Calmette-Guérin (BCG, TheraCys, others) is an active bacterial strain that can be administered systemically as a vaccine against tuberculosis. This drug, however, may not be effective in the most common strains of mycobacterium that cause tuberculosis, and its use as a vaccine may also be limited by other side effects.[96] Alternatively, this agent can be administered locally within the bladder (intravesicularly) and can initiate an immune reaction that is helpful in treating certain forms of superficial bladder cancer.[97]

Mechanism of Action. The exact reason that this agent is effective in treating cancer is unknown. Some evidence suggests that it may activate macrophages locally at the site of the cancer and that these macrophages engulf and destroy tumor cells.[97]

Adverse Effects. When administered directly into the bladder, common side effects include bladder irritation and infection. Systemic administration (immunization) may also cause dermatological reactions (e.g., peeling or scaling of the skin), allergic reactions, inflammation of lymph nodes, and local irritation or ulceration at the injection site.

Immune Globulin

Clinical Use. Immune globulin (Gamimune, Gammagard, others) is prepared by extracting immunoglobulins from donated human blood.[18] These preparations contain all subclasses of immunoglobulin (Ig) but consist primarily of IgG. Immune globulin is administered intravenously to boost immune function in several conditions, including primary immunodeficiency syndromes (e.g., congenital agammaglobulinemia, common variable immunodeficiency, and severe combined immunodeficiency), idiopathic thrombocytopenic purpura, Kawasaki disease, chronic lymphocytic leukemia, and HIV infection in children.[98-100] Other potential indications for immune globulin include dermatomyositis,

Guillain-Barré syndrome, demyelinating polyneuropathies, Lambert-Eaton myasthenia syndrome, and relapsing-remitting multiple sclerosis.

Mechanism of Action. Commercial preparations of immune globulin mimic the normal role of endogenous immunoglobulins. These preparations therefore directly act as antibodies against infectious agents. They can also help modulate the activity of T lymphocytes, macrophages, and other immune system cells to maintain immune system competence.[98]

Adverse Effects. Immune globulin may cause several side effects, such as joint and muscle pain, headache, general malaise, and GI disturbances (e.g., nausea, vomiting).[101] Although rare, allergic reactions, including anaphylaxis, can occur in some individuals. Because immune globulin is obtained from human blood, care must also be taken to prevent transmission of hepatitis and HIV from infected donors.

OTHER IMMUNOMODULATORS

Cytokines are a potential way to modify the immune system in several situations because of their ability to act as immunoregulatory chemicals. For example, cytokines such as interferon-alpha and interleukin-2 can be administered to treat certain forms of cancer (see Chapter 36). Likewise, certain interferons can help control viral infections, and interferon-beta may be helpful in autoimmune diseases such as multiple sclerosis (see Chapter 34). Researchers continue to investigate how immune function can be manipulated to treat various diseases, and additional immune system modulators will almost certainly be forthcoming.

Finally, vaccines have perhaps been the most significant advancement in modulating immune responses. As addressed in Chapter 34, these agents are typically manufactured by modifying certain antigenic substances, such as a virus, and administering the vaccine prior to viral exposure. This action enables the immune system to manufacture virus-specific antibodies that are able to attack the virus when it enters the body. Vaccines have been instrumental in eliminating certain viral diseases such as smallpox and in offering a method for dealing with other viral infections and certain cancers. Vaccines have likewise prevented plagues that had devastating effects on the world's population throughout the course of human history. Hence, the benefits of existing vaccines cannot be overstated. The development of new and more effective vaccines for various infectious and neoplastic diseases continues, and these agents will certainly be a welcome addition to the immunomodulatory drug armamentarium.

Special Concerns for Rehabilitation Patients

Physical therapists and occupational therapists are often involved in the rehabilitation of patients who have received heart, liver, kidney, and other organ transplants. Therapists also frequently deal with patients who have received autologous grafts, such as skin grafts for treating burns, and bone marrow transplants during the treatment of certain cancers. All of these patients may be taking drugs to prevent tissue rejection.

Therapists also deal with the rehabilitation of patients with musculoskeletal disorders that are caused by an autoimmune response. Many of these diseases attack connective tissues, and autoimmune diseases such as rheumatoid arthritis, dermatomyositis, and SLE are often the primary reason that patients undergo rehabilitation. Patients with a compromised immune system may develop musculoskeletal problems related to their immunodeficient state. Hence, many patients receiving physical therapy and occupational therapy are frequently using immunomodulating drugs.

Immunosuppressant drugs can have a positive impact on rehabilitation if they slow or arrest the progression of autoimmune diseases. A patient with rheumatoid arthritis, for example, will be better able participate in strengthening, range-of-motion,

Continued on following page

Special Concerns for Rehabilitation Patients (Continued)

and cardiovascular conditioning exercises if immunosuppressant drugs reduce the immune-mediated damage to joints and other tissues. Likewise, drugs that stimulate immune function will help prevent infections in patients who are immunocompromised, thereby enabling these patients to remain healthy enough to engage in exercise and other rehabilitation interventions.

These drugs can also have a negative impact on rehabilitation because of their numerous side effects, especially those of the immunosuppressants. These drugs are typically used in high doses to produce immunosuppressive effects, which are often achieved at the expense of serious toxic effects on the musculoskeletal system, CNS, and other organs and tissues. Many immunosuppressants, especially the glucocorticoids, exert catabolic effects on bone, muscle, and other tissues. Other immunosuppressants, such as cyclosporine and tacrolimus, are neurotoxic and may cause peripheral neuropathies and CNS-related problems in balance and posture.

Therefore, rehabilitation specialists can play a critical role in offsetting some of these adverse effects. Therapists can institute strengthening and general conditioning exercises to prevent breakdown of muscle, bone, and other tissues, as well as to maintain cardiovascular function. Problems associated with peripheral neuropathies, such as pain and weakness, may respond to transcutaneous electric nerve stimulation (TENS) and other electrotherapeutic treatments. Balance and gait training may help patients overcome problems caused by CNS toxicity and vestibular problems. Thus, therapists can implement specific strategies as required to help patients cope with the adverse drug effects associated with immunomodulating agents.

CASE STUDY

IMMUNOMODULATING AGENTS

Brief History. A.S. is a 47-year-old concert musician who experienced a progressive decline in renal function that ultimately led to renal failure. Kidney function was maintained artificially through renal dialysis until a suitable kidney transplant became available from a donor who died in an automobile accident. The kidney was transplanted successfully, and A.S. was placed on a prophylactic regimen of three different immunosuppressive drugs to prevent the rejection of the transplanted kidney. At the time of the transplant, cyclosporine was initiated at a dosage of 10 mg/kg of body weight each day. After 15 days, the dosage was decreased to 8 mg/kg per day and was progressively decreased over the next 2 months until a maintenance dosage of 4 mg/kg per day was achieved. On the day of surgery, he also received an intravenous dose of 0.5 g of methylprednisolone. Oral doses of methylprednisolone were then administered in dosages of 16 mg/d for the first 3 months, 12 mg/d for the next 3 months, and 8 mg/d thereafter. A loading dose of 6 mg of sirolimus (Rapamune) was administered orally after the transplant, and sirolimus was then maintained at a dosage of 2 mg per day throughout the post-transplant period. Physical therapy was initiated in the intensive care unit (ICU) 1 day after the transplant to increase strength and to facilitate recovery from the surgery.

CASE STUDY (Continued)

Problem/Influence of Medication. The therapist noted that several drugs were being used to prevent rejection, including rather high doses of methylprednisolone, a glucocorticoid agent. Glucocorticoids are notorious for their catabolic effects, and the therapist was concerned that muscle wasting and bone demineralization could impair this patient's recovery from the transplant.

1. *What interventions can the therapist administer to help offset the catabolic effects of the glucocorticoids?*
2. *How can the initial rehabilitation sessions transition to a long-term exercise program for this patient?*

See Appendix C, "Answers to Case Study Questions."

SUMMARY

Our knowledge of how the immune system functions in both normal and disease states has increased dramatically over the last several decades, and we now have drugs that can moderate the effects of the immune response in certain clinical situations. Immunosuppressants are a mainstay in preventing tissue rejection, and much of the current success of organ transplants is due to the judicious use of immunosuppressive drugs. These drugs are also beneficial in a number of diseases that have an autoimmune basis, and immunosuppressants can help alleviate symptoms or possibly even reverse the sequelae of certain diseases, such as rheumatoid arthritis. A few agents are also available that can augment or stimulate immune function in certain situations. The use of these immunostimulants will continue to expand as more is learned about how we can enhance the immune response in conditions such as cancer and certain immunocompromised states. However, immunomodulating drugs are not without problems, because many agents cause a rather nonspecific effect on immune function, which leads to serious side effects. As more is learned about the details of immune function, new drugs will be developed that are more selective in their ability to modify immune responses without causing a generalized suppression or activation of the immune system.

REFERENCES

1. Chaplin DD. Overview of the immune response. *J Allergy Clin Immunol.* 2010;125(suppl 2):S3-23.
2. Sirisinha S. Insight into the mechanisms regulating immune homeostasis in health and disease. *Asian Pac J Allergy Immunol.* 2011;29:1-14.
3. Alpdogan O. Advances in immune regulation in transplantation. *Discov Med.* 2013;15:150-159.
4. Hartono C, Muthukumar T, Suthanthiran M. Immunosuppressive drug therapy. *Cold Spring Harb Perspect Med.* 2013;3:a015487.
5. Cárdenas-Roldán J, Rojas-Villarraga A, Anaya JM. How do autoimmune diseases cluster in families? A systematic review and meta-analysis. *BMC Med.* 2013;11:73.
6. Selmi C. Autoimmunity in 2012. *Clin Rev Allergy Immunol.* 2013;45:290-301.
7. Kovarik J. From immunosuppression to immunomodulation: current principles and future strategies. *Pathobiology.* 2013;80:275-281.
8. Nussbaum C, Sperandio M. Innate immune cell recruitment in the fetus and neonate. *J Reprod Immunol.* 2011;90:74-81.
9. Bonilla FA, Oettgen HC. Adaptive immunity. *J Allergy Clin Immunol.* 2010;125(suppl 2):S33-40.
10. Dunkelberger JR, Song WC. Complement and its role in innate and adaptive immune responses. *Cell Res.* 2010;20:34-50.
11. Hu W, Pasare C. Location, location, location: tissue-specific regulation of immune responses. *J Leukoc Biol.* 2013;94:409-421.
12. Farache J, Zigmond E, Shakhar G, Jung S. Contributions of dendritic cells and macrophages to intestinal homeostasis and immune defense. *Immunol Cell Biol.* 2013;91:232-239.
13. Flannagan RS, Cosío G, Grinstein S. Antimicrobial mechanisms of phagocytes and bacterial evasion strategies. *Nat Rev Microbiol.* 2009;7:355-366.

14. Guilliams M, Lambrecht BN, Hammad H. Division of labor between lung dendritic cells and macrophages in the defense against pulmonary infections. *Mucosal Immunol.* 2013;6: 464-473.
15. Yin L, Scott-Browne J, Kappler JW, et al. T cells and their eons-old obsession with MHC. *Immunol Rev.* 2012;250:49-60.
16. Zeng WP. "All things considered": transcriptional regulation of T helper type 2 cell differentiation from precursor to effector activation. *Immunology.* 2013;140:31-38.
17. Kishiyama JL. Disorders of the immune system. In: McPhee SJ, Hammer GD, eds. *Pathophysiology of Disease. An Introduction to Clinical Medicine.* 6th ed. New York: Lange/McGraw-Hill; 2010.
18. Krensky AM, Bennett WM, Vincenti F. Immunosuppressants, tolerogens, and immunostimulants. In: Brunton L, et al, eds. *The Pharmacological Basis of Therapeutics.* 12th ed. New York: McGraw-Hill; 2011.
19. Yu D, Vinuesa CG. The elusive identity of T follicular helper cells. *Trends Immunol.* 2010;31:377-383.
20. Snyder PW. Immunology for the toxicologic pathologist. *Toxicol Pathol.* 2012;40:143-147.
21. Halleck F, Friedersdorff F, Fuller TF, et al. New perspectives of immunosuppression. *Transplant Proc.* 2013;45:1224-1231.
22. Schaefer SM, Süsal C, Sommerer C, et al. Current pharmacotherapeutical options for the prevention of kidney transplant rejection. *Expert Opin Pharmacother.* 2013;14:1029-1041.
23. Kumbala D, Zhang R. Essential concept of transplant immunology for clinical practice. *World J Transplant.* 2013;3:113-118.
24. Aliabadi A, Cochrane AB, Zuckermann AO. Current strategies and future trends in immunosuppression after heart transplantation. *Curr Opin Organ Transplant.* 2012;17:540-545.
25. Witt CA, Hachem RR. Immunosuppression: what's standard and what's new? *Semin Respir Crit Care Med.* 2013;34:405-413.
26. Carter PH, Zhao Q. Clinically validated approaches to the treatment of autoimmune diseases. *Expert Opin Investig Drugs.* 2010;19:195-213.
27. Wahren-Herlenius M, Dörner T. Immunopathogenic mechanisms of systemic autoimmune disease. *Lancet.* 2013;382:819-831.
28. Canivell S, Gomis R. Diagnosis and classification of autoimmune diabetes mellitus. *Autoimmun Rev.* 2014;13:403-407.
29. Cavalcante P, Bernasconi P, Mantegazza R. Autoimmune mechanisms in myasthenia gravis. *Curr Opin Neurol.* 2012;25: 621-629.
30. Frei P, Biedermann L, Nielsen OH, Rogler G. Use of thiopurines in inflammatory bowel disease. *World J Gastroenterol.* 2013;19:1040-1048.
31. Kim MJ, Choe YH. Monitoring and safety of azathioprine therapy in inflammatory bowel disease. *Pediatr Gastroenterol Hepatol Nutr.* 2013;16:65-70.
32. Colombo D, Ammirati E. Cyclosporine in transplantation—a history of converging timelines. *J Biol Regul Homeost Agents.* 2011;25:493-504.
33. Czaja AJ. Autoimmune hepatitis: focusing on treatments other than steroids. *Can J Gastroenterol.* 2012;26:615-620.
34. Hebert LA, Rovin BH. Oral cyclophosphamide is on the verge of extinction as therapy for severe autoimmune diseases (especially lupus): should nephrologists care? *Nephron Clin Pract.* 2011;117:c8-14.
35. Mehta SJ, Silver AR, Lindsay JO. Review article: strategies for the management of chronic unremitting ulcerative colitis. *Aliment Pharmacol Ther.* 2013;38:77-97.
36. Raut AS, Prabhu RH, Patravale VB. Psoriasis clinical implications and treatment: a review. *Crit Rev Ther Drug Carrier Syst.* 2013;30:183-216.
37. Anghel D, Tanasescu R, Campeanu A, et al. Neurotoxicity of immunosuppressive therapies in organ transplantation. *Maedica.* 2013;8:170-175.
38. Issa N, Kukla A, Ibrahim HN. Calcineurin inhibitor nephrotoxicity: a review and perspective of the evidence. *Am J Nephrol.* 2013;37:602-612.
39. Leet A, Richardson M, Senior JA, et al. A bioavailability study of cyclosporine: comparison of Neoral versus Cysporin in stable heart transplant recipients. *J Heart Lung Transplant.* 2009;28:894-898.
40. Jadhav KR, Shaikh IM, Ambade KW, Kadam VJ. Applications of microemulsion based drug delivery system. *Curr Drug Deliv.* 2006;3:267-273.
41. Castroagudín JF, Molina E, Varo E. Calcineurin inhibitors in liver transplantation: to be or not to be. *Transplant Proc.* 2011;43:2220-2223.
42. de Mare-Bredemeijer EL, Metselaar HJ. Optimization of the use of Calcineurin inhibitors in liver transplantation. *Best Pract Res Clin Gastroenterol.* 2012;26:85-95.
43. Kaminuma O. Selective inhibitors of nuclear factor of activated T cells: potential therapeutic drugs for the treatment of immunological and inflammatory diseases. *Inflamm Allergy Drug Targets.* 2008;7:35-40.
44. Pallet N, Legendre C. Deciphering calcineurin inhibitor nephrotoxicity: a pharmacological approach. *Pharmacogenomics.* 2010;11:1491-1501.
45. Hoorn EJ, Walsh SB, McCormick JA, et al. Pathogenesis of calcineurin inhibitor-induced hypertension. *J Nephrol.* 2012; 25:269-275.
46. Baschant U, Lane NE, Tuckermann J. The multiple facets of glucocorticoid action in rheumatoid arthritis. *Nat Rev Rheumatol.* 2012;8:645-655.
47. Bergmann TK, Barraclough KA, Lee KJ, Staatz CE. Clinical pharmacokinetics and pharmacodynamics of prednisolone and prednisone in solid organ transplantation. *Clin Pharmacokinet.* 2012;51:711-741.
48. Luijten RK, Fritsch-Stork RD, Bijlsma JW, Derksen RH. The use of glucocorticoids in systemic lupus erythematosus. After 60 years still more an art than science. *Autoimmun Rev.* 2013;12:617-628.
49. Vandevyver S, Dejager L, Tuckermann J, Libert C. New insights into the anti-inflammatory mechanisms of glucocorticoids: an emerging role for glucocorticoid-receptor-mediated transactivation. *Endocrinology.* 2013;154:993-1007.
50. Zanchi NE, Filho MA, Felitti V, et al. Glucocorticoids: extensive physiological actions modulated through multiple mechanisms of gene regulation. *J Cell Physiol.* 2010;224: 311-315.
51. Ponticelli C. Present and future of immunosuppressive therapy in kidney transplantation. *Transplant Proc.* 2011;43: 2439-2440.
52. Joseph A, Brasington R, Kahl L, et al. Immunologic rheumatic disorders. *J Allergy Clin Immunol.* 2010;125(suppl 2):S204-215.
53. Weinblatt ME. Methotrexate in rheumatoid arthritis: a quarter century of development. *Trans Am Clin Climatol Assoc.* 2013;124:16-25.
54. Kaltenborn A, Schrem H. Mycophenolate mofetil in liver transplantation: a review. *Ann Transplant.* 2013;18:685-696.

55. Fallatah HI, Akbar HO. Mycophenolate mofetil as a rescue therapy for autoimmune hepatitis patients who are not responsive to standard therapy. *Expert Rev Gastroenterol Hepatol.* 2011;5:517-522.
56. Feng L, Deng J, Huo DM, et al. Mycophenolate mofetil versus azathioprine as maintenance therapy for lupus nephritis: a meta-analysis. *Nephrology*. 2013;18:104-110.
57. Chiarelli LR, Molinaro M, Libetta C, et al. Inosine monophosphate dehydrogenase variability in renal transplant patients on long-term mycophenolate mofetil therapy. *Br J Clin Pharmacol.* 2010;69:38-50.
58. Meier FM, Frerix M, Hermann W, Müller-Ladner U. Current immunotherapy in rheumatoid arthritis. *Immunotherapy*. 2013;5:955-974.
59. Halleck F, Duerr M, Waiser J, et al. An evaluation of sirolimus in renal transplantation. *Expert Opin Drug Metab Toxicol.* 2012;8:1337-1356.
60. Keating GM, Lyseng-Williamson KA. Everolimus: a guide to its use in liver transplantation. *BioDrugs*. 2013;27:407-411.
61. Veroux M, Tallarita T, Corona D, et al. Sirolimus in solid organ transplantation: current therapies and new frontiers. *Immunotherapy*. 2011;3:1487-1497.
62. Flechner SM, Kobashigawa J, Klintmalm G. Calcineurin inhibitor-sparing regimens in solid organ transplantation: focus on improving renal function and nephrotoxicity. *Clin Transplant.* 2008;22:1-15.
63. Helal I, Chan L. Steroid and calcineurin inhibitor-sparing protocols in kidney transplantation. *Transplant Proc.* 2011;43: 472-477.
64. Piccolo R, Cassese S, Galasso G, et al. Long-term clinical outcomes following sirolimus-eluting stent implantation in patients with acute myocardial infarction. A meta-analysis of randomized trials. *Clin Res Cardiol.* 2012;101:885-893.
65. Townsend JC, Rideout P, Steinberg DH. Everolimus-eluting stents in interventional cardiology. *Vasc Health Risk Manag.* 2012;8:393-404.
66. Klintmalm GB, Nashan B. The role of mTOR inhibitors in liver transplantation: reviewing the evidence. *J Transplant.* 2014;2014:845438.2
67. Säemann MD, Haidinger M, Hecking M, et al. The multifunctional role of mTOR in innate immunity: implications for transplant immunity. *Am J Transplant.* 2009;9:2655-2661.
68. Soliman GA. The role of mechanistic target of rapamycin (mTOR) complexes signaling in the immune responses. *Nutrients*. 2013;5:2231-2257.
69. Sudarsanam S, Johnson DE. Functional consequences of mTOR inhibition. *Curr Opin Drug Discov Devel.* 2010;13:31-40.
70. Kaplan B, Qazi Y, Wellen JR. Strategies for the management of adverse events associated with mTOR inhibitors. *Transplant Rev.* 2014;28:126-133.
71. Nashan B, Citterio F. Wound healing complications and the use of mammalian target of rapamycin inhibitors in kidney transplantation: a critical review of the literature. *Transplantation*. 2012;94:547-561.
72. Lake DF, Briggs AD, Akporiaye ET. Immunopharmacology. In: Katzung BG, ed. *Basic and Clinical Pharmacology.* 12th ed. New York: Lange Medical Books/McGraw Hill; 2012.
73. Provenzani A, Santeusanio A, Mathis E, et al. Pharmacogenetic considerations for optimizing tacrolimus dosing in liver and kidney transplant patients. *World J Gastroenterol.* 2013;19: 9156-9173.
74. Rath T. Tacrolimus in transplant rejection. *Expert Opin Pharmacother.* 2013;14:115-122.
75. Penninga L, Møller CH, Gustafsson F, et al. Tacrolimus versus cyclosporine as primary immunosuppression after heart transplantation: systematic review with meta-analyses and trial sequential analyses of randomised trials. *Eur J Clin Pharmacol.* 2010;66:1177-1187.
76. Penninga L, Penninga EI, Møller CH, et al. Tacrolimus versus cyclosporin as primary immunosuppression for lung transplant recipients. *Cochrane Database Syst Rev.* 2013;5:CD008817.
77. Frankel HC, Qureshi AA. Comparative effectiveness of topical calcineurin inhibitors in adult patients with atopic dermatitis. *Am J Clin Dermatol.* 2012;13:113-123.
78. Wu Q, Marescaux C, Wolff V, et al. Tacrolimus-associated posterior reversible encephalopathy syndrome after solid organ transplantation. *Eur Neurol.* 2010;64:169-177.
79. Gnatta D, Keitel E, Heineck I, et al. Use of tacrolimus and the development of posttransplant diabetes mellitus: a Brazilian single-center, observational study. *Transplant Proc.* 2010;42: 475-478.
80. Carter PH, Zhao Q. Clinically validated approaches to the treatment of autoimmune diseases. *Expert Opin Investig Drugs.* 2010;19:195-213.
81. Lee S, Ballow M. Monoclonal antibodies and fusion proteins and their complications: targeting B cells in autoimmune diseases. *J Allergy Clin Immunol.* 2010;125:814-820.
82. Crowther CA, Middleton P, McBain RD. Anti-D administration in pregnancy for preventing Rhesus alloimmunisation. *Cochrane Database Syst Rev.* 2013;2:CD000020.
83. Chinen J, Buckley RH. Transplantation immunology: solid organ and bone marrow. *J Allergy Clin Immunol.* 2010;125(suppl 2): S324-335.
84. Page E, Kwun J, Oh B, Knechtle S. Lymphodepletional strategies in transplantation. *Cold Spring Harb Perspect Med.* 2013;3. pii: a015511.
85. Campara M, Tzvetanov IG, Oberholzer J. Interleukin-2 receptor blockade with humanized monoclonal antibody for solid organ transplantation. *Expert Opin Biol Ther.* 2010;10:959-969.
86. van den Hoogen MW, Hilbrands LB. Use of monoclonal antibodies in renal transplantation. *Immunotherapy*. 2011;3:871-880.
87. Aliabadi A, Grömmer M, Cochrane A, Salameh O, Zuckermann A. Induction therapy in heart transplantation: where are we now? *Transpl Int.* 2013;26:684-695.
88. Rostaing L, Saliba F, Calmus Y, et al. Review article: use of induction therapy in liver transplantation. *Transplant Rev.* 2012;26:246-260.
89. Dinarello CA, Simon A, van der Meer JW. Treating inflammation by blocking interleukin-1 in a broad spectrum of diseases. *Nat Rev Drug Discov.* 2012;11:633-652.
90. Koné-Paut I, Piram M. Targeting interleukin-1β in CAPS (cryopyrin-associated periodic) syndromes: what did we learn? *Autoimmun Rev.* 2012;12:77-80.
91. Chen M, Doherty SD, Hsu S. Innovative uses of thalidomide. *Dermatol Clin.* 2010;28:577-586.
92. Cortés-Hernández J, Torres-Salido M, Castro-Marrero J, et al. Thalidomide in the treatment of refractory cutaneous lupus erythematosus: prognostic factors of clinical outcome. *Br J Dermatol.* 2012;166:616-623.
93. Wolff D, Schleuning M, von Harsdorf S, et al. Consensus conference on clinical practice in chronic GVHD: second-line treatment of chronic graft-versus-host disease. *Biol Blood Marrow Transplant.* 2011;17:1-17.

94. Majumder S, Sreedhara SR, Banerjee S, Chatterjee S. TNF α signaling beholds thalidomide saga: a review of mechanistic role of TNF-α signaling under thalidomide. *Curr Top Med Chem*. 2012;12:1456-1467.
95. Helbig ET, Opitz B, Sander LE. Adjuvant immunotherapies as a novel approach to bacterial infections. *Immunotherapy*. 2013;5:365-381.
96. Mollica A, Stefanucci A, Costante R. Strategies for developing tuberculosis vaccines: emerging approaches. *Curr Drug Targets*. 2013;14:938-951.
97. Gandhi NM, Morales A, Lamm DL. Bacillus Calmette-Guérin immunotherapy for genitourinary cancer. *BJU Int*. 2013;112:288-297.
98. Ballow M. The IgG molecule as a biological immune response modifier: mechanisms of action of intravenous immune serum globulin in autoimmune and inflammatory disorders. *J Allergy Clin Immunol*. 2011;127:315-323.
99. Gwilliam NR, Lazar DA, Brandt ML, et al. An analysis of outcomes and treatment costs for children undergoing splenectomy for chronic immune thrombocytopenia purpura. *J Pediatr Surg*. 2012;47:1537-1541.
100. Katz U, Shoenfeld Y, Zandman-Goddard G. Update on intravenous immunoglobulins (IVIg) mechanisms of action and off-label use in autoimmune diseases. *Curr Pharm Des*. 2011;17:3166-3175.
101. Cheng MJ, Christmas C. Special considerations with the use of intravenous immunoglobulin in older persons. *Drugs Aging*. 2011;28:729-736.

CHAPTER 38

Complementary and Alternative Medications

In addition to the medications used routinely in modern medicine, consumers have access to many substances that are not considered a part of conventional or mainstream pharmacotherapeutics. These substances often consist of natural products such as herbal preparations, vitamins, minerals, and other nutritional substances that consumers take to promote optimal health or to treat various conditions. These products are usually classified as dietary supplements by the U.S. Food and Drug Administration (FDA) and are therefore not subjected to the rigorous testing and scrutiny required for prescription drugs and many over-the-counter medications.

These nontraditional products are often described as complementary and alternative medications (CAMs), to differentiate them from the more conventional medications that are classified as drugs by the FDA. To be specific, a complementary medication is a substance that is used in addition to a conventional treatment, whereas an alternative medication is used as a substitute for a more traditional or mainstream treatment.[1,2] Other terms are applied to specific interventions, such as herbal remedies, naturopathic treatments, phytomedicines, and so forth. However, for the purpose of this chapter, the term *CAM* will be used to encompass the array of substances that fall outside conventional pharmacotherapeutic regimens.

CAMs and other healing philosophies (meditation, yoga, acupuncture, etc.) have been a mainstay in certain cultures and societies. Western cultures, however, have generally been more aligned with conventional treatments and medications. Nonetheless, the interest and use of CAMs in persons living in the United States has increased dramatically over the past several years. Although it is difficult to determine the exact prevalence of CAM use, it is estimated that around 38 percent of adults in the United States use some form of CAM.[3] Interest in CAMs will almost certainly continue to increase as the popular media, the Internet, and other resources promote their potential benefits.

Because CAMs represent such a broad range of substances and interventions, it is difficult to address this topic in a single chapter. This chapter will present a general overview of the topic and will then describe some of the common CAMs that are taken by persons undergoing physical rehabilitation. This chapter's intent is to alert you to some of the more pertinent and unique aspects of CAM use and to help you understand how these substances can affect how patients respond to rehabilitation interventions.

PROBLEMS ASSOCIATED WITH CAMS

Misconceptions About CAM Safety

Many CAMs are derived from natural sources such as herbs and other plants. Therefore, some consumers assume that a "natural" product is inherently safer than a synthetic or manufactured chemical.[4,5] These individuals may likewise believe that they can take an unlimited amount of a CAM—that is, they may exceed dose limits with the idea that the product can do no harm. These misconceptions can lead to tragic consequences, as was the case with ephedra. Ephedra, derived from an evergreen shrub, also contains epinephrine (adrenaline). As discussed in Chapter 20, epinephrine is a powerful agonist (stimulant) of alpha and beta receptors on various tissues throughout the body. People took ephedra to capitalize on these effects, especially its adrenaline-like effects in promoting weight loss and enhancing athletic performance.[6,7] Unfortunately, ephedra is also a powerful cardiovascular stimulant of beta-1 receptors on the heart and alpha-1 receptors on the peripheral vasculature. Hence, some well-documented cases of heart attack and stroke were attributed to ephedra, especially when it was taken in high doses to promote weight loss.[8] In 2004, concerns about the safety of ephedra prompted the FDA to ban dietary supplements containing ephedra.[9] Unfortunately, ephedra and other banned substances can still be obtained from illicit sources via the Internet, and their use may still cause problems when they are used inappropriately for weight loss and other reasons.[7]

Patients should be reminded that CAMs are subject to all the same restrictions and potential problems as conventional medications. The case of ephedra serves as a primary example of how a product can produce powerful physiological effects regardless of whether it is derived from natural or synthetic sources. It might also help to remind patients that some very important and powerful medications such as opioids (Chapter 14), digoxin (Chapter 24), and certain anticancer drugs (Chapter 36) were originally derived from plant sources. Hence, patients should adhere to proper dosages even if the CAM originated from a natural source.

Failure to Report CAM Use

Patients are sometimes reluctant to tell their physician, nurse, pharmacist, or therapist that they are using CAMs.[10,11] These patients are often afraid that health-care providers will criticize the use of these products as being unscientific and not consistent with conventional health care. This lack of reporting may result in an adverse interaction if a specific traditional medication is administered with a CAM. Likewise, CAMs can alter the metabolism of other medications (see "Potential Adverse Effects of CAMs," below), necessitating a change in the dose of the traditional medication to maintain efficacy or avoid an adverse drug reaction. Therefore, patients should be encouraged to disclose CAM use and the use of any other nontraditional interventions, and clinicians should maintain a constructive, nonjudgmental dialogue with patients about the potential benefits and adverse effects of CAMs.[11]

Lack of Standards for Quality and Purity of CAMs

Because many CAMs are classified as food or dietary supplements, these substances are not subject to the same standards for quality and purity as traditional medications.[5,12] As a result, the active ingredients in certain products may vary considerably or may be inadequate to exert a therapeutic effect.[5,13] This seems especially true for CAMs that are derived from plant sources. Plants that grow under different environmental or soil conditions will invariably contain different amounts of the active ingredients. In addition, some CAMs may inadvertently contain toxins that are sequestered by the plant when it is growing in its natural environment. There is also the possibility that the wrong plants will be harvested and subsequently marketed as a specific type of CAM. Hence, consumers should be aware that the quality of CAMs may vary from product to product and that poor quality can result in a lack of therapeutic effects or an increased risk of toxic effects.

Delayed Use of Conventional Medications

A major concern among health-care providers is that the use of ineffective alternative medications can delay or postpone the use of effective conventional interventions.[14,15] Consumers may begin to self-treat various conditions with alternative medications, hoping that these treatments will provide relief and that they can forgo conventional or mainstream treatments. If the alternative treatment is not effective, however, the condition can worsen to the point where conventional treatment is no longer effective or takes much longer to achieve beneficial effects. Consumers should be counseled to avoid overreliance on these alternative medications and to seek conventional medical treatment if symptoms fail to resolve quickly or if they worsen during alternative medication use.

POTENTIAL ADVERSE EFFECTS OF CAMS

CAMs are often safe and are not typically associated with severe adverse effects when taken as recommended by reasonably healthy persons.[16,17] CAMs, however, can interact with conventional medications and directly increase or decrease these medications' effects.[18,19] Moreover, CAMs often influence the absorption, distribution, metabolism, and excretion of conventional medications.[19,20] In particular, CAMs can directly inhibit enzymes that normally metabolize conventional medications, thus resulting in increased levels of the active form of the conventional drugs.[21,22] On the other hand, some CAMs can stimulate the liver to synthesize more drug-metabolizing enzymes, a process known as *enzyme induction* (see "Enzyme Induction" in Chapter 3).[23,24] During enzyme induction, the liver is capable of metabolizing conventional drugs faster than normal, and the conventional medications fail to reach therapeutic levels because they are broken down too quickly.[22] Hence, conventional medications may fail to exert beneficial effects, and the disease can continue to progress even though the patient is taking the conventional medication as directed.

The extent of CAM-induced pharmacokinetic changes depends on many factors, such as the exact dose and type of CAM, the specific conventional medications being administered, and the health and comorbidities of each patient. Consequently, results from in vitro and animal studies on the interaction between CAMs and conventional medications may not be reflected by actual clinical outcomes when these drugs are used appropriately in humans.[17] Clearly, additional clinical research is needed to clarify the possible interactions between specific CAMs and traditional agents. Nonetheless, physicians must be aware of whether patients are consuming CAMs so that doses of conventional medications can be adjusted to maintain therapeutic effects if CAMs alter the effects of these medications.

Excessive or prolonged dosages of CAMs can also produce toxic effects on various tissues and organs. In particular, the liver may be damaged, and cases of acute liver failure have been documented during inappropriate CAM use or in patients with preexisting liver disease.[25,26] This makes sense considering that the liver often metabolizes CAMs in the same way that it deals with other drugs and toxins.[20,27] Other organs, including the heart, kidneys, and lungs, can also be subjected to toxic effects of high doses of CAMs much in the same way that these organs are vulnerable to untoward effects of conventional medications.

Finally, CAMs can produce side effects and adverse reactions similar to conventional medications.[28,29] Gastrointestinal (GI) disturbances (e.g., nausea, vomiting, diarrhea), headache, allergic responses, and various other reactions are possible even when CAMs are taken at appropriate doses. The type and severity of these reactions depends on many factors, including the type of CAM and the individual characteristics of each patient (genetic factors, diseases, other medications, etc.). Clearly, CAMs can produce the same types of problems as conventional medications, and consumers must be reminded that these products are actual drugs even though they may be derived from natural or nontraditional sources.

SPECIFIC CAMS

The array of CAMs is so vast that even a partial listing is difficult. Some of the more common CAMs are listed in Table 38-1 and are addressed briefly below to provide some indication of their source, primary indications, and potential adverse effects. These discussions are not intended to advocate the use of these substances or to provide a detailed evaluation of the evidence supporting or refuting their use. For more information about these or other CAMs, please refer to other sources, including those listed at the end of the chapter.[30-32]

Bee Venom

Bee venom, administered in the form of actual bee stings from the common honeybee, is occasionally used to treat people with multiple sclerosis, rheumatoid arthritis, and other disease that have an autoimmune basis.[33,34] This treatment is supposed to modulate the immune response and suppress the damage caused by the activation and attack of immune cells on specific tissues.[35] There is some evidence that bee sting therapy can produce beneficial effects in selected patients, but these treatments are certainly painful and may produce harmful effects in other individuals.[33] Additional research is needed to determine whether these treatments can promote short- or long-term benefits in persons with various autoimmune diseases.

Table 38-1
COMPLEMENTARY AND ALTERNATIVE MEDICATIONS

Common Name	Scientific Name	Original Source	Primary Indications/Effects
Bee venom	—	Live bees	Multiple sclerosis; rheumatoid arthritis; other diseases with an autoimmune basis
Chondroitin	Chondroitin sulfate	Bovine tracheal cartilage	Osteoarthritis (combined with glucosamine)
Echinacea	*Echinacea* species (*E. angustifolia; E. pallida; E. purpurea)*	Roots and seeds from the echinacea plant	Immune stimulant; treatment of colds and upper respiratory tract infections; applied topically to promote wound healing
Garlic	*Allium sativum L.*	Bulb of the garlic plant	Decrease cholesterol and other plasma lipids; anti-inflammatory; antimicrobial; antioxidant; other effects
Ginger	*Zingiber officinale*	Root of the ginger plant	Antiemetic; anti-inflammatory; antioxidant; migraine headaches; indigestion; infection; fever; other effects
Ginkgo	*Ginkgo biloba*	Leaf of the gingko tree	Improve memory and cognition; increase vascular perfusion of brain and other tissues; antioxidant; anti-inflammatory
Ginseng	*Panax ginseng*	Root of the ginseng plant	Increase well-being; reduce fatigue; used in the treatment of cancer, diabetes, cardiovascular dysfunction, and various other diseases
Glucosamine	2-amino-2-deoxyglucose; glucosamine sulfate	Manufactured synthetically from sugar-protein precursors	Osteoarthritis (combined with chondroitin)
Kava	*Piper methysticum*	Root of the kava plant	Sedative-hypnotic and antianxiety effects
Melatonin	N-acetyl-5-methoxytryptamine	Manufactured synthetically to mimic the endogenous hormone	Sedative-hypnotic; regulate sleep-wake cycles; used in various other conditions because of antioxidant and immunomodulating effects
Saw palmetto	*Serenoa repens*	Fruit of the saw palmetto palm	Benign prostatic hypertrophy
St. John's wort	*Hypericum perforatum L.*	Flowers of the St. John's wort plant	Antidepressant
Valerian	*Valeriana officinalis*	Root of the valerian plant	Sedative-hypnotic and antianxiety effects

Echinacea

Echinacea is derived from the root and seeds of several echinacea plant species that grow in parts of the Midwestern United States. This herb is used primarily to stimulate or support the immune system and is often used to treat cold symptoms and other relatively minor respiratory tract infections.[36] Although the exact reasons for beneficial effects are unclear, there is considerable evidence that echinacea can reduce symptoms of the common cold when taken soon after symptoms appear.[37,38] This product may also help prevent colds when taken on a regular basis.[36,38] Echinacea can also be administered topically to treat burns and other localized wounds. The most common side effects associated with echinacea are GI upset, skin rash, and other allergic or hypersensitivity reactions.[39]

Garlic

Garlic (*Allium sativum L*) is a bulb that grows throughout the world; its potential health benefits have been extolled for ages. Evidence suggests that garlic extract may reduce the risk of cardiovascular disease by reducing plasma lipids, lowering blood pressure, and inhibiting platelet aggregation.[40,41] Other purported benefits include antineoplastic, antimicrobial, anti-inflammatory, antihyperglycemic, and antioxidant effects.[42,43] The exact reasons for these effects are not clear but are usually attributed to allicin, a chemical that is considered to be the active component of garlic. Side effects are generally mild, consisting primarily of garlic breath odor and GI upset. Serious bleeding problems could occur, however, if patients experience antiplatelet effects from the garlic and are taking other anticoagulants such as heparin, warfarin, or aspirin.

Ginger

Ginger is extracted from the root of the ginger plant (*Zingiber officinale*); the plant originated in Asia but now grows throughout other parts of the world. Ginger is noted for its substantial antiemetic effects and can be used to control the nausea and vomiting that occurs during pregnancy, after surgery, or during cancer chemotherapy.[44-46] It also produces anti-inflammatory effects by inhibiting prostaglandin synthesis in a manner similar to aspirin and other NSAIDs (see Chapter 15).[47,48] Ginger may likewise inhibit leukotriene production (see Chapter 26), and it may affect specific genes to reduce the production of other pro-inflammatory products.[47,48] Ginger has been used for other conditions, including the treatment of sore throats, migraine headaches, indigestion, infection, and fever. Side effects of ginger are usually minor, consisting primarily of GI problems (e.g., nausea, vomiting) and allergic reactions.

Ginkgo Biloba

Ginkgo biloba is extracted from the leaves of the gingko tree (*Ginkgo biloba*) that originated in Japan and China. This herb has become synonymous with attempts to increase memory and cognition. Hence, gingko products are used extensively by many older adults, especially as a complementary or alternative treatment for Alzheimer disease.[49] Gingko is reported to improve circulation, and its effects on cognitive function may be due in part to increased cerebral perfusion. Gingko may also exert antioxidant effects, and some of its therapeutic benefits have been attributed to its ability to limit free-radical damage on vascular and other tissues.[49] There is limited or inconsistent evidence that gingko can improve memory and cognition in people with Alzheimer disease,[50] although a subset of patients may show some benefits in activities of daily living and other behaviors.[51,52] Long-term use, however, does not seem to prevent the onset of Alzheimer disease.[53] Gingko biloba and related products are generally well tolerated. Although past reports indicated that these products may inhibit blood coagulation in some patients,[54] more recent analyses indicated that bleeding problems related to gingko are not clinically relevant.[55] Nevertheless, some practitioners still suggest that gingko biloba should be used cautiously in people at risk for bleeding events or who are taking anticoagulants (e.g., heparin, warfarin, aspirin, and other NSAIDs).[56]

Ginseng

Ginseng, derived from the root of the Panax plant, is renowned as an herbal remedy for various conditions. It is often administered to increase general well-being, reduce fatigue, improve mental acuity, and promote optimal health.[57,58] Ginseng has likewise been advocated in the prevention and treatment of many diseases, including cancer, diabetes, neurodegenerative disorders, and cardiovascular disease.[57,59,60] Although the exact effects of ginseng are not well understood, there is growing evidence that ginseng and related compounds can directly influence antioxidant enzymes and various cells involved in immune responses.[61,62] The potential benefits of ginseng products are therefore typically attributed to its antioxidant properties and ability to support the immune system.[61,63] Ginseng is well tolerated when taken in moderate amounts, but it can reduce the effectiveness of anticoagulant medications such as warfarin, and it can exaggerate the effects of antihyperglycemic medications such as insulin and oral antidiabetic drugs.[19,64]

Glucosamine and Chondroitin

As discussed in Chapter 16, glucosamine and chondroitin are dietary supplements obtained from natural sources or manufactured synthetically. The primary rationale for taking glucosamine and chondroitin is to treat osteoarthritis by supplying the ingredients needed to build healthy articular cartilage and to maintain synovial fluid viscosity.[65] That is, these supplements can provide glycosaminoglycans, proteoglycans, and hyaluronic acid, which comprise the fundamental constituents needed to repair damaged cartilage, increase synovial viscosity, and exert other beneficial effects that help control inflammation and joint destruction in osteoarthritic joints.[66,67]

The potential benefits of glucosamine and chondroitin have been studied extensively in several clinical trials.[68,69] It appears that these supplements may not be helpful in reducing pain or in improving function in all patients with osteoarthritis, but certain patients with more severe pain or an increased rate of cartilage turnover may experience some beneficial effects.[70] These substances are generally well tolerated, although headache and GI problems (e.g., nausea, cramping, heartburn) may occur. Researchers continue to study the long-term effects of glucosamine and chondroitin, and future studies may provide better insight into how this CAM treatment can benefit certain subpopulations of people with osteoarthritis.

Kava

Kava originates from the root of the *Piper methysticum* (kava) plant that grows predominately in the South Pacific islands. This drug has been used for centuries by various local cultures because of its sedative and antianxiety effects. Kava has gained popularity in Western societies, and studies suggest that kava extracts can be used as an alternative to traditional sedative-hypnotic and anxiolytic drugs, such as benzodiazepines (see Chapter 6).[71,72] Kava may also produce analgesic and muscle relaxant effects, and some patients may use this product for self-treatment of back pain and other musculoskeletal injuries. Although the exact mechanism of action is unclear, kava extracts probably affect receptors within the limbic system and enhance the inhibitory effects of GABA and other neurotransmitters. Liver toxicity is the most serious effect associated with kava, but it is not clear if liver damage is caused directly by the active kava ingredients or by mold and other contaminants that occur in the raw materials from the kava plant if it is not processed properly.[73,74] Nonetheless, kava products are banned in many countries throughout Europe because of the risk of liver toxicity.[75]

Melatonin

Melatonin is an endogenous neurohormone that is produced primarily by the pineal gland. In humans, melatonin is normally released at night, with plasma levels tending to peak between 2:00 and 4:00 a.m.[76] Melatonin is associated with the ability to regulate sleep-wake cycles and perhaps other circadian rhythms.[77] Because of this effect, individuals have been using synthetic melatonin supplements primarily to treat insomnia, especially in those with disturbed sleep cycles, including people who work at night and must sleep during the day. Persons who are blind and cannot regulate melatonin release because they are unable to respond visually to normal light-dark cycles also may be taking synthetic melatonin.[78,79]

Melatonin is also associated with antioxidant effects; these effects may be beneficial in several situations, including neurodegenerative diseases such as Parkinson disease and Alzheimer disease.[80] Melatonin may have positive effects on cell division and differentiation and may therefore be helpful in treating certain forms of cancer.[81,82] Likewise, melatonin and related compounds can lower blood pressure and can exert other beneficial effects on cardiovascular function.[83,84] Melatonin is also being used to reduce migraine headaches[85] and to improve insulin responses in type 2 diabetes mellitus.[86] Clearly, melatonin has the ability to regulate a number of important physiological functions, and researchers continue to investigate the potential benefits of melatonin supplements in a number of conditions. Side effects of melatonin are usually minor, consisting primarily of headache, change in sleep cycles, vivid dreams, GI disturbances, and allergic reactions (skin rashes and itching).

Saw Palmetto

Saw palmetto (*Serenoa repens*) is a palm that grows in the southern United States, and extracts from the fruit of this palm are used primarily to treat benign prostatic hypertrophy (BPH).[87] Randomized controlled trials, however, have generally failed to find any differences in the effects of saw palmetto compared to placebo, even at double or triple the recommended doses.[88] That is, there is little evidence to support the use of this product in decreasing prostate size and improving urine flow in men with BPH. Still, some men believe saw palmetto can improve their symptoms, and possible benefits in a subset of men with BPH cannot be completely ruled out.[87] Possible side effects include headache, GI upset, and allergic reactions. Saw palmetto treatments are generally well tolerated, especially when compared to conventional medications such as finasteride (Proscar) (see Chapter 30).[89]

St. John's Wort

St. John's wort is derived from the flowers of the *Hypericum perforatum* plant that grows throughout England, Europe, Asia, and parts of the United States. This herbal supplement has been used extensively to treat symptoms of depression and anxiety. Although the details are unclear, St. John's wort probably contains several chemicals that alter the balance of central nervous system (CNS) neurotransmitters that affect mood and behavior.[90,91] As discussed in Chapter 7, depression seems to be associated with a fundamental defect in amine neurotransmitters such as serotonin, norepinephrine, and dopamine. St. John's wort may promote changes in these neurotransmitters in a manner similar to conventional prescription antidepressants.[90] Many people therefore use St. John's wort as an alternative medication to help improve mood and resolve the symptoms of depression.[92]

Several studies have suggested that products containing adequate amounts of the active chemicals from St. John's wort may be successful in treating depression, including moderate to severe cases of this disease.[93,94] St. John's wort is generally well tolerated,[92,95] but use of this product can accelerate the metabolism of other therapeutic medications such as warfarin (Chapter 25), reverse transcriptase inhibitors (Chapter 34), cyclosporine (Chapter 37), and certain anticancer agents (Chapter 36).[96] Hence, St. John's wort can prevent these other medications from reaching therapeutic levels, and dosages of other medications may have to be adjusted to maintain their efficacy when administered with St. John's wort.[95]

Valerian

Valerian is derived from the root of the *Valeriana officinalis* plant that grows throughout many parts of the world. It is generally used to treat mild cases of anxiety and to promote normal sleep. As a sleep aid, valerian may need to be taken for a week or so before beneficial effects become apparent.[97] Nonetheless, this product can be an alternative long-term treatment for people with mild-to-moderate cases of insomnia and restlessness.[98,99] Valerian appears to exert sedative and antianxiety effects in a manner similar to benzodiazepines—that is, it enhances GABA inhibition in specific parts of the brain that control sleep (see Chapter 6).[100] Side effects of valerian are generally mild and consist of headache and GI problems (e.g., nausea, vomiting).

VITAMINS AND MINERALS

Vitamins and minerals are not considered medications, but these substances are essential for maintaining physiological function and homeostasis throughout the body. Many individuals consume these substances to complement other medications and to help promote optimal health. It is beyond the scope of this chapter to address all the pertinent issues related to vitamin and mineral metabolism. Nonetheless, a brief overview of these substances and their use as dietary supplements is provided here and summarized later in Tables 38-2 and 38-3. Please refer to other sources, including those listed at the end of the chapter, for a more detailed discussion of vitamins and minerals.[101,102]

Vitamins

Vitamins comprise a diverse group of organic chemicals that the body needs to facilitate specific metabolic and biosynthetic processes.[102,103] In many cases, vitamins act as enzymatic cofactors; the vitamin works directly with the enzyme to catalyze a specific chemical reaction. In other situations, the vitamin forms an essential component of a chemical structure or species that is needed for a specific chemical reaction. The body typically needs small amounts of vitamins to promote normal growth and development and to maintain optimal health throughout adulthood.[103,104]

Table 38-2 summarizes the key aspects of vitamins needed throughout the body. Most of these vitamins cannot be synthesized within the body and must be ingested from an outside source.[105] Eating certain foods on a regular basis will provide the body with an adequate supply of the specific vitamins it needs. Fruits and vegetables, for example, often serve as a source of dietary vitamins. Alternatively, there are a myriad of vitamin supplements that consumers can purchase and self-administer to ensure adequate daily vitamin intake.

Vitamin supplements are usually required if the dietary supply of vitamins is inadequate to meet the body's daily requirements.[103] In most cases, a relatively balanced diet will provide adequate amounts of all the vitamins needed. People with diets that are extremely poor in nutrients or lacking in certain foods may benefit from vitamin supplements. Certain metabolic disorders or procedures, such as gastric bypass surgery, may likewise impair the absorption or utilization of specific

Table 38-2
VITAMINS

Vitamin	RDA/AI*	Physiological Function	Adverse Effects of Excessive Consumption**
Biotin	Men & women: 30 μg/d	Coenzyme in the synthesis of fat, glycogen, and amino acids	No adverse effects have been reported
Folic acid	Men & women: 400 μg/d	Coenzyme in the metabolism of nucleic acids and amino acids; prevents megaloblastic anemia	Adverse effects have not been documented, but high doses may mask neurological complications in people with vitamin B_{12} deficiency
Niacin	Men: 16 mg/d Women: 14 mg/d	Coenzyme or cosubstrate in many biological reactions required for energy metabolism	GI distress; vasomotor reactions (flushing)
Pantothenic acid	Men & women: 5 mg/d	Coenzyme in fatty acid metabolism	No adverse effects have been reported
Vitamin A (retinol)	Men: 900 μg/d Women: 700 μg/d	Required for normal vision, gene expression, reproduction, embryonic development, and immune function	Teratological effects; liver toxicity
Vitamin B_1 (thiamin)	Men: 1.2 mg/d Women: 1.1 mg/d	Coenzyme in the metabolism of carbohydrates and certain amino acids; prevents beriberi	No adverse effects have been reported
Vitamin B_2 (riboflavin)	Men: 1.3 mg/d Women: 1.1 mg/d	Coenzyme in numerous oxidative metabolic reactions	No adverse effects have been reported
Vitamin B_6 (pyridoxine)	Men: 1.3–1.7 mg/d Women: 1.3–1.5 mg/d	Coenzyme in the metabolism of amino acids and glycogen	No adverse effects have been reported
Vitamin B_{12} (cobalamin)	Men & women: 2.4 μg/d	Coenzyme in nucleic acid metabolism; prevents megaloblastic/pernicious anemia	No adverse effects have been reported
Vitamin C (ascorbic acid)	Men: 90 mg/d Women: 75 mg/d	Cofactor for reactions requiring reduced copper or iron metalloenzyme and as a protective antioxidant; prevents scurvy	GI disturbances, kidney stones, excess iron absorption
Vitamin D (calciferol)	Men & women: 15–20 μg/d	Maintain serum calcium and phosphorus concentrations; prevents rickets	Hypercalcemia secondary to elevated vitamin D metabolites in plasma
Vitamin E (α-tocopherol)	Men & women: 15 mg/d	Antioxidant effects	Hemorrhagic toxicity
Vitamin K	Men: 120 μg/d Women: 90 μg/d	Coenzyme during the synthesis of many proteins involved in blood clotting and bone metabolism	No adverse effects have been reported

**Recommended daily requirement (RDA) or adequate intake (AI) for men and nonpregnant women over 20 years old. Recommended values for certain vitamins (e.g., folic acid) may be higher in women who are pregnant. Values for children are typically lower and are adjusted according to the child's age.*

***Absence of reported adverse effects does not mean that there is no potential for adverse effects from high intake. Caution should still be used when taking doses well in excess of the recommended daily amounts.*

Adapted from: Institute of Medicine of the National Academies (www.iom.edu): Food & Nutrition > Dietary Reference Intakes > DRI Tables > Vitamins.

vitamins, and supplements can help resolve a potential vitamin imbalance in these situations.[106,107] In other situations, the body's demand for certain vitamins may increase, and dietary sources may be unable to provide enough of a specific vitamin. During pregnancy, for example, a supplement with folic acid may be helpful in supplying an adequate source of this vitamin for the mother and developing fetus.[108]

Hence, vitamin supplements should be administered to make up any differences between the dietary supply and the body's demand for specific vitamins. Some individuals, however, self-administer large dosages of vitamins on a regular basis with the misconception that these supplements will promote better health and offer protection from disease. Excessive dosages of vitamins are unnecessary and can be harmful if they begin to accumulate in certain tissues and organs. This is especially true for the fat-soluble vitamins A, D, E, and K.[103] Water-soluble vitamins (e.g., B complex, vitamin C) are generally less problematic because excess doses of these vitamins are excreted in the urine. Fat-soluble vitamins, however, can accumulate in adipose tissue, the liver, and various other sites throughout the body. Excess vitamin administration can result in various signs of toxicity, including drowsiness, headache, fatigue, nausea, muscle weakness, kidney dysfunction, and enlargement of the liver and spleen (see Table 38-2).[109,110]

Clinicians should therefore advise patients about the need for adequate dietary vitamin intake but should also caution patients about the indiscriminate or excessive use of vitamin supplements. Patients with specific questions can also be referred to a registered dietician who can analyze the person's vitamin needs and suggest whether supplements may be helpful.

Minerals

Minerals are small chemical substances that play key roles in various physiological processes.[103] Consider, for example, the ways that minerals such as sodium, potassium, chloride, and calcium influence the function and homeostasis of virtually every cell in the body. These minerals and several other major minerals are essential for life. Other minerals, known commonly as *trace minerals,* are not as abundant in the body but are still needed to promote the function of specific cells and tissues.

The primary roles and the recommended daily intake of major and trace minerals are listed in Table 38-3. Similar to vitamins, these minerals are typically obtained from dietary sources. Specific minerals may likewise be included in various multivitamins and other dietary supplements, with the intent that they will promote good health and prevent disease. Again, there is generally no need for mineral supplements for most people eating a reasonably balanced diet. On the other hand, mineral supplements can be helpful in specific situations where the body's need for a mineral may exceed dietary supply. Some examples of appropriate supplementation include calcium supplements for people with osteoporosis (see Chapter 31), potassium supplements for people on diuretics (see Chapter 21), and iron supplements for people with certain anemias. Hence, mineral supplements may be helpful in certain individuals, but the dose and type of supplement should be adjusted carefully.

Table 38-3
MINERALS

Mineral	Primary Physiological Function(s)	RDA/AI*
Major Minerals (Greater Than 0.005% Body Weight)		
Calcium	Mineralization of bone and teeth; synaptic transmission; muscle contraction; blood clotting	Men & women: 1,000 mg/d
Chloride	With sodium and potassium, helps maintain electrochemical and water balance across cell membrane	Men & women: 2.3 g/d
Magnesium	Cofactor for enzyme systems	Men: 420 mg/d Women: 320 mg/d
Phosphate	Facilitates energy storage and release, nucleotide synthesis, and maintenance of acid-base balance in body fluids	Men & women: 700 mg/d

Continued

Table 38-3
MINERALS—cont'd

Mineral	Primary Physiological Function(s)	RDA/AI*
Potassium	With sodium and chloride, helps maintain electrochemical and water balance across cell membrane; promotes repolarization of nerve and muscle tissues	Men & women: 4.7 g/d
Sodium	With potassium and chloride, helps maintain electrochemical and water balance across cell membrane; initiates depolarization of nerve and muscle tissues	Men & women: 1.5 g/d
Inorganic Sulfate	Provides precursors for sulfur-containing compounds	Unknown
Trace Minerals (Less Than 0.005% Body Weight)		
Chromium	Helps maintain normal blood glucose levels	Men: 35 μg/d Women: 25 μg/d
Copper	Component of enzymes in iron metabolism	Men & women: 900 μg/d
Fluoride	Stimulates new bone formation; prevents formation of dental cavities	Men: 4 mg/d Women: 3 mg/d
Iodine	Component of the thyroid hormones; prevents goiter and cretinism	Men & women: 150 μg/d
Iron	Component of hemoglobin and numerous enzymes; prevents certain anemias	Men: 8 mg/d Women: 18 mg/d
Manganese	Involved in bone formation and in enzymes involved in amino acid, cholesterol, and carbohydrate metabolism	Men: 2.3 mg/d Women: 1.8 mg/d
Molybdenum	Cofactor for enzymes involved in catabolism of certain amino acids and nucleic acids	Men & women: 45 μg/d
Selenium	Defense against oxidative stress; regulates thyroid hormone action and metabolism of vitamin C and other molecules	Men & women: 55 μg/d
Zinc	Component of many enzymes and proteins; involved in the regulation of gene expression	Men: 11 mg/d Women: 8 mg/d

**Recommended daily requirement (RDA) or adequate intake (AI) for men and nonpregnant women 30–50 years old. Values may differ for children, older adults, and pregnant women.*

Adapted from: Institute of Medicine of the National Academies (www.iom.edu): Food & Nutrition > Dietary Reference Intakes > DRI Tables > Electrolytes and Water; Elements.

Special Concerns for Rehabilitation Patients

Considering the extensive use of CAMs, many patients receiving physical therapy or occupational therapy will be taking these products to promote their health and to prevent disease. CAMs are likewise used as part of the treatment for many conditions seen in patients receiving rehabilitation, including back pain, fibromyalgia, rheumatoid arthritis, osteoarthritis, and a myriad of other systemic diseases and conditions.

Patients may feel empowered to take a more active role in controlling their health and well-being, especially if they experience beneficial effects from exercise and other rehabilitation interventions. Hence, these patients may be interested in how

Special Concerns for Rehabilitation Patients (Continued)

nutritional and dietary supplements can be used in a safe and effective manner, and they may ask therapists about various CAMs. Rehabilitation specialists will therefore be in an optimal position to serve as health-care educators in discussing the appropriate uses of CAMs and dispelling myths about unproven or improbable claims about these products' benefits.

Therapists should query their patients about CAM use as part of the evaluation process. In fact, patients may be more willing to divulge their use of CAMs to therapists as opposed to physicians and other health-care practitioners. Therapists may identify potential problems in patients taking excessive or inappropriate CAMs and can refer such patients to a physician, nurse practitioner, or registered dietician for further evaluation of the risks of using CAMs. However, therapists should not advise patients to take specific CAMs because ingestion of any chemical may cause untoward effects that are simply not apparent given the therapists' knowledge of the patient's medical background, comorbidities, diet, other medications, and so forth. Patients who are interested in taking CAMs should always be referred to other practitioners who are experts in the use of these products.

Finally, therapists should look for signs that might indicate excessive use of CAMs, such as muscle weakness, incoordination, excessive fatigue, balance problems, skin rashes or bruising, neuropathic changes, and cardiovascular impairments (increased blood pressure, arrhythmias, etc.). These signs or any unexplained change in function should be brought to the attention of the physician so that the potential risks of CAMs can be evaluated and dealt with accordingly.

CASE STUDY

COMPLEMENTARY AND ALTERNATIVE MEDICATIONS

Brief History. S.G. is a 75-year-old man who began experiencing osteoarthritic changes in his right knee when he was in his 50s. This condition worsened progressively, necessitating a total knee arthroplasty, which was performed 2 years ago. The initial knee replacement became unstable and was recently revised surgically to decrease pain and to promote better function. While in the hospital for this revision, the patient developed a deep vein thrombosis and was placed on heparin followed by warfarin (Coumadin) to control excessive coagulation. He continued taking the warfarin when he was discharged, and a physical therapist began providing home care on a regular basis. During the initial visit, the therapist asked the patient if he was taking any additional medications. He replied that he had recently started taking a nonprescription product that contained St. John's wort. Apparently, this patient had become very discouraged and despondent because of problems with his knee replacement and his inability to resume his hobbies and social activities, such as playing golf and gardening. A friend had recommended he take St. John's wort as an alternative way to improve his mood while recovering from the most recent knee surgery.

Continued on following page

CASE STUDY (Continued)

Problem/Influence of Medication. St. John's wort can cause enzyme induction, which results in an increase in the liver's ability to metabolize other medications, including warfarin. This process could result in the warfarin being metabolized too rapidly and therefore failing to reach therapeutic levels. Lack of adequate anticoagulant effects would place the patient at increased risk for subsequent thrombosis and pulmonary embolism.

Questions to Consider

1. ***What should the therapist do to resolve concerns about the interaction of St. John's wort and warfarin?***
2. ***What additional monitoring might be helpful to assess whether warfarin is still effective?***

See Appendix C, "Answers to Case Study Questions."

SUMMARY

CAMs represent a diverse array of nutritional supplements and other products that are used to promote health and prevent disease. Because CAMs are often derived from natural sources, patients may have certain misconceptions about the safety and efficacy of these products. CAMs are likewise not subjected to the scrutiny and control of traditional medications, and patient responses may be influenced by problems with the product's purity and quality. Many patients undergoing physical rehabilitation will self-administer CAMs to help treat various conditions or to maintain optimal health. Therapists should query their patients about CAM use, serve as a source of information about the potential benefits and detriments of these products, and remain alert for any untoward reactions that might indicate toxic effects of CAMs.

REFERENCES

1. Kiefer D, Pitluk J, Klunk K. An overview of CAM: components and clinical uses. *Nutr Clin Pract.* 2009;24:549-559.
2. Staud R. Effectiveness of CAM therapy: understanding the evidence. *Rheum Dis Clin North Am.* 2011;37:9-17.
3. Harris PE, Cooper KL, Relton C, Thomas KJ. Prevalence of complementary and alternative medicine (CAM) use by the general population: a systematic review and update. *Int J Clin Pract.* 2012;66:924-939.
4. Ernst E, Hung SK. Great expectations: what do patients using complementary and alternative medicine hope for? *Patient.* 2011;4:89-101.
5. Lu WI, Lu DP. Impact of Chinese herbal medicine on American society and health care system: perspective and concern. *Evid Based Complement Alternat Med.* 2014;2014:251891.
6. Chen CK, Muhamad AS, Ooi FK. Herbs in exercise and sports. *J Physiol Anthropol.* 2012;31:4.
7. Yen M, Ewald MB. Toxicity of weight loss agents. *J Med Toxicol.* 2012;8:145-152.
8. Andraws R, Chawla P, Brown DL. Cardiovascular effects of ephedra alkaloids: a comprehensive review. *Prog Cardiovasc Dis.* 2005;47:217-225.
9. Keisler BD, Hosey RG. Ergogenic aids: an update on ephedra. *Curr Sports Med Rep.* 2005;4:231-235.
10. Davis EL, Oh B, Butow PN, et al. Cancer patient disclosure and patient-doctor communication of complementary and alternative medicine use: a systematic review. *Oncologist.* 2012;17:1475-1481.
11. Frenkel M, Cohen L. Effective communication about the use of complementary and integrative medicine in cancer care. *J Altern Complement Med.* 2014;20:12-18.
12. Moquin B, Blackman MR, Mitty E, Flores S. Complementary and alternative medicine (CAM). *Geriatr Nurs.* 2009;30:196-203.
13. Ben-Arye E, Attias S, Tadmor T, Schiff E. Herbs in hemato-oncological care: an evidence-based review of data on efficacy, safety, and drug interactions. *Leuk Lymphoma.* 2010;51:1414-1423.
14. Ayers SL, Kronenfeld JJ. Delays in seeking conventional medical care and complementary and alternative medicine utilization. *Health Serv Res.* 2012;47:2081-2096.
15. Yoon SL, Grundmann O, Koepp L, Farrell L. Management of irritable bowel syndrome (IBS) in adults: conventional and complementary/alternative approaches. *Altern Med Rev.* 2011;16:134-151.
16. De Silva V, El-Metwally A, Ernst E, et al. Evidence for the efficacy of complementary and alternative medicines in the management of fibromyalgia: a systematic review. *Rheumatology.* 2010;49:1063-1068.

17. Hermann R, von Richter O. Clinical evidence of herbal drugs as perpetrators of pharmacokinetic drug interactions. *Planta Med.* 2012;78:1458-1477.
18. Chen XW, Serag ES, Sneed KB, et al. Clinical herbal interactions with conventional drugs: from molecules to maladies. *Curr Med Chem.* 2011;18:4836-4850.
19. Shi S, Klotz U. Drug interactions with herbal medicines. *Clin Pharmacokinet.* 2012;51:77-104.
20. Na DH, Ji HY, Park EJ, et al. Evaluation of metabolism-mediated herb-drug interactions. *Arch Pharm Res.* 2011;34: 1829-1842.
21. Mooiman KD, Maas-Bakker RF, Hendrikx JJ, et al. The effect of complementary and alternative medicines on CYP3A4-mediated metabolism of three different substrates: 7-benzyloxy-4-trifluoromethyl-coumarin, midazolam and docetaxel. *J Pharm Pharmacol.* 2014;66:865-874.
22. Mukherjee PK, Ponnusankar S, Pandit S, et al. Botanicals as medicinal food and their effects on drug metabolizing enzymes. *Food Chem Toxicol.* 2011;49:3142-3153.
23. Chen XW, Sneed KB, Pan SY, et al. Herb-drug interactions and mechanistic and clinical considerations. *Curr Drug Metab.* 2012;13:640-651.
24. Goey AK, Mooiman KD, Beijnen JH, et al. Relevance of in vitro and clinical data for predicting CYP3A4-mediated herb-drug interactions in cancer patients. *Cancer Treat Rev.* 2013;39:773-783.
25. Bunchorntavakul C, Reddy KR. Review article: herbal and dietary supplement hepatotoxicity. *Aliment Pharmacol Ther.* 2013;37:3-17.
26. Frazier TH, Krueger KJ. Hepatotoxic herbs: will injury mechanisms guide treatment strategies? *Curr Gastroenterol Rep.* 2009;11:317-324.
27. Shord SS, Shah K, Lukose A. Drug-botanical interactions: a review of the laboratory, animal, and human data for 8 common botanicals. *Integr Cancer Ther.* 2009;8:208-227.
28. Posadzki P, Watson LK, Ernst E. Adverse effects of herbal medicines: an overview of systematic reviews. *Clin Med.* 2013;13:7-12.
29. Ventura MT, Viola M, Calogiuri G, et al. Hypersensitivity reactions to complementary and alternative medicine products. *Curr Pharm Des.* 2006;12:3393-3399.
30. Micozzi MS. *Fundamentals of Complementary and Alternative Medicine.* 4th ed. St. Louis: Elsevier/Saunders; 2011.
31. Thomson Healthcare. *PDR for Herbal Medicine.* 4th ed. Montvale, NJ: Thompson Healthcare; 2007.
32. Skidmore-Roth L. *Mosby's Handbook of Herbal and Natural Supplements.* 4th ed. St Louis: Mosby; 2010.
33. Chen J, Lariviere WR. The nociceptive and anti-nociceptive effects of bee venom injection and therapy: a double-edged sword. *Prog Neurobiol.* 2010;92:151-183.
34. Mirshafiey A. Venom therapy in multiple sclerosis. *Neuropharmacology.* 2007;53:353-361.
35. Son DJ, Lee JW, Lee YH, et al. Therapeutic application of anti-arthritis, pain-releasing, and anti-cancer effects of bee venom and its constituent compounds. *Pharmacol Ther.* 2007;115: 246-270.
36. Schapowal A. Efficacy and safety of Echinaforce® in respiratory tract infections. *Wien Med Wochenschr.* 2013;163:102-105.
37. Nahas R, Balla A. Complementary and alternative medicine for prevention and treatment of the common cold. *Can Fam Physician.* 2011;57:31-36.
38. Woelkart K, Linde K, Bauer R. Echinacea for preventing and treating the common cold. *Planta Med.* 2008;74:633-637.
39. Huntley AL, Thompson Coon J, Ernst E. The safety of herbal medicinal products derived from Echinacea species: a systematic review. *Drug Saf.* 2005;28:387-400.
40. Khatua TN, Adela R, Banerjee SK. Garlic and cardioprotection: insights into the molecular mechanisms. *Can J Physiol Pharmacol.* 2013;91:448-458.
41. Rahman K, Lowe GM. Garlic and cardiovascular disease: a critical review. *J Nutr.* 2006;136(suppl):736S-740S.
42. Capasso A. Antioxidant action and therapeutic efficacy of Allium sativum L. *Molecules.* 2013;18:690-700.
43. Yun HM, Ban JO, Park KR, et al. Potential therapeutic effects of functionally active compounds isolated from garlic. *Pharmacol Ther.* 2014;142:183-195.
44. Ding M, Leach M, Bradley H. The effectiveness and safety of ginger for pregnancy-induced nausea and vomiting: a systematic review. *Women Birth.* 2013;26:e26-30.
45. Haniadka R, Rajeev AG, Palatty PL, et al. Zingiber officinale (ginger) as an anti-emetic in cancer chemotherapy: a review. *J Altern Complement Med.* 2012;18:440-444.
46. Palatty PL, Haniadka R, Valder B, et al. Ginger in the prevention of nausea and vomiting: a review. *Crit Rev Food Sci Nutr.* 2013;53:659-669.
47. Butt MS, Sultan MT. Ginger and its health claims: molecular aspects. *Crit Rev Food Sci Nutr.* 2011;51:383-393.
48. Grzanna R, Lindmark L, Frondoza CG. Ginger—an herbal medicinal product with broad anti-inflammatory actions. *J Med Food.* 2005;8:125-132.
49. Diamond BJ, Bailey MR. Ginkgo biloba: indications, mechanisms, and safety. *Psychiatr Clin North Am.* 2013;36:73-83.
50. Birks J, Grimley Evans J. Ginkgo biloba for cognitive impairment and dementia. *Cochrane Database Syst Rev.* 2009;1:CD003120.
51. Janssen IM, Sturtz S, Skipka G, et al. Ginkgo biloba in Alzheimer's disease: a systematic review. *Wien Med Wochenschr.* 2010;160:539-546.
52. Weinmann S, Roll S, Schwarzbach C, et al. Effects of Ginkgo biloba in dementia: systematic review and meta-analysis. *BMC Geriatr.* 2010;10:14.
53. Vellas B, Coley N, Ousset PJ, et al. Long-term use of standardised Ginkgo biloba extract for the prevention of Alzheimer's disease (GuidAge): a randomised placebo-controlled trial. *Lancet Neurol.* 2012;11:851-859.
54. Bent S, Goldberg H, Padula A, Avins AL. Spontaneous bleeding associated with ginkgo biloba: a case report and systematic review of the literature. *J Gen Intern Med.* 2005;20:657-661.
55. Kellermann AJ, Kloft C. Is there a risk of bleeding associated with standardized Ginkgo biloba extract therapy? A systematic review and meta-analysis. *Pharmacotherapy.* 2011;31: 490-502.
56. Bone KM. Potential interaction of Ginkgo biloba leaf with antiplatelet or anticoagulant drugs: what is the evidence? *Mol Nutr Food Res.* 2008;52:764-771.
57. Christensen LP. Ginsenosides chemistry, biosynthesis, analysis, and potential health effects. *Adv Food Nutr Res.* 2009;55:1-99.
58. Geng J, Dong J, Ni H, et al. Ginseng for cognition. *Cochrane Database Syst Rev.* 2010;12:CD007769.
59. Karmazyn M, Moey M, Gan XT. Therapeutic potential of ginseng in the management of cardiovascular disorders. *Drugs.* 2011;71:1989-2008.
60. Nah SY. Ginseng ginsenoside pharmacology in the nervous system: involvement in the regulation of ion channels and receptors. *Front Physiol.* 2014;5:98.

61. Jiao L, Li B, Wang M, et al. Antioxidant activities of the oligosaccharides from the roots, flowers and leaves of Panax ginseng C.A. Meyer. *Carbohydr Polym.* 2014;106:293-298.
62. Wan D, Jiao L, Yang H, Liu S. Structural characterization and immunological activities of the water-soluble oligosaccharides isolated from the Panax ginseng roots. *Planta.* 2012;235:1289-1297.
63. Kang S, Min H. Ginseng, the "immunity boost": the effects of Panax ginseng on immune system. *J Ginseng Res.* 2012;36:354-368.
64. Prabhakar PK, Doble M. Mechanism of action of natural products used in the treatment of diabetes mellitus. *Chin J Integr Med.* 2011;17:563-574.
65. Henrotin Y, Lambert C. Chondroitin and glucosamine in the management of osteoarthritis: an update. *Curr Rheumatol Rep.* 2013;15:361.
66. Henrotin Y, Lambert C, Richette P. Importance of synovitis in osteoarthritis: evidence for the use of glycosaminoglycans against synovial inflammation. *Semin Arthritis Rheum.* 2014;43:579-587.
67. Sherman AL, Ojeda-Correal G, Mena J. Use of glucosamine and chondroitin in persons with osteoarthritis. *PM R.* 2012; 4(suppl):S110-116.
68. Black C, Clar C, Henderson R, et al. The clinical effectiveness of glucosamine and chondroitin supplements in slowing or arresting progression of osteoarthritis of the knee: a systematic review and economic evaluation. *Health Technol Assess.* 2009;13:1-148.
69. Wandel S, Jüni P, Tendal B, et al. Effects of glucosamine, chondroitin, or placebo in patients with osteoarthritis of hip or knee: network meta-analysis. *BMJ.* 2010;341:c4675.
70. Bruyere O, Reginster JY. Glucosamine and chondroitin sulfate as therapeutic agents for knee and hip osteoarthritis. *Drugs Aging.* 2007;24:573-580.
71. Lakhan SE, Vieira KF. Nutritional and herbal supplements for anxiety and anxiety-related disorders: systematic review. *Nutr J.* 2010;9:42.
72. Sarris J, Kavanagh DJ. Kava and St. John's wort: current evidence for use in mood and anxiety disorders. *J Altern Complement Med.* 2009;15:827-836.
73. Rowe A, Ramzan I. Are mould hepatotoxins responsible for kava hepatotoxicity? *Phytother Res.* 2012;26:1768-1770.
74. Teschke R, Sarris J, Lebot V. Contaminant hepatotoxins as culprits for kava hepatotoxicity—fact or fiction? *Phytother Res.* 2013;27:472-474.
75. Teschke R, Wolff A. Kava hepatotoxicity: regulatory data selection and causality assessment. *Dig Liver Dis.* 2009;41:891-901.
76. Bedrosian TA, Herring KL, Walton JC, et al. Evidence for feedback control of pineal melatonin secretion. *Neurosci Lett.* 2013;542:123-125.
77. Fisher SP, Foster RG, Peirson SN. The circadian control of sleep. *Handb Exp Pharmacol.* 2013;217:157-183.
78. Lyseng-Williamson KA. Melatonin prolonged release: in the treatment of insomnia in patients aged ≥55 years. *Drugs Aging.* 2012;29:911-923.
79. Rios ER, Venâncio ET, Rocha NF, et al. Melatonin: pharmacological aspects and clinical trends. *Int J Neurosci.* 2010;120:583-590.
80. Pandi-Perumal SR, BaHammam AS, Brown GM, et al. Melatonin antioxidative defense: therapeutical implications for aging and neurodegenerative processes. *Neurotox Res.* 2013;23:267-300.
81. Cutando A, López-Valverde A, Arias-Santiago S, et al. Role of melatonin in cancer treatment. *Anticancer Res.* 2012;32:2747-2753.
82. Proietti S, Cucina A, Reiter RJ, Bizzarri M. Molecular mechanisms of melatonin's inhibitory actions on breast cancers. *Cell Mol Life Sci.* 2013;70:2139-2157.
83. Lochner A, Huisamen B, Nduhirabandi F. Cardioprotective effect of melatonin against ischaemia/reperfusion damage. *Front Biosci.* 2013;5:305-315.
84. Paulis L, Simko F, Laudon M. Cardiovascular effects of melatonin receptor agonists. *Expert Opin Investig Drugs.* 2012;21:1661-1678.
85. Guglielmo R, Martinotti G, Di Giannantonio M, Janiri L. A possible new option for migraine management: agomelatine. *Clin Neuropharmacol.* 2013;36:65-67.
86. Peschke E, Mühlbauer E. New evidence for a role of melatonin in glucose regulation. *Best Pract Res Clin Endocrinol Metab.* 2010;24:829-841.
87. Kane CJ, Raheem OA, Bent S, Avins AL. What do I tell patients about saw palmetto for benign prostatic hyperplasia? *Urol Clin North Am.* 2011;38:261-277.
88. Tacklind J, Macdonald R, Rutks I, et al. Serenoa repens for benign prostatic hyperplasia. *Cochrane Database Syst Rev.* 2012;12:CD001423.
89. MacDonald R, Tacklind JW, Rutks I, Wilt TJ. Serenoa repens monotherapy for benign prostatic hyperplasia (BPH): an updated Cochrane systematic review. *BJU Int.* 2012;109:1756-1761.
90. Bukhari IA, Dar A. Behavioral profile of Hypericum perforatum (St. John's wort) extract. A comparison with standard antidepressants in animal models of depression. *Eur Rev Med Pharmacol Sci.* 2013;17:1082-1089.
91. Butterweck V. Mechanism of action of St John's wort in depression: what is known? *CNS Drugs.* 2003;17:539-562.
92. Nahas R, Sheikh O. Complementary and alternative medicine for the treatment of major depressive disorder. *Can Fam Physician.* 2011;57:659-663.
93. Anghelescu IG, Kohnen R, Szegedi A, et al. Comparison of Hypericum extract WS 5570 and paroxetine in ongoing treatment after recovery from an episode of moderate to severe depression: results from a randomized multicenter study. *Pharmacopsychiatry.* 2006;39:213-219.
94. Linde K, Berner MM, Kriston L. St John's wort for major depression. *Cochrane Database Syst Rev.* 2008;4:CD000448.
95. Gastpar M. Hypericum extract WS ® 5570 for depression—an overview. *Int J Psychiatry Clin Pract.* 2013;17(suppl 1):1-7.
96. Madabushi R, Frank B, Drewelow B, et al. Hyperforin in St. John's wort drug interactions. *Eur J Clin Pharmacol.* 2006;62:225-233.
97. Hadley S, Petry JJ. Valerian. *Am Fam Physician.* 2003;67:1755-1758.
98. Fernández-San-Martín MI, Masa-Font R, Palacios-Soler L, et al. Effectiveness of Valerian on insomnia: a meta-analysis of randomized placebo-controlled trials. *Sleep Med.* 2010;11:505-511.
99. Salter S, Brownie S. Treating primary insomnia—the efficacy of valerian and hops. *Aust Fam Physician.* 2010;39:433-437.
100. You JS, Peng M, Shi JL, et al. Evaluation of anxiolytic activity of compound Valeriana jatamansi Jones in mice. *BMC Complement Altern Med.* 2012;12:223.

101. Binder HJ, Reuben A. Nutrient digestion and absorption. In: Boron E, Boulpaep EL, eds. *Medical Physiology*. 2nd ed. Philadelphia, PA: Elsevier/Saunders; 2012.
102. Chawla J, Kvarnberg D. Hydrosoluble vitamins. *Handb Clin Neurol.* 2014;120:891-914.
103. Chessman KH, Kumpf VJ. Assessment of nutrition status, and nutritional requirements. In: DiPiro JT, et al, eds. *Pharmacotherapy: A Pathophysiologic Approach*. 8th ed. New York: McGraw-Hill; 2011.
104. Suskind DL. Nutritional deficiencies during normal growth. *Pediatr Clin North Am.* 2009;56:1035-1053.
105. Slavin JL, Lloyd B. Health benefits of fruits and vegetables. *Adv Nutr.* 2012;3:506-516.
106. Saltzman E, Karl JP. Nutrient deficiencies after gastric bypass surgery. *Annu Rev Nutr.* 2013;33:183-203.
107. Vavricka SR, Rogler G. Intestinal absorption and vitamin levels: is a new focus needed? *Dig Dis.* 2012;30(suppl 3):73-80.
108. De-Regil LM, Fernández-Gaxiola AC, Dowswell T, Peña-Rosas JP. Effects and safety of periconceptional folate supplementation for preventing birth defects. *Cochrane Database Syst Rev.* 2010;10:CD007950.
109. Bell DA, Crooke MJ, Hay N, Glendenning P. Prolonged vitamin D intoxication: presentation, pathogenesis and progress. *Intern Med J.* 2013;43:1148-1150.
110. Rutkowski M, Grzegorczyk K. Adverse effects of antioxidative vitamins. *Int J Occup Med Environ Health.* 2012;25:105-121.

APPENDIX A

Drugs Administered by Iontophoresis and Phonophoresis

Drugs that may be administered by iontophoresis and phonophoresis are listed here. Administration of these agents by these techniques is largely empirical. The use of these substances in the conditions listed is based primarily on clinical observation and anecdotal reports in the literature. Likewise, the preparation strengths given here are merely suggestions based on currently available information.

Drug	Principal Indication(s)	Treatment Rationale	Iontophoresis	Phonophoresis
Acetic acid	Calcific tendinitis	Acetate is believed to increase solubility of calcium deposits in tendons and other soft tissues	2%–5% aqueous solution from negative pole	—
Calcium chloride	Skeletal muscle spasms	Calcium stabilizes excitable membranes; appears to decrease excitability threshold in peripheral nerves and skeletal muscle	2% aqueous solution from positive pole	—
Dexamethasone	Inflammation	Synthetic steroidal anti-inflammatory agent (see Chapter 29)	4 mg/mL in aqueous solution from negative pole	0.4% ointment
Hydrocortisone	Inflammation	Anti-inflammatory steroid (see Chapter 29)	0.5% ointment from positive pole	0.5%–1.0% ointment
Hyaluronidase	Local edema (subacute and chronic stage)	Appears to increase permeability in connective tissue by hydrolyzing hyaluronic acid, thus decreasing encapsulation and allowing disbursement of local edema	Reconstitute with 0.9% sodium chloride to provide a 150 mcg/ml solution from positive pole	—
Iodine	Adhesive capsulitis and other soft-tissue adhesions; microbial infections	Iodine is a broad-spectrum antibiotic, hence its use in infections, etc.; the sclerolytic actions of iodine are not fully understood	5%–10% solution or ointment from negative pole	10% ointment
Lidocaine	Soft-tissue pain and inflammation (e.g., bursitis, tenosynovitis)	Local anesthetic effects (see Chapter 12)	4%–5% solution or ointment from positive pole	5% ointment
Magnesium sulfate	Skeletal muscle spasms; myositis	Muscle relaxant effect may be caused by decreased excitability of the skeletal muscle membrane and decreased transmission at the neuromuscular junction	2% aqueous solution or ointment from positive pole	2% ointment
Salicylates	Muscle and joint pain in acute and chronic conditions (e.g., overuse injuries, rheumatoid arthritis)	Aspirinlike drugs with analgesic and anti-inflammatory effects (see Chapter 15)	10% trolamine salicylate ointment or 2%–3% sodium salicylate solution from negative pole	10% trolamine salicylate ointment or 3% sodium salicylate ointment
Tolazoline hydrochloride	Indolent cutaneous ulcers	Increases local blood flow and tissue healing by inhibiting vascular smooth muscle contraction	2% aqueous solution or ointment from positive pole	—
Zinc oxide	Skin ulcers; other dermatologic disorders	Zinc acts as a general antiseptic; may increase tissue healing	20% ointment from positive pole	20% ointment

APPENDIX B

Drugs of Abuse

Some of the more frequently abused drugs are listed here. Agents such as cocaine and the psychedelics are illicit drugs with no major pharmacotherapeutic value. Other drugs such as barbiturates, benzodiazepines, and opioids are used routinely for therapeutic reasons but have a strong potential for abuse when taken indiscriminately. Finally, drugs such as alcohol, caffeine, and nicotine are readily available in various commercial products but may also be considered drugs of abuse when consumed in large quantities for prolonged periods.

Drug(s)	Classification/Action	Route/Method of Administration	Effect Desired by User	Principal Adverse Effects	Additional Information
Alcohol	Sedative-hypnotic	Oral, from various beverages (wine, beer, other alcoholic drinks)	Euphoria; relaxed inhibitions; decreased anxiety; sense of escape	Physical dependence; impaired motor skills; chronic degenerative changes in the brain, liver, and other organs	See Chapter 6
Barbiturates Nembutal Seconal Others	Sedative-hypnotic	Oral or injected (IM, IV)	Relaxation and a sense of calmness; drowsiness	Physical dependence; possible death from overdose; behavior changes (irritability, psychosis) following prolonged use	See Chapter 6
Benzodiazepines Valium Librium Others	Similar to barbiturates	Similar to barbiturates	Similar to barbiturates	Similar to barbiturates	Similar to barbiturates
Caffeine	CNS stimulant	Oral; from coffee, tea, other beverages	Increased alertness; decreased fatigue; improved work capacity	Sleep disturbances; irritability; nervousness; cardiac arrhythmias	See Chapter 26
Cannabinoids Hashish Marijuana	Psychoactive drugs with mixed (stimulant and depressant) activity	Smoked; possible oral ingestion	Initial response: euphoria, excitement, increased perception; later response: relaxation, stupor, dreamlike state	Endocrine changes (decreased testosterone in males) and changes in respiratory function similar to chronic cigarette smoking are associated with heavy use	—
Cocaine	CNS stimulant (when taken systemically)	"Snorted" (absorbed via nasal mucosa); smoked (in crystalline form)	Euphoria; excitement; feelings of intense pleasure and well-being	Physical dependence; acute CNS and cardiac toxicity; profound mood swings	See Chapter 12
Narcotics Demerol Morphine Heroin Others	Natural and synthetic opioids; analgesics	Oral or injected (IM, IV)	Relaxation; euphoria; feelings of tranquility; prevent onset of opiate withdrawal	Physical dependence; respiratory depression; high potential for death due to overdose	See Chapter 14
Nicotine	CNS toxin; produces variable effects via somatic and autonomic nervous system interaction	Smoked or absorbed from tobacco products (cigarettes, cigars, chewing tobacco)	Relaxation; calming effect; decreased irritability	Physical dependence; possible carcinogen; associated with pathological changes in respiratory function during long-term tobacco use	
Psychedelics LSD Mescaline Phencyclidine (PCP) Psilocybin	Hallucinogens	Oral; may also be smoked or inhaled	Altered perception and insight; distorted senses; disinhibition	Severe hallucinations; panic reaction; acute psychotic reactions	

APPENDIX C

Answers to Case Study Questions

CHAPTER 6 CASE STUDY

Sedative-Hypnotic Drugs

1. What is the most likely reason for R.S.'s poor performance in the morning rehabilitation sessions?
   The sedative-hypnotic (flurazepam) appeared to be producing a hangover-like effect, which limited the patient's cognitive skills during the early daily activities. Flurazepam is a benzodiazepine drug with a half-life of 2.3 hours and a duration of action of 7 to 8 hours. This drug, however, is metabolized in the liver to active metabolites with half-lives ranging from 30 to 200 hours. It seems likely that R.S. was continuing to experience sedative effects from these active metabolites well into the next morning.

2. What would be the likely solution?
   The therapists can deal with this problem initially by reserving the early morning session for stretching and ROM activities and then gradually moving into upper-body strengthening. Activities that require more patient learning and comprehension can be done later in the morning or in the afternoon. The hangover-like problem should also be brought to the attention of the physician. In this case, the physician switched the hypnotic drug to zolpidem (Ambien), 10 mg administered at bedtime. Zolpidem has a half-life of 2.5 hours and a duration of action of 6 to 8 hours, so R.S. should still get the benefit of a full night's sleep. Because zolpidem is not metabolized to active metabolites, it is unlikely that it will continue to exert sedative-hypnotic effects into the next morning. Zolpidem also affects neuronal GABA receptors differently than benzodiazepines such as flurazepam. This difference might reduce the risk of problems, such as rebound insomnia, when it is time to discontinue the drug.

CHAPTER 7 CASE STUDY

Antidepressant Drugs

1. How can the therapist reduce the risk of orthostatic hypotension during rehabilitation sessions?
   To reduce orthostatic hypotension, the therapist decided to place the patient on the tilt table for the first day after imipramine was started and to monitor blood pressure regularly. The therapist had the patient perform weight shifting and upper-extremity facilitation activities while he was on the tilt table. The patient tolerated this well, so the therapist had him resume ambulation activities using the parallel bars on the following day. With the patient standing inside the bars, the therapist carefully watched for any subjective signs of dizziness or syncope in the patient (i.e., facial pallor, inability to follow instructions). Standing bouts were also limited in duration. By the third day, ambulation training

continued with the patient outside the parallel bars, but the therapist made a point of having the patient's wheelchair close at hand in case the patient began to appear faint. These precautions of careful observation and short, controlled bouts of ambulation were continued throughout the remainder of the patient's hospital stay, and the therapist observed no incident of orthostatic hypotension during physical therapy.

2. Will clinicians notice an immediate improvement in J.G.'s mood after starting this?
It is unlikely that J.G.'s mood will improve immediately when he starts taking imipramine. Antidepressants typically take at least 1 to 2 weeks to begin exerting beneficial effects and may take up to 6 weeks to reach peak effects. Moreover, clinicians should be alert for a worsening in depression or other adverse behavioral changes during the initial treatment period.

CHAPTER 8 CASE STUDY

Antipsychotic Drugs

1. Why might antipsychotic drugs cause these abnormal movements?
Antipsychotic drugs block dopamine receptors in the limbic system, but they may also decrease dopamine influence in the basal ganglia and other areas of the CNS that control movement. These abnormal movements are often classified as extrapyramidal symptoms because it appears that the drug causes changes in extrapyramidal motor pathways.

2. What specific movement disorder might be indicated by these symptoms?
Extraneous movements around the face, jaw, and tongue may indicate a specific extrapyramidal symptom called *tardive dyskinesia*.

3. Why is it critical to resolve this situation as soon as possible?
Tardive dyskinesia can be irreversible in some patients, so the therapist should notify the physician as soon as these symptoms are observed. In this case, drug therapy was progressively shifted from haloperidol to clozapine (Clozaril), 450 mg/d. Clozapine is classified as an atypical antipsychotic that is less likely to cause tardive dyskinesia than traditional agents such as haloperidol. The extrapyramidal symptoms in this patient gradually diminished over the next 8 weeks and ultimately disappeared.

CHAPTER 9 CASE STUDY

Antiepileptic Drugs

1. What factors may have precipitated F.B.'s seizure?
The seizure may have been precipitated by a number of factors, including the recent decrease in drug dosage and the fact that he was nearing the end of a dosing interval. (He had taken his last dose at lunch and would take his next dose after he went home and had dinner.) The fact that he was tired and fell asleep during the treatment probably played a role. He reported later that when seizures do occur, they tend to be when he is asleep.

2. What precautions can be taken to prevent additional seizures and guard against injuries if a seizure occurs during a rehabilitation session?
To prevent the recurrence of F.B.'s seizures during therapy, the session should be scheduled earlier in the day. In this case, his schedule was flexible enough that he could attend therapy before going to work. Also, he should take his first dose of the day approximately 1 hour before arriving at physical therapy. Other precautions that should be employed include not leaving the patient unattended in positions of risk. Treatments, for example, should be provided on a mat table or a wide, low adjustable plinth rather than a high, narrow treatment plinth from which the patient could fall during a seizure.

CHAPTER 10 CASE STUDY

Anti-Parkinson Drugs

1. What is the likely reason for the poor response to anti-Parkinson drugs on certain days?
A possible reason for the poor response on certain days is that the patient took her morning dose with a breakfast that included a large amount of protein. Levodopa is derived from an amino acid (tyrosine) and must compete with other amino acids when being absorbed from the GI tract. If there is a large amount of protein in

the patient's breakfast, the levodopa must wait until the amino acids from the dietary proteins are absorbed before the levodopa is absorbed.

2. What can be done to resolve this problem and improve the patient's response to drug therapy?
This problem might be resolved by having the patient take the morning dose with a light breakfast that contained primarily carbohydrates (levodopa can cause GI upset, so patients may not be able to take this drug on an empty stomach). Some experts recommend taking this drug with soda crackers and ginger tea (because it can settle the stomach). Levodopa medications can be taken with fruit juice, but this may not be a good option for some patients because fruit juices are typically acidic and can increase stomach upset. Patients should try to find a light meal that works best with their medications and then wait about 30 to 60 minutes before eating a larger meal. Patients should also be encouraged to take their anti-Parkinson medications at the same time each day to help provide a more consistent and predictable response to these drugs.

CHAPTER 11 CASE STUDY

General Anesthetics

1. How can the therapist safely begin rehabilitation given this patient's confusion?
It is probably not safe to attempt ambulation activities if the patient is very confused and unable to understand partial weight-bearing instructions. The therapist might limit the initial session to passive- and active-assisted exercises of both lower extremities.

2. Can any interventions help the patient overcome the residual anesthetic effects?
Active upper-extremity exercises should be encouraged within the limitations of the patient's ability to follow instructions. These exercises can help increase metabolism and excretion of the remaining anesthesia. The patient should also be placed on a program of breathing exercises in an effort to facilitate excretion of the anesthesia and to maintain respiratory function and prevent the accumulation of mucus in the airways. As the patient's mental disposition gradually improves, the therapist can initiate partial weight bearing in the parallel bars. From there, the patient can progress to a walker with a goal of independent ambulation using the device.

CHAPTER 12 CASE STUDY

Local Anesthetics

1. What should the therapist tell this patient about applying heat over the lidocaine patch?
The therapist should state emphatically that heat should never be applied on or near the lidocaine patch. The patient must be informed that heat will enhance lidocaine absorption through the skin, and that lidocaine absorption into the systemic circulation can produce serious adverse effects on the heart and CNS.

2. What are the typical recommendations for applying and changing the patch?
The therapist can also remind the patient that lidocaine patches should only be applied to intact and unbroken skin and that patches are typically worn for no more than 12 hours each day. The therapist should, of course, encourage the patient to contact her physician with any remaining questions about the use of this patch.

CHAPTER 13 CASE STUDY

Muscle Relaxants

1. How does baclofen work, and why does oral baclofen affect F.D.'s nonspastic muscles?
Baclofen mimics the effects of GABA, an inhibitory neurotransmitter in the CNS. This effect is helpful in people with spasticity because baclofen can reduce neuronal activity of spinal neurons that supply the spastic muscles. Oral administration of this drug, however, does not discriminate between neurons affecting spastic and nonspastic muscles—that is, the drug will reach the spinal cord through the systemic circulation and inhibit neurons that innervate F.D.'s arms and upper trunk as well as the neurons that affect the spastic muscles in his lower extremities. Oral baclofen will also reach the brain, resulting in sedation and cognitive impairment, especially at higher doses.

2. Is there an alternative way to administer this drug to better focus its effects on the spastic

lower extremity muscles with less effect on F.D.'s trunk and upper extremities?
Intrathecal administration is an alternative way to administer baclofen. The intrathecal route places the drug into subarachnoid space between the middle (arachnoid) and inner (pia mater) meningeal layers surrounding the spinal cord. The drug is therefore delivered more directly to the area around a specific spinal cord level rather than into the systemic circulation where it will ultimately reach all tissues in the body, including the entire spinal cord and brain. Intrathecal baclofen can potentially reduce spasticity more selectively with fewer side effects, such as sedation and reduced strength in nonspastic muscles.

3. How can the therapist address alternative administration methods with the physician and patient?
The therapist should confer with the physician and discuss the decreased voluntary muscle power and potential loss of function ability that is likely to occur with an increase in the oral baclofen dose. Intrathecal baclofen can then be addressed as an alternative treatment. If intrathecal baclofen is feasible, the physician and therapist should discuss this procedure with the patient and explain that a trial injection is typically used to assess efficacy before a pump and catheter is implanted surgically to deliver the drug into the subarachnoid space. In F.D.'s case, he agreed to an intrathecal baclofen trial, and he ultimately received a baclofen pump that was implanted into his lower left abdomen; the drug was delivered via a small catheter into the subarachnoid space at the second lumbar vertebral level. The initial infusion rate was 150 mcg/day, and this dose was gradually increased to 600 mcg/day to achieve optimal antispasticity effects with minimal effects on nonspastic muscles and cognition.

CHAPTER 14 CASE STUDY

Opioid Analgesics

1. When should the therapist schedule the treatment session so that meperidine is reaching peak effects?
The therapist should try to treat this patient approximately 1 hour following administration of the drug. Meperidine typically reaches peak effects 60 minutes after oral administration and has a 2- to 4-hour duration of action. Scheduling the initial treatment sessions about an hour after administration will take advantage of the drug's peak effects while still providing adequate analgesic effects for a few hours after the treatment.

2. What precautions should the therapist use during the initial treatments given the potential side effects of this drug?
Precautions should focus on meperidine's effects on balance, sedation, hypotension, and respiratory depression. If possible, the initial session should be scheduled at the patient's bedside because the patient will still be woozy from the combined effects of the anesthesia and the opioid analgesia. If treatment is provided in the physical therapy department, it might be best to transport the patient on a stretcher to prevent an episode of dizziness brought on directly by the drug's effects on vestibular function or indirectly by orthostatic hypotension. The therapist should likewise watch for signs of respiratory depression, including decreased respiratory rate, difficult/labored breathing (dyspnea), and bluish color of the skin and mucous membranes (cyanosis). Ideally, hemoglobin saturation should be monitored continuously with a pulse oximeter, and excessive respiratory depression should be reported to the medical staff immediately.

CHAPTER 15 CASE STUDY

Nonsteroidal Anti-Inflammatory Drugs

1. How does acetaminophen differ from NSAIDs such as aspirin and ibuprofen, and why is this difference important in this case?
Aspirin, ibuprofen, and other NSAIDs decrease pain and inflammation, decrease fever (antipyresis), and inhibit platelet activity (anticoagulant effect). Acetaminophen only has analgesic and antipyretic effects, and it lacks significant anti-inflammatory or anticoagulant effects. In this case, the patient would probably benefit from the dual effects of analgesia and anti-inflammation that is provided by aspirin, ibuprofen, and other over-the-counter NSAIDs such as ketoprofen and naproxen.

2. What should the therapist tell D.B. about taking over-the-counter pain medications?
The therapist should explain the difference between NSAIDs and acetaminophen to the patient,

and point out that acetaminophen lacks any significant anti-inflammatory effects. The therapist must also consult with the patient's physician to confirm that an NSAID was recommended. If the patient was advised to take an over-the-counter NSAID, the therapist should remind him to take the recommended dose at regular intervals to help decrease the inflammation in the bursa and to provide analgesia. Finally, the therapist should caution the patient to contact his physician if any adverse effects are noted, including GI distress and allergic reactions.

CHAPTER 16 CASE STUDY

Rheumatoid Arthritis

1. What is causing the skin changes and muscle wasting?
   Prednisone is likely causing A.T.'s muscle wasting and skin changes. This drug is a glucocorticoid, and a primary side effect of these drugs is that they break down proteins such as collagen in muscle, skin, bone, and other tissues to liberate amino acids, which are transported to the liver and transformed into glucose. Hence, her skin and skeletal muscles clearly showed evidence of wasting due to this protein catabolism. Because of her arthritic changes, A.T. has not been very active physically, so the catabolic effects of this drug combined with her rather sedentary lifestyle have also contributed to her substantial muscle loss. It is likely she has also lost considerable bone density, a fact that could be confirmed by specific bone densitometry techniques.

2. What might be an alternative drug strategy to modify disease progression in rheumatoid arthritis?
   An alternative strategy involves drugs such as etanercept (Enbrel) or adalimumab (Humira), which inhibit a specific inflammatory mediator in rheumatoid arthritis known as *tumor necrosis factor*. Whereas glucocorticoids such as prednisone inhibit virtually all aspects of the inflammatory response, tumor necrosis factor inhibitors provide a much more specific inhibition of the autoimmune response underlying rheumatoid arthritis. Moreover, these drugs do not typically cause the catabolic effects associated with glucocorticoids, so skin, muscle, bone, and other joint tissues are not adversely affected.

3. What can the therapist do to try to offset the general loss of muscle mass and strength?
   A gradual strengthening and ambulation program may help restore some muscle strength, muscle mass, and bone mineral density. The therapist should, of course, design this program according to A.T.'s current level of strength and function, and progress the program very carefully to avoid further damage to her weakened skin and musculoskeletal structures. An aquatic program, for example, might be a logical starting point, with the intention to transition to land-based activities as her strength improves and her arthritis is controlled by her drug regimen.

CHAPTER 17 CASE STUDY

Patient-Controlled Analgesia

1. How can PCA cause respiratory problems?
   The PCA was delivering an opioid (meperidine), and excessive doses of these drugs are notorious for decreasing the rate and depth of breathing. Opioids decrease respiratory drive at the brainstem level, and a larger increase in plasma CO_2 or decrease in plasma O_2 is needed to increase respiration. At high doses, these drugs essentially shut down the respiratory control center in the brainstem, and this effect is usually the cause of death in opioid overdose.

2. What are some possible reasons for the apparent overdose observed in this case?
   One possible reason for this overdose is that the PCA device was programmed incorrectly, or the pump simply malfunctioned and administered more drug than intended. Fortunately, most of the modern PCA pumps have protocols and safety features that reduce the risk of incorrect programming or will sound alarms if the pump has a mechanical malfunction. A second reason is that the pump is being activated by someone other than the patient, especially without the patient's knowledge or if the patient is asleep. This unauthorized activation by someone else is often called PCA by proxy, as opposed to the authorized activation by a nurse or caregiver. In S.G.'s case, family members had been activating the pump while he was asleep because they did not want him to wake up in pain. Even though the pump was programmed correctly, the doses were

administered repeatedly as soon as each lockout period ended. The high doses sedated this patient so that he remained asleep and immobile, which reduced drug clearance and allowed the opioid to accumulate in his bloodstream. The nurses admonished the family; they had been instructed to not activate the PCA but had evidently decided they were acting in the patient's best interest. PCA was later resumed according to the original dosing parameters, with clear instructions to family members to not activate the PCA. The remainder of the patient's recovery was uneventful, and he was able to participate actively and enthusiastically in the rehabilitation sessions.

CHAPTER 21 CASE STUDY

Hypertension

1. How would the combination of the drug regimen and the vasodilation caused by the therapeutic pool affect H.C.'s cardiovascular system?
   Because H.C. was taking a vasodilating drug (hydralazine), the additive effect of the warm pool and vasodilating agent might cause profound hypotension because of a dramatic decrease in total peripheral resistance. Also, because this patient was taking a cardioselective beta blocker (metoprolol), his heart would not be able to sufficiently increase cardiac output to offset the decreased peripheral resistance.
2. What precautions should the therapist take to avoid adverse cardiovascular changes during the pool interventions?
   When the patient is in the pool, the therapist should monitor heart rate and blood pressure at frequent, regular intervals. In this case, H.C.'s blood pressure did decrease when he was ambulating in the pool, but not to a point of concern because his active leg muscle contractions facilitated venous return, and the buoyancy of the water decreased the effects of gravity on venous pooling in the lower extremities. In fact, only at the end of the rehabilitation session, when the patient came out of the pool, did hypotension became a potential problem. H.C. was still experiencing peripheral vasodilation because of the residual effects of the warm water, but he no longer had the advantage of active muscle contractions and water buoyancy to help maintain his blood pressure.

   To prevent a hypotensive episode in a patient like H.C. at the end of the session, the therapist would place the patient supine on a stretcher as soon as he comes out of the water. Also, the patient's legs would be quickly toweled dry, and vascular support stockings could be placed on the patient's legs. In this case, these precautions allowed H.C. to progress rapidly through his rehabilitation without any adverse incidents. When he was eventually discharged from the hospital, he was ambulating with crutches, with partial weight bearing on the side of the pelvic fracture.

CHAPTER 22 CASE STUDY

Antianginal Drugs

1. What immediate action should the therapist take to help this patient during an angina attack?
   The therapist should immediately contact the nursing floor and request that the patient's medication be rushed to the physical therapy department. While waiting for the nitroglycerin to arrive, the patient's vital signs should be monitored while he is placed in a supine position on a mat table. When the nitroglycerin is brought to the patient, the patient or nurse should administer the drug sublingually while the patient remains supine. If his chest pain does not subside after 5 minutes, the patient or nurse should administer a second tablet sublingually. If angina is still present after 5 more minutes (10 minutes after the first tablet), a third sublingual tablet can be administered. If the angina attack has not subsided 5 minutes after the third tablet, the patient may be having a heart attack, and the therapist should call for emergency medical care.
2. Why did T.M. experience angina before even beginning any exercises or other rehabilitation regimens?
   Evidently, merely being transported to the physical therapy department caused this patient sufficient concern and apprehension to trigger an angina attack. The fact that his medication was not readily available created a rather anxious situation, which accentuated the angina.
3. What can be done to prevent similar situations in the future?
   To prevent a repeat of this predicament, the therapist should contact the nursing staff and request that the patient always bring his medication with

him to physical therapy. If the patient experiences angina in the future, he should be placed immediately in a supine position, and he should administer the drug sublingually. Placing the patient supine will help prevent any orthostatic hypotension that may occur with nitroglycerin. In this case, the patient was eventually fitted with a temporary prosthesis and transferred to an extended-care facility to continue rehabilitation.

CHAPTER 23 CASE STUDY

Antiarrhythmic Drugs

1. Can M.R.'s current drug regimen be contributing to the bronchoconstrictive symptoms?
Propranolol is a nonselective beta blocker, meaning that this drug will affect beta-1 receptors on the heart as well as beta-2 receptors on bronchial smooth muscle. Blockade of myocardial beta-1 receptors will be helpful in reducing his supraventricular arrhythmias. Simultaneous blockade of respiratory beta-2 receptors, however, will facilitate bronchoconstriction in patients with diseases such as emphysema, asthma, and chronic bronchitis. Likewise, bronchoconstriction may not be obvious when he is at rest but will be exacerbated as he begins to exercise.

2. What potential change in drug therapy might reduce the risk of bronchoconstriction?
A switch to a more cardioselective beta blocker, such as esmolol or metoprolol, might reduce the risk of bronchoconstriction while still effectively treating his arrhythmias. In this case, the therapist should document the patient's symptoms and perform pulmonary function tests to quantify bronchoconstriction during the exercise bout. This information can then be given to the physician, who will ultimately make the decision about whether to switch to a more cardioselective drug or consider a different type of antiarrhythmic intervention.

CHAPTER 24 CASE STUDY

Congestive Heart Failure

1. Could D.S.'s drug regimen be contributing to her current symptoms?
The therapist realized that the patient was still taking digitalis for the treatment of heart failure and that these symptoms were consistent with digitalis toxicity.

2. Why did the symptoms probably begin to emerge at this point in time?
Apparently, the stroke had sufficiently altered the metabolism and excretion of the digitalis so that the therapeutic dosage was now accumulating in the patient's body. The altered pharmacokinetic profile was probably caused in part by the decrease in the patient's mobility and level of activity that occurred after the stroke.

3. What should the therapist do?
The therapist should notify the physician immediately about the change in the patient's status. In D.S.'s case, she was admitted to the hospital, where a blood test confirmed the presence of digitalis toxicity (i.e., blood levels of digitalis were well above the therapeutic range). The digitalis dosage was reduced, and a diuretic was added to manage the congestive heart failure. The patient was soon discharged from the hospital and resumed physical therapy at home. Her rehabilitation progressed without further incident.

CHAPTER 25 CASE STUDY

Clotting Disorders

1. What effect would the drugs administered to resolve the thromboembolic episode have on this patient's physical rehabilitation?
The drugs used to resolve the thromboembolic episode greatly facilitated the patient's recovery. The use of a thrombolytic agent (alteplase) enabled the patient to resume her normal course of rehabilitation within 2 days of the pulmonary embolism. Thus, the use of these drugs directly facilitated physical therapy and occupational therapy by allowing the patient to resume therapy much sooner than if the embolism had been treated more conservatively (i.e., rest and anticoagulants) or more radically (i.e., surgery).

2. What precautions should be considered when this patient is administered thrombolytic and anticoagulant drugs?
Blood pressure should be assessed regularly, especially for the first few days after thrombolytic (alteplase) treatment. In cases where the

patient, such as C.W., remains on anticoagulant drugs (heparin, warfarin) for an extended period of time, the therapists dealing with the patient should look for signs of excessive bleeding such as skin bruising, nosebleeds, bleeding gums, and hematuria. Physical interventions that could increase bleeding, such as chest percussion, joint mobilization, application of local heat, and wound care, must be used cautiously. In C.W.'s case, she remained free from any further thromboembolic episodes and was eventually discharged to an extended-care rehabilitation facility to continue her progress.

CHAPTER 26 CASE STUDY

Respiratory Drugs

1. What additional physical interventions can be used to complement drug therapy?
   In addition to the neuromuscular facilitation activities, the physical therapist should consider a program of chest physical therapy, including postural drainage and deep-breathing exercises.
2. When should these physical interventions be administered to take optimal advantage of the effects of the pulmonary drugs?
   Chest physical therapy techniques should ideally be administered when drugs are reaching peak effects. For example, physical therapy interventions can be coordinated with the respiratory therapy treatments so that the patient receives a treatment of the mucolytic agent (acetylcysteine) 5 to 10 minutes before beginning chest physical therapy. Also, the physical therapist can have the patient self-administer a dose of the inhaled beta-2 bronchodilator approximately 1 hour prior to the chest therapy session, thus allowing the bronchodilator to produce maximal airway dilation and permit optimal clearance of bronchial secretions. In this case, the therapist implemented these additional physical interventions, and V.C. was able to make considerable progress toward motor recovery without any further respiratory problems before being discharged to an extended care facility.

CHAPTER 27 CASE STUDY

Gastrointestinal Drugs

1. How is M.B.'s current behavior contributing to his constipation?
   This patient is taking two nonprescription products that can cause constipation. The antacid product contains aluminum, which often causes constipation, and magnesium, which tends to cause diarrhea. Although these two effects often balance out, the constipating effect may be more predominate in this patient. Likewise, ibuprofen may cause constipation in some people because this drug inhibits prostaglandins that regulate GI motility. It is likely that his poor diet and lack of exercise are also contributing to reduced GI motility and constipation.
2. What advice should the therapist provide to reduce the chance of constipation and exacerbation of back pain?
   The physical therapist should consult with the patient's physician and discuss whether a brief trial with a bulk-forming laxative might be helpful during the acute episode of back pain. The therapist should also explain to the patient that straining during defecation exacerbated his back problems. In this case, M.B.'s physician recommended that he take a bulk-forming laxative to avoid constipation and straining while he was being treated for his acute back pain. His back pain improved substantially, and no additional exacerbations occurred due to straining during bowel movements. The therapist should warn the patient, however, that laxative dependence can occur during chronic use. To prevent the recurrence of this problem, he should be encouraged to ingest a high-fiber diet and adequate amounts of water to prevent constipation. Regular exercise can likewise improve GI function and can be incorporated into a regimen designed to manage his back pain. Finally, the patient should be advised that frequent or long-term use of antacid products is not typically beneficial; the patient should consult his or her physician for more effective pharmacological methods of treating and preventing gastric hyperacidity.

CHAPTER 29 CASE STUDY

Adrenocorticosteroids

1. What possible negative effects can glucocorticoids have on joint tissues?
Glucocorticoids can weaken ligaments, tendons, and other supporting structures because of an inhibitory effect on collagen formation. This catabolic effect can be substantial after intra-articular injection because the drug is localized within the joint.
2. How long can the effects of a single injection affect E.M.'s joints?
Glucocorticoids are highly lipid soluble and can therefore be retained locally within fat and other intra- and peri-articular joint tissues. Consequently, even a single glucocorticoid injection can continue to exert a catabolic effect on knee joint structures for some time.
3. How can the therapist increase joint movement without causing injury to the joint?
The therapist should administer low-intensity, prolonged-duration stretching forces that are adequate to reduce knee flexion contractures without causing injury to the weakened knee muscles, tendons, and ligaments. Extra caution should be used during the initial stretching session, at least until the therapist gets a sense of how much the patient's knees are affected by the glucocorticoid injection. Physical agents, massage, and other manual techniques should also be administered as needed to help achieve full active and passive knee extension. The patient will hopefully be able to begin a gradual strengthening program as the drugs exert their anti-inflammatory effects. Strengthening the muscles around the knee will help offset some of the catabolic effects on musculotendinous tissues, thus further reducing the chance of injury to these tissues.

CHAPTER 30 CASE STUDY

Male and Female Hormones

1. What concerns should the therapist have about this patient's recent symptoms?
Because the patient is taking an oral contraceptive and is also a cigarette smoker, the therapist should be concerned that she might have deep vein thrombosis (DVT). The tenderness, swelling, and cramping in the patient's calf certainly support this concern. Her increased headache might be unrelated, but might also be caused by elevated blood pressure that resulted from the combined effects of the contraceptive and cigarette smoking.
2. What should the therapist do about these concerns?
The therapist should immediately contact the patient's physician and explain the concern about a possible DVT. Blood pressure and pulse should also be monitored and reported to the physician. In S.K.'s case, she was referred immediately to the local hospital for further evaluation. Venous plethysmography revealed a large DVT that began in the calf but extended proximally into the popliteal vein. She was admitted to the hospital to begin anticoagulant therapy.
3. What additional medical interventions might be considered in this case?
In S.K.'s case, she was placed immediately on a low-molecular-weight heparin (enoxaparin), which was administered by subcutaneous injection (see Chapter 25). She also wore graduated compression stockings to reduce the risk of further thromboembolic disease. The oral contraceptive medication was discontinued, and she was counseled on strategies to quit smoking. The patient was eventually discharged to her home with instructions for continuing the subcutaneous heparin. After approximately 10 days, an oral anticoagulant (warfarin) was substituted for the heparin. She resumed physical therapy as an outpatient, where her neck problem was ultimately resolved without further incident.

CHAPTER 31 CASE STUDY

Agents Affecting Bone Mineral Metabolism

1. Which physical agent might help stimulate vitamin D production in this patient?
Ultraviolet radiation could help stimulate the production of endogenous vitamin D in this patient.

2. How can this physical agent affect bone metabolism?
Ultraviolet light catalyzes the conversion of a cholesterol-like precursor (7-dehydrocholesterol) to vitamin D_3 within the skin. Vitamin D_3 then undergoes conversion in the kidneys and other tissues to form specific vitamin D metabolites (i.e., 1,25-dihydroxyvitamin D), which enhances intestinal calcium absorption.

3. How can the therapist incorporate the physical agent into the comprehensive treatment for this patient?
The therapist should confer with the physician about the possibility of ultraviolet treatments for this patient. If indicated, the therapist can incorporate a program of therapeutic ultraviolet radiation into the treatment regimen. The appropriate dose of ultraviolet exposure must first be determined, followed by daily application of whole-body irradiation. In the case of this patient, ultraviolet therapy was continued throughout the remainder of the patient's hospitalization, and callus formation at the fracture site was progressing well at the time of discharge.

CHAPTER 32 CASE STUDY

Diabetes Mellitus

1. What instructions should the therapist give W.S. about monitoring and adjusting her blood glucose levels?
The therapist should remind the athlete to monitor her blood glucose levels before and after each practice session and to adjust her insulin dosage accordingly. During some of the initial practice sessions, blood glucose should also be monitored during practice to ensure that insulin dosages are adequate.

2. What precautions should the therapist have in place during practices?
On practice days, insulin should be injected into abdominal sites rather than around exercising muscles (thighs), in order to prevent the insulin from being absorbed too rapidly from the injection site. The therapist should also remind the athlete to eat a light meal before each practice and to be sure to eat again afterward. The therapist should maintain a supply of glucose tablets and fruit juice on the practice field. The athlete must be questioned periodically to look for early signs of hypoglycemia (confusion, nausea, etc.), and ingestion of carbohydrates should be encouraged whenever appropriate.

3. How can the therapist help guard against any problems that might arise after practice?
The therapist should assign a teammate to check on the athlete within an hour after practice to ensure that no delayed effects of hypoglycemia were apparent. In this case, these precautions enabled the athlete to successfully complete preseason training and compete for the entire soccer season without any serious incident.

CHAPTER 33 CASE STUDY

Antibacterial Drugs

1. Why should the therapist be concerned about the effects of ciprofloxacin on P.M.'s Achilles tendon?
The therapist should be concerned because ciprofloxacin and other fluoroquinolone antibacterials can cause tendinopathy and possible tendon rupture. The risk of tendon damage is likewise increased in this patient because she has a history of Achilles pain, and she has been increasing her training and stress on the tendon. Although she is not currently taking the drug (her prescription ended several days previously), the residual effects could still increase her risk of tendinopathy.

2. What should the therapist do in this situation?
The therapist should protect the tendon by placing the left ankle in a walking boot and having the patient use crutches with partial weight bearing on the left leg. Weight bearing should be increased gradually as tendon pain decreases, with the patient progressing to only one crutch on the right side and finally to no crutches while wearing the boot. A program of gentle stretching and strengthening should be initiated as tendon pain decreases, with the program gradually increasing to include more weight bearing and functional activities, and finally a return to running. In this patient's case, she was able to resume running after 10 weeks of rehabilitation and gradually returned to her former weekly training regimen.

CHAPTER 34 CASE STUDY

Antiviral Drugs

1. How can the therapist intervene to reduce R.K.'s pain and improve his functional ability?
   The therapist can initiate a program of transcutaneous electrical nerve stimulation (TENS) along the affected nerve pathways. The patient should be instructed in the use of the TENS unit, and intensity and other stimulation parameters can be adjusted to the patient's tolerance. The therapist should also consider other physical agents; cold neon laser, for example, may help decrease pain and increase function along the more severely affected nerves. An assistive device such as a cane, crutches, or a walker may be needed to improve safety during ambulation and reduce the risk of a fall. Strengthening exercises should be performed as tolerated to help maintain as much strength and function as possible. In this patient, the combination of physical agents (TENS, laser) and exercises helped to temporarily decrease pain and maintain function, thus improving his well-being without the use of additional pharmacological agents (pain medications).
2. Given this patient's lack of adherence to anti-HIV drugs, what is the likely outcome in this case?
   Because this patient failed to adhere carefully to the anti-HIV drug regimen, the virus reduced his lymphocyte function to a point where his immune system was unable to deal with opportunistic infections that caused severe respiratory involvement. Likewise, peripheral neuropathies progressed until he was severely debilitated and unable to ambulate or participate in other functional activities. Unfortunately, he continued to decline and ultimately died because of respiratory failure.

CHAPTER 35 CASE STUDY

Antifungal Drugs

1. What additional instructions can the therapist give the athlete about administering the antifungal agent?
   The physical therapist should make sure that the athlete is applying the antifungal medication twice each day as directed. He should also remind the athlete to continue to apply the medication for the full 4 weeks and not stop application even though the infection might appear to be resolved. The therapist should also instruct the athlete in proper skin hygiene, such as thoroughly washing and drying his feet and wearing clean socks at each practice and game.
2. What can the therapist do to reduce the chance of teammates getting this infection?
   The physical therapist should have the locker room floors and shower areas thoroughly disinfected to prevent transmission of the fungus to other team members. Athletes can likewise be encouraged to wear shower sandals rather than walk barefoot through the locker room and shower areas. In this case, the tinea pedis infection was isolated to one athlete and was resolved without further incident.

CHAPTER 36 CASE STUDY

Cancer Chemotherapy

1. Why does R.K.'s drug regimen contribute to her GI problems?
   Anticancer drugs impair cell division in cancerous cells, but many of these drugs also affect the growth and function of normal cells, especially the cells lining the GI tract. Hence, GI problems are very common with drugs like doxorubicin and other anticancer drugs. In addition, opioids and aspirin can also cause nausea and GI upset. This patient's GI problems are therefore likely caused by the analgesic drugs or by the combination of the analgesics and the anticancer antimetabolite.
2. How might the therapist intervene to help decrease the patient's pain and reduce the need for analgesic medications?
   The therapist should consider a program of local heat (hot packs) and TENS to help control pain in the lumbosacral region. This approach can provide a nonpharmacological means of alleviating pain, thereby decreasing the patient's analgesic drug requirements and related GI problems. In this patient's case, she was able to actively participate in a rehabilitation program throughout the course of her hospitalization, thus maintaining her overall strength and physical condition.

CHAPTER 37 CASE STUDY

Immunomodulating Agents

1. What interventions can the therapist administer to help offset the catabolic effects of the glucocorticoids?
   The therapist should be aware that a program of strengthening and weight-bearing exercise can help offset the breakdown of muscle and bone that can often occur with prolonged glucocorticoid administration. The therapist should therefore begin gentle resistance exercises in the ICU as soon as the patient is alert and can follow basic instructions. Strengthening exercises can be progressively increased using manual resistance, and various weights and exercise machines should be incorporated into the strengthening regimen as tolerated by the patient. The therapist should also initiate weight-bearing activities as soon as the patient is able to tolerate standing. The patient should progressively walk longer distances on level surfaces and begin to climb stairs as tolerated.
2. How can the initial rehabilitation sessions transition to a long-term exercise program for this patient?
   The therapist should work closely with the patient and the patient's family to make sure that strengthening exercises and a progressive ambulation program are continued at home. Daily walks should be encouraged, and a supervised strength-training program can be continued at a local health club or YMCA. In this case, the patient did not experience any problems related to tissue rejection, and he was able to resume his musical career and maintain an active lifestyle.

CHAPTER 38 CASE STUDY

Complementary and Alternative Medications

1. What should the therapist do to resolve concerns about the interaction of St. John's wort and warfarin?
   The therapist should contact the physician and relate the fact that the patient had recently started taking St. John's wort. The therapist can also be more vigilant for signs of thrombosis (tender, red, swollen lower extremities) and pulmonary embolism (shortness of breath, labored breathing).
2. What additional monitoring might be helpful to assess whether warfarin is still effective?
   To get an indication of warfarin efficacy, the physician can order blood tests to assess the patient's clotting times. In this patient, these tests revealed that clotting times were indeed slightly decreased, indicating that the blood was clotting too rapidly and that the dose of warfarin needed to be increased. The dose of warfarin was adjusted accordingly, and clotting time was monitored periodically to ensure that the new dose was appropriate. The patient recovered from the surgery without any further thrombotic events.

Glossary

Common terms related to pharmacology and a brief definition of each term are listed here. Synonyms (SYN), antonyms (ANT), and common abbreviations are also included, whenever applicable.

Acetylcholine: A neurotransmitter in the somatic and autonomic nervous systems; principal synapses using acetylcholine include the skeletal neuromuscular junction, autonomic ganglia, and certain pathways in the brain.

Adenylate cyclase: An enzyme located on the inner surface of many cell membranes; it is important in mediating biochemical changes in the cell in response to drug and hormone stimulation (SYN: adenyl cyclase).

Adrenergic: Refers to synapses or physiological responses involving epinephrine and norepinephrine.

Adrenocorticosteroids: The group of steroid hormones produced by the adrenal cortex. These drugs include the glucocorticoids (cortisol, cortisone), mineralocorticoids (aldosterone), and sex hormones (androgens, estrogens, progestins).

Affinity: The mutual attraction between a drug and a specific cellular receptor.

Agonist: A drug that binds to a receptor and causes some change in cell function (ANT: antagonist).

Akathisia: A feeling of extreme motor restlessness and an inability to sit still; may occur because of antipsychotic drug therapy.

Aldosterone: A steroid (mineralocorticoid) hormone produced by the adrenal cortex that acts on the kidney to increase sodium reabsorption, thereby retaining sodium in the body.

Allergy: A state of hypersensitivity to foreign substances (e.g., environmental antigens and certain drugs), manifested by an exaggerated response of the immune system.

Allosteric modulators: Substances that bind to a cell receptor and alter the receptor's affinity for specific drugs; common allosteric modulators include guanine nucleotides, ammonium ions, calcium, and other divalent cations.

Alpha receptors: A primary class of receptors that are responsive to epinephrine and norepinephrine. Alpha receptors are subclassified into alpha-1 and alpha-2 receptors based on their sensitivity to various drugs.

Amylin: A hormone released with insulin from pancreatic beta cells that helps suppress a rise in blood glucose by inhibiting glucagon release, delaying gastric emptying, and reducing food intake by increasing feelings of fullness.

Anabolic steroids: Natural and synthetic male hormones that may be misused in an attempt to increase muscle size and improve athletic performance (SYN: androgens).

Analgesia: To lessen or relieve pain. Drugs with this ability are known as *analgesics.*

Androgen: A male steroid such as testosterone.

Angina pectoris: Severe pain and constriction in the chest region, usually associated with myocardial ischemia.

Angiogenesis: The development of new blood vessels. Drugs that inhibit this effect can be useful in limiting the growth and proliferation of certain tumors.

Antagonist: A drug that binds to a receptor but does not cause a change in cell activity (SYN: blocker).

Anthelmintics: Drugs that destroy parasitic worms (e.g., tapeworms, roundworms) in the GI tract and elsewhere in the body.

Anticholinergics: Drugs that decrease activity at acetylcholine synapses. These agents are often used to diminish activity in the parasympathetic nervous system (SYN: parasympatholytic).

Anticoagulation: A decrease in the blood's capacity to coagulate (clot). Drugs with the ability to decrease coagulation are known as *anticoagulants*.

Antimetabolite: The general term for drugs that impair function in harmful cells and microorganisms by antagonizing or replacing normal metabolic substrates in those cells. Certain anti-infectious and antineoplastic agents function as antimetabolites.

Antineoplastic: A drug that prevents or attenuates the growth and proliferation of cancerous cells.

Antipyresis: The reduction of fever. Drugs with the ability to reduce fevers are known as *antipyretics*.

Antitussive: A drug that reduces coughing.

Aromatase: An enzyme responsible for estrogen biosynthesis.

Arrhythmia: A significant deviation from normal cardiac rhythm that results in a heart rate that is slower or faster than normal, or irregular (SYN: dysrhythmia).

Asthma: A chronic disease of the respiratory system characterized by bronchoconstriction, airway inflammation, and the formation of mucous plugs in the airway.

Bactericidal: An agent that kills or destroys bacteria.

Bacteriostatic: An agent that inhibits the growth and proliferation of bacteria.

Beta lactamase: An enzyme produced by certain bacteria that destroys antibacterial drugs, such as the penicillins and carbapenems. Drugs that inhibit this enzyme are known as *beta-lactamase inhibitors*, and these drugs can be administered to treat resistant bacteria that produce this enzyme.

Beta-receptor: A primary class of the receptors that are responsive to epinephrine and (to a lesser extent) norepinephrine. Beta receptors are subclassified into beta-1 and beta-2 receptors based on their sensitivity to various drugs.

Bioavailability: The extent to which a drug reaches the systemic circulation following administration by various routes.

Biotransformation: Biochemical changes that occur to the drug within the body, usually resulting in the breakdown and inactivation of the drug (SYN: drug metabolism).

Bipolar disorder: A psychological disorder characterized by mood swings ranging from excitable (manic) periods to periods of depression (SYN: manic-depression).

Bisphosphonate: A drug that promotes calcium deposition in bone and stabilizes bone by preventing excessive bone turnover and breakdown (SYN: diphosphonate).

Blood-brain barrier: The specialized anatomic arrangement of cerebral capillary walls that serves to restrict the passage of some drugs into the brain.

Blood dyscrasia: A pathological condition of the blood, usually referring to a defect in one or more of the blood's cellular elements.

Brain derived neurotrophic factor (BDNF): A protein produced in the brain that helps sustain neuronal activity and growth; BDNF may be important in mediating the effects of antidepressants and other CNS drugs.

Buccal: Referring to the cheek. Drugs administered buccally are placed between the cheek and gum and are absorbed into the circulation from the mucosa lining the gums and inner cheek.

Carcinogens: Substances that cause cancer or increase the risk of developing cancer.

Catecholamine: A group of chemically similar compounds that are important in the modulation of cardiovascular activity and many other physiological functions. Common catecholamines include epinephrine, norepinephrine, and dopamine.

Catechol-O-methyltransferase (COMT): An enzyme that degrades levodopa to an inactive metabolite in the bloodstream and other tissues. Drugs that inhibit this enzyme are known as *COMT inhibitors*, and these drugs can protect levodopa so that it is not degraded prematurely in patients with Parkinson disease.

Cathartic: An agent that causes a relatively rapid evacuation of the bowels.

Ceiling effect: The point at which no further increase in response occurs as a drug dose is progressively increased; this effect is represented by a plateau on the drug's dose-response curve (SYN: maximal efficacy).

Chemical name: A drug name that is derived from the specific chemical structure of the compound. Chemical names are not used clinically but are shortened in some way to form the drug's generic name.

Chemotherapy: The use of chemical agents to treat infectious or neoplastic disease.

Cholinergic: Refers to synapses or physiological responses involving acetylcholine.

Cholinesterase: The enzyme that breaks down acetylcholine (SYN: acetylcholinesterase).

Clearance: The process by which the active form of the drug is removed from the bloodstream by either metabolism or excretion.

Congestive heart failure: A clinical syndrome of cardiac disease that is marked by decreased myocardial contractility, peripheral edema, shortness of breath, and decreased tolerance for physical exertion.

Controlled substances: Drugs designated by the federal government as having increased potential for abuse and illegal use. These substances are grouped into five categories (schedules), with schedule I substances having the highest abuse potential and schedule V substances having a relatively low potential for abuse.

Cretinism: A congenital syndrome of mental retardation, decreased metabolism, and impaired physical development secondary to insufficient production of thyroid hormones.

Cyclic adenosine monophosphate (cAMP): The ring-shaped conformation of adenosine monophosphate, which is important in acting as a second messenger in mediating the intracellular response to drug stimulation.

Cyclooxygenase (COX): The key enzyme involved in prostaglandin biosynthesis. This enzyme converts arachidonic acid into prostaglandin G_2, thereby providing the precursor for the cell to synthesize additional prostaglandins.

Cytokine: The general term used to describe proteins produced by various immune and inflammatory cells. These proteins act as intercellular chemical signals that help orchestrate immune and inflammatory responses. Common cytokines include the interferons, interleukins, and certain growth factors.

Demand dose: Amount of drug administered when a patient activates certain drug delivery systems, such as those used during patient-controlled analgesia.

Desensitization: A brief and transient decrease in the responsiveness of cellular receptors to drug effects.

Diabetes insipidus: A disease marked by increased urination (polyuria) and excessive thirst (polydipsia) due to inadequate production of antidiuretic hormone (ADH) and/or a decrease in the renal response to ADH.

Diabetes mellitus: A disease marked by abnormal metabolism of glucose and other energy substrates caused by a defect in the production of insulin and/or a decrease in the peripheral response to insulin.

Diuretic: A drug that increases the formation and excretion of urine.

Dopa decarboxylase: The enzyme that converts dihydroxyphenylalanine (dopa) into dopamine.

Dopamine: A neurotransmitter located in the central nervous system (CNS) that is important in motor control and in certain aspects of behavior. The presence of endogenous or exogenous dopamine in the periphery also affects cardiovascular function.

Dosage: The amount of medication that is appropriate for treating a given condition or illness.

Dose: The amount of medication that is administered at one time.

Dose-response curve: The relationship between incremental doses of a drug and the magnitude of the reaction that those doses will cause.

Down-regulation: A prolonged decrease in the number and/or sensitivity of drug receptors, usually occurring as a compensatory response to overstimulation of the receptor.

Drug holidays: Periods of several days to several weeks in which medications are withdrawn from the patient to allow recovery from drug tolerance or toxicity; sometimes used in patients with advanced cases of Parkinson disease.

Drug microsomal metabolizing system (DMMS): A series of enzymes located on the smooth endoplasmic reticulum that are important in catalyzing drug biotransformation.

Dysentery: The general term for severe GI distress (diarrhea, cramps, bloody stools) that is usually associated with the presence of infectious microorganisms in the intestines.

Dyskinesia: An involuntary movement ranging from minor tremors and tics to severe uncoordinated movements of the trunk and extremities. Dyskinesias are associated with certain movement disorders and can also be a side effect of specific medications, such as antiparkinson drugs and antipsychotic medications.

Eicosanoids: The general term for the group of 20-carbon fatty acids that includes the prostaglandins, thromboxanes, and leukotrienes. These substances are involved in mediating inflammation and other pathological responses.

Emetic: A drug that initiates or facilitates vomiting.

End-of-dose akinesia: A phenomenon in Parkinson disease in which the effectiveness of the medication wears off toward the end of the dosing interval, resulting in a virtual lack of volitional movement from the patient.

Enteral administration: Administration of drugs by way of the alimentary canal.

Enzyme induction: The process wherein some drugs provoke cells to synthesize more drug-metabolizing enzymes, thus leading to accelerated drug biotransformation.

Epidural nerve block: Administration of local anesthesia into the spinal canal between the bony vertebral column and the dura mater (i.e., the injection does not penetrate the spinal membranes but remains above the dura).

Epigenetic factors: Processes that affect gene activity by chemically modifying genetic material rather than changing the actual DNA sequence. Typical epigenetic modifications include adding or removing methyl or acetyl groups to DNA, RNA, or the proteins (histones) that surround and package the DNA molecule. Certain anticancer drugs may inhibit mitosis by affecting epigenetic factors that influence cell division.

Epilepsy: A chronic neurological disorder characterized by recurrent seizures that are manifested as brief periods of altered consciousness, involuntary motor activity, or vivid sensory phenomena.

Epinephrine: A hormone synthesized primarily in the adrenal medulla, mimicking the peripheral effects of norepinephrine. Epinephrine is involved in the sympathetic nervous system response to stress and is especially effective in stimulating cardiovascular function (SYN: adrenaline).

Estrogens: The general term for natural and synthetic female hormones such as estradiol and estrone.

Expectorant: A drug that facilitates the production and discharge of mucous secretions from the respiratory tract.

First-pass effect: The phenomenon in which drugs absorbed from the stomach and small intestine must pass through the liver before reaching the systemic circulation. Certain drugs undergo extensive hepatic metabolism because of this first pass through the liver.

Food and Drug Administration (FDA): Government agency the regulates the pharmaceutical industry in the United States.

Gamma-aminobutyric acid (GABA): An inhibitory neurotransmitter in the brain and spinal cord.

Generic name: The name applied to a drug, which is not protected by a trademark; usually a shortened version of the drug's chemical name (SYN: nonproprietary name).

Glucocorticoids: The general class of steroid agents that affect glucose metabolism and are used pharmacologically to decrease inflammation and suppress the immune system. Principle examples include cortisol and corticosterone.

Glycosuria: The presence of glucose in the urine.

Gonadotropin: A hormone that produces a stimulatory effect on the gonads (ovaries and testes); primary gonadotropins include luteinizing hormone (LH) and follicle-stimulating hormone (FSH).

G proteins: Proteins that bind with guanine nucleotides and regulate cell activity. G proteins often serve as a link between surface receptors and ion channels or intracellular enzymes such as adenylate cyclase.

Half-life: The time required to eliminate 50 percent of the drug existing in the body.

Hemostasis: The process of preventing blood loss from the circulation following injury to blood vessels (ANT: hemorrhage).

Histamine: A chemical produced by various cells in the body that is involved in the modulation of certain physiological responses (e.g., secretion of gastric acid) and in the mediation of hypersensitivity (allergic) responses.

Hypercalcemia: An excessive concentration of calcium in the bloodstream (ANT: hypocalcemia).

Hyperglycemia: An excessive concentration of glucose in the bloodstream (ANT: hypoglycemia).

Hyperlipidemia: Abnormal elevation of any or all lipids (fats) in the bloodstream.

Hypersensitivity: An exaggerated response of the immune system to a foreign substance (SYN: allergic response).

Hypertension: A pathological condition characterized by a sustained, reproducible increase in blood pressure.

Hypnotic: A drug that initiates or maintains a relatively normal state of sleep.

Hypokalemia: An abnormally low concentration of potassium in the bloodstream (ANT: hyperkalemia).

Hyponatremia: An abnormally low concentration of sodium in the bloodstream (ANT: hypernatremia).

Immunosuppressants: Drugs used to attenuate the body's immune response. These agents are often used to prevent rejection of organ transplants or to treat diseases caused by overactivity in the immune system (ANT: immunostimulant).

Incretins: Hormones released from the GI tract that stimulate insulin release and exert other effects on pancreatic hormone production and GI function. The primary incretins in humans are glucagon-like peptide and glucose-dependent insulinotropic polypeptide.

Inotropic: Refers to a substance that increases muscular contraction force (positive inotrope) or decreases contraction force (negative inotrope). Certain cardiac drugs are considered positive inotropes because they increase the force of cardiac contractions.

Interferon: A member of the group of proteins that exert a number of physiological and pharmacological effects, including antiviral and antineoplastic activity.

Interleukins (IL): A family of small proteins (cytokines) produced by leukocytes that regulate immune function. Specific interleukins are designated by numbers (IL-1, IL-2, etc.), and drugs that inhibit or mimic the effects of ILs can help resolve conditions caused by excessive or deficient IL production, respectively.

Intrathecal: Administration of substances within a sheath; typically refers to injection into the subarachnoid space surrounding the spinal cord.

Laxative: An agent that promotes peristalsis and evacuation of the bowel in a relatively slow manner (as opposed to a cathartic).

Leukotriene (LT): One of the 20-carbon fatty acid compounds (eicosanoids) formed from arachidonic acid by the lipoxygenase enzyme. Leukotrienes are important in mediating certain allergic and inflammatory responses, especially in respiratory tissues.

Lipoxygenase (LOX): The enzyme that initiates leukotriene biosynthesis. This enzyme converts arachidonic acid into precursors that the cell uses to synthesize specific leukotrienes.

Loading dose: Amount of drug administered at the onset of treatment to rapidly bring the amount of drug in the body to therapeutic levels.

Lockout interval: The minimum amount of time that must expire between each dose of medication that is administered by patient-controlled analgesia (PCA). The PCA pump is inactivated during the lockout interval so that the patient cannot self-administer excessive amounts of drugs.

Lymphokines: Chemicals released from activated lymphocytes that help mediate various aspects of the immune response. Common lymphokines include the interleukins and gamma interferon.

Malignancy: A term usually applied to cancerous tumors that tend to become progressively worse.

Maximal efficacy: The maximum response a drug can produce; the point at which the response does not increase even if the dosage continues to increase (SYN: ceiling effect).

Median effective dose (ED_{50}): The drug dose that produces a specific therapeutic response in 50 percent of the patients in whom it is tested.

Median lethal dose (LD_{50}): The drug dose that causes death in 50 percent of the experimental animals in which it is tested.

Median toxic dose (TD_{50}): The drug dose that produces a specific adverse (toxic) response in 50 percent of the patients in whom it is tested.

Metabolic syndrome: A condition characterized by insulin resistance, high blood pressure, abdominal obesity, and hyperlipidemia (SYN: Syndrome X).

Metabolite: The compound that is formed when the drug undergoes biotransformation and is chemically altered by some metabolic process.

Metastasize: The transfer or spread of diseased (i.e., cancerous) cells from a primary location to other sites in the body.

Mineralocorticoids: Steroid hormones (e.g., aldosterone) that are important in regulating fluid and electrolyte balance by increasing the reabsorption of sodium from the kidneys.

Monoamine oxidase (MAO): An enzyme that breaks down monoamine neurotransmitters such as dopamine, norepinephrine, and serotonin. Drugs that suppress this enzyme are known as *MAO inhibitors*, and these drugs will prolong the effects of monoamine neurotransmitters.

Monoclonal antibody (MAB): An antibody created biosynthetically from specific cells; MABs are designed to recognize specific cell-surface antigens on cancer cells or other tissues to target the drug directly to that tissue.

Mucolytic: A drug that decreases the viscosity and increases the fluidity of mucous secretions in the respiratory tract, thus making it easier for the patient to cough up secretions.

Muscarinic receptor: A primary class of cholinergic receptors that are named according to their affinity for the muscarine toxin. Certain cholinergic agonists and antagonists also have a relatively selective affinity for muscarinic receptors.

Mycosis: A fungal infection in humans and animals.

Myxedema: The adult or acquired form of hypothyroidism characterized by decreased metabolic rate, lethargy, decreased mental alertness, weight gain, and other somatic changes.

Neuroleptic: A term frequently used to describe antipsychotic drugs, referring to the tendency of these drugs to produce a behavioral syndrome of apathy, sedation, decreased initiative, and decreased responsiveness (SYN: antipsychotic).

Nicotinic receptor: A primary class of cholinergic receptors, named according to their affinity for nicotine, as well as certain other cholinergic agonists and antagonists.

Nonproprietary name: A drug name that is usually a shortened version of the drug's chemical name and is recognized as the standard name for that drug regardless of the drug's trade or brand names (SYN: generic name).

Norepinephrine: A neurotransmitter that is important in certain brain pathways and in the terminal synapses of the sympathetic nervous system (SYN: noradrenaline).

Off-label prescribing: A drug is prescribed to treat conditions other than those approved by the FDA.

On-off phenomenon: The fluctuation in response seen in certain patients with Parkinson disease, in which the effectiveness of medications may suddenly diminish at some point between dosages.

Opioid: An analgesic drug with morphinelike effects; commonly refers to the synthetic forms of these analgesics (SYN: narcotic).

Orphan drugs: Drugs that are designed and approved to treat rare diseases. Because these drugs are only used in a small patient population (usually less that 200,000 people), financial and other incentives are often provided by various sources to encourage a drug company to develop and market the drug.

Orthostatic hypotension: A sudden fall in blood pressure that occurs when the patient stands erect; this is a frequent side effect of many medications.

Ototoxicity: The harmful side effect of some drugs and toxins influencing the ear's hearing and balance functions.

Over-the-counter drugs (OTC): Drugs that can be purchased directly by the consumer without a prescription (SYN: nonprescription drugs).

Parenteral administration: Administration of drugs by routes other than via the alimentary canal: by injection, transdermally, topically, and so on.

Parkinson disease or parkinsonism: The clinical syndrome of bradykinesia, rigidity, resting tremor, and postural instability associated with neurotransmitter abnormalities within the basal ganglia.

Patient-controlled analgesia (PCA): A technique that allows the patient to self-administer an opioid or other analgesic medication, typically by activating a pump or other electronic device that provides a small amount of drug during a certain time interval and is programmed to prevent overdose.

Pharmacodynamics: The study of how drugs affect the body—that is, the physiological and biochemical mechanisms of drug action.

Pharmacogenetics: The study of the how genetic variability can influence drug responses and metabolism.

Pharmacokinetics: The study of how the body handles drugs—that is, the manner in which drugs are absorbed, distributed, metabolized, and excreted.

Pharmacological dose: An amount of drug given that is much greater than the amount of a similar substance produced within the body; this increased dose is used to exaggerate the beneficial effects normally provided by the endogenous compound.

Pharmacotherapeutics: The study of how drugs are used in the prevention and treatment of disease.

Pharmacy: The professional discipline dealing with the preparation and dispensing of medications.

Phosphodiesterase (PDE): An enzyme that breaks down phosphodiester bonds in organic compounds. Certain phosphodiesterases are important clinically because they break down second messengers such as cyclic AMP, and drugs that inhibit these enzymes prolong the effects of cyclic AMP in the lungs and other tissues.

Physical dependence: A phenomenon that develops during prolonged use of addictive substances, signified by the onset of withdrawal symptoms when the drug is discontinued.

Physiological dose: The amount of drug given that is roughly equivalent to the amount of a similar substance normally produced within the body;

this dose is typically used to replace the endogenous substance the body is no longer able to produce.

Placebo: A medication that contains inert or inactive ingredients; used to pacify a patient or test a patient's psychophysiological response to treatment.

Potency: The dose of a drug that produces a given response in a specific amplitude. When two drugs are compared, the more potent drug will produce a given response at a lower dose.

Progestins: The general term for the natural and synthetic female hormones, such as progesterone.

Prostaglandin: A member of the family of 20-carbon fatty acid compounds (eicosanoids) formed from arachidonic acid by the cyclooxygenase enzyme. Prostaglandins help regulate normal cell activity and may help mediate certain pathological responses, including pain, inflammation, fever, and abnormal blood coagulation.

Protease: An enzyme that catalyzes several steps in the synthesis and maturation of HIV in infected cells. Drugs that suppress this enzyme are known as *protease inhibitors*, and these drugs can be used as part of the treatment of HIV infection.

Proton pump: An enzyme that moves hydrogen ions (protons) across the cell membrane. The gastric proton pump transports hydrogen ions into the stomach; drugs that inhibit this enzyme are known as *proton pump inhibitors*, and these drugs are used to reduce the formation and effects of excess gastric acid.

Psychosis: A relatively severe form of mental illness characterized by marked thought disturbances and an impaired perception of reality.

Receptor: The component of the cell (usually a protein) to which the drug binds, thus initiating a change in cell function.

Reverse transcriptase: An HIV enzyme that catalyzes the conversion of viral RNA into viral DNA in infected cells. Drugs that inhibit this enzyme are known as *reverse transcriptase inhibitors*, and these drugs can be used as part of the treatment of HIV infection.

Salicylate: The chemical term commonly used to denote compounds such as aspirin that have anti-inflammatory, analgesic, antipyretic, and anticoagulant properties.

Second messenger: The term applied to compounds formed within the cell, such as cyclic AMP. The second messenger initiates a series of biochemical changes within the cell following stimulation of a receptor on the cell's outer surface by drugs, hormones, and so on.

Sedative: A drug that produces a calming effect and serves to pacify the patient. These agents are sometimes referred to as *minor tranquilizers.*

Seizure: A sudden attack of symptoms usually associated with diseases such as epilepsy. Epileptic seizures are due to the random, uncontrolled firing of a group of cerebral neurons, which results in a variety of sensory and motor manifestations.

Selective estrogen receptor modulator (SERM): A drug that activates estrogen receptors on bone and vascular tissues, while blocking estrogen receptors on breast and uterine tissues. These drugs can be used to enhance bone mineralization and to prevent certain cancers.

Selective toxicity: A desired effect of antineoplastic and anti-infectious agents, wherein the drug kills the pathogenic organism or cells without damaging healthy tissues.

Serotonin: A neurotransmitter located in the CNS that is important in many functions, including mood, arousal, and inhibition of painful stimuli (SYN: 5-hydroxytryptamine).

Side effect: Any effect produced by a drug that occurs in addition to the principal therapeutic response.

Spinal nerve block: Administration of local anesthesia into the spinal canal between the arachnoid membrane and the pia mater (i.e., the subarachnoid space).

Statins: The class of drugs designed to lower blood cholesterol by inhibiting an enzyme (HMG-CoA reductase) that synthesizes cholesterol in the liver. Drugs in this class share a common *-statin* suffix at the end of their generic name.

Status epilepticus: An emergency characterized by a rapid series of epileptic seizures that occur without any appreciable recovery between seizures.

Steroid: The general term used to describe a group of hormones and their analogs that have a common chemical configuration but are divided into several categories depending on their primary physiological effects. Common types of steroids include the glucocorticoids (cortisone, prednisone, many others), mineralocorticoids (aldosterone), androgens/anabolic steroids (testosterone), and steroids related to female physiological function (estrogen, progesterone).

Sublingual: Under the tongue; drugs administered sublingually are absorbed into the systemic circulation via the venous drainage from underneath the tongue.

Supersensitivity: An increased response to drugs and endogenous compounds caused by an increase in the number and/or sensitivity of receptors for that drug.

Sympatholytics: Drugs that inhibit or antagonize function within the sympathetic nervous system.

Sympathomimetics: Drugs that facilitate or increase activity within the sympathetic nervous system.

Tardive dyskinesia: A movement disorder characterized by involuntary, fragmented movements of the mouth, face, and jaw (i.e., chewing, sucking, tongue protrusion, etc.). This disorder may occur during the prolonged administration of antipsychotic drugs.

Therapeutic index (TI): A ratio used to represent the relative safety of a particular drug; the larger the therapeutic index, the safer the drug. It is calculated as the median toxic dose divided by the median effective dose. (In animal trials, the median lethal dose is often substituted for the median toxic dose.)

Therapeutic window: The range of drug concentrations in the body that will promote optimal beneficial effects. Drug concentrations less than the lower end of this range will be ineffective, and concentrations greater than the upper end of this range will create excessive side effects.

Thromboxane (TX): A 20-carbon lipid compound similar to the prostaglandins and leukotrienes. Thromboxanes are especially important in regulating platelet activity and blood clotting.

Thrombus: A blood clot formed by the activation of fibrin and platelets. Excessive thrombus formation (thrombosis) can be controlled by drugs that affect various aspects of the clotting mechanisms.

Thyrotoxicosis: Abnormally high production of thyroid hormones resulting in symptoms such as nervousness, weight loss, and tachycardia (SYN: hyperthyroidism).

Tolerance: The acquired phenomenon associated with some drugs, in which larger dosages of the drug are needed to achieve a given effect when the drug is used for prolonged periods.

Toxicology: The study of the harmful effects of drugs and other chemicals.

Trade name: The name given to a drug by the pharmaceutical company; it is protected by a trademark and used by the company for marketing the drug (SYN: brand name or proprietary name).

Tumor necrosis factor (TNF): A small protein (cytokine) produced by macrophages and other cells that helps regulate inflammation and immune reactions. Drugs that suppress this factor are known as TNF inhibitors, which can help prevent TNF's destructive effects on joints and other tissues in autoimmune diseases such as rheumatoid arthritis.

Vaccine: A substance typically consisting of a modified infectious microorganism that is administered to help prevent disease by stimulating the endogenous immune defense mechanisms against infection.

Viscosupplementation: Injection of a polysaccharide (hyaluronan) into osteoarthritic joints to help restore the viscosity of synovial fluid.

Volume of distribution (V_d): A ratio used to estimate the distribution of a drug within the body relative to the total amount of fluid in the body. It is calculated as the amount of drug administered divided by the plasma concentration of the drug.

Withdrawal syndrome: The clinical syndrome of somatic and psychological manifestations that occur when a drug is removed from a patient who has become physically dependent on a drug (SYN: abstinence syndrome).

Xanthine: A category of compounds that includes stimulants such as caffeine and theophylline.

Index

Note: *f* indicates figure, and *t* indicates table.

A

Abacavir, 562*t*, 566, 572
Abarelix, 470, 610*t*
Abatacept, 240*t*, 244*t*, 247–248, 633, 633*t*
Abbokinase, 378*t*
Abciximab, 341, 378*t*, 382, 383
Abelcet, 584
Abilify, 104*t*, 106–107
Abortion, drug-induced, 479–480
ABP (androgen-binding protein), 466, 466*f*
Abreva, 560*t*, 563
Abscess, 547*t*
Acarbose, 518*t*, 520
Access port, 266
Accolate, 409–410
Accupril, 324*t*, 363*t*
Acebutolol, 310*t*, 311, 321, 321*t*, 338*t*, 353*t*, 363*t*
ACE inhibitors. *See* Angiotensin-converting enzyme (ACE) inhibitors
Aceon, 324*t*
Acetaminophen
  biotransformation, 32*t*
  half-life, 35, 35*f*
  liver damage, 25
  metabolism, 231*f*
  osteoarthritis, 251
  pain and inflammation, 230–232
  rheumatoid arthritis, 240
Acetylcholine, 62*t*, 63
  chemical structure, 294*f*
  Parkinson disease and, 296
  pre- and postganglionic neurons, 283*f*
  receptors for (*See* Cholinergic receptors)
Acetylcholine inhibitors, 158, 294–297, 295*t*
Acetylcysteine, 403
Acetylsalicylic acid. *See* Aspirin
Acid-fast bacilli, 533*t*
Acid-rebound phenomenon, 422
AcipHex, 424, 424*t*
Aclovate, 453*t*
Actemra, 240*t*, 244*t*, 249
ACTH (adrenocorticotropic hormone), 449, 449*f*, 454
Actifed, 402*t*
Actimmune, 569*t*
Actinomycetes, 533*t*
Action potential, cardiac, 349–350, 350*f*
Activase, 378*t*, 385
Active transport, 21*f*, 22–23
Actonel, 498*t*
Actos, 518*t*, 519–520
Acyclovir, 560*t*, 561
Aczone, 543*t*
Adalat, 324*t*, 339–340, 339*t*
Adalimumab, 240*t*, 244*t*, 247, 248*f*, 632, 633*t*
Addiction, opioid, 211–212, 214
Addison disease, 454
Adefovir, 560*t*
Adenosine, 355
Adenosine diphosphate (ADP) receptor inhibitors, 378*t*, 382
Adenylate cyclase-cyclic adenosine monophosphate (cAMP) system, 45–46, 46*f*, 510
Adipose tissue
  drug storage in, 24
  effect of insulin, 508
Adrenal gland, 437*t*, 438–439
Adrenal medulla, 282, 439
Adrenalin, 307
Adrenergic drugs, 301–313
  agonists, 302*t*, 303–307
  antagonists (*See* Beta blockers)
Adrenergic receptors, 48, 283*f*, 284
  classification and types, 286–287
  locations and responses, 285–286*t*
  specificity, 302*t*
  subclassifications, 284*f*, 302*t*
Adrenocortical suppression, 456
Adrenocorticosteroids, 447–462
  adrenocortical hormone biosynthesis inhibitors, 457
  anticancer agents, 609*t*
  case study, 461–462
  glucocorticoids, 449–457 (*See also* Glucocorticoids)
  mineralocorticoids, 437*t*, 439, 447, 457–459
  rehabilitation patients, 460–461
  steroid synthesis, 447–449, 448*f*
Adrenocorticotropic hormone (ACTH), 436*t*, 449, 449*f*, 454
Adriamycin RDF, 607*t*

Adrucil, 606*t*
Advair Diskus, 411*t*
Advair HFA, 411*t*
Advil, 229*t*
AeroBid, 408*t*, 453*t*
Affective disorders. *See* Antipsychotic drugs; Bipolar syndrome; Depression
Affinity, 49
Afrin, 303, 401*t*
Aftate, 587
Age, effects on drug response, 38
Agenerase, 562*t*
Aggrastat, 378*t*, 382
Agonist-antagonists, mixed, 50, 203, 206
Agonists, 49, 49*f*. *See also* Beta-adrenergic agonists
  adrenergic, 302, 303–307
  alpha, 303–305
  biased, 50
  dopamine, 140–141, 140*t*
  inverse, 50–51
  mineralocorticoid, 437*t*, 439, 447, 457–459
  mixed alpha and beta, 306–307
  opioid, 203, 204–205*t*, 205–206
  partial, 50
AIDS. *See* Human immunodeficiency virus (HIV), treatment of AIDS
Akathisia, antipsychotics and, 108*f*, 109
Akinesia, end-of-dose, 139
Akineton, 135*t*
Albendazole, 593–594, 593*t*
Albenza, 593–594
Albuterol, 306, 405*t*
Alclometasone, 453*t*
Alcohol
  baclofen for alcohol abuse, 184
  sedative effects of, 73
Aldactone, 320*t*, 369, 460
Aldara, 560*t*, 565
Aldesleukin, 611*t*
Aldex AN, 402*t*
Aldomet, 304–305, 321*t*
Aldosterone, 325, 457–458
  ACE inhibitors and, 367–368
  biosynthesis and structure, 448*f*
  effects, 439, 458–459, 458*f*
  release, 325, 325*f*, 458
Alefacept, 633, 633*t*
Alemtuzumab, 611*t*
Alendronate, 498*t*, 499
Alesse, 481*t*
Aleve, 229*t*
Alfentanil, 204*t*, 263, 263*t*
Alferon N, 569*t*
Alfuzosin, 308
Alimta, 606*t*
Alinia, 592
Aliskiren, 324*t*, 326, 363*t*, 368
Alitretinoin, 614*t*, 616
Alkaloids, 312–313
Alkeran, 604*t*
Alkylating agents, 602–603, 603*f*, 604*t*
Allegra, 401, 402*t*
Allergy
  insulin, 516–517
  penicillins, 537
Allergy treatment
  antihistamines, 401–402, 402*t*
  decongestants, 400–401, 401*t*
Alloantibody inhibitors, 386
All-trans-retinoic acid, 616
Aloxi, 602
Alpha-1 and -2 receptors, 48, 284*f*, 285–286*t*, 286–287, 302, 302*t*
Alpha agonists, 302, 302*t*, 303–305, 400, 401*t*
Alpha antagonists. *See under* Antagonists
Alphagan, 304
Alpha-glucosidase inhibitors, 518*t*, 520
Alpha-methylnorepinephrine, 304–305
Alpha-tocopherol, 648*t*
Alprazolam, 76*t*
Alrex, 454*t*
Altace, 324*t*, 363*t*
Alteplase, 378*t*, 385
Alternative medicine. *See* Complementary and alternative medications (CAMs)
Altretamine, 604*t*
Alupent, 306, 405*t*
Alzheimer disease
  adrenergic antagonists, 309
  antipsychotics, 107
  cholinergic stimulants, 292
  estrogen replacement, 476
  gingko biloba, 645
Amantadine, 135*t*, 141, 560*t*, 561–562
Amaryl, 518*t*
Ambenonium, 291*t*, 293
Ambien, 70*t*, 74*t*
AmBisome, 584
Amcinonide, 453*t*
Americaine, 166*t*
Amevive, 633, 633*t*
Amicar, 386
Amidate, 152*t*, 154
Amikacin (Amikin), 540*t*
Amiloride, 320*t*
Amino acids, 62*f*, 63, 439
Aminocaproic acid, 386
Aminoglutethimide, 457
Aminoglycosides, 539–540, 540*t*
Aminopenicillins, 536*t*
Aminophylline, 407*t*
Aminosalicylic acid, 543, 543*t*
Amiodarone, 353*t*, 354, 355
Amitriptyline, 86*t*, 91*t*, 93*t*
Amlodipine, 324*t*, 327, 339*t*
Amnesia, drug-induced, 74
Amobarbital, 70*t*, 157*t*
Amoxapine, 86*t*, 91*t*, 93*t*
Amoxicillin, 536*t*
Amoxil, 536*t*
Amphetamines, 306
Amphocin, 584
Amphotec, 584
Amphotericin B, 582*t*, 584, 588*t*
Ampicillin, 536*t*
Amprenavir, 562*t*
Amrinone, 365–366
Amrix, 181*t*
Amylin analog, 518*t*, 520
Amyl nitrite, 338, 363*t*
Amytal, 70*t*
Anabolic steroids, abuse of, 470–472, 470*t*, 471*t*
Anadrol, 469*t*, 470*t*, 471*t*
Anafranil, 86*t*, 93*t*
Anakinra, 240*t*, 244*t*, 248, 633*t*
Analgesics. *See* Anesthetic drugs; Nonsteroidal anti-inflammatory drugs (NSAIDs); Opioid analgesic drugs; Patient-controlled analgesia (PCA)
Anandron, 470
Anaprox, 228*t*, 229*t*, 240*t*
Anastrozole, 609*t*, 610
Anavar, 470*t*, 471*t*
Ancalixir, 70*t*
Ancef, 536*t*
Ancobon, 584–585
Androderm, 469*t*
AndroGel, 469*t*
Androgen-binding protein (ABP), 466, 466*f*
Androgen receptor blockers, 610
Androgens, 465
  abuse, 470–472, 470*t*, 471*t*
  adverse effects, 469
  antineoplastics, 609*t*
  clinical use, 467–470, 469*t*
  effects on athletic performance, 471
  physiological effects, 467
  source and regulation, 465–467
  specific drugs, 468, 469*t*
Android, 469*t*, 470*t*
Anectine, 158*t*
Anemia, 468
Anesthetic drugs
  general, 149–161, 151–152*t*
    adjuvants, 156–159
    case study, 160–161
    epilepsy, 126
    inhalation anesthetics, 150, 151*t*, 152–153, 153*f*
    intravenous anesthetics, 150, 151*t*, 153–154
    mechanisms, 154–156, 155*f*
    pharmacokinetics, 154
    rehabilitation patient, 160
    requirements, 149–150

route of administration, 150, 152–154
specific agents, 151–152*t*
stages of anesthesia, 150
local, 165–174
case study, 174
clinical use, 167–170
common, 166*t*
differential nerve block, 171–172, 171*t*
mechanism of action, 170–171, 170*f*
patient-controlled analgesia (PCA) (*See* Patient-controlled analgesia (PCA)
pharmacokinetics, 167
rehabilitation patients, 173
systemic effects, 172
types, 165–167
Angina pectoris, 335, 346
anticoagulants, 341
beta-adrenergic blockers, 338–339, 338*t*
calcium channel blockers, 339–340, 339*t*
case study, 345
myocardial ischemia equation, 336*f*
myocardial oxygen balance, 340–341
nonpharmacologic management, 344
organic nitrates, 335–338, 336*t*
rehabilitation patients, 344–345
types and treatments, 341–344, 342*t*
Angioedema, hereditary, 468
Angiogenesis inhibitors, 612
Angiomax, 378*t*
Angiotensin-converting enzyme (ACE) inhibitors, 324*t*, 326, 363*t*, 367–368
Angiotensin I, 325
Angiotensin II, 325, 325*f*
aldosterone release, 325, 325*f*
receptor blockers, 326
antihypertensives, 324–326, 324*t*
congestive heart failure, 363*t*, 368
Angiotensinogen, 325
Anidulafungin, 586
Animal bite, 547*t*
Animal studies, 6, 6*t*
Annexins, 242, 452
Ansaid, 228*t*, 229*t*, 240*t*
Antacids, 422–423, 422*f*
Antagonists, 49, 49*f*. *See also* Beta blockers
alpha, 307–309, 321–322, 321*t*
antihypertensives, 321–322
competitive and noncompetitive, 49–50
interleukin-1 and -2 receptor, 632, 633*t*
opioid, 206
Anterior pituitary, 436–437
Anthelmintic drugs, 593–595, 593*t*
Anthrax, 547*t*
Antiandrogens, 469–470, 609*t*
Antianginal drugs, 338*t*, 339*t*. *See also* Angina pectoris
Antianxiety drugs, 69, 75–79, 80
antidepressants, 76–77, 77t
benzodiazepines, 75–76, 76*t*, 78–79
buspirone, 76
other drugs, 77–78
problems and side effects, 78
rehabilitation patients, 78–79
Antiarrhythmic drugs, 349, 352–357, 353*t*
case study, 356–357
classification, 352–355, 353*t*
rehabilitation patients, 356
Antibacterial drugs, 531, 533–552
case study, 551–552
common infections and agents, 546, 547–549*t*, 549
inhibitors
cell wall synthesis and function, 534, 535–539, 536*t*
DNA/RNA synthesis and function, 535, 535*f*, 543–545, 543*t*
protein synthesis, 534–535, 539–542, 540*t*
mechanism, 533–535, 534*f*
other antibacterials, 545–546
rehabilitation patients, 551
resistance, 549–550, 550*f*
spectrum and activity, 533
Antibiotics, 37, 531
anticancer, 605, 607*t*
cystic fibrosis-related respiratory problems, 413
stewardship, 550
Antibodies
anti-T-cell, 632
immunosuppressant, 628*t*, 632–633, 633*t*
inhibitory (alloantibodies), 386
monoclonal, 520–521, 610, 611*t*, 612, 618
Anticholinergic drugs, 293–298
clinical applications, 294–297
common drugs, 295*t*
COPD-related respiratory problems, 296–297, 407–408, 412
gastric ulcers, 294–296, 425
nausea, 296, 430
Parkinson disease, 135*t*, 141
preoperative medications, 156, 157*t*
problems and adverse effects, 297
reversal of toxicity, 293
source and mechanism, 294
tardive dyskinesia, 109
Anticholinesterase agents (indirect-acting cholinergic stimulants), 65, 290*f*, 291–292, 291*t*
Anticoagulant drugs
angina pectoris, 341, 343
coagulation disorders, 377–381, 378*t*
Antidepressant drugs, 86
anxiety, 76–77, 77*t*
case study, 97
chronic pain, 92–93, 93*t*
common drugs, 86*t*
effects on amine synapses, 87*f*
monoamine oxidase (MAO) inhibitors, 87*t*, 88, 90, 91*t*, 92
pharmacokinetics, 90
problems and adverse effects, 90–92, 91*t*
rehabilitation patients, 95–96
second-generation drugs, 89*t*
tricyclics, 86–87*t*, 88, 91*t*, 92
Antidiabetic drugs. *See under* Diabetes mellitus
Antidiarrheal agents, 426–428, 426*t*
Antidiuretic hormone (ADH), 436*t*, 437
Antiemetic drugs, 429–430, 602
antipsychotics, 107
Antiepileptic drugs, 115–116, 118–128
case study, 127–128
chemical classification and actions, 119*t*
dosages, 125*t*
pharmacokinetics, 125
pregnancy, 125–126
rehabilitation patients, 127
second-generation drugs, 121–124, 122*t*
selection of, 124, 124*t*
status epilepticus, 126
withdrawal of medications, 126
Antiestrogens, 479, 609*t*
Antifibrinolytic drugs, 386
Antiflex, 181*t*
Antifungal drugs, 581–587
case study, 596
fungal infections, 581–582, 582*t*
mechanism, 583*f*
rehabilitation patients, 595
systemic, 582*t*, 584–586
topical, 582–583*t*, 586–587
use in mycoses, 581, 582*t*
Antigen-presenting cell (APC), 632–633
Antigens, immune response and, 626, 626*f*
Antihistamines
nausea, 430
parkinsonism, 141
preoperative medications, 156, 157*t*
respiratory problems, 401–402, 402*t*
Antihypertensive drugs, 315–330
angiotensin II receptor blockers, 324–326, 324*t*
calcium channel blockers, 319*t*, 324*t*, 326–327
case study, 329–330
categories, 319*t*
diuretics, 318–320, 319*t*, 320*t*
rehabilitation patients, 329
stepped-care treatment, 327–328
sympatholytics, 319*t*, 320–323, 321*t*
vasodilators, 319*t*, 323–324, 324*t*
Anti-inflammatory drugs. *See* Glucocorticoids; Nonsteroidal anti-inflammatory drugs (NSAIDs)
Antilirium, 291*t*
Antimalarial drugs
adverse side effects, 245
malaria, 588–591, 588*t*
mechanism of action, 244–245
rheumatoid arthritis, 243–245, 243*t*

Antimanic drugs, 94–95, 96
Antimetabolites, 603, 605, 605*f*, 606–607*t*
Antimicrobial drugs, 531
Antimicrotubule agents, 605, 608*t*
Antiminth, 595
Antimuscarinic drugs, 294–297
Antinausea agents, 602
Antineoplastic drugs. *See* Cancer chemotherapy
Antinicotinic drugs, 294
Antioxidants, 134, 619
Antiparasitic drugs
  anthelmintics, 593–595, 593*t*
  antifungals, 581–587
  antiprotozoals, 588–593
  rehabilitation patients, 595
Antiparkinson drugs. *See* Parkinson disease
Antiplatelet drugs, 377, 378*f*, 381–383. *See also* Aspirin
Antiprogestins, 479–480
Antiprotozoal drugs
  antimalarials, 588–591, 588*t*
  other protozoal infections and treatment, 588*t*, 591–593
  rehabilitation patients, 595
Antipsychotic drugs, 103–111
  bipolar disorder, 93–95
  case study, 111
  common drugs, 103*t*
  dosage, 104–105*t*
  mechanism, 103–105, 104*f*
  other uses, 106–107
  pharmacokinetics, 106
  problems and adverse effects, 107–110
  rehabilitation patients, 110
Antirheumatic drugs. *See under* Rheumatoid arthritis
Antiseizure drugs, 118–124, 118*f*. *See also* Antiepileptic drugs
  bipolar disorder, 95
Antispasm drugs, 180–182, 181*t*
  side effects, 182, 182*t*
Antispasticity drugs, 183–187, 183*t*
Anti-T-cell antibodies, 632
Antithrombin, 377
Antithrombotic drugs, 378*t*, 380
Antithymocyte globulin, 633*t*
Antithyroid drugs, 493, 502
Antitussive drugs, 399–400, 400*t*
Antiviral drugs, 557, 560–577
  case study, 576–577
  HIV and AIDS treatment, 563, 564, 571–575
  interferons, 568–570, 569*f*, 569*t*
  rehabilitation patients, 576
  resistance, 568
  specific drugs, 560–561*t*, 560–568
  vaccines, 570–571
Anxiety, 75, 77. *See also* Antianxiety drugs
Anzemet, 602
Apidra, 514*t*
Apixaban, 378*t*, 380
Apokyn, 140*t*
Apomorphine, 140*t*, 429
Apo-Quin, 353*t*
Apo-Quinidine, 353*t*
Aprepitant, 602
Apresoline, 324, 324*t*, 363*t*
Aptivus, 572
Aquatesen, 320*t*
Aquazide, 320*t*
Ara-C, 606*t*
Aralen, 240*t*, 243–244, 243*t*, 588–589
Aramine, 307
Arava, 240*t*, 243*t*, 245–246
Arbinoxa, 402*t*
Arcalyst, 633*t*
Arcapta Neohaler, 405*t*
Arduan, 158*t*
Aredia, 498*t*, 499, 500
Arfonad, 321*t*
Arformoterol, 405*t*
Argatroban, 378*t*
Aricept, 291*t*, 292
Arimidex, 610
Aripiprazole, 103*t*, 104*t*, 106–107
Aristocort, 240*t*, 454*t*
Arixtra, 380378*t*
Armour Thyroid, 494*t*
Aromasin, 610
Aromatase inhibitors, 609*t*, 610
Arranon, 606*t*
Arrhythmia. *See* Cardiac arrhythmias
Arsenic trioxide, 614–615, 614*t*
Artane, 135*t*
Artemisinin-based combination therapy (ACT), 591
Artemisinin derivatives, 590–591
Arthritis, 548*t*. *See* Rheumatoid arthritis
Arthritis-dermatitis syndrome, 548*t*
Articaine, 166*t*
Arzerra, 611*t*
Ascorbic acid, 648*t*
Asendin, 86*t*, 93*t*
Asparaginase, 614*t*, 615
Aspart, 514*t*, 515
Aspartate, 62*t*, 63
Aspirin, 219, 223, 240*t*
  angina pectoris, 341
  biotransformation of, 32*t*
  cancer treatment, 613–614
  chemical structure, 220*f*
  clearance, 34–35
  clinical applications, 224
  coagulation disorders, 378*t*
  comparison with other NSAIDs, 227–229, 227*t*
  dosage, 229*t*
  enteric-coated, 225
  interaction with methotrexate, 37
  intoxication (poisoning), 226
  overactive clotting, 378*t*, 381–382
  problems and adverse effects, 224–227, 383
  uses, 381–382
Astelin, 402*t*
Asthma, 410–412
  cromones, 409
  drugs for airway patency, 403–410, 405*t*
  leukotriene inhibitors, 410
  nonpharmacological interventions, 412
Atacand, 324*t*, 363*t*
Atarax, 402*t*
Atazanavir, 562*t*, 572
Atenolol, 287, 310*t*, 311, 321*t*, 338*t*, 339, 353*t*, 363*t*
Atherosclerosis, 375, 387
Ativan, 76*t*, 119*t*, 151*t*
Atorvastatin, 387, 388*t*
Atovaquone, 591
Atracurium, 158*t*
Atrioventricular junctional arrhythmias, 352*t*
AtroPen, 295*t*
Atropine
  cardiovascular disease, 295*t*
  clinical uses, 295*t*, 296, 297
  gastric ulcers, 425
  preoperative medication, 157*t*
  respiratory problems, 407
  respiratory tract, 296–297
  structure, 294*f*
Atrovent, 295*t*, 407
Attapulgite, 427–428
Atypical agents. *See* Second-generation (atypical) agents
Auranofin, 240*t*, 243*t*, 245
Aurolate, 243*t*
Aurothioglucose, 245
Autoimmune disease, 290
Autonomic nervous system (ANS), 279–288
  adrenal medulla, 282
  anatomy, 279–282
  integration and control, 282–283
  neurotransmitters and receptors, 283–284
  pharmacology, 287
  receptors, 284–287, 284*f*, 285–286*t*
Autophosphorylation, 508
Avandia, 518*t*, 519–520
Avapro, 324*t*, 363*t*
Avastin, 611*t*, 612
Avelox, 543*t*
Aventyl, 87*t*, 93*t*
Avlosulfon, 543, 543*t*
Avodart, 470
Avonex, 569*t*, 570
Axid, 423*t*
Aygestin, 477*t*
Azacitidine, 606*t*
Azactam, 536*t*
Azasan, 243*t*, 245

Azatadine, 402*t*
Azathioprine, 240*t*, 243*t*, 245, 627–628, 628*t*
Azelastine, 402*t*
Azidothymidine (AZT), 566, 572
Azilect, 135*t*, 141–142
Azilsartan, 324*t*
Azithromycin, 413, 540*t*
Azmacort, 408*t*, 454*t*
Azoles, 582*t*, 586–587
Aztreonam, 536*t*, 538
Azulfidine, 240*t*, 244*t*, 249, 628*t*, 631

B

Baci-IM, 536*t*
Bacille Calmette-Guérin, 634
Bacilli, gram-positive and -negative, 533*t*
Bacitracin, 536*t*, 538
Background infusion, 262–263
Baclofen, 183–185, 183*t*, 184, 184*f*, 191
Bacteremia, 547*t*, 548*t*
Bacteria. *See also* Antibacterial drugs
  basic concepts, 532
  common infections and treatment, 547–549*t*
  nomenclature, 532
  types, 533*t*
Bactericidal drugs *vs.* bacteriostatic drugs, 533. *See also* Antibacterial drugs
Bactocill, 536*t*
Bactrim, 543*t*
Bactroban, 543*t*, 544
Balanced anesthesia, 150
Banan, 536*t*
Banzel, 122*t*, 123
Baraclude, 560*t*
Barbiturates
  antiepileptics, 119–120, 119*t*
  general anesthetic, 151*t*, 153
  preoperative medications, 157*t*
  sedative-hypnotics, 70*t*, 71*f*, 72
Baroreceptor reflex, 282
Basal ganglia, 59–60, 60*f*
Basiliximab, 632, 633*t*
BayRho-D, 633*t*
B cells, 239, 239*f*
BCG, 634
BCNU, 604*t*
Beclomethasone, 408, 408*t*, 453*t*
Beclovent, 453*t*
Beepen-VK, 536*t*
Bee venom, 643, 644*t*
Belatacept, 633, 633*t*
Belladonna, 294, 295*t*
Benadryl, 135*t*, 400*t*, 402*t*
Benazepril, 324*t*
Bendamustine, 604*t*
Bendroflumethiazide, 320*t*
Beneficial effect, 11, 11*f*
Benicar, 324*t*
Benign prostatic hyperplasia (BPH), 308, 646
Benserazide, 137
Bentyl, 295*t*
Benzocaine, 166*t*
Benzodiazepines
  anesthetics, 151*t*
  antianxiety drugs, 75–76, 76*t*, 78–79
  antiepileptics, 119*t*, 120, 126
  muscle spasms, 180–181, 181*t*
  preoperative medications, 153
  rehabilitation patients, 78–79
  sedative-hypnotics, 69–72, 70*t*, 71*f*, 73–75, 74*t*, 78–79
  tardive dyskinesia, 107–109
Benzoic acid, 32*t*
Benzonatate, 400*t*
Benztropine mesylate, 135*t*, 296
Besifloxacin, 543*t*
Besivance, 543*t*
Beta-1 and -2 receptors, 48, 284*f*, 285–286*t*, 287, 302, 302*t*
Beta-2 agonist, glucocorticoids with, 410–411, 411*t*, 412
Beta-3 receptors, 286*t*, 287
Beta-adrenergic agonists, 305–306
  airway obstruction (COPD), 403–406, 404*f*, 405*t*
  asthma, 403–406, 404*f*, 405*t*
Beta blockers (adrenergic antagonists), 307–313
  antianginals, 338–339, 338*t*, 342, 343
  antiarrhythmics, 353*t*, 354
  antihypertensives, 320–321, 321*t*
  anxiolytic effects, 77
  common, 310*t*
  congestive heart failure, 363*t*, 368–369
  hyperthyroidism, 493–494
  uses according to receptor receptivity, 302*t*
Betaject, 408*t*
Beta-lactam antibiotics, 536
  carbapenems, 536*t*, 538
  cephalosporins, 536*t*, 537
  penicillins, 536–537, 536*t*
Beta-lactamase, 537, 539
Beta-lactamase inhibitors, 536*t*, 539
Betamethasone, 240*t*, 408*t*, 453*t*
Betapace, 310*t*, 311, 321*t*, 338*t*, 353*t*
Betaseron, 569*t*, 570
Betaxolol, 310*t*, 311, 321*t*
Bethanechol, 290, 291*t*, 293
Bevacizumab, 611*t*, 612, 619
Bexarotene, 614*t*, 616
Bextra, 230
Biased agonist, 50
Biaxin, 540*t*
Bicalutamide, 470, 609*t*
BiCNU, 604*t*
Bier block, 170
Biguanides, 518*t*
Bile acid binding drugs, 388*t*, 389
Bile acid sequestrants, 427, 518*t*, 520
Bile salts, 429
Biltricide, 594
Bioavailability, 19
Bioequivalence, 5
Biological response modifiers, 610, 611–612*t*, 612–613
Biotin, 648*t*
Biotransformation, 31–33
Biperiden, 135*t*, 296
Biphasic insulins, 515
Bipolar disorder, 93–95, 106–107
Birth control pill, 480
Bisacodyl, 428*t*
Bismuth salicylate, 426*t*, 427
Bisoprolol, 310*t*, 311, 321*t*, 363*t*
Bisphosphonates, 497*t*, 498*t*, 499–500
Bivalirudin, 341, 378*t*
Bladder atony
  antimuscarinic drugs, 296
  cholinergic stimulants, 292
Bleeding. *See* Hemorrhage
Blennorrhea, 549*t*
Blenoxane, 607*t*
Bleomycin, 607*t*
Blocadren, 310*t*, 311, 321*t*, 338*t*, 353*t*
Blockers. *See* Antagonists; Beta blockers (adrenergic antagonists); Neuromuscular blockers
Blocks. *See* Anesthetic drugs, local
Blood-brain barrier, 61–62
Blood coagulation. *See* Coagulation disorders; Hemostasis
Blood flow, drug distribution and, 23
Blood pressure, 315
  autonomic control, 282
  classification, 316*t*
  normal control, 316
Body temperature, 438, 491
Boldenone, 470*t*
Bolus injection, 384
Bone
  calcitonin's effect on pain, 500
  drug storage in, 24
  glucocorticoid effects on, 456–457
  mineral homeostasis
    case study, 502–503
    drugs, 498*t*, 499–502
    pharmacological control, 497, 499–502
    regulation, 496–497
    rehabilitation patients, 502
    specific bone diseases, 497, 497*t*
Boniva, 498*t*
Bortezomib, 614*t*, 615
Botulinum toxin, 65, 187–191, 188*f*
Bradycardia, 352, 352*t*
Bradykinin, 368
Brain, 59–61, 60*f*
  opioid effects on, 208, 208*f*

Brain-derived neurotrophic factor (BDNF), 85–86
Brainstem, 60
Brain stimulation, Parkinson disease and, 143
Brand (trade) name, 5
Breast cancer, 468, 478, 479, 483
Breast-feeding, drug excretion and, 34
Brethaire, 306, 405*t*
Bretylium (Bretylol), 312
Brevibloc, 310*t*, 311, 321*t*, 353*t*
Brevicon, 481*t*
Brevital sodium, 151*t*
Bricanyl, 306, 405*t*
Brimonidine, 304
Broad-spectrum agents, 533
Bromfenac, 402*t*
Bromocriptine, 140*t*
Brompheniramine, 402*t*
Bronchial asthma. *See* Asthma
Bronchiole smooth muscle, 403, 404*f*
Bronchitis, airway-patency drugs for, 403–410, 405*t*
Bronchodilators, 305, 306, 405*t*, 411*t*
  anticholinergics, 407–408
  beta-adrenergic agonists, 403–406, 405*t*
  xanthine derivatives, 406–407
Bronkaid, 401*t*
Bronkaid Mist, 307
Brovana, 405*t*
B-type natriuretic peptide (BNP), 370
Buccal administration, 16–17, 16*t*
Budesonide, 408, 408*t*, 411*t*, 453*t*
Bulk flow, 22
Bumetanide, 320*t*
Bumex, 320*t*
Bundle of His, 351, 351*f*
Bupivacaine, 166*t*, 264
Buprenex, 205*t*
Buprenorphine, 205*t*, 206, 214, 263*t*
Bupropion, 87*t*, 89*t*, 90, 91*t*
Buspirone (BuSpar), 76
Busulfan (Busulfex), 604*t*
Butamben, 166*t*
Butenafine, 583*t*, 587
Butesin Picrate, 166*t*
Butoconazole, 582*t*
Butorphanol, 151*t*, 157*t*, 205*t*
Butrans patch, 206
Byetta, 518*t*, 519
Bystolic, 310*t*, 311, 321*t*, 369

C

Cabazitaxel, 608*t*
Cabergoline, 140*t*
Caffeine, 406, 406*f*
Calan, 324*t*, 339*t*, 340, 353*t*
Calciferol, 498*t*, 648*t*
Calcijex, 498*t*
Calcimimetics, 501–502
Calcineurin inhibitors, 629, 632
Calciparin, 378*t*
Calcitonin, 496–497, 497*t*, 498*t*, 500–501
Calcitriol, 495, 498*t*, 499
Calcium, 649*t*
  bone mineral homeostasis, 496, 497
  effects of digitalis, 364
  homeostasis and metabolism, 495, 495*f*, 502
Calcium channel blockers
  antianginals, 339–340, 339*t*, 342, 343
  antiarrhythmics, 353*t*, 355
  antihypertensives, 319*t*, 324*t*, 326–327
  tardive dyskinesia, 109
Calcium supplements, 497*t*, 498*t*, 499
Campath, 611*t*
Camptosar, 609*t*
Canakinumab, 633*t*
Cancer chemotherapy, 599–621
  adjuvant therapy, 617
  case study, 620
  combination drugs, 616, 616*t*
  general principles, 600–602
  miscellaneous drugs, 614*t*
  mortality rates, 617*t*
  new strategies, 618–619
  rehabilitation patients, 619–620
  resistance to drugs, 618
  specific drugs, 602–616
  success of drugs, 617–618
  types of drugs
    alkylating agents, 602–603, 603*f*, 604*t*
    antibiotics, 605, 607*t*
    antimetabolites, 603, 605, 605*f*, 606–607*t*
    antimicrotubule agents, 605, 608*t*
    aspirin and other NSAIDs, 613–614
    classification according to cell cycle specificity, 600, 601*f*
    hormones, 608, 609–610*t*, 610
      androgens, 609*t*
      estrogen, 609*t*
      estrogen receptor blockers, 610
      selective estrogen receptor modulators (SERMs), 610
    miscellaneous, 614–616, 614*t*
    platinum coordination complexes, 613, 613*t*
    targeted and biological therapies, 610, 611–612*t*, 612–613
    topoisomerase inhibitors, 608, 609*t*
    tyrosine kinase inhibitors, 611–612*t*
Cancer prevention, aspirin and, 224
Cancer(s), 599
  breast, 468, 478, 479, 483
  hormone sensitive, 608
  prostate, 470
  thyroid, 493
Cancidas, 586
Candesartan, 324*t*, 363*t*, 368
Candida infections, 586–587
Cannabinoids, 430
Cantil, 295*t*
Capastat, 545
Capecitabine, 606*t*
Capoten, 324*t*, 363*t*, 367
Capreomycin, 545
Capsid, 558
Captopril, 324*t*, 363*t*, 367
Carafate, 426
Carbachol, 291*t*
Carbacot, 181*t*
Carbamazepine, 119*t*, 120, 124*t*, 125*t*
Carbapenems, 536*t*, 538
Carbidopa, 135*t*, 137, 137*f*, 139
Carbinoxamine, 402*t*
Carbocaine, 166*t*
Carbohydrate metabolism, 508
Carboplatin, 613*t*
Carboptic, 291*t*
Carcinogens, 599. *See also* Cancer chemotherapy
Carcinomas, 476, 599. *See also* Cancer chemotherapy
Cardene, 324*t*, 339, 339*t*
Cardiac arrhythmias, 349–357
  antiarrhythmics, 352–357, 353*t*
  cardiac action potential, 349–350, 350*f*
  cardiac electrophysiology, 349–351, 350*f*
  conduction system, 351, 351*f*
  mechanisms, 351–352
  nonpharmacological treatment, 355–356
  normal rhythm, 350–351
  types, 352, 352*t*
Cardiovascular system. *See also* Angina pectoris; Cardiac arrhythmias; Congestive heart failure
  antimuscarinic drugs, 296
  effects of aldosterone, 459
  effects of COX-2 drugs, 230
  effects of levodopa, 137–138
  effects of NSAIDs, 225–226
  estrogen and progesterone therapy, 476, 477–478
  thyroid hormones, 491
Cardizem, 324*t*, 339, 339*t*, 353*t*
Cardura, 308, 321*t*, 322
Carisoprodol, 181*t*, 182*t*
Carmustine, 604*t*
Carrier-mediated (active) transport, 21*f*, 22–23
Carteolol (Cartrol), 310*t*, 311, 321*t*, 338*t*, 363*t*
Carvedilol, 310*t*, 311, 321, 321*t*, 338, 338*t*, 363*t*, 369
Casodex, 470
Caspofungin, 586
Cassette system, 264
Castor oil, 428*t*
Catapres, 187, 304, 321*t*, 427
Catechol-O-methyl transferase inhibitors, 135*t*, 142

Cathartics, 428
Caudal block, 168–169, 169*f*
Causalgia, 169–170
C cells, 496
CCNU, 604*t*
Ceclor, 536*t*
Cedax, 536*t*
CeeNU, 604*t*
Cefaclor, 536*t*
Cefadroxil, 536*t*
Cefazolin, 536*t*
Cefdinir, 536*t*
Cefditoren, 536*t*
Cefepime, 536*t*
Cefixime, 536*t*
Cefizox, 536*t*
Cefobid, 536*t*
Cefoperazone, 536*t*
Cefotan, 536*t*
Cefotaxime, 536*t*
Cefotetan, 536*t*
Cefoxitin, 536*t*
Cefpodoxime, 536*t*
Cefprozil, 536*t*
Ceftaroline, 536*t*
Ceftazidime, 536*t*
Ceftibuten, 536*t*
Ceftin, 536*t*
Ceftizoxime, 536*t*
Ceftriaxone, 536*t*
Cefuroxime, 536*t*
Cefzil, 536*t*
Ceiling effect, 10, 10*f*
Celebrex, 227*t*, 229*t*, 230, 240*t*, 241
Celecoxib, 227*t*, 229*t*, 230, 240*t*, 241
Celestone, 240*t*, 408*t*, 453*t*
Celexa, 86*t*, 89*t*
CellCept, 628*t*, 630–631
Cell junction, 22
Cell kill hypothesis, 600
Cell membrane, 19–20, 20*f*
Cellular drug delivery, 26
Cellulitis, 548*t*
Cenestin, 477*t*
Central nervous system (CNS)
  blood-brain barrier, 61–62
  effects of drugs, 64–66, 64*f*
  effects of opioids, 207–208, 207*f*, 208*f*, 209–210
  neurotransmitters, 62–64, 62*t*
  organization, 59–61, 60*f*
  receptors, 155–156, 155*f*
Central venous access device (CVAD), 266, 266*f*
Cephalexin, 536*t*
Cephalosporins, 536*t*, 537
Cerebellum, 60–61, 60*f*
Cerebrum, 59, 60*f*
Cerebyx, 119*t*
Certolizumab, 240*t*, 244*t*, 247
Cerubidine, 607*t*
Cetirizine, 401, 402*t*
Cetuximab, 611*t*
Channel blockers, sodium, 352–354, 353*t*. *See also* Calcium channel blockers
Cheese effect, 92
Chemical names, 5
Chemical synapse, 64–65, 64*f*
Chemotherapy, cancer. *See* Cancer chemotherapy
Chemotherapy-induced nausea and vomiting (CINV), 602
Chenodeoxycholic acid (chenodiol), 430
Chernobyl nuclear accident, 493
Child birth, hormones in, 475
Children, drug metabolism and, 38
Chirocaine, 166*t*
Chloral hydrate, 70*t*
Chlorambucil, 604*t*, 634
Chloramphenicol, 540*t*, 541–542
Chlordiazepoxide, 76*t*
Chloride, 649*t*
Chlorodehydromethyltestosterone, 470*t*
Chloromycetin, 540*t*, 541–542
Chloroprocaine, 166*t*
Chloroquine, 240*t*, 243–244, 243*t*, 245, 588–589, 588*t*
Chlorothiazide, 320*t*
Chlorpheniramine, 402*t*
Chlorpromazine, 103*t*, 104*t*, 105
Chlorpropamide, 518*t*
Chlorthalidone, 320*t*
Chlor-Trimeton, 401*t*, 402*t*
Chlorzoxazone, 181*t*, 182*t*
Cholac, 428*t*
Cholecalciferol, 498*t*
Cholelitholytic drugs, 430
Cholesterol, 448*f*
Cholestyramine, 388*t*, 389, 427
Cholinergic poisoning, 297
Cholinergic receptors, 44, 44*f*, 48, 283*f*, 289–290
  classifications, 284–285, 284*f*
  locations and responses, 285*t*
Cholinergic stimulants, 290–293
  adverse effects, 293
  clinical applications, 292–293
  direct-acting, 290–291, 290*f*, 291*t*
  indirect-acting (cholinesterase inhibitor), 65, 290*f*, 291–292, 291*t*
  mechanism, 290*f*
  specific drugs, 291*t*
Cholinesterase inhibitors (indirect-acting cholinergic stimulants), 65, 290*f*, 291–292, 291*t*, 293
Chondroitin, 252, 644*t*, 645–646
Chromium, 650*t*
Chronic bronchitis, 412
Chronic obstructive pulmonary disease (COPD)
  anticholinergics, 407–408
  drugs for airway patency, 403–410, 405*t*
  glucocorticoids, 408–409, 408*t*
  leukotriene inhibitors, 410
Chronic pain treatment, 92–93, 93*t*
Ciclesonide, 453*t*
Ciclopirox, 583*t*, 587
Cidofovir, 560*t*, 562–563
Cilastatin, 536*t*
Cilostazol, 378*t*, 383
Cimetidine, 157*t*, 407, 423*t*
Cimzia, 240*t*, 244*t*, 247
Cinacalcet, 498*t*, 502
Ciprofloxacin (Cipro), 407, 543–544, 543*t*
Circadian rhythm, 449, 449*f*
Cisatracurium, 158*t*
Cisplatin, 613*t*
Citalopram, 86*t*, 89*t*, 91*t*
Citanest, 166*t*
Citracal, 498*t*
Citrucal, 428*t*
Cladribine, 606*t*
Claforan, 536*t*
Clarinex, 401, 402*t*
Clarithromycin, 540*t*
Claritin, 401, 402*t*
Clavulanate, 536*t*
Clearance, 34
Clemastine, 402*t*
Cleocin, 540*t*, 542
Clevidipine, 324*t*
Cleviprex, 324*t*
Clidinium, 295*t*
Clindamycin, 540*t*, 542
Clinical (human) studies, 6–7, 6*t*
Clinoril, 228*t*, 229*t*, 240*t*
Clobetasol, 453*t*
Clocortolone, 453*t*
Cloderm, 453*t*
Clofarabine, 606*t*
Clofazimine, 543, 543*t*
Clolar, 606*t*
Clomid, 479
Clomiphene, 479
Clomipramine, 86*t*, 91*t*, 93*t*
Clonazepam, 32*t*, 76*t*, 119*t*, 124*t*, 125*t*
Clonidine, 187, 304, 321*t*, 323, 427
Clopidogrel, 341, 378*t*, 382, 383
Clorazepate, 76*t*, 119*t*
Clotrimazole, 582*t*, 586–587
Clotting. *See* Coagulation disorders; Hemostasis
Clotting factors
  for hemophilia, 385–386
  vitamin K-dependent, 379, 379*f*, 386
Cloxacillin, 536*t*
Cloxapen, 536*t*
Clozapine, 103*t*, 104*t*
Clozaril, 104*t*
Coagulation disorders, 377–386, 391–392
  case study, 391
  clotting deficiencies and treatment, 385–386

coagulation mechanism, 376–377, 376f
drug treatment
anticoagulants, 377–381, 378t
antiplatelets, 378f, 381–383
antithrombotics, 378t, 380
fibrinolytics, 378t, 383–385
thrombolytics, 377–380, 378t
rehabilitation patients, 390
Cobalamin, 648t
Cocaine, 166–167
Cocci
infections and treatment, 548–549t
types, 533t
Codeine, 205t, 400, 400t
Cogentin, 135t
Cognex, 291t, 292
Cognitive function, hormone replacement therapy and, 476–477
Colace, 428t
Colesevelam, 388t, 389, 427, 518t, 520
Colestipol (Colistid), 388t, 389, 427
Colistimethate, 538
Colistin, 536t, 538
Colitis, 547t
Coly-Mycin S, 536t
Common cold, treatment for
antihistamines, 401–402, 402t
antitussives, 399–400, 400t
decongestants, 400–401, 401t
mucolytics and expectorants, 402–403
Compazine, 104t
Competitive antagonist, 49–50
Complementary and alternative medications (CAMs), 641–652
case study, 651–652
chemotherapy-induced nausea and vomiting (CINV), 602
minerals, 647, 649–650t
potential adverse effects, 643
problems associated with, 641–642
rehabilitation patients, 650–651
specific CAMs, 643–647, 644t
vitamins, 647, 648t, 649
Complex regional pain syndrome (CRPS), 169–170
Comprehensive Drug Abuse Prevention and Control Act, 9
Comtan, 135t, 142
COMT inhibitors, 135t, 142
Concentration gradient, 20
Congestion, 400–401, 401t
Congestive heart failure, 359–372
case study, 371
drug therapy
agents that decrease cardiac workload, 363t, 367–370
positive inotropic agents, 362, 363t, 364–367
primary drugs, 363t
rehabilitation patients, 371
effects of, 361–362, 362f
vicious cycle, 360–361, 361f
Conjugated estrogens, 477t, 498t
Conjugation, 31, 32, 32t
Constilac, 428t
Constipation, 421
Constulose, 428t
Contraceptives, hormonal
adverse effects, 482–483
mechanism of action, 482
types, 480–482, 481t
Controlled-release preparation, 25
Controlled substances, 9
Convulsions, epileptic, 115
Copper, 650t
Cordarone, 353t
Cordran, 453t
Coreg, 310t, 311, 321t, 338, 338t, 363t, 369
Corgard, 310t, 311, 321t, 338t, 353t
Corlopam, 324, 324t
Corpus luteum, 473–474, 475
Correctol, 428t
Cortef, 240t, 408t, 454t
Corticosteroids. *See* Glucocorticoids (corticosteroids)
Corticotropin-releasing hormone (CRH), 436t, 449, 449f
Cortisol (hydrocortisone), 454t
biosynthesis and structure, 447–449, 448f, 449f
depression, 85
effects, 450–453, 451f
obstructive pulmonary disease, 408t
production, 449–450, 449f
rheumatoid arthritis, 240t
Cortisone, 240t, 408t, 453t
Cortone, 240t, 408t, 453t
Corvert, 353t
Cosmegen, 607t
Co-stimulation, 632–633
Cough, antitussives for, 399–400, 400t
Coumadin, 377, 378t, 379–380
Coumarin drugs, 377, 378t
Cozaar, 324t, 363t
Craniosacral nervous system, 280
Crestor, 387, 388t
Crixivan, 562t, 572
Cromolyn sodium, 409
Cromones, 409
Cruex, 582t
Cryopyrin-associated periodic syndromes (CAPS), 632
Cubicin, 546
Cultivate, 453t
Cumulative (quantal) dose-response curve, 11, 11f
Cuprimine, 240t, 244t, 246–247
Cushing syndrome
drug-induced, 456
glucocorticoids, 454
Cuvposa, 295t
Cyclic adenosine monophosphate (cAMP), 210, 365–366, 403
Cyclic guanosine monophosphate (cGMP), 336
Cyclobenzaprine, 181, 181t, 182t
Cyclocort, 453t
Cyclogyl, 295t
Cyclomen, 469t
Cyclooxygenase (COX) enzymes, 220
COX-2 selective drugs, 229–230
adverse side effects, 230
cancer, 613
cardiovascular risks, 225–226, 230
osteoarthritis, 227
rheumatoid arthritis, 241
COX-3, 231
NSAIDs' inhibition of, 222–223, 231
Cyclopentolate, 295t
Cyclophosphamide, 240t, 249, 604t, 616, 628t, 629
Cycloserine, 536t, 538
Cyclosporine, 240t, 243t, 249, 520, 628t, 629
Cycrin, 477t
Cyklokapron, 386
Cymbalta, 77t, 86t, 89t, 93t
Cyproheptadine, 402t
Cystic fibrosis
digestion problems, 429
respiratory problems, 412–413
Cystospaz, 295t
Cytadren, 457
Cytarabine, 606t
Cytokines, 611t, 612, 635
Cytomel, 494t
Cytosar-U, 606t
Cytosolic hormone receptors, 441f, 442–443
Cytotec, 225, 426
Cytovene, 560t, 564–565
Cytoxan, 240t, 249, 604t, 628t, 629

D

Dabigatran, 378t, 380
Dacarbazine, 604t
Daclizumab, 632, 633t
Dactinomycin, 607t
Dalacin, 540t
Dalfopristin, 540t, 542
Dalmane, 70t, 74t
Dalteparin, 378, 378t
Danazol, 469t
Danocrine, 469t
Dantrium, 183t, 185–186, 186f
Dantrolene, 32t, 191
Dantrolene sodium, 183t, 185–186, 186f
Dapsone, 543, 543t
Daptomycin, 546
Daraprim, 590

Darbeptoetin, 468
Darifenacin, 295*t*
Darunavir, 562*t*, 572
Darvon, 205*t*
Daunorubicin, 607*t*
DaunoXome, 607*t*
Dayhist, 402*t*
Daypro, 228*t*, 229*t*, 240*t*
Decadron, 240*t*, 453*t*
Deca-Durabolin, 470*t*, 471*t*
Decarboxylase, peripheral inhibitor, 136–137, 137*f*
Declomycin, 540*t*
Decongestants, 400–401, 401*t*
Deep vein thrombosis (DVT). *See* Venous thrombosis
Degarelix, 470
Delatestryl, 469*t*
Delavirdine, 562*t*, 566, 572–573
Delta opioid receptor, 203*t*
Deltasone, 240*t*
Demadex, 320*t*
Demeclocycline, 540*t*
Demerol, 151*t*, 204*t*
Demser, 312
Demulen, 481*t*
Denavir, 560*t*, 564
Denileukin Diftitox, 614*t*, 615
Denosumab, 498*t*, 502
Deoxyribonucleases, 413
Deoxyribonucleic acid. *See* DNA
Depacon, 119*t*
Depakene, 119*t*
Depakote, 119*t*
Depen, 240*t*, 244*t*
Dependence
  opioid analgesics, 212–213
  sedative-hypnotics, 74–75
DepoCyt, 606*t*
Depolarizing blockers, 158*t*, 159
Depo-Provera, 481, 481*t*
Depo-Testosterone, 469*t*
Depot administration, 106
Deprenyl, 141–142
Depression, 83–86. *See also* Antidepressant drugs
  bipolar disorder, 93–95
  drug treatment, 86–95
  pathophysiology, 84–86
  rehabilitation patients, 95–96
Dermacort, 454*t*
Dermatop, 454*t*
Dermovate, 453*t*
Desensitization of receptors, 51, 51*f*, 52
Deserpidine, 312
Desflurane, 151*t*
Desipramine, 86*t*, 91*t*
Desirudin, 378*t*
Desloratadine, 401, 402*t*
Desogen, 481*t*
Desogestrel, 481*t*
Desonide, 453*t*
DesOwen, 453*t*
Desoximatasone, 453*t*
Desoxyn, 306
Desvenlafaxine, 86*t*, 89*t*, 91*t*
Desyrel, 87*t*, 89*t*, 90, 93*t*
Detemir, 514*t*
Detrol, 295*t*
Dexamethasone, 240*t*, 408*t*, 443, 453*t*
Dexchlorpheniramine, 402*t*
Dexedrine, 306
Dexlansoprazole, 424, 424*t*
Dexmedetomidine, 152*t*, 154, 156
DexPak, 408*t*, 453*t*
Dextroamphetamine, 306
Dextromethorphan, 400*t*
D. H. E. 45, 308–309
DiaBeta, 518*t*
Diabetes insipidus, 510
Diabetes mellitus, 510–523
  agents for type 2 diabetes, 517, 518*t*, 519–520
  case study, 523
  complications, 512–513
  insulin preparations, 513–515, 514*t*
  insulin therapy, 513–517, 518*t*
  nonpharmacological treatment, 521–522
  rehabilitation patiènts, 522
  type 1 and type II compared, 511–512, 511*t*
  type 1 prevention, 520–521
Diabinese, 518*t*
Dianabol, 470*t*, 471*t*
Diarrhea, 421
Diastole, 350
Diastolic heart failure, 360–361
Diazepam
  anxiety, 75–76, 76*t*
  biotransformation of, 32*t*
  chemical structure, 75*f*
  epilepsy, 119*t*
  general anesthesia, 151*t*
  muscle spasms, 180–181, 181*t*
  preoperative use, 157*t*
  spasticity, 183*t*, 186, 191
Diazoxide, 324, 324*t*
Dibenzyline, 309, 321*t*
Dibucaine, 166*t*
Diclofenac, 227*t*, 229*t*, 240*t*, 251
Dicyclomine, 295*t*
Didanosine, 562*t*, 566, 572
Didronel, 498*t*, 500
Diencephalon, 60, 60*f*
Diet
  diabetes mellitus, 521
  effects on drug response, 38
  hypertension, 328
  rheumatoid arthritis, 250
Dietary supplements. *See* Complementary and alternative medications (CAMs)
Diethylcarbamazine, 593*t*, 594
Diethylstilbestrol, 609*t*
Differential nerve block, 171–172, 171*t*
Diffusion
  between cell junctions, 22
  facilitated, 21*f*, 23
  passive, 20–22, 21*f*
Diffusion trapping, 21–22
Diflorasone, 453*t*
Diflucan, 584
Diflunisal, 227*t*, 229*t*, 240*t*
Difluprednate, 453*t*
Diflupyl, 291*t*
Digestant drugs, 429
Digitalis glycosides
  adverse effects, 365, 366*t*
  cardiac arrhythmias, 355
  congestive heart failure, 362–364, 365*f*
  effects and mechanism of action, 364, 365*f*
Digitek, 363*t*
Digitoxin, 362
Digoxin, 362, 363*t*
Dihydroergotamine, 308–309
Dihydropyridines, 327, 339–340, 355
Dihydrotestosterone, 470
Diiodotyrosine, 489, 490*f*
Dilacor, 324*t*, 339, 339*t*, 353*t*
Dilantin, 119*t*, 120
Dilaudid, 204*t*
Dilaudid Cough, 400*t*
Dilor, 407*t*
Diltiazem, 324*t*, 327, 339, 339*t*, 353*t*, 355
Dimenhydrinate, 402*t*, 430
Dimetapp Allergy, 402*t*
Diovan, 324*t*, 363*t*
Dipeptidyl peptidase (DPP)-4 inhibitors, 518*t*, 519
Diphenhydramine, 135*t*, 400*t*, 402*t*
Diphenoxylate, 426*t*, 427
Diphosphonates. *See* Bisphosphonates
Diphtheria, 547*t*
Diprivan, 152*t*, 153–154
Diprolene, 453*t*
Dipyridamole, 378*t*, 383
Diquinol, 591
Direct renin inhibitor, 326, 363*t*, 368
Disease, effects on drug response, 37
Disease-modifying antirheumatic drugs (DMARDs), 239, 242–250, 243–244*t*
  biological, 244*t*, 247–249
  combination drugs, 249–250
  glucocorticoid supplementation, 241
  other DMARDs, 249
  specific drugs, 240*t*, 243–244*t*
  traditional (nonbiological), 243–244*t*, 243–247
Disease-modifying osteoarthritic drugs (DMOADs), 251
Disinhibition, 63

Disopyramide, 353*t*
Dissociative anesthesia, 153
Ditropan, 295*t*
Diucardin, 320*t*
Diuretics
  adverse effects, 319–320
  antihypertensives, 318–320, 319*t*, 320*t*
  congestive heart failure, 363*t*, 369–370
Diuril, 320*t*
Divalproex, 119*t*
DNA
  bacterial, 535
  effects of alkylating agents, 602, 603*f*
DNA viruses, 557, 558*t*
Dobutamine, 305, 363*t*, 366–367
Dobutrex, 305, 363*t*
Docetaxel, 605, 608*t*
Docosanol, 560*t*, 563
Docusate, 428*t*
Dofetilide, 353*t*
Dolasetron, 602
Dolobid, 227*t*, 229*t*, 240*t*
Dolutegravir, 562*t*, 563, 573
Donepezil, 291*t*, 292
Dopa decarboxylase, 136, 136*f*
Dopamine, 62*t*, 63, 305
  blockers, 430
  congestive heart failure, 363*t*, 366–367
  Parkinson disease, 132–133
  schizophrenia and antipsychotics, 102–105, 104*f*
  synthesis, 136, 136*f*
Dopamine agonists, for Parkinson disease, 140–141, 140*t*, 143
Dopar, 135*t*
Doral, 70*t*, 74*t*
Doribax, 536*t*
Doripenem, 536*t*
Dornase alfa, 413
Dosage
  median effective, 11, 11*f*
  median lethal, 12
  median toxic, 11–12, 11*f*
  patient-controlled analgesia (PCA), 262–263, 263*t*
  schedule and plasma concentration, 35–36, 35*f*
Dose error reduction system (DERS), 264, 264*t*
Dose-response curve, 9–10, 10*f*
  quantal, 11, 11*f*
  receptors and, 48–49
Dostinex, 140*t*
Down-regulation of receptors, 51–52, 51*f*
Doxacurium, 158*t*
Doxazosin, 308, 321*t*, 322
Doxazosin gastrointestinal therapeutic system (GITS), 322
Doxepin, 87*t*, 91*t*, 93*t*
Doxercalciferol, 498*t*
Doxorubicin, 607*t*, 616
Doxycycline, 540*t*
Doxylamine, 402*t*
DPI (dry powder inhaler), 405
Dramamine, 402*t*
Drenison, 453*t*
Drisdol, 498*t*
Dristan 12-Hr Nasal Spray, 401*t*
Drixoral, 303
Dronedarone, 353*t*, 355
Droperidol, 153, 263
Drospirenone, 481*t*
Drostanolone, 470*t*
Droxia, 614*t*
Drug infusion. *See* Patient-controlled analgesia (PCA)
Drug microsomal metabolizing system (DMMS), 32, 32*f*
Drug-receptor interaction, 43, 46–47
Drug receptors, 43–53
  interactions, 43, 46–51
  intracellular receptors, 46
  regulation, 51–52, 51*f*
  surface receptors, 43–46
Drug reservoir, 25–26
Drug(s)
  absorption across cell membrane, 19–23
  administration, 15–19, 16*t*
  basic concepts of therapy, 9–11
  central nervous system and, 59–62
  classification, 49
  definition of, 3
  delivery of
    newer techniques of, 25–26
    targeted, 26
  development and approval, 6–9, 6*t*
  distribution within body, 23–24
  elimination, 31–39
  interactions, 37
  nomenclature, 4–5, 5*t*
  nonreceptor-mediated mechanisms, 52
  orphan, 7–8
  over-the-counter (OTC), 8–9
  safety, 11–12
  schedules, 9
  selectivity, 47–48, 48*f*
  storage in body, 24–25
  testing, 6*t*
  variations in response, 36–39
Dry powder inhaler (DPI), 405
DTIC-Dome, 604*t*
Dulcolax, 428*t*
Dulera, 411*t*
Duloxetine, 77*t*, 86*t*, 89*t*, 91*t*, 93*t*
Duraclon, 304
Duragesic patch, 206
Duranest, 166*t*
Durezol, 453*t*
Duricef, 536*t*
Dutasteride, 470
Duvoid, 291*t*
DynaCirc, 324*t*, 339, 339*t*
Dynapen, 536*t*
Dynorphins, 202
Dyphylline, 407*t*
Dyrenium, 320*t*
Dyskinesias
  antipsychotics, 109
  levodopa, 138
Dysmenorrhea, 222
Dystonias
  antipsychotics, 108*f*, 109
  muscle relaxants, 189

E

Echinacea, 644, 644*t*
Echinocandins, 586
Echothiophate, 291*t*
Econazole, 582*t*
Edarbi, 324*t*
Edecrin, 320*t*
Edrophonium, 291*t*
Efalizumab, 633*t*
Efavirenz, 562*t*, 566, 572–573
Effexor, 77*t*, 86*t*, 89*t*
Efficacy, 49
Effient, 341, 378*t*, 382
Effort angina. *See* Stable angina
Efudex, 606*t*
Eicosanoids, 220
  NSAIDs' inhibition of, 222–223
  physiological effects, 220–222, 221*t*
  synthesis, 220, 221*f*
Elavil, 86*t*, 93*t*
Eldepryl, 135*t*, 141–142
Electrolytes, antacids and, 422–423
Elidel, 632
Elimination, drug, 31–39
  biotransformation, 31–33
  excretion, 33–34, 34*f*
  plasma concentration, 35–36, 36*f*
  rates, 34–35
Eliphos, 498*t*
Eliquis, 378*t*, 380
Elixohyllin, 407*t*
Ella, 481*t*, 482
Ellence, 607*t*
Elocon, 454*t*
Eloxatin, 613*t*
Elspar, 614*t*, 615
Elvitegravir, 562*t*, 563
Emcyt, 614*t*, 615
Emend, 602
Emergency contraceptives, 481–482
Emesis, 421
Emetic drugs, 429
Emphysema, 412
  drugs for airway patency, 403–410, 405*t*
Emsam, 142
Emtricitabine, 562*t*, 566, 572
Emtriva, 562*t*, 566, 572
E-Mycin, 540*t*

Enablex, 295*t*
Enalapril, 324*t*, 363*t*, 367
Enbrel, 240*t*, 244*t*, 247, 632, 633*t*
Endep, 86*t*, 93*t*
Endocarditis, 548*t*
Endocrine system
  clinical use of endocrine drugs, 443–444
  feedback control, 440–441, 440*f*
  glands and hormones, 435–439, 436*f*, 436*t*, 437*t*
  glucocorticoid treatment of disorders, 454
  hormone effects on target cell, 441–443, 441*f*
  hormone receptors, 441–442, 441*f*
  hormone synthesis and release, 440
  hormone transport, 441
  pancreas, 438
  parathyroid, 438
  physiology and pharmacology, 439–443
  thyroid, 437–438
Endocytosis, 21*f*, 23
End-of-dose akinesia, 139
Endometriosis, 476
Endorphins, 202
Enduron, 320*t*
Enflurane, 151*t*
Enfuvirtide, 562*t*, 563–564, 573
Enjuvia, 477*t*
Enkephalins, 62*t*, 202
Enlon, 291*t*
Enoxaparin, 341, 378, 378*t*
Entacapone, 135*t*, 142
Entecavir, 560*t*
Enteral administration, 15–17, 16*t*
Enteric-coated aspirin, 225
Enteric nervous system, 279
Entocort, 453*t*
Enzymes
  induction, 33, 642
  surface receptors, 44, 45*f*
Ephedra, 642
Ephedrine, 306–307, 401*t*
Epidural nerve blockade, 168–169, 169*f*
Epigenetic modification, 615
Epilepsy, 115
Epileptic seizures. *See also* Antiepileptic drugs
  classification of, 116–117, 116*t*
  initiation and spread of, 117*f*
  rational of drug treatment for, 117–118
Epinephrine, 282, 301, 302, 306, 307, 405*t*
  effects of, 437*t*, 439
Epirubicin, 607*t*
Epivir, 562*t*, 566, 572
Eplerenone, 369, 460
Epoetin, 468
Epsom salts, 428*t*
Epstein-Barr virus, 561
Eptifibatide, 341, 378*t*, 382, 383
Equipoise, 470*t*
Eraxis, 586
Erbitux, 611*t*
Ergocalciferol, 498*t*
Ergoloid mesylate, 309
Ergomar, 308–309
Ergometrine, 308–309
Ergonovine, 308–309
Ergot alkaloids, 308–309
Ergotamine, 308–309
Ergotrate, 308–309
Erlotinib, 611*t*, 613
Ertaczo, 583*t*
Ertapenem, 536*t*
Eryc, 540*t*
Erythromycin, 540–541, 540*t*
Erythropoietin, 468
Escitalopram, 77*t*, 86*t*, 89*t*, 91*t*
Eserine, 291*t*
Esmolol, 310*t*, 311, 321*t*, 353*t*
Esomeprazole, 424, 424*t*
Estazolam, 70*t*, 74*t*
Esterified estrogens, 477*t*
Estrace, 477*t*, 498*t*
Estradiol, 465, 477*t*, 498*t*, 609*t*. *See also* Estrogen
  biosynthesis and structure, 448*f*
Estramustine, 614*t*, 615
Estratab, 477*t*
Estrogen, 465, 472–475, 498*t*
  adverse effects, 477–488
  antineoplastic indications, 609*t*
  clinical use, 475–477, 477*t*, 501
  effects, 437*t*, 439
  menstrual cycle, 473–475, 474*f*
  receptor blockers, 610
  replacement for bone loss, 457, 497*t*
Estropipate, 477*t*, 498*t*
Eszopiclone, 70*t*, 74*t*
Etanercept, 240*t*, 244*t*, 247, 248*f*, 632, 633*t*
Ethacrynic acid, 320*t*
Ethambutol, 536*t*, 538
Ethanol, sedative effects of, 73
Ethinyl estradiol, 480, 481*t*
Ethionamide, 540*t*, 542
Ethosuximide, 119*t*, 121, 124*t*, 125*t*
Ethrane, 151*t*
Ethynodiol diacetate, 481*t*
Etidocaine, 166*t*
Etidronate, 498*t*, 500
Etodolac, 227*t*, 229*t*, 240*t*
Etomidate, 152*t*, 154
Etonogestrel, 477*t*, 481*t*
Etoposide, 609*t*
Etravirine, 562*t*, 566, 572–573
Eulexin, 470
Everolimus, 628*t*, 631
Evista, 478–479, 498*t*, 501
Excretion, drug, 31, 33–34, 34*f*
Exelderm, 583*t*
Exelon, 291*t*, 292
Exemestane, 609*t*, 610
Exenatide, 518*t*, 519
Ex-Lax, 428*t*
Exocytosis, 23, 560
Expectorant drugs, 402–403
Extavia, 569*t*
Extended-release preparation, 25
Extraction ratio, 34
Extrapyramidal side effects, antipsychotics and, 107, 108
Exubera, 515
Eye
  antimuscarinic drugs, 297
  drops for, 292, 297
  infections of, 547*t*, 548*t*
Ezetimibe, 388*t*, 389
Ezetrol, 388*t*

F

Facilitated diffusion, 21*f*, 23
Factive, 543*t*
Factor Xa inhibitors, 377, 378*t*, 380
Famciclovir, 560*t*, 564
Famotidine, 423*t*
Famvir, 560*t*, 564
Fanapt, 104*t*
Fansidar, 590
Fareston, 478
Faslodex, 479
"Fast track" drug development, 7
Fat cells, 450*f*. *See also* Adipose tissue
Feen-A-Mint, 428*t*
Felbamate (Felbatol), 121–122, 122*t*, 125*t*
Feldene, 228*t*, 229*t*, 240*t*
Felodipine, 324*t*, 339, 339*t*
Femara, 610
FemCare, 582*t*
Femcon FE, 481*t*
Femtrace, 477*t*, 498*t*
Fenofibrate, 388, 388*t*
Fenoldopam, 324, 324*t*
Fenoprofen, 227*t*, 229*t*, 240*t*
Fentanyl, 153, 157*t*, 204*t*, 206, 207, 263, 263*t*, 268
Fentanyl derivatives, 151*t*
Fesoterodine, 295*t*
Fetal cells, Parkinson disease and, 143
Fever
  aspirin and, 224
  eicosanoids' effects on, 222
Fexofenadine, 401, 402*t*
Fiberall, 428*t*
Fiber Lax, 428*t*
Fibric acids (fibrates), 388–389, 388*t*
Fibricor, 388*t*
Fibrin, 377
Fibrinolysin, 377
Fibrinolytics, 377, 378*t*, 383–385
Fight-or-flight, 281, 439

Finasteride, 470
Firmagon, 470
5-FU, 606*t*
First-pass effect, 16
Flagyl, 543*t*, 544, 591–592
Flaxedil, 158*t*
Flecainide, 353*t*
Fleet Glycerin Laxative, 428*t*
Fleet Mineral Oil, 428*t*
Fleet Phospho-Soda, 428*t*
Flexeril, 181*t*
Flomax, 309
Flonase, 453*t*
Florinef, 459
Florone, 453*t*
Flovent Diskus, 453*t*
Floxin, 543*t*
Floxuridine, 606*t*
Fluconazole, 582*t*, 584
Flucytosine, 584–585
Fludara, 606*t*
Fludarabine, 606*t*
Fludrocortisone, 459
Flumadine, 560*t*, 561–562
Flunisolide, 408, 408*t*, 453*t*
Fluocin, 453*t*
Fluocinolone, 453*t*
Fluoride, 650*t*
Fluorometholone, 453*t*
Fluor-Op, 453*t*
Fluoroplex, 606*t*
Fluoroquinolones, 543–544, 543*t*
Fluorouracil, 606*t*, 616
Fluothane, 151*t*
Fluoxetine, 86*t*, 89*t*, 91*t*, 93*t*
Fluoxymesterone, 469*t*, 470*t*, 609*t*
Fluphenazine, 103*t*, 104*t*
Flurandrenolide, 453*t*
Flurazepam, 70*t*, 74*t*
Flurbiprofen, 228*t*, 240*t*
Flutamide, 470, 609*t*, 610
Fluticasone, 411*t*, 453*t*
Fluvastatin, 388*t*
Fluvoxamine, 86*t*, 89*t*, 91*t*
FML S.O.P., 453*t*
Folex, 246, 628*t*, 630
Folic acid, 246, 535, 535*f*, 603, 648*t*
Follicle-stimulating hormone (FSH), 436*t*, 465–466, 466*f*
Follicular development, 473, 474*f*
Folotyn, 607*t*
Fondaparinux, 341, 378*t*, 380
Food and Drug Administration (FDA), drug development and approval process of, 6–9, 6*t*
Food-drug interactions, 38
Foradil, 405*t*
Forane, 151*t*
Formoterol, 405*t*, 411*t*
Fortaz, 536*t*
Forteo, 498*t*, 501
Fortical, 498*t*, 500
Fortovase, 562*t*, 572
Fosamax, 498*t*, 499
Fosamprenavir, 562*t*, 572
Fosaprepitant, 602
Foscarnet (Foscavir), 560*t*, 564
Fosfomycin, 536*t*, 539
Fosinopril, 324*t*, 363*t*
Fosphenytoin, 119*t*, 126
Fospropofol, 152*t*
Fragmin, 378, 378*t*
Free radicals, 619
FUDR, 606*t*
Fukushima nuclear accident, 493
Fulvestrant, 479, 609*t*, 610
Fulvicin, 585
Fungi, 581
Fungizone, 584
Furadantin, 546
Furosemide, 320*t*
Fusion proteins, 632–633, 633*t*
Fuzeon, 562*t*, 563–564, 573

G

Gabapentin, 122, 122*t*, 124*t*, 125*t*, 183*t*, 186–187
Gabitril, 122*t*, 123
Galantamine, 291*t*, 292
Gallamine, 158*t*, 293
Gallstones, 430
Gamimune, 634–635
Gamma-aminobutyric acid (GABA)
  anesthesia and, 155
  antiepileptics and, 122
  benzodiazepines and, 70–71, 71*f*
  effects on central nervous system, 62*t*, 63
  muscle relaxants and, 180, 183
  in receptor-ion channel system, 44
  role in schizophrenia, 102
Gammagard, 634–635
Ganciclovir, 560*t*, 564–565
Ganglionic blockers, 321*t*, 323
Gantrisin, 543*t*
Garamycin, 540*t*
Garlic, 644–645, 644*t*
Gas gangrene, 547*t*
Gastric acids, 421
Gastroesophageal reflux, 421, 423
Gastrointestinal drugs, 421–431
  antacids, 422–423
  antidiarrheal agents, 426–428, 426*t*
  antimuscarinic anticholinergics, 294–296
  case study, 430–431
  H_2 receptors blockers, 157*t*, 423, 423*t*
  H. Pylori infection, 425
  laxatives and cathartics, 428–429, 428*t*
  miscellaneous drugs, 429–430
  other agents for gastric ulcers, 425–426
  proton pump inhibitors, 423–425, 424*t*
  rehabilitation patients, 430
Gastrointestinal tract (GI), 421
  drug excretion, 34
  effects of levodopa, 137
  effects of NSAIDs, 224–225
  gastric acidity and secretion, 421
  intestinal peristalsis, 292
Gaucher disease, 498*t*
Gefitinib, 611*t*, 613
Gemcitabine, 606*t*
Gemfibrozil, 388, 388*t*, 389
Gemifloxacin, 543*t*
Gemtuzumab, 611*t*
Gemzar, 606*t*
Gender and effects on drug response, 38–39
General anesthetics. *See under* Anesthetic drugs
Generic drugs, substitution of, 5–6
Generic name, 5
Gene therapy
  cystic fibrosis, 413
  diabetes mellitus, 521–522
Genetic polymorphisms, 36
Genetics
  arrhythmias, 351
  and effects on drug response, 36–37
  Parkinson disease and, 133–134
Gengraf, 629
Genital infection, 548*t*
Genora, 481*t*
Gentamicin, 540*t*
Geodon, 105*t*
Gesterol, 477*t*
Ghrelin, 507
Ginger, 644*t*, 645
Ginkgo biloba, 644*t*, 645
Ginseng, 644*t*, 645
Glargine, 514*t*
Glaucoma, 290, 292
Gleevec, 612*t*, 613
Gliadel, 604*t*
Glimepiride, 518*t*
Glipizide, 518*t*
Glitazones, 519–520
Glucagon, 437*t*, 438, 509–510
Glucagon-like peptide (GLP) 1, 519
  receptor agonists, 518*t*, 519
Glucocorticoids (corticosteroids), 444, 447, 449–457, 453–454*t*. *See also* Adrenocorticosteroids
  adverse effects, 455–457
  asthma, 408–409, 408*t*, 410–411
  circadian rhythm release, 449–450, 449*f*
  clinical uses, 453–455
  COPD-related respiratory problems, 408–409, 408*t*, 412
  cystic fibrosis-related respiratory problems, 412
  depression, 85
  immunosuppressants, 628*t*, 629–630, 632
  mechanism of action, 450

nonendocrine disorders, 454–455, 455*t*
physiological effects, 437*t*, 438–439, 450–453, 451*f*
rheumatoid arthritis, 239, 240*t*, 241–242
route of administration, 454–455
specific drugs, 453–454*t*
synthesis, 449, 449*f*
Gluconeogenesis, 509
Glucophage, 518*t*, 519
Glucosamine, 252, 644*t*, 645–646
Glucose
effects of insulin, 510
metabolism, 450–451, 451*f*
transporters, 509, 509*f*
Glucose transporter (GLUT) proteins, 509, 509*f*
Glucotrol, 518*t*
Glulisine, 514*t*
Glutamate, 62*t*, 63, 102, 213
Glutathione (GHS), 231, 231*f*
Glyburide, 518*t*
Glycerin, 428*t*
Glycine, 62*t*, 63, 155
Glycoprotein (GP) IIb-IIIa receptor inhibitors, 378*t*, 382–383
Glycoprotein pump, 618
Glycopyrrolate, 157*t*, 295*t*
Glycosuria, 512
Glyset, 518*t*, 520
Goiter. *See also* Thyroid
enlarged, 494
toxic, 492–493
Gold compounds, 243*t*, 245
Gold sodium thiomalate, 240*t*, 243*t*, 245
Golimumab, 240*t*, 244*t*, 247
Gonadotropin-releasing hormone (GnRH), 436*t*
androgen synthesis, 466
anti-cancer drugs, 470, 610*t*
Goserelin, 470, 610*t*
G protein-coupled receptors (GPCRs), 45, 459
G proteins, 44–46, 46*f*, 209–210, 212
Gradient, diffusion, 20
Gram-negative and -positive bacilli, 533*t*, 547–548*t*
Gram-negative and -positive cocci, 533*t*, 548–549*t*
Grand mal seizures, 116*t*
Granisetron, 157*t*, 602
Granisol, 602
Grapefruit juice, 38
Graves disease, 492–493
Grisactin, 585
Griseofulvin, 582*t*, 585
Growth and development, 491
Growth fraction, 600
Growth hormone, 436*t*
Growth hormone-releasing hormone (GHRH), 436*t*, 437
Guaifenesin, 403
Guanabenz, 304, 321*t*, 323
Guanethidine, 312
Guanfacine, 304, 321*t*, 323
Guanine, 603*f*
Gyne-Lotrimin, 582*t*
Gynezole-1, 582*t*
Gynodiol, 477*t*

H

H_2 blockers, 225
H_2 receptor blockers, 157*t*, 423, 423*t*
H_2 receptors, 401
H_3 receptor, 401
H_4 receptor, 401
HAART (highly active antiretroviral therapy), 573–574
Halcinonide, 453*t*
Halcion, 70*t*, 74*t*
Haldol, 104*t*
Half-life, 35, 35*f*
Halobetasol, 453*t*
Halog, 453*t*
Haloperidol, 103*t*, 104*t*
Halotestin, 469*t*, 470*t*
Halothane, 151*t*, 155
Harmonyl, 312
Health Products and Food Branch (Canada), 6
Heart. *See also* Congestive heart failure
cardiac action potentials, 349–350, 350*f*
conduction system, 351, 351*f*
normal rhythm, 350–351
Heart attack, 230, 322
Heart disease. *See* Angina pectoris; Congestive heart failure; Heart attack
Heavy metal compounds (platinum coordination complexes), 613, 613*t*
Hectorol, 498*t*
Helicobacter pylori, 422, 423, 425
Helminths, infections of, 593, 593*t*
Hemophilia, 385–386
Hemorrhage
anticoagulant drugs, 380
fibrinolytics, 385
Hemostasis, 375–377. *See also* Coagulation disorders
Heparin
angina pectoris, 341
coagulation disorders, 377–379, 378*t*
heparin-induced thrombocytopenia (HIT), 380–381
low molecular weight heparins (LWMH), 341, 378–379
Heparin lock, 377
Hepatitis, 570
Hepsera, 560*t*
Herbal remedies. *See* Complementary and alternative medications (CAMs)
Herceptin, 611*t*
Hetrazan, 594
Hexalen, 604*t*
Hexastat, 604*t*
High-density lipoproteins (HDLs), 387
Highly active antiretroviral therapy (HAART), 573–574
Hiprex, 546
Hirudin, 341
Histamine, 401
Histone deacetylase inhibitors, 614*t*, 615
HIV. *See* Human immunodeficiency virus (HIV)
HIV entry inhibitors, 573
HIV integrase, 563, 573
HIV protease, 565
HMG-CoA reductase inhibitors (statins), 387–388, 388*t*
adverse effects, 389–390
Homatropine, 295*t*
Hormone replacement therapy (HRT), 443
androgens, 467
estrogen and progesterone, 475–478
estrogen, for bone mineral homeostasis, 501
glucocorticoids, 454
mineralocorticoids, 459
thyroid hormones, 494
Hormone(s), 435. *See also* Endocrine system; Steroids
androgens, 465–467
abuse, 470–472, 470*t*
clinical use, 467–470, 469*t*
cancer treatment and (*See under* Cancer chemotherapy)
chemistry of, 439–440
definition of, 435
as drug therapy, 444
effects on target cell, 441–443, 441*f*
estrogen and progesterone, 472–475
pharmacological use, 475–478
hypothalamus, 436*t*
male and female, 465–475, 484
case study, 483–484
contraceptives, 480–483, 481*t*
rehabilitation patients, 484
other endocrine glands, 437–439, 437*t*
pancreatic, 437*t*
parathyroid, 437*t*, 495, 495*f*
peptide, 439
pituitary gland, 436–437, 436*t*
receptors, 46, 441–443, 441*f*
synthesis and release, 440
thyroid, 437*t*, 489–492, 494*t*
transport, 441
Hospital-acquired infections, 547*t*, 548*t*
H. Pylori.*See**Helicobacter pylori*
H. pylori infection, 425
Humalog, 514*t*
Human chorionic gonadotropin (HCG), 475
Human immunodeficiency virus (HIV)
case study, 576–577
clotting factor and, 386

enfuvirtide, 563
inhibitors, 562*t*
opportunistic infections, 574–575, 575*t*
protease inhibitors, 565
rehabilitation patients, 576
replication, 566–567, 567*f*
reverse transcriptase inhibitors (RTIs), 566
treatment for muscle wasting, 468
treatment of AIDS, 562, 564, 571–575
Human studies, 6–7, 6*t*
Humatin, 592
Humira, 240*t*, 244*t*, 247, 632, 633*t*
Humulin, 514*t*
Hyaluronan, 252
Hycamtin, 609*t*
Hycodan, 205*t*, 400*t*
Hydantoins, 119*t*, 120
Hydralazine, 324, 324*t*, 363*t*, 370
Hydrea, 614*t*, 615
Hydrochloric acid, antacids and, 422*f*
Hydrochlorothiazide, 320*t*
Hydrocodone, 205*t*, 400*t*
Hydrocortisone. *See* Cortisol (hydrocortisone)
Hydroflumethiazide, 320*t*
Hydrolysis, 31, 32, 32*t*
Hydromorphone, 204*t*, 263*t*, 400*t*
Hydromox, 320*t*
Hydrostat, 204*t*
Hydroxychloroquine, 240*t*, 243–244, 243*t*, 245, 589
Hydroxyprogesterone, 477*t*, 609*t*
Hydroxyurea, 614*t*, 615
Hydroxyzine, 157*t*, 402*t*
Hygroton, 320*t*
Hylutin, 477*t*
Hyoscyamine, 295*t*
Hyperaldosteronism, 460
Hyperalgesia, opioid-induced, 213–214
Hypercalcemia, 498*t*, 499
Hyperfibrinolysis, 386
Hyperglycemia, 510, 512
Hyperlipidemia, 375, 387–390, 388*t*, 391–392
Hyperosmotic laxatives, 429
Hyperparathyroidism, 497*t*
Hyperstat, 324, 324*t*
Hypertension, 315, 330. *See also* Antihypertensive drugs
angiotensin II, 325–326
blood pressure classification, 316*t*
case study, 329–330
drug therapy, 318–327
nonpharmacologic treatment, 328
pathogenesis, 316–318
possible mechanisms, 317–318, 318*f*
rehabilitation patients, 329
secondary, 316
Hyperthyroidism, 492–494, 502
symptoms, 492*t*
types, 492*t*
Hypnotic drugs. *See* Sedative-hypnotic agents
Hypoglycemia, 510, 516
Hypogonadism, 475
Hypokalemia, 320
Hypoparathyroidism, 497*t*
Hypotension, 110, 138, 322
Hypothalamus, 60, 436–437, 436*f*
Hypothyroidism, 494, 502
symptoms, 492*t*
thyroid hormone preparations, 494*t*
types, 492*t*
Hytrin, 309, 321*t*, 322

I

Ibandronate, 498*t*
Ibritumomab, 611*t*
Ibuprofen, 32*t*, 228*t*, 229*t*, 240*t*
Ibutilide, 353*t*
Idamycin, 607*t*
Idarubicin, 607*t*
IFEX, 604*t*
Ifosfamide, 604*t*
Ilaris, 633*t*
Iloperidone, 103*t*, 104*t*
Imatinib, 612*t*, 613
Iminostilbenes, 119*t*, 120
Imipenem, 536*t*, 538
Imipramine, 87*t*, 91*t*, 93*t*
Imiquimod, 560*t*, 565
Imitrex, 309
Immune globulin, 633*t*, 634–635
Immune system, 625, 626–627. *See also* immunomodulating drugs
cancer treatment and, 618–619
Immunoglobulins, 627
Immunomodulating drugs, 625–637
case study, 636
immunostimulants, 634–635
immunosuppressants, 627–632, 628*t*
antibodies, 628*t*, 632–633, 633*t*
diabetes mellitus, 520–521
fusion proteins, 632–633, 633*t*
glucocorticoids, 452, 629–630
other immunomodulators, 635
rehabilitation patients, 635–636
Imodium, 426*t*
Implanon, 477*t*
Implantable drug delivery system, 25–26
analgesics, 265, 265*f*
insulin, 515
Imuran, 240*t*, 243*t*, 245, 627–628, 628*t*
Inactive drug. *See* Biotransformation
Inamrinone, 363*t*, 365–366
IncobotulinumtoxinA, 189, 190
Indacaterol, 405*t*
Indapamide, 320*t*
Inderal, 310*t*, 311, 321*t*, 338*t*, 353*t*
Indinavir, 562*t*, 572
Indocin, 228*t*, 229*t*, 240*t*
Indomethacin, 228*t*, 229*t*, 240*t*
Indwelling IV cannula, 17
Infections and treatments
anthelmintics, 593–595, 593*t*
antibacterials, 533–552, 547–549*t* (*See also* Antibacterial drugs)
antifungals, 581–587
antiprotozoals, 588–593
antivirals, 557, 560–577 (*See also* Antiviral drugs)
Infergen, 569*t*
Infertility, 479
Inflammation. *See also* Aspirin; Glucocorticoids; Nonsteroidal anti-inflammatory drugs
aspirin, 224
physiological effect of eicosanoids, 222
Infliximab, 240*t*, 244*t*, 247, 248*f*, 632, 633*t*
Infundibulum, 436
Infusion, drug. *See* Patient-controlled analgesia (PCA)
Infusion pumps, 264–265, 264*t*, 265*f*
INH, 546
Inhalation of drugs, 17
Injection of drugs, 16*t*, 17–18
vs. patient-controlled analgesia (PCA), 261–262, 262*f*
Innohep, 378, 378*t*
Inocor, 363*t*
Inorganic sulfate, 650*t*
Inosine monophosphate dehydrogenase, 630–631
Insomnia, 69
Inspra, 369, 460
Insulin, 437*t*, 438, 508–509, 509*f*, 510, 514*t*. *See also under* Diabetes mellitus
Insulin-dependent diabetes mellitus (IDDM). *See* Type 1 diabetes
Insulin receptors, 44, 508, 509*f*
Insulin receptor substrates (IRSs), 508–509
Insulin resistance, 512
Intal, 409
Integrase inhibitors, 562*t*, 563, 573
Integrilin, 378*t*, 382
Intelence, 562*t*, 566, 572–573
Interactions
drug-drug, 37
drug-receptor, 43, 46–51
food-drug, 38
Interferons, 568–570
adverse effects, 570
antiviral effects, 568–569, 569*f*
cancer treatment, 611*t*, 612
pharmacologic applications, 569–570
types, 569*t*
Interleukins
antagonists of, 632, 633*t*
interleukin-2, 611*t*, 612
interleukin-6, 249
rheumatoid arthritis, 249

Intermediate-density lipoproteins (IDLs), 387
Intermediate pituitary, 437
Intra-arterial injection, 17–18
Intracellular receptor, 46
Intramuscular (IM) injection, 18
  antipsychotics, 106
  vs. patient-controlled analgesia (PCA), 261–262, 262*f*
Intrathecal administration, 266–267, 266*f*
Intrathecal anesthesia, 168–169, 169*f*
Intrathecal injection, 8
Intrauterine device, 481
Intravenous (IV) injection, 17
Intron A, 569*t*
Intropin, 305, 363*t*
Intuniv, 321*t*
Invanz, 536*t*
Invega, 105*t*
Inverse agonist, 50–51
Inversine, 321*t*
Investigational new drug (IND), 6–7
Invirase, 562*t*, 572
Iodide, 493
Iodine, 493, 650*t*
Iodoquinol, 591
Ionization, 21, 21*f*
Iontophoresis, 19, 167–168, 206–207
  patient-controlled transdermal analgesia, 267–268
Ipecac, 429
Ipratropium, 295*t*, 297, 407, 412
Iprivask, 378*t*
Irbesartan, 324*t*, 363*t*
Iressa, 611*t*, 613
Irinotecan, 609*t*
Iron, 650*t*
Irreversible antagonist. *See* Noncompetitive antagonist
Irritable bowel syndrome (IBS), 295
Isentress, 562*t*, 563, 573
Islets of Langerhans, 507
Ismelin, 312
Isocarboxazid, 87*t*
Isoflurane, 151*t*
Isoflurophate, 291*t*
Isoniazid, 533, 546
Isophane insulin, 514*t*
Isoproterenol, 306, 405*t*
Isoptin, 324*t*, 339*t*, 340, 353*t*
Isopto Carbachol, 291*t*
Isopto Carpine, 291*t*
Isopto Homapin, 295*t*
Isosorbide dinitrate, 337–338, 342, 363*t*, 370
Isosorbide mononitrate, 338, 342, 363*t*
Isradipine, 324*t*, 339, 339*t*
Istodax, 614*t*, 615
Isuprel, 306, 405*t*
Itraconazole, 582*t*, 584, 585
Ivermectin, 593*t*, 594
Ixabepilone, 608*t*
Ixempra, 608*t*

J

Januvia, 518*t*, 519
Jevtana, 608*t*
Jimsonweed, 294
Joint disease. *See* Osteoarthritis; Rheumatoid arthritis
Juvenile arthritis, 237
Juvenile diabetes, 511

K

Kaletra, 562*t*, 572
Kanamycin, 540*t*
Kantrex, 540*t*
Kaolin, 427–428
Kaopectate, 426*t*, 427
Kapidex, 424, 424*t*
Kappa opioid receptor, 203*t*
Kava, 644*t*, 646
Keflex, 536*t*
Kefzol, 536*t*
Kemstro, 183*t*
Keppra, 122*t*, 123
Kerlone, 310*t*, 311, 321*t*
Ketalar, 152*t*
Ketamine, 152*t*, 263
Ketek, 540*t*, 542
Ketoacidosis, 512
Ketoconazole, 457, 584, 585–586
Ketolide antibacterials, 542
Ketoprofen, 228*t*, 229*t*, 240*t*
Ketorolac, 224, 228*t*, 263
Kidneys
  drug excretion and, 33–34, 34*f*
  effects of aldosterone, 458
Kidrolase, 614*t*
Kineret, 240*t*, 244*t*, 248, 633*t*
Klonopin, 76*t*, 119*t*
Korlym, 480
Kytril, 156, 602

L

Labetalol, 310*t*, 311, 321, 321*t*, 338*t*, 363*t*
Lacosamide, 122, 122*t*, 125*t*
Lactation, drug excretion and, 34
Lactulose, 428*t*
Lamictal, 122–123, 122*t*
Lamisil, 586
Lamivudine, 562*t*, 566, 572
Lamotrigine, 122–123, 122*t*, 124*t*, 125*t*
Lamprene, 543, 543*t*
Laniazid, 546
Lanoxin, 363*t*
Lansoprazole, 424, 424*t*
Lantus, 514*t*
Lanvis, 607*t*
Lariam, 589
Larodopa, 135*t*
Lasix, 320*t*
Latuda, 104*t*
Laudanum, 427
Laxatives, 428–429, 428*t*
Leflunomide, 240*t*, 243*t*, 245–246
Left heart failure, 361, 362*f*
Legionnaires' disease, 547*t*
Lenalidomide, 616, 634
Lepirudin, 378*t*, 380
Lescol, 388*t*
Letrozole, 609*t*, 610
Leukeran, 604*t*, 634
Leukotrienes, 220
  inhibitors, 409–410, 411
  physiologic effects, 220–222, 221*t*
  synthesis, 220, 221*f*
Leuprolide, 470, 610*t*
Leustatin, 606*t*
Levalbuterol, 405*t*
Levaquin, 543–544, 543*t*
Levatol, 310*t*, 311, 321*t*, 338*t*
Levemir, 514*t*
Levetiracetam, 122*t*, 123, 124*t*, 125*t*
Levlen, 481*t*
Levobupivacaine, 166*t*
Levocetirizine, 402*t*
Levodopa, 134–135, 135*t*
  adverse effects, 137–139
  carbidopa and levodopa preparation, 136–137, 137*f*, 138–139
  drug holiday, 139–140
  pharmacokinetics, 135–136, 136*f*
  timing of administration, 142–143
Levo-dromoran, 204*t*
Levofloxacin, 543–544, 543*t*
Levonorgestrel, 477*t*, 481*t*, 482
Levophed, 307
Levorphanol, 204*t*
Levothroid, 494*t*
Levothyroxine (T_4), 494, 494*t*
Levsin, 295*t*
Lexapro, 77*t*, 86*t*, 89*t*
Lexiva, 562*t*, 572
Librax, 296
Librium, 76*t*
Lidex, 453*t*
Lidocaine, 32*t*, 166*f*, 166*t*, 353*t*
Limbic system, 61
Linagliptin, 518*t*, 519
Lincocin, 540*t*, 542
Lincomycin, 540*t*, 542
Lincorex, 540*t*, 542
Linezolid, 540*t*, 542
Lioresal, 183*t*
Liothyronine (T_3), 494, 494*t*
Liotrix, 494*t*
Lipid bilayer, 20, 20*f*
Lipid rafts, 20
Lipid rescue, 172

Lipids
diffusion, 21
metabolism, 450–451, 451*f*, 508
Lipitor, 387, 388*t*
Lipocortins. *See* Annexins
Lipoproteins, 387
Liquaemin, 378*t*
Liraglutide, 518*t*, 519
Lisinopril, 324*t*, 363*t*
Lispro, 514*t*, 515
Listeriosis, 547*t*
Lithium, 94–95, 95*t*
Livalo, 388*t*
Liver
drug biotransformation and, 33
effects of androgens, 472
effects of insulin, 508
Local anesthetics. *See under* Anesthetic drugs
Local anesthetic systemic toxicity (LAST), 172
Lodine, 227*t*, 229*t*, 240*t*
Loestrin, 481*t*
Lomotil, 426*t*
Lomustine, 604*t*
Loniten, 324, 324*t*
Loop diuretics, 319, 320*t*
Lo-Ovral, 481*t*
Loperamide, 426*t*, 427
Lopid, 388*t*
Lopinavir, 562*t*, 572
Lopressor, 310*t*, 311, 321*t*, 338*t*, 339, 353*t*, 363*t*
Loprox, 583*t*
Loratadine, 401, 402*t*
Lorazepam, 76*t*, 119*t*, 151*t*, 157*t*
Lorox, 587
Losartan, 324*t*, 363*t*, 368
Lotemax, 454*t*
Lotensin, 324*t*
Loteprednol, 454*t*
Lotriderm, 582*t*
Lotrimin, 583*t*
Lovastatin, 388*t*
Lovenox, 341, 378, 378*t*
Low-density lipoproteins (LDLs), 387
Low molecular weight heparins (LMWH), 341, 378–379
Loxapine, 103*t*, 104*t*
Loxitane, 104*t*
Lozol, 320*t*
Lufyllin, 407*t*
Luminal, 70*t*
Lunesta, 70*t*, 74*t*
Lungs, drug excretion and, 33–34
Lupron, 470
Lurasidone, 104*t*
Lusedra, 152*t*
Luteal phase, 473
Luteinizing hormone (LH), 436*t*, 441, 465, 466*f*
Luvox, 86*t*, 89*t*
Lyme disease, 549*t*
Lymphogranuloma venereum, 549*t*
Lymphokines, 626–627
Lyrica, 122*t*, 123
Lysodren, 457, 614*t*, 615

M

Macroangiopathy, 513
Macrodantin, 546
Macrolide antibiotics, 540–541, 540*t*
Madopar, 137
Magnesium, 355, 649*t*
Magnesium hydroxide, 428*t*
Magnesium sulfate, 428*t*
Major histocompatibility complex (MHC) proteins, 626
Major tranquilizers, 101
Makena, 477*t*
Malaria, 587, 588*t*
Mammalian target of rapamycin (mTOR) inhibitor, 631
Mandelamine, 546
Manganese, 650*t*
Manic-depressive disorder. *See* Bipolar disorder
MAO inhibitors. *See* Monoamine oxidase (MAO) inhibitors
Maraviroc, 562*t*, 563
Marcaine, 166*t*
Marplan, 87*t*
Masteron, 470*t*
Matulane, 604*t*
Mavik, 324*t*, 363*t*
Maxair, 306, 405*t*
Maxalt, 309
Maximal effect, 10, 10*f*
Maxipime, 536*t*
MDIs (metered-dose inhalers), 404
Mebendazole, 593*t*, 594
Mecamylamine, 294, 321*t*, 323
Mechlorethamine, 604*t*
Meclizine, 430
Meclofenamate, 228*t*, 229*t*, 240*t*
Meclomen, 228*t*, 229*t*, 240*t*
Median effective dose, 11, 11*f*
Median lethal dose, 12
Median toxic dose, 11–12, 11*f*
Medihaler-Iso, 405*t*
Medrol, 240*t*, 408*t*, 454*t*
Medroxyprogesterone, 477*t*, 481, 481*t*, 609*t*
Mefloquine, 589
Mefoxin, 536*t*
Megace, 477*t*
Megestrol, 477*t*, 609*t*
Meglitinides, 517, 518*t*, 519
Melanocortin system, 437
Melanocyte-stimulating hormone (MSH), 437
Melarsoprol, 588*t*
Melatonin, 72, 644*t*, 646
Mellaril, 104*t*, 105
Meloxicam, 228*t*, 229*t*, 240*t*
Melphalan, 604*t*
Membrane, cell, 19–20, 20*f*
Membrane proteins, 19–20, 20*f*
Membrane(s)
effects of drugs, 66
structure and function, 19–20, 20*f*
Menest, 477*t*, 498*t*
Meningitis, 547*t*, 548*t*
Menopause, replacement therapy and, 476–477
Menstrual cycle, 473–475, 474*f*
dysmenorrhea, 222
irregularities, 475–476
Mental illness. *See* Antipsychotic drugs; Bipolar syndrome; Depression
Mentax, 583*t*, 587
Mepenzolate, 295*t*
Meperidine, 151*t*, 157*t*, 204*t*, 263, 263*t*
Mephenteramine, 303
Mepivacaine, 166*t*
Meprobamate, 77
Mepron, 591
Mercaptopurine, 606*t*, 634
Meropenem, 536*t*
Merrem I.V., 536*t*
Mesencephalon, 60
Mestinon, 291*t*
Mestranol, 481*t*
Metabolic syndrome, 317, 512
Metabolism, drug. *See* Biotransformation
Metabolite, 31
Metahydrin, 320*t*
Metamucil, 428*t*
Metaproterenol, 306, 405*t*
Metaraminol, 307
Metaxalone, 181*t*, 182*t*
Metered-dose inhalers (MDIs), 404
Metformin, 518*t*, 519
Methacholine, 290–291, 291*t*
Methadone, 32*t*, 204*t*, 214, 263*t*
Methadose, 204*t*
Methamphetamine, 306
Methandrostenolone, 470*t*, 471*t*
Methenamine, 546
Methenolone, 470*t*
Methimazole, 493
Methocarbamol, 181*t*, 182*t*, 191
Methohexital, 151*t*
Methotrexate, 37, 240*t*, 243*t*, 246, 603, 606*t*
combination with DMARDs, 250
immunosuppressants, 628*t*, 630
Methoxamine, 303
Methscopolamine, 295*t*
Methyclothiazide, 320*t*
Methylcellulose, 428*t*
1-methyl-4-phenyl-1,2,3, 6-tetrahydropyridine (MPTP), 134
Methyldopa, 304–305, 321*t*

Methylprednisolone, 240*t*, 408*t*, 454*t*
Methyltestosterone, 469*t*, 470*t*
Metoclopramide, 425–426
Metocurine, 158*t*
Metolazone, 320*t*
Metopirone, 457
Metoprolol, 287, 310*t*, 311, 321*t*, 338*t*, 339, 353*t*, 363*t*
Metronidazole, 543*t*, 544, 588*t*, 591–592
Metubine, 158*t*
Metyrapone, 457
Metyrosine, 65, 312
Mevacor, 388*t*
Mexiletine, 353*t*
Mexitil, 353*t*
Miacalcin, 498*t*, 500
Micafungin, 586
Micardis, 324*t*, 363*t*
Micazole, 583*t*
Miconazole, 37, 583*t*, 586–587
Microangiopathy, 513
Micronase, 518*t*
Micronor, 477*t*, 481*t*
Midamor, 320*t*
Midazolam, 151*t*, 157*t*
Midbrain, 60
Midrodrine, 303
Mifepristone, 479–480
Miglitol, 518*t*, 520
Migranal, 308–309
Milrinone, 363*t*, 365–366
Miltown, 77
Mineralocorticoids, 437*t*, 439, 447, 457–459
Mineral oil, 428*t*
Minerals, 649–650*t*
Minipills, 480–481
Minipress, 309, 321*t*, 322, 363*t*
Minocin, 540*t*
Minocycline, 540*t*
Minoxidil, 324, 324*t*
Mintezol, 595
MiraLax, 428*t*
Mirapex, 140*t*
Mircette, 481*t*
Mirena, 477*t*
Mirtazapine, 87*t*, 89*t*, 91*t*
Misoprostol, 225, 241, 426
MitoExtra, 607*t*
Mitomycin, 607*t*
Mitotane, 457, 614*t*, 615
Mitoxantrone, 607*t*
Mivacron, 158*t*
Mivacurium, 158*t*
Mixed agonist-antagonist opioids, 203
Mixed agonist-antagonists, 50
Moban, 104*t*
Mobic, 228*t*, 229*t*, 240*t*
Moexipril, 324*t*
Molindone, 103*t*, 104*t*
Molybdenum, 650*t*
Mometasone, 411*t*, 454*t*
Monistat, 583*t*
Monitan, 338*t*, 353*t*, 363*t*
Monoamine oxidase (MAO) inhibitors
  depression, 87*t*, 88, 90, 91*t*, 92
  interactions with foods, 38
  Parkinson disease, 135*t*, 141–142, 143
Monoamines, 62*t*, 63
Monoclonal antibodies, 520–521, 610, 611*t*, 612, 618
Monocor, 363*t*
Monodox, 540*t*
Monoiodotyrosine, 489, 490*f*
Monopril, 324*t*, 363*t*
Montelukast, 220, 409–410
Monurol, 536*t*, 539
Morning-after pill, 481–482
Morphine, 201, 202*f*, 204*t*, 263, 263*t*
Motion sickness, 296
Motrin, 228*t*, 229*t*
Moxifloxacin, 543*t*
Moxonidine, 323
MPTP (1-methyl-4-phenyl-1,2,3, 6-tetrahydropyridine), 134
MTOR inhibitor, 631
Mucolytic drugs, 402–403
Mucomyst, 403
Mucosil, 403
Multaq, 353*t*
Multiple sclerosis (MS), 184, 570
Mu opioid receptor, 203*t*
Mupirocin, 543*t*, 544
Mureins, 534
Muromonab-CD3 monoclonal antibody, 633*t*
Muscarine
  cholinergic antagonists, 294–297, 295*t*, 407, 421, 425
  cholinergic stimulants, 290–293
  receptors, 48, 283*f*, 284–285, 284*f*, 285*t*, 289
Muscle
  catabolism and androgen treatment, 467–468
  drug storage in, 24–25
  effects of cortisol, 451, 451*f*
  effects of insulin, 508
  glucocorticoid effects on, 456
  hypertonicity and topical anesthesia, 167
  stretch reflex, 179, 180*f*
Muscle relaxants. *See* Skeletal muscle relaxant drugs
Mustargen, 604*t*
Mutamycin, 607*t*
Myambutol, 536*t*, 538
Myasthenia gravis, 65, 292–293
Mycamine, 586
Mycelex, 582*t*
Mycobutin, 543*t*, 544–545
Mycophenolate mofetil, 628*t*, 630–631
Mycoplasmas, 533*t*
Mycosis(es), 581, 582*t*
Mycostatin, 583*t*
Mykrox, 320*t*
Myleran, 604*t*
Mylocel, 614*t*
Mylotarg, 611*t*
Myobloc, 189
Myocardium. *See also* Angina pectoris
  cells of, 360
  infarction, 310, 343, 381
  ischemia equation, 336*f*
Myochrysine, 240*t*, 245
Mysoline, 119*t*
Mytelase, 291*t*
Myxedema. *See* Hypothyroidism

N

Nabumetone, 228*t*, 229*t*, 240*t*
N-acetyl-p-benzoquinoneimine (NAPQI), 231–232, 231*f*
Nadolol, 310*t*, 311, 321*t*, 338*t*, 353*t*
Nafarelin, 470
Nafcillin, 536*t*
Naftifine (Naftin), 583*t*, 587
Nalbuphine, 151*t*, 205*t*, 263*t*
Nalfon, 227*t*, 229*t*, 240*t*
Nallpen, 536*t*
Naloxone, 206
Naltrexone, 206
Nandrolone, 469*t*, 470*t*, 471*t*
Nanotechnology, in drug delivery, 26, 618
Naprosyn, 228*t*, 229*t*, 240*t*
Naproxen, 228*t*, 229*t*, 240*t*
Naqua, 320*t*
Narcan, 206
"Narcotic," as a term, 201
Narcotics. *See* Opioid analgesic drugs
Nardil, 87*t*
Nasacort, 454*t*
Nasalcrom, 409
Nasalide, 453*t*
Nasonex, 454*t*
Nateglinide, 517, 518*t*, 519
Natrecor, 363*t*, 370
Natulan, 604*t*
Natural remedies. *See* Complementary and alternative medications (CAMs)
Naturetin, 320*t*
Nausea, 602
Navane, 104*t*
Navelbine, 608*t*
Nebcin, 540*t*
Nebivolol, 310*t*, 311, 321, 321*t*, 369
Nebulizer, 404–405
NebuPent, 592
Nefazodone, 87*t*, 89*t*, 90, 91*t*
Nelarabine, 606*t*
Nelfinavir, 562*t*, 572
Nembutal, 70*t*, 119*t*
Neoadjuvant therapy, 617
Neo-Fradin, 540*t*

Neomycin, 538, 540*t*
Neoplasms, 599
Neoplastic disease. *See* Cancer chemotherapy
Neoral, 240*t*, 243*t*, 628*t*, 629
Neosar, 604*t*, 628*t*, 629
Neostigmine, 291*t*, 292, 293
Neo-Synephrine, 303
Nephron. *See* Kidneys
Nerve blocks. *See also* Anesthetic drugs
  Bier, 170
  central, 168–169, 169*f*, 173
  continuous, 168, 267, 269–270
  differential, 171–172, 171*t*
  peripheral, 168
  sympathetic, 169–170
Nervous system. *See* Autonomic nervous system (ANS)
Nesacaine, 166*t*
Nesiritide, 363*t*, 370
Neupro, 140*t*
Neurogenesis hypothesis of depression, 85, 85*f*
Neuroleptanesthesia, 153
Neuroleptic drugs. *See* Antipsychotic drugs
Neuroleptic malignant syndrome (NMS), 109, 186
Neuromuscular blockage, reversal, 293
Neuromuscular blockers, 157–159, 158*t*
Neurontin, 122, 122*t*, 183*t*, 186–187
Neurotransmitters
  amine, 84
  autonomic, 283–284, 283*f*
  central, 62–64, 62*t*, 65
  depression and, 84
Neutral protamine Hagedorn (NPH) insulins, 514, 515
Nevirapine, 562*t*, 566, 572–573
New drug application (NDA), 6–7
Nexavar, 612*t*
Nexium, 424, 424*t*
Niacin, 388*t*, 389, 648*t*
Niacor, 388*t*
Niaspan, 388*t*, 389
Nicardipine, 324*t*, 339, 339*t*
Niclosamide, 593*t*, 595
Nicotinic acid, 389
Nicotinic receptors, 48, 283*f*, 284, 284*f*, 285*t*, 289
Nifedipine, 324*t*, 327, 339–340, 339*t*, 355
Nilandron, 470
Nilstat, 583*t*
Nilutamide, 470, 609*t*
Nimbex, 158*t*
Nipent, 607*t*
Nipride, 324
Nisoldipine, 324*t*
Nitazoxanide, 592
Nitrates. *See* Organic nitrates
Nitric oxide, 324
Nitro-Bid, 336–337
Nitro-Dur, 336–337
Nitrofurantoin, 546
Nitrogen monoxide, 151*t*
Nitrogen mustard, 604*t*
Nitroglycerin
  angina pectoris, 336–337, 336*t*, 342
  congestive heart failure, 370
  stable angina, 342
Nitropress, 324, 324*t*
Nitroprusside, 324, 324*t*
Nitrostat, 336–337
Nitrous oxide, 151*t*
Nizatidine, 423*t*
Nizoral, 457, 585–586
N-methyl-D-aspartate (NMDA) receptor, 155–156
Noctec, 70*t*
Nolahist, 402*t*
Nolvadex, 478
Nomenclature, drug, 4–5, 5*t*
Nonalimentary administration. *See* Parenteral administration
Nonbenzodiazepines, 70*t*, 72–75, 74*t*, 80
Noncompetitive antagonist, 50
Nondepolarizing blockers, 158*t*, 159
Non-insulin-dependent diabetes mellitus (NIDDM). *See* Type 2 diabetes
Nonlipid-soluble compounds, 21
Nonnucleoside reverse transcriptase inhibitors (NNRTIs), 562*t*, 566, 572–573
Nonprescription drugs. *See* Over-the-counter (OTC) drugs
Nonproprietary (generic) name, 5
Nonsedating antihistamines, 401–402, 402*t*
Nonsteroidal anti-inflammatory drugs (NSAIDs), 219–233
  acetaminophen, 230–232, 231*f*
  aspirin, 219, 220*f*, 223, 613–614 (*See also* Aspirin)
  cancer treatment, 613–614
  case study, 233
  clinical applications, 224
  common drugs, 227–228*t*
  comparison with aspirin, 227–229
  COX-2 selective drugs, 229–230
  cystic fibrosis-related respiratory problems, 412–413
  dosages, 229*t*
  eicosanoids, 220–223, 221*f*, 221*t*
  mechanism of action, 222–223
  muscle spasms, 182
  osteoarthritis, 227, 251
  pharmacokinetics, 232
  problems and adverse effects, 224–227
  rehabilitation patients, 232
  rheumatoid arthritis, 239, 240–241, 240*t*
Norcuron, 158*t*
Nordette, 481*t*
Norelgestromin, 480, 481*t*
Norepinephrine, 62*t*, 63, 282, 283, 301, 306, 307
  effects, 437*t*, 439
  receptors for (*See* Adrenergic receptors)
  serotonin-norepinephrine reuptake inhibitors (SNRIs), 88, 89*t*, 91–92
Norethindrone, 477*t*, 481*t*
Norflex, 181*t*
Norfloxacin, 543*t*
Norfranil, 87*t*, 93*t*
Norgestrel, 481*t*
Norinyl, 481*t*
Normodyne, 310*t*, 311, 321*t*, 363*t*
Noroxin, 543*t*
Norpace, 353*t*
Norplant, 481, 481*t*
Norpramin, 86*t*
Nor-QD, 481*t*
Nortriptyline, 87*t*, 91*t*, 93*t*
Norvasc, 324*t*, 339*t*
Norvir, 562*t*, 572
Novantrone, 607*t*
Novocain, 166*t*
Novolin, 514*t*
NovoLog, 514*t*
Novoreserpine, 321*t*
Novosecobarb, 70*t*
NPH insulins, 514, 515
NSAIDs. *See* Nonsteroidal anti-inflammatory drugs (NSAIDs)
Nubain, 151*t*, 205*t*
Nuclear hormone receptors, 441*f*, 443
Nucleic acid, bacterial, 535
Nucleocapsid, 558
Nucleoside reverse transcriptase inhibitors (NRTIs), 562*t*
Nucynta, 205*t*
Nujol, 428*t*
Nulojix, 633, 633*t*
Nupercainal, 166*t*
Nuprin, 229*t*
Nuromax, 158*t*
NuvaRing, 481*t*
Nyaderm, 583*t*
Nydrazid, 546
Nystatin, 583*t*, 587
Nystop, 583*t*
Nytol, 402*t*

O

Octreotide, 427
OcuClear, 303
Ocu-Pentolate, 295*t*
Ofatumumab, 611*t*
Official (generic) name, 5
Off-label prescribing, 8
Ofloxacin, 543*t*
Ogen, 477*t*, 498*t*
Olanzapine, 103*t*, 105*t*
Olmesartan, 324*t*

Olopatadine, 402*t*
Omeprazole, 241, 424, 424*t*
Omnaris, 453*t*
Omnicef, 536*t*
Omnipen, 536*t*
Oncovin, 608*t*, 634
Ondansetron, 157*t*, 602
Onglyza, 518*t*, 519
On-off phenomenon, 139
Ontak, 614*t*, 615
Onxol, 608*t*
Opana, 151*t*, 204*t*
Opioid analgesic drugs, 201–216, 204–205*t*
  addiction, 211–212
  anesthesia, 153
  case study, 215
  classification of specific agents, 203, 205–206
  clinical applications, 210–211
  dependence and withdrawal symptoms, 212–213, 212*t*
  endogenous opioids, 202
  mechanism of action, 207–210, 207*f*
  patient-controlled analgesia (PCA), 261–262, 262*f*, 263, 270
  peripheral-acting, 208–209, 209*f*
  pharmacokinetics, 206–207
  problems and adverse effects, 211
  receptors, 202–203, 203*t*
  rehabilitation patients, 214–215
  route of administration, 210
  sources, 201–202
  tolerance, 212, 213
  treatment of addiction, 213–214
Opioids
  antidiarrheals, 426–428, 426*t*
  endogenous, 63, 202
  general anesthetics, 151*t*
  preoperative medications, 157*t*
Opium, 202
Optimine, 402*t*
Oral administration, 15–16, 16*t*
Orencia, 240*t*, 244*t*, 247–248, 633, 633*t*
Oreton, 469*t*
Organic nitrates
  angina pectoris, 335–338, 336*t*, 342
  congestive heart failure, 363*t*, 370
  stable angina, 342
Organs, drug storage in, 25
Orinase, 518*t*
Orphan drugs, 7–8
Orphenadrine citrate, 181*t*, 182*t*, 191
Ortho-Cept, 481*t*
Orthoclone OKT3, 633*t*
Ortho-Cyclen, 481*t*
Ortho-Est, 477*t*, 498*t*
Ortho Evra, 481*t*
Ortho-Novum, 481*t*
Orthostatic hypotension, 110, 138, 322
Orudis, 228*t*, 229*t*, 240*t*
Oruvail, 228*t*
Os-Cal 498, 498*t*
Oseltamivir, 560*t*, 565
Osmosis, 22
Osteoarthritis, 227, 250–254
Osteomalacia, 497*t*
Osteomyelitis, 548*t*
Osteoporosis, 242, 457, 475, 478–479, 497*t*, 499, 500, 501
Otitis media, 547*t*, 548*t*
Otrivin, 303, 401*t*
Over-the-counter (OTC) drugs, 8–9
Ovral, 481*t*
Ovrette, 481*t*
Ovulation, 473
Oxacillin, 536*t*
Oxaliplatin, 613*t*
Oxamniquine, 593*t*, 595
Oxandrin, 469*t*
Oxandrolone, 469*t*, 470*t*, 471*t*
Oxaprozin, 228*t*, 229*t*, 240*t*
Oxazepam, 76*t*
Oxcarbazepine, 119*t*, 120, 124*t*, 125*t*
Oxiconazole, 583*t*
Oxidation, 31, 32, 32*t*
Oxistat, 583*t*
Oxybutynin, 295*t*
Oxycodone, 205*t*
OxyContin, 205*t*
Oxygen free radicals, 133–134
Oxymetazoline, 303, 401*t*
Oxymetholone, 469*t*, 470*t*, 471*t*
Oxymorphone, 151*t*, 204*t*, 263*t*
Oxytocin, 436*t*
Oxytrol, 295*t*

P

P2Y12 blockers, 341
Pacemaker cells, 351
Pacerone, 353*t*
Paclitaxel, 605, 608*t*
Paget disease, 497*t*, 500
Pain
  calcitonin and bone pain, 500
  chronic, 92–93, 93*t*
  eicosanoids' effects on, 222
Pain relief. *See* Aspirin; Opioid analgesic drugs
Paliperidone, 103*t*, 105*t*
Palivizumab, 560*t*
Pallidotomy, 143
Palonosetron, 602
Pamelor, 87*t*, 93*t*
Pamidronate, 498*t*, 499, 500
Pamine, 295*t*
Pancreas, 438, 507–508
  enzymes, 429
  hormones, 437*t*
Pancuronium, 158*t*, 293
Panitumumab, 611*t*
Panretin, 614*t*, 616
Pantoloc, 424*t*
Pantoprazole, 424, 424*t*
Pantothenic acid, 648*t*
Paracetamol. *See* Acetaminophen
Paraflex, 181*t*
Parafollicular cells, 496
Parafon, 181*t*
Paraplatin, 613*t*
Parasites, 581
  anthelmintic infections and treatments, 593–595, 593*t*
  fungal infections and treatments, 581–587
  protozoal infections and treatments, 587–593
  rehabilitation patients, 595
Parasympathetic nervous system, 279–282, 281*t*
Parathyroid, 438
Parathyroid hormone (PTH), 437*t*, 438, 495, 495*f*, 496
Paratyphoid fever, 548*t*
Parcopa, 135*t*
Paregoric, 426*t*, 427
Parenteral administration, 15, 16*t*, 17–18
Paricalcitol, 498*t*
Pariet, 424*t*
Parkinson disease, 131, 145
  antimuscarinic drugs, 296
  antipsychotics, 107
  case study, 144–145
  environmental factors, 134
  genetic factors, 133–134
  levodopa, 134–140, 135*t*, 136*f*, 142–143
  neurosurgical interventions, 143
  other drugs, 140–142
  pathophysiology, 132–133, 132*f*
  rehabilitation patients, 144
  timing of drug therapy, 142–143
Parlodel, 140*t*
Parnate, 87*t*
Paromomycin, 592
Paroxetine, 77*t*, 86*t*, 91*t*
Partial agonist, 50
Parturition, hormones in, 475
PAS, 543
Paser, 543, 543*t*
Passive diffusion, 20–22, 21*f*
Patanase, 402*t*
Patch, transdermal. *See* Transdermal patch
Pathocil, 536*t*
Patient-controlled analgesia (PCA), 261–272
  administration routes
    epidural, 266–267, 266*f*
    intravenous, 263*t*, 265–266, 266*f*
    other potential routes, 268
    PCA pumps, 264–265, 264*t*, 265*f*
    regional, 267
    transdermal, 267–268

case study, 272
comparison with traditional methods, 268–270
dosing strategies and parameters, 262–263, 263*t*
opioids, 211
pharmacokinetic basis, 261–262, 262*f*
problems and side effects, 270–271, 270*t*
rehabilitation patients, 271
types of analgesics, 263–264
Paveral, 205*t*
Pavulon, 158*t*
Paxil, 77*t*, 86*t*
PBZ, 402*t*
Pectin, 427–428
Pediapred, 454*t*
Pediatex, 402*t*
Pegasys, 569*t*
Pegintron, 569*t*
Pemetrexed, 606*t*
Penbutolol, 310*t*, 311, 321*t*, 338*t*
Penciclovir, 560*t*, 564
Penicillamine, 240*t*, 244*t*, 246–247
Penicillinase, 537
Penicillin-binding proteins (PBPs), 537
Penicillins, 536–537, 536*t*
Penlac, 583*t*
Pentam, 592
Pentamidine, 588*t*, 592
Pentazocine, 151*t*, 205*t*, 263*t*
Pentobarbital, 70*t*, 119*t*, 157*t*
Pentostatin, 607*t*
Pentothal, 151*t*
Pentoxifylline, 378*t*, 383
Pen-Vee, 536*t*
Pepcid, 423*t*
Peptic ulcer, 295–296, 421
Peptide hormones, 439, 441*f*
Peptides, 62*t*, 63–64, 439
Peptidoglycans, 534
Pepto-Bismol, 426*t*, 427
Performance anxiety, 77
Perforomist, 405*t*
Periactin, 402*t*
Perindopril, 324*t*
Peripheral decarboxylase inhibitors, 136–137, 137*f*
Permitil, 104*t*
Peroxisome proliferator activated receptor, 388–389
Perphenazine, 103*t*, 104*t*
Persantine, 378*t*, 383
Personalized oncology, 619
Pethidine, 204*t*
Petit mal seizures, 116*t*
pH, lipid diffusion and, 21, 21*f*
Pharmacodynamics, 4, 4*f*
Pharmacogenetics, 4, 37
Pharmacokinetics, 4, 4*f*
drug absorption, 19–23
drug administration, 15–19, 16*t*
drug distribution within body, 23–24
drug elimination, 31–39
drug storage, 24–25
newer drug delivery techniques, 25–26
Pharmacological dose, 447
Pharmacology
areas of study in, 3–4, 4*f*
basic principles of, 3–11
Pharmacotherapeutics, 3–4, 4*f*
Pharmacy, 4
Phenelzine, 87*t*, 91*t*
Phenindamine, 402*t*
Phenobarbital, 157*t*
antiepileptic, 119*t*, 124*t*, 125*t*, 126
sedative-hypnotic, 70*t*
Phenoxybenzamine, 309, 321*t*
Phentolamine, 309
Phenylephrine, 302, 303, 401*t*
Phenytek, 120
Phenytoin, 119*t*, 120, 124*t*, 125*t*, 126
Pheochromocytoma, 308
Phillips' Milk of Magnesia, 428*t*
Phonophoresis, 19, 167–168
PhosLo, 498*t*
Phosphate, 496, 649*t*
Phosphodiesterase (PDE) inhibitors, 365–366, 370, 406
Phospholine iodide, 291*t*
Phospholipids, 19–20, 20*f*
Phyllocontin, 407*t*
Physical dependence. *See* Dependence
Physiological dose, 447
Physostigmine, 291*t*, 293
Pilocar, 291*t*
Pilocarpine, 290, 291*t*
Pimecrolimus, 632
Pindolol, 310*t*, 311, 321, 321*t*, 338*t*
Pioglitazone, 518*t*, 519–520
Pipecuronium, 158*t*
Piperacillin, 536*t*
Piperazine, 593*t*, 595
Pirbuterol, 306, 405*t*
Pirenzepine, 425
Piroxicam, 228*t*, 229*t*, 240*t*
Pitavastatin, 388*t*
Pituitary gland, 436–437, 436*f*
Plan B, 481*t*, 482
Plaquenil, 240*t*, 243*t*, 244, 589
Plasma concentration, 35–36, 36*f*
Plasma lipids. *See also* Lipids
effects of androgens, 472
effects of hormone replacement therapy (HRT), 476
Plasma proteins, 23. *See also* Protein(s)
Plasmin, 376*f*, 377, 383
Platelet inhibitors, 378*t*
Platinol, 613*t*
Platinum coordination complexes, 613, 613*t*
Plavix, 341, 378*t*, 382
Plenaxis, 470
Plendil, 324*t*, 339, 339*t*
Pletal, 378*t*, 383
Pneumonia, 547*t*, 548*t*, 549*t*
Podactin, 583*t*
Poisoning
aspirin, 226
cholinergic, 297
Polaramine, 402*t*
Polocaine, 166*t*
Polycarbophil, 428*t*
Polycillin, 536*t*
Polyethylene glycol, 428*t*
Polymyxin B, 536*t*, 538, 539
Polymyxin E, 538
Polysynaptic inhibitors, 181
Polythiazide, 320*t*
Pomalidomide, 634
Pontocaine, 166*t*
Positive inotropic effect, 362
Posterior pituitary, 437
Postganglionic neuron, 280, 283*f*
Postmarketing surveillance, 7
Postsynaptic receptor, 65
Posture (calcium supplement), 498*t*
Potassium, 650*t*
Potassium-sparing diuretics, 319, 320*t*
Potency, 10–11, 10*f*
PPIs (proton pump inhibitors), 225, 423–425, 424*t*
Pradaxa, 378*t*, 380
Pralatrexate, 607*t*
Pramipexole, 140*t*
Pramlintide, 518*t*, 520
Pramoxine, 166*t*
Prandin, 517, 518*t*, 519
Prasugrel, 341, 378*t*, 382
Pravachol, 388*t*
Pravastatin, 388*t*
Prax, 166*t*
Praziquantel, 593*t*, 594
Prazosin, 309, 321*t*, 322, 363*t*, 370
Precedex, 152*t*, 154
Preclinical (animal) studies, 6, 6*t*
Precose, 518*t*, 520
Prednicarbate, 454*t*
Prednisolone, 240*t*, 408*t*, 454*t*, 609*t*
Prednisone, 240*t*, 408*t*, 454*t*, 609*t*
Pregabalin, 122*t*, 123, 125*t*
Preganglionic neuron, 280, 283*f*
Pregnancy
epilepsy and, 125–126
hormones in, 475
termination, 479–480
Prelone, 240*t*, 408*t*, 454*t*
Premarin, 477*t*, 498*t*
Preoperative medication, 156, 157*t*, 296
Prescribing, off-label, 8
Pressure gradient, 20
Presynaptic action potential, 64–65
Presynaptic adrenergic inhibitors
antihypertensives, 321*t*, 322–323
Presynaptic autoreceptor, 85

Presynaptic inhibition, 65
Prevacid, 424, 424*t*
Prezista, 562*t*, 572
Priftin, 543*t*, 544–545
Prilocaine, 166*t*
Prilosec, 424, 424*t*
Primacor, 363*t*
Primaquine, 589–590
Primatene Mist, 307, 405*t*
Primaxin, 536*t*
Primidone, 119*t*, 125*t*
Primobolan, 470*t*
Primsol, 543*t*
Prinivil, 324*t*, 363*t*
Prinzmetal ischemia (variant angina), 342*t*, 343
Pristiq, 86*t*, 89*t*
ProAmatine, 303
Probanthel, 295*t*
Pro-Banthine, 295*t*
Procainamide, 353*t*
Procaine, 166*t*
Procarbazine, 604*t*
Procardia, 324*t*, 339–340, 339*t*
Prochlorperazine, 103*t*, 104*t*
Prodrox, 477*t*
Prodrug, 26, 31
Progesterone, 472–475, 477*t*
  adverse effects, 477–478
  pharmacological use, 475–477, 477*t*
Progestins, 437*t*, 439, 465, 477*t*, 609*t*
Prograf, 628*t*, 631–632
Prolactin-inhibitory factor (PIF), 436*t*
Proleukin, 611*t*
Prolia, 498*t*, 502
Proliferative phase, 473
Prolixin, 104*t*
Prolonged-action preparation, 25
Proloprim, 543*t*, 545
Promethazine, 157*t*
Prometrium, 477*t*
Pronestyl, 353*t*
Propafenone, 353*t*
Propantheline, 295*t*
Propecia, 470
Propofol, 152*t*, 153–154
Propoxyphene, 205*t*
Propranolol, 302, 310*t*, 311, 321, 321*t*, 338*t*, 353*t*
Propylthiouracil (Propyl-Thyracil), 493
Proquin XR, 543*t*
Proscar, 470
ProSom, 70*t*, 74*t*
Prostaglandins, 219, 220
  gastric ulcers, 426
  heat attack and stroke, 230
  NSAIDs' inhibition of, 222–223, 225, 381
  physiological effects, 220–222, 221*t*
  rheumatoid arthritis and, 240–241
  synthesis, 220, 221*f*
Prostanoid, 220
Prostate cancer, 470
Prostigmin, 291*t*
Protease-inhibitor boosting, 566
Protease inhibitors, 562*t*, 565–566, 572
Protein(s)
  fusion, 632–633, 633*t*
  membrane, 19–20, 20*f*
  metabolism, 450–451, 451*f*, 508
  regulatory (G), 44–46, 46*f*
Protonix, 424, 424*t*
Proton pump, 423, 424*f*
Proton pump inhibitors (PPIs), 225, 241, 423–425, 424*t*
Protostat, 543*t*, 544, 591–592
Protozoa, 587
Protriptyline, 87*t*, 91*t*
Proventil, 306, 405*t*
Provera, 477*t*
Provocholine, 291*t*
Prozac, 86*t*, 89*t*, 93*t*
Pseudoephedrine, 303, 401*t*
Pseudoparkinsonism, 108*f*, 109
Psorcon, 453*t*
Psychosis, 101
  levodopa-induced, 138–139
Psyllium, 428*t*
Puberty, delayed, 468
Pulmicort, 408*t*, 453*t*
Pulmonary administration, 17
Pulmonary embolism (PE), 384
Pulmophyllin, 407*t*
Pulmozyme, 413
Pumps
  infusion, 264–265, 264*t*, 265*f*
  insulin, 515
Purine nucleotides, 603
Purines, 64
Purinethol, 606*t*
Puri-nethol, 634
Purkinje fibers, 349, 351*f*
Pyrantel pamoate, 593*t*, 595
Pyrazinamide, 546
Pyridostigmine, 291*t*, 292, 293
Pyridoxine, 648*t*
Pyrilamine, 402*t*
Pyrimethamine, 590
Pyrimethamine/sulfadoxine, 588*t*, 590
Pyrimidine nucleotides, 603
Pyrlex, 402*t*

Q

Quantal dose-response curve, 11, 11*f*
Quarzan, 295*t*
Quazepam, 70*t*, 74*t*
Quelicin, 158*t*
Questran, 388*t*, 389, 427
Quetiapine, 103*t*, 105*t*
Quinapril, 324*t*, 363*t*
Quinethazone, 320*t*
Quinidine, 353*t*, 588*t*
Quinine, 590
Quinupristin, 540*t*, 542
Qvar, 408*t*

R

Rabeprazole, 424, 424*t*
Ralivia, 205*t*
Raloxifene, 478–479, 498*t*, 501, 610
Raltegravir, 562*t*, 563, 573
Ramelteon, 70*t*, 72–73, 74*t*
Ramipril, 324*t*, 363*t*
Ranexa, 340–341, 355
Raniclor, 536*t*
Ranitidine, 157*t*, 423*t*
Ranolazine, 340–341, 342, 355
Rapaflo, 309
Rapamune, 628*t*, 631
Rapifen, 204*t*
Raptiva, 633*t*
Rasagiline, 135*t*, 141–142
Rauwolfia alkaloids, 312–313
Razadyne, 291*t*
Reactive oxygen species (ROS), 133–134
Rebif, 569*t*, 570
Rebound anxiety, 78
Receptor-enzyme system, 44, 45*f*
Receptor internalization, 51
Receptor-ion channel system, 43–44, 44*f*
Receptors. *See also* Drug receptors
  adrenergic, 283*f*, 284, 284*f*, 285–286*t*, 286–287
  anesthesia and, 155, 155*f*
  autonomic, 283–287, 284*f*
  cholinergic, 44, 44*f*, 48, 283*f*, 284–285, 284*f*, 285*t*, 289–290
  depression and, 84–85
  hormone, 441–443, 441*f*
  opioid, 202–203, 203*t*
  supersensitivity, 52, 84–85
  toll-like, 245
Receptor selectivity, 302–303
Receptor sensitivity theory of depression, 84, 84*f*
Receptor tyrosine kinase, 44, 45*f*
Reclast, 498*t*
Recombinant human deoxyribonuclease (rhDNAse), 413
Recombinant tissue plasminogen activator (rt-PA), 385
Rectal administration, 16*t*, 17
Reduction, 31, 32, 32*t*
Reflex sympathetic dystrophy syndrome (RSDS), 169–170
Reflex tachycardia, 322, 324
Refludan, 378*t*, 380
Regitine, 309
Reglan, 425–426
Regonol, 291*t*
Relafen, 228*t*, 229*t*, 240*t*

Relaxants, muscle. *See* Skeletal muscle relaxants
Relenza, 561*t*, 565
Remeron, 87*t*, 89*t*
Remicade, 240*t*, 244*t*, 247, 632, 633*t*
Remifentanil, 205*t*, 263
Reminyl, 291*t*, 292
Renal osteodystrophy, 498*t*
Renedil, 339*t*
Renese, 320*t*
Renin, 325
Renin-angiotensin system, 324–325, 325*f*. *See also* Angiotensin-converting enzyme (ACE) inhibitors; Angiotensin II
  antihypertensive drugs affecting, 325–326
  cardiac drugs affecting, 367–368
ReoPro, 378*t*, 382
Repaglinide, 517, 518*t*, 519
Replacement therapy, hormone. *See* Hormone replacement therapy (HRT)
Replesta, 498*t*
Repolarization, drugs that prolong, 353*t*, 354–355
Requip, 140*t*
Rescriptor, 562*t*, 566, 572–573
Reserfia, 312, 321*t*
Reserpine, 65, 312, 321*t*, 322–323
Resistance
  antibacterials, 549–550, 550*f*
  antineoplastics, 618
  antivirals, 568
Respiratory drugs, 399–415
  airway obstruction in COPD, 403
  anticholinergics, 296–297, 407–408
  antihistamines, 401–402, 402*t*
  antitussives, 399–400, 400*t*
  beta-adrenergic agonists, 403–406, 404*f*, 405*t*
  bronchial asthma, 410–412
  bronchospasms, 296–297
  case study, 414–415
  coughing and respiratory trace irritation, 399–400, 400*t*
  cromones, 409
  cystic fibrosis-related respiratory problems, 412–413
  decongestants, 400–401, 401*t*
  expectorants, 402–403
  glucocorticoids, 408–409, 408*t*
  leukotriene inhibitors, 409–410
  mucolytics, 402–403
  rehabilitation patients, 413–414
  reversible bronchospasm in COPD, 412
  xanthine derivatives, 406–407, 406*f*, 407*t*
Respiratory system, 399
Restoril, 70*t*, 74*t*
Retavase, 378*t*, 385
Reteplase, 378*t*, 385
Reticular formation, 60
Retinoids, 614*t*, 616
Retinol, 648*t*
Retrovir, 562*t*, 566, 572
Reuptake, 65
Revatio, 363*t*, 370
Reverse transcriptase inhibitors, 566–567, 567*f*
Reversol, 291*t*
ReVia, 206
Revimine, 363*t*
Revlimid, 616
Reyataz, 562*t*, 572
Reye syndrome, 226, 231
Rheumatoid arthritis, 237–250, 253–254
  case study, 253–254
  corticosteroids, 240*t*
  criteria for classification, 238*t*
  dietary implications, 250
  disease-modifying antirheumatic drugs (DMARDs), 242–250, 243–244*t*
  drug categories, 240*t*
  glucocorticoids, 241–242
  immune basis, 239, 239*f*
  nonsteroidal anti-inflammatory drugs (NSAIDs), 240–241
  rehabilitation patients, 253
Rheumatrex, 240*t*, 243*t*, 246, 628*t*, 630
Rhinocort, 453*t*
Rho(D) immunoglobulin, 632
RhoGAM, 633*t*
Ribavirin, 560*t*, 567–568
Riboflavin, 648*t*
Rickets, 497*t*
Rickettsiae, 533*t*
Ridactate, 498*t*
Ridaura, 240*t*, 243*t*, 245
Rifabutin, 543*t*, 544–545
Rifadin, 543*t*, 544–545
Rifampin, 543*t*, 544–545
Rifamycins, 543*t*, 544–545
Rifapentine, 543*t*, 544–545
Right heart failure, 361–362, 362*f*
Rilmenidine, 323
Rilonacept, 633*t*
Rimactane, 543*t*, 544–545
Rimantadine, 560*t*, 561–562
Rimexolone, 454*t*
Risedronate, 498*t*
Risperdal, 105*t*
Risperidone, 103*t*, 105*t*
Ritonavir, 562*t*, 566, 572
Rituxan, 248–249, 611*t*
Rituximab, 248–249, 611*t*
Rivaroxaban, 341, 378*t*, 380
Rivastigmine, 291*t*, 292
Rizatriptan, 309
RNA, bacterial, 535
RNA viruses, 557, 558*t*
Robaxin, 181*t*
Robinul, 295*t*
Rocaltrol, 498*t*
Rocephin, 536*t*
Rocuronium, 158*t*
Rofact, 543*t*
Rofecoxib, 225–226, 230
Rogaine, 324
Romidepsin, 614*t*, 615
Ropinirole, 140*t*
Ropivacaine, 264
Rosiglitazone, 518*t*, 519–520
Rosuvastatin, 387, 388*t*
Rotigotine, 140*t*
Routes of administration, 15–19, 16*t*
Roxicodone, 205*t*
Rozerem, 70*t*, 72–73, 74*t*
RU486, 479–480
Rubex, 607*t*
Rufinamide, 122*t*, 123
Rythmodan, 353*t*
Rythmol, 353*t*

S

Sabril, 122*t*, 123–124
Salicylates, 223
Salmeterol, 306, 405*t*, 411*t*
Saluron, 320*t*
Sanctura, 295*t*
Sandimmune, 240*t*, 249, 628*t*, 629
Sandostatin, 427
Sani-Supp, 428*t*
Saquinavir, 562*t*, 572
Sarcomas, 599. *See also* Cancer chemotherapy
Saw palmetto, 644*t*, 646
Saxagliptin, 518*t*, 519
Schedules, drug, 9
Schizophrenia, 101–103
Scopolamine, 157*t*, 295*t*, 296, 430
Seasonal allergies, 401–402, 402*t*
Secobarbital, 70*t*, 157*t*
Seconal, 70*t*
Second-generation (atypical) agents
  antidepressants, 89*t*
  antiepileptics, 121–124, 122*t*
  antihistamines, 401–402
  antipsychotics, 103–104, 103*t*, 104–105*t*, 105–106
  cephalosporins, 537
Second messenger, 45–46, 46*f*
Sectral, 310*t*, 311, 321*t*, 338*t*, 353*t*, 363*t*
Sedative-hypnotic agents, 69–75, 70*t*, 80
  antipsychotics, 110
  barbiturates, 70*t*, 72
  benzodiazepines, 69–72, 70*t*, 73–75, 74*t*, 78–79
  case study, 79
  common drugs, 70*t*
  nonbenzodiazepines, 70*t*, 72–75, 74*t*, 80
  pharmacokinetics, 73, 74*t*
  problems and side effects, 73–75
  rehabilitation patients, 78–79

Sedative, preoperative, 156, 157*t*
Seizures, epileptic. *See* Epileptic seizures
Selective estrogen receptor modulators (SERMs), 50, 478–479, 497*t*, 501, 610
Selective serotonin reuptake inhibitors (SSRIs), 88, 89*t*, 91–92, 91*t*
Selective toxicity, 531
Selectivity, drug, 47–48, 48*f*
Selegiline, 135*t*, 141–142
Selenium, 650*t*
Selzentry, 562*t*, 563–564, 573
Senna, 428*t*
Senokot, 428*t*
Sensipar, 498*t*, 502
Sensorcaine, 166*t*
Septocaine, 166*t*
Serax, 76*t*
Serevent, 306, 405*t*
Seromycin, 536*t*
Serophene, 479
Seroquel, 105*t*
Serotonin, 62*t*, 63
  blockers, 430
  receptor antagonists, 157*t*
  reuptake inhibitors, 86*t*, 88, 89*t*, 91–92
Serotonin syndrome, 92
Sertaconazole, 583*t*
Sertoli cells, 466, 466*f*
Sertraline, 77*t*, 86*t*, 89*t*, 91*t*
Serzone, 87*t*, 89*t*, 90
Sevoflurane, 151*t*
Sex characteristics
  female, 473
  male, 467
Sex (gender), effects on drug response, 38–39
Sex hormones. *See* Hormones, male and female
Sildenafil, 363*t*, 370
Silodosin, 309
Silvadene, 543*t*
Simple replacement therapy. *See* Hormone replacement therapy (HRT)
Simponi, 240*t*, 244*t*, 247
Simulect, 632, 633*t*
Simvastatin, 388*t*
Sinemet, 135*t*, 137
Sinequan, 87*t*, 93*t*
Singulair, 409–410
Sinus arrhythmias, 352*t*
Sinusitis, 547*t*, 548*t*
Sirolimus, 628*t*, 631
Sitagliptin, 518*t*, 519
Skelaxin, 181*t*
Skeletal muscle relaxant drugs, 179–193
  agents for spasticity, 183–187, 183*t*
  antispasm agents, 180–182
  botulinum toxin, 65, 187–191, 188*f*
  case study, 193
  pharmacokinetics, 191
  rehabilitation patients, 191–192
  spasticity *vs.* spasms, 179–180
Skyla, 477*t*
Sodium, 650*t*
  anesthetics and, 170–171, 170*f*
  digitalis and, 364
  mineralocorticoids and, 458–459, 458*f*
Sodium channel blockers, 352–354, 353*t*
Sodium nitroprusside, 370
Sodium phosphate, 428*t*
Sodium-potassium exchange protein, 364
Sodium-potassium pump, 364
Solfoton, 70*t*, 119*t*
Solganal, 245
Solifenacin, 295*t*
Soma, 181*t*
Somatostatin, 507
Sonata, 70*t*, 74*t*
Sonophoresis (phonophoresis), 19
Sorafenib, 612*t*
Sorine, 311, 321*t*, 353*t*
Sotacor, 353*t*
Sotalol, 310*t*, 311, 321*t*, 338*t*, 353*t*
Spasms, 180
Spasticity, 179–180
Spectazole, 582*t*
Spectracef, 536*t*
Spermatogenesis, 465, 466*f*, 467
Spinal cord, 60*f*, 61
  opioid effects on, 207–208, 207*f*
Spinal nerve blockade, 168–169, 169*f*
Spiriva, 295*t*, 408
Spirochetes, 533*t*
Spironolactone, 320*t*, 369, 460
Sporanox, 585
Sprintec, 481*t*
Stable angina, 341–343, 342*t*
Stadol, 151*t*, 205*t*
Stage fright, 77
Stanozolol, 470*t*
Starlix, 517, 518*t*, 519
Statins
  adverse effects, 389–390
  hyperlipidemia, 387–388, 388*t*
  unstable angina, 387–388
Status epilepticus, 126
Stavudine, 562*t*, 566, 572
Stelazine, 104*t*
Stem cells, Parkinson disease and, 143
Sterapred, 408*t*, 454*t*
Steroids, 439, 441*f*, 442–443, 442*f*. *See also* Adrenocorticosteroids; Glucocorticoids; Mineralocorticoids
  male and female hormones, 465–475, 483–484
  synthesis, 447–449, 448*f*
Stimulants. *See also* Cholinergic stimulants
  immunostimulants, 634–635
  laxatives, 428–429, 428*t*
  sympathomimetic, 90
St. John's wort, 644*t*, 647
Stool softeners, 428*t*, 429
Streptokinase, 384–385
Streptomycin, 540*t*
Streptozocin, 607*t*
Stretch reflex, 179, 180*f*
Striant, 469*t*
Stribild, 562*t*, 563, 573
Stroke, 230, 381, 384
Stromectol, 594
Subcutaneous (SC) injection, 18
Sublimaze, 151*t*, 204*t*
Sublingual administration, 16–17, 16*t*
Substance P, 62*t*, 63
Succinimides, 119*t*, 121
Succinylcholine, 36, 158*t*
Sudafed, 303, 401*t*
Sufentanil, 205*t*, 263, 263*t*
Sugammedex, 158–159
Sular, 324*t*
Sulbactam, 536*t*
Sulconazole, 583*t*
Sulcrate, 426
Sulfadiazine, 543*t*, 545
Sulfamethoxazole, 545
Sulfasalazine, 240*t*, 244*t*, 249, 628*t*, 631
Sulfate, inorganic, 650*t*
Sulfatrim, 543*t*
Sulfisoxazole, 543*t*, 545
Sulfonamides, 543*t*, 545
Sulfonylureas, 517, 518*t*
Sulindac, 228*t*, 229*t*, 240*t*
Sumatriptan, 309
Sunitinib, 612*t*
Supersensitivity of receptors, 52
  depression and, 84–85
Suppositories. *See* Rectal administration
Suprane, 151*t*
Supraventricular arrhythmias, 352*t*
Suprax, 536*t*
Surface membrane receptors, 43–44, 44*f*, 441*f*, 442
Surmontil, 87*t*
Surveillance, postmarketing, 7
Sustained-release preparation, 25
Sustiva, 562*t*, 566, 572–573
Sutent, 612*t*
Symadine, 560*t*
Symbicort, 411*t*
Symlin, 518*t*, 520
Symmetrel, 135*t*, 141, 560*t*, 561–562
Sympathetic block, 169–170
Sympathetic nervous system, 279–282, 281*t*
  beta blockers, 368–369
  digitalis, 364
  hypertension, 317–318, 318*f*
Sympatholytic drugs
  alpha blockers, 307–309, 321–322, 321*t*
  antihypertensives, 319*t*, 320–323, 321*t*
  beta blockers, 309–312, 310*t*, 320–321, 321*t*
  centrally acting agents, 321*t*, 323

ganglionic blockers, 321*t*, 323
presynaptic adrenergic inhibitors, 312–313, 322–323
Sympathomimetic stimulants, 90
Synagis, 560*t*
Synapse, 64–65, 64*f*
Synarel, 470
Syndrome X (metabolic syndrome), 317, 512
Synercid, 540*t*, 542
Synovitis. *See* Rheumatoid arthritis
Synthroid, 494*t*
Syphilis, 549*t*
Syringe driver pump, 264, 265*f*
Systole, 350

T

Tachycardia, 352, 352*t*
Tacrine, 291*t*, 292
Tacrolimus, 628*t*, 629, 631–632
Tagamet, 423*t*
Talwin, 151*t*, 205*t*
Tambocor, 353*t*
Tamiflu, 560*t*, 565
Tamofen, 478
Tamoxifen, 478, 609*t*, 610
Tamsulosin, 309
Tapazole, 493
Tapentadol, 205*t*
Tarceva, 611*t*, 613
Tardive dyskinesia, antipsychotics and, 107–109, 108*f*
Targretin, 614*t*, 616
Tasmar, 135*t*, 142
Tavist, 402*t*
Taxanes, 605
Taxol, 608*t*
Taxotere, 608*t*
Tazicef, 536*t*
Tazobactam, 536*t*
T cells, 239, 239*f*, 626–627, 626*f*
Teflaro, 536*t*
Tegretol, 119*t*, 120
Tekturna, 324*t*, 326, 363*t*, 368
Telachlor, 402*t*
Telbivudine, 560*t*
Telenzepine, 425
Telithromycin, 540*t*, 542
Telmisartan, 324*t*, 363*t*
Temazepam, 70*t*, 74*t*
Temodar, 604*t*
Temovate, 453*t*
Temozolomide, 604*t*
Temperature, body, 438, 491
Temsirolimus, 628*t*, 631
Tenecteplase, 378*t*, 385
Tenex, 304, 321*t*
Teniposide, 609*t*
Tenofovir, 562*t*, 566, 572
Tenormin, 310*t*, 311, 321*t*, 338*t*, 339, 353*t*, 363*t*
Tensilon, 291*t*
Terazol, 583*t*
Terazosin, 309, 321*t*, 322
Terbinafine, 582*t*, 586
Terbutaline, 306, 405*t*
Terconazole, 583*t*
Teriparatide, 498*t*, 501
Tessalon, 400*t*
Testim, 469*t*
Testoderm, 469*t*
Testopel pellets, 469*t*
Testosterone
abuse, 470*t*
agents for clinical use, 469*t*
antineoplastic indications, 609*t*
biosynthesis and structure, 448*f*
cypionate, 471*t*
effects, 437*t*, 439, 467
synthesis, 465–467, 466*f*
Testred, 469*t*
Tetracaine, 166*t*
Tetracycline(s), 35, 540*t*, 541, 588*t*
Thalamotomy, 143
Thalamus, 60, 60*f*
Thalidomide, 614*t*, 615–616, 634
Thalidone, 320*t*
Theobromine, 406, 406*f*
Theophylline, 36*f*, 406, 406*f*, 407, 407*t*, 411
TheraCys, 634
Therapeutic index (TI), 12
Thermogenesis, 438, 491
Thiabendazole, 593*t*, 595
Thiamin, 648*t*
Thiazide diuretics, 319, 320*t*
Thiazolidinediones, 518*t*, 519–520
Thioguanine, 607*t*
Thiopental, 151*t*
Thioplex, 604*t*
Thioridazine, 103*t*, 104*t*, 105
Thiotepa, 604*t*
Thiothixene, 103*t*, 104*t*
Third-generation agents
beta blockers, 321, 369
cephalosporins, 537
Thoracolumbar nervous system. *See* Sympathetic nervous system
Thorazine, 104*t*, 105
Threshold dose, 10, 10*f*
Thrombin, 377
Thrombin inhibitors, direct, 341, 377, 378*t*, 380
Thrombocytopenia, 380–381
Thrombogenesis, 375, 382
Thrombolytic drugs, 377–380, 378*t*
Thrombosis, 343
Thromboxane, 220
NSAIDs' inhibition of, 222–223, 381
physiological effects of, 220–222, 221*t*
synthesis of, 220, 221*f*
Thrombus, 222, 224. *See also* Thrombogenesis
Thyroglobulin (TGB), 490–491, 490*f*
Thyroid
drugs
hyperthyroidism, 492–494
hypothyroidism, 494, 494*t*
rehabilitation patients, 502
gland, 437–438
hormones, 437*t*, 443, 489–492
synthesis, 489–491, 490*f*
Thyroid cancer, 493
Thyroid-stimulating hormone (TSH), 436*t*, 491
Thyrolar, 494*t*
Thyrotoxicosis. *See* Hyperthyroidism
Thyrotropin-releasing hormone (TRH), 436*t*, 491
Thyroxine, 437*t*, 438, 489, 490*f*
Tiagabine, 122*t*, 123, 124*t*, 125*t*
Ticar, 536*t*
Ticarcillin, 536*t*
Ticlid, 378*t*, 382
Ticlopidine, 378*t*, 382
Tigecycline, 541
Tight glycemic control, 513
Tight junctions, 22
Tikosyn, 353*t*
Timed-release preparation, 25
Timentin, 536*t*
Timolol, 310*t*, 311, 321*t*, 338*t*, 353*t*
Tinactin, 583*t*, 587
Tinidazole, 588*t*
Tinzaparin, 378, 378*t*
Tioconazole, 583*t*
Tiotropium, 295*t*, 297, 407, 408, 412
Tipranavir, 572
Tirofiban, 341, 378*t*, 382, 383
Tissue factor, 376–377, 376*f*
Tissue healing, NSAIDs and, 227
Tissue plasminogen activator (t-PA), 376*f*, 377, 385
Tissue transplants
diabetes mellitus, 521
Parkinson disease, 143
Tivicay, 562*t*, 563, 573
Tizanidine, 183*t*, 187, 305
TNF-a, 247, 248*f*. *See also* Tumor necrosis factor inhibitors
TNKase, 378*t*, 385
TOBI, 540*t*
Tobramycin, 540*t*
Tocainide, 353*t*
Tocilizumab, 240*t*, 244*t*, 249
Tofranil, 87*t*, 93*t*
Tolazamide, 518*t*
Tolbutamide, 518*t*
Tolcapone, 135*t*, 142
Tolectin, 228*t*, 229*t*, 240*t*
Tolerance, drug, 33
intrathecal baclofen, 185
nitrate, 337
opioid analgesics, 212, 213

receptor sensitivity, 52
sedative-hypnotics, 74–75
Tolinase, 518*t*
Toll-like receptors (TLRs), 245
Tolmetin, 228*t*, 229*t*, 240*t*
Tolnaftate, 583*t*, 587
Tolterodine, 295*t*
Tonocard, 353*t*
Topamax, 122*t*, 123
Topical administration, 16*t*, 18
Topicort, 453*t*
Topiramate, 122*t*, 123, 124*t*, 125*t*
Topoisomerase inhibitors, 608, 609*t*
Topotecan, 609*t*
Toprol-XL, 310*t*, 311
Toradol, 224, 228*t*
Toremifene, 478, 609*t*, 610
Torisel, 628*t*, 631
Torsades de pointes, 354
Torsemide, 320*t*
Tositumomab, 611*t*
Toviaz, 295*t*
Toxicity, selective, 531
Toxicology, 4, 4*f*
Toxins
cholinergic poisoning, 297
Parkinson disease and, 134
Trachoma, 549*t*
Tracrium, 158*t*
Trade name, 5
Tradjenta, 518*t*, 519
Tramadol, 205*t*, 263
Trandate, 310*t*, 311, 321*t*, 338*t*, 363*t*
Trandolapril, 324*t*, 363*t*
Tranexamic acid, 386
Tranquilizers, 101
Transdermal patch, 16*t*, 18–19
anesthetics, 168
contraception, 480
nitroglycerin, 337, 337*f*
opioids, 206
Transderm-Scop, 295*t*
Transplants, tissue. *See* Tissue transplants
Transport, active, 21*f*, 22–23
Tranxene, 76*t*, 119*t*
Tranylcypromine, 87*t*, 91*t*
Trazodone, 87*t*, 89*t*, 90, 91*t*, 93*t*
Treanda, 604*t*
Trecator, 540*t*, 542
Trental, 378*t*, 383
Tretinoin, 614*t*, 616
Triamcinolone, 240*t*, 408, 408*t*, 454*t*
Triaminic, 401*t*
Triamterene, 320*t*
Triazolam, 70*t*, 74*t*
Trichlormethiazide, 320*t*
Tricor, 388*t*
Tricyclics, 86–87*t*, 88, 91*t*, 92
Tridesilon, 453*t*
Trifluoperazine, 103*t*, 104*t*
Triflupromazine, 103*t*
Trifluridine, 560*t*, 565
Trihexyphenidyl, 135*t*, 296
Triiodothyronine, 437*t*, 438, 489, 490*f*
Trilafon, 104*t*
Trileptal, 119*t*, 120
Trimethaphan, 294, 321*t*, 323
Trimethoprim, 543*t*, 545
Trimipramine, 87*t*, 91*t*
Trimpex, 543*t*, 545
Tripelennamine, 402*t*
Triphasil, 481*t*
Triprolidine, 402*t*
Triptorelin, 610*t*
Trisenox, 614*t*
Tronolane, 166*t*
Trospium, 295*t*
Truphylline, 407*t*
Tubarine, 158*t*
Tubocurarine, 158*t*, 293
Tumor necrosis factor inhibitors, 244*t*, 247, 248*f*, 250, 632, 633*t*
Tums, 498*t*
Turinabol, 470*t*
Tussigon, 400*t*
Tygacil, 540*t*
Type 2 diabetes, 511–512, 511*t*. *See also* Diabetes mellitus
Type-5 phosphodiesterase enzyme (PDE5), 370
Type I diabetes, 511, 511*t*. *See also* Diabetes mellitus
Typhoid fever, 548*t*
Tyramine, 92
Tyrosine, 489
chemical structure, 490*f*
hydroxylase, 136*f*
kinase inhibitors, 611–612*t*, 612–613, 619
thyroid hormone synthesis, 489
Tyzeka, 560*t*

U

Ulcers, gastric, 425–426
Ulipristal, 481*t*, 482
Ultane, 151*t*
Ultiva, 205*t*
Ultram, 205*t*
Ultravate, 453*t*
Unasyn, 536*t*
Unipen, 536*t*
Unipolar depression, 93. *See also* Depression
Unisom Nighttime Sleep-Aid, 402*t*
Univasc, 324*t*
Unstable angina, 342*t*, 343–344
Upper respiratory tract infections, 399–400, 400*t*
Urecholine, 290, 291*t*
Urethritis, 549*t*
Urex, 546
Urinary tract infection and bladder atony, 547*t*, 548*t*
antimuscarinic drugs, 296
cholinergic stimulants, 292
Urokinase, 378*t*, 384
Uroxatral, 308
Ursodeoxycholic acid (ursodiol), 430
Uterus, beta-2-selective drugs and, 306

V

Vaccines, 570–571, 574, 635
Vaginal ring, 480
Vagistat, 583*t*
Valacyclovir, 561, 561*t*
Valcyte, 561*t*, 564–565
Valdecoxib, 225–226, 230
Valerian, 644*t*, 647
Valganciclovir, 561*t*, 564–565
Valium, 75–76, 75*f*, 76*t*, 151*t*
epilepsy, 119*t*
spasms, 180–181, 181*t*
spasticity, 183*t*
Valproates, 119*t*, 121
Valproate sodium, 119*t*
Valproic acid, 119*t*, 124*t*, 125*t*, 126
Valsartan, 324*t*, 363*t*, 368
Valtrex, 561, 561*t*
Vanadom, 181*t*
Vanceril, 453*t*
Vancocin, 536*t*
Vancomycin, 536*t*, 539
Vantin, 536*t*
Variant angina, 342*t*, 343
Vasodilators
antihypertensives, 319*t*, 323–324, 324*t*
congestive heart failure, 363*t*, 370
Vasotec, 324*t*, 363*t*, 367
Vasoxyl, 303
Vecamyl, 321*t*
Vectibix, 611*t*
Vecuronium, 158*t*
Velban, 608*t*, 634
Velbe, 608*t*
Velcade, 614*t*, 615
Venlafaxine, 77*t*, 86*t*, 89*t*, 91*t*
Venous thrombosis, 377
Ventolin, 306, 405*t*
Ventricular arrhythmias, 352*t*
VePesid, 609*t*
Verapamil, 324*t*, 327, 339*t*, 340, 353*t*, 355
Verdeso, 453*t*
Verelan, 339*t*, 353*t*
Vermox, 594
Versed, 151*t*
Very-low-density lipoproteins (VLDLs), 387
Vesanoid, 614*t*, 616
Vesicare, 295*t*
Vexol, 454*t*
Vfend, 586

Viagra, 363*t*, 370
Vibramycin, 540*t*
Victoza, 519
Vidaza, 606*t*
Videx, 562*t*, 566, 572
Vigabatrin, 122*t*, 123–124, 125*t*
Vimpat, 122, 122*t*
Vinblastine, 605, 608*t*, 634
Vinca alkaloids, 605
Vincasar, 608*t*, 634
Vincristine, 605, 608*t*, 634
Vinorelbine, 605, 608*t*
Vioxx, 230
Viracept, 562*t*, 572
Viral replication, 559–560, 559*f*
Viral resistance, 568
Viral thymidine kinase, 561
Viramune, 562*t*, 566, 572–573
Virazole, 560*t*, 567–568
Viread, 562*t*, 566, 572
Virilon, 469*t*
Viroptic, 560*t*, 565
Viruses, 557–560. *See also* Antiviral drugs
  basic components, 558, 559*f*
  classification, 557, 558*t*
  replication, 559–560, 559*f*
  resistance, 568
  structure and function, 558–560, 559*f*
Viscosupplementation, 251–252
Visken, 310*t*, 311, 321*t*, 338*t*
Vistaril, 402*t*
Vistide, 560*t*, 562–563
Vitamin D
  bone mineral homeostasis, 496, 497*t*, 498*t*, 499
  calcium absorption, 495
Vitamins
  alternative medications, 647, 648*t*, 649
  vitamin B_3, 389
  vitamin K, 379, 379*f*, 386
Vitrasert, 564–565
Vivactil, 87*t*
Vivitrol, 206
Voltaren, 227*t*, 229*t*, 240*t*
Volume of distribution, 24, 24*t*, 35
Voriconazole, 582*t*, 586
Vorinostat, 614*t*, 615
Vumon, 609*t*

W

Warfarin, 37, 377, 378*t*, 379–380
Welchol, 388*t*, 389, 427, 518*t*, 520
Wellbutrin, 87*t*, 89*t*, 90
Winstrol, 470*t*
Women's Health Initiative (WHI), 476
Wyamine, 303
Wycillin, 536*t*
Wymox, 536*t*
Wytensin, 304, 321*t*

X

Xanax, 76*t*
Xanthine derivatives, 406–407, 406*f*, 407*t*
Xarelto, 378*t*, 380
Xeloda, 606*t*
Xeomin, 189
Xopenex, 405*t*
Xylocaine, 166*t*, 353*t*
Xylometazoline, 303, 401*t*
Xyzal, 402*t*

Y

Yasmin, 481*t*
Yaz, 481*t*
Yodoxin, 591

Z

Zafirlukast, 220, 409–410
Zaleplon, 70*t*, 74*t*
Zanaflex, 183*t*, 187, 305
Zanamivir, 561*t*, 565
Zanosar, 607*t*
Zantac, 423*t*
Zarontin, 119*t*, 121
Zaroxolyn, 320*t*
Zebeta, 310*t*, 311, 321*t*, 363*t*
Zemplar, 498*t*
Zemuron, 158*t*
Zenapax, 632, 633*t*
Zerit, 562*t*, 566, 572
Zestril, 324*t*, 363*t*
Zetia, 388*t*, 389
Zevalin, 611*t*
Ziagen, 562*t*, 566, 572
Zidovudine, 562*t*, 566, 572
Zileuton, 220, 409–410
Zinacef, 536*t*
Zinc, 650*t*
Ziprasidone, 103*t*, 105*t*
Zithromax, 540*t*
Zmax, 540*t*
Zocor, 388*t*
Zofran, 156, 602
Zoladex, 470
Zoledronic acid, 498*t*
Zolinza, 614*t*, 615
Zoloft, 77*t*, 86*t*, 89*t*
Zolpidem, 70*t*, 74*t*
Zonegran, 122*t*, 124
Zonisamide, 122*t*, 124, 124*t*, 125*t*
Zortress, 628*t*, 631
Zosyn, 536*t*
Zovia, 481*t*
Zovirax, 560*t*, 561
Zyban, 89*t*, 90
Zyflo, 409–410
Zyprexa, 105*t*
Zyrtec, 401, 402*t*
Zyvox, 540*t*, 542

COMMON DRUG SUFFIXES

Medications that are chemically and functionally similar often have generic names that share a common ending or suffix. Listed here are some drug classes that contain groups of drugs that share a common suffix. Please note that some members of a drug class may have a suffix that is different from the one indicated; for instance, not all benzodiazepines end with *-epam* or *-olam*.

Drug Class	Suffix	Common Examples	Primary Indication or Desired Effect (Chapter in Parentheses)
Angiotensin-converting enzyme (ACE) inhibitors	*-pril*	Captopril, enalapril	Antihypertensive (21), congestive heart failure (24)
Angiotensin-II receptor blockers	*-sartan*	Candesartan, losartan	Antihypertensive (21), congestive heart failure (24)
Azole antifungals	*-azole*	Fluconazole, miconazole	Fungal infections (35)
Barbiturates	*-barbital*	Phenobarbital, secobarbital	Sedative-hypnotic (6), antiseizure (9), anesthetic (11)
Benzodiazepines	*-epam* or *-olam*	Diazepam, temazepam, alprazolam, triazolam	Sedative-hypnotic (6), antianxiety (6), antiseizure (9), anesthetic (11)
Beta blockers	*-olol*	Metoprolol, propranolol	Antihypertensive (21), antianginal (22), antiarrhythmic (23), congestive heart failure (24)
Bisphosphonates	*-dronate*	Alendronate, pamidronate	Osteoporosis (31)
Bronchodilators (adrenergic)	*-erol*	Albuterol, pirbuterol	Bronchodilation (26)
Bronchodilators (xanthine derivatives)	*-phylline*	Theophylline, aminophylline	Bronchodilation (26)
Calcium channel blockers (dihydropyridine group)	*-ipine*	Nifedipine, nicardipine	Antihypertensive (21), antianginal (22)
Cyclooxygenase type 2 (COX-2) inhibitors	*-coxib*	Celecoxib	Pain, inflammation (15)
Glucocorticoids	*-sone* or *-olone**	Cortisone, dexamethasone, prednisone, prednisolone, triamcinolone	Anti-inflammatory (16, 29), immunosuppressants (37)
Histamine H_2-receptor blockers	*-idine*	Cimetidine, ranitidine	Gastric ulcers (27)
HIV protease inhibitors	*-avir*	Ritonavir, saquinavir	HIV infection (34)
HMG-CoA reductase inhibitors (statins)	*-statin*	Pravastatin, simvastatin	Hyperlipidemia (25)
Local anesthetics	*-caine*	Lidocaine, bupivicaine	Local anesthetic (12), antiarrhythmics (23)
Low-molecular-weight heparins	*-parin*	Dalteparin, enoxaparin	Anticoagulants (25)
Oral antidiabetics (sulfonylurea group)	*-amide*	Chlorpropamide, tolbutamide	Antidiabetic (type 2 diabetes mellitus) (32)
Penicillin antibiotics	*-cillin*	Penicillin, ampicillin, amoxicillin	Bacterial infections (33)
Proton pump inhibitors	*-prazole*	Omeprazole, lansoprazole	Gastric ulcers (27)
Tetracycline antibiotics	*-cycline*	Tetracycline, doxycycline	Bacterial infections (33)
Various other antibacterials	*-micin* or *-mycin*†	Streptomycin, gentamicin, erythromycin	Bacterial infections (33)

**Some anabolic steroids also end with* -olone, *such as nandrolone and oxymetholone (Chapter 30).*
†*Some antibiotics ending with* -mycin *or* -rubicin *are used as antineoplastics (Chapter 36).*